NUTRITION AND HEALTH

Adrianne Bendich, PhD, FACN, SERIES EDITOR

For further volumes:
http://www.springer.com/series/7659

Gregory J. Anderson · Gordon D. McLaren
Editors

Iron Physiology and Pathophysiology in Humans

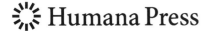

Editors
Gregory J. Anderson
Iron Metabolism Laboratory
Queensland Institute of Medical Research
Brisbane, QLD 4006, Australia
greg.anderson@qimr.edu.au

Gordon D. McLaren
Hematology/Oncology Section
Veterans Affairs Long Beach Healthcare System
Long Beach, CA 90822, USA

Division of Hematology/Oncology
Department of Medicine
University of California, Irvine
Chao Family Comprehensive Cancer Center
UC Irvine Medical Center
Orange, CA 92868, USA
gordon.mclaren@va.gov

ISBN 978-1-60327-484-5 e-ISBN 978-1-60327-485-2
DOI 10.1007/978-1-60327-485-2
Springer New York Dordrecht Heidelberg London

Library of Congress Control Number: 2011940768

Printed on acid-free paper

Humana Press is part of Springer Science+Business Media (www.springer.com)

Gregory J. Anderson dedicates this book to Karen L. and Ian G. Anderson for their support and understanding and to members of his laboratory and close colleagues for their stimulating discussions over many years.

Gordon D. McLaren dedicates this volume to Christine E. McLaren, Ph.D., and Graham D. McLaren for their encouragement and to his younger colleagues for their continued inspiration.

We would also like to dedicate this book to several key investigators in the iron field who have passed away in recent years. They have made enormous contributions to the study of iron metabolism, and the iron community is much diminished by the loss of these distinguished friends and colleagues.

John Beard
Ernest Beutler
Clement Finch
Hiromi Gunshin
Dick van der Helm
Giuliana Zanninelli

Series Editor Page

The great success of the *Nutrition and Health* series is the result of the consistent overriding mission of providing health professionals with texts that are essential because each includes: (1) a synthesis of the state of the science, (2) timely, in-depth reviews by the leading researchers in their respective fields, (3) extensive, up-to-date fully annotated reference lists, (4) a detailed index, (5) relevant tables and figures, (6) identification of paradigm shifts and the consequences, (7) virtually no overlap of information between chapters, but targeted, inter-chapter referrals, (8) suggestions of areas for future research, and (9) balanced, data-driven answers to patients' as well as health professionals' questions which are based upon the totality of evidence rather than the findings of any single study.

The series volumes are not the outcome of a symposium. Rather, each editor has the potential to examine a chosen area with a broad perspective, both in subject matter as well as in the choice of chapter authors. The editor(s), whose training(s) is (are) both research and practice oriented, has the opportunity to develop a primary objective for their book, define the scope and focus, and then invite the leading authorities to be part of their initiative. The authors are encouraged to provide an overview of the field, discuss their own research, and relate the research findings to potential human health consequences. Because each book is developed de novo, the chapters are coordinated so that the resulting volume imparts greater knowledge than the sum of the information contained in the individual chapters.

Iron Physiology and Pathophysiology in Humans, edited by Gregory J. Anderson, Ph.D., and Gordon D. McLaren, M.D., fully exemplifies the goals of the *Nutrition and Health* series. Iron is an essential micronutrient for humans. It is critical for the synthesis of DNA and proteins and serves as a cofactor for numerous enzymes, including those involved in energy metabolism and a range of other biochemical functions in cells. Iron also is an essential component of hemoglobin and myoglobin and thereby plays a critical role in oxygen transport and delivery. Iron is also the most abundant transition metal in the human body. Yet, many nutritionists are more aware of the adverse effects of iron overload than its critical role in brain development, kidney function, immune responses, and growth, as examples. This volume is very timely as there is currently only one other up-to-date volume for professionals concerning the role of iron in nutrition and clinical medicine. The *Nutrition and Health* series includes the volume *Iron Deficiency and Overload: From Basic Biology to Clinical Practice*, edited by Shlomo Yehuda, Ph.D., and David Mostofsky, Ph.D., that was published in 2010 and emphasized the critical role of iron in the brain and the clinical consequences of its deficiency as well as overload. Dr. Anderson served as a coauthor of the first chapter in this 2010 volume. The current volume reflects the newest research on the molecular biology as well as the genetics behind the most critical aspects of iron physiology and pathology. This important text provides a timely review of the latest science concerning iron metabolism as well as practical, data-driven options to manage at-risk populations with the best accepted therapeutic nutritional and medical interventions. The overarching goal of the editors is to provide fully referenced information to health professionals so they may enhance the nutritional welfare and overall health of clients and patients who are at risk for less than optimal iron status. This excellent, up-to-date volume will add great value to the practicing health professional as well as those professionals and students who have an interest in the latest information on the science behind iron requirements during the life span, and the potential for iron to modulate the effects of chronic diseases and conditions that are widely seen in the majority of patient populations.

Drs. Anderson and McLaren are internationally recognized leaders in the field of iron research and hematology. Both editors are excellent communicators and they have worked tirelessly to develop a book on iron that will be the benchmark in the field. In-depth chapters cover the most important aspects of the complex interactions between cellular functions, diet, and iron requirements as well as genetic mutations that affect iron metabolism. The links between iron and chronic inflammatory diseases and the acute conditions that can adversely affect the quality of life and health are also considered. Dr. Anderson, Ph.D., is the Head of the Iron Metabolism Laboratory, Queensland Institute of Medical Research; Associate Professor, Department of Medicine, University of Queensland; and Head, Cancer and Cell Biology Division as well as NHMRC Senior Research Fellow at the Queensland Institute of Medical Research. He also serves as an Adjunct Professor at the School of Molecular and Microbial Sciences, University of Queensland. Dr. Anderson is currently the President-Elect of the International Bioiron Society. He is a member of the Editorial Board of Biometals. Dr. McLaren, M.D., is a physician in the Hematology/Oncology Section of the Veteran's Affairs (VA) Long Beach Healthcare System, Long Beach, CA, and is also Professor in the Division of Hematology/Oncology, Department of Medicine and Chao Family Comprehensive Cancer Center, University of California, Irvine, CA. He has served as the Chair, CDC/NCHM, Review Panel "Diagnosis and Treatment of Hereditary Hemochromatosis," as well as the Chair, Iron Overload Education Session at the American Society of Hematology's Annual Meeting. In 2010, Dr. McLaren was a member of the NIH/NIDDK Special Emphasis Panel on "Centers of Excellence in Molecular Hematology." He currently serves as Vice-Chair, American Society of Hematology, Scientific Committee on Iron and Heme. Dr. McLaren is a member of the Medical and Scientific Advisory Board of the Iron Disorders Institute (www.irondisorders.org).

This comprehensive, in-depth volume is logically organized into six sections. The first section reviews cellular iron metabolism. The four introductory chapters provide readers with an overview of the proteins involved in iron metabolism and the basic pathways by which iron is utilized and stored in cells and how these processes are regulated. The chapters in the first section of the volume concerned with iron biochemistry and metabolism provide the reader with a clear understanding of the state of the science and where gaps in knowledge still remain so that the clinically related chapters can be more easily understood. The proteins involved in iron homeostasis, including transferrin, the transferrin receptors, ferritin, ferroportin, hepcidin, divalent metal-ion transporter 1, mitoferrin in mitochondria, and others, are described. The importance of heme as well as iron metabolism is emphasized. The movement of iron in the ferrous and ferric ionic states is clearly explained, and when further research is required to fully understand the metabolic processes, these are pointed out to the reader. There is also an introduction to the diversity of genetic mutations that result in inherited defects in iron metabolism.

Section II, on iron physiology, contains eight chapters and, comprehensively reviews the basics of iron metabolism, beginning with the sources of iron in the human diet and the different requirements during the life stages, including pre-term birth, as well as the differences between the iron requirements of men and women. Dietary sources of iron can be classified as either from heme iron sources or non-heme iron sources, and the absorption as well as regulation of iron is described. The major iron transport protein in the blood is transferrin, and this protein, as well as its receptor, and the fates of non-transferrin-bound iron are discussed in detail. The majority of iron in the body is conserved during the breakdown of red blood cells containing iron bound to hemoglobin, and the recycling of heme-derived iron is reviewed. The proteins involved in the salvage pathways, including hemopexin and haptoglobin, are described. Serum iron concentrations are normally maintained within a narrow range of 10–30 μM, and transferrin's saturation is usually between 20–40%, providing an adequate buffer for an unexpected influx of iron into the systemic circulation. Regulation of serum iron involves the liver, spleen, duodenum, and the reticuloendothelial system, hormones, and genetic factors. The majority of the body's iron is in its red blood cells, and erythropoiesis is explained in detail, as are the incorporation of iron into heme and the formation of the hemoglobin molecule. The reticuloendothelial system is responsible for recycling and redistributing erythrocyte iron as well as the other components of the red blood cell. Although in the past the macrophage was considered the only immune cell involved in iron metabolism, there is now evidence that T lymphocytes and other immune cells also may be involved in regulating iron homeostasis. Iron status also affects the ability of the immune system to fight infection and modulate inflammatory responses. Most human pathogens require iron for replication, and the immune system's unique proteins protect against bacterial iron acquisition, resulting in better control of infectious diseases. These complex interactions are explained in depth in the last two chapters of this section.

The next two sections examine in detail the effects of disorders in iron homeostasis, considering first the anemias and then iron-overload conditions. The essentiality of iron for hemoglobin production and the consequences of iron deficiency as well as iron deficiency anemia are described in detail including the peripheral effects of iron deficiency. In addition to the adverse effects of iron deficiency on oxygen-carrying capacity of the blood, there are many non-hematological clinical manifestations of iron deficiency. Often, the skin color will be reduced and this may be due to vasoconstriction; there may be increased cardiac output and breathing may be labored; muscle fatigue and cramping are often seen. Endurance is compromised and may be the consequence of reduction in any of the 200+ iron-requiring enzymes. Temperature regulation may be impaired which may be related to iron's requirement for neuron myelination in the spinal cord and white matter. New data linking Restless Legs Syndrome with iron deficiency are included. Iron deficiency in pregnancy is linked to low birth weight and pre-term delivery and maternal morbidity as well as mortality. The adverse consequences of low iron status in the neonatal brain may be the result of lower than normal formation of the protective myelin sheath covering critical brain neurons. Important new studies also examine the interaction between zinc and iron and provide further evidence of the complexity of nutrient–nutrient interactions. The nongenetically related causes of anemia are outlined including a chapter describing anemia due to chronic inflammatory diseases. There is also a separate chapter on the iron-loading anemias, an important class of hematological disorders.

The pathologies associated with iron overload are systematically reviewed in eight comprehensive and clinically relevant chapters. The critical importance of the liver in iron homeostasis is reviewed and liver pathology associated with iron overload is examined in detail in its own chapter. A second, related chapter examines the mechanisms behind the pathological effects of iron in the liver and heart, emphasizing the cellular, biochemical, and inflammatory responses and the damaging effects of reactive oxygen species. Chronic liver disease associated with excessive alcohol intake, hepatitis C infection, and obesity is associated with disturbances in iron homeostasis, and this topical area is also covered. The chapter that describes hereditary hemochromatosis and the discovery in only 1996 of the *HFE* gene provides an extensive discussion of the pathology, diagnosis, and treatment of this common disorder. The following chapter discusses the non-HFE-related hemochromatoses and concentrates on the defining clinical features and treatments with emphasis on juvenile hemochromatosis and ferroportin disease.

There is a unique additional chapter that describes some of the other iron-related disorders including hereditary hyperferritinemia-cataract syndrome, aceruloplasminemia, and atransferrinemia. The neuropathology associated with iron overload is described in the next chapter. Iron is required for the optimal functioning of the enzymes responsible for the synthesis and degradation of the major brain neuropeptides including dopamine, serotonin, and noradrenalin. Iron is found in specific sites within the brain and there are many neurotransmitters that require iron for their synthesis. Excess iron within the brain has been associated with a number of neurodegenerative diseases including Parkinson's disease, Alzheimer's disease, Friedreich's ataxia, Wilson's disease, Restless Legs Syndrome, and others. Additionally, as we age, there is an accumulation of iron in the brain that may participate in oxidative damage to neural tissues. Enhanced synthesis of enzymes that result in increased iron in mitochondria and concomitant increased oxidative damage has been seen in tissues from affected human brains. Under normal conditions, cellular iron concentrations in the brain are tightly controlled. When iron levels are abnormally high, the brain reduces the level of iron intake and is resistant to the adverse effects of iron overload initially, but peripheral changes may result in secondary damage to the brain that results in oxidative damage. The new classification of neurodegeneration with brain iron accumulation is highlighted with a consideration of pantothenate kinase deficiency; however, it is not clear if this is a cause and effect relationship or that the iron excess occurs after some initiating event. The final chapter in the iron overload part examines the association of iron status and cancer risk and concludes that, for most cancers, there is insufficient consistent evidence of an association of higher iron status and greater cancer risk. The same chapter includes an extensive review of the importance of iron to bacterial and viral pathogenicity. Tuberculosis, HIV, malaria, and other infectious organisms are included in this review.

Section V includes critical clinical information on diagnoses and therapies related to defects in iron homeostasis. It begins with a chapter on methods for assessing iron status in the body, something which is essential for both diagnosing disorders of iron metabolism and monitoring their therapy. The chapter on genetic testing, with 333 references and 12 tables, describes in detail the known genetic defects associated with mutations affecting iron physiology. More than 100 genetic mutations are described and the race/ethnicities that are most affected are tabulated. The full scope of genetic testing procedures is described including sample collection, methods of mutation analysis, and the process of selection of genes for analysis. The ethical, legal, and social ramifications of genetic testing are objectively discussed. There is a chapter devoted to the chemistry and biochemistry of the iron chelators currently used to treat iron overload that includes 13 figures to assist in understanding the structure/function relationships of these medicines. A separate chapter examines the clinical aspects of using the chelators including their effects on the heart, use in children, dosing, tolerability, and toxicity.

Section VI of this comprehensive volume contains three unique chapters that examine some of the model systems available to study iron metabolism. The most well-recognized mammalian models are genetically altered mice, including knockouts of the major proteins involved in iron transport and its regulation discussed in earlier chapters. Tables are provided that describe most of the mouse and rat genetic models for hereditary hemochromatosis and other inherited defects in iron homeostasis. Yeasts have also proved extremely valuable as models for studying basic cellular iron metabolism, as they can synthesize heme and other iron-containing proteins. The pros and cons of using a yeast model system are objectively described. Zebrafish are also used as the fish are transparent, and the formation of heme and globin and the binding of iron to form hemoglobin as well as the formation of the red blood cell can be visualized in this model. Genetic models of anemia have been developed using this model.

It is abundantly clear that the editors have developed an excellent comprehensive volume that will be a valuable asset for clinicians in many fields as well as cell biologists, geneticists, biochemists, and advanced students in clinical nutrition. The editors have chosen 40 of the most well-recognized and respected authors who are internationally distinguished researchers, clinicians, and epidemiologists who provide a broad foundation for understanding the role of iron in the molecular, genetic, cellular, and clinical aspects of nutritional and therapeutic management of iron status. Hallmarks of all of the 31 chapters include complete explanations of terms with the abbreviations fully defined for the reader and consistent use of terminology between chapters. Key features of the volume include informative key words that are at the beginning of each chapter as well as an in-depth index. Recommendations and practice guidelines are included in relevant chapters. The volume contains more than 100 detailed tables and informative figures and more than 4,500 up-to-date references that provide the reader with excellent sources of worthwhile information about the critical role of iron nutrition, optimal iron status, and the adverse clinical consequences of altered iron homeostasis.

In conclusion, *Iron Physiology and Pathophysiology in Humans*, edited by Gregory J. Anderson and Gordon D. McLaren provides health professionals in many areas of research and practice with the most up-to-date, well-referenced volume on the importance of iron status in determining the health of an individual. This volume will serve the reader as the benchmark in this complex area of interrelationships between the essentiality of iron, its functions throughout the body including its critical role in erythropoiesis, and the biochemistry and clinical relevance of iron-containing enzymes and other active molecules involved in iron absorption, transport, metabolism, and excretion; and bring forth the importance of optimal iron status on immune function, the function of the liver, heart, lungs, kidney, muscle, bone, and the brain. Moreover, the interactions between genetic and environmental factors and the numerous comorbidities seen with both iron deficiency and iron overload in the most at-risk populations are clearly delineated so that students as well as practitioners can better understand the complexities of these interactions. Drs. Anderson and McLaren are applauded for their efforts to develop the most authoritative resource in the field to date, and this excellent text is a very welcome addition to the *Nutrition and Health* series.

Adrianne Bendich, Ph.D., FACN
Series Editor

Preface

The inspiration for this volume was the outstanding book *Iron Metabolism in Man* by Thomas Bothwell and his colleagues. Although it was published more than three decades ago in 1979, it remains a valuable reference today. The basic outline of *Iron Physiology and Pathophysiology in Humans* is not dissimilar to the work of Bothwell et al. It begins with a focus on normal iron metabolism in humans, then progresses to mechanisms of altered iron metabolism in disease. Other chapters cover methods for assessing iron status, the role of iron chelators as therapeutic agents, and various model systems for studying iron homeostasis. Our hope is that this new book will serve both as a resource for workers in the field and a starting point for readers who wish to pursue further study.

By 1979, the fundamental concepts of iron physiology in humans were understood, including the iron cycle within the body, plasma iron kinetics and exchange with the tissues, and iron storage. It was also recognized that intestinal iron absorption is controlled to maintain body iron balance. The state of the art at the cellular and molecular level had advanced to the stage of studying iron transport by transferrin and iron storage in ferritin and hemosiderin, but in retrospect it is now apparent that most of the proteins of iron transport and regulation were then unknown. Similarly, the pathophysiology of a number of disease processes had been described, including iron deficiency and several forms of iron overload such as hereditary hemochromatosis and hemosiderosis resulting from transfusions of red blood cells. Approaches to the diagnosis of various disorders of iron metabolism were established, based on the availability of well-validated tests for the assessment of iron status. These methods have subsequently been supplemented by newer tests and technological advances. On the other hand, efficacious treatment for disorders such as iron deficiency and iron overload had already become relatively standardized, using oral iron replacement and iron removal by therapeutic phlebotomy and iron chelation, respectively.

Over the intervening years, there has been a great expansion of knowledge about iron metabolism and its disorders, and it has become obvious that an update of the field is long overdue. In thinking about the need for a new overview, we quickly realized that the best approach would be to enlist the help of various experts. We asked them to focus on current advances, as recent years have seen a renaissance in the field, fueled by new techniques in molecular biology and genetics. Given the breadth and complexity of the field, we recognized that it would be impractical to attempt to do justice to every facet of iron metabolism in a single volume. Rather, we encouraged the chapter authors to highlight many of the most important areas, with the dual aims of presenting basic principles about the state of the art and providing the reader with a basis for additional research.

One of the primary areas of focus concerns the proteins that transport and store iron and those that play a role in regulating these processes. Much new information has become available about the function and regulation of the previously known and highly evolutionarily conserved molecules transferrin and ferritin. In addition, the last few years have seen the discovery of many previously unknown proteins of iron metabolism, in what is generally considered a new golden age in the field.

Examples include membrane iron transport proteins such as divalent metal-ion transporter 1 and ferroportin 1, enzymes such as the iron oxidase hephaestin and the iron reductase duodenal cytochrome B, and regulatory molecules such as hepcidin, HFE, transferrin receptor 2, and hemojuvelin. Intertwined with these discoveries have been significant advances in understanding disorders of iron metabolism. Novel inherited etiologies of iron deficiency have been discovered, and more is known about the etiology of some previously described causes such as achlorhydria in atrophic gastritis, now recognized as a frequent complication of *H. pylori* infection. The discovery of the hemochromatosis gene (*HFE*) has made it possible to study the prevalence of *HFE*-related hemochromatosis in different populations, and the recognition of the role of HFE and other proteins in regulating hepcidin expression has led to an understanding of the mechanisms underlying both primary and secondary forms of iron overload. Advances in diagnosis of disorders of iron metabolism and assessment of body iron stores have added significantly to the tools available to clinicians. The serum transferrin receptor assay and noninvasive imaging modalities have been notable achievements. Genetic testing for mutations in *HFE* and other genes facilitates the diagnosis of hemochromatosis, and the development of oral iron chelators has been a major advance in treatment of patients with transfusional iron overload. Future advances foreshadowed by recent work may include the ability to modify the expression or action of hepcidin and thereby make it feasible to control dysregulated intestinal iron absorption, whether inappropriately increased, as in hemochromatosis and ineffective erythropoiesis, or decreased in inflammation.

We would like to recognize all the investigators who have made the many important contributions to the field that have created the need for this book, and especially the authors of the individual chapters, without whose efforts creation of the book would not have been possible. It is equally important to acknowledge Adrianne Bendich, editor of the *Nutrition and Health* series, and her dedicated team at Humana/Springer (notably Amanda Quinn in the later stages) for their great patience and guidance as this volume came together. Without their support and encouragement it would have been very difficult to see his project through to completion.

Brisbane, QLD, Australia — Gregory J. Anderson, Ph.D.
Long Beach, CA, USA — Gordon D. McLaren, M.D.

Contents

Section III Disorders of Iron Homeostasis: Anemias

Section IV Disorders of Iron Homeostasis: Iron Overload and Related Conditions

Section V Clinical Diagnosis and Therapy

Contributors

Gregory J. Anderson, BSc, MSc, PhD Iron Metabolism Laboratory, Queensland Institute of Medical Research, Brisbane, QLD, Australia

Bruce R. Bacon, MD Division of Gastroenterology and Hepatology, Department of Internal Medicine, Saint Louis University School of Medicine, St. Louis, MO, USA

James C. Barton, MD Southern Iron Disorders Center, Department of Medicine, University of Alabama at Birmingham, Birmingham, AL, USA

John L. Beard Department of Nutritional Sciences, Pennsylvania State University, University Park, PA, USA

Carole Beaumont, PhD INSERM U773, Centre de Recherche Biomédicale Bichat-Beaujon (CRB3), Université Paris Diderot, Paris, France

Robert S. Britton, PhD Division of Gastroenterology and Hepatology, Department of Internal Medicine, Saint Louis University School of Medicine, St. Louis, MO, USA

Anita C. G. Chua, PhD School of Medicine and Pharmacology and Western Australian Institute for Medical Research, University of Western Australia, Fremantle Hospital, Fremantle, WA, Australia

Darrell H.G. Crawford, MD Discipline of Medicine, The University of Queensland
The Gallipoli Medical Research Foundation, Greenslopes Hospital, Brisbane, QLD, Australia

Maria de Sousa, MD, PhD, FRCPath GABBA Program/ICBAS, IBMC, Molecular and Cellular Biology Institute, University of Porto, Porto, Portugal

Yves Deugnier, MD Liver Unit and CIC INSERM 0203, Pontchaillou University Hospital, Rennes, France

Hal Drakesmith, BA, PhD Molecular Immunology Group, Weatherall Institute of Molecular Medicine, John Radcliffe Hospital, Oxford University, Oxford, UK

Carrie Durward Department of Nutritional Sciences, Pennsylvania State University, University Park, PA, USA

Corwin Q. Edwards, MD Departments of Medicine, Intermountain Medical Center and University of Utah, Salt Lake City, USA

Robert E. Fleming, MD Department of Pediatrics, Cardinal Glennon Children's Medical Center

Department of Biochemistry & Molecular Biology, Saint Louis University School of Medicine, St. Louis, MO, USA

Linda M. Fletcher, PhD Discipline of Medicine, The University of Queensland

The Gallipoli Medical Research Foundation, Greenslopes Hospital, Brisbane, QLD, Australia

Paula Goodman Fraenkel, MD Division of Hematology/Oncology, Department of Medicine, Beth Israel Deaconess Medical Center and Harvard Medical School, Boston, MA, USA

Tomas Ganz, MD, PhD Departments of Medicine and Pathology, David Geffen School of Medicine, University of California, Los Angeles, CA, USA

Victor R. Gordeuk, MD Sickle Cell Center, Division of Hematology and Oncology, Department of Medicine, University of Illinois at Chicago, Chicago, IL, USA

Ross M. Graham, PhD School of Medicine and Pharmacology and Western Australian Institute for Medical Research, University of Western Australia, Fremantle Hospital, Fremantle, WA, Australia

Z. Leah Harris, MD Department of Pediatrics, Vanderbilt University, Nashville, TN, USA

Chaim Hershko, MD Department of Hematology, Shaare Zedek Medical Center and Hebrew University of Jerusalem, Jerusalem, Israel

Robert C. Hider, PhD Department of Pharmacy, Institute of Pharmaceutical Science, King's College London, UK

Kris V. Kowdley, MD Center for Liver Disease, Digestive Disease Institute, Virginia Mason Medical Center, Seattle, WA, USA

Pauline L. Lee, PhD Department of Molecular and Experimental Medicine, The Scripps Research Institute, La Jolla, CA, USA

Weng-In Leong, RD, PhD Department of Nutrition, University of California Davis, Davis, CA, USA

Roland Lill, PhD Institut für Zytobiologie, Philipps-Universität Marburg, Marburg, Germany

Bo Lönnerdal, PhD Department of Nutrition, University of California Davis, Davis, CA, USA

Yong Min Ma, PhD Institute of Pharmaceutical Science, King's College London, London, UK

Andrew T. McKie, PhD Division of Nutritional Sciences, Kings College London, London, UK

Martina U. Muckenthaler, PhD Molecular Medicine Partnership Unit, Heidelberg, Germany

Department of Pediatric Oncology, Hematology and Immunology, Heidelberg, Germany

Gordon D. McLaren Hematology/Oncology Section, Department of Medicine, Veterans Affairs Long Beach Healthcare System, Long Beach, CA, USA

Division of Hematology/Oncology, Department of Medicine, University of California, Irvine, Chao Family Comprehensive Cancer Center, UC Irvine Medical Center, Orange, CA, USA

Sergei Nekhai, PhD Center for Sickle Cell Disease, Division of Hematology and Oncology, Department of Medicine, Howard University, Washington, DC, USA

Caroline C. Philpott, MD Genetics and Metabolism Section, Liver Diseases Branch, NIDDK, NIH, National Institute of Diabetes and Digestive and Kidney Diseases, National Institutes of Health, Bethesda, MD, USA

Sokhon Pin, BS, MBiotech Department of Anesthesiology and Critical Care Medicine, Johns Hopkins University, Baltimore, MD, USA

Prem Ponka, MD, PhD Departments of Physiology and Medicine, Lady Davis Institute for Medical Research, Jewish General Hospital, McGill University, Montreal, QC, Canada

John B. Porter, MA, MD, FRCP, FRCPath Department of Hematology, University College London, London, UK

Graça Porto, MD, PhD GABBA Program/ICBAS, IBMC, Molecular and Cellular Biology Institute, University of Porto, Porto, Portugal

Lawrie W. Powell, AC, MD, PhD Department of Gastroenterology and Hepatology

The Centre for the Advancement of Clinical Research, Royal Brisbane and Women's Hospital, Brisbane, QLD, Australia

Grant A. Ramm, PhD Hepatic Fibrosis Group, Queensland Institute of Medical Research, Brisbane, QLD, Australia

Stefano Rivella, PhD Department of Pediatric Hematology-Oncology, Children's Cancer and Blood Foundation Laboratories, Weill Medical College of Cornell University, New York, NY, USA

Tracey A. Rouault, MD Molecular Medicine Program, Eunice Kennedy Shriver National Institutes of Child Health and Human Development, Bethesda, MD, USA

Cindy N. Roy, PhD Division of Geriatric Medicine and Gerontology, Johns Hopkins University, Baltimore, MD, USA

Richard G. Ruddell, PhD Hepatic Fibrosis Group, Queensland Institute of Medical Research, Brisbane, QLD, Australia

Paul Sharp, PhD Nutritional Sciences Division, King's College London, London, UK

Alex D. Sheftel, PhD University of Ottawa, Ottawa Heart Institute, Ottawa, ON, Canada

Robert J. Simpson, PhD Division of Nutritional Sciences, Kings College London, London, UK

Barry Skikne, MD Celgene Corporation, Overland Park, KS, USA

Richard Skoien, MD Department of Gastroenterology and Hepatology, Centre for Liver Disease Research, Princess Alexandra Hospital, The University of Queensland, Woolloongabba, QLD, Australia

Ann Smith, PhD School of Biological Sciences, University of Missouri-K.C., Kansas City, MO, USA

Surjit Kaila Srai, PhD Institute of Structural and Molecular Biology, University College London, London, UK

V. Nathan Subramaniam, PhD Membrane Transport Laboratory, Queensland Institute of Medical Research, Brisbane, QLD, Australia

Sarah J. Texel, MS Department of Neuroscience, Johns Hopkins University, Baltimore, MD, USA

Elizabeth C. Theil, PhD Children's Hospital of Oakland Research Institute (CHORI), Oakland, CA, USA

Nutritional Sciences & Toxicology, University of California, Berkeley, CA, USA

Molecular & Structural Biochemistry, North Carolina State University, Raleigh, NC, USA

Debbie Trinder, PhD School of Medicine and Pharmacology and Western Australian Institute for Medical Research, University of Western Australia, Fremantle Hospital, Fremantle, WA, Australia

Bruno Turlin, MD Department of Pathology, Pontchaillou University Hospital, Rennes, France

Sophie Vaulont, PhD Institut Cochin, INSERM U567, CNRS, Paris, France

Daniel F. Wallace, PhD Membrane Transport Laboratory, Queensland Institute of Medical Research, Brisbane, QLD, Australia

Günter Weiss, MD Department of Internal Medicine I, Clinical Immunology and Infectious Diseases, Medical University, Innsbruck, Austria

Mark Worwood, MD Emeritus Professor, Cardiff University, Cardiff, Wales, UK

Xueying Xu, MD, PhD Department of Anesthesiology and Critical Care Medicine, Johns Hopkins University, Baltimore, MD, USA

Section I
Cellular Iron Metabolism

Chapter 1
Proteins of Iron Homeostasis

Surjit Kaila Srai and Paul Sharp

Keywords DMT1 • Ferroportin • Heme • Hepcidin • HFE • Iron regulation • Iron storage • Iron transport

1 Introduction

Iron is essential for a number of biochemical functions in the body including the transport of oxygen in the blood and energy production in the mitochondria. Therefore, humans require an abundant and regular source of dietary iron to maintain normal health. This is amply demonstrated by data indicating that as many as a third of the world's population suffer from iron deficiency, making it the most common nutrient deficiency disorder. In addition to pathologies associated with iron deficiency, excess iron is highly toxic and can lead to cell and organ damage. Interestingly, while the body levels of other dietary metals can be regulated by excretion in the feces and urine, humans do not possess the capacity to remove excess iron from the body. As a consequence, a number of proteins have evolved which tightly regulate mammalian iron homeostasis. The actions of these proteins control the rate of duodenal iron absorption, its delivery, utilization and storage by metabolically active tissues, and its recycling by reticuloendothelial macrophages. The purpose of this chapter is to introduce the reader to some of the key proteins that maintain iron balance in humans. We have divided these proteins into families based on their function. This includes (1) the proteins that are involved in iron transport across cellular membranes; (2) the reductases and oxidases that facilitate the movement of iron across cell membranes; (3) iron transport in the circulation and its intracellular storage; and (4) the proteins that control iron homeostasis by regulating all of the above processes. Mutations in the genes encoding many of these proteins lead to a wide range of diseases highlighting the varied role that iron plays in human metabolism. Many of these diseases will be discussed in depth in subsequent chapters.

S.K. Srai, Ph.D.
Institute of Structural and Molecular Biology, University College London, London, UK
e-mail: k.srai@biochem.ucl.ac.uk

P. Sharp, Ph.D. (✉)
Nutritional Sciences Division, King's College London, London, UK
e-mail: paul.a.sharp@kcl.ac.uk

G.J. Anderson and G. McLaren (eds.), *Iron Physiology and Pathophysiology in Humans*, Nutrition and Health, DOI 10.1007/978-1-60327-485-2_1,

2 Proteins Mediating Iron Transport Across Cellular Membranes

2.1 Divalent Metal-Ion Transporter 1

The divalent metal transporter, DMT1 – also known as the divalent cation transporter, DCT1 [1], natural resistance–associated macrophage protein, NRAMP2 [2, 3] and solute-linked carrier family 11 (proton-coupled divalent metal ion transporters), member 2 (SLC11A2) – transports ferrous iron across the apical membrane of the intestinal epithelium [1, 4] (Fig. 1.1). In addition to its essential role in dietary non-heme iron absorption, DMT1 is also required for the endosomal release of transferrin-bound iron. The targeted disruption of DMT1 in mice has confirmed its obligate role in both intestinal iron absorption and in the development of erythroid precursors into mature erythrocytes [5]. This function is further underlined by evidence showing that mutations in DMT1 in the *mk/mk* mouse [3] and the Belgrade rat [6] and humans [1, 7–10] lead to the development of microcytic anemia.

At least four DMT1 isoforms exist through alternate splicing in exon 16 [11] and the presence of two transcription start sites – in exon 1A and 1B, respectively [12]. Exon 16 splicing gives rise to two variants that differ in their terminal 19–25 amino acids and their 3′ untranslated region (UTR); one variant contains an iron responsive element (IRE) in its 3′ UTR whereas the other lacks this sequence [11]. Isoforms containing a 3′ IRE may be subject to iron-sensitive post-transcriptional regulation via the IRE–IRP system (discussed later in this chapter). All four isoforms can be detected

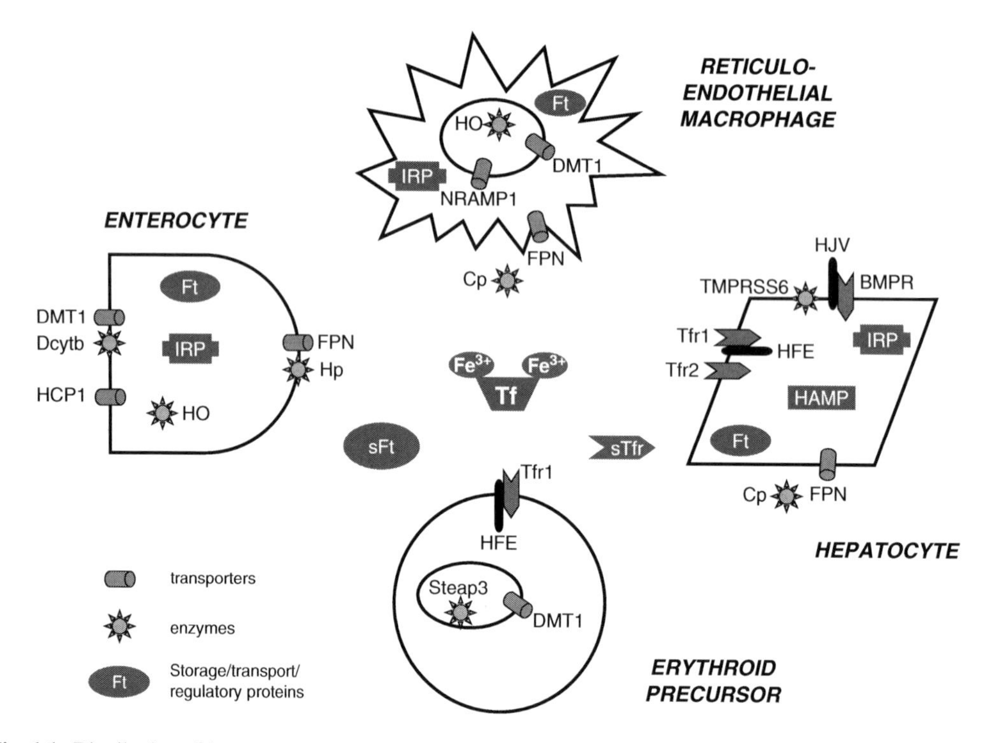

Fig. 1.1 Distribution of iron transport, storage and regulatory proteins in various cell types. *Abbreviations*: *BMPR* bone morphogenetic protein receptor, *Cp* ceruloplasmin, *Dcytb* duodenal cytochrome b, *DMT1* divalent metal transporter 1, *Ft* ferritin, *FPN* ferroportin, *HAMP* hepcidin antimicrobial peptide, *HCP1* heme carrier protein 1, *HFE* hereditary hemochromatosis protein, *HJV* hemojuvelin, *HO* heme oxygenase, *Hp* hephaestin, *IRP* iron regulatory proteins (IRP1/IRP2), *NRAMP1* natural resistance–associated macrophage protein 1, *sFt* serum ferritin, *STEAP3* six transmembrane epithelial antigen of the prostate 3, *sTfr* serum transferrin receptor, *Tf* transferrin, *Tfr1* transferrin receptor 1, *Tfr2* transferrin receptor 2, *TMPRSS6* transmembrane serine protease family member 6 (matriptase 2)

at varying levels in intestinal epithelial cells [12]; and while the exon 1A/IRE-containing variant has been suggested to be the predominant functional isoform with respect to intestinal iron absorption, all four isoforms can transport iron with equal efficiency [13]. Within intracellular endosomes, there appears to be differential localisation of the different DMT1 isoform. The IRE-containing variants are localized to the late endosomes and lysosomes [14–17] whereas non-IRE isoforms are associated with the transferrin receptor-containing early endosomes [15, 17].

In the intestine, DMT1 expression is increased when body iron levels are depleted [1, 18, 19]. This may reflect the presence of the IRE in the 3′ UTR [1] which can bind cytosolic IRP [20]. In addition to these longer term changes in expression, there is good evidence that DMT1 levels respond more rapidly to changes in dietary composition. The so-called "mucosal block" hypothesis was formulated more than 50 years ago following studies which demonstrated that a large oral dose of iron could reduce subsequent iron absorption ([21, 22]; reviewed in [23]). It was argued that due to the short time interval between doses, the initial dose must have acted directly on the mature enterocytes rather than the crypt cells. More recent studies with rodents given an iron bolus [24–26] and in cell culture models [16, 27] suggest that the primary mechanism for mucosal block arises from redistribution of DMT1 between the plasma membrane and intracellular compartments. Our evidence suggests that DMT1 is trafficked from the apical membrane of intestinal epithelial cells to late endosomes/lysosomes [16]. Such a mechanism may be important physiologically for optimizing iron absorption from a meal so that it matches the body's metabolic requirements.

Rapid transcriptional control of iron transport genes may also be important in regulating intestinal iron homeostasis. In this context, two recent studies have identified a role for hypoxia-inducible factors – in particular HIF2α – as important local regulators that respond to decreased intracellular iron levels and low oxygen tension by up-regulating the expression of DMT1 and the ferric reductase Dcytb [28, 29].

2.2 Heme Transporters

In addition to non-heme iron, the iron contained within heme also makes an important contribution to dietary iron absorption. Heme is absorbed intact [30] and the iron is liberated intracellularly under the action of heme oxygenase [31]. While there is a great deal of information regarding the mechanisms involved in non-heme iron absorption, much less is known about potential heme transport mechanisms. A number of candidate heme transport proteins have been identified in the intestinal epithelium including the Breast Cancer Resistance Protein, ABCG2 [32], the feline leukemia virus C receptor protein, FLVCR [33] and the heme carrier protein, HCP1 [34]. Of these candidate transporters, only HCP1 acts as a heme importer (Fig. 1.1), while both ABCG2 and FLVCR mediate heme efflux. The high duodenal expression of HCP1 supports a potential role in heme absorption from the diet; however, this has been complicated by recent evidence suggesting that HCP1 may function primarily as a proton-coupled folate transporter [35]. In an interesting recent development, the heme-regulated gene (HRG) family of proteins has been identified in *C. elegans* [36]. These proteins play an essential role in heme transport and homeostasis in nematodes and their orthologues are also expressed in vertebrates, including humans, suggesting that HRG proteins may also play an important role in heme biology in mammals.

2.3 Ferroportin

Iron efflux from all tissues is mediated by ferroportin [37] – also known as Iron Regulated Transporter 1 (IREG1) [38], Metal Transporter Protein 1 (MTP1) [39] and solute-linked carrier family 40 (iron-regulated transporter) member 1 (SLC40A1) (Fig. 1.1). To date, ferroportin is the only identified iron efflux protein and is particularly important for iron release into the circulation from absorptive enterocytes, iron recycling macrophages, hepatocytes and the placental syncytiotrophoblast. Not surprisingly therefore, global deletion of ferroportin in mice is embryonically lethal [37]. Furthermore, mice with intestine-specific ferroportin deletions (achieved by expression of an inducible intestine-restricted villin-cre-ferroportin transgene) develop iron deficiency highlighting the essential role of ferroportin in dietary iron assimilation [40].

Studies with *Xenopus laevis* oocytes overexpressing ferroportin indicate that this protein mediates the unidirectional efflux of ferrous iron [37, 38]. However, in order for exported iron to be loaded onto transferrin for transport in the circulation, it must be oxidized to its ferric form. Therefore, ferroportin forms only half of the iron efflux pathway, working in concert with the ferroxidases hephaestin and ceruloplasmin (discussed later). Ferroportin is primarily localized to the plasma membrane of cells; in polarized epithelia such as the duodenum and placenta, it is expressed at the basolateral membrane of cells [37, 38] which is consistent with its function as an iron export protein. Interestingly, there have been reports of ferroportin protein expression on the apical membrane of enterocytes [41], but this remains controversial. In iron-recycling macrophages, ferroportin appears to reside in intracellular vesicles but following iron loading [42] or erythrophagocytosis [43, 44], ferroportin is rapidly translocated to the plasma membrane. A recent study has suggested that the trafficking of ferroportin in macrophages may be under the control of Mon1A which plays a fundamental role in the macrophages secretory apparatus [45].

The regulation of ferroportin expression is complex. Ferroportin mRNA contains a single IRE in the 5′ UTR [38, 39] which is predicted to raise protein expression under high iron conditions. In agreement with this hypothesis, iron loading increases ferroportin expression in the liver [39], lung [46] and macrophage [44]. However, the response to changes in iron status is tissue specific. In the duodenum, ferroportin is elevated by iron deficiency but not by iron loading [38]. Recently, a second ferroportin transcript (termed FPN1B) has been identified which lacks the IRE and is not repressed in iron-deficient conditions [47]. While the FPN1A and FPN1B transcripts give rise to identical protein products, their tissue distribution is different; FPN1B is more highly expressed in the duodenum and in erythroid precursors. The identification of the FPN1B transcript provides an explanation of the lack of IRE/IRP-dependent regulation of duodenal iron absorption in the face of systemic iron deficiency.

In addition to regulation by iron, it is now know that ferroportin is the cellular target for the regulatory actions of hepcidin (discussed in detail in subsequent chapters). However, recent work suggests that there may also be subtle tissue-specific differences in ferroportin–hepcidin interactions in the duodenum and macrophage [48–50].

The original identification of ferroportin arose from a study of mutations associated with impaired iron metabolism in zebrafish (*Danio rerio*). One of these fish with impaired hematopoiesis, named *weissherbst*, resulted from mutations in the zebrafish homologue of mammalian ferroportin [37]. Subsequently, a number of mutations have been identified in human ferroportin that give rise to an iron loading syndrome that has been referred to as either type IV hemochromatosis or ferroportin disease (see Chap. 20).

2.4 *Transferrin Receptors*

Transferrin receptors are the main route for iron entry into most cells. To date, two distinct transferrin receptors have been identified, TfR1 (the subject of many reviews) which is expressed on all proliferating cells to permit iron acquisition for the cell cycle and TfR2 [51] which is expressed mainly on hepatocytes [52] (Fig. 1.1).

TfR1 exists on the surface of cells as a disulfide-bonded homodimer of 760-residue subunits (reviewed in [53]). At physiological pH (7.4), TfR1 binds circulating transferrin (either mono-ferric or di-ferric) at the cell surface and the receptor-transferrin complex is endocytosed via a clathrin-mediated mechanism (reviewed in [54]). The transferrin-containing endosome is acidified by recruitment of a V-type proton ATPase permitting the release of iron from transferrin (apotransferrin remains bound to its receptor at the acid pH of the endosome). In erythroid precursors, the iron is reduced by STEAP3 ([55], discussed below) and exits the endosome through DMT1 [6]. The apo-transferrin/TfR1 complex is recycled back to the cell surface where at pH 7.4 it dissociates from its receptor and re-enters the circulation. Iron uptake via this pathway may be regulated by the HFE protein, which competes with transferrin for a common binding site on TfR1 [56, 57].

Studies with Tfr1 knockout mice and zebrafish expressing the *chianti* phenotype highlight the essential role of Tfr1, particularly in development and functioning of erythroid tissue. Murine Tfr1 deletion is embryonically lethal and is characterized by severely disrupted erythropoiesis and neurological development [58]. Furthermore, heterozygous mice carrying only one copy of the Tfr1 allele exhibit impaired erythroid development and abnormal iron homeostasis [58]. Zebrafish, unlike humans and mice, contain two Tfr1-like genes. A mutation in Tfr1a, which is highly expressed in erythroid tissue, gives rise to the *chianti* phenotype characterized by microcytic hypochromic anemia [59]. Interestingly, over-expression of mouse Tfr1, mouse Tfr2 and zebrafish Tfr1b partly rescued the *chianti* phenotype, suggesting that they could permit transferrin-bound iron uptake by erythroid precursors for hemoglobin synthesis [59].

Tfr1 mRNA expression is highly regulated by iron status and this is mediated by the presence of five IRE motifs in the 3′ UTR of the mRNA sequence [60]. Under iron-deficient conditions, the IRE sequences are bound by iron regulatory proteins, protecting the mRNA from endonucleolytic degradation and thus increasing mRNA half-life. As a consequence, Tfr1 protein expression is up-regulated in iron deficiency. In contrast, IRE are unbound under iron replete conditions, leading to rapid degradation of Tfr1 mRNA and a reduction in cellular protein expression [60–62].

Tfr2 has significant sequence homology to Tfr1 and can also bind and transport transferrin-bound iron, albeit with a much lower affinity than Tfr1 [51, 63]. Unlike Tfr1 which is ubiquitously expressed, the expression of Tfr2 is restricted to the liver, and normal and neoplastic hematopoietic cells [51, 64]. Interestingly, mutations in Tfr2 lead to severe hepatic iron overload, termed type III hemochromatosis [65], highlighting its importance in iron homeostasis. These findings have been further confirmed by disruption of the Tfr2 gene in mice [66–68], which also leads to hepatic iron loading.

Tfr2 mRNA expression does not appear to be regulated in response to changes in iron status and its transcript does not contain the IRE motifs that are characteristic of Tfr1 mRNA [51]. Studies using cell culture models [63, 64] as well as in vivo studies in mice [69] report no changes in Tfr2 mRNA levels in response to altered iron status. However, Tfr2 protein expression is up-regulated in response to elevated levels of di-ferric transferrin [70, 71], which binds to Tfr2and increases its membrane stability [70, 72]. Binding of di-ferric transferrin also alters the cellular fate of Tfr2; increasing the levels associated with recycling endosomes and decreasing the fraction of Tfr2 targeted to the lysosomes for degradation [73]. Because of this tight regulation by di-ferric transferrin, Tfr2 has been proposed as a sensor of iron status that monitors changes in circulating transferrin saturation. Intriguingly, two recent studies suggest that the HFE protein interacts with Tfr2 and may therefore be an important component of this iron-sensing pathway [74, 75].

In addition to membrane-associated cellular Tfr1, a soluble form (sTfr) exists in human serum. During the maturation process, erythroid precursors shed transferrin receptors from their cell surface into the circulation [76, 77]. The shedding process is primarily mediated by an integral membrane protease belonging to the disintegrin and metalloprotease (ADAM) family [78] and results in the proteolytic cleavage of Tfr1 at Arg-100 within the transmembrane stalk [79, 80]. Serum transferrin receptor concentrations are increased in patients with elevated levels of immature erythroid cells and in individuals with iron deficiency, but are not altered (or are lower than normal) in patients with the anemia of chronic disease [81, 82]. As such, sTfr has emerged as a powerful biomarker to distinguish between these two forms of anemia (especially when used in conjunction with measurement of serum ferritin). Interestingly, recent data have shown that increasing transferrin saturation decreases the release of sTfr and this effect is mediated by a direct molecular interaction between transferrin and its receptor, indicating that sTfr does not only reflect the iron demand of the cells but also the iron availability in the bloodstream [83].

2.5 *Mitoferrin*

Once taken up by cells in its various forms, iron is utilized for a number of metabolic functions including the synthesis of heme, the production of hemoglobin and the assembly of iron-sulfur clusters. Many of these processes take place in the mitochondrion but the mechanisms by which mitochondria accumulate and store iron has only recently been discovered. Mitoferrin, a member of the vertebrate mitochondrial solute carrier family (SLC25A37) was identified by positional cloning, and is highly expressed in hematopoietic tissue [84]. A mutation in the mitoferrin gene in zebrafish is responsible for the *frascati* phenotype that shows profound hypochromic anemia and the arrest of erythroid maturation owing to defects in mitochondrial iron uptake. Mitoferrin orthologues (MRS3 and MRS4) also exist in yeast and disruption of these genes causes defects in hemoprotein production and the mitochondrial synthesis of iron-sulfur clusters [85–88]. Interestingly, work by Shaw et al. [84] indicates that expression of murine mitoferrin can rescue the defects in iron metabolism exhibited in the *frascati* zebrafish, and furthermore that introduction of zebrafish mitoferrin can complement the yeast MRS3/4 mutant, indicating that the function of the gene may be highly conserved.

2.6 *Natural Resistance–Associated Macrophage Protein 1*

The NRAMP family of proteins has two mammalian members; NRAMP1 (SLC11A1) which confers resistance to infection by mycobacteria [89]; and NRAMP2 (DMT1 or SLC11A2) [2] which transports iron across the apical membrane of duodenal enterocytes and the membrane of transferrin-containing endosomes [1, 3, 6] (Fig. 1.1). NRAMP orthologues exist in yeast (SMF1 and SMF2) [90] and in *Drosophila melanogaster* (malvolio) [91] and are all thought to act as metal ion transporters [92].

NRAMP1 is almost exclusively expressed in macrophages and neutrophils where upon activation it is recruited to phagosomal membranes [93]. In inbred mouse models, increased susceptibility to infections by intracellular pathogens is associated with a single amino acid substitution (glycine to aspartic acid) at position 169, which lies in the predicted fourth transmembrane domain of the protein [94]. Like other members of the NRAMP family, NRAMP1 is a metal ion transport protein but its mode of action remains unclear. Gros and colleagues have proposed that NRAMP1 acts as a membrane efflux pump in phagosomes, thereby restricting the availability of essential metals such as Mn^{2+} and Fe^{2+} to the pathogen [95–97]. In contrast, there is evidence from other groups that NRAMP1 acts as a metal influx pump to increase the production of oxygen radicals through Fenton-type chemistry [98, 99]. Furthermore, studies in Xenopus oocytes have suggested that NRAMP1 could act as proton-coupled antiporter [100], unlike its family member DMT1 which acts as a symporter [1, 4]. Interestingly, recent evidence suggests that both NRAMP1 and DMT1 are required for efficient macrophage iron recycling following erythrophagocytosis [101, 102].

NRAMP1 polymorphisms are distributed along the entire NRAMP1 genomic sequence and a complex linkage disequilibrium pattern exists within and around the NRAMP1 locus [103, 104].

It is becoming increasingly apparent (>100 papers) that NRAMP1 polymorphisms may predispose individuals to a number of human infections (some of the evidence is reviewed in [105, 106]). We have recently shown that hypoxia inducible factor (HIF-1) regulates allelic variation in SLC11A1 expression by directly binding to microsatellite (GT/AC)n dinucleotides during macrophage activation by infection. Therefore it is assumed that HIF-1 influences heritable variation in SLC11A1-dependent innate resistance to infection and inflammation within and between populations [107]. Determining the rationale for these associations remains a major challenge for the future.

3 Iron Reductases and Oxidases That Facilitate the Movement of Iron Across Membranes

3.1 Duodenal Cytochromes b (Dcytb)

Non-heme iron is present in the diet mainly as ferric salts and oxides. However, these compounds are not bioavailable and iron must be reduced to the ferrous form prior to absorption by duodenal enterocytes. A number of dietary factors contribute to the conversion of Fe(III) to Fe(II), notably ascorbic acid [108] and a number of meat digestion products [109–112]. In addition, several studies have demonstrated that the brush-border surface of duodenal enterocytes and cultured intestinal cells possess ferric reductase enzymic activity [113–115]. The enzyme responsible for this process, named Dcytb (duodenal cytochrome b) (Fig. 1.1), a homologue of cytochrome b_{561}, was cloned from mouse duodenal mRNA using a subtractive hybridisation strategy [116]. Dcytb is expressed at the apical membrane of duodenal enterocytes, the major site for the absorption of dietary iron and like other members of the cytochrome b_{561} family is a heme-containing, ascorbate requiring protein [116, 117].

The mRNA expression of Dcytb is highly regulated by dietary iron status, hypoxia and in hemochromatosis [116, 118], suggesting that it plays an important role in the maintenance of body iron homeostasis. In vitro studies show a dramatic increase in iron uptake in cultured cell lines over-expressing Dcytb [119, 120]. In contrast, the targeted disruption of the *Cybrd1* gene (which encodes Dcytb) in mice does not lead to an iron-deficient phenotype [121], casting doubt on the absolute requirement of Dcytb for intestinal iron absorption. An important caveat to these studies is that humans rely totally on the diet to provide vitamin C, whereas mice can synthesize abundant quantities of vitamin C *de novo* from glucose, and as such may have less need for a duodenal surface ferric reductase. However, it is interesting to note that, unlike DMT1 and ferroportin where a number of disease-causing mutations have been identified, only one recent report has linked a single nucleotide polymorphism in Dcytb to impaired iron metabolism [122].

3.2 The Six Transmembrane Epithelial Antigen of the Prostate (STEAP) Family

A second family of reductase proteins – the STEAP family – has recently been identified and, with the exception of STEAP1, these proteins act as iron reductases in vitro [55, 123]. One of these proteins, STEAP 3, acts as the endosomal ferric reductase in erythroid precursors, converting iron liberated from transferrin from ferric to ferrous so that it can exit endosomes via DMT1 [55] (Fig. 1.1). A mutation in STEAP 3 in *nm1054* mice leads to hypochromic, microcytic anemia due to the inability of erythroid precursors to utilize transferrin-bound iron. This essential role of STEAP 3 was confirmed following the generation of STEAP 3 knockout mice, which like their spontaneous mutant (*nm1054*) counterparts also exhibited anemia.

3.3 Ceruloplasmin

The essential role played by copper in the regulation of iron metabolism has been recognized for many years (reviewed extensively by [124, 125]). However, it is only relatively recently that we have begun to understand the molecular basis for the biological interactions between these two metals. In experimental animals, it is possible to generate anemia by both copper deficiency and iron deficiency, which display remarkably similar hematological features [126, 127]. The common factor in the etiology of both of these diseases was identified as ceruloplasmin, a multicopper binding protein with serum oxidase activity [128]. Subsequent studies revealed that ceruloplasmin acted as a ferroxidase converting Fe^{2+} to Fe^{3+} [129] and increased the rate of loading of iron onto transferrin [130] (Fig. 1.1). Further studies with perfused liver preparations showed that ceruloplasmin markedly stimulated iron efflux from the liver suggesting that it is a crucial factor for the mobilization of iron from the body stores for metabolic utilization [131]. More recently, the key role of ceruloplasmin in iron metabolism has been confirmed in studies on human patients and mice displaying disrupted ceruloplasmin production. In patients with aceruloplasminemia, and in ceruloplasmin-null mice, there is accumulation of iron in a number of organs, including the liver and various regions of the brain [132], as well as hypoferremia and impaired erythropoiesis.

While ceruloplasmin is often thought of as a plasma protein, synthesized and secreted by the liver, a second form of the enzyme, which is bound to the cell membrane by a glycosylphosphatidylinositol (GPI)-anchor (GPI-ceruloplasmin), is localized to the surface of astrocytes in the central nervous system (CNS) [133]. GPI-ceruloplasmin is produced by alternative splicing of the ceruloplasmin gene [134, 135] and is essential for iron efflux from cells in the CNS [136]. Mechanistically, GPI-ceruloplasmin and soluble ceruloplasmin may be important for the stabilization of the ferroportin efflux transporter at the plasma membrane. Recent studies have shown that the loss of ceruloplasmin activity prevents ferroportin-mediated iron export in cultured cells [137].

The essential role of copper in the regulation of iron metabolism is also evident in lower eukaryotic species. Genetic studies of iron metabolism in the yeast *Saccharomyces cerevisiae* have shown that a copper-binding protein Fet3, which has sequence homology to ceruloplasmin, is required for high-affinity iron uptake [138, 139]. Like ceruloplasmin, Fet3 has ferroxidase activity suggesting that oxidation and reduction of iron are crucial to its movement across biological membranes in yeast as well as in mammals.

3.4 Hephaestin

The link between copper and iron metabolism has been further enhanced by studies carried out in *sla* (sex-linked anemia) mice. The *sla* phenotype is characterized by normal iron absorption from the diet but defective transfer of iron into the plasma. The *sla* locus is present on the X-chromosome; this region has subsequently been mapped [140] and the candidate gene mutated in the *sla* mice identified. The gene encodes the protein hephaestin [141], a copper-containing protein with homology to ceruloplasmin (Fig. 1.1). Hephaestin expression is not limited to the duodenum, and is widely expressed along the length of the gastrointestinal tract, suggesting that it may have other physiological functions in addition to the regulation of iron absorption [141–143]. Recent work has confirmed that hephaestin, like ceruloplasmin, exhibits significant ferroxidase activity [144]. Further modeling of the protein predicts that the mutation present in the *sla* mice would lead to protein misfolding and reduced ferroxidase activity [144, 145]. The cellular localisation of the hephaestin protein is intriguing. Based on the actions of ceruloplasmin, one would predict that hephaestin would localize to the basolateral membrane of duodenal enterocytes where it could interact with ferroportin to oxidise iron leaving the enterocytes so that it could be loaded onto transferrin. However, in normal enterocytes, in addition to some staining on the basolateral membrane [146], there is abundant expression of hephaestin protein within intracellular structures [142]. Taken together, these studies suggest that in normal enterocytes hephaestin may traffic between intracellular organelles and the cell surface. In contrast, in *sla* mice, hephaestin is localized exclusively to the supranuclear compartment of enterocytes [146] suggesting that the mutation leads to mislocalisation of hephaestin protein and results in the functional deficiency in iron efflux from the *sla* intestine.

4 Iron Transport and Storage Proteins

4.1 *Transferrin*

Approximately 3–4 mg of iron circulates in the plasma bound to a specific binding protein, transferrin (Tf) (Fig. 1.1). Serum Tf is a member of the Tf superfamily of proteins that includes lactoferrin (found in milk and other secretory fluids), ovotransferrin (found in avian egg white) and melanotransferrin. Whereas the primary function of serum transferrin – the transport of iron to sites of utilization and storage within the body – is clearly defined, the functions of the other major members of Tf superfamily are less clear [147]. There are approximately 19 Tf variants, however only Tf C can be found in the majority of humans [148]. The Tfs are synthesized primarily in the liver and are formed of single polypeptide chains of approximately 80 kDa, which can bind two atoms of ferric iron [149]. The binding of iron to transferrin is reversible and pH-dependent, with complete association above pH 7 but increasing dissociation at acid pH (below pH 6.5). The equilibrium constant for iron–transferrin binding is 10^{26}–10^{30} [150].

Tf concentration in the circulation is of the order of 30 μM and it is approximately 30–35% saturated with iron in people with normal iron status. Given that there are two iron binding sites on the protein, Tf can exist as iron-free apo-Tf, in the monoferric form, or as di-ferric- or holo-Tf. At normal circulating levels, the majority of iron-bound transferrin is present as mono-Tf, whereas di-ferric-Tf predominates in iron-loading disorders such as hemochromatosis [151]. Interestingly, the binding of di-ferric-Tf to Tfr1 is at least one order of magnitude greater than for monoferric-Tf [152].

4.2 *Ferritin*

The ferritin molecule is a hollow protein shell, composed of 24 polypeptide subunits, with an overall molecular weight of approximately 500 kDa that can store up to 4,500 ferric iron atoms (reviewed in [153]). Ferritins are the main iron storage molecules in all mammalian tissues and consist of a mixture of two subunits referred to as L- and H- ferritin (Fig. 1.1). In general, L-rich ferritins are characteristic of organs storing iron for a prolonged period (e.g., liver and spleen) and these ferritins usually have relatively high average iron content (1,500 Fe atoms/molecule or more). H-rich ferritins which are characteristic of heart and brain have relatively low average iron contents (less than 1,000 Fe atoms/molecule). H-ferritin chains are important for Fe(II) oxidation whereas L-chains assist in the formation of the ferritin core. Ferritins are not inert and are constantly turned over [154]. The iron stored in ferritin is available for utilization by other functional proteins and can be mobilized following lysosomal degradation of the ferritin complex [155]. The mechanisms by which iron is donated to ferritin for storage have remained elusive. However, a recent study has identified the poly(rC)-binding protein 1 (PCBP1) as a key component of this pathway [156]. PCBP1 binds iron, and can also bind directly to ferritin to facilitate iron loading. Furthermore, knocking down PCBP1 with siRNA in human cells decreases ferritin–iron levels, increasing the cytosolic iron pool.

Induction of ferritin synthesis in response to iron administration was first observed by Granick [157] in the gastrointestinal mucosa of guinea pigs after iron feeding. The response is rapid and this may reflect the need to limit the cell's exposure to pro-oxidant free iron. The iron-mediated induction of ferritin expression is largely post-transcriptional and involves IRP binding to a stem-loop IRE present in the 5′ untranslated region of both H- and L-ferritin mRNAs [158–161]. Under iron replete conditions, ferritin mRNA is efficiently translated. However, when cellular iron levels decrease, ferritin protein levels are also lowered. This decrease in ferritin is directly attributable to the position of the IRE in the 5′ UTR. The IRE in both ferritin H and L chain is less than 40 bases from the AUG site and binding of IRP to these IRE sequences prevents the binding of the eukaryotic initiation factor (eIF4F) complex to the 43S ribosomal subunit that is necessary for protein translation [162].

Small amounts of ferritin normally circulate in the serum [163, 164]. In humans, serum ferritin appears to consist largely of a glycosylated form of L-ferritin [165, 166], which has a low iron content [167, 168]. In normal healthy subjects, there is a close correlation between serum ferritin and the body iron stores with 1 μg/L serum ferritin being equivalent to approximately 8–10 mg tissue iron [169, 170]. Serum ferritin levels range from 30 to 300 μg/L in men and 15 to 150 μg/L in women. Serum ferritin derives from tissue ferritin and can be secreted from the liver [171, 172] and from lymphoid cells [173]. Interestingly, it was recently observed that glycosylated L-ferritin, akin to that present in serum, can be actively secreted from human hepatoma cells [174].

In 2001, a novel form of ferritin was identified that localized to the mitochondria [175]. Mitochondrial ferritin is encoded by an intronless gene on chromosome 5q23 [175, 176]; however, unlike cytosolic ferritin, the mitochondrial form lacks a 5′ IRE. Mitochondrial ferritin is 79% identical to cytosolic H-ferritin, but has a long amino acid N-terminal mitochondrial import sequence which is cleaved during processing, and exhibits ferroxidase activity [175]. The expression of mitochondrial ferritin mRNA is highest in metabolically active tissues such as the testis and is noticeably absent from tissues associated explicitly with iron storage such as the liver and spleen [175, 177]. While mitochondrial ferritin does sequester iron, these data suggest that the primary role of the protein might be to protect cells that generate high mitochondrial levels of reactive oxygen species during metabolism from the pro-oxidant effects of iron.

Under conditions of iron excess, some cellular ferritin can be converted into another storage form known as hemosiderin [178], which can be clearly identified in tissues associated with iron storage, including the liver, spleen and bone marrow [178–180]. Both ferritin and hemosiderin are found in lysosomal structures that have been termed siderosomes. Hemosiderin is typically insoluble [181] and is generally considered to be a degradation product of ferritin [178, 179]. Hemosiderin particle sizes are smaller than those of cytosolic ferritin cores [182] and are formed following lysosomal degradation of ferritin. The enzymes causing the cleavage have not been identified.

5 Proteins Involved in the Regulation of Iron Status

5.1 Iron Regulatory Proteins

A number of genes associated with the maintenance of iron homeostasis are tightly regulated in response to the prevailing intracellular iron levels through post-transcriptional mechanisms that involve interactions between cytosolic iron regulatory proteins (IRP) and stem-loop structures known as iron responsive elements (IRE). These IRE motifs exist in either the 5′ or 3′ untranslated region (UTR) of several target mRNA species. Two cytosolic iron regulatory proteins, IRP-1 and IRP-2, are known to exist in most cells and both of these proteins can bind to IRE structures when cellular iron levels are depressed. However, under iron replete conditions, RNA binding is quickly inactivated by either post-translational modification of IRP-1 or degradation of IRP-2.

The mechanism underlying the iron-dependent inactivation of IRP-1 has been studied extensively. Structurally, IRP-1 is very similar to the mitochondrial aconitase [183] that converts citrate to isocitrate in the tricarboxylic acid cycle. Under conditions of iron deficiency, IRP-1 binds avidly to IRE sequences, but when cells are iron replete, IRP-1 acts as a cytoplasmic aconitase. This dual function is controlled by the presence or absence of an iron-sulfur cluster. When cellular iron is high, a 4Fe-4S cluster is inserted into the IRE-binding pocket of IRP-1 and is held in place by three conserved cysteine residues (these residues are also present in the mitochondrial aconitase). Under these conditions, IRP-1 has a closed conformation and cannot bind IREs. The fourth position iron in the cluster is highly labile and is readily removed when cellular iron levels fall, leading to disassembly of the Fe-S cluster, which permits the apoprotein to bind IRE sequences (reviewed in [184–186]).

IRP-2 is less abundant in cells than IRP-1 and is subject to *de novo* synthesis when cellular iron levels are low but is targeted for proteosomal degradation when iron levels are high [187]. IRP-2 contributes significantly to the total IRP RNA binding activity in several tissues but particularly in the brain [188] and intestine [189]. Both IRP-1 and IRP-2 bind successfully to the consensus IRE sequence; however, evidence suggests that IRP-2 may be able to recognize exclusively a specific subset of IRE sequences [190, 191].

5.2 HFE

Hereditary hemochromatosis is a common inborn error of iron metabolism (approximately 1:200 people mainly of northern European decent are affected) that is characterized by excess iron accumulation and deposition within several tissues, especially the liver. The most common form of hemochromatosis arises from an autosomal recessive mutation that leads to the substitution of tyrosine for cysteine at amino acid 282 (C282Y) of the HFE protein [192]. Other mutations, such as H63D, which is more prevalent than C282Y, and S65C may be associated with mild iron loading. Other rarer mutations include missense mutations in exon 2 of the *HFE* gene (I105T and G93R) and a splice-site mutation (IVS3+1G/T) that may contribute to the classical hemochromatosis phenotype (reviewed in [193]).

The HFE protein is a member of the MHC class 1 family of molecules that are involved in antigen presentation to T-cells [192]. Like other class I proteins, HFE contains three extracellular loops ($\alpha 1$, $\alpha 2$, $\alpha 3$) which are essential for its function [194]. The $\alpha 3$ domain is required for HFE to associate with β_2-microglobulin for normal intracellular processing and cell surface expression [195–197]. Recent evidence also suggests that the $\alpha 3$ loop is also the site for HFE/Tfr2 interactions [72]. In addition to its interaction with β_2-microglobulin, HFE also binds to Tfr1, via its $\alpha 2$ loop, regulating the rate at which transferrin-bound iron can enter the cell [195, 198]. Given these interactions, it is not surprising therefore that the HFE protein is highly expressed in a number of tissues that have major roles in body iron metabolism, principally the liver (in Kupffer cells and hepatocytes) [52, 199] (Fig. 1.1) but also the duodenum (where it is found exclusively in the crypts of Lieberkühn) [200], and in tissue macrophages and circulating monocytes [201]. The involvement of HFE in iron metabolism has been further confirmed using Hfe knockout mice, which develop liver iron overload and resemble the human hereditary hemochromatosis phenotype [202].

5.3 Hepcidin

Hepcidin is a major regulator of body iron homeostasis. The HAMP (hepcidin antimicrobial peptide) gene is expressed predominantly in the liver and its mRNA encodes an 84 amino acid pre-pro-peptide which undergoes cellular cleavage [203] to release the active 25 amino acid peptide into the circulation [204, 205]. The mature peptide contains eight cysteine residues that yield four disulphide bonds originally thought to confer a distorted hairpin-like structure [206]. However, more recent analysis has produced an updated structure for hepcidin, comprising a stable β-sheet together with a β-hairpin loop [207]. Hepcidin was first identified as an antimicrobial peptide in human plasma ultrafiltrate and urine [204, 205]. However, it became apparent that hepcidin expression is also associated with the regulation of body iron status in both health and disease. Studies revealed that hepcidin expression is dramatically increased when liver iron is high (following dietary iron loading) [208], and is down-regulated by feeding a low-iron diet [19]. In addition to its modulation by iron, hepcidin expression also responds dramatically to changes in the erythroid requirement for iron. Phlebotomy [209], hemolysis [209, 210] and elevated erythropoietin levels [209], major stimuli for reticulocytosis, all inhibit hepcidin production, and result in increased iron assimilation from the diet.

A role for hepcidin in iron metabolism was first established using knockout mice in which the USF2 transcription factor had been deleted. These animals developed a severe iron overload, strikingly similar to that found in human hemochromatosis and in the *Hfe* $^{-/-}$ mouse [211]. Subsequent examination of the *Usf2* $^{-/-}$ mice revealed that the hepcidin gene had also been disrupted (the two mouse genes are only 1,240 bp apart) [208] and an alternative gene-targeting strategy confirmed that it was the disruption of the hepcidin gene and not USF2 that resulted in the iron overloading phenotype [212]. Recent studies have demonstrated a further link between hepcidin expression and the regulation of human iron metabolism. HAMP gene mutations (93delG and C166T – both homozygous recessive mutations) give rise to a severe iron loading disease that typically affects people in their late teens and early twenties, termed juvenile hemochromatosis (also known as HFE Type 2B) [213]. Further mutations in the hepcidin gene have also been identified which alter the structure and function of the mature peptide (reviewed in [214]).

In addition to null animals, transgenic mice over-expressing hepcidin have also been generated [212]. These animals have severe body iron deficiency and microcytic hypochromic anemia, suggesting a reciprocal relationship between hepcidin expression and iron accumulation. Furthermore, studies in humans have demonstrated that elevated expression of hepcidin is associated with the anemia of chronic disease [205, 209, 215, 216], indicating that pathological changes in hepcidin expression have severe consequences for body iron metabolism.

Hepcidin is thought to exert its effects on iron metabolism by inhibiting iron efflux through the ferroportin transporter. A number of in vitro studies suggest that hepcidin binds directly to ferroportin, rapidly (within 1–4 h) inducing the internalization and degradation of transporter protein [217–220]. This in turn impairs the release of iron from its target cells (namely, the reticuloendothelial macrophages and the duodenal enterocytes) into the circulation. While both in vivo and in vitro studies support this rapid mode of action in macrophages [42, 43, 48, 49], recent data from our laboratory [48, 50] and others [49] suggest that intestinal iron transport is not affected by hepcidin over the same time scale. We have proposed that upon its release into the circulation, hepcidin initially targets iron recycling macrophages resulting in down-regulation of ferroportin protein levels and as a consequence hypoferremia. The inhibitory effects of hepcidin on duodenal iron transport and enterocyte ferroportin levels are only evident following chronic exposure to hepcidin. Since the reticuloendothelial macrophages recycle some 20–25 mg Fe/day from senescent red blood cells, compared with only 1–2 mg Fe/day assimilated from the diet by the duodenal enterocytes, we believe the fact that macrophages respond more acutely to a hepcidin challenge is fully consistent with their paramount importance in maintaining body iron homeostasis.

5.4 TMPRSS6

A number of investigators have identified iron-deficient individuals that do not respond to iron supplementation therapy. Recent studies [221–223] have identified several mutations in the TMPRSS6 gene which gives rise to this phenotype. TMPRSS6 encodes a member of the type II transmembrane serine protease family known as matriptase-2. Its full role in controlling body iron status is unclear; however, two mouse models have recently been used to address this issue – the *mask* mouse (which arose from a chemically induced recessive mutation in *Tmprss6*) [224], and the *Tmprss6* knockout mouse [225]. Both models are characterized by microcytic anemia and a progressive loss of hair from the body but not the face of the mouse. TMPRSS6 appears to be a suppressor of hepcidin expression [224], possibly acting via the cleavage of the regulatory protein hemojuvelin [226]. In *mask* and *Tmprss6–/–* mice [224, 225], or in human subjects with TMPRSS6 mutations [223, 227–229], the lack of functional matriptase 2 results in inappropriately high hepcidin levels. Modulation of hepcidin expression in turn leads to downstream effects on intestinal iron absorption and macrophage iron recycling. Recent genome-wide association studies have also identified TMPRSS6 as a strong candidate gene for determining iron status [230–233].

5.5 Hemojuvelin

Juvenile hemochromatosis can be divided into two distinct subtypes; type 2B is associated with mutations in hepcidin, while type 2A occurs as a consequence of mutations in hemojuvelin (HJV). The HJV protein is attached to the surface of hepatocytes and skeletal and cardiac myocytes through a GPI anchor and shares significant homology to the repulsive guidance molecule family. Interestingly, HJV expression is greatest in skeletal and cardiac muscle, suggesting that these organs also may play a major role in regulating body iron metabolism. While a number of mutations in HJV have been identified (reviewed in [214]), one particular mutation (G320V) is significantly more frequent than others [234–240]. Iron overload associated with HJV mutations is accompanied by greatly diminished hepcidin levels in human patients [236] and in mice [241, 242].

Interestingly, there is evidence that HJV can be shed from the cell surface through the action of a pro-protein convertase [243–245]. Intriguingly soluble HJV (sHJV) when added to hepatoma cells can decrease hepcidin expression, suggesting that sHJV may regulate the effects of the cell-associated HJV protein on hepcidin expression [246]. HJV, like other members of the repulsive guidance molecule family, acts as a co-receptor for bone morphogenetic protein (BMP) receptors [247]. Activation of BMP receptor/HJV with BMP2/4 leads to phosphorylation of SMAD proteins (SMAD 1, 5 and 8 are involved in the HJV pathway) which form heteromeric complexes with SMAD 4 and act as transcription factors. Disruption of this pathway via the liver-specific deletion of Smad 4 in mice recapitulates the juvenile hemochromatosis phenotype [248]. In addition, mutations in HJV impair BMP signaling and down-regulate hepcidin expression in hepatocytes [247]. While several BMPs can interact with HJV to regulate hepcidin expression, BMP6 has emerged as the major regulator of iron homeostasis. BMP6 expression in hepatocytes is regulated by iron status [249]. Furthermore, deletion of the BMP6 gene in mice results in massive iron overload with markedly reduced hepcidin expression [250, 251], suggesting that other endogenous BMPs cannot compensate for the loss of BMP6.

5.6 *Frataxin*

Friedreich's ataxia is an autosomal recessive neuro- and cardio-degenerative disorder affecting 1 in 40,000 Caucasians. The majority of patients have trinucleotide repeat (GAA) within the first intron of the gene encoding frataxin, which leads to iron accumulation within the mitochondria (reviewed in [252–254]). Frataxin is a 210-amino acid protein located predominantly within the mitochondria – associated with the mitochondrial membrane and present as a free soluble protein [255]. The initial link between frataxin and iron metabolism was established in studies using the yeast frataxin homologue (Yfh1) [256]. Yeast lacking Yfh1p accumulate iron [256] and exhibit decreased ability to synthesize iron-sulfur clusters [257]. Interestingly, frataxin can substitute for Yfh1p in yeast, suggesting that they are functional homologues [256, 258]. Human metabolism is reliant on a number of enzymes containing iron-sulfur clusters and frataxin has been suggested to act as a chaperone for iron in mitochondrial iron-sulfur cluster assembly [259, 260]. One key iron-sulfur protein is ferrochelatase, the enzyme responsible for insertion of iron into protoporphyrin IX to form heme. Recent work has suggested that frataxin may act as a high-affinity binding partner for ferrochelatase [261], indicating that frataxin is central to both iron-sulfur and heme protein synthesis.

It is noteworthy that the identification and characterisation of many of the genes and proteins discussed in this chapter has taken place in the past 10–15 years. The roles of these proteins in maintaining iron homeostasis, and the pathological implications of gene mutations will be discussed in more depth in subsequent chapters. Novel proteins and regulatory pathways continue to be identified, for example growth differentiation factor 15 (GDF15) [262, 263] and twisted gastrulation (TWSG1) [264], both members of the TGF-β superfamily that are proposed to act as negative regulators of hepcidin expression; and neogenin which is a putative regulator of membrane HJV levels [265–267]. It seems likely that the next 15 years will be an equally productive era in unraveling the complex pathways that regulate iron homeostasis.

References

1. Gunshin H, Mackenzie B, Berger UV, Gunshin Y, Romero MF, Boron WF, et al. Cloning and characterization of a mammalian proton-coupled metal-ion transporter. Nature. 1997;388:482–8.
2. Gruenheid S, Cellier M, Vidal S, Gros P. Identification and characterization of a second mouse Nramp gene. Genomics. 1995;25:514–25.
3. Fleming MD, Trenor III CC, Su MA, Foernzler D, Beier DR, Dietrich WF, et al. Microcytic anaemia mice have a mutation in Nramp2, a candidate iron transporter gene. Nat Genet. 1997;16:383–6.
4. Tandy S, Williams M, Leggett A, Lopez-Jimenez M, Dedes M, Ramesh B, et al. Nramp2 expression is associated with pH-dependent iron uptake across the apical membrane of human intestinal Caco-2 cells. J Biol Chem. 2000;275:1023–9.
5. Gunshin H, Fujiwara Y, Custodio AO, Direnzo C, Robine S, Andrews NC. Slc11a2 is required for intestinal iron absorption and erythropoiesis but dispensable in placenta and liver. J Clin Invest. 2005;115:1258–66.
6. Fleming MD, Romano MA, Su MA, Garrick LM, Garrick MD, Andrews NC. Nramp2 is mutated in the anemic Belgrade (b) rat: evidence of a role for Nramp2 in endosomal iron transport. Proc Natl Acad Sci USA. 1998;95:1148–53.
7. Mims MP, Guan Y, Pospisilova D, Priwitzerova M, Indrak K, Ponka P, et al. Identification of a human mutation of DMT1 in a patient with microcytic anemia and iron overload. Blood. 2005;105:1337–42.
8. Beaumont C, Delaunay J, Hetet G, Grandchamp B, de Montalembert M, Tchernia G. Two new human DMT1 gene mutations in a patient with microcytic anemia, low ferritinemia, and liver iron overload. Blood. 2006;107:4168–70.
9. Iolascon A, d'Apolito M, Servedio V, Cimmino F, Piga A, Camaschella C. Microcytic anemia and hepatic iron overload in a child with compound heterozygous mutations in DMT1 (SCL11A2). Blood. 2006;107:349–54.
10. Lam-Yuk-Tseung S, Camaschella C, Iolascon A, Gros P. A novel R416C mutation in human DMT1 (SLC11A2) displays pleiotropic effects on function and causes microcytic anemia and hepatic iron overload. Blood Cells Mol Dis. 2006;36:347–54.

11. Lee PL, Gelbart T, West C, Halloran C, Beutler E. The human Nramp2 gene: characterization of the gene structure, alternative splicing, promoter region and polymorphisms. Blood Cells Mol Dis. 1998;24:199–215.
12. Hubert N, Hentze MW. Previously uncharacterized isoforms of divalent metal transporter (DMT)-1: implications for regulation and cellular function. Proc Natl Acad Sci USA. 2002;99:12345–50.
13. Mackenzie B, Takanaga H, Hubert N, Rolfs A, Hediger MA. Functional properties of multiple isoforms of human divalent metal-ion transporter 1 (DMT1). Biochem J. 2007;403:59–69.
14. Canonne-Hergaux F, Gruenheid S, Ponka P, Gros P. Cellular and subcellular localization of the Nramp2 iron transporter in the intestinal brush border and regulation by dietary iron. Blood. 1999;93:4406–17.
15. Tabuchi M, Tanaka N, Nishida-Kitayama J, Ohno H, Kishi F. Alternative splicing regulates the subcellular localization of divalent metal transporter 1 isoforms. Mol Biol Cell. 2002;13:4371–87.
16. Johnson DM, Yamaji S, Tennant J, Srai SK, Sharp PA. Regulation of divalent metal transporter expression in human intestinal epithelial cells following exposure to non-haem iron. FEBS Lett. 2005;579:1923–9.
17. Lam-Yuk-Tseung S, Gros P. Distinct targeting and recycling properties of two isoforms of the iron transporter DMT1 (NRAMP2, Slc11A2). Biochemistry. 2006;45:2294–301.
18. Trinder D, Oates PS, Thomas C, Sadleir J, Morgan EH. Localisation of divalent metal transporter 1 (DMT1) to the microvillus membrane of rat duodenal enterocytes in iron deficiency, but to hepatocytes in iron overload. Gut. 2000;46:270–6.
19. Frazer DM, Wilkins SJ, Becker EM, Vulpe CD, McKie AT, Trinder D, et al. Hepcidin expression inversely correlates with the expression of duodenal iron transporters and iron absorption in rats. Gastroenterology. 2002;123:835–44.
20. Wardrop SL, Richardson DR. The effect of intracellular iron concentration and nitrogen monoxide on Nramp2 expression and non-transferrin-bound iron uptake. Eur J Biochem. 1999;263:41–9.
21. Hahn PF, Bale WF, Ross JF, Balfour WM, Whipple GH. Radioactive iron absorption by gastro-intestinal tract: influence of anemia, anoxia, and antecedent feeding distribution in growing dogs. J Exp Med. 1943;78:169–88.
22. Hahn PF, Bale WF, Ross JF, Balfour WM, Whipple GH. Radioiron absorption in anemic dogs; fluctuations in the mucosal block and evidence for a gradient of absorption in the gastrointestinal tract. J Exp Med. 1950;92:375–82.
23. Beutler E. History of iron in medicine. Blood Cells Mol Dis. 2002;29:297–308.
24. Oates PS, Trinder D, Morgan EH. Gastrointestinal function, divalent metal transporter-1 expression and intestinal iron absorption. Pflugers Arch. 2000;440:496–502.
25. Yeh KY, Yeh M, Watkins JA, Rodriguez-Paris J, Glass J. Dietary iron induces rapid changes in rat intestinal divalent metal transporter expression. Am J Physiol Gastrointest Liver Physiol. 2000;279:G1070–9.
26. Frazer DM, Wilkins SJ, Becker EM, Murphy TL, Vulpe CD, McKie AT, et al. A rapid decrease in the expression of DMT1 and Dcytb but not Ireg1 or hephaestin explains the mucosal block phenomenon of iron absorption. Gut. 2003;52:340–6.
27. Sharp P, Tandy S, Yamaji S, Tennant J, Williams M, Srai SKS. Rapid regulation of divalent metal transporter (DMT1) protein but not mRNA expression by non-haem iron in human intestinal Caco-2 cells. FEBS Lett. 2002;510:71–6.
28. Mastrogiannaki M, Matak P, Keith B, Simon MC, Vaulont S, Peyssonnaux C. HIF-2alpha, but not HIF-1alpha, promotes iron absorption in mice. J Clin Invest. 2009;119:1159–66.
29. Shah YM, Matsubara T, Ito S, Yim SH, Gonzalez FJ. Intestinal hypoxia-inducible transcription factors are essential for iron absorption following iron deficiency. Cell Metab. 2009;9:152–64.
30. Wheby MS, Suttle GE, Ford III KT. Intestinal absorption of hemoglobin iron. Gastroenterology. 1970;58:647–54.
31. Raffin SB, Woo CH, Roost KT, Price DC, Schmid R. Intestinal absorption of hemoglobin iron-heme cleavage by mucosal heme oxygenase. J Clin Invest. 1974;54:1344–52.
32. Krishnamurthy P, Ross DD, Nakanishi T, Bailey-Dell K, Zhou S, Mercer KE, et al. The stem cell marker Bcrp/ABCG2 enhances hypoxic cell survival through interactions with heme. J Biol Chem. 2004;279:24218–25.
33. Quigley JG, Yang Z, Worthington MT, Phillips JD, Sabo KM, Sabath DE, et al. Identification of a human heme exporter that is essential for erythropoiesis. Cell. 2004;118:757–66.
34. Shayeghi M, Latunde-Dada GO, Oakhill JS, Laftah AH, Takeuchi K, Halliday N, et al. Identification of an intestinal heme transporter. Cell. 2005;122:789–801.
35. Qiu A, Jansen M, Sakaris A, Min SH, Chattopadhyay S, Tsai E, et al. Identification of an intestinal folate transporter and the molecular basis for hereditary folate malabsorption. Cell. 2006;127:917–28.
36. Rajagopal A, Rao AU, Amigo J, Tian M, Upadhyay SK, Hall C, et al. Haem homeostasis is regulated by the conserved and concerted functions of HRG-1 proteins. Nature. 2008;453:1127–31.
37. Donovan A, Brownlie A, Zhou Y, Shepard J, Pratt SJ, Moynihan J, et al. Positional cloning of zebrafish ferroportin1 identifies a conserved vertebrate iron exporter. Nature. 2000;403:776–81.
38. McKie AT, Marciani P, Rolfs A, Brennan K, Wehr K, Barrow D, et al. A novel duodenal iron-regulated transporter, IREG1, implicated in the basolateral transfer of iron to the circulation. Mol Cell. 2000;5:299–309.

39. Abboud S, Haile DJ. A novel mammalian iron-regulated protein involved in intracellular iron metabolism. J Biol Chem. 2000;275:19906–12.
40. Donovan A, Lima CA, Pinkus JL, Pinkus GS, Zon LI, Robine S, et al. The iron exporter ferroportin/Slc40a1 is essential for iron homeostasis. Cell Metab. 2005;1:191–200.
41. Thomas C, Oates PS. Ferroportin/IREG-1/MTP-1/SLC40A1 modulates the uptake of iron at the apical membrane of enterocytes. Gut. 2004;53:444–9.
42. Delaby C, Pilard N, Goncalves AS, Beaumont C, Canonne-Hergaux F. Presence of the iron exporter ferroportin at the plasma membrane of macrophages is enhanced by iron loading and down-regulated by hepcidin. Blood. 2005;106:3979–84.
43. Knutson MD, Oukka M, Koss LM, Aydemir F, Wessling-Resnick M. Iron release from macrophages after erythrophagocytosis is up-regulated by ferroportin 1 overexpression and down-regulated by hepcidin. Proc Natl Acad Sci USA. 2005;102:1324–8.
44. Delaby C, Pilard N, Puy H, Canonne-Hergaux F. Sequential regulation of ferroportin expression after erythrophagocytosis in murine macrophages: early mRNA induction by haem, followed by iron-dependent protein expression. Biochem J. 2008;411:123–31.
45. Wang F, Paradkar PN, Custodio AO, McVey WD, Fleming MD, Campagna D, et al. Genetic variation in Mon1a affects protein trafficking and modifies macrophage iron loading in mice. Nat Genet. 2007;39:1025–32.
46. Yang F, Wang X, Haile DJ, Piantadosi CA, Ghio AJ. Iron increases expression of iron-export protein MTP1 in lung cells. Am J Physiol Lung Cell Mol Physiol. 2002;283:L932–9.
47. Zhang DL, Hughes RM, Ollivierre-Wilson H, Ghosh MC, Rouault TA. A ferroportin transcript that lacks an iron-responsive element enables duodenal and erythroid precursor cells to evade translational repression. Cell Metab. 2009;9:461–73.
48. Chaston T, Chung B, Mascarenhas M, Marks J, Patel B, Srai SK, et al. Evidence for differential effects of hepcidin in macrophages and intestinal epithelial cells. Gut. 2008;57:374–82.
49. Mena NP, Esparza A, Tapia V, Valdes P, Nunez MT. Hepcidin inhibits apical iron uptake in intestinal cells. Am J Physiol Gastrointest Liver Physiol. 2008;294:G192–8.
50. Chung B, Chaston T, Marks J, Srai SK, Sharp PA. Hepcidin decreases iron transporter expression in vivo in mouse duodenum and spleen and in vitro in THP-1 macrophages and intestinal Caco-2 cells. J Nutr. 2009;139:1457–62.
51. Kawabata H, Yang R, Hirama T, Vuong PT, Kawano S, Gombart AF, et al. Molecular cloning of transferrin receptor 2. A new member of the transferrin receptor-like family. J Biol Chem. 1999;274:20826–32.
52. Zhang AS, Xiong S, Tsukamoto H, Enns CA. Localization of iron metabolism-related mRNAs in rat liver indicate that HFE is expressed predominantly in hepatocytes. Blood. 2004;103:1509–14.
53. Aisen P. Transferrin receptor 1. Int J Biochem Cell Biol. 2004;36:2137–43.
54. Hentze MW, Muckenthaler MU, Andrews NC. Balancing acts: molecular control of mammalian iron metabolism. Cell. 2004;117:285–97.
55. Ohgami RS, Campagna DR, Greer EL, Antiochos B, McDonald A, Chen J, et al. Identification of a ferrireductase required for efficient transferrin-dependent iron uptake in erythroid cells. Nat Genet. 2005;37:1264–9.
56. Lebron JA, West Jr AP, Bjorkman PJ. The hemochromatosis protein HFE competes with transferrin for binding to the transferrin receptor. J Mol Biol. 1999;294:239–45.
57. Roy CN, Penny DM, Feder JN, Enns CA. The hereditary hemochromatosis protein, HFE, specifically regulates transferrin-mediated iron uptake in HeLa cells. J Biol Chem. 1999;274:9022–8.
58. Levy JE, Jin O, Fujiwara Y, Kuo F, Andrews NC. Transferrin receptor is necessary for development of erythrocytes and the nervous system. Nat Genet. 1999;21:396–69.
59. Wingert RA, Brownlie A, Galloway JL, Dooley K, Fraenkel P, Axe JL, et al. The chianti zebrafish mutant provides a model for erythroid-specific disruption of transferrin receptor 1. Development. 2004;131:6225–35.
60. Casey JL, Hentze MW, Koeller DM, Caughman SW, Rouault TA, Klausner RD, et al. Iron-responsive elements: regulatory RNA sequences that control mRNA levels and translation. Science. 1988;240:924–8.
61. Mullner EW, Kuhn LC. A stem-loop in the 3′ untranslated region mediates iron-dependent regulation of transferrin receptor mRNA stability in the cytoplasm. Cell. 1988;53:815–25.
62. Mullner EW, Neupert B, Kuhn LC. A specific mRNA binding factor regulates the iron-dependent stability of cytoplasmic transferrin receptor mRNA. Cell. 1989;58:373–82.
63. Kawabata H, Germain RS, Vuong PT, Nakamaki T, Said JW, Koeffler HP. Transferrin receptor 2-alpha supports cell growth both in iron-chelated cultured cells and in vivo. J Biol Chem. 2000;275:16618–25.
64. Kawabata H, Nakamaki T, Ikonomi P, Smith RD, Germain RS, Koeffler HP. Expression of transferrin receptor 2 in normal and neoplastic hematopoietic cells. Blood. 2001;98:2714–9.
65. Camaschella C, Roetto A, Cali A, De GM, Garozzo G, Carella M, et al. The gene TFR2 is mutated in a new type of haemochromatosis mapping to 7q22. Nat Genet. 2000;25:14–5.
66. Fleming RE, Ahmann JR, Migas MC, Waheed A, Koeffler HP, Kawabata H, et al. Targeted mutagenesis of the murine transferrin receptor-2 gene produces hemochromatosis. Proc Natl Acad Sci USA. 2002;99:10653–8.

67. Wallace DF, Summerville L, Subramaniam VN. Targeted disruption of the hepatic transferrin receptor 2 gene in mice leads to iron overload. Gastroenterology. 2007;132:301–10.
68. Wallace DF, Summerville L, Crampton EM, Frazer DM, Anderson GJ, Subramaniam VN. Combined deletion of Hfe and transferrin receptor 2 in mice leads to marked dysregulation of hepcidin and iron overload. Hepatology. 2009;50:1992–2000.
69. Fleming RE, Migas MC, Holden CC, Waheed A, Britton RS, Tomatsu S, et al. Transferrin receptor 2: continued expression in mouse liver in the face of iron overload and in hereditary hemochromatosis. Proc Natl Acad Sci USA. 2000;97:2214–9.
70. Johnson MB, Enns CA. Diferric transferrin regulates transferrin receptor 2 protein stability. Blood. 2004;104:4287–93.
71. Robb A, Wessling-Resnick M. Regulation of transferrin receptor 2 protein levels by transferrin. Blood. 2004;104:4294–9.
72. Chen J, Enns CA. The cytoplasmic domain of transferrin receptor 2 dictates its stability and response to holo-transferrin in Hep3B cells. J Biol Chem. 2007;282:6201–9.
73. Johnson MB, Chen J, Murchison N, Green FA, Enns CA. Transferrin receptor 2: evidence for ligand-induced stabilization and redirection to a recycling pathway. Mol Biol Cell. 2007;18:743–54.
74. Goswami T, Andrews NC. Hereditary hemochromatosis protein, HFE, interaction with transferrin receptor 2 suggests a molecular mechanism for mammalian iron sensing. J Biol Chem. 2006;281:28494–8.
75. Chen J, Chloupkova M, Gao J, Chapman-Arvedson TL, Enns CA. HFE modulates transferrin receptor 2 levels in hepatoma cells via interactions that differ from transferrin receptor 1-HFE interactions. J Biol Chem. 2007;282:36862–70.
76. Pan BT, Johnstone RM. Fate of the transferrin receptor during maturation of sheep reticulocytes in vitro: selective externalization of the receptor. Cell. 1983;33:967–78.
77. Pan BT, Teng K, Wu C, Adam M, Johnstone RM. Electron microscopic evidence for externalization of the transferrin receptor in vesicular form in sheep reticulocytes. J Cell Biol. 1985;101:942–8.
78. Kaup M, Dassler K, Weise C, Fuchs H. Shedding of the transferrin receptor is mediated constitutively by an integral membrane metalloprotease sensitive to tumor necrosis factor alpha protease inhibitor-2. J Biol Chem. 2002;277:38494–502.
79. Shih YJ, Baynes RD, Hudson BG, Flowers CH, Skikne BS, Cook JD. Serum transferrin receptor is a truncated form of tissue receptor. J Biol Chem. 1990;265:19077–81.
80. Fuchs H, Lucken U, Tauber R, Engel A, Gessner R. Structural model of phospholipid-reconstituted human transferrin receptor derived by electron microscopy. Structure. 1998;6:1235–43.
81. Ferguson BJ, Skikne BS, Simpson KM, Baynes RD, Cook JD. Serum transferrin receptor distinguishes the anemia of chronic disease from iron deficiency anemia. J Lab Clin Med. 1992;119:385–90.
82. Weiss G, Goodnough LT. Anemia of chronic disease. N Engl J Med. 2005;352:101110–23.
83. Dassler K, Zydek M, Wandzik K, Kaup M, Fuchs H. Release of the soluble transferrin receptor is directly regulated by binding of its ligand ferritransferrin. J Biol Chem. 2006;281:3297–304.
84. Shaw GC, Cope JJ, Li L, Corson K, Hersey C, Ackermann GE, et al. Mitoferrin is essential for erythroid iron assimilation. Nature. 2006;440:96–100.
85. Foury F, Roganti T. Deletion of the mitochondrial carrier genes MRS3 and MRS4 suppresses mitochondrial iron accumulation in a yeast frataxin-deficient strain. J Biol Chem. 2002;277:24475–83.
86. Muhlenhoff U, Stadler JA, Richhardt N, Seubert A, Eickhorst T, Schweyen RJ, et al. A specific role of the yeast mitochondrial carriers MRS3/4p in mitochondrial iron acquisition under iron-limiting conditions. J Biol Chem. 2003;278:40612–20.
87. Li L, Kaplan J. A mitochondrial-vacuolar signaling pathway in yeast that affects iron and copper metabolism. J Biol Chem. 2004;279:33653–61.
88. Zhang Y, Lyver ER, Knight SA, Lesuisse E, Dancis A. Frataxin and mitochondrial carrier proteins, Mrs3p and Mrs4p, cooperate in providing iron for heme synthesis. J Biol Chem. 2005;280:19794–807.
89. Vidal SM, Malo D, Vogan K, Skamene E, Gros P. Natural resistance to infection with intracellular parasites: isolation of a candidate for Bcg. Cell. 1993;73:469–85.
90. West AH, Clark DJ, Martin J, Neupert W, Hartl FU, Horwich AL. Two related genes encoding extremely hydrophobic proteins suppress a lethal mutation in the yeast mitochondrial processing enhancing protein. J Biol Chem. 1992;267:24625–33.
91. Rodrigues V, Cheah PY, Ray K, Chia W. malvolio, the Drosophila homologue of mouse NRAMP-1 (Bcg), is expressed in macrophages and in the nervous system and is required for normal taste behaviour. EMBO J. 1995;14:3007–20.
92. Nevo Y, Nelson N. The NRAMP family of metal-ion transporters. Biochim Biophys Acta. 2006;1763:609–20.
93. Fortier A, Min-Oo G, Forbes J, Lam-Yuk-Tseung S, Gros P. Single gene effects in mouse models of host: pathogen interactions. J Leukoc Biol. 2005;77:868–77.

94. Vidal S, Gros P, Skamene E. Natural resistance to infection with intracellular parasites: molecular genetics identifies Nramp1 as the Bcg/Ity/Lsh locus. J Leukoc Biol. 1995;58:382–90.
95. Jabado N, Jankowski A, Dougaparsad S, Picard V, Grinstein S, Gros P. Natural resistance to intracellular infections: natural resistance-associated macrophage protein 1 (Nramp1) functions as a pH-dependent manganese transporter at the phagosomal membrane. J Exp Med. 2000;192:1237–48.
96. Forbes JR, Gros P. Divalent-metal transport by NRAMP proteins at the interface of host–pathogen interactions. Trends Microbiol. 2001;9:397–403.
97. Forbes JR, Gros P. Iron, manganese, and cobalt transport by Nramp1 (Slc11a1) and Nramp2 (Slc11a2) expressed at the plasma membrane. Blood. 2003;102:1884–92.
98. Kuhn DE, Baker BD, Lafuse WP, Zwilling BS. Differential iron transport into phagosomes isolated from the RAW264.7 macrophage cell lines transfected with Nramp1Gly169 or Nramp1Asp169. J Leukoc Biol. 1999;66:113–9.
99. Kuhn DE, Lafuse WP, Zwilling BS. Iron transport into mycobacterium avium-containing phagosomes from an Nramp1(Gly169)-transfected RAW264.7 macrophage cell line. J Leukoc Biol. 2001;69:43–9.
100. Goswami T, Bhattacharjee A, Babal P, Searle S, Moore E, Li M, et al. Natural-resistance-associated macrophage protein 1 is an H+/bivalent cation antiporter. Biochem J. 2001;354:511–9.
101. Soe-Lin S, Apte SS, Mikhael MR, Kayembe LK, Nie G, Ponka P. Both Nramp1 and DMT1 are necessary for efficient macrophage iron recycling. Exp Hematol. 2010;38:609–17.
102. Soe-Lin S, Apte SS, Andriopoulos Jr B, Andrews MC, Schranzhofer M, Kahawita T, et al. Nramp1 promotes efficient macrophage recycling of iron following erythrophagocytosis in vivo. Proc Natl Acad Sci USA. 2009;106:5960–5.
103. Shaw MA, Collins A, Peacock CS, Miller EN, Black GF, Sibthorpe D, et al. Evidence that genetic susceptibility to Mycobacterium tuberculosis in a Brazilian population is under oligogenic control: linkage study of the candidate genes NRAMP1 and TNFA. Tuber Lung Dis. 1997;78:35–45.
104. Yip SP, Leung KH, Lin CK. Extent and distribution of linkage disequilibrium around the SLC11A1 locus. Genes Immun. 2003;4:212–21.
105. Blackwell JM, Goswami T, Evans CA, Sibthorpe D, Papo N, White JK, et al. SLC11A1 (formerly NRAMP1) and disease resistance. Cell Microbiol. 2001;3:773–84.
106. McDermid JM, Prentice AM. Iron and infection: effects of host iron status and the iron-regulatory genes haptoglobin and NRAMP1 (SLC11A1) on host–pathogen interactions in tuberculosis and HIV. Clin Sci (Lond). 2006;110:503–24.
107. Bayele HK, Peyssonnaux C, Giatromanolaki A, Arrais-Silva WW, Mohamed HS, Collins H, et al. HIF-1 regulates heritable variation and allele expression phenotypes of the macrophage immune response gene SLC11A1 from a Z-DNA forming microsatellite. Blood. 2007;110:3039–48.
108. Han O, Failla ML, Hill AD, Morris ER, Smith Jr JC. Reduction of Fe(III) is required for uptake of nonheme iron by Caco-2 cells. J Nutr. 1995;125:1291–9.
109. Taylor PG, Martinez-Torres C, Romano EL, Layrisse M. The effect of cysteine-containing peptides released during meat digestion on iron absorption in humans. Am J Clin Nutr. 1986;43:68–71.
110. Huh EC, Hotchkiss A, Brouillette J, Glahn RP. Carbohydrate fractions from cooked fish promote iron uptake by Caco-2 cells. J Nutr. 2004;134:1681–9.
111. Hurrell RF, Reddy MB, Juillerat M, Cook JD. Meat protein fractions enhance nonheme iron absorption in humans. J Nutr. 2006;136:2808–12.
112. Armah CN, Sharp P, Mellon FA, Pariagh S, Lund EK, Dainty JR, et al. L-Alpha-glycerophosphocholine contributes to meat's enhancement of nonheme iron absorption. J Nutr. 2008;138:873–7.
113. Raja KB, Simpson RJ, Peters TJ. Investigation of a role for reduction in ferric iron uptake by mouse duodenum. Biochim Biophys Acta. 1992;1135:141–6.
114. Riedel HD, Remus AJ, Fitscher BA, Stremmel W. Characterization and partial purification of a ferrireductase from human duodenal microvillus membranes. Biochem J. 1995;309(Pt 3):745–8.
115. Ekmekcioglu C, Feyertag J, Marktl W. A ferric reductase activity is found in brush border membrane vesicles isolated from Caco-2 cells. J Nutr. 1996;126:2209–17.
116. McKie AT, Barrow D, Latunde-Dada GO, Rolfs A, Sager G, Mudaly E, et al. An iron-regulated ferric reductase associated with the absorption of dietary iron. Science. 2001;291:1755–9.
117. Su D, Asard H. Three mammalian cytochromes b561 are ascorbate-dependent ferrireductases. FEBS J. 2006;273:3722–34.
118. Muckenthaler M, Roy CN, Custodio AO, Minana B, deGraaf J, Montross LK, et al. Regulatory defects in liver and intestine implicate abnormal hepcidin and Cybrd1 expression in mouse hemochromatosis. Nat Genet. 2003;34:102–7.
119. Latunde-Dada GO, Simpson RJ, McKie AT. Duodenal cytochrome B expression stimulates iron uptake by human intestinal epithelial cells. J Nutr. 2008;138:991–5.
120. Wyman S, Simpson RJ, McKie AT, Sharp PA. Dcytb (Cybrd1) functions as both a ferric and a cupric reductase in vitro. FEBS Lett. 2008;582:1901–6.

121. Gunshin H, Starr CN, Direnzo C, Fleming MD, Jin J, Greer EL, et al. Cybrd1 (duodenal cytochrome b) is not necessary for dietary iron absorption in mice. Blood. 2005;106:2879–83.
122. Constantine CC, Anderson GJ, Vulpe CD, McLaren CE, Bahlo M, Yeap HL, et al. A novel association between a SNP in CYBRD1 and serum ferritin levels in a cohort study of HFE hereditary haemochromatosis. Br J Haematol. 2009;147:140–9.
123. Ohgami RS, Campagna DR, McDonald A, Fleming MD. The Steap proteins are metalloreductases. Blood. 2006;108:1388–94.
124. Fox PL. The copper–iron chronicles: the story of an intimate relationship. Biometals. 2003;16:9–40.
125. Sharp P. The molecular basis of copper and iron interactions. Proc Nutr Soc. 2004;63:563–9.
126. Smith SE, Medlicott M. The blood picture of iron and copper deficiency anemias in the rat. Am J Physiol. 1944;141:354–8.
127. Cartwright GE, Gubler CJ, Bus JA, Wintrobe MM. Studies of copper metabolism. XVII. Further observations on the anemia of copper deficiency in swine. Blood. 1956;11:143–53.
128. Holmberg CG, Laurell CB. Investigations in serum copper. II. Isolation of the copper containing protein and a description of some of its properties. Acta Chem Scand. 1948;2:550–6.
129. Curzon G, Vallet L. The purification of human ceruloplasmin. Biochem J. 1960;74:279–87.
130. Osaki S, Johnson DA, Frieden E. The possible significance of the ferrous oxidase activity of ceruloplasmin in normal human serum. J Biol Chem. 1966;241:2746–51.
131. Osaki S, Johnson DA. Mobilization of liver iron by ferroxidase (ceruloplasmin). J Biol Chem. 1969;244:5757–8.
132. Harris ZL. Aceruloplasminemia. J Neurol Sci. 2003;207:108–9.
133. Patel BN, David S. A novel glycosylphosphatidylinositol-anchored form of ceruloplasmin is expressed by mammalian astrocytes. J Biol Chem. 1997;272:20185–90.
134. Patel BN, Dunn RJ, David S. Alternative RNA splicing generates a glycosylphosphatidylinositol-anchored form of ceruloplasmin in mammalian brain. J Biol Chem. 2000;275:4305–10.
135. Hellman NE, Gitlin JD. Ceruloplasmin metabolism and function. Annu Rev Nutr. 2002;22:439–58.
136. Jeong SY, David S. Glycosylphosphatidylinositol-anchored ceruloplasmin is required for iron efflux from cells in the central nervous system. J Biol Chem. 2003;278:27144–8.
137. De Domenico I, Ward DM, di Patti MC, Jeong SY, David S, Musci G, et al. Ferroxidase activity is required for the stability of cell surface ferroportin in cells expressing GPI-ceruloplasmin. EMBO J. 2007;26:2823–31.
138. Askwith C, Eide D, Van HA, Bernard PS, Li L, vis-Kaplan S, et al. The FET3 gene of *S. cerevisiae* encodes a multicopper oxidase required for ferrous iron uptake. Cell. 1994;76:403–10.
139. Dancis A, Haile D, Yuan DS, Askwith C, Eide D, Moehle C, et al. Molecular characterization of a copper transport protein in *S. cerevisiae*: an unexpected role for copper in iron transport. Cell. 1994;76:393–402.
140. Anderson GJ, Murphy TL, Cowley L, Evans BA, Halliday JW, McLaren GD. Mapping the gene for sex-linked anemia: an inherited defect of intestinal iron absorption in the mouse. Genomics. 1998;48:34–9.
141. Vulpe CD, Kuo YM, Murphy TL, Cowley L, Askwith C, Libina N, et al. Hephaestin, a ceruloplasmin homologue implicated in intestinal iron transport, is defective in the sla mouse. Nat Genet. 1999;21:195–9.
142. Frazer DM, Vulpe CD, McKie AT, Wilkins SJ, Trinder D, Cleghorn GJ, et al. Cloning and gastrointestinal expression of rat hephaestin: relationship to other iron transport proteins. Am J Physiol Gastrointest Liver Physiol. 2001;281:G931–9.
143. Rolfs A, Bonkovsky HL, Kohlroser JG, McNeal K, Sharma A, Berger UV, et al. Intestinal expression of genes involved in iron absorption in humans. Am J Physiol Gastrointest Liver Physiol. 2002;282:G598–607.
144. Chen H, Attieh ZK, Su T, Syed BA, Gao H, Alaeddine RM, et al. Hephaestin is a ferroxidase that maintains partial activity in sex-linked anemia mice. Blood. 2004;103:3933–9.
145. Syed BA, Beaumont NJ, Patel A, Naylor CE, Bayele HK, Joannou CL, et al. Analysis of the human hephaestin gene and protein: comparative modelling of the N-terminus ecto-domain based upon ceruloplasmin. Protein Eng. 2002;15:205–14.
146. Kuo YM, Su T, Chen H, Attieh Z, Syed BA, McKie AT, et al. Mislocalisation of hephaestin, a multicopper ferroxidase involved in basolateral intestinal iron transport, in the sex linked anaemia mouse. Gut. 2004;53:20120–6.
147. Syed BA, Sargent PJ, Farnaud S, Evans RW. An overview of molecular aspects of iron metabolism. Hemoglobin. 2006;30:69–80.
148. Giblett ER, Hickman CG, Smithies O. Serum transferrins. Nature. 1959;183:1589–90.
149. Crichton RR. Proteins of iron storage and transport. Adv Protein Chem. 1990;40:281–363.
150. Saltman P, Charley PJ. The regulation of iron metabolism by equilibrium binding and chelation. In: Seven MJ, editor. Metal-binding in medicine. Philadelphia: Lippincott; 1960. p. 241–4.
151. Fletcher J. Iron transport in the blood. Proc R Soc Med. 1970;63:1216–8.
152. Huebers HA, Finch CA. The physiology of transferrin and transferrin receptors. Physiol Rev. 1987;67:520–82.
153. Harrison PM, Arosio P. The ferritins: molecular properties, iron storage function and cellular regulation. Biochim Biophys Acta. 1996;1275:161–203.

154. Drysdale JW, Munro HN. Regulation of synthesis and turnover of ferritin in rat liver. J Biol Chem. 1966;241:3630–7.
155. Roberts S, Bomford A. Ferritin iron kinetics and protein turnover in K562 cells. J Biol Chem. 1988;263:19181–7.
156. Shi H, Bencze KZ, Stemmler TL, Philpott CC. A cytosolic iron chaperone that delivers iron to ferritin. Science. 2008;320:1207–10.
157. Granick S. Protein apoferritin and ferritin in iron feeding and absorption. Science. 1946;103:107.
158. Aziz N, Munro HN. Iron regulates ferritin mRNA translation through a segment of its 5 untranslated region. Proc Natl Acad Sci USA. 1987;84:8478–82.
159. Hentze MW, Rouault TA, Caughman SW, Dancis A, Harford JB, Klausner RD. A *cis*-acting element is necessary and sufficient for translational regulation of human ferritin expression in response to iron. Proc Natl Acad Sci USA. 1987;84:6730–4.
160. Hentze MW, Caughman SW, Rouault TA, Barriocanal JG, Dancis A, Harford JB, et al. Identification of the iron-responsive element for the translational regulation of human ferritin mRNA. Science. 1987;238:1570–3.
161. Leibold EA, Munro HN. Characterization and evolution of the expressed rat ferritin light subunit gene and its pseudogene family. Conservation of sequences within noncoding regions of ferritin genes. J Biol Chem. 1987;262:7335–41.
162. Muckenthaler M, Gray NK, Hentze MW. IRP-1 binding to ferritin mRNA prevents the recruitment of the small ribosomal subunit by the cap-binding complex eIF4F. Mol Cell. 1998;2:383–8.
163. Addison GM, Beamish MR, Hales CN, Hodgkins M, Jacobs A, Llewellin P. An immunoradiometric assay for ferritin in the serum of normal subjects and patients with iron deficiency and iron overload. J Clin Pathol. 1972;25:326–9.
164. Jacobs A, Worwood M. Ferritin in serum. Clinical and biochemical implications. N Engl J Med. 1975;292:95195–6.
165. Cragg SJ, Wagstaff M, Worwood M. Sialic acid and the microheterogeneity of human serum ferritin. Clin Sci (Lond). 1980;58:259–62.
166. Cragg SJ, Wagstaff M, Worwood M. Detection of a glycosylated subunit in human serum ferritin. Biochem J. 1981;199:565–71.
167. Worwood M, Dawkins S, Wagstaff M, Jacobs A. The purification and properties of ferritin from human serum. Biochem J. 1976;157:97–103.
168. Arosio P, Yokota M, Drysdale JW. Characterization of serum ferritin in iron overload: possible identity to natural apoferritin. Br J Haematol. 1977;36:199–207.
169. Walters GO, Miller FM, Worwood M. Serum ferritin concentration and iron stores in normal subjects. J Clin Pathol. 1973;26:770–2.
170. Cook JD. Defining optimal body iron. Proc Nutr Soc. 1999;58:489–95.
171. Mack U, Cooksley WG, Ferris RA, Powell LW, Halliday JW. Regulation of plasma ferritin by the isolated perfused rat liver. Br J Haematol. 1981;47:403–12.
172. Tran TN, Eubanks SK, Schaffer KJ, Zhou CY, Linder MC. Secretion of ferritin by rat hepatoma cells and its regulation by inflammatory cytokines and iron. Blood. 1997;90:4979–86.
173. Dorner MH, Silverstone A, Nishiya K, de Sostoa A, Munn G, de Sousa M. Ferritin synthesis by human T lymphocytes. Science. 1980;209:1019–21.
174. Ghosh S, Hevi S, Chuck SL. Regulated secretion of glycosylated human ferritin from hepatocytes. Blood. 2004;103:2369–76.
175. Levi S, Corsi B, Bosisio M, Invernizzi R, Volz A, Sanford D, et al. A human mitochondrial ferritin encoded by an intronless gene. J Biol Chem. 2001;276:24437–40.
176. Drysdale J, Arosio P, Invernizzi R, Cazzola M, Volz A, Corsi B, et al. Mitochondrial ferritin: a new player in iron metabolism. Blood Cells Mol Dis. 2002;29:376–83.
177. Santambrogio P, Biasiotto G, Sanvito F, Olivieri S, Arosio P, Levi S. Mitochondrial ferritin expression in adult mouse tissues. J Histochem Cytochem. 2007;55:1129–37.
178. Wixom RL, Prutkin L, Munro HN. Hemosiderin: nature, formation, and significance. Int Rev Exp Pathol. 1980;22:193–225.
179. Richter GW. Studies of iron overload. Rat liver siderosome ferritin. Lab Invest. 1984;50:26–35.
180. Iancu TC. Ultrastructural pathology of iron overload. Baillieres Clin Haematol. 1989;2:475–95.
181. Weir MP, Gibson JF, Peters TJ. Biochemical studies on the isolation and characterization of human spleen haemosiderin. Biochem J. 1984;223:31–8.
182. Andrews SC, Brady MC, Treffry A, Williams JM, Mann S, Cleton MI, et al. Studies on haemosiderin and ferritin from iron-loaded rat liver. Biol Met. 1988;1:33–42.
183. Rouault TA, Stout CD, Kaptain S, Harford JB, Klausner RD. Structural relationship between an iron-regulated RNA-binding protein (IRE-BP) and aconitase: functional implications. Cell. 1991;64:881–3.
184. Hentze MW, Kuhn LC. Molecular control of vertebrate iron metabolism: mRNA-based regulatory circuits operated by iron, nitric oxide, and oxidative stress. Proc Natl Acad Sci USA. 1996;93:8175–82.

185. Eisenstein RS, Blemings KP. Iron regulatory proteins, iron responsive elements and iron homeostasis. J Nutr. 1998;128:2295–8.
186. Cairo G, Pietrangelo A. Iron regulatory proteins in pathobiology. Biochem J. 2000;352:241–50.
187. Iwai K, Drake SK, Wehr NB, Weissman AM, LaVaute T, Minato N, et al. Iron-dependent oxidation, ubiquitination, and degradation of iron regulatory protein 2: implications for degradation of oxidized proteins. Proc Natl Acad Sci USA. 1998;95:4924–8.
188. Samaniego F, Chin J, Iwai K, Rouault TA, Klausner RD. Molecular characterization of a second iron-responsive element binding protein, iron regulatory protein 2. Structure, function, and post-translational regulation. J Biol Chem. 1994;269:30904–10.
189. Henderson BR, Seiser C, Kuhn LC. Characterization of a second RNA-binding protein in rodents with specificity for iron-responsive elements. J Biol Chem. 1993;268:27327–34.
190. Butt J, Kim HY, Basilion JP, Cohen S, Iwai K, Philpott CC, et al. Differences in the RNA binding sites of iron regulatory proteins and potential target diversity. Proc Natl Acad Sci USA. 1996;93:4345–9.
191. Henderson BR, Menotti E, Kuhn LC. Iron regulatory proteins 1 and 2 bind distinct sets of RNA target sequences. J Biol Chem. 1996;271:4900–8.
192. Feder JN, Gnirke A, Thomas W, Tsuchihashi Z, Ruddy DA, Basava A, et al. A novel MHC class I-like gene is mutated in patients with hereditary haemochromatosis. Nat Genet. 1996;13:399–408.
193. Sebastiani G, Walker AP. HFE gene in primary and secondary hepatic iron overload. World J Gastroenterol. 2007;13:4673–89.
194. Lebron JA, Bennett MJ, Vaughn DE, Chirino AJ, Snow PM, Mintier GA, et al. Crystal structure of the hemochromatosis protein HFE and characterization of its interaction with transferrin receptor. Cell. 1998;93:111–23.
195. Feder JN, Tsuchihashi Z, Irrinki A, Lee VK, Mapa FA, Morikang E, et al. The hemochromatosis founder mutation in HLA-H disrupts beta2-microglobulin interaction and cell surface expression. J Biol Chem. 1997;272:14025–8.
196. Waheed A, Parkkila S, Zhou XY, Tomatsu S, Tsuchihashi Z, Feder JN, et al. Hereditary hemochromatosis: effects of C282Y and H63D mutations on association with beta2-microglobulin, intracellular processing, and cell surface expression of the HFE protein in COS-7 cells. Proc Natl Acad Sci USA. 1997;94:12384–9.
197. Waheed A, Grubb JH, Zhou XY, Tomatsu S, Fleming RE, Costaldi ME, et al. Regulation of transferrin-mediated iron uptake by HFE, the protein defective in hereditary hemochromatosis. Proc Natl Acad Sci USA. 2002;99:3117–22.
198. Parkkila S, Waheed A, Britton RS, Bacon BR, Zhou XY, Tomatsu S, et al. Association of the transferrin receptor in human placenta with HFE, the protein defective in hereditary hemochromatosis. Proc Natl Acad Sci USA. 1997;94:13198–202.
199. Bastin JM, Jones M, O'Callaghan CA, Schimanski L, Mason DY, Townsend AR. Kupffer cell staining by an HFE-specific monoclonal antibody: implications for hereditary haemochromatosis. Br J Haematol. 1998;103:931–41.
200. Parkkila S, Waheed A, Britton RS, Feder JN, Tsuchihashi Z, Schatzman RC, et al. Immunohistochemistry of HLA-H, the protein defective in patients with hereditary hemochromatosis, reveals unique pattern of expression in gastrointestinal tract. Proc Natl Acad Sci USA. 1997;94:2534–9.
201. Parkkila S, Parkkila AK, Waheed A, Britton RS, Zhou XY, Fleming RE, et al. Cell surface expression of HFE protein in epithelial cells, macrophages, and monocytes. Haematologica. 2000;85:340–5.
202. Zhou XY, Tomatsu S, Fleming RE, Parkkila S, Waheed A, Jiang J, et al. HFE gene knockout produces mouse model of hereditary hemochromatosis. Proc Natl Acad Sci USA. 1998;95:2492–7.
203. Valore EV, Ganz T. Posttranslational processing of hepcidin in human hepatocytes is mediated by the prohormone convertase furin. Blood Cells Mol Dis. 2008;40:132–8.
204. Krause A, Neitz S, Magert HJ, Schulz A, Forssmann WG, Schulz-Knappe P, et al. LEAP-1, a novel highly disulfide-bonded human peptide, exhibits antimicrobial activity. FEBS Lett. 2000;480:147–50.
205. Park CH, Valore EV, Waring AJ, Ganz T. Hepcidin, a urinary antimicrobial peptide synthesized in the liver. J Biol Chem. 2001;276:7806–10.
206. Hunter HN, Fulton DB, Ganz T, Vogel HJ. The solution structure of human hepcidin, a peptide hormone with antimicrobial activity that is involved in iron uptake and hereditary hemochromatosis. J Biol Chem. 2002;277:37597–603.
207. Jordan JB, Poppe L, Haniu M, Arvedson T, Syed R, Li V, et al. Hepcidin revisited, disulfide connectivity, dynamics, and structure. J Biol Chem. 2009;284:24155–67.
208. Pigeon C, Ilyin G, Courselaud B, Leroyer P, Turlin B, Brissot P, et al. A new mouse liver-specific gene, encoding a protein homologous to human antimicrobial peptide hepcidin, is overexpressed during iron overload. J Biol Chem. 2001;276:7811–9.
209. Nicolas G, Chauvet C, Viatte L, Danan JL, Bigard X, Devaux I, et al. The gene encoding the iron regulatory peptide hepcidin is regulated by anemia, hypoxia, and inflammation. J Clin Invest. 2002;110:1037–44.

210. Frazer DM, Inglis HR, Wilkins SJ, Millard KN, Steele TM, McLaren GD, et al. Delayed hepcidin response explains the lag period in iron absorption following a stimulus to increase erythropoiesis. Gut. 2004;53:1509–15.
211. Nicolas G, Bennoun M, Devaux I, Beaumont C, Grandchamp B, Kahn A, et al. Lack of hepcidin gene expression and severe tissue iron overload in upstream stimulatory factor 2 (USF2) knockout mice. Proc Natl Acad Sci USA. 2001;98:8780–5.
212. Nicolas G, Bennoun M, Porteu A, Mativet S, Beaumont C, Grandchamp B, et al. Severe iron deficiency anemia in transgenic mice expressing liver hepcidin. Proc Natl Acad Sci USA. 2002;99:4596–601.
213. Roetto A, Papanikolaou G, Politou M, Alberti F, Girelli D, Christakis J, et al. Mutant antimicrobial peptide hepcidin is associated with severe juvenile hemochromatosis. Nat Genet. 2003;33:21–2.
214. Wallace DF, Subramaniam VN. Non-HFE haemochromatosis. World J Gastroenterol. 2007;13:4690–8.
215. Weinstein DA, Roy CN, Fleming MD, Loda MF, Wolfsdorf JI, Andrews NC. Inappropriate expression of hepcidin is associated with iron refractory anemia: implications for the anemia of chronic disease. Blood. 2002;100:3776–81.
216. Nemeth E, Rivera S, Gabayan V, Keller C, Taudorf S, Pedersen BK, et al. IL-6 mediates hypoferremia of inflammation by inducing the synthesis of the iron regulatory hormone hepcidin. J Clin Invest. 2004;113:1271–6.
217. Nemeth E, Tuttle MS, Powelson J, Vaughn MB, Donovan A, Ward DM, et al. Hepcidin regulates cellular iron efflux by binding to ferroportin and inducing its internalization. Science. 2004;306:2090–3.
218. De Domenico I, Ward DM, Nemeth E, Vaughn MB, Musci G, Ganz T, et al. The molecular basis of ferroportin-linked hemochromatosis. Proc Natl Acad Sci USA. 2005;102:8955–60.
219. Drakesmith H, Schimanski LM, Ormerod E, Merryweather-Clarke AT, Viprakasit V, Edwards JP, et al. Resistance to hepcidin is conferred by hemochromatosis-associated mutations of ferroportin. Blood. 2005;106:1092–7.
220. De Domenico I, Ward DM, Langelier C, Vaughn MB, Nemeth E, Sundquist WI, et al. The molecular mechanism of hepcidin-mediated ferroportin down-regulation. Mol Biol Cell. 2007;18:2569–78.
221. Finberg KE, Heeney MM, Campagna DR, Aydinok Y, Pearson HA, Hartman KR, et al. Mutations in TMPRSS6 cause iron-refractory iron deficiency anemia (IRIDA). Nat Genet. 2008;40:569–71.
222. Guillem F, Lawson S, Kannengiesser C, Westerman M, Beaumont C, Grandchamp B. Two nonsense mutations in the TMPRSS6 gene in a patient with microcytic anemia and iron deficiency. Blood. 2008;112:2089–91.
223. Melis MA, Cau M, Congiu R, Sole G, Barella S, Cao A, et al. A mutation in the TMPRSS6 gene, encoding a transmembrane serine protease that suppresses hepcidin production, in familial iron deficiency anemia refractory to oral iron. Haematologica. 2008;93:1473–9.
224. Du X, She E, Gelbart T, Truksa J, Lee P, Xia Y, et al. The serine protease TMPRSS6 is required to sense iron deficiency. Science. 2008;320:1088–92.
225. Folgueras AR, de Martin LF, Pendas AM, Garabaya C, Rodriguez F, Astudillo A, et al. Membrane-bound serine protease matriptase-2 (Tmprss6) is an essential regulator of iron homeostasis. Blood. 2008;112:2539–45.
226. Silvestri L, Pagani A, Nai A, De Domenico I, Kaplan J, Camaschella C. The serine protease matriptase-2 (TMPRSS6) inhibits hepcidin activation by cleaving membrane hemojuvelin. Cell Metab. 2008;8:502–11.
227. De Falco L, Totaro F, Nai A, Pagani A, Girelli D, Silvestri L, et al. Novel TMPRSS6 mutations associated with iron-refractory iron deficiency anemia (IRIDA). Hum Mutat. 2010;31:E1390–405.
228. Edison ES, Athiyarath R, Rajasekar T, Westerman M, Srivastava A, Chandy M. A novel splice site mutation c.2278 (−1) G>C in the TMPRSS6 gene causes deletion of the substrate binding site of the serine protease resulting in refractory iron deficiency anaemia. Br J Haematol. 2009;147:766–9.
229. Ramsay AJ, Quesada V, Sanchez M, Garabaya C, Sarda MP, Baiget M, et al. Matriptase-2 mutations in iron-refractory iron deficiency anemia patients provide new insights into protease activation mechanisms. Hum Mol Genet. 2009;18:3673–83.
230. Tanaka T, Roy CN, Yao W, Matteini A, Semba RD, Arking D, et al. A genome-wide association analysis of serum iron concentrations. Blood. 2010;115:94–6.
231. Benyamin B, Ferreira MA, Willemsen G, Gordon S, Middelberg RP, McEvoy BP, et al. Common variants in TMPRSS6 are associated with iron status and erythrocyte volume. Nat Genet. 2009;41:1173–5.
232. Chambers JC, Zhang W, Li Y, Sehmi J, Wass MN, Zabaneh D, et al. Genome-wide association study identifies variants in TMPRSS6 associated with hemoglobin levels. Nat Genet. 2009;41:1170–2.
233. Beutler E, Van GC, te Loo DM, Gelbart T, Crain K, Truksa J, et al. Polymorphisms and mutations of human TMPRSS6 in iron deficiency anemia. Blood Cells Mol Dis. 2010;44:16–21.
234. Lee PL, Barton JC, Brandhagen D, Beutler E. Hemojuvelin (HJV) mutations in persons of European, African-American and Asian ancestry with adult onset haemochromatosis. Br J Haematol. 2004;127:224–9.
235. Lee PL, Beutler E, Rao SV, Barton JC. Genetic abnormalities and juvenile hemochromatosis: mutations of the HJV gene encoding hemojuvelin. Blood. 2004;103:4669–71.
236. Papanikolaou G, Samuels ME, Ludwig EH, MacDonald ML, Franchini PL, Dube MP, et al. Mutations in HFE2 cause iron overload in chromosome 1q-linked juvenile hemochromatosis. Nat Genet. 2004;36:77–82.
237. Daraio F, Ryan E, Gleeson F, Roetto A, Crowe J, Camaschella C. Juvenile hemochromatosis due to G320V/Q116X compound heterozygosity of hemojuvelin in an Irish patient. Blood Cells Mol Dis. 2005;35:174–6.

238. Gehrke SG, Pietrangelo A, Kascak M, Braner A, Eisold M, Kulaksiz H, et al. HJV gene mutations in European patients with juvenile hemochromatosis. Clin Genet. 2005;67:425–8.
239. Wallace DF, Dixon JL, Ramm GA, Anderson GJ, Powell LW, Subramaniam N. Hemojuvelin (HJV)-associated hemochromatosis: analysis of HJV and HFE mutations and iron overload in three families. Haematologica. 2005;90:254–5.
240. Aguilar-Martinez P, Lok CY, Cunat S, Cadet E, Robson K, Rochette J. Juvenile hemochromatosis caused by a novel combination of hemojuvelin G320V/R176C mutations in a 5-year old girl. Haematologica. 2007;92:421–2.
241. Huang FW, Pinkus JL, Pinkus GS, Fleming MD, Andrews NC. A mouse model of juvenile hemochromatosis. J Clin Invest. 2005;115:2187–91.
242. Niederkofler V, Salie R, Arber S. Hemojuvelin is essential for dietary iron sensing, and its mutation leads to severe iron overload. J Clin Invest. 2005;115:2180–6.
243. Kuninger D, Kuns-Hashimoto R, Nili M, Rotwein P. Pro-protein convertases control the maturation and processing of the iron-regulatory protein, RGMc/hemojuvelin. BMC Biochem. 2008;9:9.
244. Lin L, Nemeth E, Goodnough JB, Thapa DR, Gabayan V, Ganz T. Soluble hemojuvelin is released by proprotein convertase-mediated cleavage at a conserved polybasic RNRR site. Blood Cells Mol Dis. 2008;40:122–31.
245. Silvestri L, Pagani A, Camaschella C. Furin-mediated release of soluble hemojuvelin: a new link between hypoxia and iron homeostasis. Blood. 2008;111:924–31.
246. Lin L, Goldberg YP, Ganz T. Competitive regulation of hepcidin mRNA by soluble and cell-associated hemojuvelin. Blood. 2005;106:2884–9.
247. Babitt JL, Huang FW, Wrighting DM, Xia Y, Sidis Y, Samad TA, et al. Bone morphogenetic protein signaling by hemojuvelin regulates hepcidin expression. Nat Genet. 2006;38:531–5349.
248. Wang RH, Li C, Xu X, Zheng Y, Xiao C, Zerfas P, et al. A role of SMAD4 in iron metabolism through the positive regulation of hepcidin expression. Cell Metab. 2005;2:399–409.
249. Kautz L, Meynard D, Monnier A, Darnaud V, Bouvet R, Wang RH, et al. Iron regulates phosphorylation of Smad1/5/8 and gene expression of Bmp6, Smad7, Id1, and Atoh8 in the mouse liver. Blood. 2008;112:1503–9.
250. Meynard D, Kautz L, Darnaud V, Canonne-Hergaux F, Coppin H, Roth MP. Lack of the bone morphogenetic protein BMP6 induces massive iron overload. Nat Genet. 2009;41:478–81.
251. Andriopoulos Jr B, Corradini E, Xia Y, Faasse SA, Chen S, Grgurevic L, et al. BMP6 is a key endogenous regulator of hepcidin expression and iron metabolism. Nat Genet. 2009;41:482–7.
252. Napier I, Ponka P, Richardson DR. Iron trafficking in the mitochondrion: novel pathways revealed by disease. Blood. 2005;105:1867–74.
253. Bencze KZ, Kondapalli KC, Cook JD, McMahon S, Millan-Pacheco C, Pastor N, et al. The structure and function of frataxin. Crit Rev Biochem Mol Biol. 2006;41:269–91.
254. Wilson RB. Iron dysregulation in Friedreich ataxia. Semin Pediatr Neurol. 2006;13:166–75.
255. Gibson TJ, Koonin EV, Musco G, Pastore A, Bork P. Friedreich's ataxia protein: phylogenetic evidence for mitochondrial dysfunction. Trends Neurosci. 1996;19:465–8.
256. Babcock M, de Silva D, Oaks R, vis-Kaplan S, Jiralerspong S, Montermini L, et al. Regulation of mitochondrial iron accumulation by Yfh1p, a putative homolog of frataxin. Science. 1997;276:1709–12.
257. Chen OS, Hemenway S, Kaplan J. Inhibition of Fe-S cluster biosynthesis decreases mitochondrial iron export: evidence that Yfh1p affects Fe-S cluster synthesis. Proc Natl Acad Sci USA. 2002;99:12321–6.
258. Cavadini P, Gellera C, Patel PI, Isaya G. Human frataxin maintains mitochondrial iron homeostasis in *S. cerevisiae*. Hum Mol Genet. 2000;9:2523–30.
259. Gerber J, Muhlenhoff U, Lill R. An interaction between frataxin and Isu1/Nfs1 that is crucial for Fe/S cluster synthesis on Isu1. EMBO Rep. 2003;4:906–11.
260. Yoon T, Cowan JA. Iron-sulfur cluster biosynthesis. Characterization of frataxin as an iron donor for assembly of [2Fe-2S] clusters in ISU-type proteins. J Am Chem Soc. 2003;125:6078–84.
261. Yoon T, Cowan JA. Frataxin-mediated iron delivery to ferrochelatase in the final step of heme biosynthesis. J Biol Chem. 2004;279:25943–6.
262. Tanno T, Bhanu NV, Oneal PA, Goh SH, Staker P, Lee YT, et al. High levels of GDF15 in thalassemia suppress expression of the iron regulatory protein hepcidin. Nat Med. 2007;13:1096–101.
263. Finkenstedt A, Bianchi P, Theurl I, Vogel W, Witcher DR, Wroblewski VJ, et al. Regulation of iron metabolism through GDF15 and hepcidin in pyruvate kinase deficiency. Br J Haematol. 2009;144:789–93.
264. Tanno T, Porayette P, Sripichai O, Noh SJ, Byrnes C, Bhupatiraju A, et al. Identification of TWSG1 as a second novel erythroid regulator of hepcidin expression in murine and human cells. Blood. 2009;114:181–6.
265. Zhang AS, Yang F, Meyer K, Hernandez C, Chapman-Arvedson T, Bjorkman PJ, et al. Neogenin-mediated hemojuvelin shedding occurs after hemojuvelin traffics to the plasma membrane. J Biol Chem. 2008;283:17494–502.
266. Zhang AS, Anderson SA, Meyers KR, Hernandez C, Eisenstein RS, Enns CA. Evidence that inhibition of hemojuvelin shedding in response to iron is mediated through neogenin. J Biol Chem. 2007;282:12547–56.
267. Zhang AS, West Jr AP, Wyman AE, Bjorkman PJ, Enns CA. Interaction of hemojuvelin with neogenin results in iron accumulation in human embryonic kidney 293 cells. J Biol Chem. 2005;280:33885–94.

Chapter 2
Cellular Iron Physiology

Martina U. Muckenthaler and Roland Lill

Keywords CIA machinery • Cysteine desulfurase • DMT1 • Ferredoxin • Ferroportin • Iron export • Iron uptake • Iron–sulfur protein • ISC machinery • Transferrin

1 Introduction

As a component of heme and iron–sulfur cluster-containing proteins, iron is essential for oxygen transport, cellular respiration, DNA synthesis, and numerous other biochemical activities. If iron is limiting, cellular growth arrest and cell death may be a consequence. Conversely, iron excess and "free" reactive iron is toxic. Ferrous iron reacts with hydrogen- or lipid-peroxides to generate hydroxyl or lipid radicals, respectively. These radicals damage lipid membranes, proteins, and nucleic acids. Because a narrow range of cellular iron levels needs to be maintained to assure cell survival, processes balancing cellular iron homeostasis are tightly controlled. These include iron uptake, iron release, intracellular iron distribution, iron utilization in the cytoplasm, mitochondria or other organelles, and intracellular iron storage. In this chapter, we discuss mechanisms of cellular iron uptake and release, follow iron through the cell to the places of storage and utilization, and elaborate on the mechanisms involved in two major iron-utilizing processes, heme and Fe/S protein biogenesis.

2 Mechanisms of Cellular Iron Uptake

Within the circulation ferric iron (Fe^{3+}) is bound to transferrin, which is the principle source of iron for all mammalian tissues. Some cell types, however, have developed specialized iron acquisition routes. These include the uptake of iron or heme directly from the diet by absorptive duodenal enterocytes or the recycling of iron from effete red blood cells by specialized macrophages.

M.U. Muckenthaler, Ph.D. (✉)
Molecular Medicine Partnership Unit, Heidelberg, Germany

Department of Pediatric Oncology, Hematology and Immunology, Heidelberg, Germany
e-mail: martina.muckenthaler@med.uni-heidelberg.de

R. Lill, Ph.D.
Institut für Zytobiologie, Philipps-Universität Marburg, Marburg, Germany
e-mail: lill@staff.uni-marburg.de

G.J. Anderson and G. McLaren (eds.), *Iron Physiology and Pathophysiology in Humans*, Nutrition and Health, DOI 10.1007/978-1-60327-485-2_2,

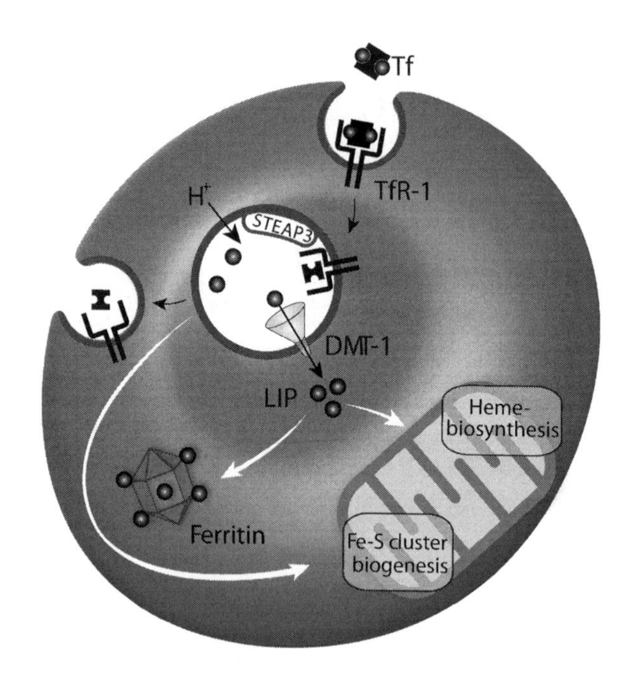

Fig. 2.1 Erythroid precursors in the bone marrow acquire iron via transferrin receptor 1 (*TfR1*)-dependent endocytosis of diferric transferrin (*Tf*). Iron is reduced by the ferrireductase STEAP3 and exported out of the endosome via DMT1 to contribute to the cytoplasmic labile iron pool (*LIP*). In addition, iron may be delivered to the mitochondria by direct contact with the endosomes. Iron that is not stored in ferritin within the cytosol is available for Fe/S cluster biogenesis and heme synthesis in mitochondria. This figure is a modified version of a figure previously published in Muckenthaler et al., Annu. Rev. Nutr. 2008. 28:3.1–3.17

2.1 *Transport of Iron-Loaded Transferrin Across Cellular Membranes*

In the blood, iron circulates bound to transferrin (Tf), an abundant liver-derived protein with extremely high affinity for iron. Tf provides iron to most cell types of the body. Iron saturation of serum Tf is mainly determined by the amount of iron (a) absorbed from the diet, (b) recycled from senescent red blood cells and released by macrophages, and (c) utilized for erythropoiesis, the most important iron consumer [1]. Cells have evolved several mechanisms to utilize iron-loaded Tf. Best understood is the uptake of diferric-Tf via transferrin receptor 1 (TfR1) which is expressed ubiquitously on the surface of many cell types. Tf–TfR1 complexes localize to clathrin-coated pits, which are internalized into endosomes via receptor-mediated endocytosis. Early Tf-containing endosomes are acidified by a proton pump, leading to a conformational change in both Tf and TfR1 to release iron. The recently identified ferrireductase STEAP3 (six-transmembrane epithelial antigen of the prostate-3), or related proteins, then reduce Fe^{3+} and the resulting ferrous iron is imported into the cytosol via divalent metal-ion transporter 1 (DMT1) [2, 3] and into mitochondria for heme and Fe/S cluster biosynthesis. Apo-Tf and TfR1 are recycled back to the cell surface for further cycles of iron binding and uptake. The Sec15l1 protein of erythroid cells is homologous to a yeast protein of the exocyst complex and assists Tf-cycling [4–6]. Excess cytoplasmic iron may then be stored within the iron storage protein ferritin (Fig. 2.1).

The special importance of Tf-mediated iron uptake during erythropoiesis is revealed by several mouse models and human diseases and is consistent with the enormous need of iron by erythroid precursor cells for hemoglobin synthesis (a) Tf-deficient mice and hypotransferrinemia patients develop severe microcytic hypochromic anemia with tissue iron deposition [7, 8]; (b) TfR1-deficient mice succumb to severe anemia with microcytic hypochromic erythrocytes and decreased iron stores at mid gestation [9]; (c) DMT1 deficient mice and patients present with impaired iron uptake in erythroid precursors [2, 10]; and (d) mutations in the ferrireductase STEAP3 [3] and the exocyst complex protein Sec15l1 [4] contribute to an anemic phenotype in mice. TfR1 and DMT1 contain regulatory RNA structures, iron responsive elements (IRE) [11], within their 3′ untranslated regions [12] that confer iron regulation to these mRNAs (see also Chap. 3). In iron deficiency, iron regulatory proteins (IRP) 1 and 2 bind to multiple IREs located within the TfR1 3′UTR to increase TfR1 mRNA stability [13]. The importance of the IRE/IRP system in regulating TfR1 expression during erythropoiesis was recently underlined by the finding that IRP2-deficient mice fail to protect TfR1 mRNA sufficiently against degradation. This in turn reduces TfR1 protein levels, hampers iron uptake and hemoglobinization of the red cells, and leads to microcytosis [14, 15].

More recently, a protein with high homology to TfR1 was discovered and named transferrin receptor-2 (TfR2) [16]. Its expression is restricted to hepatocytes, duodenal crypt cells, and erythroid cells, suggesting a more specialized role for this protein. TfR2 also binds Tf but with approximately 30-fold lower affinity than TfR1. Unlike TfR1, TfR2 expression is not regulated by the IRE/IRP regulatory system but rather at the level of protein stability, involving receptor stabilization upon ligand binding [17–19]. A link to iron homeostasis was established by the finding that mutations in the human TfR2 result in a rare form of the iron overload disorder hemochromatosis [20]. A third, Tf-bound iron uptake mechanism is operational in polarized epithelial cells of the kidney. Here, Tf uptake occurs through megalin-dependent, cubilin-mediated endocytosis and was suggested to supply iron for renal proximal tubules [12].

2.2 *Transport of Heme and Hemoglobin*

Under conditions of intravascular hemolysis, which is observed in disorders such as sickle cell anemia or thalassemia, hemoglobin (Hb) and heme are released into the circulation. Heme is highly toxic due to oxidative and proinflammatory effects and therefore detoxification must occur fast. Free Hb can be sequestered by the acute phase protein haptoglobin (HP). Both free Hb as well as Hb/HP complexes are then transported into monocytes and macrophages by the hemoglobin scavenger receptor CD163 [21, 22] (Fig. 2.2). Alternatively, heme can be sequestered from hemoglobin by a second acute phase protein, hemopexin (HPX), which provides a backup mechanism for heme clearance [23]. HPX–heme complexes are absorbed by cells via the low-density lipoprotein receptor-related protein (LRP/CD91), which is expressed in several cell types including macrophages, hepatocytes, neurons, and syncytiotrophoblasts [24] (Fig. 2.2). During hemolysis, the functions of HPX and HP are only partially redundant because mice deficient in the HP and HPX genes are more sensitive to hemolytic stress when both genes are inactivated [25, 26]. Within the cell, toxic effects of heme are prevented by the activity of the heme oxygenases which break down the porphyrin ring into biliverdin, carbon monoxide, and iron [27].

Under physiological conditions, a substantial amount of iron is taken up by tissue macrophages of the spleen, bone marrow, and liver by phagocytosis of old and damaged red blood cells. Red cells are engulfed within the phagosome where they are lysed. Hemoglobin is catabolized and heme is degraded via heme oxygenase to release iron [1] (Fig. 2.2). Iron then can be either stored within ferritin or exported via the iron exporter ferroportin to be bound to Tf and made available for a new cycle of erythropoiesis (Fig. 2.2).

2.3 *Iron Absorption of Dietary Iron by Intestinal Absorptive Cells*

Dietary iron is absorbed from the lumen of the gut across the apical membrane of absorptive enterocytes. It is then translocated through the cell and released basolaterally into the blood stream where it is loaded onto apo-Tf. The intestinal mucosa mainly absorbs two forms of iron: inorganic iron and heme (Fig. 2.3). A more extensive coverage of intestinal iron absorption is provided in Chap. 6, but some of the major points are highlighted here.

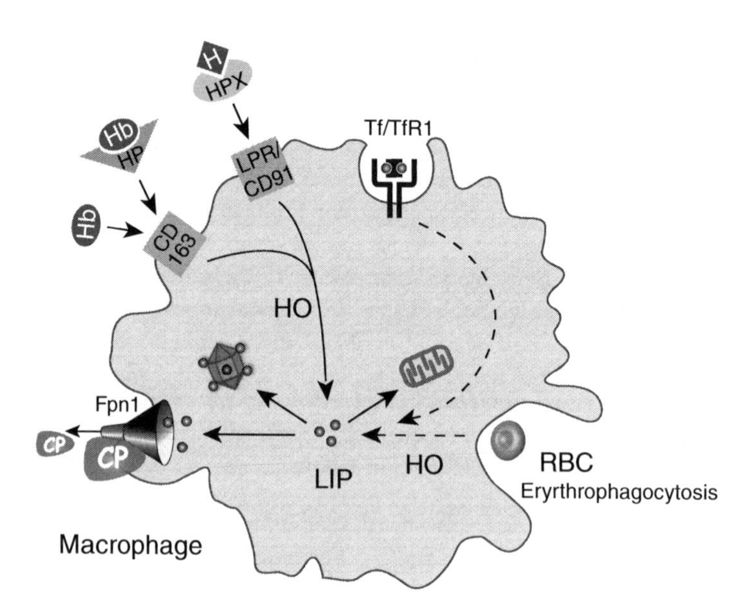

Fig. 2.2 Macrophages acquire iron via transferrin receptor 1 (*TfR1*)-dependent endocytosis of diferric transferrin (*Tf*), the uptake of heme (*H*), hemoglobin (*Hb*), or through erythrophagocytosis. Heme is sequestered by hemopexin (*HPX*) and is absorbed via the low-density lipoprotein receptor-related protein (*LRP/CD91*). Both free hemoglobin as well as Hb/haptoglobin (*HP*) complexes are transported into the cell by the hemoglobin scavenger receptor CD163. Red blood cells (*RBC*) may enter macrophages via erythrophagocytosis. The heme moiety of hemoglobin is then degraded by the heme oxygenase (*HO*) to release iron. Intracellular iron traffics toward mitochondria, is stored within ferritin in the cytosol, or can be exported via ferroportin 1 (*FPN1*). Ceruloplasmin (*CP*) oxidizes Fe^{2+} after cellular iron export for loading onto transferrin. This figure is a modified version of a figure previously published in Muckenthaler et al., Annu. Rev. Nutr. 2008. 28:3.1–3.17

Dietary non-heme iron exists primarily in the poorly bioavailable and insoluble Fe^{3+} form, which must be reduced to Fe^{2+} for transport across the intestinal epithelium. It was widely believed that DCYTB (ferrireductase duodenal cytochrome *b*; also known as CYBRD1 [cytochrome *b* reductase 1]), whose expression is increased by iron deficiency and hypoxia, would fulfil this function [28]. Ablation of the Dcytb gene in the mouse suggests that it may be dispensable for iron absorption; however, this has yet to be resolved [29]. Ferrous iron then enters the cell through DMT1. Mice with a selective ablation of DMT1 in the intestinal mucosa develop a severe iron-deficiency anemia demonstrating the important role of this transporter [30]. In addition to its intestinal iron transport function, DMT1 is also implicated in Fe^{2+} recapture in the kidney [31–33] and in brain iron transport [34]. How iron is transferred intracellularly from the apical side of epithelial cells to the basolateral iron export machinery is still largely unknown (Fig. 2.3).

In diets rich in meat, two thirds of the dietary iron supply is accounted for by heme. Intact heme is translocated across the brush-border membrane. To release the iron moiety, heme is degraded by heme oxygenase (HO) to feed the cellular low-molecular-weight iron pool (Fig. 2.3). HCP1 (also named solute carrier family 46 member A1, SlC46A1) was recently suggested as a putative apical heme carrier. It is expressed in the intestine, responds to stimuli that affect iron absorption (e.g., hypoxia, dietary or systemic iron loading), and was shown to transport heme into cells [35]. However, a function of this protein in heme transport was recently challenged by the description of a major function of SlC46A1 in proton-coupled folate transport [36].

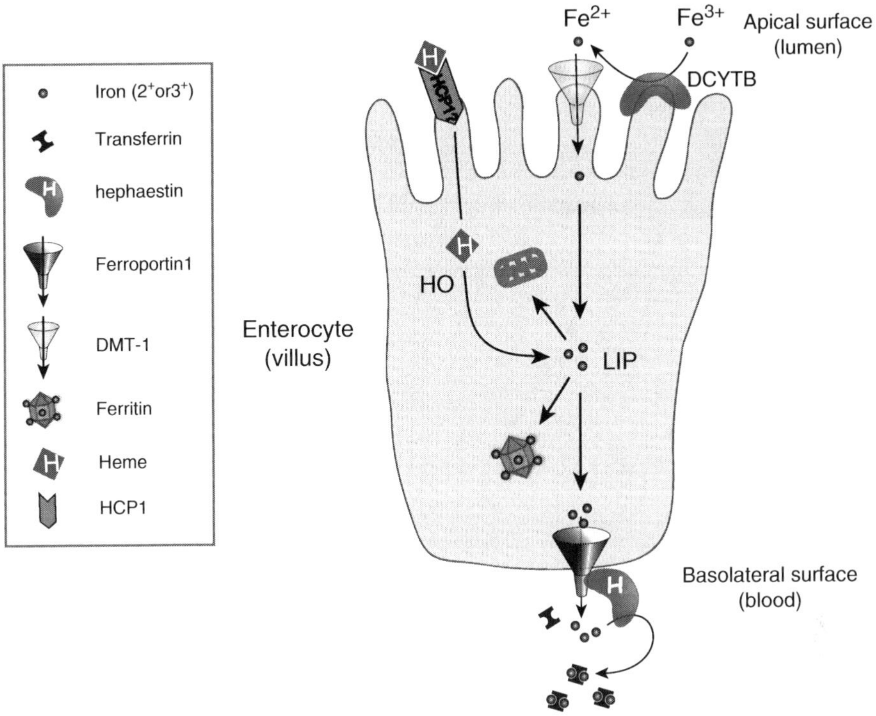

Fig. 2.3 Dietary iron that exists mainly in the insoluble Fe^{3+} form is reduced to Fe^{2+} by DCYTB (ferrireductase duodenal cytochrome *b*). Ferrous iron then enters the duodenal enterocyte through divalent metal-ion transporter, DMT1. Alternatively, heme is translocated across the brush-border membrane via the putative apical heme carrier protein 1 (*HCP1*). To release the iron, the heme moiety is degraded by heme oxygenase (*HO*) to feed the cytosolic labile iron pool (*LIP*). Iron that is not stored in ferritin is transported through the basolateral surface of the enterocyte via ferroportin 1. Hephaestin (*H*) oxidizes Fe^{2+} after cellular iron export for loading onto transferrin. This figure is a modified version of a figure previously published in Muckenthaler et al., Annu. Rev. Nutr. 2008. 28:3.1–3.17

2.4 *Alternative Pathways of Iron Transport Across Cellular Membranes*

In healthy individuals, Tf-dependent iron uptake is the most important cellular iron uptake pathway. However, several observations in conditions of pathological iron overload suggest distinct transport pathways for non-Tf bound iron. First, massive iron overload develops in nonhematopoietic tissues (e.g., liver and pancreas) in mice and humans lacking Tf [7]. Second, TfR1-deficient mice show normal embryonic organ development before they succumb to severe anemia in mid-gestation [9]. Third, iron is rapidly cleared from plasma in iron overload diseases like hereditary hemochromatosis where the iron-binding capacity of Tf is exceeded.

An alternative iron transport mechanism is the sequestration of iron by the neutrophil gelatinase-associated lipocalin (NGAL/24p3). Lipocalins are expressed and secreted by immune cells, hepatocytes, and renal tubular cells. They play a role in innate immunity by binding bacterial siderophores, thus participating in iron depletion to limit bacterial growth [37, 38]. Consistently, 24p3-deficient mice develop bacteremia more easily than their wild-type counterparts [39]. Recently, two cell surface receptors for 24p3 have been identified. One receptor, called 24p3R, was suggested to internalize apo-24p3 that then sequesters intracellular iron, possibly bound to a yet unidentified mammalian siderophore. Iron-bound 24p3 may then exit the cell and cause apoptosis as a result of iron depletion [40]. A second molecule that acts as a 24p3 receptor is the well-characterized multiprotein receptor megalin–cubilin that binds 24p3 with high affinity [41]. Megalin is expressed by proximal tubule cells in the kidney, which are known target cells of 24p3. Mice with a genetic 24p3R deficiency excrete 24p3 into the urine. Thus, megalin/cubilin-type receptors participate in taking up iron-binding proteins including α1-microglobulin [42], free hemoglobin [43], and Tf [12] in tubular cells, preventing their excretion into the urine.

Under iron overload conditions, ferrous iron (Fe^{2+}) uptake occurs in cardiomyocytes and possibly other excitable cells, such as pancreatic beta cells, anterior pituitary cells and neurons, by voltage-dependent L-type Ca^{2+} channels (LTCC) and promiscuous divalent metal transporters. Treatment of mice subjected to experimental iron overload by drugs that block LTCC function reduced myocardial iron accumulation and oxidative stress and protected from cardiac dysfunction [44–46].

Alternatively, iron may enter cells bound to acidic isoferritin [47]. But the mechanisms involved in this process as well as the responsible receptor are incompletely understood.

3 Mechanisms of Cellular Iron Release

3.1 Ferroportin-Mediated Iron Release

Duodenal enterocytes, macrophages, hepatocytes, placenta syncytiotrophoblasts, and cells of the central nervous system (CNS) release iron in a controlled fashion so that the metal is available when it is needed. Ferroportin (FPN1), a ferrous iron Fe^{2+} transporter is the only iron exporter identified to date [48–50].

FPN1 expression at the basolateral side of duodenal enterocytes assures iron efflux of dietary iron into the blood stream (Fig. 2.3). For efficient iron export, Fpn1 acts together with the multi-copper ferroxidase hephaestin that oxidizes Fe^{2+} for binding to Tf [51]. While hephaestin can be substituted under some stress conditions (e.g., acute bleeding) by the other known multi-copper ferroxidase ceruloplasmin [52], FPN1 is indispensable for iron export from enterocytes. Mice lacking intestinal FPN1 retain iron in the mucosa and develop hypochromic anemia [53]. The regulation of iron absorption involves complex transcriptional, posttranscriptional, and posttranslational mechanisms conferred by signals transmitted from the size of the body iron store, the erythropoietic activity, and by recent dietary iron intake. The FPN1 mRNA bears a functional IRE motif in its 5′UTR, which mediates IRP-dependent translational control [54, 55]. A critical role for the IRE/IRP regulatory system in securing physiological intestinal FPN1 expression was recently demonstrated in mice with simultaneous ablation of the two IRP isoforms, which caused a marked increase in FPN1 expression [56]. In addition, the central systemic regulator of iron metabolism, hepcidin, controls intestinal iron export via FPN1 [57]. This regulatory circuit is disrupted in the frequent iron overload disorder hereditary hemochromatosis that is characterized by increased intestinal iron export. In the current model, inappropriately low hepatic hepcidin expression in hemochromatosis leads high intestinal FPN1 protein levels that then facilitate increased iron absorption [58].

Most serum iron is derived from internal recycling of damaged and senescent erythrocytes and this takes place within specialized tissue macrophages of the reticuloendothelial system (RES), which phagocytose and lyse the red cells. In addition, macrophages can scavenge hemoglobin or heme that escape from cells under conditions of intravascular hemolysis. The heme moiety is then catabolized by heme oxygenase 1 to liberate inorganic iron. Iron is then released from the macrophages in a controlled fashion that positively correlates with the iron requirements of the bone marrow [59]. While cells of the RES can release iron in the form of hemoglobin, heme, or ferritin, targeted mutagenesis experiments in the mouse suggest that FPN1 is the major conduit of iron release [53].

Many disorders of iron metabolism are closely linked to alterations in FPN1 expression. For example, hereditary iron overload diseases can be explained by inappropriately low expression of the iron-regulated hormone hepcidin or by mutations in FPN1. Conversely, increased hepcidin expression in response to inflammatory mediators decreases FPN1 cell surface expression [60]. The clearance of FPN1 prevents iron export from the RES and leads to a drop in plasma iron (hypoferremia). If the inflammatory or autoimmune condition persists, anemia will develop. It is of note that IRP2-deficient mice display an unexpected iron deficiency in spleen and bone marrow macrophages. This is associated with diminished expression of FPN1, suggesting that FPN1 levels in macrophages are also controlled by the key cellular iron regulatory system [15].

Cellular iron export is impaired in mice and humans with aceruloplasminemia, an iron overload disease due to mutations in the ferroxidase ceruloplasmin (Cp). A possible molecular mechanism underlying these observations was recently uncovered where an absence of Cp triggered the rapid internalization and degradation of FPN1 [61]. In this study, depletion of extracellular iron could maintain cell surface expression of FPN1 even in the absence of Cp, suggesting that Cp is important for removing the iron that is exported by FPN1. Indeed, in the absence of Cp, iron remains bound to FPN1, which is then recognized by an ubiquitin ligase and targeted for degradation. The requirement for a ferroxidase to maintain iron transport activity represents a novel mechanism of regulating cellular iron export. The same mechanism is operational on the surface of glioma cells and astrocytes, providing an explanation for brain iron overload in patients with aceruloplasminemia [61].

3.2 Heme Export by the Feline Leukemia Virus, Subgroup C, Receptor (FLVCR)

Specialized cell types like erythroid progenitor cells need to export excess heme to prevent maturation arrest and apoptosis. Heme export is mediated by the feline leukemia virus, subgroup C receptor (FLVCR) [62]. FLVCR-null mice die in mid-gestation and show a lack of definitive erythropoiesis and craniofacial and limb deformities resembling those of patients with Diamond-Blackfan anemia [63]. By contrast, mice with FLVCR deleted neonatally develop macrocytic anemia with proerythroblast maturation arrest, suggesting an essential role for heme export in cell survival. Additionally, FLVCR is required for heme export from macrophages that phagocytose senescent red cells, suggesting that heme trafficking is an important component of systemic iron homeostasis.

4 Nature of Intracellular Iron

While in recent years our understanding of cellular iron transport and its regulation has increased considerably, still relatively little is known about the fate of intracellular iron. Free iron is dangerous because it catalyzes the formation of reactive oxygen species. Therefore most iron is bound to proteins like the iron storage protein ferritin. However, there seems to be a small amount of iron that appears to be unbound and available for regulation of iron homeostasis. This labile iron pool (LIP) amounts to less than 5% of the total cellular iron and is accessible to chelation. The LIP is composed of Fe^{2+} and Fe^{3+} and thought to be associated with a variety of small molecules such as organic anions, polypeptides, and phospholipids. It is a dynamic entity that can change rapidly and must be managed by intracellular homeostatic mechanisms [64]. Lysosomes seem to be an important source of the cellular LIP [65], most likely by degrading macromolecules such as ferritin. The LIP also contributes to the formation of dinitrosyl non-heme iron complexes (DNIC) that are detected in many nitric oxide–producing tissues and play a role in NO-dependent cellular processes [66]. It is commonly assumed that the LIP has two functions (a) a rapidly adjustable iron source for immediate metabolic utilization and (b) the control of gene expression by post-translationally regulating the major control system of cellular homeostasis, the iron regulatory proteins.

Most iron entering the cell that is not utilized immediately is stored and detoxified by ferritin, a ubiquitous and highly conserved iron-binding protein [67]. Ferritin maintains cellular iron homeostasis by sequestering the metal from the intracellular LIP. In vertebrates, ferritin is a multimeric protein comprised of 24 subunits of two types, termed H and L. The ratio of H to L subunits can vary depending on tissue type and physiologic status, and in response to inflammation or infection. Ferritin has enzymatic properties, converting Fe^{2+} to Fe^{3+} as iron is internalized and sequestered in its mineral core. This ferroxidase activity is an inherent feature of the H subunit. Ferritin can accumulate up to 4,500 iron atoms as a ferrihydrite mineral in a protein shell [68]. Coordinated degradation of ferritin and the concomitant release of iron help mobilize iron for cellular functions. However, the underlying mechanisms are poorly understood. Ferritin synthesis is regulated at multiple levels. Hormones and cytokines control ferritin gene transcription [13]. This pool of mRNA is then regulated at the level of translation by the IRE/IRP regulatory system in response to iron bioavailability [13]. The levels of intracellular ferritin are determined by the balance between synthesis and degradation that occurs both within the cytosol and lysosomes [67].

A unique H-type ferritin homopolymer with a putative function in iron storage is located in mitochondria [mitochondrial ferritin (MtF)] [69]. Under physiological conditions, mitochondrial ferritin is mainly expressed in the testis [70]. Like its cytosolic counterpart, MtF readily incorporates and oxidizes iron in vitro. Experimental overexpression of MtF results in mitochondrial iron accumulation, decreased cytosolic ferritin, and increased TfR1 expression [71]. Interestingly, the level of MtF is increased in association with mitochondrial iron accumulation in sideroblastic anemias, suggesting a protective role of MtF against iron-mediated toxicity [72].

Under terminal erythropoiesis when iron demand is extremely high, iron that enters the cell may not be seen by the cytoplasm but may rather be transferred to the mitochondria directly to efficiently satisfy the needs for erythropoiesis [73]. This hypothesis received further support by a recent finding in cultured primary murine erythroid progenitor cells from fetal liver. Within these cells, IRP activity strongly declines during terminal differentiation and appears no longer to be regulated by the cellular iron content. Consistently, expression of IRE-containing mRNAs, like ferritin and TfR1 escapes the control by the IRPs. These data were interpreted such that massive mitochondrial iron import for heme biosynthesis may involve mechanism(s) whereby iron is not sensed within the cytosol [74].

5 Mitochondrial Iron Metabolism

Mitochondria are doubtless the major sites of iron consumption in the cell as they harbor the major iron-requiring biosynthetic processes, namely, heme formation and iron-sulfur (Fe/S) protein maturation. Conspicuously, mitochondria not only produce heme and Fe/S proteins for their own needs, but also supply heme for integration into extra-mitochondrial hemoproteins and they play a crucial role in the maturation of Fe/S proteins outside mitochondria. Therefore it is not surprising that mitochondria are major regulatory elements for cellular iron homeostasis. Dysfunction of heme synthesis in erythroid cells or of mitochondrial Fe/S protein biogenesis in possibly all cell types leads to complex signaling events, resulting in increased iron uptake into the cell and into mitochondria. The consequences of malfunctions in these processes are often connected to various hematological disorders and iron storage diseases. The two biosynthetic processes are intimately linked due to multiple functional connections and changes in one process often affect the other pathway. We will briefly review the molecular mechanisms of heme biosynthesis and of cellular Fe/S protein maturation before we turn to the regulatory influences of mitochondrial function on iron homeostasis. More extensive reviews on heme biosynthesis and Fe/S protein biogenesis have been published elsewhere [75–79].

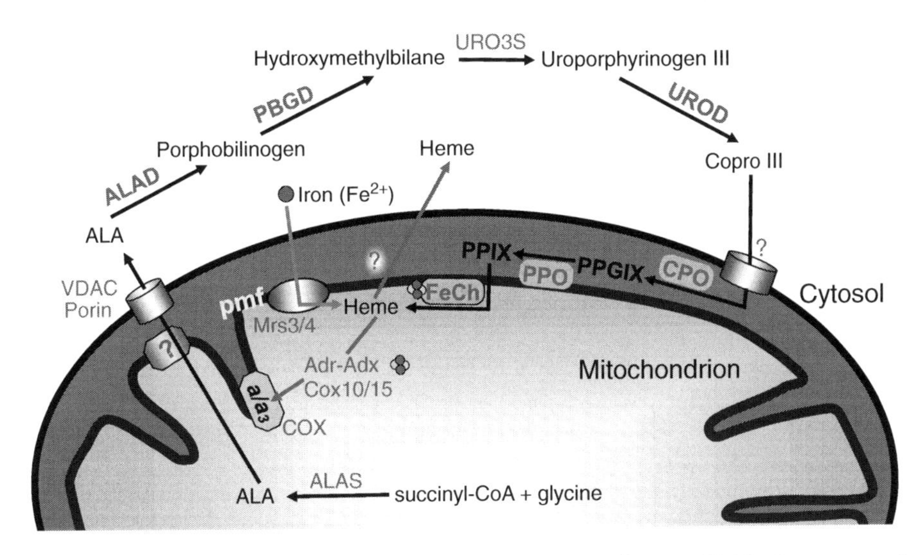

Fig. 2.4 The pathway of heme biosynthesis and its connection to Fe/S cluster metabolism. Mitochondria host the first and the last three reactions of heme production in eukaryotes, while four intermediate steps are performed in the cytosol. The reaction starts with the condensation of succinyl-CoA and glycine by δ-aminolaevulinate synthase (*ALAS*) to generate δ-aminolaevulinate (*ALA*). This compound leaves the mitochondria via unknown transporters in the inner membrane and possibly VDAC (also termed porin) in the outer membrane. Four enzymes (see text) convert ALA to coproporphyrinogen III (*Copro III*) which enters the mitochondrial intermembrane space, where it is converted to protoporphyrinogen IX (*PPGIX*) by the enzyme coproporphyrinogen oxidase (*CPO*). Protoporphyrinogen oxidase (*PPO*) bound to the outer face of the inner membrane converts PPGIX to protoporphyrin IX (*PPIX*) which then crosses the inner membrane to reach ferrochelatase (FeCh). This enzyme contains a [2Fe–2S] cluster in most organisms, and inserts ferrous iron (Fe^{2+}) into the porphyrin ring to produce heme. Iron is imported into mitochondria via the carrier proteins Mrs3/4 (also termed mitoferrin) in a membrane potential-dependent fashion (*pmf*). The production of heme A (for generation of cytochromes *a* and a_3 of cytochrome oxidase; COX) depends on the farnesyl transferase Cox10 and the hydroxylase consisting of Cox15 and the Fe/S protein adrenodoxin (Adx; yeast Yah1) and its reductase Adr (yeast Arh1). Other abbreviations: *VDAC* voltage-dependent anion channel, *ALAD* ALA dehydratase, *PBGD* porphobilinogen deaminase, *URO3S* uroporphyrinogen III synthase, *UROD* uroporphyrinogen decarboxylase

5.1 A General Overview on Heme Biosynthesis

The first and last three steps of heme biosynthesis take place inside mitochondria with the intermediate steps occurring in the cytosol (Fig. 2.4). The pathway is well conserved in eukaryotes. The first enzyme, δ-aminolevulinate synthase (ALAS) condenses glycine and succinyl-CoA to generate δ-aminolevulinate (ALA). In higher eukaryotes, there are two isoforms of this enzyme. ALAS1 is present in virtually all non-erythroid cells and is involved in supplying heme for housekeeping functions, whereas ALAS2 (also termed eALAS) is resident to the erythroid system and mainly supplies the heme required for cytosolic hemoglobin. The synthesis of ALAS2 is regulated by iron availability via the IRP system, as its mRNA contains a 5′-IRE stem-loop structure recognized by IRP1 and IRP2 [80] serving to decrease its synthesis at low iron availability, thereby decreasing the production of heme. The efficiency of ALAS import into mitochondria is regulated by heme-binding to heme regulatory elements (so-called CPV tripeptide motifs) present in the mitochondrial targeting sequence (presequence) of the precursor form of the enzyme. This may provide a fine-tuning mechanism for the overall efficiency of heme synthesis [81]. Moreover, ALAS1 and ALAS2 are transcriptionally regulated by quite different mechanisms, thus adjusting the level of the enzymes to the cellular needs of heme [75].

ALA is exported to the cytosol where the next four steps of synthesis take place (Fig. 2.4). The ALA transporter in the mitochondrial inner membrane is still unknown, but could be a member of the mitochondrial carrier family. In the cytosol, ALA dehydratase combines two molecules of ALA to the monopyrrole porphobilinogen. Four of these molecules are then combined by porphobilinogen deaminase and uroporphyrinogen III synthase, resulting in the cyclic tetrapyrrole uroporphyrinogen III. After decarboxylation by uroporphyrinogen decarboxylase, the product, coproporphyrinogen III, is transported back to mitochondria, where coproporphyrinogen oxidase located in the intermembrane space catalyzes its oxygen-dependent decarboxylation to protoporphyrinogen IX (Fig. 2.4). Targeting of coproporphyrinogen III into the mitochondrial intermembrane space is a matter of debate. It recently has been claimed that the ABC transporter of the mitochondrial outer membrane, ABCB6, may be involved in importing this porphyrin derivative into the organelle [82]. In yeast, ABCB6 can functionally replace the yeast counterpart Atm1 which is located in the mitochondrial inner membrane and plays a role in cytosolic Fe/S protein biogenesis [83] (see also below). Both the yeast protein and ABCB6 are similar in amino acid sequence to the mammalian ABCB7 transporter of the mitochondrial inner membrane which is the functional orthologue of Atm1 [84–86]. It is unclear how active transport of a low-molecular-mass compound into the intermembrane space could be achieved given that the outer membrane possesses two large openings which allow the free passage of molecules of up to 5 kDa, namely, the voltage-dependent anion carrier VDAC (also termed porin) [87] and the translocase of the mitochondrial outer membrane (TOM complex) [88]. Moreover, recent findings have found that ABCB6 is also located in the plasma membrane and Golgi [89–91]. Therefore, more functional studies are needed to solve the question of mitochondrial targeting of coproporphyrinogen III and the putative role of ABCB6 in this step [92].

The last two steps take place at the mitochondrial inner membrane and are performed by protoporphyrinogen oxidase to produce protoporphyrin IX which is then converted to heme by the insertion of an iron ion by the enzyme ferrochelatase (Fig. 2.4). The first reaction requires oxygen and creates the conjugated planar ring system. Protoporphyrinogen oxidase is a functional dimer and located in the inner membrane with major parts exposed to the intermembrane space where it interacts with coproporphyrinogen oxidase. The crystal structures of protoporphyrinogen oxidase and the matrix-exposed peripheral inner membrane protein ferrochelatase [93, 94] suggest an interaction of both proteins through the inner membrane (Fig. 2.4). This interaction could also provide the molecular basis for the transfer of protoporphyrin IX across the inner membrane so that no specific transporter is required. Both crystal structures show putative channels for substrate transfer from the active site of protoporphyrinogen oxidase to that of ferrochelatase. Lateral openings of this channel might explain the exit of the product heme from the enzymes and also why, in vitro, it is possible to supply protoporphyrin IX to intact mitochondria for efficient heme formation [95]. Ferrochelatase operates as a dimer and in most organisms, but not in *Saccharomyces cerevisiae*, contains a C-terminal Fe/S cluster which is essential for its function [96]. This cofactor underlines the intimate link between the two major iron-consuming pathways in mitochondria. Iron is necessary in its reduced (ferrous) form and is supplied to ferrochelatase via the putative iron transporters Mrs3/4 (in Zebrafish designated mitoferrin), members of the mitochondrial carrier family [97–100]. Iron import across the inner membrane requires a membrane potential [95]. Heme is finally either used inside mitochondria, e.g., in cytochromes *b* and *c*, or exported to the cytosol via unknown transport pathways for attachment to various proteins, e.g., catalase (Fig. 2.4). A fraction of the ferrochelatase product, heme B, is further modified by farnesylation and hydroxylation to form the heme A required for cytochrome oxidase (respiratory complex IV) insertion [101, 102]. These steps have been studied extensively in yeast and shown to require Cox10 (for farnesylation) as well as the hydroxylase consisting of Cox15 together with the [2Fe–2S] cluster-containing ferredoxin Yah1 and its reductase Arh1 (see below). The mammalian counterparts of the latter two enzymes are the well-known adrenodoxin and adrenodoxin reductase (Fig. 2.4).

Several diseases are associated with functional defects in heme biosynthesis [75]. For instance, mutations in ALAS2 are causative for X-linked sideroblastic anemia (XLSA) which is characterized by a microcytic hypochromic anemia and the presence of ring sideroblasts, i.e., iron-loaded mitochondria surrounding the nucleus in ring-shaped structures. While numerous different mutations have been identified in ALAS2, no disease-relevant genetic alterations of ALAS1 have been reported, indicating the indispensable character of heme synthesis for housekeeping functions of each cell. Mutations in the enzymes of the intermediate steps typically result in accumulation of the intermediate precursor products and consequently various specific porphyrias such as hereditary coproporphyria for coproporphyrinogen oxidase or variegate porphyria for protoporphyrinogen oxidase. Finally, ferrochelatase mutations elicit the classical form of erythropoietic protoporphyria (EPP). Protoporphyrin accumulates mainly in bone marrow reticulocytes from which it reaches the liver via transport through the plasma. Excess protoporphyrin is then excreted with bile and finally in feces. In the patients with EPP, the residual ferrochelatase activity is between 10% and 25% of normal, indicating the need for a substantial amount of residual heme synthesis for life. In yeast, deletion of ferrochelatase is lethal unless the cells are grown in the presence of the detergent Tween and ergosterol to supply the cells with this sterol. Synthesis of ergosterol in yeast occurs in a heme-dependent fashion.

5.2 A General Overview on Fe/S Protein Biogenesis

In this chapter, we provide a general overview on the basic concepts underlying Fe/S protein maturation in (non-plant) eukaryotes. More detailed reviews can be found elsewhere [77–79]. Since the majority of the studies on this process so far have been performed in *S. cerevisiae*, our summary will concentrate mainly on this model organism. However, virtually all components identified in yeast are conserved in higher eukaryotes [103] and hence it seems likely that biogenesis follows similar mechanisms. Initial studies performed in these higher organisms support this expectation and will be mentioned briefly.

5.2.1 The Mitochondrial Iron–Sulfur Cluster (ISC) Assembly Machinery

Mitochondria perform a central role in Fe/S protein maturation in eukaryotes in that they are required for biogenesis of all cellular Fe/S proteins. They harbor the "ISC assembly machinery" which was inherited from bacteria during endosymbiosis. To date, 15 ISC assembly proteins are known to assist this complex biosynthetic process. Their functions can be assigned to one of two major sub-reactions of the biosynthesis process [104] (Fig. 2.5). First, an Fe/S cluster is transiently assembled on the scaffold protein Isu1, a central component of Fe/S cluster assembly [105, 106]. In some fungi such as *S. cerevisiae*, a functional homologue termed Isu2 arose through a gene duplication. Since Isu1 and Isu2 are functionally redundant, we will refer to Isu1 only in the following. Second, the Fe/S cluster is transferred from Isu1 to recipient apoproteins and assembled into the polypeptide chain by coordination with specific amino acid residues. Both partial reactions require the assistance of specific ISC components.

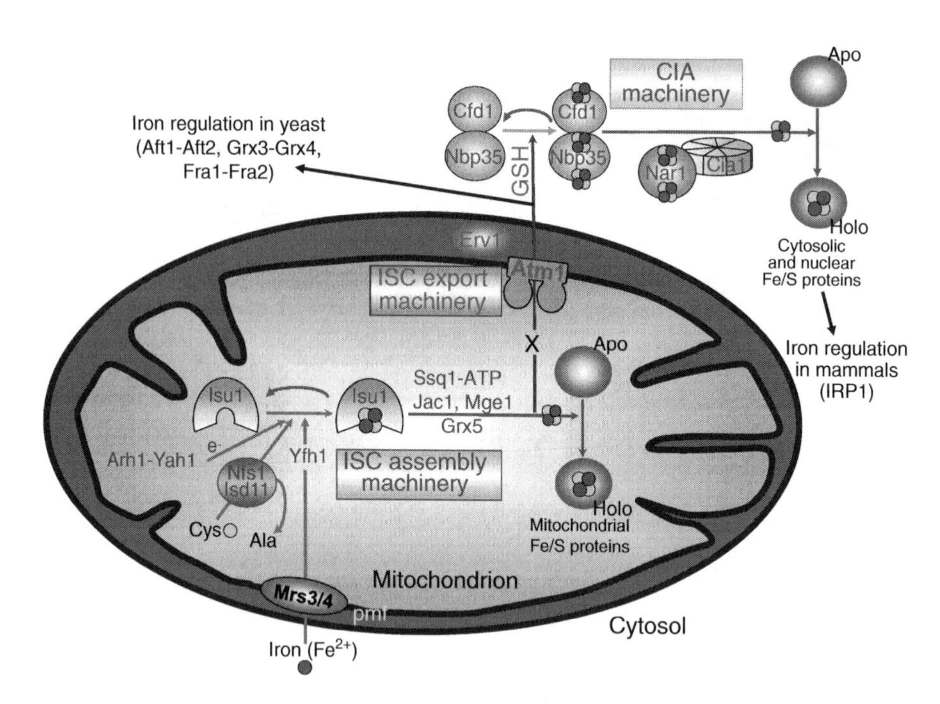

Fig. 2.5 A model for Fe/S protein biosynthesis in yeast and higher eukaryotes and its role in iron homeostasis. The mitochondrial ISC assembly machinery is required for maturation of all cellular Fe/S proteins. The ISC export and CIA machineries are specifically involved in the assembly of extra-mitochondrial Fe/S proteins. Biosynthesis of Fe/S clusters inside mitochondria can be divided into two major steps: the generation of a transient Fe/S cluster on the scaffold protein Isu1 and the transfer of the Fe/S cluster to apoproteins. The first step depends on several proteins including the cysteine desulfurase complex Nfs1–Isd11 as the sulfur donor, Yfh1 (frataxin) as the iron donor, and the electron (e^-) transfer chain consisting of ferredoxin reductase (Arh1) and ferredoxin (Yah1). Fe/S cluster transfer from Isu1 to apoproteins is facilitated by a dedicated chaperone system and the monothiol glutaredoxin Grx5. The ISC export system, including the ABC transporter Atm1, exports an unknown compound (X) to the cytosol, where it supports Fe/S protein maturation on Cfd1–Nbp35. The assembled Fe/S clusters on Cfd1–Nbp35 are then transferred to apoproteins via the assistance of Nar1 and Cia1. In addition, mitochondria play a decisive role in cellular iron homeostasis by regulating iron uptake, storage, and distribution in the cell. In yeast, this regulatory process requires the function of the two ISC machineries including the ABC transporter Atm1, but not the CIA components. Presumably, the substrate exported by Atm1 provides a signal for the transcription factors Aft1–Aft2 and additional proteins (see text) to indicate the iron status of mitochondria. This means that iron homeostasis in yeast is critically controlled by Fe/S protein assembly inside mitochondria. In mammals, both the ISC and CIA machineries are involved in maturation of the cytosolic Fe/S protein IRP1 which together with the non-Fe/S protein IRP2 (not shown) regulates iron uptake, distribution, and storage within the cell by a posttranscriptional mechanism. For further details see text. Other abbreviations: *pmf* proton-motive force, *GSH* glutathione

Fe/S cluster assembly on Isu1 critically depends on the function of the cysteine desulfurase complex comprised of Nfs1 and Isd11 [107–110] (Fig. 2.5). Even though Nfs1 contains the enzymatic activity as a cysteine desulfurase and releases sulfur to form a Nfs1-bound persulfide, the Nfs1–Isd11 complex is the functional entity for sulfur transfer from Nfs1 to Isu1 in vivo. This reaction is facilitated by a direct interaction of Nfs1 and Isu1 [111, 112]. Upon binding of iron to Isu1, the Fe/S cluster is formed by a still unknown chemical mechanism. The functional importance of mammalian

Nfs1 and Isu1 for cellular Fe/S protein biogenesis has recently been demonstrated by RNAi depletion techniques in human HeLa cells [113, 114]. Yfh1 (termed frataxin in higher eukaryotes) undergoes an iron-stimulated interaction with Isu1-Nfs1 [111]. Since the protein binds iron in vitro, frataxin is thought to serve as the iron donor of the reaction [115]. As demonstrated by RNAi-mediated depletion, human frataxin plays a general role in Fe/S protein maturation in cultured cells [116]. Fe/S protein maturation may be the primary function of frataxin, explaining all or most of the (secondary) phenotypes arising from a frataxin deficiency. Iron is imported into the mitochondrial matrix by the same mitochondrial carrier proteins, Mrs3 and Mrs4, which supply iron to heme [97–100, 117]. Fe/S cluster assembly on Isu1 further depends on an electron transfer chain comprised of the ferredoxin reductase Arh1 and the [2Fe–2S] ferredoxin Yah1, which likely receives its electrons from NADH [118, 119] (Fig. 2.5). The electrons are believed to be used for reduction of the sulfane sulfur (S^0) liberated from cysteine to the sulfide (S^{2-}) present in Fe/S clusters, but experimental proof for this assumption is lacking. Interestingly, the mammalian homologues of yeast Arh1 and Yah1 are adrenodoxin reductase (ADR) and adrenodoxin (ADX) which are well known for their role in steroid biogenesis inside mitochondria in adrenal gland cells [120, 121]. No experimental confirmation has been obtained so far for a general function of these factors in Fe/S protein biogenesis of higher eukaryotes.

The second major step of biogenesis involves the release of the Isu1-bound Fe/S cluster, its transfer to apoproteins, and its assembly into the apoprotein by coordination with the specific amino acid ligands. To date, four yeast proteins are known to specifically assist this process [104]. The dedicated chaperone system comprised of the Hsp70 family member Ssq1, the DnaJ-like co-chaperone Jac1 and the nucleotide exchange factor Mge1 is critical for these steps [122, 123]. Ssq1 undergoes a highly specific protein interaction with Isu1 which is thought to labilize Fe/S cluster binding to Isu1, thus facilitating cluster dissociation and transfer to apoproteins [124]. Jac1 can also bind to Isu1 itself, but this interaction is not essential [125]. Another important function in this partial reaction is performed by the mitochondrial monothiol glutaredoxin Grx5, yet its precise role is unknown [126]. Functional inactivation of the zebrafish homologue of Grx5 is linked to a strong defect in erythroid heme biosynthesis, which is the result of impaired biosynthesis of the cytosolic Fe/S protein IRP1 and consequently a defective synthesis of ALAS2 [127].

While all the ISC proteins appear to be required as general biogenesis factors, some of the ISC proteins play a more specialized role. A recent combination of genetic, cell biological, and biochemical approaches has shown that the function of Isa1 and Isa2 proteins is critical for the enzymatic activity of mitochondrial aconitase-like proteins (yeast Aco1 and Lys4) and the mitochondrial S-adenosylmethionine (SAM)-dependent proteins biotin synthase (yeast Bio2) and lipoic acid synthase (yeast Lip5) [128, 129]. These proteins are required in addition and after the function of the ISC assembly proteins described above. While their involvement in the functional activation of the above-mentioned four mitochondrial enzymes is well supported by auxotrophies for glutamate, lysine, biotin, and lipoic acid developed by Isa1- and/or Isa2-deficient cells, their precise molecular function remains to be clarified. Recently, another protein termed Iba57 has been identified that physically interacts with both Isa1 and Isa2 [129]. Disruption of its gene elicits a highly similar phenotype as *ISA1* and/or *ISA2* deletion mutants, suggesting that all three proteins are operating in the same pathway. The eukaryotic Isa1/2 proteins and Iba57 are the first examples of ISC components which show specificity for the maturation of a subset of Fe/S proteins.

5.2.2 The Role of the Mitochondrial ISC System for Extra-Mitochondrial Fe/S Protein Assembly

All evidence available so far indicates that Fe/S protein maturation in both the cytosol and nucleus is strictly dependent on the function of the ISC assembly machinery. While this observation was first made in yeast, similar observations have recently been obtained for the human ISC proteins Nfs1, Isu1, and frataxin [113, 114, 116, 130, 131]. Apparently, the function of the mitochondrial ISC machinery is critical for the ability of the cell to generate extra-mitochondrial Fe/S proteins, but the molecular details of this dependence are still enigmatic. For yeast and human Nfs1 and yeast Isu1, it has been shown that these proteins are required inside mitochondria to perform this task [113, 132, 133]. There is ample evidence for the fact that mitochondria export a (still unknown) component from the mitochondrial matrix to the cytosol where it performs an essential function in the Fe/S maturation process. The export reaction is accomplished by the ABC transporter Atm1 of the mitochondrial inner membrane or its mammalian counterpart ABCB7 [85, 107, 134, 135] (Fig. 2.5). Atm1/ABCB7 is the central component of the so-called ISC export machinery which encompasses two other components, the sulfhydryl oxidase Erv1 of the intermembrane space and glutathione (GSH). Depletion of either of these three components in yeast results in a highly similar phenotype i.e. normal biogenesis of mitochondrial Fe/S proteins, impairment of extra-mitochondrial Fe/S protein maturation, stimulation of the Aft1-dependent iron regulon (see below), and iron accumulation inside mitochondria [136, 137]. The latter three phenotypes are also observed upon depletion of the major components of the ISC assembly machinery, indicating that Fe/S protein maturation and iron homeostasis are tightly coordinated in yeast, and that mitochondria are a major regulatory system for iron homeostasis.

5.2.3 The Cytosolic Fe/S Protein Assembly (CIA) Machinery

Maturation of the cytosolic and nuclear Fe/S proteins is catalyzed by the cytosolic iron–sulfur protein assembly (CIA) system comprised of four known proteins (Fig. 2.5). These proteins are conserved in higher eukaryotes. According to recent in vivo and in vitro studies, this process can also be subdivided into two major partial reactions [138]. First, an Fe/S cluster is assembled on the P-loop NTPases Cfd1 and Nbp35 which serve as a scaffold. Second, the transiently bound Fe/S cluster is transferred from the Cfd1–Nbp35 complex to apoproteins by a process requiring the CIA proteins Nar1 and Cia1. Unlike the mitochondrial Isu1 scaffold, Cfd1 and Nbp35 do not directly interact with a sulfur-donating protein such as the extra-mitochondrial version of Nfs1, as genetic and biochemical studies have not established a role for this protein in the process. Since the mitochondrial version Nfs1 and other mitochondrial ISC assembly components are needed for extra-mitochondrial Fe/S cluster formation [113, 132, 133], mitochondria appear to serve as the sulfur donor for extra-mitochondrial Fe/S protein biogenesis. This is further supported by biochemical reconstitution of the Fe/S cluster assembly process on Cfd1-Nbp35 under anaerobic conditions (Dutkiewicz et al., unpublished). Fe/S cluster assembly requires intact mitochondria, cysteine, iron, matrix ATP, and a membrane potential. The P-loop NTPases Cfd1 and Nbp35 form a heterotetramer and bind up to three [4Fe–4S] clusters in vitro [138]. Both proteins possess four conserved cysteine residues at their C-termini. Mutagenesis experiments have identified the central cysteine pair forming the CPxC motif of particular importance for Fe/S cluster assembly on these proteins (Netz et al., unpublished).

Cfd1 and Nbp35 are involved in the activation of the CIA protein Nar1 by assembly of two Fe/S clusters on this iron-only hydrogenase-like protein (Fig. 2.5). The Nar1 holoprotein, activated this way, will then assist the second partial reaction, the Fe/S cluster transfer to target apoproteins [139]. In this reaction, it interacts and collaborates with Cia1, a WD40 repeat protein with seven β-propellers forming a doughnut-shaped structure [140, 141]. Interestingly, Cia1 is not needed to assemble the Fe/S clusters on Nar1, indicating its late role in the process. The molecular roles of Nar1 and Cia1 are still unclear. The close similarity of Nar1 to iron-only hydrogenases, including the conservation of the two Fe/S clusters, may indicate a role in electron transfer. It is tempting to speculate that this may help to dissociate the Fe/S cluster from the Cfd1–Nbp35 complex, thus facilitating transfer to target proteins. Cia1, like other WD40 repeat proteins, may serve as a docking platform for the other CIA proteins. None of the known CIA proteins has been shown to directly interact with the apoform of target Fe/S proteins.

Nuclear Fe/S proteins show a similar dependence on the mitochondrial ISC and the CIA proteins for maturation [140]. However, it is still unclear where maturation of the nuclear Fe/S proteins occurs. Either they are assembled in the cytosol and then imported as a holoprotein, or the assembly process takes place in the nucleus, requiring the import of the apoprotein into the nucleus. Since small amounts of the CIA proteins Cfd1, Nbp35, and Nar1 and the majority of Cia1 have been localized in the nucleus, both scenarios seem possible. Additionally, or alternatively, the nuclear CIA components could be involved in repair of damaged Fe/S clusters in this compartment, but virtually nothing is known about this potential process.

As mentioned above, virtually all eukaryotes contain close sequence relatives of the yeast CIA proteins, suggesting a conserved function and similar pathways of biogenesis. However, the mammalian proteins are proposed to participate in rather diverse cellular functions. For instance, the Cia1 relative Ciao1 has been shown to interact with the Wilms tumor protein and this has a potential role in transcription regulation [142]. The yeast Nar1 homologue IOP1 may modulate the activity of hypoxia-inducible factor 1α [143]. The mouse counterparts of yeast Nbp35 and Cfd1 interact with kinesin 5A in murine cells, suggesting a function in centrosome duplication [144].

Recent experimental tests have shown a direct function of the homologues of Nar1 (termed IOP1) and Nbp35 in Fe/S protein assembly in mammalian cells. Using the RNAi technique to deplete these proteins, a specific role in cytosolic, but not mitochondrial Fe/S protein maturation could be shown [145, 146]. Useful target Fe/S proteins for these studies are the cytosolic aconitase, i.e., the holoform of iron regulatory protein 1 (IRP1) which contains a [4Fe–4S] cluster, glutamine phosphoribosylpyrophosphate amidotransferase (GPAT) which is stable in the cytosol only in the presence of its Fe/S cluster, and xanthine oxidase which contains a molybdenum cofactor in addition to its Fe/S cluster. In addition, the binding of the apoform of IRP1 to iron responsive elements (IRE) of certain mRNAs involved in iron metabolism can be used as an (indirect) indication of Fe/S cluster assembly. Even though a role for the mammalian counterparts of Cfd1 and Ciao1 in Fe/S protein biogenesis seems likely from these studies, only complementation of the yeast *cia1*-defective mutant by human Ciao1 provides direct experimental evidence for this notion so far.

5.3 *The Regulatory Connection Between Fe/S Protein Biogenesis and Iron Homeostasis*

5.3.1 The Role of the Yeast Mitochondrial ISC Systems in the Regulation of Cellular Iron Homeostasis

Work over the past decade has established the important role of mitochondria in cellular iron homeostasis [76, 79, 147, 148]. Yeast Yfh1 (frataxin) and Atm1 were the first ISC proteins for which such a function was identified, in fact long before their primary function in Fe/S protein biogenesis was ascertained [149, 150]. It is now clear that virtually the entire ISC machinery (with the exception of the Isa1/2 and Iba57 proteins) has a strong impact on iron homeostasis in yeast. The molecular foundations underlying this regulatory role are not clear yet. It is believed that mitochondria produce and export, presumably via the ISC export component Atm1 (Fig. 2.5), a component which interacts, directly or indirectly, with the iron-responsive transcription factors Aft1–Aft2 which activate genes of the so-called iron regulon. These genes are involved in cellular uptake, storage, intracellular distribution, and utilization of iron. The relationship of the iron regulatory component produced by mitochondria to the factor facilitating Fe/S cluster assembly on Cfd1–Nbp35 (X in Fig. 2.5) is unknown. The regulatory compound can inhibit Aft1–Aft2 target gene activation, possibly by interfering with the shuttling of the proteins between the nucleus and the cytosol. Aft1 was shown to depend on the importin Pse1 for nuclear import, while the exportin Msn5 and iron are necessary to translocate Aft1 back to the cytosol under iron-replete conditions [151, 152].

Aft1 interacts with several other proteins which are important determinants of iron regulation (Fig. 2.5). First, a role of the monothiol glutaredoxins Grx3 and Grx4 has been noted in that both proteins bind to Aft1 in an iron-independent fashion [153–155]. Deletion of the two Grx proteins results in accumulation of Aft1 in the nucleus and transcriptional activation of the iron regulon. It has been speculated that either Aft1 or the Grx proteins bind an Fe/S cluster, thus explaining the ISC dependence of the regulatory mechanism. However, so far no Fe/S cluster has been found on any of these proteins under in vivo conditions. Further, the lack of a detectable role of the CIA machinery in cellular iron homeostasis [156] supports the notion that regulation is not triggered by binding of a generic Fe/S cluster. Recently, two additional proteins termed Fra1 and Fra2 were shown to interact with the Grx proteins in an iron-independent fashion [155]. Deletion of either of the *FRA1* or *FRA2* genes leads to nuclear localization of Aft1 and the induction of the Aft1-dependent iron regulon, indicating that these proteins belong to the signaling pathway leading from the mitochondrial ISC machinery to the Aft1 transcription factor. How the complex between the Grx and Fra proteins affects Aft1 activity is currently unknown. In addition to this transcriptional level of iron regulation, a posttranscriptional mechanism via stimulated mRNA degradation is used to fine-tune iron homeostasis [156, 157]. The protein Cth2 binds to 3′-ends of mRNAs encoding proteins involved in iron-dependent processes and downregulates these mRNAs by degradation. This mechanism helps in fine-tuning intracellular iron distribution and utilization under iron-limiting conditions.

5.3.2 The Role of Both the ISC and CIA Machineries in the Regulation of Cellular Iron Homeostasis in Mammals

In contrast to the striking similarities of Fe/S protein biogenesis in yeast and mammalian cells, iron regulation is achieved by radically different mechanisms in these organisms, mainly because in mammals IRP1 and IRP2 are the key regulators of this process by a posttranscriptional mechanism [1, 80, 158]. Nevertheless, recent findings indicate that the two mitochondrial ISC systems also play a decisive role in mammalian iron regulation. This is due to their role in the assembly of the Fe/S cluster on cytosolic IRP1. Since this step also involves the function of the mammalian CIA machinery, it is not surprising that recently a role for human Nar1 and Nbp35 in iron homeostasis was defined [145, 146]. This is in contrast to yeast where CIA proteins have no detectable role in iron homeostasis (see Fig. 2.5).

As mentioned above, depletion of human frataxin, Isu1 or Nfs1 proteins by RNAi results in impaired IRP1 Fe/S cluster maturation [113, 114, 116]. In turn, Isu1-depleted cells showed iron accumulation, at least in the presence of additional ferric iron in the growth medium. A similar impact of the ISC assembly machinery on cellular iron status was shown for the zebrafish mutant *shiraz* which is defective in mitochondrial glutaredoxin Grx5 [127]. This defect resulted in lower heme levels which were shown to be caused by low expression of ALAS2 (see above). This effect was caused by the increase of the IRP1 apoform secondary to the Grx5 defect, thus leading to decreased translation of ALAS2 in erythroid cells. The studies suggest an intimate connection between Fe/S cluster biogenesis and heme biosynthesis in erythroid precursors via the regulatory function of IRP1 on mitochondrial ALAS2 translation. This connection also explains why Fe/S protein biogenesis defects frequently elicit a hematological disease phenotype (see Table 2.1).

A crucial function in the regulation of iron homeostasis has been assigned to ABCB7, a member of the mammalian ISC export machinery which is mutated in patients with X-linked sideroblastic anemia and cerebellar ataxia (XLSA/A) [134, 159] (see also above). A conditional knock-out of the murine *ABCB7* gene in liver caused a marked iron accumulation in hepatocytes [85] mimicking the disease phenotype of patients with XLSA/A. The increased IRE binding capacity of IRP1 in ABCB7-deficient cells

Table 2.1 Diseases linked to iron–sulfur proteins and their biogenesis

Human protein	Yeast protein	Function	Associated disease
ISC assembly machinery			
Frataxin	Yfh1	Iron donor	Friedreich's ataxia
huGrx5	Grx5	Fe/S cluster transfer	Microcytic anemia with ring sideroblasts
ADR	Arh1	Reduction	Tumor suppressor
huIsu1	Isu1	Scaffold for Fe/S cluster assembly	Myopathy with exercise tolerance
ISC export machinery			
ABCB7	Atm1	ABC transporter	X-linked sideroblastic anemia and cerebellar ataxia (XLSA/A)
ALR	Erv1	Sulfhydryl oxidase	Liver regeneration?
Iron trafficking			
Mitoferrin	Mrs3-Mrs4	Iron transporter	Erythropoietic protoporphyria (EPP)
Fe/S proteins			
Complex I	–	Respiration	MELAS, Leigh syndrome, LHON
Complex II	Succinate dehydrogenase	Respiration	Tumor suppressor
XPD	Rad3	ATP-dependent DNA helicase	Xeroderma pigmentosum, Cockayne syndrome, trichothiodystrophy
FancJ	Rad3	ATP-dependent DNA helicase	Fanconi anemia, breast cancer
MYH	Ntg2	DNA glycosylase	Colon cancer

is consistent with the increased iron uptake seen in these cells, presumably to counteract the primary defect in cytosolic Fe/S protein maturation. Similarly, silencing of *ABCB7* expression by RNAi in human cell culture causes massive iron accumulation in mitochondria with an apparent concomitant iron depletion in the cytosol [135]. These findings underline the important role of mitochondria in mammalian iron regulation.

Finally, depletion of the CIA components huNbp35 and huNar1 by RNAi causes a decrease in ferritin and an increase in the expression of TfR1 as a result of the increased IRP1–IRE binding subsequent to impaired IRP1 Fe/S cluster maturation [145, 146]. These findings indicate that the CIA machinery, via its role in the maturation of IRP1, has an effect on iron metabolism in higher eukaryotes, thus distinguishing it from *S. cerevisiae*. Together, all these studies document the important role of the ISC assembly, ISC export, and CIA machineries for the regulation of the iron metabolism in mammalian cells. This regulatory effect is mediated through the increased IRE-binding activity of IRP1 upon an impairment of Fe/S cluster assembly.

5.4 Diseases Associated with Fe/S Protein Biogenesis

The importance of Fe/S protein biogenesis for cell viability explains why mutations in some of its genes are associated with various diseases, some of which have been mentioned above (Table 2.1). For instance, depletion of frataxin in human cells by more than 70% causes the neurodegenerative disorder Friedreich's ataxia, the most common autosomal recessive ataxia [160]. Patients show mitochondrial Fe/S protein defects and accumulate iron in mitochondria. Mouse models with targeted deletion of the frataxin gene in muscle, neuronal or liver tissues reproduce many of the phenotypes of patients, including the deficiencies in Fe/S enzymes and mitochondrial iron accumulation [161]. Two other members of the ISC assembly machinery are associated with hematological phenotypes.

A functional defect in the human glutaredoxin Grx5 was found in a patient with microcytic anemia with iron overload (ring sideroblasts) [162]. Consistent with a primary defect in Fe/S protein biogenesis and hence increased IRE-binding activity of IRP1, patient cells showed low levels of aconitase and H-ferritin, but increased TfR1. This phenotype reproduces some features found in the zebrafish mutant *shiraz* described above. A splicing defect in the gene encoding the scaffold protein Isu1 leads to severely reduced expression of this essential ISC assembly protein and is associated with myopathy with exercise intolerance [163, 164]. The adrenodoxin reductase ADR was identified as a tumor suppressor [165]. Finally, a functional defect of the human erythroid isoform of mitoferrin (the homolog of yeast Mrs3/4) elicits a variant form of erythropoietic protoporphyria (EPP) [100].

Human diseases connected to Fe/S proteins include components in mitochondria and the nucleus (Table 2.1). Mitochondrial succinate dehydrogenase (complex II) was proposed to function as a tumor suppressor [166]. Likewise, mutations in subunits of mitochondrial respiratory complex I (NADH-ubiquinone oxidoreductase) are associated with a number of mitochondrial diseases including MELAS (mitochondrial encephalomyopathy, lactic acidosis and stroke-like episodes), Leigh syndrome, and LHON (Leber's hereditary optic atrophy). Nuclear Fe/S proteins relevant for human disease encompass the ATP-dependent DNA helicase XPD and related proteins such as FancJ involved in DNA repair (nucleotide excision repair) [167]. Mutations in XPD are found in Fe/S cluster-coordinating residues and are associated with diseases such as Xeroderma pigmentosum, Cockayne syndrome, and trichothiodystrophy [168]. FancJ mutations are the hallmark of Fanconi anemia patients. As a final example, the MutY homologue MYH performs a function as a DNA glycosylase in base excision repair, and has been associated with colon cancer [169].

6 Conclusion

The last 20 years were hallmarked by the discovery of proteins involved in iron transport and iron handling within cells. However, we are just beginning to understand how these transport proteins function and how their expression is regulated by environmental signals like iron requirements, hypoxia, or infectious and inflammatory stimuli. We still know very little how iron traffics and how it is distributed within the cell to avoid toxic effects and to assure specific intracellular delivery and insertion into iron binding sites of proteins and cofactors. We must learn how iron metabolism differs between organs and how it is affected by cell–cell interactions. A major future challenge will be to understand how iron homeostasis is maintained within the central nervous system and how iron deficiency and iron overload affect brain physiology. We further will need to address how disease states affect basic cellular iron physiology to allow exploration of novel therapeutic concepts.

Recent years also uncovered numerous components of Fe/S protein assembly, and first ideas exist how Fe/S proteins might be assembled in both mitochondria and the cytosol. However, it is clear that not all ISC and CIA components have been identified yet. Their future discovery and the molecular investigation of the biochemical mechanisms underlying biosynthesis represent exciting challenges. Further, the regulatory connection between Fe/S protein biogenesis, heme synthesis, and intracellular iron homeostasis needs to be better understood to get a more comprehensive picture of the physiology of intracellular iron. Here, we need to identify regulatory compounds that assure the cross talk between these three iron-related processes and understand their function at the molecular level.

Acknowledgments We gratefully acknowledge Dr. A.D. Sheftel and Dr. S. Altamura for helpful comments on our manuscript. MM is generously supported by the Deutsche Forschungsgemeinschaft (MU 1108/4-1), EEC Framework 6 (LSHM-CT-2006037296 EuroIron1), Landesstiftung Baden Württemberg and the BMBF (HepatoSy-Iron_liver). RL acknowledges generous support from Deutsche Forschungsgemeinschaft (SFB 593 and TR1, Gottfried-Wilhelm Leibniz program, and GRK 1216), the German-Israeli foundation GIF, Rhön Klinikum AG, and Fonds der chemischen Industrie.

References

1. Hentze MW, Muckenthaler MU, Andrews NC. Balancing acts: molecular control of mammalian iron metabolism. Cell. 2004;117:285–97.
2. Fleming MD, Romano MA, Su MA, Garrick LM, Garrick MD, Andrews NC. Nramp2 is mutated in the anemic Belgrade (b) rat: evidence of a role for Nramp2 in endosomal iron transport. Proc Natl Acad Sci USA. 1998;95:1148–53.
3. Ohgami RS, Campagna DR, Greer EL, et al. Identification of a ferrireductase required for efficient transferrin-dependent iron uptake in erythroid cells. Nat Genet. 2005;37:1264–9.
4. Lim JE, Jin O, Bennett C, et al. A mutation in Sec15l1 causes anemia in hemoglobin deficit (hbd) mice. Nat Genet. 2005;37:1270–3.
5. White RA, Boydston LA, Brookshier TR, et al. Iron metabolism mutant hbd mice have a deletion in Sec15l1, which has homology to a yeast gene for vesicle docking. Genomics. 2005;86:668–73.
6. Zhang AS, Sheftel AD, Ponka P. The anemia of "haemoglobin-deficit" (hbd/hbd) mice is caused by a defect in transferrin cycling. Exp Hematol. 2006;34:593–8.
7. Trenor 3rd CC, Campagna DR, Sellers VM, Andrews NC, Fleming MD. The molecular defect in hypotransferrinemic mice. Blood. 2000;96:1113–8.
8. Ponka P. Rare causes of hereditary iron overload. Semin Hematol. 2002;39:249–62.
9. Levy JE, Jin O, Fujiwara Y, Kuo F, Andrews NC. Transferrin receptor is necessary for development of erythrocytes and the nervous system. Nat Genet. 1999;21:396–9.
10. Mims MP, Guan Y, Pospisilova D, et al. Identification of a human mutation of DMT1 in a patient with microcytic anemia and iron overload. Blood. 2005;105:1337–42.
11. Zimmerman C, Klein KC, Kiser PK, et al. Identification of a host protein essential for assembly of immature HIV-1 capsids. Nature. 2002;415:88–92.
12. Kozyraki R, Fyfe J, Verroust PJ, et al. Megalin-dependent cubilin-mediated endocytosis is a major pathway for the apical uptake of transferrin in polarized epithelia. Proc Natl Acad Sci USA. 2001;98:12491–6.
13. Muckenthaler M, Galy B, Hentze MW. Systemic iron homeostasis and the iron-responsive element/iron-regulatory protein (IRE/IRP) regulatory network. Annu Rev Nutr. 2008;28:197–213.
14. Cooperman SS, Meyron-Holtz EG, Olivierre-Wilson H, Ghosh MC, McConnell JP, Rouault TA. Microcytic anemia, erythropoietic protoporphyria, and neurodegeneration in mice with targeted deletion of iron-regulatory protein 2. Blood. 2005;106:1084–91.
15. Galy B, Ferring D, Minana B, et al. Altered body iron distribution and microcytosis in mice deficient in iron regulatory protein 2 (IRP2). Blood. 2005;106:2580–9.
16. Kawabata H, Yang R, Hirama T, et al. Molecular cloning of transferrin receptor 2. A new member of the transferrin receptor-like family. J Biol Chem. 1999;274:20826–32.
17. Johnson MB, Enns CA. Diferric transferrin regulates transferrin receptor 2 protein stability. Blood. 2004;104:4287–93.
18. Robb A, Wessling-Resnick M. Regulation of transferrin receptor 2 protein levels by transferrin. Blood. 2004;104:4294–9.
19. Chen J, Enns CA. The cytoplasmic domain of transferrin receptor 2 dictates its stability and response to holo-transferrin in Hep3B cells. J Biol Chem. 2007;282:6201–9.
20. Camaschella C, Roetto A, Cali A, et al. The gene TFR2 is mutated in a new type of haemochromatosis mapping to 7q22. Nat Genet. 2000;25:14–5.
21. Kristiansen M, Graversen JH, Jacobsen C, et al. Identification of the haemoglobin scavenger receptor. Nature. 2001;409:198–201.
22. Schaer DJ, Schaer CA, Buehler PW, et al. CD163 is the macrophage scavenger receptor for native and chemically modified hemoglobins in the absence of haptoglobin. Blood. 2006;107:373–80.
23. Hrkal Z, Vodrazka Z, Kalousek I. Transfer of heme from ferrihemoglobin and ferrihemoglobin isolated chains to hemopexin. Eur J Biochem. 1974;43:73–8.
24. Hvidberg V, Maniecki MB, Jacobsen C, Hojrup P, Moller HJ, Moestrup SK. Identification of the receptor scavenging hemopexin-heme complexes. Blood. 2005;106:2572–9.
25. Tolosano E, Hirsch E, Patrucco E, et al. Defective recovery and severe renal damage after acute hemolysis in hemopexin-deficient mice. Blood. 1999;94:3906–14.
26. Tolosano E, Fagoonee S, Hirsch E, et al. Enhanced splenomegaly and severe liver inflammation in haptoglobin/hemopexin double-null mice after acute hemolysis. Blood. 2002;100:4201–8.
27. Otterbein LE, Soares MP, Yamashita K, Bach FH. Heme oxygenase-1: unleashing the protective properties of heme. Trends Immunol. 2003;24:449–55.
28. McKie AT, Barrow D, Latunde-Dada GO, et al. An iron-regulated ferric reductase associated with the absorption of dietary iron. Science. 2001;291:1755–9.

29. Gunshin H, Starr CN, Direnzo C, et al. Cybrd1 (duodenal cytochrome b) is not necessary for dietary iron absorption in mice. Blood. 2005;106(8):2879–83.
30. Gunshin H, Fujiwara Y, Custodio AO, Direnzo C, Robine S, Andrews NC. Slc11a2 is required for intestinal iron absorption and erythropoiesis but dispensable in placenta and liver. J Clin Invest. 2005;115:1258–66.
31. Ferguson CJ, Wareing M, Ward DT, Green R, Smith CP, Riccardi D. Cellular localization of divalent metal transporter DMT-1 in rat kidney. Am J Physiol Renal Physiol. 2001;280:F803–14.
32. Hubert N, Hentze MW. Previously uncharacterized isoforms of divalent metal transporter (DMT)-1: implications for regulation and cellular function. Proc Natl Acad Sci USA. 2002;99:12345–50.
33. Ludwiczek S, Theurl I, Muckenthaler MU, et al. Ca2+ channel blockers reverse iron overload by a new mechanism via divalent metal transporter-1. Nat Med. 2007;13:448–54.
34. Jeong SY, David S. Glycosylphosphatidylinositol-anchored ceruloplasmin is required for iron efflux from cells in the central nervous system. J Biol Chem. 2003;278:27144–8.
35. Shayeghi M, Latunde-Dada GO, Oakhill JS, et al. Identification of an intestinal heme transporter. Cell. 2005;122:789–801.
36. Qiu A, Jansen M, Sakaris A, et al. Identification of an intestinal folate transporter and the molecular basis for hereditary folate malabsorption. Cell. 2006;127:917–28.
37. Yang J, Goetz D, Li JY, et al. An iron delivery pathway mediated by a lipocalin. Mol Cell. 2002;10:1045–56.
38. Richardson DR. 24p3 and its receptor: dawn of a new iron age? Cell. 2005;123:1175–7.
39. Berger T, Togawa A, Duncan GS, et al. Lipocalin 2-deficient mice exhibit increased sensitivity to Escherichia coli infection but not to ischemia–reperfusion injury. Proc Natl Acad Sci USA. 2006;103:1834–9.
40. Devireddy LR, Gazin C, Zhu X, Green MR. A cell-surface receptor for lipocalin 24p3 selectively mediates apoptosis and iron uptake. Cell. 2005;123:1293–305.
41. Hvidberg V, Jacobsen C, Strong RK, Cowland JB, Moestrup SK, Borregaard N. The endocytic receptor megalin binds the iron transporting neutrophil-gelatinase-associated lipocalin with high affinity and mediates its cellular uptake. FEBS Lett. 2005;579:773–7.
42. Leheste JR, Rolinski B, Vorum H, et al. Megalin knockout mice as an animal model of low molecular weight proteinuria. Am J Pathol. 1999;155:1361–70.
43. Gburek J, Verroust PJ, Willnow TE, et al. Megalin and cubilin are endocytic receptors involved in renal clearance of hemoglobin. J Am Soc Nephrol. 2002;13:423–30.
44. Oudit GY, Sun H, Trivieri MG, et al. L-type Ca2+ channels provide a major pathway for iron entry into cardiomyocytes in iron-overload cardiomyopathy. Nat Med. 2003;9:1187–94.
45. Mwanjewe J, Grover AK. Role of transient receptor potential canonical 6 (TRPC6) in non-transferrin-bound iron uptake in neuronal phenotype PC12 cells. Biochem J. 2004;378:975–82.
46. Oudit GY, Trivieri MG, Khaper N, Liu PP, Backx PH. Role of L-type Ca2+ channels in iron transport and iron-overload cardiomyopathy. J Mol Med. 2006;84:349–64.
47. Meyron-Holtz EG, Vaisman B, Cabantchik ZI, et al. Regulation of intracellular iron metabolism in human erythroid precursors by internalized extracellular ferritin. Blood. 1999;94:3205–11.
48. Abboud S, Haile DJ. A novel mammalian iron-regulated protein involved in intracellular iron metabolism. J Biol Chem. 2000;275:19906–12.
49. Donovan A, Brownlie A, Zhou Y, et al. Positional cloning of zebrafish ferroportin1 identifies a conserved vertebrate iron exporter. Nature. 2000;403:776–81.
50. McKie AT, Marciani P, Rolfs A, et al. A novel duodenal iron-regulated transporter, IREG1, implicated in the basolateral transfer of iron to the circulation. Mol Cell. 2000;5:299–309.
51. Vulpe CD, Kuo YM, Murphy TL, et al. Hephaestin, a ceruloplasmin homologue implicated in intestinal iron transport, is defective in the sla mouse. Nat Genet. 1999;21:195–9.
52. Cherukuri S, Potla R, Sarkar J, Nurko S, Harris ZL, Fox PL. Unexpected role of ceruloplasmin in intestinal iron absorption. Cell Metab. 2005;2:309–19.
53. Donovan A, Lima CA, Pinkus JL, et al. The iron exporter ferroportin/Slc40a1 is essential for iron homeostasis. Cell Metab. 2005;1:191–200.
54. Lymboussaki A, Pignatti E, Montosi G, Garuti C, Haile DJ, Pietrangelo A. The role of the iron responsive element in the control of ferroportin1/IREG1/MTP1 gene expression. J Hepatol. 2003;39:710–5.
55. Liu XB, Hill P, Haile DJ. Role of the ferroportin iron-responsive element in iron and nitric oxide dependent gene regulation. Blood Cells Mol Dis. 2002;29:315–26.
56. Galy B. Iron regulatory proteins are essential for intestinal function and control key iron absorption molecules in the duodenum. Cell Metab. 2008;7:79–85.
57. Nemeth E, Tuttle MS, Powelson J, et al. Hepcidin regulates cellular iron efflux by binding to ferroportin and inducing its internalization. Science. 2004;306:2090–3.
58. Pietrangelo A. Hemochromatosis: an endocrine liver disease. Hepatology. 2007;46:1291–301.
59. Knutson M, Wessling-Resnick M. Iron metabolism in the reticuloendothelial system. Crit Rev Biochem Mol Biol. 2003;38:61–88.

60. Ganz T. Molecular control of iron transport. J Am Soc Nephrol. 2007;18:394–400.
61. De Domenico I, Vaughn MB, Li L, et al. Ferroportin-mediated mobilization of ferritin iron precedes ferritin degradation by the proteasome. EMBO J. 2006;25:5396–404.
62. Quigley JG, Yang Z, Worthington MT, et al. Identification of a human heme exporter that is essential for erythropoiesis. Cell. 2004;118:757–66.
63. Keel SB, Doty RT, Yang Z, et al. A heme export protein is required for red blood cell differentiation and iron homeostasis. Science. 2008;319:825–8.
64. Andrews NC. Probing the iron pool. Focus on "detection of intracellular iron by its regulatory effect". Am J Physiol Cell Physiol. 2004;287:C1537–8.
65. Kurz T, Gustafsson B, Brunk UT. Intralysosomal iron chelation protects against oxidative stress-induced cellular damage. FEBS J. 2006;273:3106–17.
66. Zhang Y, Hogg N. S-nitrosothiols: cellular formation and transport. Free Radic Biol Med. 2005;38:831–8.
67. Torti FM, Torti SV. Regulation of ferritin genes and protein. Blood. 2002;99:3505–5316.
68. Harrison PM. Ferritin: an iron-storage molecule. Semin Hematol. 1977;14:55–70.
69. Levi S, Corsi B, Bosisio M, et al. A human mitochondrial ferritin encoded by an intronless gene. J Biol Chem. 2001;276:24437–40.
70. Santambrogio P, Biasiotto G, Sanvito F, Olivieri S, Arosio P, Levi S. Mitochondrial ferritin expression in adult mouse tissues. J Histochem Cytochem. 2007;55:1129–37.
71. Nie G, Sheftel AD, Kim SF, Ponka P. Overexpression of mitochondrial ferritin causes cytosolic iron depletion and changes cellular iron homeostasis. Blood. 2005;105:2161–7.
72. Cazzola M, Invernizzi R, Bergamaschi G, et al. Mitochondrial ferritin expression in erythroid cells from patients with sideroblastic anemia. Blood. 2003;101:1996–2000.
73. Sheftel AD, Zhang AS, Brown C, Shirihai OS, Ponka P. Direct interorganellar transfer of iron from endosome to mitochondrion. Blood. 2007;110:125–32.
74. Schranzhofer M, Schifrer M, Cabrera JA, et al. Remodeling the regulation of iron metabolism during erythroid differentiation to ensure efficient heme biosynthesis. Blood. 2006;107:4159–67.
75. Ajioka RS, Phillips JD, Kushner JP. Biosynthesis of heme in mammals. Biochim Biophys Acta. 2006;1763:723–36.
76. Napier I, Ponka P, Richardson DR. Iron trafficking in the mitochondrion: novel pathways revealed by disease. Blood. 2005;105:1867–74.
77. Rouault TA, Tong WH. Iron–sulphur cluster biogenesis and mitochondrial iron homeostasis. Nat Rev Mol Cell Biol. 2005;6:345–51.
78. Lill R, Mühlenhoff U. Iron–sulfur protein biogenesis in eukaryotes: components and mechanisms. Annu Rev Cell Dev Biol. 2006;22:457–86.
79. Lill R, Mühlenhoff U. Maturation of iron–sulfur proteins in eukaryotes: mechanisms, connected processes, and diseases. Annu Rev Biochem. 2008;77:669–700.
80. Wallander ML, Leibold EA, Eisenstein RS. Molecular control of vertebrate iron homeostasis by iron regulatory proteins. Biochim Biophys Acta. 2006;1763(7):668–89.
81. Lathrop JT, Timko MP. Regulation by heme of mitochondrial protein transport through a conserved amino acid motif. Science. 1993;259:522–5.
82. Krishnamurthy PC, Du G, Fukuda Y, et al. Identification of a mammalian mitochondrial porphyrin transporter. Nature. 2006;443:586–9.
83. Mitsuhashi N, Miki T, Senbongi H, et al. MTABC3, a novel mitochondrial ATP-binding cassette protein involved in iron homeostasis. J Biol Chem. 2000;275:17536–40.
84. Csere P, Lill R, Kispal G. Identification of a human mitochondrial ABC transporter, the functional orthologue of yeast Atm1p. FEBS Lett. 1998;441:266–70.
85. Pondarre C, Antiochos BB, Campagna DR, et al. The mitochondrial ATP-binding cassette transporter Abcb7 is essential in mice and participates in cytosolic iron-sulphur cluster biogenesis. Hum Mol Genet. 2006;15:953–64.
86. Pondarre C, Campagna DR, Antiochos B, Sikorski L, Mulhern H, Fleming MD. Abcb7, the gene responsible for X-linked sideroblastic anemia with ataxia, is essential for hematopoiesis. Blood. 2007;109:3567–9.
87. Colombini M. Measurement of VDAC permeability in intact mitochondria and in reconstituted systems. Methods Cell Biol. 2007;80:241–60.
88. Künkele KP, Heins S, Dembowski M, et al. The preprotein translocation channel of the outer membrane of mitochondria. Cell. 1998;93:1009–19.
89. Paterson JK, Shukla S, Black CM, et al. Human ABCB6 localizes to both the outer mitochondrial membrane and the plasma membrane. Biochemistry. 2007;46:9443–52.
90. Tsuchida M, Emi Y, Kida Y, Sakaguchi M. Human ABC transporter isoform B6 (ABCB6) localizes primarily in the golgi apparatus. Biochem Biophys Res Commun. 2008;369:369–75.
91. Jalil YA, Ritz V, Jakimenko A, et al. Vesicular localization of the rat ATP-binding cassette half-transporter rAbcb6. Am J Physiol Cell Physiol. 2008;294:C579–90.

92. Hamza I. Intracellular trafficking of porphyrins. ACS Chem Biol. 2006;1:627–9.
93. Koch M, Breithaupt C, Kiefersauer R, Freigang J, Huber R, Messerschmidt A. Crystal structure of protoporphyrinogen IX oxidase: a key enzyme in haem and chlorophyll biosynthesis. EMBO J. 2004;23:1720–8.
94. Wu CK, Dailey HA, Rose JP, Burden A, Sellers VM, Wang BC. The 2.0 A structure of human ferrochelatase, the terminal enzyme of heme biosynthesis. Nat Struct Biol. 2001;8:156–60.
95. Lange H, Kispal G, Lill R. Mechanism of iron transport to the site of heme synthesis inside yeast mitochondria. J Biol Chem. 1999;274:18989–96.
96. Dailey HA. Terminal steps of haem biosynthesis. Biochem Soc Trans. 2002;30:590–5.
97. Foury F, Roganti T. Deletion of the mitochondrial carrier genes MRS3 and MRS4 suppresses mitochondrial iron accumulation in a yeast frataxin-deficient strain. J Biol Chem. 2002;277:24475–83.
98. Mühlenhoff U, Stadler J, Richhardt N, et al. A specific role of the yeast mitochondrial carriers Mrs3/4p in mitochondrial iron acquisition under iron-limiting conditions. J Biol Chem. 2003;278:40612–20.
99. Li L, Kaplan J. A mitochondrial-vacuolar signaling pathway in yeast that affects iron and copper metabolism. J Biol Chem. 2004;279(32):33653–61.
100. Shaw GC, Cope JJ, Li L, et al. Mitoferrin is essential for erythroid iron assimilation. Nature. 2006;440:96–100.
101. Barros MH, Nobrega FG, Tzagoloff A. Mitochondrial ferredoxin is required for heme A synthesis in Saccharomyces cerevisiae. J Biol Chem. 2002;277:9997–10002.
102. Barros MH, Carlson CG, Glerum DM, Tzagoloff A. Involvement of mitochondrial ferredoxin and Cox15p in hydroxylation of heme O. FEBS Lett. 2001;492:133–8.
103. Lill R, Mühlenhoff U. Iron–sulfur protein biogenesis in eukaryotes. Trends Biochem Sci. 2005;30:133–41.
104. Mühlenhoff U, Gerber J, Richhardt N, Lill R. Components involved in assembly and dislocation of iron–sulfur clusters on the scaffold protein Isu1p. EMBO J. 2003;22:4815–25.
105. Schilke B, Voisine C, Beinert H, Craig E. Evidence for a conserved system for iron metabolism in the mitochondria of Saccharomyces cerevisiae. Proc Natl Acad Sci USA. 1999;96:10206–11.
106. Garland SA, Hoff K, Vickery LE, Culotta VC. Saccharomyces cerevisiae ISU1 and ISU2: members of a well-conserved gene family for iron–sulfur cluster assembly. J Mol Biol. 1999;294:897–907.
107. Kispal G, Csere P, Prohl C, Lill R. The mitochondrial proteins Atm1p and Nfs1p are required for biogenesis of cytosolic Fe/S proteins. EMBO J. 1999;18:3981–9.
108. Wiedemann N, Urzica E, Guiard B, et al. Essential role of Isd11 in iron-sulfur cluster synthesis on Isu scaffold proteins. EMBO J. 2006;25:184–95.
109. Adam AC, Bornhövd C, Prokisch H, Neupert W, Hell K. The Nfs1 interacting protein Isd11 has an essential role in Fe/S cluster biogenesis in mitochondria. EMBO J. 2006;25:174–83.
110. Shan Y, Napoli E, Cortopassi G. Mitochondrial frataxin interacts with ISD11 of the NFS1/ISCU complex and multiple mitochondrial chaperones. Hum Mol Genet. 2007;16(8):929–41.
111. Gerber J, Mühlenhoff U, Lill R. An interaction between frataxin and Isu1/Nfs1 that is crucial for Fe/S cluster synthesis on Isu1. EMBO Rep. 2003;4:906–11.
112. Li K, Tong WH, Hughes RM, Rouault TA. Roles of the mammalian cytosolic cysteine desulfurase, ISCS, and scaffold protein, ISCU in iron–sulfur cluster assembly. J Biol Chem. 2006;281:12344–51.
113. Biederbick A, Stehling O, Rösser R, et al. Role of human mitochondrial Nfs1 in cytosolic iron–sulfur protein biogenesis and iron regulation. Mol Cell Biol. 2006;26:5675–87.
114. Tong WH, Rouault TA. Functions of mitochondrial ISCU and cytosolic ISCU in mammalian iron–sulfur cluster biogenesis and iron homeostasis. Cell Metab. 2006;3:199–210.
115. Bencze KZ, Yoon T, Millan-Pacheco C, et al. Human frataxin: iron and ferrochelatase binding surface. Chem Commun (Camb). 2007;14:1798–800.
116. Stehling O, Elsässer HP, Brückel B, Mühlenhoff U, Lill R. Iron–sulfur protein maturation in human cells: evidence for a function of frataxin. Hum Mol Genet. 2004;13:3007–15.
117. Zhang Y, Lyver ER, Knight SA, Pain D, Lesuisse E, Dancis A. Mrs3p, Mrs4p, and frataxin provide iron for Fe–S cluster synthesis in mitochondria. J Biol Chem. 2006;281:22493–502.
118. Lange H, Kispal G, Kaut A, Lill R. A mitochondrial ferredoxin is essential for biogenesis of intra- and extra-mitochondrial Fe/S proteins. Proc Natl Acad Sci USA. 2000;97:1050–5.
119. Li J, Saxena S, Pain D, Dancis A. Adrenodoxin reductase homolog (Arh1p) of yeast mitochondria required for iron homeostasis. J Biol Chem. 2001;276:1503–9.
120. Lambeth JD, Seybert DW, Lancaster JRJ, Salerno JC, Kamin H. Steroidogenic electron transport in adrenal cortex mitochondria. Mol Cell Biochem. 1985;45:13–31.
121. Stocco DM. Intramitochondrial cholesterol transfer. Biochim Biophys Acta. 2000;1486:184–97.
122. Craig EA, Marszalek J. A specialized mitochondrial molecular chaperone system: a role in formation of Fe/S centers. Cell Mol Life Sci. 2002;59(10):1658–65.
123. Dutkiewicz R, Marszalek J, Schilke B, Craig EA, Lill R, Mühlenhoff U. The Hsp70 chaperone Ssq1p is dispensable for iron–sulfur cluster formation on the scaffold protein Isu1p. J Biol Chem. 2006;281:7801–8.

124. Dutkiewicz R, Schilke B, Cheng S, Knieszner H, Craig EA, Marszalek J. Sequence-specific interaction between mitochondrial Fe–S scaffold protein Isu and Hsp70 Ssq1 is essential for their in vivo function. J Biol Chem. 2004;279:29167–74.
125. Andrew AJ, Dutkiewicz R, Knieszner H, Craig EA, Marszalek J. Characterization of the interaction between the J-protein Jac1 and the scaffold for Fe–S cluster biogenesis, Isu1. J Biol Chem. 2006;281:14580–7.
126. Rodriguez-Manzaneque MT, Tamarit J, Belli G, Ros J, Herrero E. Grx5 is a mitochondrial glutaredoxin required for the activity of iron/sulfur enzymes. Mol Biol Cell. 2002;13:1109–21.
127. Wingert RA, Galloway JL, Barut B, et al. Deficiency of glutaredoxin 5 reveals Fe–S clusters are required for vertebrate haem synthesis. Nature. 2005;436:1035–9.
128. Mühlenhoff U, Gerl MJ, Flauger B, et al. The ISC proteins Isa1 and Isa2 are required for the function but not for the de novo synthesis of the Fe/S clusters of biotin synthase in Saccharomyces cerevisiae. Eukaryot Cell. 2007;6:495–504.
129. Gelling C, Dawes IW, Richhardt N, Lill R, Mühlenhoff U. Mitochondrial Iba57p is required for Fe/S cluster formation on aconitase and activation of radical-SAM enzymes. Mol Cell Biol. 2007;28:1851–61.
130. Martelli A, Wattenhofer-Donzé M, Schmucker S, Bouvet S, Reutenauer L, Puccio H. Frataxin is essential for extramitochondrial Fe–S cluster proteins in mammalian tissues. Hum Mol Genet. 2007;16:2651–8.
131. Lu C, Cortopassi G. Frataxin knockdown causes loss of cytoplasmic iron-sulfur cluster functions, redox alterations and induction of heme transcripts. Arch Biochem Biophys. 2007;457:111–22.
132. Gerber J, Neumann K, Prohl C, Mühlenhoff U, Lill R. The yeast scaffold proteins Isu1p and Isu2p are required inside mitochondria for maturation of cytosolic Fe/S proteins. Mol Cell Biol. 2004;24:4848–57.
133. Mühlenhoff U, Balk J, Richhardt N, et al. Functional characterization of the eukaryotic cysteine desulfurase Nfs1p from Saccharomyces cerevisiae. J Biol Chem. 2004;279:36906–15.
134. Bekri S, Kispal G, Lange H, et al. Human ABC7 transporter: gene structure and mutation causing X-linked sideroblastic anemia with ataxia (XLSA/A) with disruption of cytosolic iron-sulfur protein maturation. Blood. 2000;96:3256–64.
135. Cavadini P, Biasiotto G, Poli M, et al. RNA silencing of the mitochondrial ABCB7 transporter in HeLa cells causes an iron-deficient phenotype with mitochondrial iron overload. Blood. 2007;109:3552–9.
136. Lange H, Lisowsky T, Gerber J, Mühlenhoff U, Kispal G, Lill R. An essential function of the mitochondrial sulfhydryl oxidase Erv1p/ALR in the maturation of cytosolic Fe/S proteins. EMBO Rep. 2001;2:715–20.
137. Sipos K, Lange H, Fekete Z, Ullmann P, Lill R, Kispal G. Maturation of cytosolic iron-sulfur proteins requires glutathione. J Biol Chem. 2002;277:26944–9.
138. Netz DJ, Pierik AJ, Stümpfig M, Mühlenhoff U, Lill R. The Cfd1-Nbp35 complex acts as a scaffold for iron–sulfur protein assembly in the yeast cytosol. Nat Chem Biol. 2007;3:278–86.
139. Balk J, Pierik AJ, Aguilar Netz D, Mühlenhoff U, Lill R. The hydrogenase-like Nar1p is essential for maturation of cytosolic and nuclear iron–sulphur proteins. EMBO J. 2004;23:2105–15.
140. Balk J, Aguilar Netz DJ, Tepper K, Pierik AJ, Lill R. The essential WD40 protein Cia1 is involved in a late step of cytosolic and nuclear iron–sulfur protein assembly. Mol Cell Biol. 2005;25:10833–41.
141. Srinivasan V, Netz DJA, Webert H, et al. Structure of the yeast WD40 domain protein Cia1, a component acting late in iron–sulfur protein biogenesis. Structure. 2007;15:1246–57.
142. Johnstone RW, Wang J, Tommerup N, Vissing H, Roberts T, Shi Y. Ciao1 is a novel WD40 protein that interacts with the tumor suppressor protein WT1. J Biol Chem. 1998;273:10880–7.
143. Huang J, Song D, Flores A, et al. IOP1, a novel hydrogenase-like protein that modulates hypoxia-inducible factor-1alpha activity. Biochem J. 2007;401:341–52.
144. Christodoulou A, Lederer CW, Surrey T, Vernos I, Santama N. Motor protein KIFC5A interacts with Nubp1 and Nubp2, and is implicated in the regulation of centrosome duplication. J Cell Sci. 2006;119:2035–47.
145. Song D, Lee FS. A role for IOP1 in mammalian cytosolic iron–sulfur protein biogenesis. J Biol Chem. 2008;283:9231–8.
146. Stehling O, Netz DJA, Niggemeyer B, et al. Human Nbp35 is essential for both cytosolic iron-sulfur protein assembly and iron homeostasis. Mol Cell Biol. 2008;28:5517–28.
147. Philpott CC. Iron uptake in fungi: a system for every source. Biochim Biophys Acta. 2006;1763:636–45.
148. Kaplan J, McVey War D, Crisp RJ, Philpott CC. Iron-dependent metabolic remodeling in S. cerevisiae. Biochim Biophys Acta. 2006;1763:646–51.
149. Babcock M, De Silva D, Oaks R, et al. Regulation of mitochondrial iron accumulation by Yfh1p, a putative homolog of frataxin. Science. 1997;276:1709–12.
150. Kispal G, Csere P, Guiard B, Lill R. The ABC transporter Atm1p is required for mitochondrial iron homeostasis. FEBS Lett. 1997;418:346–50.
151. Ueta R, Fujiwara N, Iwai K, Yamaguchi-Iwai Y. Mechanism underlying the iron-dependent nuclear export of the iron-responsive transcription factor Aft1p in Saccharomyces cerevisiae. Mol Biol Cell. 2007;18:2980–90.
152. Ueta R, Fukunaka A, Yamaguchi-Iwai Y. Pse1p mediates the nuclear import of the iron-responsive transcription factor Aft1p in Saccharomyces cerevisiae. J Biol Chem. 2003;278:50120–7.

153. Ojeda L, Keller G, Mühlenhoff U, Rutherford JC, Lill R, Winge DR. Role of glutaredoxin-3 and glutaredoxin-4 in the iron-regulation of the Aft1 transcriptional activator in Saccharomyces cerevisiae. J Biol Chem. 2006;281:17661–9.
154. Pujol-Carrion N, Belli G, Herrero E, Nogues A, de la Torre-Ruiz MA. Glutaredoxins Grx3 and Grx4 regulate nuclear localisation of Aft1 and the oxidative stress response in Saccharomyces cerevisiae. J Cell Sci. 2006;119:4554–64.
155. Kumanovics A, Chen O, Li L, et al. Identification of FRA1 and FRA2 as genes involved in regulating the yeast iron regulon in response to decreased mitochondrial iron–sulfur cluster synthesis. J Biol Chem. 2008;283:10276–86.
156. Hausmann A, Samans B, Lill R, Mühlenhoff U. Cellular and mitochondrial remodeling upon defects in iron–sulfur protein biogenesis. J Biol Chem. 2008;283:8318–30.
157. Puig S, Askeland E, Thiele DJ. Coordinated remodeling of cellular metabolism during iron deficiency through targeted mRNA degradation. Cell. 2005;120:99–110.
158. Rouault TA. The role of iron regulatory proteins in mammalian iron homeostasis and disease. Nat Chem Biol. 2006;2:406–14.
159. Allikmets R, Raskind WH, Hutchinson A, Schueck ND, Dean M, Koeller DM. Mutation of a putative mitochondrial iron transporter gene (ABC7) in X-linked sideroblastic anemia and ataxia (XLSA/A). Hum Mol Genet. 1999;8:743–9.
160. Puccio H, Koenig M. Friedreich ataxia: a paradigm for mitochondrial diseases. Curr Opin Genet Dev. 2002;12:272–7.
161. Puccio H, Simon D, Cossee M, et al. Mouse models for Friedreich ataxia exhibit cardiomyopathy, sensory nerve defect and Fe–S enzyme deficiency followed by intramitochondrial iron deposits. Nat Genet. 2001;27:181–6.
162. Camaschella C, Campanella A, De Falco L, et al. The human counterpart of zebrafish shiraz shows sideroblastic-like microcytic anemia and iron overload. Blood. 2007;110:1353–8.
163. Olsson A, Lind L, Thornell LE, Holmberg M. Myopathy with lactic acidosis is linked to chromosome 12q23.3–24.11 and caused by an intron mutation in the ISCU gene resulting in a splicing defect. Hum Mol Genet. 2008;17:1666–72.
164. Mochel F, Knight MA, Tong WH, et al. Splice mutation in the iron–sulfur cluster scaffold protein ISCU causes myopathy with exercise intolerance. Am J Hum Genet. 2008;82:652–60.
165. Hwang PM, Bunz F, Yu J, et al. Ferredoxin reductase affects p53-dependent, 5-fluorouracil-induced apoptosis in colorectal cancer cells. Nat Med. 2001;7:1111–7.
166. Gottlieb E, Tomlinson IP. Mitochondrial tumour suppressors: a genetic and biochemical update. Nat Rev Cancer. 2005;5:857–66.
167. Rudolf J, Makrantoni V, Ingledew WJ, Stark MJ, White MF. The DNA repair helicases XPD and FancJ have essential iron–sulfur domains. Mol Cell. 2006;23:801–8.
168. Andressoo JO, Hoeijmakers JH, Mitchell JR. Nucleotide excision repair disorders and the balance between cancer and aging. Cell Cycle. 2006;5:2886–8.
169. Lukianova OA, David SS. A role for iron–sulfur clusters in DNA repair. Curr Opin Chem Biol. 2005;9:145–51.

Chapter 3
Regulation of Iron Metabolism in Mammalian Cells

Tracey A. Rouault

Keywords Ferritin • Ferroportin • IRE • IRP1 • IRP2 • Posttranscriptional regulation • TfR

1 Introduction

Iron is an essential nutrient for all mammalian cells, and numerous proteins are dedicated to the uptake and distribution of iron within cells. As discussed in previous chapters, there are proteins that facilitate iron uptake, including transferrin receptors 1 and 2 (TfR1 and TfR2) [1] and DMT1 [2], proteins dedicated to iron storage, including ferritin H and L chains [3, 4], and an iron exporter, ferroportin [5, 6]. Most cellular proteins are synthesized in the cytosol and those that require an iron cofactor generally acquire their iron from the cytosolic iron pool. The nature of the cytosolic iron pool remains uncharacterized, as the iron is not associated with a specific known iron carrier molecule. The iron in this accessible iron pool may be bound with low affinity to abundant negatively charged molecules, including citrate and ATP. Because the cytosol of cells is a reducing environment, most cellular iron is likely in the ferrous (Fe^{2+}) rather than in the ferric (Fe^{3+}) state. Iron that enters the endosome in the transferrin cycle is initially in the ferric state, but an endosomal reductase, Steap3 [7], reduces it to ferrous iron, the form that is transported into cytosol by DMT1. When iron is taken up by ferritin, it is oxidized by ferroxidase activity of the ferritin H chain [3, 4], which facilitates precipitation and storage of iron in the ferritin heteropolymer.

To ensure that iron supplies are sufficient to support synthesis of new proteins and growth, cells coordinate iron uptake, storage, and export activities by regulating expression levels of the proteins responsible for these activities. Iron regulatory proteins 1 and 2 (IRP1 and IRP2) are homologous proteins that sense cytosolic iron levels and regulate expression of TfR1, one isoform of DMT1, ferritin H and L chains, ferroportin and several other iron metabolism proteins (reviewed in 8–10). In cells that are iron starved, IRP1 and IRP2 bind to conserved stem-loop structures found in the mRNAs that encode these proteins, which are known as iron-responsive elements (IREs). In the ferritin and ferroportin transcripts, the IREs are found in the 5′UTR near the cap-binding site where translation factors initially assemble. In TfR1 and DMT1, the IREs are found in the 3′UTR, a region of mRNA that is often important in determining the half-life of transcripts. The mechanism by which IRPs sense cytosolic iron levels and accordingly increase or decrease their capacity to bind to IREs is the major subject of this chapter.

T.A. Rouault, M.D. (✉)
Molecular Medicine Program, Eunice Kennedy Shriver National Institutes of Child Health and Human Development, Bethesda, MD 20892, USA
e-mail: rouault@mail.nih.gov

G.J. Anderson and G. McLaren (eds.), *Iron Physiology and Pathophysiology in Humans*, Nutrition and Health, DOI 10.1007/978-1-60327-485-2_3,

2 The IRE–IRP Regulatory System

The IRE–IRP regulatory system is based on the ability of cytosolic IRPs to affect the stability of a previously synthesized mRNA, or to alter the efficiency with which a given transcript is translated. Unlike many cellular regulatory systems, most of the regulatory activity in the IRE–IRP system occurs post-transcriptionally [8–10]. An important key to the system is that target transcripts have evolved to contain one or more IREs. An IRE consists of conserved sequence and structural features [11–13]. It contains an upper stem composed of five base-paired residues that assume a helical structure, which is generally separated from a lower base-paired stem by an unpaired "bulged" cytosine near the 5′ end. The bulged C divides the upper from the lower stem, functioning as a hinge that enables the upper and lower stems to flexibly alter their relative alignments. In some IREs, such as those found in ferritin, the lower stem contains a second characteristic bulged "U" residue, which may further facilitate bending of the lower stem relative to the upper stem. In addition, IREs contain a six-membered loop, which contains a base-pair between residues 1 and 5 that structures the loop, enabling the A, G, and U residues at positions 2, 3, and 4 to protrude out (Fig. 3.1). The "bulged" C and the "AGU" pseudotriloop of the loop are distinctive molecular features that are separated from one another by a fixed distance and angle. They constitute the two major recognition features for binding by iron regulatory proteins [13, 14]. The bulged C fits into a binding pocket of domain 4 of IRP1, and the AGU residues fit into a binding pocket that opens between domains 2 and 3 of apo-IRP1.

Mammalian cells contain two iron regulatory proteins, IRP1 and IRP2, which differ in the mechanism by which they sense cellular iron status. IRP1 is a bifunctional protein, which, like IRP2, is expressed in virtually all mammalian cells. In cells that are iron replete, IRP1 contains a cubane iron–sulfur cluster and is a functional aconitase enzyme that interconverts citrate and isocitrate in cytosol, similar to the reaction catalyzed by mitochondrial aconitase in the citric acid cycle. Two distinct but homologous genes encode the cytosolic and mitochondrial aconitase genes. As there is also a distinct cytosolic isocitrate dehydrogenase, active cytosolic aconitase likely contributes to

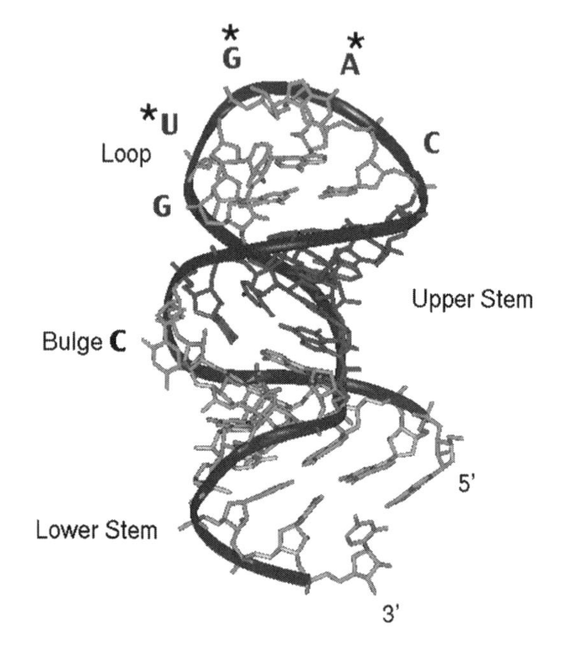

Fig. 3.1 The IRE is an RNA stem-loop structure. The upper and lower stems are composed of Watson–Crick base-pairs which are in a helical conformation. In the six-membered loop, the C at position 1 of the loop forms a base-pair with the G at position 5. The C–G base-pair structures the loop, allowing the A, G, and U residues (denoted by *asterisks*) to form a pseudotriloop of residues that can form multiple hydrogen bonds with protein(s). The upper and lower stems are separated by an unpaired "bulge" C that confers flexibility on the structure by interrupting the helix

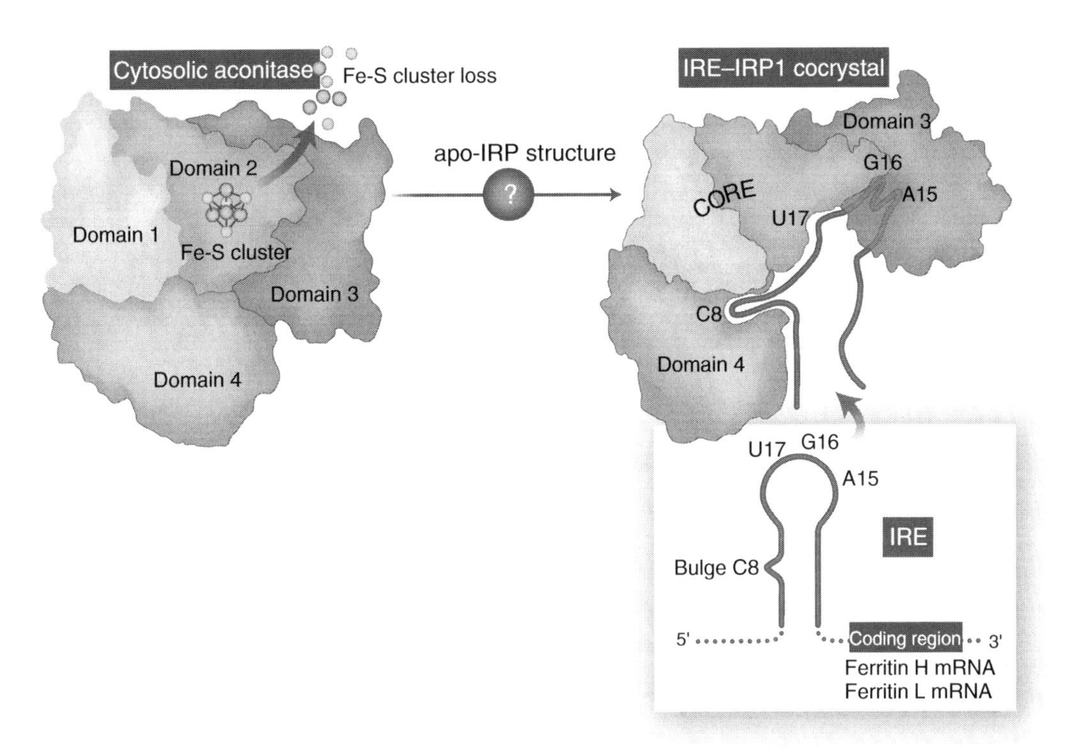

Fig. 3.2 IRP1 functions as a cytosolic aconitase or an IRE-binding protein. When IRP1 contains an iron–sulfur cluster, it functions as a cytosolic aconitase, whereas upon loss of the cluster, it undergoes a significant conformational change that enables it to bind IREs with high affinity. The bulged C of the IRE fits into a pocket in domain 4, whereas residues of the pseudotriloop reach into a pocket opened by movement of domain 3 relative to domain 2

extra-mitochondrial metabolism in several ways, particularly perhaps by facilitating NADPH synthesis by cytosolic isocitrate dehydrogenase [15]. The iron–sulfur cluster of cytosolic aconitase is crucial for aconitase activity, as it is one of the ligands for the substrates citrate and isocitrate, along with over 23 amino acid residues that line that enzymatic active site cleft [16, 17].

The status of the iron–sulfur cluster is also the key to transformation of IRP1 into an IRE-binding protein, as the IRE-binding form lacks the cluster. The mechanism by which IRP1 converts into the apo-form devoid of an iron–sulfur cluster may involve the fundamental chemical properties of exposed iron–sulfur clusters. Iron–sulfur clusters are notoriously sensitive to oxidation events, which can cause spontaneous disassembly of the cluster. In the aconitases, iron–sulfur clusters are unusually sensitive to oxidation because the cluster is exposed to solvent [18]. Although disassembly of iron–sulfur clusters may depend on random oxidation events, it is also thought that disassembly of the cluster is facilitated when IRP1 is phosphorylated at serine 138 [19, 20]. In contrast to cluster disassembly, numerous proteins dedicated to assembly of iron–sulfur clusters are expressed in mammalian cells and it is likely that the iron–sulfur cluster of cytosolic aconitase is reconstituted by reassembly after spontaneous degradation in cells, but only when cells contain sufficient iron to resynthesize the cluster [21–23].

Loss of the iron–sulfur cluster of IRP1 permits IRP1 to undergo a conformational change that transforms it into an IRE-binding protein. Solution of the structure of the IRE bound to IRP1 confirmed that major conformational changes were required for acquisition of IRE-binding activity [13, 14] (Fig. 3.2). The bulged C fits into a pocket within domain 4 of IRP1, which the RNA can access because domain 4 of apo-IRP1 (apo-IRP1 refers to IRP1 devoid of an iron–sulfur cluster) rotates on a hinge linker that connects it to domains 1–3. Opening of the active site cleft allows the residues that normally face into the aconitase active-site cleft to interact with large molecules that would otherwise be excluded from the narrow cleft. Another important change occurs between domains 2 and 3 in apo-IRP1, where conformational changes create a pocket that accommodates the unpaired AGU residues of the loop. Most of the important RNA–protein interactions occur between the bulged C and its binding pocket, and the AGU pseudotriloop and its pocket, and the multiple hydrogen bonds at both sites (about 12 per site) account for the very high-affinity binding (in the picomolar range) that has been observed [13]. Thus, IRP1 functions as an aconitase when it contains an intact iron–sulfur cluster, whereas it functions as an IRE-binding protein when it lacks an iron–sulfur cluster.

IRP2 is a second IRE-binding protein that is highly homologous to IRP1 and binds with high affinity to IREs [24, 25]. However, unlike IRP1, IRP2 does not appear to have another function or to bind an iron–sulfur cluster. In addition, IRP2 is very difficult to find in iron-replete cells, because it undergoes iron-dependent degradation in vivo [26, 27]. Complicating matters further, IRP2 is subject to rapid degradation in lysates that contain iron and are exposed to oxygen, and analysis of IRP2 levels and binding activity can be misleadingly low unless assays are performed in lysates that contain a strong iron chelator such as desferrioxamine, or in lysates that are made and tested under anaerobic conditions [28]. The initial step of iron-dependent degradation of IRP2 in cells likely involves some type of iron-dependent oxidation, but its exact nature is not known [29]. Although there is agreement that the degradation pathway of IRP2 involves ubiquitination and proteasomal degradation, the initial identification of the ubiquitin ligase [30] has been disputed [31]. IRP2 contains a 73 amino acid insertion relative to IRP1 that was initially thought to be important for degradation [26], but it appears that features outside of this cysteine- and proline-rich domain are more important for iron-dependent degradation [32, 33]. Thus, much remains to be discovered about the intracellular iron-dependent degradation pathway of IRP2. Nevertheless, IRP2 levels and binding activity appear to accurately reflect cytosolic iron status, and since the intracellular iron pool that is sensed by IRP2 cannot be directly measured, IRP2 levels often are used to indirectly assess intracellular iron levels.

Thus, in iron-replete cells, IRE-binding activities of both IRP1 and IRP2 are reduced, either because insertion of an iron–sulfur cluster promotes a conformational change, or an iron-dependent modification promotes degradation by the ubiquitin–proteasome system. In each case, IRE-binding activity correlates with levels of iron in the cytosolic pool of iron. Both IRP1 and IRP2 bind to most IREs with similar affinity and they therefore each have the potential to provide backup to a system that relies on their combined binding activity. In iron-starved cells, IRP binding represses translation of mRNAs that contain IREs near the 5′ end of the transcript, including ferritin and ferroportin [34], whereas it stabilizes the transcript of TfR1 and thereby increases expression of TfR1 protein. These changes are appropriate for intracellular iron homeostasis, as expression of ferritin should be diminished in cells that are iron starved, whereas expression of TfR1 should be increased to bring more iron into the cell (Fig. 3.3).

Many questions have been raised about the specificity of binding of each IRP for different IRE targets [12, 35], with the hypothesis advanced that IRP2 binds well to ferritin-type IREs that contain a complex bulge in the lower stem, but not to simple IREs in which helical base-pairs in the upper and lower stems are separated only by the bulged C. A major difference between IREs of ferritin and other IREs is that ferritin IREs have an unpaired U in a position two residues 5′ of the bulged C. Since nucleotides that are exposed and are not engaged in base-pairing mediate most contacts with RNA binding proteins, the unpaired U has the potential to be important in specificity [13]. IRP1 and IRP2 were equally efficacious in translationally repressing ferritin expression in one study [36], suggesting that both IRPs contribute to translational regulation of ferritin. Questions about specificity cannot be definitively resolved using in vitro studies, but target specificities can be assessed in animals engineered to lack either IRP1 or IRP2. These studies revealed that IRP2 has a major role in regulation not only of ferritin IREs, but also of other transcripts that contain simple IREs such as the TfR1 transcript [37] and the eALAS transcript [38], as is discussed below.

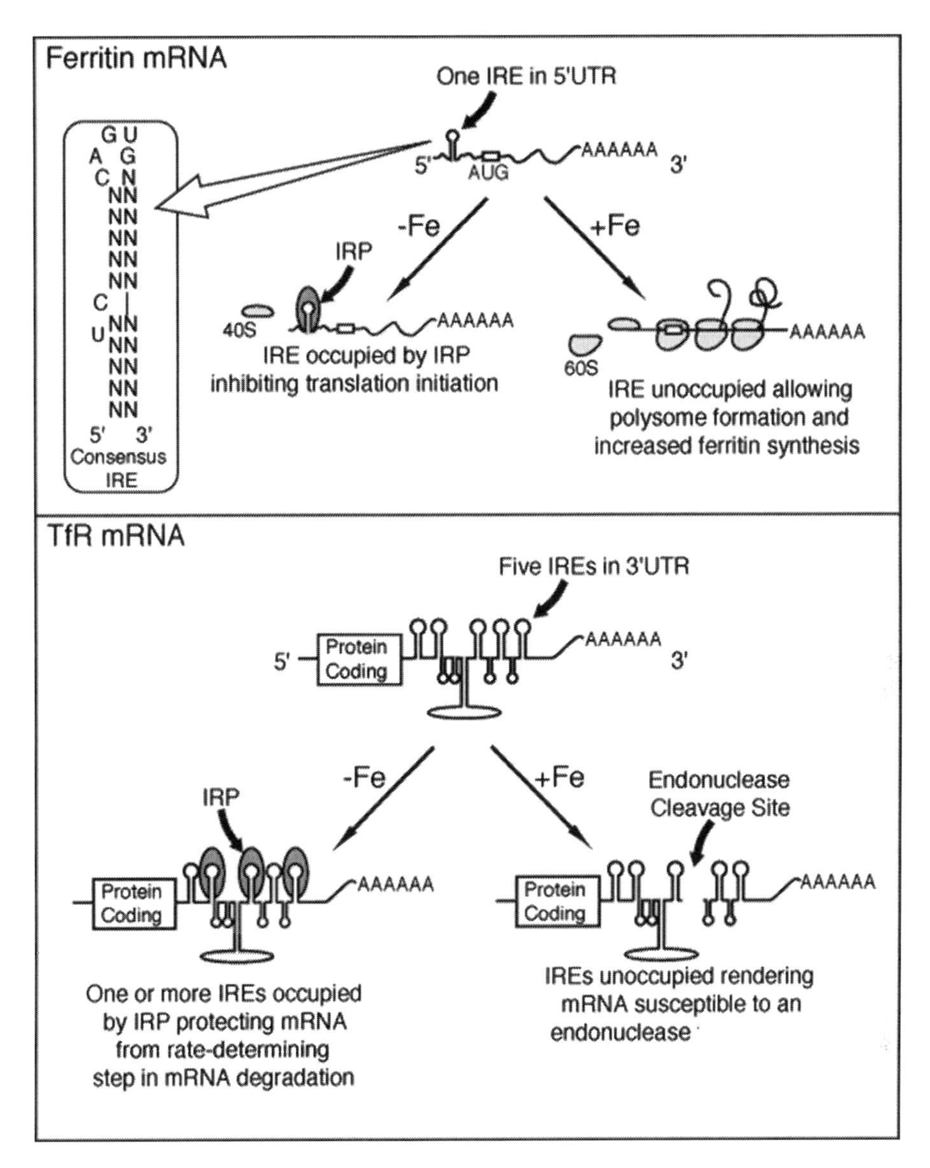

Fig. 3.3 IRP binding to IREs results in repression of translation of ferritin and stabilization of the TfR1 mRNA. In iron-depleted cells, IRPs bind to the ferritin IRE at the 5′ end of the transcript and interfere with assembly of translation initiation factors. Ferritin IREs typically have a bulged C, and an unpaired U, as depicted. In the TfR1 mRNA, there are five IREs, each of which can bind an IRP. Binding of IRPs protects the transcript from being cleaved by an endonuclease. Upon cleavage, the mRNA cleavage products are rapidly degraded

3 The Role of IRPs in Physiology

Based on experiments performed in cell lines, it was not clear what role each IRP played in physiology and it seemed likely that each IRP would have the ability to function as a backup for the other. However, targeted deletion of the IRP1 or IRP2 genes yielded very different phenotypes in mice. Somewhat unexpectedly, the IRP1 "knockout" mouse appeared to have fairly normal iron status in most tissues [28]. In contrast, the IRP2 "knockout" mouse ($Irp2^{-/-}$) developed a mild microcytic anemia [38, 39] and progressive adult-onset neurodegeneration characterized by an abnormal gait and tremor [37]. The symptoms and neuropathologic changes in $Irp2^{-/-}$ animals are subtle and progressive. One group suggested that their mice did not develop "symptomatic" neurodegeneration, although they reported a significant compromise in motor abilities of their mouse based on testing with a rotarod, which indicated that their mice were not neurologically normal [40]. In the erythroid cells and brain tissue of $Irp2^{-/-}$ mice, ferritin levels are high, whereas Tfr1 levels are low, consistent with the results expected if there is a marked decrease in IRE-binding activity. Since Irp1 is present in the affected tissues in mice, it was interesting to observe that Irp1 is mainly in the cytosolic aconitase form in mammalian tissues, and it does not readily convert to the IRE-binding form in the tissues of iron-starved mice, even in the absence of Irp2 [28].

Since activation of the IRE-binding activity of IRP1 was repeatedly observed in cell lines that were treated with iron chelators or otherwise deprived of iron, it was initially difficult to reconcile the results of multiple tissue culture experiments with the phenotypes of $Irp^{-/-}$ animals. However, culture of cells under different oxygen concentrations yielded an important insight into IRP activities. Because oxygen must be transported over significant distances to various tissues by heme in red cells, mammalian tissues are exposed to oxygen concentrations far below those in the atmosphere. At oxygen concentrations similar to those of mammalian tissues (oxygen concentrations of 3–6% compared to atmospheric concentrations of 21%), it is difficult to induce IRE-binding activity of IRP1, even by starving cells of iron. It is likely that the inability to activate IRE-binding activity of IRP1 is related to the fact that the iron–sulfur cluster is more stable at lower oxygen concentrations. Conversely, levels of IRP2 increase significantly in cells that are maintained at low oxygen concentrations, perhaps because the degradation pathway of IRP2 appears to be initiated by an oxidation event. The contrary effects of low oxygen on the IRE-binding activities of IRP1 compared to IRP2 can explain much about the phenotypes of $Irp^{-/-}$ mice [41]. At normal tissue oxygen concentrations (3–6% O_2), IRP1 mainly functions as an aconitase, contributing less than half of total IRE-binding activity in most tissues, whereas IRE-binding activity of IRP2 increases concomitantly with an increase in protein levels at low tissue oxygen concentrations.

Although the differential effects of low tissue oxygen concentrations on IRE-binding activities of the two IRPs explain much about the phenotypes of $Irp1^{-/-}$ and $Irp2^{-/-}$ animals, there is yet another feature that is crucial in developing iron misregulation and the phenotypes of these mice. In $Irp1^{-/-}$ animals, Irp2 levels increase such that total IRE-binding activity levels almost equal the IRE-binding activities contributed by both Irp1 and Irp2 in wild-type animals [41]. Increased Irp2 levels compensate for the loss of Irp1 and its IRE-binding activity. It is not clear how Irp2 levels increase, but it is possible that loss of Irp1 and its IRE-binding activity leads to a minor increase in ferritin synthesis and a concomitant decrease in Tfr1 levels, resulting in a subtle diminution of cytosolic iron pools. Since Irp2 levels appear to correlate directly with cytosolic iron levels, the increase in Irp2 levels may directly reflect and oppose this subtle iron depletion.

In animals that lack both Irp2 alleles and one functional Irp1 allele, the anemia and neurodegenerative symptoms previously observed in $Irp2^{-/-}$ are much more severe. In addition, ferritin levels are higher, and Tfr1 levels are lower than in $Irp2^{-/-}$ mice [42]. These results suggest that both IRP1 and IRP2 contribute to regulation of target transcripts, a conclusion supported by the fact that animals that are bred to lack both alleles of Irp1 and Irp2 die at the blastocyst stage of development, before embryos have developed sufficiently to implant in the uterus [43]. Thus, the IRE–IRP system is indispensable in animals at the earliest stages of development. To analyze the effects of IRPs in specific tissues, animals were generated in which IRP activity could be eliminated in specific tissues. Animals engineered to lack IRP activity in the intestinal mucosa died within weeks of birth and levels of ferroportin in the intestinal mucosa were abnormally high, indicating that ferroportin is a true target of the IRP regulatory system [44].

The reason that neurons and red cells are compromised by loss of IRPs is likely because these cells are functionally iron starved. When ferritin is over-expressed, it competes with other proteins for iron, and sequesters iron that could otherwise be used for synthesis of proteins and prosthetic groups such as heme [45]. The fact that ferritin competes with other proteins for iron and effectively sequesters iron may be the central reason that ferritin translation is repressed by IRPs in iron-deficient cells. In the absence of IRE-binding activity, not only does ferritin expression increase, but iron uptake simultaneously decreases, which contributes further to iron depletion. Thus, cells that lack sufficient IRE-binding activity can misallocate iron reserves, allowing ferritin to sequester iron that should be available to meet basic metabolic needs, even though incoming iron supplies are also diminished.

4 The Evolution and Scope of the IRE–IRP System

The IRE–IRP regulatory system coordinates iron metabolism in a sophisticated and highly sensitive manner in mammalian cells, but the regulatory system does not appear to be well developed in lower animal forms or simple eukaryotes. There is no cytosolic aconitase in *Saccharomyces cerevisiae*, and although there is a cytosolic aconitase in *Caenorhabditis elegans*, there is no evidence that the *C. elegans* aconitase can function as an IRE-binding protein [46]. Ferritin IREs are present in metazoans, including sea anemones and sponges, but these organisms do not contain IREs in other transcripts [47]. In *Drosophila melanogaster*, there are two cytosolic aconitases, one of which binds IREs [48], and there is evidence that IRE-binding activity regulates synthesis of ferritin and succinate dehydrogenase in flies [49]. Thus, flies contain a rudimentary IRE–IRP system.

Since the IRE–IRP system is highly developed in mammalian cells, many of its characteristics must have evolved in mammals. As cytosolic aconitase activity, but not IRE-binding activity, is found in worms [46], it is likely that the IRE–IRP system developed by exploiting the potential instability of the iron–sulfur cluster of cytosolic aconitase. The cubane iron–sulfur cluster of cytosolic aconitase can be readily oxidized by superoxide, oxygen, nitric oxide, and other oxidants (reviewed in [8, 9]). When these oxidants remove an electron, the entire structure of the cluster is destabilized and it spontaneously disintegrates. Proteins dedicated to the synthesis of iron–sulfur clusters likely provide replacement clusters to cytosolic aconitase when the iron–sulfur clusters undergo oxidative degradation [22, 23]. However, if these iron–sulfur cluster assembly proteins obtain their iron from the cytosolic iron pool, and the pool has become depleted of iron in the time that elapsed since initial synthesis and cluster degradation, cells may be unable to synthesize a replacement iron–sulfur cluster. Failure to replace the iron–sulfur cluster of IRP1 would result in a buildup of apoprotein. In the absence of the iron–sulfur cluster, the apoprotein form of IRP1 may assume new conformations, because the cluster constrains the conformational space. It does this by binding to three cysteines of cytosolic aconitase as well as the substrates citrate and isocitrate. The substrates bind both to the cluster and to residues on the opposite side of the active-site cleft. Accumulation of apoprotein in cells would be expected to correlate with development of iron depletion. Thus, if this apoprotein could be recruited into a process that would reverse the iron depletion, it could offer cells a competitive advantage [50].

How might accumulation of the apoprotein form of cytosolic aconitase work to reverse cellular iron depletion? Since the apoprotein accumulates in the cytosol, it could either act upon transcripts in the cytosol, or it could be transported to the nucleus to function as a transcriptional repressor or activator. Transport into the nucleus would require developing a specialized nuclear transport signal, whereas acting upon cytosolic transcripts would require no extra modifications in the apoprotein form of cytosolic aconitase. In addition, the apoprotein would be in the correct location to resume its enzymatic activities if the iron–sulfur cluster was repaired or replaced. To transform the apoprotein into an important regulatory molecule, targets that would fit the conformation of the apoprotein likely had to evolve.

In eukaryotic mRNAs, the 5′ and 3′UTRs can evolve rapidly, as these portions of the mRNA are not constrained by the specific sequence requirements of protein-coding regions. If mutations in the 5′UTR produced an RNA stem-loop that could be bound tightly by the apo form of cytosolic aconitase, that RNA stem-loop might be retained in evolution. For example, ferritin H and L chains contain an IRE near the 5′ end of the transcript, and binding by apo-IRP1 inhibits translation by interfering with assembly of the translation machinery. Repression of ferritin synthesis produces a desirable result for cells because ferritin does not compete with other proteins to bind iron. Similarly, an IRE could have evolved near the 5′ end in ferroportin, since cells that are iron depleted need to hoard iron rather than allow their iron to be exported from the cell. As 3′UTRs tend to contain elements that determine the rate of mRNA decay, binding of apoprotein in the 3′UTR could interfere with degradation processes and could lengthen the mRNA half-life in transcripts such as TfR1. Increasing the levels of TfR1 mRNA results in increased TfR1 biosynthesis, which reverses cellular iron depletion by enhancing iron uptake.

As IREs in different transcripts differ from one another, particularly in the sequences that provide base-paired stems and structure, it is reasonable to suggest that each IRE arose as an independent evolutionary selection event. This scenario is compatible with the discovery of IREs in many different transcripts in many different species [47]. A functional IRE present in the mitochondrial aconitase transcript reduces synthesis of this iron–sulfur protein when cells have diminished iron stores [51–53]. IREs that likely affect mRNA half-life have been found in one transcript of DMT1 [54] and in the cell cycle protein Cdc14a [55]. In addition, a functional IRE is present in the 5′UTR of the hypoxia inducible factor 2 α (HIF2 α) transcript [56]. The discovery of an IRE in the HIF2 α transcript is important, because HIF1 and 2 α are important oxygen sensors that regulate transcription of numerous genes involved in the switch from normoxia to hypoxia, including glycolysis enzymes and the production of erythropoietin, the major growth factor that regulates erythropoiesis [57].

5 Diseases and the IRE–IRP System

Several diseases in humans and mice are caused by problems with the IRE–IRP regulatory system. Humans that have mutations in the ferritin L chain develop hereditary hyperferritinemia and bilateral cataract syndrome [58]. They have markedly elevated serum ferritin levels and cataracts, but they do not have other more serious symptoms. The reason for high serum ferritins is that these patients have mutations in the ferritin L chain IRE that reduce the ability of IRPs to bind and to repress translation. The severity of disease correlates with the reduction of IRE-binding ability [9].

Mice that lack Irp2 develop microcytic anemia, erythropoietic protoporphyria, and adult-onset neurodegeneration. These phenotypes arise as a result of increased ferritin, decreased TfR1 expression, and misregulation of other known IRP targets such as eALAS [38], ferroportin [44], and perhaps HIF2 α. The IRP2 gene is located on human chromosome 15q25, and thus far, no mutations of IRP2 have been described that cause human disease. However, it is fairly likely that mutations or deletions of IRP2 will prove to be a cause of human disease, as many diseases characterized by anemia and neurodegeneration are not yet well understood. The incentive to find such diseases is high, because studies in the mouse $Irp2^{-/-}$ mouse have demonstrated that the neurologic compromise of $Irp2^{-/-}$ animals can be prevented. When animals are treated with the stable nitroxide, Tempol, normal regulation of ferritin and Tfr1 is restored in the brain. Tempol can be supplied by supplementation of food, as Tempol is absorbed in the duodenum and crosses the blood-brain barrier. In cells, it causes disassembly of the iron–sulfur cluster of IRP1, which converts IRP1 into the IRE-binding form and counteracts the deficiency of IRE-binding activity caused by loss of IRP2 [59].

In cancer syndromes such as Von-Hippel Lindau (VHL) disease, many of the features of the renal cancer are thought to be attributable to high levels of HIF2 α, which is normally ubiquitinated by the VHL complex in normoxic cells [60]. HIF2 α is a transcription factor that increases expression of glycolysis enzymes, erythropoietin, VEGF, and numerous other genes. In normoxic cells, an iron-dependent prolyl hydroxylase modifies HIF residues, which then enables the VHL ubiquitination complex to bind to HIF and mark it for degradation. The fact that HIF2 α has an IRE in the 5 UTR [56] links its expression to the IRE–IRP system and indicates that reagents such as Tempol might be useful in treatment of VHL renal cancer.

6 Transcriptional Regulation of Iron Metabolism Genes

Although posttranscriptional regulation of TfR1, ferritin, and other IRP targets is very important in intracellular iron homeostasis, transcription of these genes is also regulated. In TfR1, several HIF-binding sites are important in transcription [61, 62], with transcription of TfR1 increasing in cells that over-express HIF1α [63]. More recently, it has been reported that HIF2α is required to transcriptionally activate DMT1 and Dcytb in response to iron deficiency [64]. Thus, HIF1 and 2α increase transcription of targets such as TfR1, DMT1, and Dcytb. Interestingly, HIFα inhibits transcription of hepcidin [65].

In addition to the emerging role of HIF α transcription factors, other transcription factors important in iron metabolism include Stat 5, Nrf2, and SMAD4. Both TfR1 and IRP2 are transcriptional targets of the signal transducer and activator of transcription, Stat5, in erythroid cells, which enables signaling through the erythropoietin receptor to increase expression of both TfR1 and IRP2 [66]. Increased transcription of both ferritin H and L chains is mediated by the transcription factor Nrf2 in response to oxidants and prooxidant xenobiotics [67, 68], which helps cells to avert some of the damage associated with oxidative stress by sequestering iron and reducing its participation in Fenton chemistry. Much remains to be learned about transcriptional regulation of genes that are important in iron metabolism. For instance, transcriptional regulation of ferroportin is clearly important, particularly in the intestinal mucosa [69], but this is poorly understood. Studies of the hepcidin promoter demonstrate important roles for Stat 3 [70, 71], for SMAD4 [72] and for HIFα [65].

7 Posttranscriptional Modifications of IRPs

Both IRP1 and IRP2 have been observed to undergo phosphorylation and the phosphorylation status potentially affects function. In IRP1, phosphorylation at serine 138 destabilizes the iron–sulfur cluster and facilitates conversion to the IRE-binding form [19, 20]. Phosphorylation of IRP1 at serine 711 inhibits the conversion of citrate to isocitrate [19]. IRP2 also undergoes phosphorylation in cells treated with phorbol esters [73]. This phosphorylation occurs at serine 157 and is coordinated with cell cycle progression, with phosphorylation mediated by Cdk1/cyclin B and dephosphorylation mediated by Cdc14a. The phosphorylation reduces the IRE-binding activity of IRP2 during mitosis, which increases ferritin synthesis and reduces TfR1 synthesis, perhaps to diminish free iron and iron-dependent oxidation events during a time when the DNA of the cell is exposed and vulnerable to damage [74].

8 Summary

The IRE–IRP regulatory system is found in rudimentary form in flies, but its breadth and importance in regulation of cytosolic iron status is most extensive in mammalian cells. The regulatory system is based mainly on the ability of IRP1 and IRP2 to change their ability to bind to IREs in various transcripts, depending on cellular iron status. Binding to an IRE in the 5′UTR of transcripts generally represses translation, whereas binding to IREs in the 3′UTR likely generally increases mRNA stability. Functional IREs are found in numerous transcripts of iron metabolism genes and it is likely that the list of IRE-containing target transcripts will continue to grow as new genes are found and 5′ and 3′UTRs are carefully sequenced and analyzed.

References

1. Aisen P. Transferrin receptor 1. Int J Biochem Cell Biol. 2004;36:2137–43.
2. Mims MP, Prchal JT. Divalent metal transporter 1. Hematology. 2005;10:339–45.
3. Torti FM, Torti SV. Regulation of ferritin genes and protein. Blood. 2002;99:3505–16.
4. Theil EC, Matzapetakis M, Liu X. Ferritins: iron/oxygen biominerals in protein nanocages. J Biol Inorg Chem. 2006;11:803–10.
5. McKie AT, Barlow DJ. The SLC40 basolateral iron transporter family (IREG1/ferroportin/MTP1). Pflugers Arch. 2004;447:801–6.
6. Donovan A, Lima CA, Pinkus JL, et al. The iron exporter ferroportin/Slc40a1 is essential for iron homeostasis. Cell Metab. 2005;1:191–200.
7. Ohgami RS, Campagna DR, Greer EL, et al. Identification of a ferrireductase required for efficient transferrin-dependent iron uptake in erythroid cells. Nat Genet. 2005;37:1264–9.
8. Wallander ML, Leibold EA, Eisenstein RS. Molecular control of vertebrate iron homeostasis by iron regulatory proteins. Biochim Biophys Acta. 2006;1763:668–89.
9. Rouault TA. The role of iron regulatory proteins in mammalian iron homeostasis and disease. Nat Chem Biol. 2006;2:406–14.
10. Muckenthaler MU, Galy B, Hentze MW. Systemic iron homeostasis and the iron-responsive element/iron-regulatory protein (IRE/IRP) regulatory network. Annu Rev Nutr. 2008;28:197–213.
11. Addess KJ, Basilion JP, Klausner RD, Rouault TA, Pardi AJ. Structure and dynamics of the iron responsive element RNA: implications for binding of the RNA by iron regulatory proteins. J Mol Biol. 1997;274:72–83.
12. Ke Y, Wu J, Leibold EA, Walden WE, Theil EC. Loops and bulge/loops in iron-responsive element isoforms influence iron regulatory protein binding. Fine-tuning of mRNA regulation? J Biol Chem. 1998;273:23637–40.
13. Volz K. The functional duality of iron regulatory protein 1. Curr Opin Struct Biol. 2008;18:106–11.
14. Walden WE, Selezneva AI, Dupuy J, et al. Structure of dual function iron regulatory protein 1 complexed with ferritin IRE-RNA. Science. 2006;314:1903–8.
15. Tong WH, Rouault TA. Metabolic regulation of citrate and iron by aconitases: role of iron-sulfur cluster biogenesis. Biometals. 2007;20:549–64.
16. Beinert H, Kennedy MC, Stout DC. Aconitase as iron–sulfur protein, enzyme, and iron-regulatory protein. Chem Rev. 1996;96:2335–73.
17. Dupuy J, Volbeda A, Carpentier P, Darnault C, Moulis JM, Fontecilla-Camps JC. Crystal structure of human iron regulatory protein 1 as cytosolic aconitase. Structure. 2006;14:129–39.
18. Rouault TA, Klausner RD. Iron–sulfur clusters as biosensors of oxidants and iron. Trends Biochem Sci. 1996;21:174–7.
19. Brown NM, Anderson SA, Steffen DW, et al. Novel role of phosphorylation in Fe–S cluster stability revealed by phosphomimetic mutations at Ser-138 of iron regulatory protein 1. Proc Natl Acad Sci USA. 1998;95:15235–40.
20. Clarke SL, Vasanthakumar A, Anderson SA, et al. Iron-responsive degradation of iron-regulatory protein 1 does not require the Fe–S cluster. EMBO J. 2006;25:544–53.
21. Rouault TA, Tong WH. Opinion: iron–sulphur cluster biogenesis and mitochondrial iron homeostasis. Nat Rev Mol Cell Biol. 2005;6:345–51.
22. Rouault TA, Tong WH. Iron–sulfur cluster biogenesis and human disease. Trends Genet. 2008;24:398–407.
23. Lill R, Muhlenhoff U. Maturation of iron–sulfur proteins in eukaryotes: mechanisms, connected processes, and diseases. Annu Rev Biochem. 2008;77:669–700.

24. Samaniego F, Chin J, Iwai K, Rouault TA, Klausner RD. Molecular characterization of a second iron responsive element binding protein, iron regulatory protein 2 (IRP2): structure, function and post-translational regulation. J Biol Chem. 1994;269:30904–10.
25. Guo B, Yu Y, Leibold EA. Iron regulates cytoplasmic levels of a novel iron-responsive element-binding protein without aconitase activity. J Biol Chem. 1994;269:24252–60.
26. Iwai K, Klausner RD, Rouault TA. Requirements for iron-regulated degradation of the RNA binding protein, iron regulatory protein 2. EMBO J. 1995;14:5350–7.
27. Guo B, Phillips JD, Yu Y, Leibold EA. Iron regulates the intracellular degradation of iron regulatory protein 2 by the proteasome. J Biol Chem. 1995;270:21645–51.
28. Meyron-Holtz EG, Ghosh MC, Iwai K, et al. Genetic ablations of iron regulatory proteins 1 and 2 reveal why iron regulatory protein 2 dominates iron homeostasis. EMBO J. 2004;23:386–95.
29. Iwai K, Drake SK, Wehr NB, et al. Iron-dependent oxidation, ubiquitination, and degradation of iron regulatory protein 2: implications for degradation of oxidized proteins. Proc Natl Acad Sci USA. 1998;95:4924–8.
30. Yamanaka K, Ishikawa H, Megumi Y, et al. Identification of the ubiquitin-protein ligase that recognizes oxidized IRP2. Nat Cell Biol. 2003;5:336–40.
31. Zumbrennen KB, Hanson ES, Leibold EA. HOIL-1 is not required for iron-mediated IRP2 degradation in HEK293 cells. Biochim Biophys Acta. 2008;1783:246–52.
32. Wang J, Chen G, Muckenthaler M, Galy B, Hentze MW, Pantopoulos K. Iron-mediated degradation of IRP2, an unexpected pathway involving a 2-oxoglutarate-dependent oxygenase activity. Mol Cell Biol. 2004;24:954–65.
33. Hanson ES, Rawlins ML, Leibold EA. Oxygen and iron regulation of iron regulatory protein 2. J Biol Chem. 2003;278:40337–42.
34. Liu XB, Hill P, Haile DJ. Role of the ferroportin iron-responsive element in iron and nitric oxide dependent gene regulation. Blood Cells Mol Dis. 2002;29:315–26.
35. Ke Y, Sierzputowska-Gracz H, Gdaniec Z, Theil EC. Internal loop/bulge and hairpin loop of the iron-responsive element of ferritin mRNA contribute to maximal iron regulatory protein 2 binding and translational regulation in the iso-iron-responsive element/iso-iron regulatory protein family. Biochemistry. 2000;39:6235–42.
36. Kim HY, Klausner RD, Rouault TA. Translational repressor activity is equivalent and is quantitatively predicted by in vitro RNA binding for two iron-responsive element binding proteins, IRP1 and IRP2. J Biol Chem. 1995;270:4983–6.
37. LaVaute T, Smith S, Cooperman S, et al. Targeted deletion of iron regulatory protein 2 causes misregulation of iron metabolism and neurodegenerative disease in mice. Nat Genet. 2001;27:209–14.
38. Cooperman SS, Meyron-Holtz EG, Olivierre-Wilson H, Ghosh MC, McConnell JP, Rouault TA. Microcytic anemia, erythropoietic protoporphyria, and neurodegeneration in mice with targeted deletion of iron-regulatory protein 2. Blood. 2005;106:1084–91.
39. Galy B, Ferring D, Minana B, et al. Altered body iron distribution and microcytosis in mice deficient in iron regulatory protein 2 (IRP2). Blood. 2005;106:2580–9.
40. Galy B, Holter SM, Klopstock T, et al. Iron homeostasis in the brain: complete iron regulatory protein 2 deficiency without symptomatic neurodegeneration in the mouse. Nat Genet. 2006;38:967–9.
41. Meyron-Holtz EG, Ghosh MC, Rouault TA. Mammalian tissue oxygen levels modulate iron-regulatory protein activities in vivo. Science. 2004;306:2087–90.
42. Smith SR, Cooperman S, Lavaute T, et al. Severity of neurodegeneration correlates with compromise of iron metabolism in mice with iron regulatory protein deficiencies. Ann N Y Acad Sci. 2004;1012:65–83.
43. Smith SR, Ghosh MC, Ollivierre-Wilson H, Tong WH, Rouault TA. Complete loss of iron regulatory proteins 1 and 2 prevents viability of murine zygotes beyond the blastocyst stage of embryonic development. Blood Cells Mol Dis. 2006;36:283–7.
44. Galy B, Ferring-Appel D, Kaden S, Grone HJ, Hentze MW. Iron regulatory proteins are essential for intestinal function and control key iron absorption molecules in the duodenum. Cell Metab. 2008;7:79–85.
45. Cozzi A, Corsi B, Levi S, Santambrogio P, Albertini A, Arosio P. Overexpression of wild type and mutated human ferritin H-chain in HeLa cells: in vivo role of ferritin ferroxidase activity. J Biol Chem. 2000;275:25122–9.
46. Gourley BL, Parker SB, Jones BJ, Zumbrennen KB, Leibold EA. Cytosolic aconitase and ferritin are regulated by iron in *Caenorhabditis elegans*. J Biol Chem. 2003;278:3227–34.
47. Piccinelli P, Samuelsson T. Evolution of the iron-responsive element. RNA. 2007;13:952–66.
48. Lind MI, Missirlis F, Melefors O, et al. Of two cytosolic aconitases expressed in Drosophila, only one functions as an iron-regulatory protein. J Biol Chem. 2006;281:18707–14.
49. Kohler SA, Henderson BR, Kuhn LC. Succinate dehydrogenase b mRNA of *Drosophila melanogaster* has a functional iron-responsive element in its 5′-untranslated region. J Biol Chem. 1995;270:30781–6.
50. Rouault TA. Biochemistry. If the RNA fits, use it. Science. 2006;314:1886–7.
51. Kim HY, LaVaute T, Iwai K, Klausner RD, Rouault TA. Identification of a conserved and functional iron-responsive element in the 5′UTR of mammalian mitochondrial aconitase. J Biol Chem. 1996;271:24226–30.
52. Schalinske KL, Chen OS, Eisenstein RS. Iron differentially stimulates translation of mitochondrial aconitase and ferritin mRNAs in mammalian cells. Implications for iron regulatory proteins as regulators of mitochondrial citrate utilization. J Biol Chem. 1998;273:3740–6.

53. Gray NK, Pantopoulos K, Dandekar T, Ackrell BAC, Hentze MW. Translational regulation of mammalian and drosophila citric-acid cycle enzymes via iron-responsive elements. Proc Natl Acad Sci USA. 1996;93:4925–30.
54. Gunshin H, Allerson CR, Polycarpou-Schwarz M, et al. Iron-dependent regulation of the divalent metal ion transporter. FEBS Lett. 2001;509:309–16.
55. Sanchez M, Galy B, Dandekar T, et al. Iron regulation and the cell cycle: identification of an iron-responsive element in the 3′-untranslated region of human cell division cycle 14A mRNA by a refined microarray-based screening strategy. J Biol Chem. 2006;281:22865–74.
56. Sanchez M, Galy B, Muckenthaler MU, Hentze MW. Iron-regulatory proteins limit hypoxia-inducible factor-2alpha expression in iron deficiency. Nat Struct Mol Biol. 2007;14:420–6.
57. Lofstedt T, Fredlund E, Holmquist-Mengelbier L, et al. Hypoxia inducible factor-2alpha in cancer. Cell Cycle. 2007;6:919–26.
58. Hetet G, Devaux I, Soufir N, Grandchamp B, Beaumont C. Molecular analyses of patients with hyperferritinemia and normal serum iron values reveal both L ferritin IRE and 3 new ferroportin (slc11A3) mutations. Blood. 2003;102:1904–10.
59. Ghosh MC, Tong WH, Zhang D, et al. Tempol-mediated activation of latent iron regulatory protein activity prevents symptoms of neurodegenerative disease in IRP2 knockout mice. Proc Natl Acad Sci USA. 2008;105:12028–33.
60. Kaelin WGJ. The von Hippel-Lindau tumour suppressor protein: O2 sensing and cancer. Nat Rev Cancer. 2008;8:865–73.
61. Tacchini L, Bianchi L, Bernelli-Zazzera A, Cairo G. Transferrin receptor induction by hypoxia. HIF-1-mediated transcriptional activation and cell-specific post-transcriptional regulation. J Biol Chem. 1999;274:24142–6.
62. Lok CN, Ponka P. Identification of a hypoxia response element in the transferrin receptor gene. J Biol Chem. 1999;274:24147–52.
63. Alberghini A, Recalcati S, Tacchini L, Santambrogio P, Campanella A, Cairo G. Loss of the von Hippel Lindau tumor suppressor disrupts iron homeostasis in renal carcinoma cells. J Biol Chem. 2005;280:30120–8.
64. Shah YM, Matsubara T, Ito S, Yim SH, Gonzalez FJ. Intestinal hypoxia-inducible transcription factors are essential for iron absorption following iron deficiency. Cell Metab. 2009;9:152–64.
65. Peyssonnaux C, Zinkernagel AS, Schuepbach RA, et al. Regulation of iron homeostasis by the hypoxia-inducible transcription factors (HIFs). J Clin Invest. 2007;117:1926–32.
66. Kerenyi MA, Grebien F, Gehart H, et al. Stat5 regulates cellular iron uptake of erythroid cells via IRP-2 and TfR-1. Blood. 2008;112:3878–88.
67. Pietsch EC, Chan JY, Torti FM, Torti SV. Nrf2 mediates the induction of ferritin H in response to xenobiotics and cancer chemopreventive dithiolethiones. J Biol Chem. 2003;278:2361–9.
68. Tsuji Y, Ayaki H, Whitman SP, Morrow CS, Torti SV, Torti FM. Coordinate transcriptional and translational regulation of ferritin in response to oxidative stress. Mol Cell Biol. 2000;20:5818–27.
69. McKie AT, Marciani P, Rolfs A, et al. A novel duodenal iron-regulated transporter, IREG1, implicated in the basolateral transfer of iron to the circulation. Mol Cell. 2000;5:299–309.
70. Falzacappa MVV, Spasic MV, Kessler R, Stolte J, Hentze MW, Muckenthaler MU. STAT3 mediates hepatic hepcidin expression and its inflammatory stimulation. Blood. 2007;109:353–8.
71. Wrighting DM, Andrews NC. Interleukin-6 induces hepcidin expression through STAT3. Blood. 2006;108:3204–9.
72. Wang RH, Li C, Xu X, et al. A role of SMAD4 in iron metabolism through the positive regulation of hepcidin expression. Cell Metab. 2005;2:399–409.
73. Kl S, Rs E. Phosphorylation and activation of both iron regulatory proteins 1 and 2 in HL60 cells. J Biol Chem. 1996;271:7168–76.
74. Wallander ML, Zumbrennen KB, Rodansky ES, Romney SJ, Leibold EA. Iron-independent phosphorylation of iron regulatory protein 2 regulates ferritin during the cell cycle. J Biol Chem. 2008;283:23589–98.

Chapter 4
Concentrating, Storing, and Detoxifying Iron: The Ferritins and Hemosiderin

Elizabeth C. Theil

Keywords Ferritin • Gated pores • Iron • Iron mineral • Oxygen • Protein nanocage

1 Introduction

Ferritins are important in both iron and oxygen metabolism, based on patterns of gene regulation and protein function. The DNA is regulated by oxidants and is coordinated with other antioxidant response genes [1]. The mRNA function regulated by iron and oxygen [2–4] with direct sensing of ferrous ion in the repressor (IRP) complex [5], is coordinated with iron trafficking and oxygen metabolism mRNAs [6]. Ferritin protein converts both cytoplasmic iron (Fe^{2+}) and oxygen (O_2), into catalytic product, and mineral precursors in ~2:1 ratio [7]. A mineral with 2,000 Fe has consumed almost 1,500 dioxygen molecules in mineral formation, decreasing, at least locally, both iron and oxygen in the cytoplasm. The antioxidant function of ferritin mineralization is even more extreme in bacterial Dps proteins where Fe^{2+} and H_2O_2 are used to form the ferric oxy mineral. The reaction is a defense mechanism pathogenic bacteria used to resist macrophage H_2O_2 released in the oxidative burst [8]. Heme as both an oxidant and iron source induces both transcription and translation of ferritin DNA and mRNA with synergistic effects on ferritin expression [9].

Ferritins are multifunctional protein nanocages with catalytic sites, mineralization sites, and gated exit pores (Fig. 4.1). Several of the properties are shared with other protein families such as the diiron/dioxygen catalysts and gated ion channels. The first step, and some of the intermediate steps, is now understood at the molecular level (Fig. 4.2) However, almost nothing is known about where protons and electrons, involved in mineral formation or dissolution, move into or out of the protein cage.

E.C. Theil, Ph.D. (✉)
Children's Hospital of Oakland Research Institute (CHORI), Oakland, CA 94609, USA

Nutritional Sciences & Toxicology, University of California, Berkeley, CA 94609, USA

Molecular & Structural Biochemistry, North Carolina State University, Raleigh, NC 27695, USA
e-mail: etheil@chori.org

G.J. Anderson and G. McLaren (eds.), *Iron Physiology and Pathophysiology in Humans*, Nutrition and Health, DOI 10.1007/978-1-60327-485-2_4,

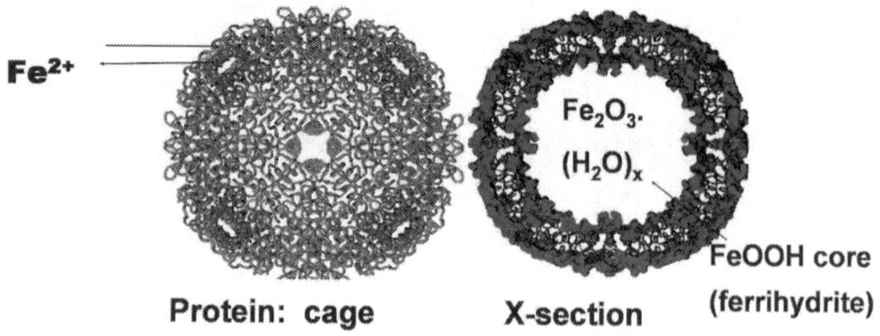

Fe2+
Fe2O3·(H2O)x
FeOOH core (ferrihydrite)
Protein: cage
X-section

Fig. 4.1 The ferritin protein cage. Sites of Fe entry, Fe exit, and the FeO mineral are indicated

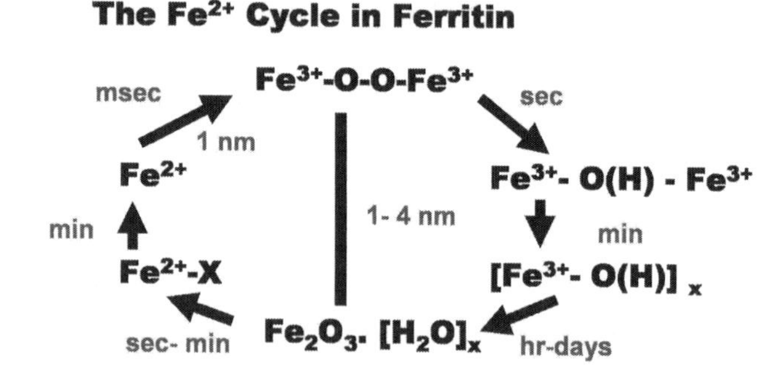

Fig. 4.2 The Fe^{2+} cycle in ferritin. The steps in the cycle of Fe^{2+} oxidation, mineralization, and reduction in ferritin are shown. All of the Fe steps are known from Mossbauer spectroscopy, but to date, only the diferric peroxo (DFP) has been fully characterized (Reviewed in [5])

2 Tissue Ferritins

2.1 *Ferritin Iron Concentration and the Detoxification of Iron and Oxygen*

Each tissue contains a specific member of the ferritin family, based on the differential expression of the two types of cytoplasmic genes in animals (H and L) and H in all other organisms form archaea to higher plants [7, 10]; nomenclature of the multiple H type subunits found in many organisms has not been standardized and they are named H, H′, M or H-1, H-2, etc. In catalytically active eukaryotic ferritins, a long, ferric post-oxidation channel has been discovered that facilitates reactions between catalytic products while still inside the protein cage, so that ferric iron emerging into the cavity is already a mineral nucleus. Iron mineralization of the different protein nanocages is accomplished by the synthesis of protein subunits, self-assembly of protein nanocages, and the reaction of Fe^{2+} with O_2 (or H_2O_2) either catalytically (ferritin H), or by mass action (ferritin L). Thus, two of the more abundant substrates for oxy radical formation, iron and oxygen, are detoxified in the same reaction. The solid mineral phase of ferritin is an iron concentrate by virtue of the fact that the water bound to Fe^{2+} ions in solution is released during linking (hydrolysis) of hydrated ferric ions during mineralization, a process similar to rust formation [the resulting bridges between the Fe^{3+} atoms are O or O(H)]. The ferritin catalytic substrates, iron and oxygen, explain why genetic regulation of ferritin expression is linked to both antioxidant and iron genes.

2.2 Structure: The Role of Subunits

The H type subunits of cytoplasmic ferritins, mitochondrial ferritins [11, 12], plastid ferritins (plants), and bacterial ferritins (± heme) are enzymatically (ferroxidase) active and named ferritin H subunits, while in humans and other animal ferritins, a second subunit type L is synthesized that is catalytically active. Animal ferritins are coassembled from H and L types subunits, in some cases, with three types of subunits H, H′(M) and L. The ratio of H:H′(M): L subunits is specific to each cell type and by prediction which is assumed to match rates of iron mineralization to specific cell metabolism. The terms H and L subunits in animals have had several definitions. First, when ferritin was studied in tissues with high ferritin abundance, H was defined as Heart, and L as Liver [13]. Later, when ferritin was studied in more animal tissues, and when biochemical methods improved, H was defined as higher and L as lower during denaturing gel electrophoresis or, based on mass, H as heavier and L as lighter. When cloning allowed sequence identification of the different electrophoretic species in ferritin, a very complex relationship was revealed between ferritin subunit mass and mobility during denaturing gel electrophoresis. In addition, the discovery of the ferroxidase (Fe/O_2 oxidoreductase) sites revealed another ferritin H and L subunit difference [7, 10]. Thus, subunit size, subunit mobility, and catalytic activity coincide with subunit mass in humans, with ferritin H the *h*eavier, the *h*ighest after denaturing gel electrophoresis, and with higher iron oxidation rates. However, the coincidence is not universal. For example, catalytically active and inactive subunits can have the same electrophoretic mobility in pig [14], or have reversed mobility in mouse [15], or have different mobilities and the same mass in frogs [16]. However, the sequence characteristics of ferritin H associated with the ferroxidase sites and high iron oxidation rate (catalysis) are constant and provide the most reliable definition of the ferritin *H* subunit. Ferritin *L*, then, is defined as low oxidation rate. The range of H:L subunits in human tissue ferritins varies from 10:1 (erythroid, heart) to 0.2:1 (in liver) and 0.12:1 in horse spleen [13, 17–21]. Physiological consequences of different H:L subunit ratios in different tissues remain obscure even with the multiple experimental approaches used, for example, genetic ablation, RNA inhibition, and solution studies of the isolated proteins. H and L subunit sequences may be a fertile area in systematic genomics exploration. There are many, many ferritin sequences known in vertebrates, for example, only some of which are known pseudogenes. Possibly among the rest that remain uncharacterized in humans, for example, is an intron-containing mitochondrial ferritin gene [11] and a cytoplasmic H′(M) gene that was obscured by different introns and exons.

2.3 Experimental Analyses of Ferritin H and L Function

Genetic alterations, experimental or spontaneous, indicate participation of both ferritin H and L genes in normal physiology. For example, ferritin H gene deletion is embryonic lethal in mice, but a mouse with ferritin L gene deletion has yet to be obtained. (Is the deletion lethal to embryonic stem cells?) In addition, mutations in ferritin H and ferritin L genes are associated with different abnormalities in the eye [22–24] and central nervous system [3, 25, 26]. In one case of a ferritin L mutation, the protein was associated with abnormal iron flux and consequent oxidative damage [27]. Further, RNA inhibition in cultured mammalian cells indicates that ferritin H enhanced resistance to oxidative stress and modified iron pools, while ferritin L influenced cell division rates [28]. Finally, recent observations indicate that ferritin can interact with microtubules [29], suggesting that one ramification of changing the H:L subunit ratio in ferritin could be integration with cell-specific features of the cytoskeleton.

Why animals have a gene encoding a catalytically inactive ferritin L subunit, in contrast to multiple, catalytically active ferritin H subunits in plant tissues and in bacteria, remains a puzzle after decades of study at the genetic, cellular, and biochemical levels. Without such information, sorting out the physiological significance of cell-specific variations in ferritin H and ferritin L expression [13, 17–21] is a formidable task. Until then, the impact of disease on ferritin H and L expression, for example, chronic exposure to excess iron [30–32] will be difficult to explain.

2.4 *Fe Uptake and Fe/O Catalysis*

Iron is concentrated in the cavity of ferritin protein nanocages by translocating ferric oxo-bridged dimers from the active sites in the middle of protein subunits to the cavity (Figs. 4.1 and 4.2), or, in L ferritins, by diffusion of Fe^{2+} into the cavity [33] where the other substrate, dioxygen, is dissolved in the buffer. After the 2 Fe^{+2}/O_2 reaction, hydrated ferric ions can bind to glutamate carboxylate side chains and react with other ferric ions to form Fe^{3+}-O-Fe^{3+} bridges by releasing H_2O and after many such reactions, building hydrated ferric oxide minerals. Mineralization in L ferritins occurs without hydrogen peroxide release [34, 35].

$Fe^{3+}O$ complexes reach the large, central, ferritin cavity, after catalytic reactions of Fe^{2+} with dioxygen at active sties of ferritin H subunits; in the mini-ferritins (Dps proteins), the oxidant is usually, but not always, hydrogen peroxide. The catalytic reaction products in eukaryotic ferritins, Fe^{3+}–O–Fe^{3+} dimers (ferritin H) react with the products of subsequent catalytic reactions, while still inside post-oxidation, nucleation channels 20 Å long; the channels connect the active sites to the cavity [36]. Phosphate, in the buffer or cell environment, is also incorporated into the mineral in rough proportion to the ambient concentration to build up the solid phase (mineral concentrate) [10, 37, 38].

The buildup of large ferritin minerals in the cavity of eukaryotic ferritins, using the mineral nuclei, is an obscure process as it is for calcium and phosphate in bone and tooth. In the ferritin biomineral, both protons and water are released as the iron mineral "hardens" similarly to "rust" or ferrihydrite. So many protons are released during ferritin mineral synthesis that unless buffer capacities are adjusted, proton release is sufficient to acidify the solution (<pH 4) and precipitate the protein. How the local acidity associated with ferritin mineralization is buffered in vivo is unknown. Since iron and oxygen are both consumed in making the mineral, ferritin is literally an antioxidant that minimizes oxidative stress and detoxifies both iron and oxidant (O_2) by the synthesis of the solid, oxy mineral; reactions at the mineral surface are blocked by the protein cage. The mineralization process is different in heme-containing bacterioferritins [39], as well as in bacterial mini-ferritins (half the number of subunits) [7, 8], also called Dps proteins. While mini-ferritins have a similar function of trapping iron and oxidants in the mineral, the different active sites are between subunits, rather than buried inside, and the substrates are often H_2O_2 and Fe^{2}+ [40]; some mini-ferritins such as those in *B. anthracis* use dioxygen with Fe^{2+} in the catalytic reactions [41]. The entry and exit pores in mini-ferritins are similar to those in eukaryotic ferritins [42].

The use of recombinant, protein nanocages composed entirely of one or the other subunit has provided some clues about H and L ferritin function. The enzymatic activity of ferritin H type subunits, for example, couples $2Fe^{2+}$ with O_2 (or H_2O_2 in mini-ferritins) to produce mineral precursors in the protein cage, Fe^{3+}–O(H)–Fe^{3+}. The reaction is very fast (ms) and rapidly removes ferrous ions and oxygen from the cytosol ($2Fe^{2+}:O_2$) (Fig. 4.2) or, in the case of bacterial mini-ferritins, ferrous ions and hydrogen peroxide from the cytoplasm and the vicinity of bacterial DNA [36]. In eukaryotic ferritins, catalysis and the ferritin active sites are related to diiron cofactor oxygenases involved in fatty acid desaturation (Δ9 desaturase), DNA synthesis (ribonucleotide reductase), and conversion of methane to methanol (methane monooxygenase), except that in ferritin, both iron and oxygen are

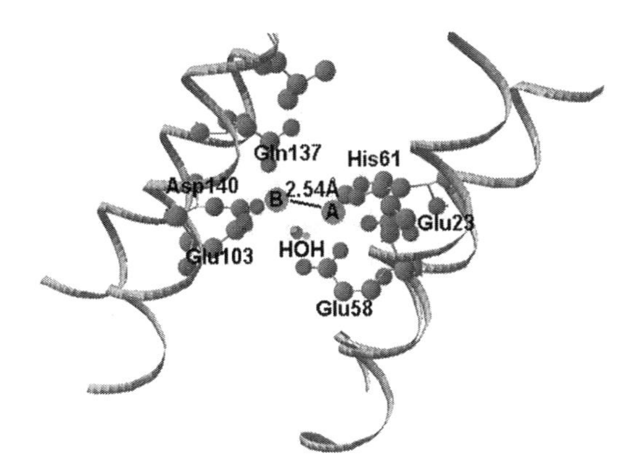

Fig. 4.3 The catalytic ferroxidase site in ferritin. Active-site metal-binding ligands, suggested by co-crystals of ferritin H subunits with Zn and with Mg, were inserted in a L ferritin cDNA, one at a time. Each mutant was expressed in *E. coli* and the protein tested to determine the residues required for Fe^{2+} oxidation with dioxygen and formation of the diferric peroxo catalytic intermediate (The figure is from [38] with permission)

substrates and the iron is released from the catalytic site (Fig. 4.3) as diferric oxo products, while in the others, iron is a cofactor and facilitates the reaction between the oxygen substrate and an organic substrate [7]. Ferritin catalysis and diiron oxygenase catalysis share a diferric peroxo intermediate. A downside of the rapid production of Fe^{3+}–O(H)–Fe^{3+} in the catalytic coupling reaction of H-type ferritin subunit catalysis is the hydrogen peroxide when the diferric peroxo intermediate decays [43]. As the iron content of ferritin increases, H_2O_2 production decreases although catalytic coupling continues [44–46].

Ferritin L cages, by contrast with ferritin H cages, are very slow to take up Fe. The diferric peroxo intermediate is absent, but can be observed in L ferritin chimeric proteins with H type active site ligands [47] (Fig. 4.3). Not only are active-site ligands absent in L ferritins, but there are different conformations of key side chains in ferritin L protein crystals [48–50]. While the overall similarity of the protein structure of ferritin L and ferritin H type subunits explains how they can coassemble [27, 51], the mechanistic advantage of cell-specific variations in ferritin H:L subunits is not clear. One possibility could relate to the cell-specific capacity for hydrogen peroxide degradation (cell-specific expression of peroxiredoxins, catalase, peroxidases) or signaling [52, 53].

Another possibility is the crystallinity of the mineral, as previously observed in vivo by comparing high L ferritin from liver, which is much more disordered than high H-type subunits ferritin from heart [54]. The absence of H-type catalytic sites and ferric post-oxidation channels in L ferritin subunits would eliminate the controlled mineral nucleation observed in H-type ferritins [36]. Rates of Fe oxidation in all H-type or all L-type ferritins differ by more than 1,000-fold [47]. The multiple intermediates in ferritins with H subunits are separated in both time and space (Fig. 4.2). While the initial coupling is vanishingly fast (ms), with the diferric peroxo intermediate decaying within seconds into the diferric oxo-bridged mineral precursor, the decay rate is variable depending on the environment [55]. Release of the ferroxidase product and pre-mineralization requires minutes, but mature formation of mineral can take hours to complete.

The difference between the active (ferroxidase) sites in ferritin and the diiron oxygenases involves two amino acids that differ by only one nucleotide in the DNA codons. The small number of mutations required to interconvert the ferritin H active sites and the diiron oxygenase sites suggest a simple evolutionary connection between the two families of active sites. Ferritin nanocages of L subunits contain all the metal sites of H subunits (pores and mineral nucleation sites) except the catalytic sites. Fe^{2+} in ferritin cages with L subunits enters the protein cage rapidly (minutes), but is oxidized over tens of minutes inside the cavity that is filled with oxygenated buffer. Possibly, the small amount of hydrogen peroxide produced in the early stages of Fe^{2+} oxidation at ferritin H subunit catalytic sites and known as an intracellular signal [52, 53], induces expression of iron uptake or iron chaperone proteins by indicating the availability of ferritin nanocages for iron/oxygen uptake.

2.5 *Ferritin Iron Uptake from Foods and Iron Deficiency Anemia*

Many seeds of nitrogen-fixing plants that take up extra iron in the nodule, such as soybeans contain large amounts of iron stored as ferritin [56], lentils, and garbanzo, also have large amounts of ferritin iron (EC Theil, unpublished observations). Often the ferritin is concentrated in the hull of the seed and is lost in many foods such as tofu and processed soy protein [57]. Soybean ferritin, as a model, binds to a specific receptor on polarized Caco-2 cells [58], and is internalized by clathrin-dependent [acid-sensitive, high sucrose-sensitive, or μ_2-(subunit of AP2)-sensitive] endocytosis. Ferritin receptors for animal ferritin occur in a variety of other cultured cell types such as kidney, erythroid, lipocytes, and brain [59–62], with binding constants comparable to soybean ferritin, in the nanomolar range. The iron transported into cells with soybean ferritin appears in the labile iron pool (LIP) [58]. Ferritin receptors in the intestine can play a role in absorption of iron from ferritin in legume seeds since ferritin is a stable protein. Evidence that ferritin survives digestion intact and is absorbed by mechanisms distinct from ferrous sulfate, ferric-chelate (nitrotriacetic acid), or heme has recently been obtained in rat intestine transport studies ex vivo, and in humans with ferrous sulfate or hemoglobin competitors, using fast (stomach) and slow (intestine) release capsules (EC Theil, MT Nunez, F Pizzarro, and K Schümann, in review). Such interactions can explain iron absorption values of >25% in rat [63] and humans fed soybeans or pure ferritin [64–66]. The efficiency of ferritin as a source of dietary iron is very high, contrasting with only one iron atom in heme or Fe^{2+} salts, since for each transport event ~1,000 iron atoms will cross the cell membrane inside the ferritin protein nanocage.

The physiological relevance of ferritin binding to the intestinal cell model is illustrated by the increase in the LIP. Immunoreactive, fluorescently or ^{131}I labeled, soybean ferritin was detectable inside the cells along with the increase in LIP iron [58]. In erythroid cells [59], the contribution of exogenous ferritin to the LIP was also observed. Ferritin uptake mechanisms distinct from iron in non-heme iron salts are illustrated by the phytate sensitivity of uptake from $FeSO_4$ and phytate resistance of iron uptake from ferritin observed in humans, even when unusually high phytate concentrations were present [64, 67]. Apparent inconsistencies in earlier data suggesting that iron is poorly absorbed from legume seeds or isolated ferritin appears related to low equilibration of iron label with preexisting iron mineral inside the ferritin protein cage, whether the label was exogenous or endogenous, and/or related to partial denaturation of ferritin, for example, [68–71]. The studies contrast with more recent studies based on increased knowledge of ferritin biochemistry, where the label was added under conditions representative of the mineralized iron in ferritin, as discussed in [63, 72–74]. Such results emphasize the complexity of non-heme iron absorption and the selective recognition by the intestinal cell surface among different iron species.

The rate of iron deficiency, the most common nutrient deficiency in the world, is rising again in industrialized countries, leading to inefficiency and work loss. In industrialized countries such as Japan, the current average rate of iron deficiency in women is 17%, with 22% for women under 50 years of age [75], and 10% in the US with values of 19–22% for Hispanic and African-American women [76]. New treatments for iron deficiency are needed since those developed over the last 500 years are failing. Iron nutrition is discussed in detail in Chap. 5. Ferritin iron, naturally in whole legume seeds or as engineered supplements, is clearly an underutilized approach to solving the iron deficiency problem.

3 Ferritin Gene Transcription and mRNA Translation

Ferritin synthesis is coordinated by DNA promoter sequences (MARE/ARE, maf responsive/antioxidant response elements) and mRNA promoter sequences (IRE, iron-responsive elements) [2–4, 29]. The MARE/ARE sequence is also present in the genes encoding β-globin, heme oxygenase1, thioredoxin reductase1, and NAD(P)H quinone oxido-reductase1, proteins involved in oxygen transport, repair of oxygen/oxidant damage, or heme degradation. The IRE is also present in mRNAs encoding transferrin receptor1, DMT1, and ferroportin, required for Fe trafficking/transport, as well as in mt-aconitase and erythroid aminolevulinate synthase, required in oxygen metabolism, and in both hypoxia-inducible factor-2α [77], and a cell-cycle phosphatase (Cdc 14a) [78]. Whether the sophistication of ferritin genetic regulation is a model for many proteins or reflects the pivotal role of ferritins in iron and oxygen metabolism remains to be seen.

The rate of ferritin biosynthesis depends on the amount of ferritin mRNA and the fraction of MARE/ARE-DNA and IRE-RNA bound to protein repressors. Since the concentrations of ferritin mRNA and both DNA and mRNA protein repressors will vary under different physiological conditions, the fraction of repressed RNA or the fraction of time the DNA is repressed will change as physiology changes. (The mRNA repressors, IRP1 and IRP2 are discussed in more detail in Chap. 3). Since DNA activity determines the rate of synthesis of ferritin H and L mRNAs, when mediated by the MARE/ARE/repressor interactions, ferritin mRNA is increased by antioxidant inducers such as t-butylperoxide, sulforophane, and heme with much greater sensitivity than by ferric ammonium citrate [1, 9, 79, 80]. Earlier studies in which chronic exposure to large, injected doses of ferric salts produced increased amounts of ferritin mRNA [16, 30, 31] may, in fact, have been the result of oxidative stress.

Bach1 has been identified as the ferritin H and L MARE/ARE repressor [1]. When heme binds to Bach1, Bach1 MARE/ARE:DNA interactions are prevented both in vivo and in vitro [1]. Bach1:MARE/ARE-DNA interactions link ferritin H and L gene regulation to that of the other phase II antioxidant response genes.

The cellular mechanism of ferritin DNA transcription induction depends on increased retention of Bach1 in the cytoplasm. Under such conditions, maf, which also interacts with the MARE/ARE sequence, binds the transcription enhancer NF-E2 or related factors, Nrf1, Nrf2, and Nrf3, to facilitate assembly of the transcription complex on MARE/ARE-DNAs [81, 82]. No structural information on Bach1:DNA complexes is available.

The cellular mechanism that induces ferritin translation depends on decreasing IRP/IRE RNA interactions. Recent studies show that ferrous iron itself weakens the IRE/IRP complex [5] allowing eIF-4G mediated assembly of the translation complex on IRE-mRNAs [83] and ribosome binding [84, 85]. The released IRP is targeted either to proteosomal degradation or iron–sulfur cluster insertion machinery, both of which minimize RNA binding. The stability of the IRE-RNA/IRP complex varies for mRNA with different IRE-RNA structures [5, 86–89]. The IRP-binding sites of each IRE-RNA (Fig. 4.4) are conserved, but the base pairs differ and combined with conserved unpaired bases can bend the RNA helix as much as 30° from the axis of a standard RNA β helix. Thus the binding specificity each IRE-mRNA reflects the base pairs in the RNA helices, which do not contact the IRP repressor. Interestingly, the differences in the IRE-RNA/IRP binding stability are analogous to the differences in the magnitude of the response to iron in vivo. When RNA and protein bind, complex structural changes occur in the IRP protein compared to the protein with a [4Fe–4S] cluster inserted (c-aconitase) or the apoprotein, based on CD, neutron scattering, and protein crystallography [90–93]. Excess Fe^{2+} enhances dissociation of the IRP from IRE-RNA, with the free IRP targeted proteosomes or to the FeS cluster insertion machinery. Evidence of Fe^{2+} binding to IRE-RNA, in the absence of evidence for Fe^{2+} binding to IRP [5], suggests that rather than a [4Fe–4S]/protein–"switch," the iron-dependent regulatory change is an Fe^{2+}-RNA "switch" that enhances IRE-RNA/IRP dissociation.

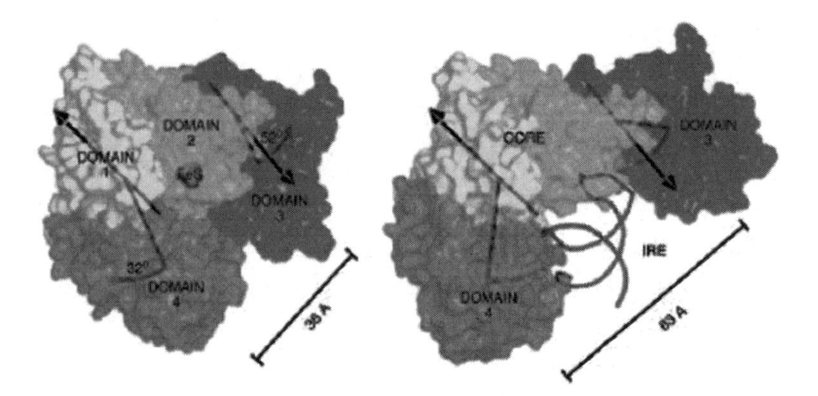

Fig. 4.4 Structure of a eukaryotic mRNA protein repressor, IRP1, complexed to the RNA regulator, IRE. Two independent sites on IRP1 bind two spatially separated, loop regions of the ferritin H-IRE RNA. The structural differences between the polypeptide bound to RNA (IRP1) or bound to an 4Fe–4S cluster (c-aconitase) are very large, indicating a huge reorganization during "switching" or, the alternative of distinct apoprotein folding pathways that depend on the relative concentrations of IRE-RNA and FeS chaperones/scaffold proteins during folding. Note the exposed RNA surface in the protein/RNA complex, which contain the sites of Fe^{2+} -binding [5] (The figure is from [82] with permission)

Coordination of gene transcription and translation by heme binding to both the DNA (Bach1) and mRNA (IRP) repressors [94, 95] is a ferritin-specific phenomenon, to date. The dual regulatory functions of heme have a synergistic effect on synthesis [9], when both the synthesis of ferritin mRNA and the translation of protein are increased. While heme can bind directly to Bach1 to regulate ferritin gene transcription, as well as binding to IRPs to regulate translation, the induction of transcription by t-butyl hydroquinone and sulforophane or induction of translation by ferric salts or H_2O_2 is less direct. One effect is the availability of Fe for FeS cluster biosynthesis, a series of complex regulated steps. Another is signal transduction of iron or other translational regulatory signals mediated by phosphorylation or dephosphorylation and/or protein turnover [2, 78, 96–98].

4 Hemosiderin

Hemosiderin is defined as non-heme, cytoplasmic iron that is insoluble [10, 99]. Hemosiderin iron can be used physiologically [100]. Since hemosiderin cannot be studied in solution, it remains difficult to study at the molecular level. A variety of studies converge on the conclusion that hemosiderin is derived from ferritin after autophagy [101–106] or translocation to lysosomes or other subcellular compartments such as mitochondria, and in plants, to plastids [12, 107].

Autophagy is used by cells to clean the cytoplasm during various types of stress by removing, relatively nonselectively, cytoplasmic components [108]. Experimentally, when cells are stressed by excess iron, the large amount of iron in lysosomes is likely the result of increased autophagy [109]. The distribution of ferritin between cytoplasm and lysosomes likely varies among normal cell types, in addition to varying with stress in a single cell type. Thus, the amount of hemosiderin, lysosomal ferritin, and cytoplasmic ferritin will depend on environmental and regulatory variables [110] that likely contribute to the apparent inconsistencies in experiments on ferritin turnover and iron release, for example, [110–112].

5 Recovery of Iron from the Ferritin Mineral

There are at least two different mechanisms for the recovery of iron from the ferritin mineral. (1) Ferritin is degraded in lysosomes and the iron dissolved and transported by unknown mechanisms. (2) Cytoplasmic, and possibly mitochondrial ferritin pores that reversibly fold and unfold control access of cytoplasmic reductants to the ferric mineral and rates of iron release from ferritin to chelators or chaperones. Ferritin has no consensus lysosomal targeting sequence [113], making autophagy the likely mechanism for entry of *endogenous* ferritin into lysosomes. However, the entry of *exogenous* soybean ferritin via AP-2 (μ_2)-dependent endocytosis [58] provides an alternative route for exogenous ferritin to reach lysosomes. Thus, the stress associated with excess iron or inflammation, which increase autophagy, may explain accumulations of ferritin in lysosomes and large increases in ferritin synthesis. Small molecules can also modulate the distributions between the cytoplasma and lysosomes as shown in a recent study [114]. In the study, desferrioxamine which enters cells by endocytosis removed ferritin iron in the lysosomes, while an oral chelator, such as desferasirox, which is in the cytoplasm, removed iron from cytosolic ferritin.

5.1 *Ferritin-Gated Pore Structure*

Releasing iron from the intact ferritin protein nanocage in the cytoplasm is supported by two types of evidence. The first type of evidence is structure/function/genomic studies of the pores at the three-fold axis of the ferritin cage. The second type of evidence is from the iron release in cultured cells.

The eight pores in the ferritin cage can unfold without unfolding the helices of the protein cage [115] (Fig. 4.5). The ferritin cage itself has long been known to be very stable to heat and denaturants [116, 117]. When the ferritin pores are unfolded, reductants such as NADH/FMN have access to more of the mineral and can reduce more of the ferric iron. The phenomenon of unfolding ferritin

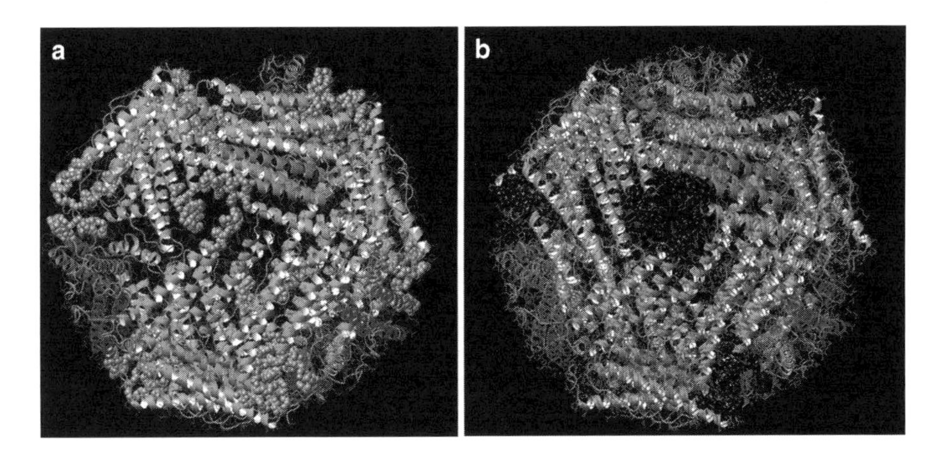

Fig. 4.5 Structure of the ferritin protein nanocage with folded or unfolded pores. Whether the ferritin pores (eight) are folded or unfolded, the polypeptide chains of each subunit are intact, but in the open pore mutant, the structural disorder associated with unfolding is so high that no electron density was observed in protein crystals. Mineral forms normally in both proteins, and the minerals are stable. When reductant (NADH/FMN) is added, the mineral is dissolved 30-times faster in the mutant with unfolded pores than in wild type under the same conditions [103]. (**a**) 1065 Wild-type ferritin nanocage (pores in "ball" format). (**b**) Open pore mutant (L134P) (The graphics were created by XS Liu and were used, with permission, from the cover of the issue with reference [106] and from [5])

pores can be measured as the increase in formation of Fe^{2+} chelated complexes, usually Fe^{2+}-bipyridyl, outside the protein cage [115] when biological reductants are added. Fe^{3+} chelators such as desferrioxamine B (DFO) can also be used [118, 119], but unless the local concentration of DFO is high, some Fe^{2+} is lost, possibly by competition between the ferroxidase binding sites and DFO [120]. Such observations explain, in part, why chelation therapies with Fe^{3+} chelators are so slow [121]. Folding of the ferritin pores is controlled by two pairs of amino acids that are highly conserved in all known ferritins. Amino acid substitution at any of the four positions increases emptying of mineral from the cage, sometimes as much as 30-fold. The pore gating amino acids were identified by searching for amino acids that were highly conserved, present near pores in 3D space and with no assigned function [115, 122]. Two of the four amino acids required for normal pore folding are the ion pair between arginine, at the end of α-helix B and an aspartate in the C/D loop; the third amino acid is a leucine in helix D. The fourth amino acid required for ferritin pore gating is a hydrophobic amino acid that can be leucine, as in human, animal, and plant ferritins, or isoleucine in some ferritins of single-celled organisms. When the ferritin pores are unfolded by mutation, they can be refolded by lowering the temperature [7, 120], suggesting a dynamic equilibrium for folding/unfolding that is temperature dependent [120].

5.2 *Ferritin Pore Properties Related to Iron Chelation Potential and In Vivo Function*

Ferritin pores melted at temperatures far below the protein nanocage itself [118], and unfolded at urea concentrations 1–5,000 times lower than needed to alter the cage structure. There are eight pores/ferritin cage. Mutation of a single gating amino acid will selectively unfold the pores, as well as heat or chaotropes (Fig. 4.5). Interestingly, 1 mM urea, which opens the pores, is in the physiological range (serum urea is 2–7 mM) and lowers the pore melting temperature (50% of the pores) to 43°C, in the physiological range. The iron content of serum ferritin is often very low [123, 124], which may relate to the normal serum urea concentrations, which are high enough to unfold ferritin pores, thus exposing the ferritin iron mineral to serum reductants. Ferritin pores in wild-type protein cages can be unfolded with peptides identified in a combinatorial phage display library (10^9 heptapeptides). Five peptides bound tightly to the ferritin proteins cage. When the five peptides were synthesized and tested for function, only one of the five peptides has a functional effect on unfolding the pores. When the synthetic peptide, which unfolded ferritin, was conjugated to desferrioxamine to increase local desferrioxamine concentrations around the ferritin pores were increased. With the desferrioxamine-peptide conjugate, the Fe chelation rate increased 3.3-fold compared to free peptide plus free desferrioxamine, and eightfold compared to controls [120]. Such data indicate potential therapeutic uses in vivo. In the synthetic peptide experiment, a second functional peptide was identified that appeared to close the pores [120]. It may be that a set of proteins exists in cells to unfold and to fold the ferritin pores, depending on the cell need for iron (or the state of inflammation).

In vivo partners that unfold the pores are suggested by the conservation of the amino acids in ferritin which "gate" iron reduction/transfer from the mineral to a chelator. If so, they are likely to be upregulated in severe iron deficiency. Support for such an idea comes from an experiment where cells were made iron deficient by overexpression of ferroportin. In such cells, iron was released from the protein in the cytoplasm before protein degradation [111], possibly through the unfolding of the protein pores by regulators similar in function to the pore-unfolding peptide [120]. In another experiment, when human wild-type ferritin or ferritin with a pore-unfolding mutation were overexpressed to the same level in separate HepG2 cultured cell transfects, the amount of iron in the open-pore mutant protein after incubation was significantly lower than in the wild-type ferritin; cell iron uptake was the same whether the overexpressed protein was wild-type or pore mutant. After incubation of the transfected cells with desferrioxamine, more of the cellular iron was in the desferrioxamine-containing medium, when cells with the mutant protein than the wild protein, indicating more iron in the LIP for cells with the pore mutant ferritin [125].

6 Perspective

Metabolic roles of ferritin family members are now understood to be integrated with antioxidant (Phase II) responses, cell cycle phosphatases, and hypoxia responses, in addition to the well-known role in concentrating iron. Still to be fully understood are metabolic roles of the two types of ferritin genes, one catalytically inactive and restricted to animals (ferritin L) and the other catalytically active (ferritin H-type subunit that are present in archaea, bacteria, higher plants and animals). Since gene deletion studies are lacking for ferritin L, and since studies that assess the impact of mRNA suppression of ferritin L-type and ferritin H-type subunits in different cell and tissue types and under oxygen and iron stress are few, the selective advantage of ferritin L in animals remains mysterious. Molecular mechanisms for gut iron absorption from exogenous ferritin and iron aggregates are also incompletely known, even though many foods such as legumes are a rich source of absorbable ferritin iron. The subdivision of iron physiology into heme and non-heme iron minimizes the range of iron speciation and the matching molecular selectivity of intestinal cell surface recognitions for ferrous, ferric chelates, protein-coated minerals (ferritin).

Structure/function studies recently completed revealed the ferritin cage as a sophisticated protein reactor that manages iron as it travels ~50 Å from entry through the pores to the active sites and through the nucleations channels to the cavity [36, 126, 127]. Very likely, the outer cage of the ferritin surface contains docking sites for chaperones that deliver or remove ferrous ions coming into or out the cage. The identification of ferritin catalytic intermediates and mechanisms is relatively recent, as is the awareness that ferritin enzyme activity is related to the diiron oxygenases important in DNA synthesis and desaturation of fatty acids. For that reason, the very earliest intermediates in ferritin catalysis, such as the Fe^{2+}-protein complexes that give rise to the diferric peroxo complex, the fate of the O in the catalytic peroxo intermediate, and mechanistic understanding of Fe as a substrate in ferritin and cofactor in the other diiron proteins, are still to be discovered. Comparisons of the similarities and differences in the protein sites and mechanisms of ferritin hold keys for fundamental understanding of differences between substrates and cofactors in enzymes while studies of ferritin channels and pres gating have a large potential impact on iron chelation therapies and on defining intracellular partners for ferritin in cells. Further, since ferritin pores are accessible for studies in the soluble protein complex, biophysical studies of ferritin pore dynamics can also model the less accessible protein pores in membranes and thus increase understanding of many ion transport processes in cells.

Gene regulation of ferritin synthesis remains one of the more complicated sets of interrelated mechanisms in biology. Specific ferritin protein repressors targeted to DNA (Bach1) and mRNA (IRP1,2) co-regulate ferritin genes with antioxidant response (Phase II) genes and with iron trafficking, hypoxia, cell cycle, and TCA cycle mRNAs. Heme is a corepressor that interacts directly with the selective repressors Bach1, IRP1, and IRP 2. But, exploration of the full complement of interactions between the ferritin DNA and RNA regulatory elements, *trans* regulatory factors, cellular signals, transcription complexes, and ribosomes is recent and incomplete. In addition, knowledge of the postsynthetic regulation of ferritin protein stability, and thus of the formation of hemosiderin is still limited. The inclusion of Fe and O_2 among the regulatory signals for ferritin synthesis, the very substrates of ferritin catalytic sites and constituents of the ferritin mineral, emphasizes the central position of ferritin in a feedback loop that links iron and oxygen metabolism. Obtaining the answers to the many questions remaining about ferritin physiology, structure/function, and gene regulation are crucial to both normal physiology and health as well as to understanding diseases related to abnormal iron and oxygen metabolism.

Acknowledgments The work of the author that is included here results from fruitful and satisfying interactions with collaborators, predoctoral students, and postdoctoral trainees, and for which the author is very grateful. Financial support to the author has been from NIH grant DK20251, CHORI, and the Cooley's Anemia Foundation, and for studies on ferritin as a nutritional iron source from NIH grant HL56169, the NCARS, and Condycet.

References

1. Hintze KJ, Theil EC. Cellular regulation and molecular interactions of the ferritins. Cell Mol Life Sci. 2006;63:591–600.
2. Wallander ML, Leibold EA, Eisenstein RS. Molecular control of vertebrate iron homeostasis by iron regulatory proteins. Biochim Biophys Acta. 2006;1763:668–89.
3. Rouault TA. The role of iron regulatory proteins in mammalian iron homeostasis and disease. Nat Chem Biol. 2006;2:406–14.
4. Hentze MW, Muckenthaler MU, Andrews NC. Balancing acts: molecular control of mammalian iron metabolism. Cell. 2004;117:285–97.
5. Khan MA, Walden WE, Goss DJ, Theil EC. Direct Fe2+ sensing by iron-responsive messenger RNA: repressor complexes weakens binding. J Biol Chem. 2009;284:30122–8.
6. Theil EC, Goss DJ. Living with iron (and oxygen): questions and answers about iron homeostasis. Chem Rev. 2009;109:4568–79.
7. Liu X, Theil EC. Ferritin: dynamic management of biological iron and oxygen chemistry. Acc Chem Res. 2005;38:167–75.
8. Chiancone E, Ceci P, Ilari A, Ribacchi F, Stefanini S. Iron and proteins for iron storage and detoxification. Biometals. 2004;17:197–202.
9. Hintze KJ, Theil EC. DNA and mRNA elements with complementary responses to hemin, antioxidant inducers, and iron control ferritin-L expression. Proc Natl Acad Sci USA. 2005;102:15048–52.
10. Harrison PM, Arosio P. The ferritins: molecular properties, iron storage function and cellular regulation. Biochim Biophys Acta. 1996;1275:161–203.
11. Drysdale J, Arosio P, Invernizzi R, et al. Mitochondrial ferritin: a new player in iron metabolism. Blood Cells Mol Dis. 2002;29:376–83.
12. Levi S, Arosio P. Mitochondrial ferritin. Int J Biochem Cell Biol. 2004;36:1887–9.
13. Drysdale JW, Adelman TG, Arosio P, et al. Human isoferritins in normal and disease states. Semin Hematol. 1977;14:71–88.
14. Collawn Jr JF, Donato Jr H, Upshur JK, Fish WW. A comparison by HPLC of ferritin subunit types in human tissues. Comp Biochem Physiol. 1985;81B:901–4.
15. Beaumont C, Torti SV, Torti FM, Massover WH. Novel properties of L-type polypeptide subunits in mouse ferritin molecules. J Biol Chem. 1996;271:7923–6.
16. Dickey LF, Sreedharan S, Theil EC, Didsbury JR, Wang Y-H, Kaufman RE. Differences in the regulation of messenger RNA for housekeeping and specialized-cell ferritin: a comparison of three distinct ferritin complementary DNAs, the corresponding subunits, and identification of the first processed in amphibia. J Biol Chem. 1987;262:7901–7.
17. Powell LW, Alpert E, Isselbacher KJ, Drysdale JW. Human isoferritins: organ specific iron and apoferritin distribution. Br J Haematol. 1975;30:47–55.
18. Arosio P, Adelman TG, Drysdale JW. On ferritin heterogeneity. Further evidence for heteropolymers. J Biol Chem. 1978;253:4451–8.
19. Lavoie DJ, Ishikawa K, Listowsky I. Correlations between subunit distribution, microheterogeneity, and iron content of human liver ferritin. Biochemistry. 1978;17:5448–54.
20. Konijn AM, Glickstein H, Vaisman B, Meyron-Holtz EG, Slotki IN, Cabantchik ZI. The cellular labile iron pool and intracellular ferritin in K562 cells. Blood. 1999;94:2128–34.
21. Vaisman B, Meyron-Holtz EG, Fibach E, Krichevsky AM, Konijn AM. Ferritin expression in maturing normal human erythroid precursors. Br J Haematol. 2000;110:394–401.
22. Girelli D, Corrocher R, Bisceglia L, et al. Molecular basis for the recently described hereditary hyperferritinemia-cataract syndrome: a mutation in the iron-responsive element of ferritin L-subunit gene (the "Verona mutation"). Blood. 1995;86:4050–3.

23. Cazzola M, Skoda RC. Translational pathophysiology: a novel molecular mechanism of human disease. Blood. 2000;95:3280–8.
24. Roetto A, Bosio S, Gramaglia E, Barilaro MR, Zecchina G, Camaschella C. Pathogenesis of hyperferritinemia cataract syndrome. Blood Cells Mol Dis. 2002;29:532–5.
25. Curtis AR, Fey C, Morris CM, et al. Mutation in the gene encoding ferritin light polypeptide causes dominant adult-onset basal ganglia disease. Nat Genet. 2001;28:350–4.
26. Levi S, Cozzi A, Arosio P. Neuroferritinopathy: a neurodegenerative disorder associated with L-ferritin mutation. Best Pract Res Clin Haematol. 2005;18:265–76.
27. Cozzi A, Santambrogio P, Corsi B, Campanella A, Arosio P, Levi S. Characterization of the l-ferritin variant 460InsA responsible of a hereditary ferritinopathy disorder. Neurobiol Dis. 2006;23:644–52.
28. Cozzi A, Corsi B, Levi S, Santambrogio P, Biasiotto G, Arosio P. Analysis of the biologic functions of H- and L-ferritins in HeLa cells by transfection with siRNAs and cDNAs: evidence for a proliferative role of L-ferritin. Blood. 2004;103:2377–83.
29. Hasan MR, Koikawa S, Kotani S, Miyamoto S, Nakagawa H. Ferritin forms dynamic oligomers to associate with microtubules in vivo: implication for the role of microtubules in iron metabolism. Exp Cell Res. 2006;312:1950–60.
30. White K, Munro HN. Induction of ferritin subunit synthesis by iron is regulated at both the transcriptional and translational levels. J Biol Chem. 1988;263:8938–42.
31. Leggett BA, Fletcher LM, Ramm GA, Powell LW, Halliday JW. Differential regulation of ferritin H and L subunit mRNA during inflammation and long-term iron overload. J Gastroenterol Hepatol. 1993;8:21–7.
32. Jenkins ZA, Hagar W, Bowlus CL, et al. Iron homeostasis during transfusional iron overload in β-thalassemia and sickle cell disease: changes in iron regulatory protein and ferritin expression. Pediatr Hematol Oncol. 2007;24:237–43.
33. Rohrer JS, Joo M-S, Dartyge E, Sayers DE, Fontaine A, Theil EC. Stabilization of iron in a ferrous form by ferritin: a study using dispersive and conventional X-ray absorption spectroscopy. J Biol Chem. 1987;262:11385–7.
34. Waldo GS, Theil EC. Ferritin and iron biomineralization. In: Suslick KS, editor. Comprehensive supramolecular chemistry, bioinorganic systems. Oxford: Pergamon; 1996. p. 65–89.
35. Sun S, Chasteen ND. Ferroxidase kinetics of horse spleen apoferritin. J Biol Chem. 1992;267:25160–6.
36. Turano P, Lalli D, Felli I, Theil E, Bertini I. NMR reveals pathway for ferric mineral precursors to the central cavity of ferritin. Proc Natl Acad Sci USA. 2010;107:545–50.
37. Rohrer JS, Islam QT, Watt GD, Sayers DE, Theil EC. Iron environment in ferritin with large amounts of phosphate, from *Azotobacter vinelandii* and horse spleen, analyzed using extended X-ray absorption fine structure (EXAFS). Biochemistry. 1990;29:259–64.
38. Waldo GS, Wright E, Whang ZH, Briat JF, Theil EC, Sayers DE. Formation of the ferritin iron mineral occurs in plastids. Plant Physiol. 1995;109:797–802.
39. Le Brun NE, Crow A, Murphy ME, Mauk AG, Moore GR. Iron core mineralisation in prokaryotic ferritins. Biochim Biophys Acta. 2010;1800:732–44.
40. Chiancone E, Ceci P. The multifaceted capacity of Dps proteins to combat bacterial stress conditions: detoxification of iron and hydrogen peroxide and DNA binding. Biochim Biophys Acta. 2010;1800:798–805.
41. Liu X, Kim K, Leighton T, Theil EC. Paired *Bacillus anthracis* Dps (mini-ferritin) have different reactivities with peroxide. J Biol Chem. 2006;281:27827–35.
42. Bellapadrona G, Stefanini S, Zamparelli C, Theil EC, Chiancone E. Iron translocation into and out of Listeria innocua Dps and size distribution of the protein-enclosed nanomineral are modulated by the electrostatic gradient at the 3-fold “ferritin-like” pores. J Biol Chem. 2009;284:19101–9.
43. Jameson GN, Jin W, Krebs C, et al. Stoichiometric production of hydrogen peroxide and parallel formation of ferric multimers through decay of the diferric-peroxo complex, the first detectable intermediate in ferritin mineralization. Biochemistry. 2002;41:13435–43.
44. Jameson GNL, Walters EM, Manieri W, Schurmann P, Johnson MK, Huynh BH. Spectroscopic evidence for site specific chemistry at a unique iron site of the [4Fe–4S] cluster in ferredoxin:thioredoxin reductase. J Am Chem Soc. 2003;125:1146–7.
45. Zhao G, Bou-Abdallah F, Arosio P, Levi S, Janus-Chandler C, Chasteen ND. Multiple pathways for mineral core formation in mammalian apoferritin. The role of hydrogen peroxide. Biochemistry. 2003;42:3142–50.
46. Waldo GS, Theil EC. Formation of iron(III)-tyrosinate is the fastest reaction observed in ferritin. Biochemistry. 1993;32:13262–9.
47. Liu X, Theil EC. Ferritin reactions: direct identification of the site for the diferric peroxide reaction intermediate. Proc Natl Acad Sci USA. 2004;101:8557–62.
48. Trikha J, Theil EC, Allewell NM. High resolution crystal structures of amphibian red-cell L ferritin: potential roles for structural plasticity and solvation in function. J Mol Biol. 1995;248:949–67.
49. Granier T, Langlois d'Estaintot B, Gallois B, et al. Structural description of the active sites of mouse L-chain ferritin at 1.2 A resolution. J Biol Inorg Chem. 2003;8:105–11.

50. Hempstead PD, Yewdall SJ, Fernie AR, et al. Comparison of the three-dimensional structures of recombinant human H and horse L ferritins at high resolution. J Mol Biol. 1997;268:424–48.
51. Otsuka S, Listowsky I, Niitsu Y, Urushizaki I. Assembly of intra- and interspecies hybrid apoferritins. J Biol Chem. 1980;255:6234–7.
52. Rhee SG, Kang SW, Jeong W, Chang TS, Yang KS, Woo HA. Intracellular messenger function of hydrogen peroxide and its regulation by peroxiredoxins. Curr Opin Cell Biol. 2005;17:183–9.
53. Giorgio M, Trinei M, Migliaccio E, Pelicci PG. Hydrogen peroxide: a metabolic by-product or a common mediator of ageing signals? Nat Rev Mol Cell Biol. 2007;8:722–8.
54. St Pierre T, Tran KC, Webb J, Macey DJ, Heywood BR, Sparks NH, et al. Organ-specific crystalline structures of ferritin cores in beta-thalassemia/hemoglobin E. Biol Met. 1991;4:162–5.
55. Tosha T, Hasan MR, Theil EC. The ferritin Fe2 site at the diiron catalytic center controls the reaction with O_2 in the rapid mineralization pathway. Proc Natl Acad Sci USA. 2008;105:18182–7.
56. Ambe S, Ambe F, Nozuki T. Mossbauer study of iron in soybean seeds. J Agric Food Chem. 1987;35:292–6.
57. National Nutrient Database for Standard Reference, Release 17. Nutrient Data Laboratory Home Page, http://www.nal.usda.gov/fnic/foodcomp. US Department of Agriculture, Agricultural Research Service; 2004.
58. San Martin CD, Garri C, Pizarro F, Walter T, Theil EC, Núñez M. Caco-2 intestinal epithelial cells absorb soybean ferritin by mu2 (AP2)-dependent endocytosis. J Nutr. 2008;138:659–66.
59. Meyron-Holtz EG, Vaisman B, Cabantchik ZI, et al. Regulation of intracellular iron metabolism in human erythroid precursors by internalized extracellular ferritin. Blood. 1999;94:3205–11.
60. Chen TT, Li L, Chung DH, et al. TIM-2 is expressed on B cells and in liver and kidney and is a receptor for H-ferritin endocytosis. J Exp Med. 2005;202:955–65.
61. Liao QK, Kong PA, Gao J, Li FY, Qian ZM. Expression of ferritin receptor in placental microvilli membrane in pregnant women with different iron status at mid-term gestation. Eur J Clin Nutr. 2001;55:651–6.
62. Ramm GA, Britton RS, O'Neill R, Bacon BR. Identification and characterization of a receptor for tissue ferritin on activated rat lipocytes. J Clin Invest. 1994;94:9–15.
63. Beard JL, Burton JW, Theil EC. Purified ferritin and soybean meal can be sources of iron for treating iron deficiency in rats. J Nutr. 1996;126:154–60.
64. Murray-Kolb LE, Welch R, Theil EC, Beard JL. Women with low iron stores absorb iron from soybeans. Am J Clin Nutr. 2003;77:180–4.
65. Davila-Hicks P, Theil EC, Lonnerdal B. Iron in ferritin or in salts (ferrous sulfate) is equally bioavailable in nonanemic women. Am J Clin Nutr. 2004;80:936–40.
66. Lonnerdal B, Bryant A, Liu X, Theil EC. Iron absorption from soybean ferritin in nonanemic women. Am J Clin Nutr. 2006;83:103–7.
67. Sayers MH, Lynch SR, Jacobs P, et al. The effects of ascorbic acid supplementation on the absorption of iron in maize, wheat and soya. Br J Haematol. 1973;24:209–18.
68. Layrisse M, Martínez-Torres C, Renzy M, Leets I. Ferritin iron absorption in man. Blood. 1975;45:689–98.
69. Martínez-Torres C, Renzi M, Layrisse M. Iron absorption by humans from hemosiderin and ferritin, further studies. J Nutr. 1976;106:128–35.
70. Lynch SR, Dassenko SA, Beard JL, Cook JD. Iron absorption from legumes in humans. Am J Clin Nutr. 1984;40:42–7.
71. Skikne B, Fonzo D, Lynch SR, Cook JD. Bovine ferritin iron bioavailability in man. Eur J Clin Invest. 1997;27:228–33.
72. Theil EC, Burton JW, Beard JL. A sustainable solution for dietary iron deficiency through plant biotechnology and breeding to increase seed ferritin control. Eur J Clin Nutr. 1997;51:S28–31.
73. Lonnerdal B, Lonnerdal B, Theil EC. Rebuttal to J. Hunt letter to the editor. Am J Clin Nutr. 2005;81:1179–80.
74. Burton JW, Harlow C, Theil EC. Evidence for reutilization of nodule iron in soybean seed development. J Plant Nutr. 1998;21:913–27.
75. Kusumi E, Shoji M, Endou S, et al. Prevalence of anemia among healthy women in 2 metropolitan areas of Japan. Int J Hematol. 2006;84:217–9.
76. Killip S, Bennett JM, Chambers MD. Iron deficiency anemia. Am Fam Physician. 2007;75:671–8.
77. Sanchez M, Galy B, Muckenthaler MU, Hentze MW. Iron-regulatory proteins limit hypoxia-inducible factor-2alpha expression in iron deficiency. Nat Struct Mol Biol. 2007;14:420–6.
78. Sanchez M, Galy B, Dandekar T, et al. Iron regulation and the cell cycle: identification of an iron-responsive element in the 3′-untranslated region of human cell division cycle 14A mRNA by a refined microarray-based screening strategy. J Biol Chem. 2006;281:22865–74.
79. Tsuji Y, Torti SV, Torti FM. Activation of the ferritin H enhancer, FER-1, by the cooperative action of members of the AP1 and Sp1 transcription factor families. J Biol Chem. 1998;273:2984–92.
80. Iwasaki K, Mackenzie EL, Hailemariam K, Sakamoto K, Tsuji Y. Hemin-mediated regulation of an antioxidant-responsive element of the human ferritin H gene and role of Ref-1 during erythroid differentiation of K562 cells. Mol Cell Biol. 2006;26:2845–56.

81. Igarashi K, Sun J. The heme-Bach1 pathway in the regulation of oxidative stress response and erythroid differentiation. Antioxid Redox Signal. 2006;8:107–18.
82. Giudice A, Montella M. Activation of the Nrf2-ARE signaling pathway: a promising strategy in cancer prevention. Bioessays. 2006;28:169–81.
83. De Gregorio E, Preiss T, Hentze MW. Translation driven by an eIF4G core domain in vivo. EMBO J. 1999;18:4865–74.
84. Zahringer J, Baliga BS, Munro HN. Subcellular distribution of total poly(A)-containing RNA and ferritin-mRNA in the cytoplasm of rat liver. Biochem Biophys Res Commun. 1976;68:1088–93.
85. Dickey LF, Wang YH, Shull GE, Wortman III IA, Theil EC. The importance of the 3 -untranslated region in the translational control of ferritin mRNA. J Biol Chem. 1988;263:3071–4.
86. Ke Y, Wu J, Leibold EA, Walden WE, Theil EC. Loops and bulge/loops in iron-responsive element isoforms influence iron regulatory protein binding: fine-tuning of mRNA regulation? J Biol Chem. 1998;273:23637–40.
87. Gunshin H, Allerson CR, Polycarpou-Schwarz M, et al. Iron-dependent regulation of the divalent metal ion transporter. FEBS Lett. 2001;509:309–16.
88. Leipuviene R, Theil EC. The family of iron responsive RNA structures (IRE) regulated by changes in cellular iron and oxygen. Cell Mol Life Sci. 2007;64:2945–55.
89. Goforth JB, Anderson SA, Nizzi CP, Eisenstein RS. Multiple determinants within iron-responsive elements dictate iron regulatory protein binding and regulatory hierarchy. RNA. 2010;16:154–69.
90. Brazzolotto X, Timmins P, Dupont Y, Moulis JM. Structural changes associated with switching activities of human iron regulatory protein 1. J Biol Chem. 2002;277:11995–2000.
91. Yikilmaz E, Rouault TA, Schuck P. Self-association and ligand-induced conformational changes of iron regulatory proteins 1 and 2. Biochemistry. 2006;44:8470–8.
92. Dupuy J, Volbeda A, Carpentier P, Darnault C, Moulis JM, Fontecilla-Camps JC. Crystal structure of human iron regulatory protein 1 as cytosolic aconitase. Structure. 2006;14:129–39.
93. Walden WE, Selezneva AI, Dupuy J, et al. Structure of dual function iron regulatory protein 1 complexed with ferritin IRE-RNA. Science. 2006;314:1903–8.
94. Goessling LS, Mascotti DP, Thach RE. Involvement of heme in the degradation of iron-regulatory protein 2. J Biol Chem. 1998;273:12555–7.
95. Jeong J, Rouault TA, Levine RL. Identification of a heme-sensing domain in iron regulatory protein 2. J Biol Chem. 2004;279:45450–4.
96. Schalinske KL, Eisenstein RS. Phosphorylation and activation of both iron regulatory protein 1 (IRP1) and IRP2 in HL60 cells. J Biol Chem. 1996;271:7168–76.
97. Fillebeen C, Chahine D, Caltagirone A, Segal P, Pantopoulos K. A phosphomimetic mutation at Ser-138 renders iron regulatory protein 1 sensitive to iron-dependent degradation. Mol Cell Biol. 2003;23:6973–81.
98. Clarke SL, Vasanthakumar A, Anderson SA, et al. Iron-responsive degradation of iron-regulatory protein 1 does not require the Fe–S cluster. EMBO J. 2006;25:544–53.
99. Theil EC. Ferritin: structure, gene regulation, and cellular function in animals, plants, and microorganisms. Annu Rev Biochem. 1987;56:289–315.
100. Shoden A, Gabrio BW, Finch CA. The relationship between ferritin and hemosiderin in rabbits and man. J Biol Chem. 1953;204:823–30.
101. Matioli GT, Baker RF. Denaturation of ferritin and its relationship with hemosiderin. J Ultrastruct Res. 1963;8:477–90.
102. Marton PF. Ultrastructural study of erythrophagocytosis in the rat bone marrow. I. Red cell engulfment by reticulum cells. II. Iron metabolism in reticulum cells following red cell digestion. Scand J Haematol. 1975;23:1–26.
103. Mann S, Wade VJ, Dickson DPE, et al. Structural specificity of haemosiderin iron cores in iron-overload diseases. FEBS Lett. 1988;234:69–72.
104. Iancu TC, Deugnier Y, Halliday JW, Powell LW, Brissot P. Ultrastructural sequences during liver iron overload in genetic hemochromatosis. J Hepatol. 1997;27:628–38.
105. St. Pierre TG, Webb J, Mann S. Ferritin and hemosiderin: structural and magnetic studies of the iron core. In: Mann S, Webb J, Williams JP, editors. Biomineralization: chemical and biochemical perspectives. New York: VCH; 1989. p. 295–344.
106. Miyazaki E, Kato J, Kobune M, et al. Denatured H-ferritin subunit is a major constituent of haemosiderin in the liver of patients with iron overload. Gut. 2002;50:413–9.
107. Curie C, Briat JF. Iron transport and signaling in plants. Annu Rev Plant Biol. 2003;2003:183–206.
108. Orvedahl A, Levine B. Viral evasion of autophagy. Autophagy. 2008;4:1–6.
109. Richter GW. The iron-loaded cell – the cytopathology of iron storage: a review. Am J Pathol. 1978; 91:363–96.
110. Kurz T, Terman A, Brunk UT. Autophagy, ageing and apoptosis: the role of oxidative stress and lysosomal iron. Arch Biochem Biophys. 2007;462:220–30.
111. De Domenico I, Vaughn MB, Li L, et al. Ferroportin-mediated mobilization of ferritin iron precedes ferritin degradation by the proteasome. EMBO J. 2006;25:5396–404.

112. Kidane TZ, Sauble E, Linder MC. Release of iron from ferritin requires lysosomal activity. Am J Physiol Cell Physiol. 2006;291:C445–55.
113. Bonifacino JS, Traub LM. Signals for sorting of transmembrane proteins to endosomes and lysosomes. Annu Rev Biochem. 2003;72:395–447.
114. De Domenico I, Ward DM, Kaplan J. Specific iron chelators determine the route of ferritin degradation. Blood. 2009;114:4546–51.
115. Takagi H, Shi D, Ha Y, Allewell NM, Theil EC. Localized unfolding at the junction of three ferritin subunits: a mechanism for iron release? J Biol Chem. 1998;273:18685–8.
116. Listowsky I, Blauer G, Enlard S, Betheil JJ. Denaturation of horse spleen ferritin in aqueous guanidinium chloride solutions. Biochemistry. 1972;11:2176–82.
117. Santambrogio P, Levi S, Arosio P, et al. Evidence that a salt bridge in the light chain contributes to the physical stability difference between heavy and light human ferritins. J Biol Chem. 1992;267:14077–83.
118. Liu X, Jin W, Theil EC. Opening protein pores with chaotropes enhances Fe reduction and chelation of Fe from the ferritin biomineral. Proc Natl Acad Sci USA. 2003;100:3653–8.
119. Crichton RR, Roman F, Roland F. Iron mobilization from ferritin by chelating agents. J Inorg Biochem. 1980;13:305–16.
120. Liu XS, Patterson LD, Miller MJ, Theil EC. Peptides selected for the protein nanocage pores change the rate of iron recovery from the ferritin mineral. J Biol Chem. 2007;282:31821–3185.
121. Vichinsky EP. Current issues with blood transfusions in sickle cell disease. Semin Hematol. 2001;38:14–22.
122. Jin W, Takagi H, Pancorbo NM, Theil EC. "Opening" the ferritin pore for iron release by mutation of conserved amino acids at interhelix and loop sites. Biochemistry. 2001;40:7525–32.
123. Worwood M, Dawkins S, Wagstaff M, Jacobs A. The purification and properties of ferritin from human serum. Biochem J. 1976;157:97–103.
124. Herbert V, Jayatilleke E, Shaw S, et al. Serum ferritin iron, a new test, measures human body iron stores unconfounded by inflammation. Stem Cells. 1997;15:291–6.
125. Hasan MR, Tosha T, Theil EC. Ferritin contains less iron (59Fe) in cells when the protein pores are unfolded by mutation. J Biol Chem. 2008;283:31394–400.
126. Tosha T, Ng HL, Bhattasali O, Alber T, Theil EC. Moving metal ions through ferritin-protein nanocages from three-fold pores to catalytic sites. J Am Chem Soc. 2010;132:14562–9.
127. Theil EC. Ferritin protein nanocages use ion channels, catalytic sites, and nucleation channels to manage iron/oxygen chemistry. Curr Opin Chem Biol. 2011;15:304–11.

Section II
Iron Physiology

Chapter 5
Iron Nutrition

Weng-In Leong and Bo Lönnerdal

Keywords Bioavailability • Dietary iron intake • Food iron • Fortification • Heme iron • Iron • Iron Requirements • Nutrition • Supplementation

1 Iron Requirements Across the Life Span

1.1 Infancy

Healthy term infants with normal birth weight are born with a considerable endowment of iron and high hemoglobin levels which together are usually sufficient to maintain their needs for growth during the first 6 months of life [1]. Infants begin life with approximately 80 mg iron/kg body weight [2], which can be compared with 55 mg iron/kg for adult men. With a concentration of hemoglobin of ~170 g/L at birth, a 3.5 kg term infant who doubles his or her weight by 6 months of age should be able to maintain a hemoglobin level of 90–110 g/L without the need for extra iron. During the first half of infancy, infants utilize their abundant iron stores for body use and growth, which then often become exhausted by 6 months of age. The low iron content in human milk is believed to be adequate to meet their iron needs, as exclusively breast-fed infants rarely show any signs of iron deficiency during the first 6 months of life [3]. With a typical milk volume of 780 mL/day and a breast milk iron concentration of ~0.35 mg/L, a daily intake of 0.27 mg of iron is believed to be adequate for infants at this stage [4]. Preterm and low-birth-weight infants, however, exhaust their iron stores at an earlier age as they have lower fetal iron stores and proportionately greater weight gain than those of term infants [1]. The size of the newborn's iron stores is strongly affected by birth weight and gestational age. The transfer of iron from maternal blood to the fetus occurs mostly during the third trimester and contributes ~4 mg daily [5]. Hence, infants born prematurely have reduced iron stores. Iron requirements of preterm and low-birth-weight infants are therefore higher and iron supplementation is necessary before 6 months of age [6, 7]. Besides prematurity and low birth weight, the timing of umbilical cord clamping and maternal iron status also affect the iron endowment of the newborn. Early cord clamping decreases iron transfer to the infants, whereas delayed cord clamping increases the red cell volume in the infants and, in turn, increases the iron endowment [8–10].

W.-I. Leong, R.D., Ph.D. • B. Lönnerdal, Ph.D. (✉)
Department of Nutrition, University of California Davis, Davis, CA 95616, USA
e-mail: bllonnerdal@ucdavis.edu

G.J. Anderson and G. McLaren (eds.), *Iron Physiology and Pathophysiology in Humans*, Nutrition and Health, DOI 10.1007/978-1-60327-485-2_5,

Delayed umbilical cord clamping for 2 min increases total body iron by about 33%, resulting in greater iron stores at 6 months of age [10]. Maternal iron deficiency does not appear to compromise the iron endowment of the infants [11, 12], but severe maternal iron deficiency, i.e., anemia, does have an adverse effect on iron status of the newborn. Infants of moderately and severely anemic mothers have lower iron stores [13] and a threefold increased risk of low birth weight [14], placing them at higher risk of iron deficiency at an early age. Indeed, the incidence of iron deficiency and anemia during later infancy is higher in infants born to mothers with iron deficiency anemia than in infants born to iron-replete mothers [15–17]. Taken together, iron requirements during the first half of infancy depend greatly on the iron endowment of the infants at birth. Providing that normal birth weight, term infants born to iron-replete mothers are exclusively breast-fed and have delayed cord clamping, the provision of iron from breast milk and their own stores is usually adequate to meet their iron needs during the first half of infancy.

The proper level of iron fortification to use in infant formulas has been a subject of controversy. Since early studies indicated that the bioavailability of iron is higher from breast milk than from cow's milk and infant formula, it was argued that formula should contain a higher level of iron than that of breast milk. For many years, most iron-fortified infant formulas contained 7–12 mg of iron/L, which appears inordinately high; this is 20–40 times more iron than in breast milk. In fact, infants fed formula with 12 mg of iron/L had lower copper status than infants fed formula with 7 mg/L [3]. The higher level of iron fortification also appeared unnecessary as infants were found to absorb as much iron from a formula with 8 mg of iron/L as from formula with 12 mg/L [18]. More recently, iron levels have been decreased to 4 mg/L in many formulas, and studies have actually shown that 1.6 mg/L is adequate to maintain normal iron status of formula-fed infants up to 6 months of age [19]. This issue is complicated, however, as infant formulas in some areas are primarily used up to 6 months of age (when the iron requirements are lower) and in other areas up to 12 months (when iron requirements become higher, see below). From an iron nutrition perspective, it may be preferable to have one level of iron for younger and another one for older infants.

During the second half of infancy, continued rapid growth and expansion of hemoglobin mass together with depleted iron stores contribute to the high iron requirement of infants. Even though iron in human milk is highly bioavailable, the iron concentration of 0.20–0.35 mg/L in human milk is low [4]. Exclusive breastfeeding alone is therefore not always adequate to meet the high iron requirement during this stage. The American Academy of Pediatrics (AAP) recommends exclusive breastfeeding for the first 6 months of age and that iron-fortified infant cereal and complementary food should be introduced to infants after 6 months of age [7, 20]. Addition of meat to infant diets has been shown to increase iron absorption considerably [21]. Infants who are not breast-fed should be given iron-fortified formula, which should contain 4–12 mg iron/L [22]. Infants weaned before 12 months of age should not receive cow's milk [7], which has a very low concentration of iron (0.1–0.2 mg/L), which is also of poor bioavailability [23]. Whole cow's milk may also cause gastrointestinal bleeding, which further increases the iron loss of the infants. The gastrointestinal bleeding is assumed to be caused by an allergic reaction to cow's milk protein. For 6–12-month-old infants, the total requirement for absorbed iron is estimated to be 0.69 mg/day. This amount of iron is needed for the basal iron loss (0.26 mg/day), increase in hemoglobin mass (0.37 mg/day), increase in non-storage iron in tissues (0.009 mg/day) and increase in storage iron (0.051 mg/day) [4]. Iron is needed to increase the storage iron as iron stores are low at this stage of infancy. The daily basal loss of iron/kg body weight is 0.03 mg [24], which includes urinary, fecal, and dermal iron losses. The increase in hemoglobin mass is a function of growth rate. With a weight increment of 13 g/day [25], a blood volume of 70 mL/kg body weight [26], a hemoglobin concentration of 120 g/L blood, and an iron content of 3.39 mg/g in hemoglobin [27], the amount of daily iron needed for the increase in hemoglobin mass is 0.37 mg. As for iron deposited in tissues, which is mainly for myoglobin and iron-containing enzymes, it is estimated to be 0.7 mg/kg body weight for a 12-month-old infant [27]. With a daily weight increment of 13 g, the amount of iron needed for tissue deposition is 0.009 mg/day, and ~12% of the total body iron deposited (hemoglobin mass and tissue iron) is needed for the increase in storage iron [28].

Even though there is no difference in the estimated iron requirement between boys and girls during infancy, substantial sex differences in iron status have been observed during infancy [29]. Hemoglobin, mean corpuscular volume, and serum ferritin concentrations were found to be lower and transferrin receptor and zinc protoporphyrin concentrations to be higher in boys than in girls at 4, 6, and 9 months of age. Moreover, boys at 9 months of age had a higher risk of being classified with iron deficiency anemia than girls [29]. The sex differences in mean corpuscular volume and zinc protoporphyrin concentrations may reflect normal physiological differences between genders. On the other hand, the differences in hemoglobin and transferrin receptors seem to reflect a higher incidence of iron deficiency in boys. Sex-specific reference values to define iron deficiency may need to be developed for some of the iron status indicators [29]. Indeed, the current reference values for iron status indicators may not be appropriate for infants as those values are extrapolated from older children and adults [30]. For instance, an increase in hemoglobin after iron treatment is used as a criterion for iron deficiency anemia in adults [31]; however, iron supplements significantly increased hemoglobin concentrations of infants younger than 6 months regardless of initial iron status, indicating that hemoglobin response to iron is not a useful criterion to define iron deficiency in infants at this age [32]. During the first year of life, dietary iron is channeled to erythropoiesis but not to iron stores even in the absence of iron deficiency, whereas surplus iron is channeled to iron stores during the second year of life [33]. Iron metabolism undergoes considerable developmental changes during infancy. In adults, iron homeostasis is primarily regulated by intestinal iron absorption, which is inversely related to iron stores. Erythropoiesis and dietary iron intake also play a part in regulating intestinal iron absorption. Unlike adults, iron absorption of 6-month-old infants is independent of iron status and dietary iron intake [34]. Iron absorption is not downregulated in 6-month-old iron-replete infants receiving iron supplements, but homeostatic downregulation of iron absorption occurs in 9-month-old infants given iron supplements [34]. On the other end of the spectrum, infants with low iron status are able to upregulate iron absorption at both 6 and 9 months of age to compensate for their inadequate iron status [35]. To date, our knowledge regarding these developmental changes in iron metabolism during infancy is limited. A better understanding of iron metabolism and the mechanisms behind these development changes during early life are likely to lead to a more complete comprehension of iron nutrition during infancy.

1.2 Childhood

Children between 1 and 3 years of age still require relatively large amounts of iron for rapid growth. Low iron stores carried from late infancy, high physiological demands, and a diet usually not rich in iron-containing foods make young children susceptible to iron deficiency. A diet containing mainly milk and excluding other foods is not able to provide enough iron and may cause problems with maintaining iron stores. Not only is the iron content of cow's milk low, both calcium and cow's milk protein inhibit iron absorption [36–38]. A recommendation to limit cow's milk consumption to less than 700 mL/day has been made [39] and a diversified diet rich in highly bioavailable iron sources and ascorbic acid is encouraged. The estimated requirement for absorbed iron is 0.54 mg/day for this age group [4], which is needed for basal iron losses, iron storage, increase in hemoglobin mass and non-storage tissues iron as growth continues. Iron requirements are believed to be similar for boys and girls during childhood. Based on total body iron losses measured in adults [40], the daily basal loss of young children is estimated to be 0.33 mg after adjusting to the children's body surface area. Increases in hemoglobin mass and non-storage tissue iron require ~0.18 and 0.004 mg of daily iron, respectively. With a weight increment of about 6.3 g/day and tissue iron deposition of 0.7 mg/kg body weight, an estimate of 0.004 mg is needed for these young children to increase their non-storage tissue iron. Similar to older infants, the amount of iron required by young children to increase their iron stores is ~12% of the total body iron deposited [28], which is ~0.023 mg/day.

As for older school-aged children, iron requirements and the risk of iron deficiency are lower because of a relatively slower growth rate and consumption of a more diverse diet. However, school-age children in developing countries with gastrointestinal blood loss from hookworm infection and consumption of diets with low iron bioavailability still have a high prevalence of iron deficiency anemia [41]. The requirement for absorbed iron in children 4–8 years old is about 0.74 mg/day, including 0.47 mg for basal losses, 0.25 mg for hemoglobin accretion, 0.004 mg for tissue deposition, and 0.015 mg for iron storage [4]. The amount of non-storage iron deposited in tissues is similar to younger children; however, the amount of iron needed for iron storage is comparatively less. Beyond 3 years of age, the percent of iron devoted to iron stores decreases progressively [4].

1.3 Adolescence

The relatively uniform growth seen in childhood is replaced by growth with increased velocity during adolescence. Iron requirement increases as a result of rapid growth, greater blood volume and erythrocyte mass, increased lean body mass, and the onset of menstruation in girls. The estimated requirements for absorbed iron in boys (1.06 mg/day) and girls (1.02 mg/day) of age 9–13 are quite similar. Daily basal iron losses are ~0.6 mg, which are derived on the basis of 14 μg basal iron losses per kg body in adults [40]. For hemoglobin mass, boys develop greater red blood cell mass than girls. The estimated weight gain per year in boys is about 4.87 kg. With a blood volume of 75 mL/kg body weight [26], an estimated hemoglobin concentration of 134.4 g/L [42] and an iron content of 3.39 mg/g hemoglobin [27], daily iron needed for the expanded hemoglobin mass in boys is about 0.46 mg. As for 9–13-year-old girls, with a weight increment of 4.77 kg/year, a blood volume of 66 mL/kg body weight [26], and a hemoglobin concentration of about 133 g/L [42], the estimated amount of iron needed to support the expansion of hemoglobin mass is 0.39 mg. Besides hemoglobin mass, lean body mass also increases. This, in turn, raises the iron requirement for myoglobin and iron-containing enzymes in muscles. Since the amount of iron deposited in tissues is ~0.13 mg/kg body weight gain [27], ~0.002 mg iron is required daily for the increase in non-storage tissue for both genders. The provision of iron stores is not as much of a concern as in infants and young children as the majority of this group is believed to have adequate stores. By age 9 and further, an increase in iron stores is therefore not considered as a component of iron needs [4].

The estimated daily iron requirements for adolescents aged 14–18 are 1.38 and 1.44 mg for boys and girls, respectively. The requirement for girls is large and higher than in boys, mainly because of the onset of menstruation. Indeed, adolescent girls are particularly prone to iron deficiency because of the increased demand for iron, menstrual iron loss, and poor dietary habits. With a 28 days menstrual cycle of 27.6 mL blood loss, an iron concentration of 3.39 mg/g hemoglobin and an average hemoglobin concentration of 135 g/L blood [42], menstrual iron loss is estimated to be 0.45 mg/day [4]. For girls who have started to menstruate before the age of 14, the amount of iron loss from menstruation should be taken into account when estimating their daily iron requirement. Besides menstrual iron loss, the daily requirement for absorbed iron also covers basal iron losses (0.85 mg/day), an increase in hemoglobin mass (0.14 mg/day), and an increase in non-storage iron in tissues (0.001 mg/day). During this stage, average weights are 70.3 kg for boys and 61.4 kg for girls. Weight increments of boys and girls average about 2.75 kg/year and 1.63 kg/year, respectively. The amount of iron deposited in tissues per body weight gain is the same as for 9–13-year-old adolescents [27]. For boys, the amount of required absorbed iron of 1.38 mg/day is needed for basal iron losses (0.98 mg/day), increase in hemoglobin mass (0.4 mg/day), and increase in non-storage iron in tissue (0.001 mg/day).

The adolescent growth spurt begins at an average age of about 10 years for girls and grows at peak velocity at about age 12, though it varies among individuals. Menstruation usually occurs

1 year after peak growth. The growth spurt starts later in boys, at around 12 years of age, but they have a higher growth peak velocity than girls. The average weight gain for boys and girls can be as high as 10 and 7 kg, respectively, during the peak year of growth spurt. This dramatic weight gain imposes an additional iron need of 0.53 mg/day for boys and 0.2 mg/day for girls [4].

1.4 Adults

Iron needs among adult men decrease after adolescence as growth ceases. The required amount of absorbed iron only needs to replace the daily basal iron losses of about 1.1 mg iron. This is estimated based on the median adult body weight of 77.4 kg reported in NHANES III and basal iron losses of 14 μg/kg body weight [40]. As a consequence of the lower iron requirements, iron stores increase throughout life in men, who rarely exhibit iron deficiency [43].

Unlike men, iron needs of adult women continue to be high even after the adolescent growth spurt. To cover menstrual losses, women have to absorb 0.51 mg iron more than adult men on a daily basis [4]. This is estimated using a 28 days menstrual cycle of 30.9 mL blood loss, an average iron concentration of 3.39 mg/g hemoglobin [27] and an average hemoglobin concentration of 135 g/L blood [42]. Women's daily basal iron loss/kg body weight is estimated to be similar to that of adult men, and with a median body weight of 64 kg reported in NHANES III, daily basal iron loss is 0.9 mg. Together with the menstrual iron loss, the total iron need of adult women is about 1.4 mg/day, which is higher than in men.

Because of smaller erythrocyte mass and iron stores in women, the body iron content of women (40 mg/kg body weight) is lower than that of men (50 mg/kg body weight) [44]. Dietary iron intake is typically lower in women than in men as men have higher total energy intake from food. Having a higher iron requirement, smaller iron stores, and lower dietary iron intake compared to that of men results in women having a higher risk for iron deficiency. On the other hand, postmenopausal women have a lower risk of iron deficiency [43] as their iron losses are small and iron stores usually increase through the rest of life. Postmenopausal women only need to replace their basal iron loss of 0.9 mg/day [4].

1.5 Pregnancy

Pregnancy is a critical period characterized by rapid growth and development accompanied by increased nutrient requirements. Maternal iron requirements increase substantially to support fetal growth and placental tissue development as well as the increased hemoglobin mass during pregnancy. Plasma volume increases until term to accommodate the need for extra blood flow to the fetus, placenta, and uterus as well as to compensate for maternal blood loss during delivery. Hemoglobin mass also expands to raise the oxygen transport capacity, which is necessary to meet the increased oxygen demand of the growing fetus and the mother. Since the plasma volume increases (45–50%) earlier in pregnancy and increases more than the red cell mass (33%), the hemoglobin concentration falls [44, 45]. This decrease continues until the end of the second trimester when the increase in the red cell mass becomes synchronized with the increase in plasma volume. Hemoglobin concentration then slightly rises to pre-pregnant levels by term. This normal physiological change in hemoglobin level is observed even in iron-sufficient women [46].

The total estimated usage of iron throughout the entire pregnancy is 1,070 mg, including 500 mg iron for the expansion of hemoglobin mass, 245 mg iron for fetal growth, 75 mg for placental and cord iron deposition, and 250 mg for basal iron losses [4]. Blood loss at delivery accounts to about

150–250 mg iron, which implies that 250–350 mg of iron is retained in the body. The net iron usage is estimated to be 720–820 mg [4]. Despite the unchanged basal iron losses of 0.9 mg/day throughout pregnancy [40], the demand for iron is not uniform during the course of pregnancy. During the first trimester, the iron need of the fetus is negligible, expansion of red cell mass has not begun and with the amenorrhea of pregnancy, little iron is required. In contrast, almost all the iron needed for hemoglobin mass expansion and deposition in the fetus and placenta is utilized during the second half of pregnancy [47]. The iron requirement of the fetus increases proportionally with the weight of the fetus, with most iron deposition during the third trimester [48]. Iron deposition in the fetus and placenta is estimated to be 25 mg (0.27 mg/day), 100 mg (1.1 mg/day), and 190 mg (2.0 mg/day) during the first, second, and third trimester, respectively. For hemoglobin mass expansion, 250 mg (2.7 mg/day) iron is needed for the second and the third trimester each. When translated into daily requirements, iron demand is thus quite large during the second and third trimester, averaging 5 and 6 mg/day, respectively, compared to about 1.2 mg/day in the first trimester [4]. For pregnant adolescents, iron requirements are even higher as the iron need for hemoglobin mass increase and tissue iron deposition during growth need to be taken into account.

With the increased iron requirement and reduced iron stores as pregnancy progresses, the efficiency of intestinal iron absorption increases during the second and the third trimester as a homeostatic response [49]. Nevertheless, iron requirements during pregnancy cannot be easily met by diet alone even with a diet with highly bioavailable iron [50]. When iron is not readily available, the iron needs of the fetus are met at the expense of maternal iron stores. Hence, iron deficiency anemia is rarely seen in infants at birth, but iron deficiency often occurs during the later stages of pregnancy even in women who enter pregnancy with relatively adequate iron stores [46]. Compared to the iron stores of 300 mg in healthy women, the extra iron of 1,070 mg required for pregnancy is a large amount. In fact, most women rarely acquire sufficient iron stores before entering pregnancy [50, 51]. Together, these considerations explain the high prevalence of iron deficiency among pregnant women. It is estimated that most pregnant women in developing countries and about 30–40% of pregnant women in developed countries are iron deficient [52]. Maternal iron deficiency anemia increases the risk for preterm labor, low birth weight, and perinatal mortality [53, 54]. Iron supplementation of pregnant women is therefore recommended and supported by the World Health Organization, Institute of Medicine, and other advisory groups to prevent iron deficiency anemia during pregnancy [4, 39, 52].

1.6 Lactation

Unlike pregnancy, the iron requirement during lactation is not increased and is in fact lower than that of nonpregnant, non-lactating women. The daily need for absorbed iron is 1.17 mg, which covers the daily basal losses of 0.9 mg and the daily secretion of 0.27 mg iron in breast milk [4]. Because of the low iron need, the recuperation of iron reserves after delivery, and the amenorrhea of lactation, iron status improves during the postpartum period. However, iron deficiency may continue in women whose iron stores are low and who have substantial blood losses during delivery.

1.7 Elderly

Iron is required to replace the daily basal losses in order to maintain iron balance in elderly. It is assumed that basal iron losses are constant with age. Hence, the daily requirement of absorbed iron is estimated to be about 0.9 and 1.0 mg for elderly women and men, respectively. With low iron

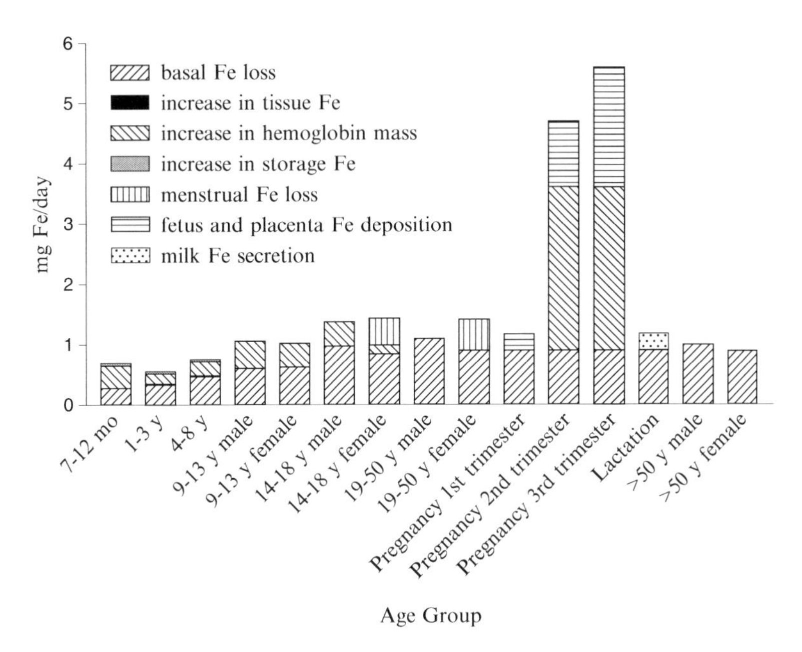

Fig. 5.1 Estimated daily average iron requirements during different life stages. Components used to estimate iron needs include basal Fe loss, increase in tissue Fe, hemoglobin mass, storage Fe, menstrual Fe loss, fetus and placenta Fe deposition, and Fe secretion in human milk (Data from [4])

requirements, iron deficiency anemia is more uncommon in elderly than in young people. Moreover, it is rarely caused by dietary iron deficiency, especially in developed countries [55]. The cases of iron deficiency anemia in the elderly are usually related to gastrointestinal blood loss caused by diseases [56] and medications or by hypochlorhydria, resulting in poor absorption of iron. The estimated daily average iron requirements during different life stages are illustrated in Fig. 5.1.

1.8 Special Considerations

Several factors impact iron requirements and deserve special considerations when estimating iron needs. Intestinal parasitic infections which are prevalent in developing countries, can cause significant blood loss, and in turn, raise iron requirements. This is worsened when the diet is inadequate in bioavailable iron, which is common in developing countries. In some cases, iron bioavailability of diets with a limited variety of foods can be as low as 5%. Compared with an estimated iron bioavailability of 18% from a mixed Western diet including meat, the iron bioavailability of a vegetarian diet is only about 10%, which makes the iron requirement of vegetarians 1.8 times higher than that of nonvegetarians [4]. Other groups having higher iron requirements include frequent blood donors and endurance athletes. Blood donations of about 500 mL/year require an addition of 0.6–0.7 mg iron daily, which is a substantial amount when compared with the 1.1 mg daily iron need in adult men. With frequent exercise and intense endurance training, the estimated iron requirement can be 30–70% higher [57, 58]. Daily iron losses are observed to be increased in male and female athletes with prolonged training [58]. Depressed iron stores and reductions in hematologic parameters are also seen with intense physical exercise [59, 60]. It has been suggested that intense physical exercise can result in increased gastrointestinal blood losses and hemoglobinuria from erythrocyte rupture in the feet during running [60, 61]. Furthermore, suboptimal dietary intake may also play a part in the marginal iron status of these individuals. In contrast to blood donors or athletes, women using oral contraceptives have lower iron needs as they have an ~60% reduction in menstrual blood loss [4]. However, postmenopausal women under hormone replacement therapy can have uterine bleeding, which increases their iron requirements [4, 62].

2 Dietary References Intakes

The Food and Nutrition Board of the Institute of Medicine developed the Dietary Reference Intakes (DRIs), which is a set of reference values that serve as standards for nutrient intakes for healthy persons in the United States and Canada [4]. Dietary Reference Intakes (DRIs) include Estimated Average Requirements (EAR), Recommended Dietary Allowances (RDA), Adequate Intakes (AI), and Tolerable Upper Intake Levels (UL).

The EAR is the average daily nutrient intake level estimated to meet the requirements of half of the healthy individuals in a particular life stage and gender group. The EAR for iron was determined using the factorial modeling method. Components including basal iron losses, increased iron requirement during growth due to blood volume expansion and increased tissue and storage iron, menstrual iron losses, fetal iron requirement and hemoglobin mass expansion during pregnancy, placenta iron concentration, and iron secretion into breast milk were used as factors in the modeling to estimate the physiological requirement for absorbed iron. Iron bioavailability was also taken into account when determining the percentage of iron absorption. Based on the assumption that 90% of dietary iron is non-heme iron with 16.8% absorption [63] and 10% of dietary iron is heme iron [64] with 25% absorption [36] in the typical diversified North American diet, an iron absorption of 18% was used to estimate EARs. For instance, the daily requirement of absorbed iron in adult men is 1.1 mg and with an absorption efficiency of 18%, the EAR is 6 mg. However, an 18% absorption efficiency does not apply to infants 7–12 months old or to pregnant women during their second and third trimesters [4]. Because the diet of infants aged 7–12 months contains less meat and more cereals and vegetables, a 10% bioavailability was used when estimating their EARs [4, 65, 66]. As for pregnant women, the iron absorption efficiency is increased as a physiological response; thus, 25% absorption efficiency was used to estimate their EAR.

Based on the EAR, the RDA is calculated so that this daily intake level meets the requirements of nearly all (97–98%) healthy individuals in a group. However, scientific evidence was considered insufficient to determine the EAR for breast-fed infants 0–6 months old. As a result, an RDA for this group was not established. Instead, the Adequate Intake (AI) is used for breast-fed infants 0–6 months old. AI is the recommended average daily nutrient intake level based on observed or estimates of nutrient intake by a group that is assumed to be adequate in this nutrient. As breast milk is the recommended sole source of food for healthy, full-term infants up to 6 months of age, the daily mean iron intake (0.27 mg/day) supplied by human milk was used to set the AI for these infants.

The Tolerable Upper Intake Level (UL) for iron is 40 mg/day for infants through 13 years old and 45 mg/day for everyone older, including pregnant and lactating women. UL is the highest level of daily intake that is likely to pose no risk of adverse health effects to almost all individuals in the general population. The UL represents total nutrient intake from food, water, and supplements. Although it is recommended not to exceed the UL intake level, intakes above the UL are appropriate for investigations during well-controlled trials and for individuals under medical supervision. The UL for iron was determined based on gastrointestinal distress including nausea, vomiting, diarrhea, and constipation as an adverse effect observed in a controlled, double-blind study in men and women receiving daily iron supplements of 60 mg. Together with the estimated mean dietary intake of 11 mg/day in these subjects, a lowest-observed-adverse-effect-level (LOAEL) of about 70 mg/day was determined, which was then divided by an uncertainly factor of 1.5, giving rise to the

Table 5.1 Dietary recommended intakes for iron

Group	EAR (mg/day)		RDA (mg/day)			
	Male	Female	Male	Female	AI (mg/day)	UL (mg/day)
0–6 months					0.27	40
7–12 months	6.9	6.3	11	11		40
1–3 years	3	3	7	7		40
4–8 years	4.1	4.1	10	10		40
9–13 years	5.9	5.7	8	8		40
14–18 years	7.7	7.9	11	15		45
19–30 years	6	8.1	8	18		45
31–50 years	6	8.1	8	18		45
51–70 years	6	5	8	8		45
>70 years	6	5	8	8		45
Pregnancy						
≤18 years		23		27		45
18–50 years		22		27		45
Lactation						
≤18 years		7		10		45
18–50 years		6.5		9		45

Abbreviations: *EAR* estimated average requirements, *RDA* recommended dietary allowances, *AI* adequate intakes, *UL* tolerable upper intake levels

UL of 45 mg/day. Only the adverse gastrointestinal effects were used to determine the UL for iron. The iron level for acute iron poisoning was not considered in setting the UL. Due to no evidence of clinically adverse effects of iron–zinc interactions and the disappearance of the impairment in zinc absorption when supplementary iron is consumed with food [67], the inhibitory effect of iron on zinc absorption was not considered when the UL was set. Other adverse effects such as increased risks of vascular disease and cancer were not used either because of the unclear relationship with dietary iron intake at that time. The 2001 DRIs for iron are shown in Table 5.1.

In the UK, estimated iron requirements are based on advice given by the Committee on Medical Aspects of Food and Nutrition Policy (COMA) in the early 1990s [68]. Reference Nutrient Intakes (RNI), which is equivalent to the RDA in the US, cover the needs of nearly all the population (97.5%). The RNI of iron for 0–3-month-old (1.7 mg/day) and 4–6-month-old (4.3 mg/day) infants are set higher than the AI (0.27 mg/day) of the DRI for 0–6-month-old infants. The RNI of iron for pregnant and lactating women is the same as that of nonpregnant and non-lactating women, whereas the RDA has a 9–12 mg/day iron increment and 5–9 mg/day iron decrement during pregnancy and lactation, respectively, compared to nonpregnant and non-lactating women. With the above exceptions, RNI and RDA of iron are quite similar during early childhood and adolescence, and in adults and elderly.

3 Dietary Sources of Iron and Iron Intake

Dietary iron exists as either heme iron or non-heme iron. Heme iron is derived from hemoglobin and myoglobin found in animal foods such as red meats, seafood, and poultry. Non-heme iron is found mainly in plant foods such as lentils, beans, rice, and maize. Heme iron absorption is efficient, ranging from 15% to 35%, and is not significantly affected by diet, although calcium has been reported to inhibit its absorption [36]. On the other hand, non-heme iron absorption ranges from 2% to 20% [69] and is influenced by inhibitors and enhancers found in the diet.

Phytates, polyphenols (e.g., tannic acid), as well as calcium decrease non-heme iron absorption [36, 70–73]. Phytate, which is present in legumes, rice, and whole grains, and tannic acid, which is found in tea and coffee, bind iron and form insoluble complexes in the intestinal lumen that inhibit iron absorption. Some proteins present in soybeans also have an inhibitory effect on non-heme iron absorption, and this is independent of the phytate effect [74]. Iron absorption from legumes such as soybeans, beans, and lentils has been reported to be as low as 0.84–1.91% [75], and vegetarians are often found to have low iron status [76]. Calcium has been suggested to interfere with the degradation of phytate and also inhibit absorption during iron transfer through the enterocyte [77]; however, the mechanism behind its inhibitory effect is not well understood. It is possible that calcium may have a transitory effect on iron absorption, thereby affecting the results from single meal isotope studies, as many studies on long-term feeding of high calcium diets or calcium supplements fail to find any adverse effects on iron status of infants, adolescents, and women. The bioavailability of non-heme iron is enhanced by ascorbic acid and meat proteins [78, 79]. Ascorbic acid reduces dietary ferric iron to ferrous iron and forms soluble complexes with iron. In addition, it helps to release non-heme iron bound to inhibitors. Likewise, low-molecular-weight peptides, released during digestion of meat proteins, bind to iron to form soluble complexes and prevent iron from binding to inhibitors [80, 81]. The enhancing effect of ascorbic acid and meat proteins is most apparent when these two enhancers are consumed with foods high in phytates or tannins, such as cereals, legumes, or tea. Vitamin A has been suggested to enhance the absorption of iron [82], but recent studies using stable isotopes fail to show such an effect [83]. The bioavailability of iron from breast milk is higher than from formulas or whole milk. Early studies indicated that infants absorb about 50% of iron in human milk, but only absorb about 10% of iron in formulas or whole milk iron [84]. Recent studies, however, suggest that the difference is not as large, although breast milk iron is better absorbed [85]. The mechanism behind this high bioavailability of breast milk iron has not been fully elucidated, but lactoferrin, which is the most abundant iron-binding proteins in human milk, has been proposed to play a role in iron absorption [86]. A specific receptor for lactoferrin has been found in the small intestine of infants [87] and as lactoferrin can resist digestion and is found intact in the stool of breast-fed infants [88], this is a plausible scenario. The fact that overexpression of the lactoferrin receptor in human intestinal cells in culture increases iron uptake [89] supports the notion of lactoferrin receptor-mediated uptake of iron from lactoferrin.

Dietary iron concentration is usually about 5–7 mg/1,000 kcal energy intake. An iron intake of about 12 mg/day is therefore expected with a typical adult diet. In general, boys and men have higher iron intakes than girls and women, and their intakes usually exceed the RDA in all age groups. The median iron intake of men is about 16–18 mg/day, whereas the median daily intake for most women is about 12 mg, which is lower than the RDA [4]. Dietary iron intake of pregnant women is approximately 15 mg/day, which is only about 56% of the RDA [4]. The low iron intake of women puts them at high risk of iron deficiency. Consumption of energy-restricted diets, low nutrient-dense diets, or diets with poorly bioavailable iron sources all contribute to an inadequate iron intake and should be discouraged.

It is helpful to include foods that enhance non-heme iron absorption when iron intakes are low and iron requirements and losses are high. Increasing ascorbic acid intake during meals and avoiding large amounts of tea and coffee with meals are helpful ways to improve iron absorption. Meat, poultry, and fish are good sources of iron as most of the iron provided is highly bioavailable heme iron. Moreover, meat proteins promote the absorption of non-heme iron [81]. Dried beans, dried fruits, and vegetables are also good food sources, although their non-heme iron is not as bioavailable as heme iron in meats. Indeed, vegetarians can also obtain adequate amounts of iron from their plant-based diets as long as their diets contain sufficient amounts of iron-rich plant foods. Some other food sources of iron are egg yolk, whole grain, cereal, and enriched breads. Milk, milk products, and corn are notoriously poor sources of iron. To be considered as high in iron, foods need to provide 20% or more of the daily value (DV), which is set as 18 mg for iron. Foods providing 10–19% of the daily value are considered good sources of iron, whereas foods providing 5% or less of the DV are low sources. Selected food sources of heme and non-heme iron are shown in Tables 5.2 and 5.3.

Table 5.2 Selected food sources of heme iron

Food	mg iron per serving	% daily value
Braunschweiger (a pork liver sausage), 3 oz	9.4	52
Breaded, fried oysters, 3 oz	6.0	33
Braised lean beef chunk, 3 oz	3.2	18
Breaded, fried clams, 3 oz	2.2	12
Roasted dark meat turkey, 3 oz	2.3	13
Roasted duck, 3 oz	2.3	13
Roasted chicken breast, 3 oz	1.1	6
Halibut, 3 oz	0.9	5
Broiled pork loin, 3 oz	0.8	4
Canned white tuna, 3 oz	0.8	4

From U.S. Department of Agriculture's Nutrient Database (http://www.nal.usda.gov/fnic/foodcomp/Data/SR20/nutrlist/sr20w303.pdf)

Table 5.3 Selected food sources of non-heme iron

Food	mg iron per serving	% daily value
Iron-fortified ready-to-eat cereal, 1 cup	18	100
Boiled soybean, 1 cup	8.8	48
Boiled lentils, 1 cup	6.6	36
Cooked spinach, 1 cup	6.4	35
Boiled kidney beans, 1 cup	5.2	29
Boiled black beans, 1 cup	3.6	20
Cooked enriched white rice, 1 cup	3.2	18
Seedless raisins, 1 cup	2.7	15
Whole egg, 1	1	6
Whole wheat bread, 1 slice	0.9	5

From U.S. Department of Agriculture's Nutrient Database (http://www.nal.usda.gov/fnic/foodcomp/Data/SR20/nutrlist/sr20w303.pdf)

4 Assessment of Iron Bioavailability

The bioavailability of iron in different foods varies depending on the food sources, composition of the diet, and physiological factors. Iron bioavailability can be assessed with the use of radioisotopes, stable isotopes, or the hemoglobin regeneration assay. For assessment using radioisotopes, the test food is either extrinsically or intrinsically labeled with the radioisotope ^{59}Fe, which is a gamma emitter. A whole body count is made shortly after the ingestion of the labeled test food using a whole body counter. The resulting count is considered a 100% value, which will subsequently decrease as a result of fecal excretion. Another count of the whole body radioactivity is made about 14 days later. After correcting the count for radioactive decay and expressing it as a percentage of the post-administration count, a direct measure of retained ^{59}Fe is determined. Whole body counting using radioisotopes is a direct, simple, and possibly the most reliable measure for iron retention. Besides, only tracer doses are required for labeling purposes and radioisotopes are easier to measure than stable isotopes. However, concern about the safety of ionizing radiation exists. Though radioisotopes are still being used, they are considered inappropriate to use in infants and children.

As an alternative to radioisotopes, stable isotopes are used, especially in studies on infants, children, and pregnant women. ^{54}Fe, ^{56}Fe, ^{57}Fe, ^{58}Fe are the four naturally occurring stable isotopes of iron, and the most commonly used stable isotopes in human nutrition studies are ^{57}Fe and ^{58}Fe [90].

The dose of the isotopes used depends on the natural abundance of the enriched isotope [90]. The natural abundance of ^{57}Fe and ^{58}Fe is 2.1% and 0.3%, respectively. Isotopes with the least natural abundance allow lower amounts of tracers to be used to achieve measurable enrichments in the samples. This is important as high doses of iron can make a significant contribution to the total iron content of the tested food, which, in turn, influences the absorption results. Unlike radioisotopes, stable isotopes do not emit radiation and thus whole body counting cannot be performed. Instead, hemoglobin incorporation of the stable isotopes is used as a direct measure of iron bioavailability. Since the majority of newly absorbed iron is incorporated into reticulocytes for hemoglobin synthesis, the proportion of the stable isotopes found in hemoglobin after ingestion of an isotopically labeled test food is used to determine iron bioavailability. Basically, a blood sample is obtained about 14 days after dosing and the isotopic enrichment of the blood sample is measured using mass spectrometry such as thermal ionization mass spectrometry (TIMS) or inductively coupled plasma mass spectrometry (ICP-MS).

The hemoglobin regeneration method was originally designed to determine iron bioavailability from different iron sources for fortification purposes. This method is rarely performed in humans and usually is used in animal models. Basically, rats are made iron depleted by feeding them an iron-deficient diet until anemia develops. They are then divided into groups and fed diets containing the iron compounds studied in different concentrations, and ferrous sulfate is used as a reference iron source. After weeks of repletion, hemoglobin levels increase and these increases reflect the bioavailability of the dietary iron sources and the iron concentrations of the diets. Iron bioavailability of the studied iron compounds is expressed relative to the effect of ferrous sulfate.

5 Iron Fortification and Iron Supplementation

Besides dietary modification and diversification to increase the iron content and bioavailability of the diet to prevent iron deficiency [91, 92], iron fortification and iron supplementation are used to improve iron nutrition of the population.

5.1 Iron Fortification

Iron fortification of commonly consumed food staples is a practical and cost-effective strategy to improve iron nutrition of a large population. Iron fortification has been used in developed countries for the last 60 years and has shown beneficial effects. The reduction in the prevalence of iron deficiency in young children in developed countries is attributed to iron fortification of infant formulas and weaning foods [93].Consumption of iron-fortified wheat flour is also thought to contribute to the low occurrence of iron deficiency anemia in female adolescents and women [94]. However, the efficacy of iron fortification in developing countries has traditionally not been high. The use of poorly bioavailable iron fortificants, low fortification levels, and inadequate consumption of the food vehicle have led to a low impact of iron fortification in developing countries [94, 95]. Recent innovative approaches ensuring the use of bioavailable iron in appropriate quantities have shown effectiveness in improving iron status of target populations.

Among all iron compounds used, ferrous sulfate is the most bioavailable with a relative bioavailability value (RBV) set as 100 and it ranks first as recommended iron compound used for food fortification by the WHO [96].Unfortunately, iron in ferrous sulfate reacts easily with other food components, causing unacceptable color and flavor changes, and often promotes fat oxidation and rancidity in the food. Therefore, it is not suitable to be used in foods with air-permeable packages

Table 5.4 Characteristics of some iron compounds used for iron fortification

Iron compounds	Characteristics	WHO recommendation	Food vehicles
Ferrous sulfate	Water soluble Most bioavailable Can cause unacceptable food sensory changes Suitable for food with fast turnover	Ranks first as the recommended iron compound used for food fortification	Cereal-based complementary foods, dry milk
Elemental iron (electrolytic iron)	Water insoluble Lower bioavailability than ferrous sulfate	Recommended levels used are twice the level of ferrous sulfate	Electrolytic iron: cereal-based complementary foods, breakfast cereals, low extraction wheat flour
Ferric pyrophosphate	Unlikely to cause unacceptable food sensory changes		Ferric pyrophosphate: rice, cocoa products, salt
NaFeEDTA	Water soluble, chelate	Recommended for high-phytate cereals and high-peptide sauces	Cereal flour, high extraction wheat flour, fish and soy sauce
	Higher bioavailability than ferrous sulfate when used in high-phytate foods	Added at half the level of ferrous sulfate in high-phytate foods	
	Does not precipitate peptides in fish and soy sauces	Added at the same level as ferrous sulfate in low-phytate foods	

and long storage time. Ferrous sulfate is, however, commonly used in infant formula and products packaged in cans and jars with short shelf life. Two other widely used iron fortificants are elemental iron (electrolytic iron) and ferric pyrophosphate. Because of their low solubility, they are unlikely to cause adverse sensory changes in food, but they have a lower RBV. To compensate for their lower bioavailability, their recommended levels used are twice as high as that for ferrous sulfate [96]. Another iron compound used is NaFeEDTA, which has a RBV two to three times higher than ferrous sulfate when used in foods with high phytic acid content. This distinct feature enables NaFeEDTA to be the recommended iron compound used in high-phytate cereals [96]. A summary of the characteristics of selected iron compounds is shown in Table 5.4. Apart from the RBV of the iron compounds, efficacy of the iron-fortified foods also depends on the amount of iron added to the food, the consumption pattern of the food vehicle by the target population, presence of dietary inhibitors or enhancers in the diet, amount of iron lacking in the diet, and the prevalence of other micronutrients deficiencies and infections, which negatively affect iron utilization.

WHO has recently issued recommendations for iron compounds to be used and guidelines to define iron fortification level and to assess iron status in order to monitor the efficacy of the fortification intervention. Most of the iron fortification studies conducted following these guidelines have shown good efficacy of the iron-fortified foods and improved iron status of the studied population. Fortification of maize flour with ferrous fumarate and other nutrients in South Africa has been shown to improve iron status and motor development and to reduce anemia in infants [97]. Moroccan children consuming ferrous sulfate or ferric pyrophosphate fortified salt [98], Vietnamese women consuming NaFeEDTA-fortified fish sauce [99], and children in Chile receiving ferrous sulfate and ascorbic acid–fortified milk powder [100] had decreased prevalence of iron deficiency anemia. Improved iron status has been observed in women receiving fortified wheat flour snack fortified with electrolytic iron or ferrous sulfate in Thailand [101] and in children consuming NaFeEDTA-fortified whole maize flour in Kenya [102]. Ferric pyrophosphate–fortified rice in India also decreased the prevalence of iron deficiency in children [103]. Though the above studies have shown good efficacy, infections or other micronutrients deficiencies can have negative impact on the efficacy of the iron fortification. For instance, the fortification of salt with ferric pyrophosphate improved the iron status of children in West Africa, but the prevalence of anemia remained unchanged. Iron utilization was believed to be impaired by the high prevalence of malaria and riboflavin deficiency in the studied children, in turn affecting the efficacy of the fortification [104]. In addition to iron fortification of commonly consumed food staples, home fortification of complementary foods with multiple micronutrient supplements has been developed in recent years. This practice had shown beneficial effects on target groups [105–109]. Supplements in the form of powders ("Sprinkles"), crushable tablets, and fat-based spreads, which were added to the weaning food just before feeding, have shown positive effects on motor development in 12-month-old Ghanaian infants [105]. Sprinkles powders have also been efficacious in treating and preventing anemia in Ghanaian [109] and Cambodian infants [106]. Iron status and growth were also improved in moderately malnourished infants in Malawi when using a fortified spread [107].

In regard to potential adverse effects of iron fortification, concern has been raised about mass iron fortification in some segments of the population who are iron sufficient or at risk of iron overload. Increased iron accumulation in individuals with hereditary hemochromatosis is a potential risk of iron fortification. In addition, iron absorption is increased in individuals with thalassemia, indicating that they would absorb more iron from fortified foods. Nevertheless, the level of iron fortification used is lower and more similar to a physiological environment than supplementation, and is considered a safe intervention. Overall, iron fortification imposed on existing food habits and the customary diet of the target population represents a cost-effective, feasible, safe, and sustainable approach in reducing the prevalence of iron deficiency.

5.2 *Iron Supplementation*

Another approach to control iron deficiency is iron supplementation. This approach is cost effective over short periods of time and efficacious if well monitored [110]. Unlike fortification, supplementation delivers a larger dose of iron, without food. Ferrous sulfate and ferrous gluconate are preferred to be used in iron supplements because of their high iron bioavailability and low cost. The recommended iron dose for supplementation is about 30 mg daily in developed countries, and can be as high as 240 mg daily in some developing countries [111]. When an iron supplement is taken on an empty stomach or with juice or water rather than with tea, coffee, or milk, absorption is enhanced. Other factors affecting the absorption of iron from the supplements include iron dosage, iron status of the recipient, and whether it is taken alone or with other supplements.

Routine iron supplementation is sometimes advised during infancy to prevent iron deficiency [39, 112]. Recommendations for iron supplementation of children in populations with high occurrence of anemia have been made [112] and shown to be effective in preventing iron deficiency. Pregnant women also have high iron requirements that are difficult to meet through diet alone; supplementation is therefore the standard recommendation and practice during pregnancy [39]. The International Nutritional Anemia Consultative Group (INACG)/WHO/UNICEF recommends daily iron supplements of 2 mg/kg weight be given to infants and young children 6–24 months of age to prevent anemia and a routine daily iron supplementation of 60 mg for 6 months for pregnant women [112]. Iron supplementation of pregnant women increased infant birth weight and reduced the incidence of preterm delivery and low-birth-weight infants, though it did not decrease the prevalence of anemia during the third trimester [54, 112]. Improved iron status and reduced impairments in cognitive and motor development were seen in iron-deficient children with iron supplementation [113]. Nonetheless, the prevalence of iron deficiency remains high in developing countries, which can be attributed to the poor compliance and logistics of supply [41, 114]. Due to negative effects such as gastric discomfort, potential toxicity, and potential interference with zinc absorption and status [67, 115], the acceptability of iron supplements is low. Individuals with undiagnosed hemochromatosis taking iron supplements is another problem, as additional iron will accumulate in tissues that are already iron overloaded. Other concerns regarding potential adverse effects of iron supplementation exist. Growth and weight gain of iron-replete infants and young children given iron supplements have been shown to be adversely affected in some studies [116, 117]. Iron supplementation lowered the gain in length and head circumference in Swedish infants with satisfactory iron status [116]. Weight gain was also lower in iron-replete young children receiving iron supplements [117]. In addition, copper status was found to be negatively affected in iron-supplemented infants as assessed by erythrocyte copper/zinc-superoxide dismutase [118]. Furthermore, the beneficial effect of zinc supplementation on growth in Indonesian infants was nullified with iron supplementation [115]. In malaria-endemic populations, iron supplementation is associated with increased risk of serious infections in children [119, 120]. Special caution with iron supplementation should therefore be exercised, especially in regions with high transmission of malaria and other serious infections. There is no doubt that iron supplementation benefits individuals at risk of iron deficiency; however, potential adverse effects to certain populations should not be neglected. Identification of individuals with iron deficiency or at risk of iron deficiency may be needed, so that iron supplementation can be targeted to individuals that will benefit from the supplementation.

References

1. Dallman PR, Siimes MA, Stekel A. Iron deficiency in infancy and childhood. Am J Clin Nutr. 1980;33:86–118.
2. Rios E, Lipschitz DA, Cook JD, Smith NJ. Relationship of maternal and infant iron stores as assessed by determination of plasma ferritin. Pediatrics. 1975;55:694–9.
3. Lönnerdal B, Hernell O. Iron, zinc, copper and selenium status of breast-fed infants and infants fed trace element fortified milk-based infant formula. Acta Paediatr. 1994;83:367–73.
4. Food and Nutrition Board, Institute of Medicine. Dietary reference intakes for vitamin A, vitamin K, arsenic, boron, chromium, copper, iodine, iron, manganese, molybdenum, nickel, silicon, vanadium, and zinc. Washington, DC: National Academy Press; 2002. p. 290–393.
5. Lukens JN. Iron metabolism and iron deficiency. St. Louis: Mosby; 1995.
6. Dewey KG, Cohen RJ, Rivera LL, Brown KH. Effects of age of introduction of complementary foods on iron status of breast-fed infants in Honduras. Am J Clin Nutr. 1998;67:878–84.
7. Gartner LM, Morton J, Lawrence RA, et al. Breastfeeding and the use of human milk. Pediatrics. 2005;115:496–506.
8. Grajeda R, Perez-Escamilla R, Dewey KG. Delayed clamping of the umbilical cord improves hematologic status of Guatemalan infants at 2 mo of age. Am J Clin Nutr. 1997;65:425–31.
9. Gupta R, Ramji S. Effect of delayed cord clamping on iron stores in infants born to anemic mothers: a randomized controlled trial. Indian Pediatr. 2002;39:130–5.
10. Chaparro CM, Neufeld LM, Tena Alavez G, Eguia-Liz Cedillo R, Dewey KG. Effect of timing of umbilical cord clamping on iron status in Mexican infants: a randomised controlled trial. Lancet. 2006;367:1997–2004.
11. Harthoorn-Lasthuizen EJ, Lindemans J, Langenhuijsen MM. Does iron-deficient erythropoiesis in pregnancy influence fetal iron supply? Acta Obstet Gynecol Scand. 2001;80:392–6.
12. Siimes AS, Siimes MA. Changes in the concentration of ferritin in the serum during fetal life in singletons and twins. Early Hum Dev. 1986;13:47–52.
13. Singla PN, Tyagi M, Shankar R, Dash D, Kumar A. Fetal iron status in maternal anemia. Acta Paediatr. 1996;85:1327–30.
14. Rasmussen K. Is there a causal relationship between iron deficiency or iron-deficiency anemia and weight at birth, length of gestation and perinatal mortality? J Nutr. 2001;131:590S–601S [discussion 601S–603S].
15. Colomer J, Colomer C, Gutierrez D, et al. Anaemia during pregnancy as a risk factor for infant iron deficiency: report from the Valencia Infant Anaemia Cohort (VIAC) study. Paediatr Perinat Epidemiol. 1990;4:196–204.
16. De Pee S, Bloem MW, Sari M, Kiess L, Yip R, Kosen S. The high prevalence of low hemoglobin concentration among Indonesian infants aged 3–5 months is related to maternal anemia. J Nutr. 2002;132:2215–21.

17. Kilbride J, Baker TG, Parapia LA, Khoury SA, Shuqaidef SW, Jerwood D. Anaemia during pregnancy as a risk factor for iron-deficiency anaemia in infancy: a case–control study in Jordan. Int J Epidemiol. 1999;28:461–8.
18. Fomon SJ, Ziegler EE, Serfass RE, Nelson SE, Frantz JA. Erythrocyte incorporation of iron is similar in infants fed formulas fortified with 12 mg/L or 8 mg/L of iron. J Nutr. 1997;127:83–8.
19. Hernell O, Lönnerdal B. Iron status of infants fed low-iron formula: no effect of added bovine lactoferrin or nucleotides. Am J Clin Nutr. 2002;76:858–64.
20. Dallman PR. Progress in the prevention of iron deficiency in infants. Acta Paediatr Scand Suppl. 1990;365:28–37.
21. Engelmann MD, Davidsson L, Sandström B, Walczyk T, Hurrell RF, Michaelsen KF. The influence of meat on nonheme iron absorption in infants. Pediatr Res. 1998;43:768–73.
22. Committee on Nutrition. American Academy of Pediatrics. Iron fortification of infant formulas. Pediatrics. 1999;104:119–23.
23. Lönnerdal B, Keen CL, Hurley LS. Iron, copper, zinc, and manganese in milk. Annu Rev Nutr. 1981;1:149–74.
24. Garby L, Sjölin S, Vuille JC. Studies on erythro-kinetics in infancy. IV. The long-term behaviour of radioiron in circulating foetal and adult haemoglobin, and its faecal excretion. Acta Paediatr. 1964;53:33–41.
25. Dibley MJ, Goldsby JB, Staehling NW, Trowbridge FL. Development of normalized curves for the international growth reference: historical and technical considerations. Am J Clin Nutr. 1987;46:736–48.
26. Hawkins WW. Iron, copper and cobalt. In: Beaton GH, McHenry EW, editors. Nutrition: a comprehensive treatise. New York: Academic; 1964. p. 309–72.
27. Smith NJ, Rios E. Iron metabolism and iron deficiency in infancy and childhood. Adv Pediatr. 1974;21:239–80.
28. Dallman PR. Iron deficiency in the weanling: a nutritional problem on the way to resolution. Acta Paediatr Scand Suppl. 1986;323:59–67.
29. Domellöf M, Lönnerdal B, Dewey KG, Cohen RJ, Rivera LL, Hernell O. Sex differences in iron status during infancy. Pediatrics. 2002;110:545–52.
30. Aggett PJ, Agostoni C, Axelsson I, et al. Iron metabolism and requirements in early childhood: do we know enough? A commentary by the ESPGHAN Committee on Nutrition. J Pediatr Gastroenterol Nutr. 2002;34:337–45.
31. Worwood M. The laboratory assessment of iron status – an update. Clin Chim Acta. 1997;259:3–23.
32. Domellöf M, Dewey KG, Lönnerdal B, Cohen RJ, Hernell O. The diagnostic criteria for iron deficiency in infants should be reevaluated. J Nutr. 2002;132:3680–6.
33. Lind T, Hernell O, Lönnerdal B, Stenlund H, Dömellof M, Persson LÅ. Dietary iron intake is positively associated with hemoglobin concentration during infancy but not during the second year of life. J Nutr. 2004;134:1064–70.
34. Domellöf M, Lönnerdal B, Abrams SA, Hernell O. Iron absorption in breast-fed infants: effects of age, iron status, iron supplements, and complementary foods. Am J Clin Nutr. 2002;76:198–204.
35. Hicks PD, Zavaleta N, Chen Z, Abrams SA, Lönnerdal B. Iron deficiency, but not anemia, upregulates iron absorption in breast-fed Peruvian infants. J Nutr. 2006;136:2435–8.
36. Hallberg L, Brune M, Erlandsson M, Sandberg AS, Rossander-Hulten L. Calcium: effect of different amounts on nonheme- and heme-iron absorption in humans. Am J Clin Nutr. 1991;53:112–9.
37. Hallberg L, Rossander-Hulten L, Brune M, Gleerup A. Bioavailability in man of iron in human milk and cow's milk in relation to their calcium contents. Pediatr Res. 1992;31:524–7.
38. Hurrell RF, Lynch SR, Trinidad TP, Dassenko SA, Cook JD. Iron absorption in humans as influenced by bovine milk proteins. Am J Clin Nutr. 1989;49:546–52.
39. CDC. Recommendations to prevent and control iron deficiency in the United States. MMWR 1998;47 (No. RR–3) p. 5.
40. Green R, Charlton R, Seftel H, et al. Body iron excretion in man: a collaborative study. Am J Med. 1968;45:336–53.
41. Yip R. Iron deficiency: contemporary scientific issues and international programmatic approaches. J Nutr. 1994;124:1479S–90S.
42. Beaton GH, Corey PN, Steele C. Conceptual and methodological issues regarding the epidemiology of iron deficiency and their implications for studies of the functional consequences of iron deficiency. Am J Clin Nutr. 1989;50:575–85.
43. Yip R. Age related changes in iron metabolism. In: Brock JH, Halliday JW, Pippard MJ, Powell LW, editors. Iron metabolism in health and disease. London: Saunders; 1994. p. 427–48.
44. Bothwell TH. Iron metabolism in man. Oxford, St. Louis: Blackwell Scientific; 1979 [distributors USA Blackwell Mosby].
45. Chamberlain G, Hytten FE. Clinical physiology in obstetrics. 2nd ed. Oxford/Boston/St. Louis: Blackwell; 1991 [Distributors USA Mosby-Year Book].

46. Puolakka J, Janne O, Pakarinen A, Järvinen PA, Vihko R. Serum ferritin as a measure of iron stores during and after normal pregnancy with and without iron supplements. Acta Obstet Gynecol Scand Suppl. 1980; 95:43–51.
47. Hallberg L. Perspectives on nutritional iron deficiency. Annu Rev Nutr. 2001;21:1–21.
48. Widdowson EM, Spray CM. Chemical development in utero. Arch Dis Child. 1951;26:205–14.
49. Barrett JF, Whittaker PG, Williams JG, Lind T. Absorption of non-haem iron from food during normal pregnancy. BMJ. 1994;309:79–82.
50. Fomon SJ, Zlotkin S. Nutritional anemias. Vevey/New York: Raven Press; 1992.
51. World Health Organization. Maternal Health and Safe Motherhood Programme, World Health Organization. Nutrition Programme. The prevalence of anaemia in women: a tabulation of available information. 2nd ed. Geneva: World Health Organization; 1992.
52. World Health Organization. Dept. of Nutrition for Health and Development. Iron deficiency anaemia: assessment, prevention and control. A guide for programme managers. Geneva: World Health Organization; 2001.
53. Brabin BJ, Hakimi M, Pelletier D. An analysis of anemia and pregnancy-related maternal mortality. J Nutr. 2001;131:604S–14S [discussion 14S–15S].
54. Cogswell ME, Parvanta I, Ickes L, Yip R, Brittenham GM. Iron supplementation during pregnancy, anemia, and birth weight: a randomized controlled trial. Am J Clin Nutr. 2003;78:773–81.
55. Rimon E, Levy S, Sapir A, et al. Diagnosis of iron deficiency anemia in the elderly by transferrin receptor-ferritin index. Arch Intern Med. 2002;162:445–9.
56. Smith DL. Anemia in the elderly. Am Fam Physician. 2000;62:1565–72.
57. Ehn L, Carlmark B, Höglund S. Iron status in athletes involved in intense physical activity. Med Sci Sports Exerc. 1980;12:61–4.
58. Weaver CM, Rajaram S. Exercise and iron status. J Nutr. 1992;122:782–7.
59. Stewart JG, Ahlquist DA, McGill DB, Ilstrup DM, Schwartz S, Owen RA. Gastrointestinal blood loss and anemia in runners. Ann Intern Med. 1984;100:843–5.
60. Magnusson B, Hallberg L, Rossander L, Swolin B. Iron metabolism and "sports anemia." II. A hematological comparison of elite runners and control subjects. Acta Med Scand. 1984;216:157–64.
61. Weight LM. 'Sports anaemia.' Does it exist? Sports Med. 1993;16:1–4.
62. Archer DF, Dorin MH, Heine W, Nanavati N, Arce JC. Uterine bleeding in postmenopausal women on continuous therapy with estradiol and norethindrone acetate. Endometrium Study Group. Obstet Gynecol. 1999;94:323–9.
63. Cook JD, Dassenko SA, Lynch SR. Assessment of the role of nonheme-iron availability in iron balance. Am J Clin Nutr. 1991;54:717–22.
64. Raper NR, Rosenthal JC, Woteki CE. Estimates of available iron in diets of individuals 1 year old and older in the nationwide food consumption survey. J Am Diet Assoc. 1984;84:783–7.
65. Davidsson L, Galan P, Cherouvrier F, et al. Bioavailability in infants of iron from infant cereals: effect of dephytinization. Am J Clin Nutr. 1997;65:916–20.
66. Skinner JD, Carruth BR, Houck KS, et al. Longitudinal study of nutrient and food intakes of infants aged 2 to 24 months. J Am Diet Assoc. 1997;97:496–504.
67. Sandström B, Davidsson L, Cederblad Å, Lönnerdal B. Oral iron, dietary ligands and zinc absorption. J Nutr. 1985;115:411–4.
68. Committee on Medical Aspects of Food Policy. Dietary reference values for food energy and nutrients for the United Kingdom. Report of the panel on dietary reference values of the Committee on Medical Aspects of Food Policy. Rep Health Soc Subj (Lond). 1991;41(1):1–210.
69. Tapiero H, Gate L, Tew KD. Iron: deficiencies and requirements. Biomed Pharmacother. 2001;55:324–32.
70. Brune M, Rossander L, Hallberg L. Iron absorption and phenolic compounds: importance of different phenolic structures. Eur J Clin Nutr. 1989;43:547–57.
71. Cook JD, Reddy MB, Burri J, Juillerat MA, Hurrell RF. The influence of different cereal grains on iron absorption from infant cereal foods. Am J Clin Nutr. 1997;65:964–9.
72. Minihane AM, Fairweather-Tait SJ. Effect of calcium supplementation on daily nonheme-iron absorption and long-term iron status. Am J Clin Nutr. 1998;68:96–102.
73. Samman S, Sandström B, Toft MB, et al. Green tea or rosemary extract added to foods reduces nonheme-iron absorption. Am J Clin Nutr. 2001;73:607–12.
74. Lynch SR, Dassenko SA, Cook JD, Juillerat MA, Hurrell RF. Inhibitory effect of a soybean-protein – related moiety on iron absorption in humans. Am J Clin Nutr. 1994;60:567–72.
75. Lynch SR, Beard JL, Dassenko SA, Cook JD. Iron absorption from legumes in humans. Am J Clin Nutr. 1984;40:42–7.
76. Donovan UM, Gibson RS. Iron and zinc status of young women aged 14 to 19 years consuming vegetarian and omnivorous diets. J Am Coll Nutr. 1995;14:463–72.
77. Hallberg L, Rossander-Hulthen L, Brune M, Gleerup A. Inhibition of haem-iron absorption in man by calcium. Br J Nutr. 1993;69:533–40.

78. Hunt JR, Gallagher SK, Johnson LK. Effect of ascorbic acid on apparent iron absorption by women with low iron stores. Am J Clin Nutr. 1994;59:1381–5.
79. Siegenberg D, Baynes RD, Bothwell TH, et al. Ascorbic acid prevents the dose-dependent inhibitory effects of polyphenols and phytates on nonheme-iron absorption. Am J Clin Nutr. 1991;53:537–41.
80. Taylor PG, Martinez-Torres C, Romano EL, Layrisse M. The effect of cysteine-containing peptides released during meat digestion on iron absorption in humans. Am J Clin Nutr. 1986;43:68–71.
81. Hurrell RF, Reddy MB, Juillerat M, Cook JD. Meat protein fractions enhance nonheme iron absorption in humans. J Nutr. 2006;136:2808–12.
82. Layrisse M, Garcia-Casal MN, Solano L, et al. New property of vitamin A and beta-carotene on human iron absorption: effect on phytate and polyphenols as inhibitors of iron absorption. Arch Latinoam Nutr. 2000;50:243–8.
83. Walczyk T, Davidsson L, Rossander-Hulthen L, Hallberg L, Hurrell RF. No enhancing effect of vitamin A on iron absorption in humans. Am J Clin Nutr. 2003;77:144–9.
84. Saarinen UM, Siimes MA, Dallman PR. Iron absorption in infants: high bioavailability of breast milk iron as indicated by the extrinsic tag method of iron absorption and by the concentration of serum ferritin. J Pediatr. 1977;91:36–9.
85. Fomon SJ, Ziegler EE, Nelson SE. Erythrocyte incorporation of ingested 58Fe by 56-day-old breast-fed and formula-fed infants. Pediatr Res. 1993;33:573–6.
86. Lönnerdal B, Iyer S. Lactoferrin: molecular structure and biological function. Annu Rev Nutr. 1995;15:93–110.
87. Kawakami H, Lönnerdal B. Isolation and function of a receptor for human lactoferrin in human fetal intestinal brush-border membranes. Am J Physiol. 1991;261:G841–6.
88. Davidson LA, Lönnerdal B. Persistence of human milk proteins in the breast-fed infant. Acta Paediatr Scand. 1987;76:733–40.
89. Suzuki YA, Shin K, Lönnerdal B. Molecular cloning and functional expression of a human intestinal lactoferrin receptor. Biochemistry. 2001;40:15771–9.
90. Abrams SA. Stable isotopes studies of mineral metabolism: calcium, magnesium, and iron. In: Wong WW, Abrams SA, editors. Stable isotopes in human nutrition. Cambridge: CAB International; 2003. p. 35–59.
91. Gibson RS, Hotz C. Dietary diversification/modification strategies to enhance micronutrient content and bioavailability of diets in developing countries. Br J Nutr. 2001;85 Suppl 2:S159–66.
92. Gibson RS, Perlas L, Hotz C. Improving the bioavailability of nutrients in plant foods at the household level. Proc Nutr Soc. 2006;65:160–8.
93. Fomon S. Infant feeding in the 20th century: formula and beikost. J Nutr. 2001;131:409S–20S.
94. Hurrell RF. The mineral fortification of foods. Surrey: Leatherhead; 1999.
95. Hurrell R, Bothwell T, Cook JD, et al. The usefulness of elemental iron for cereal flour fortification: a SUSTAIN Task Force report. Sharing United States technology to aid in the improvement of nutrition. Nutr Rev. 2002;60:391–406.
96. World Health Organization. Guidelines on food fortification with micronutrients. Geneva: World Health Organization; 2006.
97. Faber M, Kvalsvig JD, Lombard CJ, Benade AJ. Effect of a fortified maize-meal porridge on anemia, micronutrient status, and motor development of infants. Am J Clin Nutr. 2005;82:1032–9.
98. Zimmermann MB, Zeder C, Chaouki N, Saad A, Torresani T, Hurrell RF. Dual fortification of salt with iodine and microencapsulated iron: a randomized, double-blind, controlled trial in Moroccan schoolchildren. Am J Clin Nutr. 2003;77:425–32.
99. Thuy PV, Berger J, Davidsson L, et al. Regular consumption of NaFeEDTA-fortified fish sauce improves iron status and reduces the prevalence of anemia in anemic Vietnamese women. Am J Clin Nutr. 2003;78:284–90.
100. Hertrampf E, Olivares M, Pizzaro F, Walter T. Impact of iron fortified milk in infants: evaluation of effectiveness. Why iron is important and what to do about it: a new perspective. Report of the International Nutritional Anemia Consultative Group Symposium, INACG. Hanoi; 2001.
101. Zimmermann MB, Winichagoon P, Gowachirapant S, et al. Comparison of the efficacy of wheat-based snacks fortified with ferrous sulfate, electrolytic iron, or hydrogen-reduced elemental iron: randomized, double-blind, controlled trial in Thai women. Am J Clin Nutr. 2005;82:1276–82.
102. Andang'o PE, Osendarp SJ, Ayah R, et al. Efficacy of iron-fortified whole maize flour on iron status of schoolchildren in Kenya: a randomised controlled trial. Lancet. 2007;369:1799–806.
103. Moretti D, Zimmermann MB, Muthayya S, et al. Extruded rice fortified with micronized ground ferric pyrophosphate reduces iron deficiency in Indian schoolchildren: a double-blind randomized controlled trial. Am J Clin Nutr. 2006;84:822–9.
104. Wegmuller R, Camara F, Zimmermann MB, Adou P, Hurrell RF. Salt dual-fortified with iodine and micronized ground ferric pyrophosphate affects iron status but not hemoglobin in children in Cote d'Ivoire. J Nutr. 2006;136:1814–20.

105. Adu-Afarwuah S, Lartey A, Brown KH, Zlotkin S, Briend A, Dewey KG. Randomized comparison of 3 types of micronutrient supplements for home fortification of complementary foods in Ghana: effects on growth and motor development. Am J Clin Nutr. 2007;86:412–20.
106. Giovannini M, Sala D, Usuelli M, et al. Double-blind, placebo-controlled trial comparing effects of supplementation with two different combinations of micronutrients delivered as sprinkles on growth, anemia, and iron deficiency in Cambodian infants. J Pediatr Gastroenterol Nutr. 2006;42:306–12.
107. Kuusipalo H, Maleta K, Briend A, Manary M, Ashorn P. Growth and change in blood haemoglobin concentration among underweight Malawian infants receiving fortified spreads for 12 weeks: a preliminary trial. J Pediatr Gastroenterol Nutr. 2006;43:525–32.
108. Smuts CM, Dhansay MA, Faber M, et al. Efficacy of multiple micronutrient supplementation for improving anemia, micronutrient status, and growth in South African infants. J Nutr. 2005;135:653S–9S.
109. Zlotkin S, Arthur P, Schauer C, Antwi KY, Yeung G, Piekarz A. Home-fortification with iron and zinc sprinkles or iron sprinkles alone successfully treats anemia in infants and young children. J Nutr. 2003;133:1075–80.
110. Baltussen R, Knai C, Sharan M. Iron fortification and iron supplementation are cost-effective interventions to reduce iron deficiency in four subregions of the world. J Nutr. 2004;134:2678–84.
111. Sood SK, Ramachandran K, Mathur M, et al. W.H.O. sponsored collaborative studies on nutritional anaemia in India. 1. The effects of supplemental oral iron administration to pregnant women. Q J Med. 1975;44:241–58.
112. Stoltzfus RJ, Dreyfuss ML, International Nutritional Anemia Consultative Group, World Health Organization, United Nations Children's Fund. Guidelines for the use of iron supplements to prevent and treat iron deficiency anemia. Washington, DC: ILSI Press; 1998.
113. Iannotti LL, Tielsch JM, Black MM, Black RE. Iron supplementation in early childhood: health benefits and risks. Am J Clin Nutr. 2006;84:1261–76.
114. Yip R, Ramakrishnan U. Experiences and challenges in developing countries. J Nutr. 2002;132:827S–30S.
115. Lind T, Lönnerdal B, Stenlund H, et al. A community-based randomized controlled trial of iron and zinc supplementation in Indonesian infants: interactions between iron and zinc. Am J Clin Nutr. 2003;77:883–90.
116. Dewey KG, Domellöf M, Cohen RJ, Landa Rivera L, Hernell O, Lönnerdal B. Iron supplementation affects growth and morbidity of breast-fed infants: results of a randomized trial in Sweden and Honduras. J Nutr. 2002;132:3249–55.
117. Idjradinata P, Watkins WE, Pollitt E. Adverse effect of iron supplementation on weight gain of iron-replete young children. Lancet. 1994;343:1252–4.
118. Domellöf M, Dewey KG, Cohen RJ, Lönnerdal B, Hernell O. Iron supplements reduce erythrocyte copper–zinc superoxide dismutase activity in term, breastfed infants. Acta Paediatr. 2005;94:1578–82.
119. Gera T, Sachdev HP. Effect of iron supplementation on incidence of infectious illness in children: systematic review. BMJ. 2002;325:1142.
120. Oppenheimer SJ. Iron and its relation to immunity and infectious disease. J Nutr. 2001;131:616S–33S.

Chapter 6
Intestinal Iron Absorption

Andrew T. McKie and Robert J. Simpson

Keywords Dcytb • DMT1 • Duodenum • Ferroportin • HCP1 • Heme • Hepcidin • Hephaestin • HIF2 alpha • Iron • IRP1 • IRP2 • Regulation

1 Introduction

The last 15 years has seen tremendous advances made in our understanding, at the molecular level, of the proteins involved in iron transport and regulation of iron metabolism with the major players involved in intestinal non-heme iron transport now identified. This achievement comes after several decades had seen little progress in this area and it was the application of modern molecular biology techniques starting about 25 years ago that has revolutionized our understanding. Advances have also been made in understanding the regulation of iron absorption with the iron hormone hepcidin emerging as the key systemic regulator. Moreover, the regulation of hepcidin production by several well-known signal transduction pathways has been shown and the stage has now been reached where intervention treatments based on molecules which regulate hepcidin represent viable approaches to the treatment of iron disorders. The molecular regulation of the main intestinal proteins involved in iron absorption is well advanced. The present chapter will bring together recent findings on physiology, molecular biology, and biochemistry of iron absorption and attempt to provide an integrated view of the regulation of this process.

2 Overview of Iron Metabolism in Mammals

In man, the normal diet should contain 13–18 mg of iron per day, of which only 1 mg is absorbed. In iron deficiency, absorptive capacity may be increased to 2–4 mg and in iron overload it is reduced to 0.5 mg. Under normal circumstances, the intestine takes up more iron than is required and, depending on the body's demand for iron, a certain amount is transferred to the circulation, the rest being retained by the enterocyte and lost when the villus cells are exfoliated. The principle site of iron absorption is the duodenum and proximal jejunum. Once iron is absorbed into the bloodstream, it is conserved and there is little excretion via the kidneys. This was established by pioneering work of McCance and Widdowson who were the first to suggest that body iron stores were determined by

A.T. McKie, Ph.D. (✉) • R.J. Simpson, Ph.D.
Division of Nutritional Sciences, Kings College London, London SE1 9NH, UK
e-mail: andrew.t.mckie@kcl.ac.uk

G.J. Anderson and G. McLaren (eds.), *Iron Physiology and Pathophysiology in Humans*, Nutrition and Health, DOI 10.1007/978-1-60327-485-2_6,

regulation of intestinal iron absorption [1]. They found that when various transition metals were intravenously injected into the body, iron was the only metal not rapidly excreted in the urine.

The formation of red blood cells requires about 30 mg of iron daily and this is balanced by an equal flux of iron from the breakdown of senescent red blood cells by the reticuloendothelial (RE) cells in the spleen, liver (Kupffer cells), and bone marrow. Body iron losses are small in comparison and are associated with the sloughing of epithelial cells (skin, gastrointestinal cells, urinary tract cells) and the loss of fluids (e.g., tears, sweat, and particularly in menstruating women, blood). This accounts for the loss of 1 mg/day of iron. In man, dietary iron intake consists of two components: heme iron (predominantly in red meat) and non-heme or inorganic iron (also abundant in meat, but the main form of iron in vegetables, cereals, etc.). The absorption of both is discussed below.

3 Heme Iron Absorption

Intestinal absorption of heme is not yet well understood and it is not clear how heme iron enters the intestinal mucosa. Early work established that heme is released by digestion of hemoproteins in the stomach and duodenal lumen [2–4]. Heme differs from non-heme iron in its solubility and availability profile. Heme tends to form oligomeric aggregates in acid solution and this is promoted if ligands can bridge between the iron atoms chelated within the heme or if neutral molecules such as water are the iron ligands. If high enough concentrations of charged ligands are present, bridging does not occur and heme becomes soluble. Examples of good ligands for heme iron are amines such as arginate and importantly, hydroxide. Thus, solubility of heme is promoted by high concentrations of hydroxide (i.e., higher pH values) or amino acids or peptides that can act as ligands to the iron within heme. As with non-heme iron absorption (see below), the machinery for heme iron absorption is most active in the proximal intestine [5] and involves breakdown of the heme within the mucosa by heme oxygenase [6] with release of iron that is then transported to the blood, probably by the same mechanism used for non-heme iron (i.e., via ferroportin as discussed in detail below). The mucosal uptake of heme appears to involve a receptor on the brush border membrane [7] and transport of the heme into the enterocytes. HCP1 was identified as a candidate transporter for heme [8]; however, this protein was subsequently shown to be more active as a folate transporter and renamed PCFT [9, 10]. Loss of function mutations in PCFT/HCP1 are associated with hereditary folate deficiency and further work is needed to clarify whether this protein plays any significant role in heme absorption. It is noteworthy that absorption of heme iron is not regulated as tightly by iron stores as non-heme iron absorption [7], presumably relating to a less tightly regulated mucosal uptake step. The oxidation state of heme iron does not seem to affect its solubility and the absorption of heme iron is not affected by food factors that alter non-heme iron absorption. Thus, heme iron has a relatively high bioavailability (15–30%) that is relatively constant. One result of this weaker regulation and high bioavailability is that higher iron stores are associated with high intakes of heme iron [11–13].

4 Non-Heme Iron Absorption

Knowledge of non-heme iron absorption is much more extensive than that of heme absorption as the former is more highly regulated and more associated with iron deficiency. The remainder of this chapter focuses on non-heme iron absorption. Non-heme (or inorganic) iron is present in the diet as either the reduced ferrous (Fe(II), Fe^{2+}) ionic form or the oxidized ferric (Fe(III), Fe^{3+}) form. Under normal physiological conditions (i.e., neutral pH and in the presence of oxygen), ferrous iron is rapidly oxidized to the ferric form which has a strong tendency to precipitate as iron hydroxide. Several luminal factors, both in the diet and secreted by the gut, can have marked effects on the absorption of dietary iron. In studies of iron absorption in animals and humans, subjects are normally fasted before administering radioactively labeled iron into the intestine. The presence of food drastically reduces the bioavailability of non-heme iron due to components of the diet (such as phytates, polyphenols) binding the iron to form complexes that are not available for intestinal uptake [14]. In contrast, the presence of luminal reducing agents, such as ascorbate, is known to enhance iron absorption. Iron binding or complexing agents, forming weaker, soluble low-molecular-mass complexes (such as citrate, ascorbate, and perhaps some amino acids and peptides and other organic acids) can also enhance iron absorption. Non-heme iron is absorbed early in digestion mainly in the duodenum where the low pH favors solubility and reduction of iron. Further down the intestine, it is likely that the formation of insoluble ferric complexes reduces bioavailability. The transport of non-heme iron across the duodenal mucosa has been studied intensively over the years and is highly adaptive to changes in iron requirements (low iron stores, pregnancy, erythropoiesis, hypoxia). Much progress has been made in the last few years in identifying the proteins involved in this process and these will be described below.

5 Anatomical Location of Iron Absorption

It has been shown that iron in the stomach is relatively soluble and significant amounts are reduced to Fe (II) by dietary and secreted factors [15, 16]. The low pH of the stomach is a major factor in the release of ionized, soluble iron from the food, and loss of gastric acid secretion can compromise iron absorption, leading to anemia [17]. Early studies of the iron absorption mechanism and its regulation established that this process was mainly confined to the duodenum and proximal jejunum where the small intestinal lumenal pH is most suited to maintaining non-heme iron in a soluble form (reviewed in [18]). With the exception of hephaestin, whose mRNA is more uniformly expressed along the length of the gut, the duodenum and proximal jejunum coincides with highest expression of various iron transport molecules – DCYTB, DMT1, and FPN. However, more recent data have shown that the colon also expresses relatively high levels of FPN, DMT1, and hephaestin, but not DCYTB [19, 20]. This would suggest that the colon may also be important for iron metabolism and, given the low expression of FPN in the ileum, it is possible that some iron lost through ileal epithelial cell sloughing is reabsorbed in the colon. The lack of DCYTB in the colon is interesting and may reflect the fact that the environment in the colonic lumen is reducing and therefore a surface reductase is not required, that another reductase is present, or that another form of iron is absorbed. Due to its high iron absorptive capacity with a high degree of regulation, the remainder of this chapter focuses on proximal intestine and especially the duodenum.

6 Iron Absorption: A Two-Step Process

Manis and Schachter showed in 1961 that the absorption process in the proximal intestine can be divided into two steps, namely, *uptake* of lumenal iron into the mucosa and *transfer* of iron from mucosa to the blood [21]. This terminology has been almost universally adopted in subsequent work, as it fits not only with iron absorption kinetic parameters that have been extensively measured in vivo, but also with the major sites of localization of the principle proteins involved in iron absorption (below).

Early work provided evidence for the regulation of iron absorption at both the uptake and transfer steps, with a few experiments suggesting distinct mechanisms operated on the two steps. For a review of the early studies on iron absorption, please see [22]. Simple principles of metabolic regulation would lead one to expect the primary regulated step in a pathway would be the first committed step. In many metabolic pathways, this is indeed observed. In the case of a potentially toxic nutrient like iron, things get more complicated. Older ideas ("mucosal block") focused on iron as a potentially toxic metal and the body had to be protected from excess absorption. Such ideas could fit with the primary regulated step being the basolateral transfer step. However, iron is essential as well as being potentially toxic, not only for the body but also for the enterocytes responsible for absorbing it from the diet. The latter consideration means that mucosal uptake also needs to be regulated and some regulated coordination of the two steps is needed to maintain an efficient flux across the enterocyte and prevent enterocyte iron levels dropping too low or building up too high. Elegant molecular mechanisms have been identified which can bring about this complex regulation and these will be described in more detail below. Current molecular evidence supports earlier kinetic studies and indicates that the basolateral transport of iron is rate-limiting for iron entry into the circulation.

7 Proteins Involved in Uptake: DMT1 and DCYTB

7.1 DMT1

Divalent metal-ion transporter 1 (DMT1; also known as NRAMP2 or DCT1) was the first mammalian iron transporter to be identified by two groups working independently. Gunshin et al. [23] used the *Xenopus* oocyte expression cloning system to identify a cDNA that caused a rapid inward current in the presence of ferrous iron in the external medium in comparison with a water-injected control. The transport of iron into the oocyte was highly dependent on an inward-directed proton gradient. The mechanism of iron transport is therefore likely to be proton coupled and requires a pH gradient [24]. *DMT1* mRNA was shown to be highly expressed in the duodenum and strongly upregulated in iron deficiency. The mRNA was later shown to contain a functional iron responsive element (IRE) in its 3′ untranslated region which can mediate iron-dependent regulation [25]. In the other study, Fleming et al. were working on the genetic basis of the microcytic anemia (mk/mk) mouse [26]. This mouse strain has a hypochromic, microcytic anemia and affected animals have both defective intestinal iron absorption and reduced iron uptake by developing erythroid cells. The causative gene was identified as *Nramp2* [26]. The same group later showed an identical mutation was present in Dmt1 in the Belgrade rat which has a similar microcytic anemia [27]. Thus, the expression pattern along with transport data and powerful genetic evidence are consistent with DMT1 being responsible for the regulated step of duodenal iron uptake. Genetic knockout experiments have since shown that DMT1 is essential for life [28] and human DMT1 mutations that cause anemia have been identified [29–31]. DMT1 plays a role in reticulocyte iron uptake (and indeed in iron uptake by most body cells) as well as intestinal iron uptake, and mice with global Dmt1 knockout die within a few days of birth with severe anemia [28]. Complete loss of Dmt1 is more severe than the mk or Belgrade mutations mentioned above, indicating that these mutants retain some Dmt1 function. In an intestine-specific Dmt1 knockout, survival is improved but mice rapidly become iron deficient after weaning, indicating DMT1 is the major pathway for iron absorption in adults [28]. A detailed study of iron absorption in Dmt1 knockout mice has not been published; however, there are sufficient published data [28] to estimate total body iron levels (and therefore dietary iron absorption) in such mice. The fact that the mice grow normally for at least 3 days after birth strongly suggests normal iron absorption from dam's milk. Thus, neonatal iron absorption from the mother's milk seems to be Dmt1 independent. Mice start to consume adult foods at about 15 days of age and wean at about 21 days and a progressive decline in body iron seems to occur from about 15 days of age in the Dmt1 intestinal knockout. Intestine-specific Dmt1 knockout mice still grow from 4 to 8 weeks of age and therefore their calculated total body iron increases, suggesting that a non-DMT1 absorption pathway may be present [28]. The assumptions needed for the total body iron calculation, however, make this increase debatable. Suggestions have been made that in mice in which both the *Dmt1* (intestine-specific) and *Hfe* genes have been knocked out, an alternative iron absorption pathway exists [32]. However, the data supporting this possibility have not been published and the conclusion is based on the improved survival of the double knockout mice [28]. This increased survival could be explained by increased prenatal and neonatal iron absorption associated with the *Hfe* deletion, leading to increased iron stores at weaning that allow the Dmt1 intestinal knockout animals to survive a little longer. In addition, the tissue-specific gene knockout may not be 100% efficient in all the mice. The question of alternate (i.e., non-DMT1) iron absorption pathways that may make a minor contribution to adult iron absorption therefore remains to be resolved and more detailed studies of the Dmt1 intestinal knockout mouse need to be carried out.

DMT1 has been shown to transport other divalent metals such as Zn, Mn, Co, and Cd. However, whether this property of DMT1 has any physiological relevance is open to question. In the case of zinc, absorption from the diet is controlled by members of the ZIP and ZNT family. There is also evidence that ZIP4 and ZIP14 can transport iron and may play a role in iron uptake in some tissues [33, 34]. It has been demonstrated that manganese absorption is impaired in Belgrade rats (presumably as a result of the mutation in Dmt1 [35]). Iron deficiency or anemia cause increases in tissue cadmium levels, suggesting that these conditions could be risk factors for cadmium toxicity [36]. Interestingly, the increased Cd uptake may not be mediated by DMT1 [37, 38]. On the other hand, Zn and Cu have been reported to regulate DMT1 expression [39, 40], providing another possible mechanism for metal interactions with iron absorption.

7.2 DCYTB

DMT1 transports only ferrous iron whereas dietary iron is likely to be mostly in the ferric form. Thus, a ferric reductase was predicted to be present in the duodenal mucosa [41]. The presence of such a surface ferric reductase activity in the duodenum was first described some time before the discovery of DMT1 [42]. The reductase activity was strongly stimulated by hypoxia and iron deficiency, both of which stimulate iron absorption, especially of ferric iron [42]. In addition, it was found that the activity was highest in the duodenum and lowest in the ileum, compatible with the profile of iron absorption along the gut. Attempts to purify the protein responsible for this activity provided evidence that it was associated with a b-type heme center that was immunologically distinct from the NADPH oxidase GP91-Phox [43]. The protein was, however, never successfully purified using biochemical methods as the heme was lost early in the purification [44]. The gene responsible for this activity, Dcytb (for duodenal cytochrome b; also called Cybrd1), was eventually identified using a subtractive cloning strategy [45]. The protein sequence of DCYTB was homologous to cytochrome b561, a b-type heme transmembrane dehydroascorbate reductase highly expressed in chromaffin granule membranes in the adrenal medulla [46, 47]. The role of b561 is to reduce granular dehydroascorbate to ascorbate by transporting an electron donated by cytoplasmic ascorbate across the granule membrane [48]. In addition to b561, DCYTB was identical to the N terminus of a protein called P30 [49, 50]. When expressed in either *Xenopus* oocytes or cultured cells, Dcytb induces ferric reductase activity. The protein has recently been found at high concentrations in the membrane of mature red blood cells of scorbutic species such as human and guinea pig, but is absent from those of non-scorbutic species (those able to synthesize ascorbic acid) such as mice and rats [51]. This has led to the hypothesis that DCYTB plays a physiological role in ascorbate regeneration; however, this has yet to be confirmed.

7.3 *Dcytb* Knockout Mouse

In 2005, Gunshin et al. described the phenotype of a Dcytb knockout mouse in which Dcytb was deleted in all tissues [52]. The Dcytb knockout mice on the 129 background displayed a relatively mild phenotype – relative to loss of either DMT1 or FPN – with a small reduction in liver iron, normal hematological parameters with no overt anemia. The authors therefore concluded that DCYTB was not required for iron absorption in mice. However, the study was limited to measurement of liver iron and no measurements of iron absorption itself or duodenal reductase activity were made to rule out compensatory effects from other ferric reductases [53]. The study did not address possible confounding strain effects, e.g., the fact that the 129 strain are highly resistant to iron deficiency due to their high liver iron stores (relative to other strains such as C57) and do not become anemic even when chronically fed iron-restricted diets. Hence the effect of lack of DCYTB may be more obvious in another background such as C57. We have now examined the same DCYTB knockout mice used by Gunshin et al. and measured duodenal ferric reductase activity. We found that Dcytb is the only iron-regulated duodenal ferric reductase and that in Dcytb knockout mice inclusive there were significant decreases in spleen iron compared to WT mice (Choi et al. 2010, unpublished). We conclude that Dcytb is required for optimal iron metabolism likely by increasing the bioavailability of ferrous iron for the transporter DMT1, a process that is likely to be important under dietary iron-limited conditions.

7.4 Proteins Involved in Iron Transfer: Ferroportin and Hephaestin

The basolateral iron transporter was identified by three groups working independently and therefore surfaces in the literature under three different aliases: Ireg1 [54], ferroportin [55], and MTP1 [56]. The more descriptive appellation of ferroportin (FPN) is now most widely used. FPN was first isolated and reported using the same strategy which identified Dcytb [54]. The predominant mRNA for FPN contains a functional IRE sequence, is highly localized to the duodenum and is regulated by several independent stimulators of iron absorption. The presence of an alternatively spliced, non-IRE FPN mRNA has been recently described and resolves some issues regarding FPN regulation (see below) [57]. The gene encodes a highly hydrophobic membrane protein with 10–12 transmembrane spanning domains, which bears little sequence identity with any other transporter family. Transfecting polarized epithelial cells with a tagged FPN showed the protein was targeted to the basolateral membrane. This finding led to the hypothesis that FPN was an iron-regulated protein involved in the transfer of iron to the circulation across this membrane. The *Xenopus* oocyte expression system demonstrated that FPN did indeed stimulate efflux of iron [54]. Donovan et al. [55] used positional cloning to identify the gene responsible for the *wiessherbst* (weh) mutant phenotype in zebrafish, so called because their lack of hemoglobin gives them a pale appearance. The gene they identified was the zebrafish homologue of FPN. In zebrafish, FPN was found to be expressed in the yolk sac where it is likely to be responsible for transfer of iron from the maternally derived iron stores to the embryonic circulation. In the third report, an approach of enriching for cDNAs containing IREs [56] was used.

In addition to its role in the transfer of iron from the intestine to the circulation, FPN likely also plays an important role in iron transport in other cells, notably the macrophages where iron efflux is required to recycle iron back into the circulation from the breakdown of hemoglobin. These red cell recycling macrophages are found in the liver (Kupffer cells), bone marrow, and splenic red pulp. FPN knockout mice die early in life confirming that FPN is essential in mammals [58]. Selective knockout of the gene in the intestine confirmed that FPN was required for intestinal iron absorption [58].

Mutations in FPN cause type IV hemochromatosis [59–61] also known as Ferroportin disease with an autosomal dominant inheritance distinct from HFE mutations. The clinical data from these patients shows distinct differences from patients with HFE mutations [59]. In some patients with FPN mutations, serum ferritin levels are very high and reticuloendothelial (RE) cells are severely iron loaded. In contrast, in HFE patients macrophages are low in iron [59]. These data suggest a fault in the recycling of macrophage iron in patients with FPN mutations, consistent with the high expression of FPN in these cells. In other patients, transferrin saturation is high and the defect appears to be the inability of FPN to recognize hepcidin, so-called hepcidin resistance [62, 63]. Hereditary defects causing diseases of iron metabolism are discussed extensively elsewhere in this volume.

Mice with sex-linked anemia (sla) develop anemia due to a defect in the intestinal transfer of iron to the circulation. As a consequence, iron builds up in the enterocytes and the animals become anemic [64, 65]. Using a positional cloning approach, the defective gene was identified by Anderson, Vulpe, and coworkers [66]. Interestingly, the protein sequence encoded by this novel gene (hephaestin) was very similar to ceruloplasmin, a copper-containing protein with ferroxidase activity. However, unlike ceruloplasmin, which is a secreted protein, hephaestin contains a single putative transmembrane domain at its C terminus, which may serve to anchor the protein into a membrane. Hephaestin is highly expressed in small intestine, though it does not show the regional predominance in the duodenum that FPN1, Dcytb, or DMT1 display. In fact, hephaestin is expressed along the length of the gut with no obvious gradient. This suggests hephaestin may have additional roles in the intestine unrelated to iron absorption. The subcellular location of hephaestin is also puzzling for a protein implicated in transfer of iron to the circulation. Studies indicate the protein is found not only on the basolateral membrane but also in intracellular perinuclear vesicles [20, 67]. The transport of iron through the enterocyte itself is an important aspect of the absorptive process about which little has been confirmed [68]. It is possible that hephaestin has a role in this process or has a separate function in basolateral cytoplasmic vesicles (see below for further discussion of vesicle trafficking in iron absorption).

8 The Regulation of Iron Absorption

The two key membrane iron transporters, DMT1 and FPN, show remarkably complex regulation, with the critical levels of each in their respective membranes determined by a combination of transcriptional, translational/mRNA stability and protein trafficking and turnover mechanisms (Fig. 6.1). The regulation of FPN in particular shows an apparently inconsistent set of regulatory mechanisms, with transcription being increased by low iron but translation of the resulting major mRNA being blocked by IRPs under the same conditions. A third level of regulation operates through the action of hepcidin to downregulate FPN protein at the basolateral membrane when iron levels are high. The presence of multiple control mechanisms leads to some degree of redundancy and knockout and mutant mice show varying degrees of loss of iron absorption regulation. In order to understand this complexity, one needs to consider the fact that the enterocyte has intrinsic (housekeeping) iron requirements. Although these requirements may be quantitatively small compared to overall body requirements, they are nevertheless important to the enterocytes and may conflict with body iron requirements and the need to regulate flux of iron across the enterocyte. DMT1 regulation seems relatively straightforward in that the enterocyte's intrinsic need to control its housekeeping iron levels operates in the same direction as the body's iron requirements, so both enterocyte and body need to increase iron uptake at times of iron depletion. There are again three levels of regulation – transcriptional, regulation of the stability and therefore the level of translatable mRNA by IRPs, and the trafficking of the protein to/from the BBM by iron levels. DCYTB regulation seems much simpler with primarily a transcriptional regulation. Hephaestin regulation is less well understood. We will describe the various mechanisms by which iron absorption gene expression is controlled, then describe an integrated model that explains the functional significance of these various mechanisms.

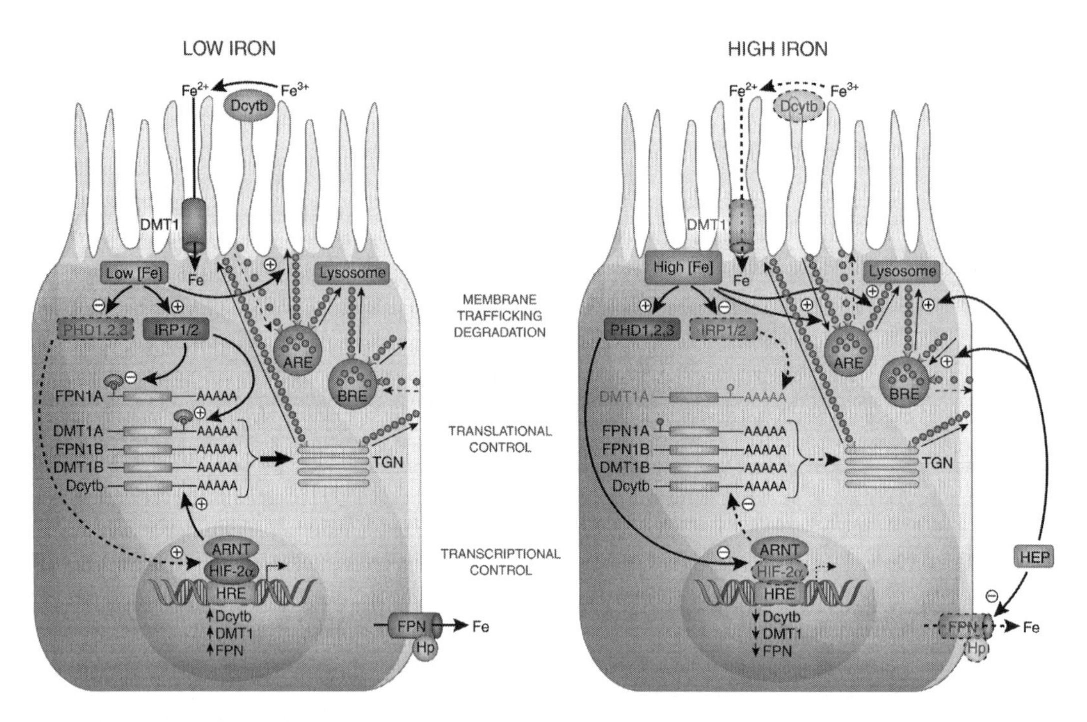

Fig. 6.1 Iron absorption regulation in enterocytes. Regulation operates at three levels (**a**) transcription of iron absorption genes in the nucleus is controlled by HIF2α; (**b**) levels and translation rates of some mRNAs are controlled by the IRP/IRE system in the cytosol and rough endoplasmic reticulum; and (**c**) the localization and degradation of some proteins in their target plasma membranes is also regulated. These differing mechanisms of regulation operate on differing timescales: transcription affects protein levels after some hours, protein turnover in membranes can be directly altered in minutes, and effects on mRNA can lead to changes in protein levels from minutes to hours later. ARE-Apical recyling endosome, BRE-basolateral recyling endosome

8.1 *Transcriptional Control of DMT1, DCYTB, and FPN by HIF2α*

Until recently, an iron-dependent mechanism for controlling transcription of the key iron absorption genes was lacking and no iron-sensitive transcription factors had been identified in the enterocyte. However, hypoxia-inducible factors (HIFs) have recently been identified as potential iron sensors in the duodenum. HIFs have long been known to be key oxygen-sensitive transcription factors identified as regulating erythropoietin expression [69], but they are now known to regulate a host of genes including many iron metabolism genes [70]. At the heart of the oxygen-sensing mechanism lie the prolyl hydroxylases, (PHDs of which there are three isoforms PHD1-3) which hydroxylate HIF and potentially respond to oxygen, iron, and ascorbate levels. Thus, these enzymes have the potential to act as iron sensors [71] and HIF could operate as an iron-sensitive transcription factor.

HIF2α has been identified as a key transcription factor that regulates genes encoding proteins involved in iron absorption in landmark studies by Shah et al. [70] and Mastrogiannaki et al. [72, 73]. Dcytb does not have a recognizable IRE and hence its strong regulation by iron and hypoxia therefore seemed likely to be transcriptionally controlled. Both studies show that DMT1 and Dcytb contain hypoxia response elements (HREs) within their promoters, which preferentially bind HIF2α, rather than HIF-1α, and activate transcription. Selective deletion of HIF2α in the enterocytes of mice results in low levels of DMT1 and Dcytb (as well as FPN1 and hephaestin, suggesting that these genes are also dependent on HIF2α), leading to low serum and liver iron and anemia. Interestingly, this effect could not be counteracted by reduced hepcidin levels in these mice. These findings help resolve a long standing observation that increased iron absorption (and in particular iron uptake) is an early (6–8 h) response to hypoxia [74, 75], preceding alterations in plasma iron, erythropoiesis, or liver iron levels.

8.2 Posttranscriptional Control by IRPs

Although several of the iron transporters (DMT1 and FPN) contain IREs, the control of iron absorption by the IRP/IRE mechanism has never been adequately explained. The IRE in the 5′ region of FPN has been shown to bind IRPs [54], and this strongly inhibits protein translation as intestinal Irp knockout mice have massive increases in FPN protein levels [76]. DMT1 protein, on the other hand, contains a 3′ IRE which stabilizes the mRNA, resulting in increased protein levels in iron deficiency [25, 76]. Dcytb and hephaestin, however, do not appear to contain IREs despite (in the case of Dcytb) being highly upregulated by iron deficiency.

However, some clarity may now be emerging with recent studies suggesting that non-IRE splice forms of DMT1 and FPN may be of greater relative importance for iron absorption. The IRE forms, on the other hand, may regulate iron for housekeeping purposes and prevent the enterocyte from becoming too iron deficient or iron loaded. Zhang and colleagues showed that two splice variants of FPN exist, one containing a 5′ IRE (FPN1A) and a non-IRE FPN1B [57]. Importantly, the FPN1B transcript appears to make up over 20% of the total duodenal FPN. The FPN1B transcript was highly responsive to iron, implying transcriptional regulation. DMT1 also exists as a non-IRE form which is upregulated by iron deficiency [76]. Hence it appears that transcriptional regulation of the non-IRE forms of FPN and DMT1, which leads to an upregulation of these genes under iron-deficient conditions and enables them to evade regulation by the IRP/IREs is of primary importance in regulating iron absorption. Precisely why FPN mRNA has a splice variant that can be translationally blocked in iron deficiency is unclear. Perhaps this mechanism prevents the enterocyte from becoming iron deficient to such an extent that its normal metabolism is compromised.

8.3 Control of Protein Trafficking by Iron (DMT1) and Hepcidin (FPN)

It has been known for many years that high oral doses of iron downregulate iron absorption. Part of this downregulation is associated with loss of DMT1 from the brush border membrane due to altered protein trafficking [77, 78]. The details of how this occurs have not been worked out. In contrast, the trafficking of ferroportin away from the basolateral membrane is known to be mediated by hepcidin binding [79] and this effect is thought to be central to the action of hepcidin to downregulate iron absorption. Hepcidin action is considered in detail in Chap. 9.

It has been suggested that some fraction of iron absorption proceeds via vesicular transport mechanisms [68]. The possibility that some or all of the intestinal absorption of iron is mediated by transcytosis, or pathways partly involving endocytosis or exocytosis of iron in vesicles was first raised by Johnson et al. [80] who showed that microtubule poisons are effective inhibitors of iron absorption in vivo in rats. We were not able to reproduce these findings in mice ([81]; also Simpson RJ, unpublished data). More recently, Peres et al. [82] showed in rats that absorption of iron complexed to caseinophosphopeptide was partially inhibited by the endocytosis inhibitor phenylarsine oxide. The inhibition was <30% and absorption of iron complexed to gluconate was not inhibited at all. It is possible that the chemical form of iron given in such experiments affects the outcome, with some iron complexes transported by vesicular transport pathways.

Much more evidence that iron transport across epithelial cells depends on vesicular transport has been obtained in studies of cultured cells [68, 83]. The limitations of such studies as predictors of in vivo iron absorption mechanisms have been discussed by Sharp and Srai [84]. It should be noted that early data on in vivo iron absorption has frequently shown low-affinity iron absorption that is regulated by iron [85–88]. It is difficult to explain such low-affinity pathways by a high-affinity membrane transporter such as DMT1. Such a low-affinity pathway might be explained by a gated pinocytotic transcytosis pathway triggered by iron interacting with DMT1, although it is difficult to envisage a requirement for FPN for such a pathway. Given the requirement that any physiological pathway in adults must involve DMT1 and FPN, one may suggest that low-affinity pathways are not of physiological interest but may be important pharmacologically and may not require DMT1 or FPN. Studies of absorption of high doses of iron have not yet been carried out in intestine-specific Dmt1 or Fpn knockout mice. Others have found that the rapid phase of iron absorption seems to proceed with iron gaining some access to cytosolic ferritin [89, 90]. On the other hand, others have found in a recent study that iron absorption was little affected by increased cytosolic ferritin [91]. In the absence of more detailed studies in vivo, it is not possible to rule out transcytosis; however, the available data remain most consistent with a membrane transport-based mechanism with iron traversing the cytosol. This latter pathway could also be affected by microtubule inhibitors if the localization of any of the key transport components (FPN, Dcytb, Heph, or DMT1) was affected by such inhibitors.

Overall, these protein trafficking regulation mechanisms can be seen as rapidly acting controls that can downregulate iron uptake or iron absorption within minutes. This contrasts with transcription regulation which likely acts on a timescale of hours to alter DMT1 and FPN levels. Translational control via IRPs can act on an intermediary timescale.

9 Systemic Regulation

9.1 Hepcidin

The identification of hepcidin as a key regulator of iron absorption and iron distribution in health and disease has greatly advanced our understanding of iron homeostasis in humans. Hepcidin, synthesized in the liver, circulates in plasma before binding to FPN on enterocytes, macrophages, and other cells, promoting degradation of the transporter and thereby inhibiting iron release from these cells [79]. Hepcidin can be regulated positively (by increased iron stores and inflammatory cytokines such as IL6) [92, 93] or negatively (by anemia and hypoxia) [93], although the mechanism(s) involved have not been fully elucidated. The relative importance and crosstalk between these factors and the signaling pathways involved in determining net levels of plasma hepcidin is not clear. Hepcidin regulation is discussed in more detail in Chap. 9.

9.2 Liver Iron Sensing (TfR2, HFE, TfR1, HJV, BMPs)

It is thought that the level of transferrin saturation or the level of diferric transferrin is an important determinant of hepcidin levels, but how this system operates is not completely understood [94]. Primary mouse hepatocytes increase hepcidin levels in response to increasing transferrin saturation [95]. TfR2 has been implicated in hepcidin regulation via changes in levels of transferrin and/or transferrin saturation. TfR2 shares 45% sequence identity with TfR1, is abundantly expressed on hepatocytes, and binds diferric transferrin with 20–30-fold lower affinity than TfR1. Whereas TfR1 is inversely regulated by iron expression, TfR2 protein is upregulated in cell lines and animal models in response to increased levels of diferric transferrin, but not apotransferrin or NTBI [96], suggesting that this receptor could serve as an iron sensor on the hepatocyte cell membrane. Furthermore, the finding that humans with mutations in TfR2 develop iron overload [97] associated with hepcidin deficiency and mouse models of whole body knockout (or targeted hepatocyte disruption) of Tfr2 [98] are also hepcidin deficient, is consistent with the idea that this receptor is an iron-sensing molecule on the pathway regulating hepcidin synthesis by the liver.

HFE is clearly involved in regulating hepcidin synthesis as hepcidin deficiency characterizes human and mouse models of HFE-related hemochromatosis [99]; however, its role in iron sensing is unclear. HFE has been shown to bind to TFR1 and to the same domain that also binds diferric transferrin; therefore, HFE and transferrin compete for binding to TfR1 [100]. HFE also binds to TfR2 and binding has been shown to stabilize the receptor [101, 102]. It has been proposed that HFE displaced from TfR1 by diferric transferrin could bind to TfR2 and signal an increase in hepcidin expression, but this mechanism has yet to be proven in vivo.

Hemojuvelin (HJV) contains a C-terminal glycosylphosphatidylinositol anchor and has been found as both cell-associated and soluble forms. The cell-associated form positively regulates hepcidin gene transcription through the BMP signal transduction pathway while the soluble form, demonstrated in cell culture medium and in the circulation in vivo, has been found to suppress hepcidin mRNA in primary cultures of mouse hepatocytes [103]. Ganz and colleagues have proposed that through competitive binding at the hepatocyte membrane, the two forms of HJV reciprocally regulate hepcidin expression in response to changes in extracellular iron concentration [103].

Hence, iron sensing in hepatocytes is likely to be extremely complex and involve HJV, BMPs, TfR2, and HFE. Recently, a liver-specific type II transmembrane serine protease (TMPRSS6, or matriptase-2) has been shown to be required for the appropriate response of hepcidin to iron deficiency [104, 105]. The enzyme has been shown to cleave membrane-bound HJV and therefore act as a negative regulator of hepcidin [106]. In addition, BMP6 has recently been shown to be essential for hepcidin production [107, 108] with Bmp6 KO mice becoming highly iron loaded due to lack of hepcidin [107]. Further work in this area is clearly required.

10 Integrated Control of Iron Flux Across the Enterocyte

Balancing iron flux across the mucosa to provide for body iron requirements and at the same time satisfy the enterocyte's own iron needs is achieved by the above control mechanisms. In addition to these, as in all cells, enterocytes possess ferritin to protect themselves from excess iron and this is regulated by IRPs via a 5′ UTR translation repression mechanism. The rapid downregulation of DMT1 from the apical membrane seems also to operate as a defense against sudden excess iron entry into enterocytes.

Making sense of all these various control mechanisms needs consideration of their differing purposes as well as the differing timescales they operate on. Regulation of iron absorption requires coordinated up/downregulation of all the primary iron-sensitive genes responsible for moving iron across the enterocytes and the HIF system plays a key role in this regulation. On the other hand, the IRP/IRE posttranscriptional control mechanisms perform a housekeeping role which serves to protect the enterocyte from becoming too iron deficient or iron loaded. This is illustrated by the findings with Irp knockout mice. Double knockout of both Irp1 and Irp2 in intestinal cells only (global double knockout is embryonic lethal) leads to severe derangement of enterocytes early in life [76], thus emphasizing the importance of the IRP system for fundamental cell metabolism. Furthermore, Galy et al. noticed that Dmt1 non-IRE mRNA was upregulated and Dmt1 IRE was only mildly decreased in these double knockout mice. This, taken with more drastic effects of the Irp knockout on other IRE-regulated proteins, implied some transcriptional upregulation of Dmt1 gene. The enterocytes of the Irp double intestinal knockout mice were likely to be severely functionally iron deficient due to upregulation of FPN and ferritin protein and the Hif2 transcriptional control provides a molecular mechanism for a compensatory increase in Dmt1 gene transcription that can balance the increased degradation of the Dmt1 IRE mRNA. Irp2 is believed to be the main IRP for iron regulation in enterocytes and selective knockout of this gene leads to increased ferritin and FPN production [91] and therefore functional enterocyte iron deficiency. Once again, Dmt1 is relatively unchanged, presumably because of increased transcription of the Dmt1 gene in response to the relative enterocyte iron deficiency. Overall iron absorption was found to be unchanged [91], suggesting that the IRP system does not affect regulation of iron absorption *per se*.

The hepcidin/FPN system acts as a signaling mechanism to communicate body iron requirements to the duodenal enterocyte. However, hepcidin itself can be seen primarily to function as the regulator of plasma iron levels. Regulating plasma iron is particularly important. This pool of iron turns over rapidly, yet must supply the erythroid marrow (and other cells) with sufficient iron for their metabolic needs while at the same time preventing excess (and potentially toxic) iron accumulating.

In situations where iron accesses the duodenum in bursts (meal feeding, as in humans, or when high doses of iron are given to animals), the varying timescales of regulatory mechanisms become more apparent. It has long been known that transfer of an oral dose of iron to the carcass of rats follows two phases, an early burst of iron transfer to the plasma and a slower phase of transfer over several hours. During the early phase, existing FPN protein acts to efflux iron to the plasma. Excess iron in the cytosol is taken up by ferritin but also stimulates translation of ferritin and FPN mRNAs and shuts down transcription of the FPN, Dcytb, and DMT1 genes. The arrival of iron in the plasma subsequently leads to increased hepcidin production that will tend to block further efflux from the enterocytes; however, the translation of more FPN1A mRNA will leave some capacity for efflux, albeit at a slower rate.

11 Conclusion

The above description highlights the complexity of iron absorption regulation and the difficulties of providing a simple explanation of this complexity. The most likely explanation is that the various regulatory mechanisms have been acquired at different times through the evolutionary history of mammals, the resulting system being, like many biological structures, not designed from scratch but a make-do-and-mend system that has evolved to meet various physiological requirements as best it can.

References

1. McCance RA, Widdowson EM. Absorption and excretion of iron. Lancet. 1937;2:680–4.
2. Conrad ME, Weintraub LR, Sears DA, Crosby WH. Absorption of hemoglobin iron. Am J Physiol. 1966;211:1123–30.
3. Conrad ME, Benjamin BI, Williams HL, Foy AL. Human absorption of hemoglobin–iron. Gastroenterology. 1967;53:5–10.
4. Weintraub LR, Conrad ME, Crosby WH. Absorption of hemoglobin iron by the rat. Proc Soc Exp Biol Med. 1965;120:840–3.
5. Uzel C, Conrad ME. Absorption of heme iron. Semin Hematol. 1998;35:27–34.
6. Raffin SB, Woo CH, Roost KT, Price DC, Schmid R. Intestinal absorption of hemoglobin iron–heme cleavage by mucosal heme oxygenase. J Clin Invest. 1974;54:1344–52.
7. Latunde-Dada GO, Takeuchi K, Simpson RJ, McKie AT. Haem carrier protein 1 (HCP1): expression and functional studies in cultured cells. FEBS Lett. 2006;580:6865–70.
8. Shayeghi M, Latunde-Dada GO, Oakhill JS, Laftah AH, Takeuchi K, Halliday N, et al. Identification of an intestinal heme transporter. Cell. 2005;122:789–801.
9. Qiu A, Jansen M, Sakaris A, Min SH, Chattopadhyay S, Tsai E, et al. Identification of an intestinal folate transporter and the molecular basis for hereditary folate malabsorption. Cell. 2006;127:917–28.
10. Zhao R, Min SH, Qiu A, Sakaris A, Goldberg GL, Sandoval C, et al. The spectrum of mutations in the PCFT gene, coding for an intestinal folate transporter, that are the basis for hereditary folate malabsorption. Blood. 2007;110:1147–52.
11. Rossi E, Bulsara MK, Olynyk JK, Cullen DJ, Summerville L, Powell LW. Effect of hemochromatosis genotype and lifestyle factors on iron and red cell indices in a community population. Clin Chem. 2001;47:202–8.

12. Cade JE, Moreton JA, O'Hara B, Greenwood DC, Moor J, Burley VJ, et al. Diet and genetic factors associated with iron status in middle-aged women. Am J Clin Nutr. 2005;82:813–20.
13. Greenwood DC, Cade JE, Moreton JA, O'Hara B, Burley VJ, Randerson-Moor JA, et al. HFE genotype modifies the influence of heme iron intake on iron status. Epidemiology. 2005;16:802–5.
14. Turnbull A, Cleton F, Finch CA. Iron absorption. IV. The absorption of hemoglobin iron. J Clin Invest. 1962;41:1897–907.
15. Bergheim O, Kirch ER. Reduction of iron in the human stomach. J Biol Chem. 1949;177:591–6.
16. Simpson RJ, Peters TJ. Forms of soluble iron in mouse stomach and duodenal lumen: significance for mucosal uptake. Br J Nutr. 1990;63:79–89.
17. Golubov J, Flanagan P, Adams P. Inhibition of iron absorption by omeprazole in rat model. Dig Dis Sci. 1991;36:405–8.
18. Miret S, Simpson RJ, McKie AT. Physiology and molecular biology of dietary iron absorption. Annu Rev Nutr. 2003;23:283–301.
19. Takeuchi K, Bjarnason I, Laftah AH, Latunde-Dada GO, Simpson RJ, McKie AT. Expression of iron absorption genes in mouse large intestine. Scand J Gastroenterol. 2005;40:169–77.
20. Frazer DM, Vulpe CD, McKie AT, Wilkins SJ, Trinder D, Cleghorn GJ, et al. Cloning and gastrointestinal expression of rat hephaestin: relationship to other iron transport proteins. Am J Physiol Gastrointest Liver Physiol. 2001;281:G931–9.
21. Manis JG, Schachter D. Active transport of iron by intestine: features of the two-step mechanism. Am J Physiol. 1962;203:73–80.
22. McKie AT, Simpson RJ. Basolateral transport of iron in mammalian intestine: from physiology to molecules. In: Templeton DM, editor. Molecular and cellular iron transport. New York: Marcel Dekker; 2002. p. 175–88.
23. Gunshin H, Mackenzie B, Berger UV, Gunshin Y, Romero MF, Boron WF, et al. Cloning and characterization of a mammalian proton-coupled metal-ion transporter. Nature. 1997;388:482–8.
24. Tandy S, Williams M, Leggett A, Lopez-Jimenez M, Dedes M, Ramesh B, et al. Nramp2 expression is associated with pH-dependent iron uptake across the apical membrane of human intestinal Caco-2 cells. J Biol Chem. 2000;275:1023–9.
25. Gunshin H, Allerson CR, Polycarpou-Schwarz M, Rofts A, Rogers JT, Kishi F, et al. Iron-dependent regulation of the divalent metal ion transporter. FEBS Lett. 2001;509:309–16.
26. Fleming MD, Trenor CC, Su MA, Foernzler D, Beier DR, Dietrich WF, et al. Microcytic anaemia mice have a mutation in Nramp2, a candidate iron transporter gene. Nat Genet. 1997;16:383–6.
27. Fleming MD, Romano MA, Su MA, Garrick LM, Garrick MD, Andrews NC. Nramp2 is mutated in the anemic Belgrade (b) rat: evidence of a role for Nramp2 in endosomal iron transport. Proc Natl Acad Sci USA. 1998;95:1148–53.
28. Gunshin H, Fujiwara Y, Custodio AO, Direnzo C, Robine S, Andrews NC. Slc11a2 is required for intestinal iron absorption and erythropoiesis but dispensable in placenta and liver. J Clin Invest. 2005;115:1258–66.
29. Mims MP, Guan Y, Pospisilova D, Priwitzerova M, Indrak K, Ponka P, et al. Identification of a human mutation of DMT1 in a patient with microcytic anemia and iron overload. Blood. 2005;105:1337–42.
30. Iolascon A, d'Apolito M, Servedio V, Cimmino F, Piga A, Camaschella C. Microcytic anemia and hepatic iron overload in a child with compound heterozygous mutations in DMT1 (SCL11A2). Blood. 2006;107:349–54.
31. Beaumont C, Delaunay J, Hetet G, Grandchamp B, de Montalembert M, Tchernia G. Two new human DMT1 gene mutations in a patient with microcytic anemia, low ferritinemia, and liver iron overload. Blood. 2006;107:4168–70.
32. Mackenzie B, Garrick MD. Iron imports. II. Iron uptake at the apical membrane in the intestine. Am J Physiol Gastrointest Liver Physiol. 2005;289:G981–6.
33. Lichten LA, Cousins RJ. Mammalian zinc transporters: nutritional and physiologic regulation. Annu Rev Nutr. 2009;29:153–76.
34. Liuzzi JP, Aydemir F, Nam H, Knutson MD, Cousins RJ. Zip14 (Slc39a14) mediates non-transferrin-bound iron uptake into cells. Proc Natl Acad Sci USA. 2006;103:13612–7.
35. Chua AC, Morgan EH. Manganese metabolism is impaired in the Belgrade laboratory rat. J Comp Physiol B. 1997;167:361–9.
36. Min KS, Ueda H, Kihara T, Tanaka K. Increased hepatic accumulation of ingested Cd is associated with upregulation of several intestinal transporters in mice fed diets deficient in essential metals. Toxicol Sci. 2008;106:284–9.
37. Raja K, Jafri S, Peters T, Simpson R. Iron and cadmium uptake by duodenum of hypotransferrinaemic mice. Biometals. 2006;19:547–53.
38. Suzuki T, Momoi K, Hosoyamada M, Kimura M, Shibasaki T. Normal cadmium uptake in microcytic anemia mk/mk mice suggests that DMT1 is not the only cadmium transporter in vivo. Toxicol Appl Pharmacol. 2008;227:462–7.
39. Yamaji S, Tennant J, Tandy S, Williams M, Singh Srai SK, Sharp P. Zinc regulates the function and expression of the iron transporters DMT1 and IREG1 in human intestinal Caco-2 cells. FEBS Lett. 2001;507:137–41.

40. Tennant J, Stansfield M, Yamaji S, Srai S, Sharp P. Effects of copper on the expression of metal transporters in human intestinal Caco-2 cells. FEBS Lett. 2002;527:239.
41. Crane FL, Sun IL, Clark MG, Grebing C, Low H. Transplasma-membrane redox systems in growth and development. Biochim Biophys Acta. 1985;811:233–64.
42. Raja KB, Simpson RJ, Peters TJ. Investigation of a role for reduction in ferric iron uptake by mouse duodenum (published erratum appears in Biochim Biophys Acta 1993; 1176: 197). Biochim Biophys Acta. 1992;1135:141–6.
43. Pountney DJ, Raja KB, Simpson RJ, Wrigglesworth JM. The ferric-reducing activity of duodenal brush–border membrane vesicles is associated with a b-type haem. Biometals. 1999;12:53–62.
44. Pountney DJ, Raja KB, Bottwood MJ, Wrigglesworth JM, Simpson RJ. Mucosal surface ferricyanide reductase activity in mouse duodenum. Biometals. 1996;9:15–20.
45. McKie AT, Barrow D, Latunde-Dada GO, Rolfs A, Sager G, Mudaly E, et al. An iron-regulated ferric reductase associated with the absorption of dietary iron. Science. 2001;291:1755–9.
46. Srivastava M, Duong LT, Fleming PJ. Cytochrome b561 catalyzes transmembrane electron transfer. J Biol Chem. 1984;259:8072–5.
47. Duong LT, Fleming PJ, Russell JT. An identical cytochrome b561 is present in bovine adrenal chromaffin vesicles and posterior pituitary neurosecretory vesicles. J Biol Chem. 1984;259:4885–9.
48. Fleming PJ, Kent UM. Secretory vesicle cytochrome b561: a transmembrane electron transporter. Ann N Y Acad Sci. 1987;493:101–7.
49. Escriou V, Laporte F, Garin J, Brandolin G, Vignais PV. Purification and physical properties of a novel type of cytochrome b from rabbit peritoneal neutrophils. J Biol Chem. 1994;269:14007–14.
50. Escriou V, Laporte F, Vignais PV, Desbois A. Differential characterization of neutrophil cytochrome p30 and cytochrome b-558 by low-temperature absorption and resonance Raman spectroscopies. Eur J Biochem. 1997;245:505–11.
51. Su D, May JM, Koury MJ, Asard H. Human erythrocyte membranes contain a cytochrome b561 that may be involved in extracellular ascorbate recycling. J Biol Chem. 2006;281:39852–9.
52. Gunshin H, Starr CN, Direnzo C, Fleming MD, Jin J, Greer EL, et al. Cybrd1 (duodenal cytochrome b) is not necessary for dietary iron absorption in mice. Blood. 2005;106:2879–83.
53. Frazer DM, Wilkins SJ, Vulpe CD, Anderson GJ. The role of duodenal cytochrome b in intestinal iron absorption remains unclear. Blood. 2005;106:4413.
54. McKie AT, Marciani P, Rolfs A, Brennan K, Wehr K, Barrow D, et al. A novel duodenal iron-regulated transporter, IREG1, implicated in the basolateral transfer of iron to the circulation. Mol Cell. 2000;5:299–309.
55. Donovan A, Brownlie A, Zhou Y, Shepard J, Pratt SJ, Moynihan J, et al. Positional cloning of zebrafish ferroportin1 identifies a conserved vertebrate iron exporter. Nature. 2000;403:776–81.
56. Abboud S, Haile DJ. A novel mammalian iron-regulated protein involved in intracellular iron metabolism. J Biol Chem. 2000;275:19906–12.
57. Zhang DL, Hughes RM, Ollivierre-Wilson H, Ghosh MC, Rouault TA. A ferroportin transcript that lacks an iron-responsive element enables duodenal and erythroid precursor cells to evade translational repression. Cell Metab. 2009;9:461–73.
58. Donovan A, Lima CA, Pinkus JL, Pinkus GS, Zon LI, Robine S, et al. The iron exporter ferroportin/Slc40a1 is essential for iron homeostasis. Cell Metab. 2005;1:191–200.
59. Montosi G, Donovan A, Totaro A, Garuti C, Pignatti E, Cassanelli S, et al. Autosomal-dominant hemochromatosis is associated with a mutation in the ferroportin (SLC11A3) gene. J Clin Invest. 2001;108:619–23.
60. Devalia V, Carter K, Walker AP, Perkins SJ, Worwood M, May A, et al. Autosomal dominant reticuloendothelial iron overload associated with a 3-base pair deletion in the ferroportin 1 gene (SLC11A3). Blood. 2002;100:695–7.
61. Roetto A, Merryweather-Clarke AT, Daraio F, Livesey K, Pointon JJ, Barbabietola G, et al. A valine deletion of ferroportin 1: a common mutation in hemochromastosis type 4. Blood. 2002;100:733–4.
62. Drakesmith H, Schimanski LM, Ormerod E, Merryweather-Clarke AT, Viprakasit V, Edwards JP, et al. Resistance to hepcidin is conferred by hemochromatosis-associated mutations of ferroportin. Blood. 2005;106:1092–7.
63. Schimanski LM, Drakesmith H, Merryweather-Clarke AT, Viprakasit V, Edwards JP, Sweetland E, et al. In vitro functional analysis of human ferroportin (FPN) and hemochromatosis-associated FPN mutations. Blood. 2005;105:4096–102.
64. Bannerman RM, Cooper RG. Sex-linked anemia: a hypochromic anemia of mice. Science. 1966;151:581–2.
65. Peppriell JE, Edwards JA, Bannerman RM. The kinetics of iron uptake by isolated intestinal cells from normal mice and mice with sex-linked anemia. Blood. 1982;60:635–41.
66. Vulpe CD, Kuo YM, Murphy TL, Cowley L, Askwith C, Libina N, et al. Hephaestin, a ceruloplasmin homologue implicated in intestinal iron transport, is defective in the sla mouse. Nat Genet. 1999;21:195–9.

67. Kuo YM, Su T, Chen H, Attieh Z, Syed BA, McKie AT, et al. Mislocalisation of hephaestin, a multicopper ferroxidase involved in basolateral intestinal iron transport, in the sex linked anaemia mouse. Gut. 2004;53:201–6.
68. Ma Y, Yeh M, Yeh Ky, Glass J. Iron imports. V. Transport of iron through the intestinal epithelium. Am J Physiol Gastrointest Liver Physiol. 2006;290:G417–22.
69. Semenza GL, Wang GL. A nuclear factor induced by hypoxia via de novo protein synthesis binds to the human erythropoietin gene enhancer at a site required for transcriptional activation. Mol Cell Biol. 1992;12:5447–54.
70. Peyssonnaux C, Nizet V, Johnson RS. Role of the hypoxia inducible factors HIF in iron metabolism. Cell Cycle. 2008;7:28–32.
71. Berra E, Ginouves A, Pouyssegur J. The hypoxia-inducible-factor hydroxylases bring fresh air into hypoxia signalling. EMBO Rep. 2006;7:41–5.
72. Shah YM, Matsubara T, Ito S, Yim SH, Gonzalez FJ. Intestinal hypoxia-inducible transcription factors are essential for iron absorption following iron deficiency. Cell Metab. 2009;9:152–64.
73. Mastrogiannaki M, Matak P, Keith B, Simon MC, Vaulont S, Peyssonnaux C. HIF-2alpha, but not HIF-1alpha, promotes iron absorption in mice. J Clin Invest. 2009;119:1159–66.
74. Hathorn MK. The influence of hypoxia on iron absorption in the rat. Gastroenterology. 1971;60:76–81.
75. Raja KB, Simpson RJ, Pippard MJ, Peters TJ. In vivo studies on the relationship between intestinal iron (Fe3+) absorption, hypoxia and erythropoiesis in the mouse. Br J Haematol. 1988;68:373–8.
76. Galy B, Ferring-Appel D, Kaden S, Grone HJ, Hentze MW. Iron regulatory proteins are essential for intestinal function and control key iron absorption molecules in the duodenum. Cell Metab. 2008;7:79–85.
77. Ma Y, Specian RD, Yeh Ky, Yeh M, Rodriguez-Paris J, Glass J. The transcytosis of divalent metal transporter 1 and apo-transferrin during iron uptake in intestinal epithelium. Am J Physiol Gastrointest Liver Physiol. 2002;283:G965–74.
78. Frazer DM, Wilkins SJ, Becker EM, Murphy TL, Vulpe CD, McKie AT, et al. A rapid decrease in the expression of DMT1 and Dcytb but not Ireg1 or hephaestin explains the mucosal block phenomenon of iron absorption. Gut. 2003;52:340–6.
79. Nemeth E, Tuttle MS, Powelson J, Vaughn MB, Donovan A, Ward DM, et al. Hepcidin regulates cellular iron efflux by binding to ferroportin and inducing its internalization. Science. 2004;306:2090–3.
80. Johnson G, Jacobs P, Purves LR. The effects of cytoskeletal inhibitors on intestinal iron absorption in the rat. Biochim Biophys Acta. 1985;843:83–91.
81. Simpson RJ, Osterloh KRS, Raja KB, Snape SD, Peters TJ. Studies on the role of transferrin and endocytosis in the uptake of Fe3+ from Fe-nitrilotriacetate by mouse duodenum. Biochim Biophys Acta. 1986; 884:166–71.
82. Peres JM, Bouhallab S, Bureau F, Neuville D, Maubois JL, Devroede G, et al. Mechanisms of absorption of caseinophosphopeptide bound iron. J Nutr Biochem. 1999;10:215–22.
83. Moriya M, Linder MC. Vesicular transport and apotransferrin in intestinal iron absorption, as shown in the Caco-2 cell model. Am J Physiol Gastrointest Liver Physiol. 2006;290:G301–9.
84. Sharp P, Srai SK. Molecular mechanisms involved in intestinal iron absorption. World J Gastroenterol. 2007;13:4716–24.
85. Beutler E, Kelly BM, Beutler F. The regulation of iron absorption: II. Relationship between iron dosage and iron absorption. Am J Clin Nutr. 1962;11:559–67.
86. Wheby MS, Jones LG, Crosby WH. Studies on iron absorption. Intestinal regulatory mechanisms. J Clin Invest. 1964;43:1433–42.
87. Gitlin D, Cruchard A. On the kinetics of iron absorption in mice. J Clin Invest. 1962;41:344–50.
88. Hahn PF, Carothers EL, Darby WJ, Martin M, Sheppard CW, Cannon RO, et al. Iron metabolism in human pregnancy as studied with radioactive isotope, Fe59. Am J Obstet Gynecol. 1951;61:477–86.
89. Snape S, Simpson RJ, Peters TJ. Subcellular localization of recently-absorbed iron in mouse duodenal enterocytes: identification of a basolateral membrane iron-binding site. Cell Biochem Funct. 1990;8:107–15.
90. Osterloh K, Snape S, Simpson RJ, Grindley H, Peters TJ. Subcellular distribution of recently absorbed iron and of transferrin in the mouse duodenal mucosa. Biochim Biophys Acta. 1988;969:166–75.
91. Galy B, Ferring D, Minana B, Bell O, Janser HG, Muckenthaler M, et al. Altered body iron distribution and microcytosis in mice deficient in iron regulatory protein 2 (IRP2). Blood. 2005;106:2580–9.
92. Pigeon C, Ilyin G, Courselaud B, Leroyer P, Turlin B, Brissot P, et al. A new mouse liver-specific gene, encoding a protein homologous to human antimicrobial peptide hepcidin, is overexpressed during iron overload. J Biol Chem. 2001;276:7811–9.
93. Nicolas G, Chauvet C, Viatte L, Danan JL, Bigard X, Devaux I, et al. The gene encoding the iron regulatory peptide hepcidin is regulated by anemia, hypoxia, and inflammation. J Clin Invest. 2002;110:1037–44.
94. Frazer DM, Anderson GJ. The orchestration of body iron intake: how and where do enterocytes receive their cues? Blood Cells Mol Dis. 2003;30:288–97.

95. Lin L, Valore EV, Nemeth E, Goodnough JB, Gabayan V, Ganz T. Iron transferrin regulates hepcidin synthesis in primary hepatocyte culture through hemojuvelin and BMP2/4. Blood. 2007;110:2182–9.
96. Robb A, Wessling-Resnick M. Regulation of transferrin receptor 2 protein levels by transferrin. Blood. 2004;104:4294–9.
97. Camaschella C, Roetto A, Cali A, De Gobbi M, Garozzo G, Carella M, et al. The gene TFR2 is mutated in a new type of haemochromatosis mapping to 7q22. Nat Genet. 2000;25:14–5.
98. Fleming RE, Ahmann JR, Migas MC, Waheed A, Koeffler HP, Kawabata H, et al. Targeted mutagenesis of the murine transferrin receptor-2 gene produces hemochromatosis. Proc Natl Acad Sci USA. 2002;99:10653–8.
99. Fleming RE, Sly WS. Mechanisms of iron accumulation in hereditary hemochromatosis. Annu Rev Physiol. 2002;64:663–80.
100. Lebron JA, West Jr AP, Bjorkman PJ. The hemochromatosis protein HFE competes with transferrin for binding to the transferrin receptor. J Mol Biol. 1999;294:239–45.
101. Chen J, Chloupkova M, Gao J, Chapman-Arvedson TL, Enns CA. HFE modulates transferrin receptor 2 levels in hepatoma cells via interactions that differ from transferrin receptor 1-HFE interactions. J Biol Chem. 2007;282:36862–70.
102. Gao J, Chen J, Kramer M, Tsukamoto H, Zhang AS, Enns CA. Interaction of the hereditary hemochromatosis protein HFE with transferrin receptor 2 is required for transferrin-induced hepcidin expression. Cell Metab. 2009;9:217–27.
103. Lin L, Goldberg YP, Ganz T. Competitive regulation of hepcidin mRNA by soluble and cell-associated hemojuvelin. Blood. 2005;106:2884–9.
104. Du X, She E, Gelbart T, Truksa J, Lee P, Xia Y, et al. The serine protease TMPRSS6 is required to sense iron deficiency. Science. 2008;320:1088–92.
105. Finberg KE, Heeney MM, Campagna DR, Aydinok Y, Pearson HA, Hartman KR, et al. Mutations in TMPRSS6 cause iron-refractory iron deficiency anemia (IRIDA). Nat Genet. 2008;40:569–71.
106. Silvestri L, Pagani A, Nai A, De Domenico I, Kaplan J, Camaschella C. The serine protease matriptase-2 (TMPRSS6) inhibits hepcidin activation by cleaving membrane hemojuvelin. Cell Metab. 2008;8:502–11.
107. Meynard D, Kautz L, Darnaud V, Canonne-Hergaux F, Coppin H, Roth MP. Lack of the bone morphogenetic protein BMP6 induces massive iron overload. Nat Genet. 2009;41:478–81.
108. Andriopoulos Jr B, Corradini E, Xia Y, Faasse SA, Chen S, Grgurevic L, et al. BMP6 is a key endogenous regulator of hepcidin expression and iron metabolism. Nat Genet. 2009;41:482–7.

Chapter 7
Plasma Iron and Iron Delivery to the Tissues

Ross M. Graham, Anita C.G. Chua, and Debbie Trinder

Keywords HFE • Iron uptake • Liver • Metal binding • Non-transferrin bound iron • Plasma iron • Receptor-mediated endocytosis • Transferrin • Transferrin receptor • Transferrin-bound iron

Abbreviations

BCEC	Brain capillary endothelial cell
DCYTB	Duodenal cytochrome B
DMT1	Divalent metal transporter 1
IRE	Iron-responsive element
IRP	Iron regulatory protein
NTBI	Non-transferrin bound iron
STEAP3	Six-transmembrane epithelial antigen of the prostate 3
TBI	Transferrin-bound iron
TFR	Transferrin receptor

1 Introduction

Iron is a transition element which has two biologically important oxidation states, +2 and +3. It is an essential trace element and, as such, takes part in a large number of varied biological processes, many of which utilize the interconversion of ferrous and ferric iron. Ferrous iron is relatively soluble but is readily oxidized to the ferric form which is sparingly soluble at physiological pH [1] and will precipitate if not solubilized. It is also possible for the electron released from the oxidation reaction to participate in the formation of reactive oxygen species which can cause oxidative damage if present in high enough concentrations. Consequently, many elegant processes have evolved which render iron both soluble and non-toxic, allowing organisms to accumulate iron in forms which are both safe and functional.

R.M. Graham, Ph.D. • A.C.G. Chua, Ph.D. • D. Trinder, Ph.D. (✉)
School of Medicine and Pharmacology and Western Australian Institute for Medical Research, University of Western Australia, Fremantle Hospital, Fremantle, WA, Australia
e-mail: debbie.trinder@uwa.edu.au

G.J. Anderson and G. McLaren (eds.), *Iron Physiology and Pathophysiology in Humans*, Nutrition and Health, DOI 10.1007/978-1-60327-485-2_7,

This chapter will provide an overview of the normal processes of iron transport in mammals, including a summary of the transport molecules and their mechanisms of iron capture and release. We will also outline the mechanisms of iron acquisition by tissues and the regulation of these processes.

2 Nature of Iron in the Plasma

Iron circulates in the plasma in a variety of forms. The major form is bound to the glycoprotein, transferrin. In addition, there is a pool of minor forms, termed "non-transferrin bound iron" (NTBI), which includes iron bound to low-molecular-weight chelators, macromolecules, and other proteins.

2.1 Transferrin-Bound Iron

The concentration of transferrin in normal adult plasma is approximately 30 μM and the concentration of iron is approximately 20 μM. Each transferrin molecule can bind up to two atoms of iron; thus, plasma transferrin is approximately one-third saturated under normal conditions [2]. The remaining, unoccupied, binding sites on transferrin provide a large buffering capacity in the case of an increase in plasma iron levels. This is important given the low solubility and potential toxicity of free iron.

There are no gender differences in plasma transferrin concentration although plasma iron concentration is slightly higher in adult men than women. Indeed, under normal conditions, plasma iron concentration is remarkably stable throughout life, initially dropping to approximately half its birth level of approximately 30 μM within the first 3–6 months of life and slowly rising to about 20 μM at puberty. Following puberty, plasma iron rises slightly again by another 25% in males only. In contrast, plasma transferrin concentration almost doubles in the first year following birth, from approximately 20 μM to approximately 35 μM, decreasing about 20% in the ensuing years until puberty, when the adult level is reached [3].

In addition to iron, transferrin is capable of binding many other metals, including Ga^{3+}, Co^{3+}, Mn^{2+}, and Cu^{2+}, but with much lower affinity [4]. It is unclear whether such binding contributes to transport of these metals *in vivo*, although it has been speculated that transferrin may play a role in detoxification of heavy metals or naturally occurring radioactive metals [5].

2.2 Non-Transferrin Bound Iron

Descriptively, NTBI refers to a heterogeneous pool of plasma iron bound to molecules other than transferrin, including low-molecular-weight chelators, macromolecules, such as heme, and proteins, such as albumin or ferritin. However, in practice, NTBI is defined more narrowly as plasma iron bound with low affinity to low-molecular-weight chelators or non-specifically to plasma proteins. It was initially postulated as a pool of iron which appeared in iron overload, when the binding capacity of plasma transferrin had been saturated [6], but in the ensuing years, it has been reported in conditions under which iron-binding sites on transferrin have not been limiting [7, 8]. The presence of NTBI in a multitude of states suggests that its presence in plasma is normal and likely to be in equilibrium with transferrin-bound iron. The major component of this pool has been identified as ferric citrate [9, 10]; however, other forms are undoubtedly present as evidenced by the variation in the levels determined by different methods, suggesting that there are sub-pools of NTBI which are accessible, either chemically or physically, by some chelators and not by others [11, 12].

The serum concentrations of NTBI are the subject of considerable debate. Normally, it is thought to represent a very small proportion of transport iron, with studies placing the concentration between

0 and 1 μM [9, 13–15]; however, in diseases of iron overload, values up to 5 μM are commonly described although values as high as 20 μM have been reported [11, 12, 16–19]. The ambiguity arises from the variety of methods employed to measure NTBI, their inherent limitations and, indeed, the lack of certainty about the chemical forms of the iron being measured. A study comparing methods used routinely and using common serum samples indicated a large variation in the values reported for each sample dependent on the method used and the laboratory conducting the assays [20].

NTBI is considered to have the potential to catalyze toxic reactions. Iron complexed to citrate has been reported to induce lipid peroxidation, DNA strand breakage, and other toxic effects [21–24], but the subject is controversial [25–27].

3 The Biology of Transferrin

Transferrin was first described as a metal-binding component in serum in the mid-1940s [28, 29]. Subsequently, it was found to be the major plasma iron transport protein [2, 30]. It is a monomeric, bilobed glycoprotein, synthesized predominantly by the liver in the normal state. Other tissues such as the brain, testes, and mammary glands can produce it, but this production is unlikely to contribute significantly to plasma levels [31–33]. In humans, it consists of 679 amino acids with a molecular weight of approximately 80 kDa. Its primary sequence is highly conserved amongst higher animals and its tertiary structure is maintained by the presence of some 19 disulfide bonds [34, 35]. The two lobes, termed N- and C-lobes, are homologous and the protein is thought to have arisen as the result of gene duplication and combination [36].

3.1 Metal Binding

Each lobe contains an iron-binding site in a cleft formed by two sub-domains linked by a hinge region [37]. The metal co-ordination sites are provided by similar conserved amino acids, aspartate, histidine, and two tyrosines (Fig. 7.1). The remaining two co-ordination bonds are provided by a carbonate anion which, itself, is co-ordinated by a conserved arginine residue [38, 39]. A number of other

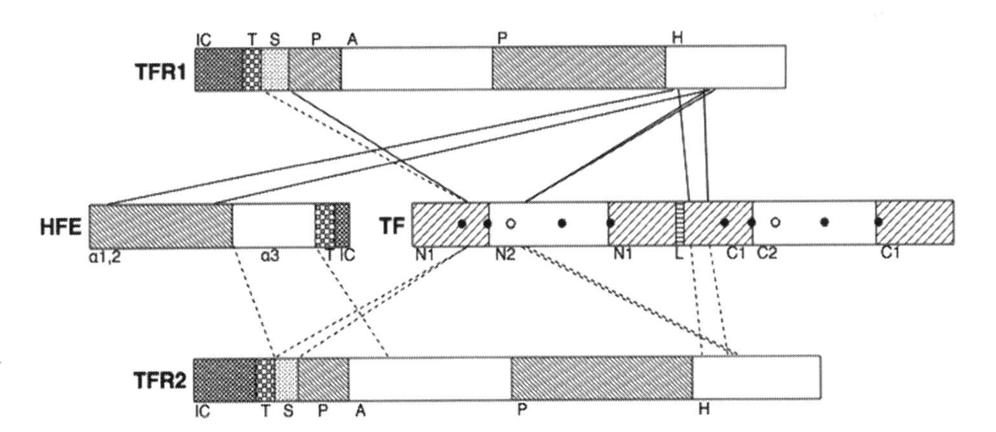

Fig. 7.1 Schematic diagram of interactions between the transferrin receptors and their ligands. Domains of the proteins are indicated by different patterns. *IC* intracellular, *T* transmembrane, *S* stalk, *P* protease-like, *A* apical, *H* helical, *α1,2* α1,2 superdomain, *α3* α3 domain, *N1* N1-lobe, *N2* N2-lobe, *C1* C1-lobe, *C2* C2-lobe, *L* linker. Residues involved in the coordination of iron or bicarbonate to transferrin are shown (*filled circle*). *Solid lines* indicate regions of known interacting residues, dotted lines indicate interacting regions where specific residues are unknown. Domains of TFR2 have been inferred from information from TFR1 as have regions of binding of TF to TFR2 (Information from [38–43])

amino acid residues act to stabilize the structure; in the N-lobe, two lysine residues form a hydrogen bond in the iron-containing structure at neutral pH [44], whereas the analogous function in the C-lobe is provided by a bridge between a lysine, an aspartate, and an arginine residue [44]. Further stabilization of the metal-containing structure is provided by another layer of interactions, principally between a number of conserved aromatic residues, which are different for each lobe [45].

Iron binding to apotransferrin is an ordered process. The initial step involves carbonate binding to each lobe which is followed by iron binding to the C-lobe only. This is followed by several rounds of proton loss and conformational changes. Iron can then bind to the N-lobe, once again followed by several rounds of proton loss and conformational changes. The protein then undergoes a final conformational change to arrive at its final structure [46].

3.2 Iron Release from Transferrin

Iron release has been studied more completely in the N-lobe. Following the decrease in pH, the synergistic carbonate anion is protonated, causing changes in hydrogen bonding and movement of side chains, resulting in reductions in the affinities of the protein for both the anion and the metal and also a partial opening of the metal binding site [47]. One of the two lysine residues which form the di-lysine bridge becomes protonated, breaking the hydrogen bond. This was postulated to result in electrostatic repulsion, causing the two domains of the binding cleft to rotate apart, exposing the metal and its binding site [44]. Recently, it has been proposed that electrostatic repulsion is not sufficient to explain the change in conformation and that the proton accepted by the lysine residue is then transferred to one of the tyrosine residues involved in coordinating the iron atom, directly destabilizing metal binding [48, 49]. Either way, exposed side chains may then bind small anions, stabilizing the open binding cleft and allowing removal of the metal [50]. The identity of the anions is unknown; many have been used *in vitro*, but whether they participate *in vivo* is uncertain. Both chloride and citric acid have been suggested based on their concentrations in physiological media [50, 51], and citric acid has also been identified in the crystal structure of apotransferrin [51], but this may simply be due to its presence in the crystallization solution rather than indicating a physiological role.

Release of the metal from the C-lobe appears to occur in a similarly elegant manner, but does so without the presence of lysines in analogous positions to those in the N-lobe. Instead, metal release appears to be triggered by protonation at low pH of an aspartic acid residue, disrupting its hydrogen bonds with a lysine and an arginine residue, which results in the required conformational change [44]. This difference also explains the long-noted observation that iron is released from the N-lobe of free transferrin prior to its release from the C-lobe as the pH is reduced [52]: the pK_a of the di-lysine system is slightly higher than that of the Lys-Asp-Arg system [44].

4 The Transferrin Receptors

Two transferrin receptors have been identified in mammals. The first, transferrin receptor (TFR) 1, is an almost ubiquitously expressed type II transmembrane homodimer. In humans, each subunit consists of 760 amino acids comprising a short, intracellular tail at the N-terminus, which contains the endocytosis signals [53], followed by a single membrane-spanning region and a large, extracellular C-terminal region. The extracellular portion, which is connected to the transmembrane region by a 38-residue stalk, is folded into three domains: a protease-like domain, an apical domain, and a helical domain (Fig. 7.1) [54, 55]. It is glycosylated, phosphorylated, and palmitylated [56–58] and the stalks of the homodimer are linked by two disulfide bonds [57]. It binds diferric transferrin with high affinity in a pH-dependent manner.

The second transferrin receptor, TFR2, is also a type II transmembrane homodimer. It shares 45% identity and 66% similarity with the primary sequence of the extracellular portion of TFR1. It is also dimerized via one or more disulfide bonds and contains multiple glycosylation sites [59]. The specific residues involved in these post-translational modifications are yet to be verified. Like TFR1, it binds diferric transferrin in a pH-dependent manner and mediates uptake of iron by receptor-mediated endocytosis [59–63]. However, the interaction of transferrin with TFR2 is up to 30-fold weaker than that with TFR1, and, in contrast to TFR1, TFR2 is predominantly expressed in hepatocytes and is not regulated by cellular iron levels [59, 61, 64].

5 Delivery of Transferrin-Bound Iron to Cells

5.1 Transferrin Receptor 1-Mediated Endocytosis

The identification of transferrin as the plasma iron-binding protein led to the discovery that the cellular uptake of transferrin-bound iron (TBI) is mediated by specific receptors on the plasma membrane [29, 65] which we now call TFR1. Cellular acquisition of TBI mediated by TFR1 involves a high-affinity receptor-mediated endocytic pathway. As shown in Fig. 7.2, this multistep process

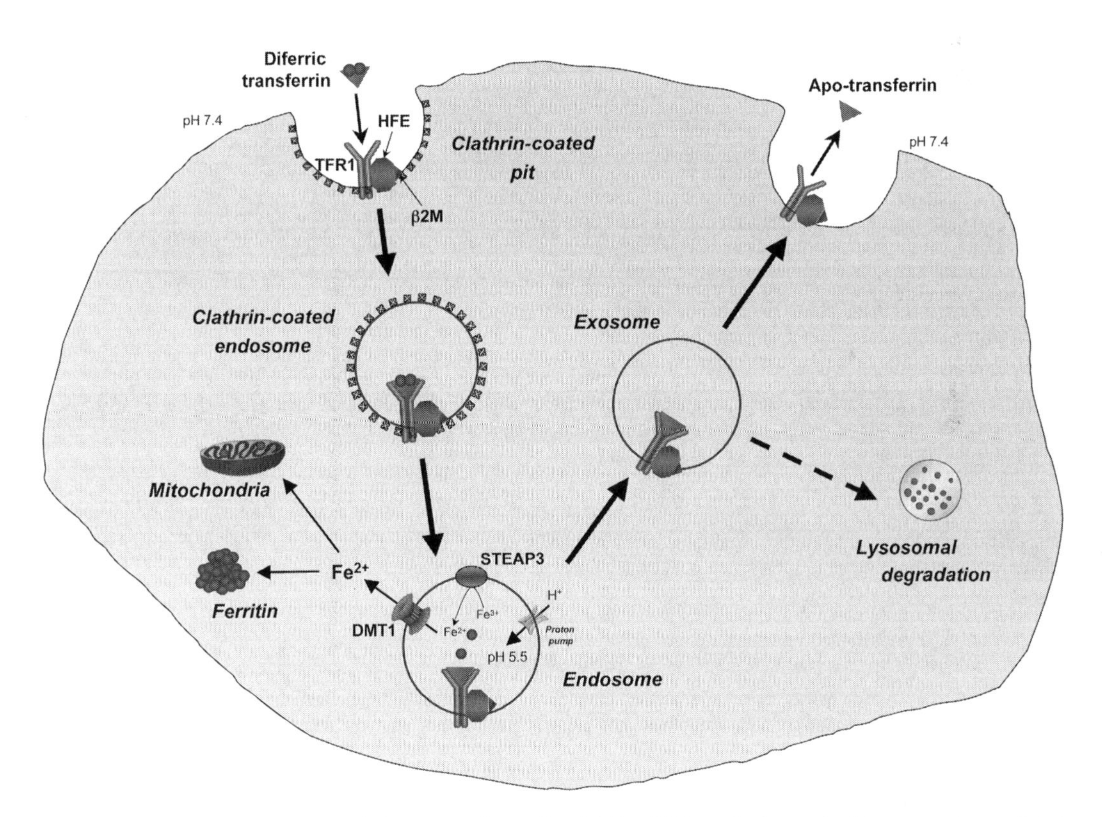

Fig. 7.2 TFR1-mediated endocytosis in mammalian cells. Cellular TBI uptake is acquired by a receptor-mediated endocytic process via TFR1 with high affinity. HFE/β2M competes with diferric transferrin for binding to TFR1 and regulates TBI uptake. Upon binding of diferric transferrin to TFR1 at the extracellular pH of 7.4, the endocytic process is initiated. TBI is internalized into the cell and iron is released from transferrin within the endosome as the pH drops to 5.5 through the action of a proton pump. The released iron is reduced from ferric to ferrous iron by a ferrireductase, possibly STEAP3, and transported across the endosomal membrane by DMT1. Cytosolic iron is either stored as ferritin or is incorporated into the mitochondria for heme protein synthesis. Apotransferrin and its receptors are recycled to the cell surface and the iron-free transferrin is released into the circulation

involves (1) transferrin-TFR1 interaction, followed by (2) endocytosis of the transferrin-TFR1 complex, (3) release of iron from the transferrin-TFR1 complex, and finally by (4) the transfer of iron across the endosomal membrane into the cytosolic compartment of the cell.

5.1.1 Transferrin–Transferrin Receptor 1 Interaction

Receptor-mediated endocytosis mediated by TFR1 is initiated when circulating transferrin binds to TFR1 at the cell surface. The transferrin–TFR1 interaction is neither temperature nor energy dependent; however, the interaction is reversible, and is dependent on the pH of the milieu and iron status of transferrin [66, 67]. This interaction has several important consequences for transferrin-bound iron uptake. The interaction of transferrin with TFR1 is stable for both the iron-containing form of the ligand at extracellular pH and apotransferrin at the lower pH in the endosome. At the extracellular pH of 7.4, TFR1 preferentially binds diferric transferrin (dissociation constant of 10^{-7}–10^{-9} M) and will also bind monoferric transferrin (dissociation constant of 10^{-6} M). Apotransferrin does not compete significantly with diferric transferrin for TFR1 binding. However, the affinity of TFR1 for apotransferrin increases and for diferric transferrin decreases as the pH drops below 6.5; at pH 5–6, the affinity of TFR1 for apotransferrin is similar to that for diferric transferrin at pH 7.4 [66, 68]. In addition, the receptor appears to reduce the release rate of iron from transferrin at neutral pH [69] and is also involved in facilitating iron release within the endosome.

Both lobes of transferrin bind to the receptor (Fig. 7.1); binding causes a straightening of transferrin and it appears that the C-lobe binds first followed by the N-lobe. A negatively charged area on the C-lobe interacts with a positively charged area on the helical domain of TFR1. The N-lobe interacts not only with the helical domain of TFR1 but also with the protease-like domain. The interactions are mixed hydrophobic and ionic in contrast to the largely ionic bonds between the C-lobe and the receptor. The arrangement between the two proteins is unusual and places the N-lobe of transferrin adjacent to the stalk region of TFR1, between the proximal surface of the receptor and the membrane [40, 69].

5.1.2 Transferrin–Transferrin Receptor 1 Endocytosis

Following the binding of transferrin to TFR1, the transferrin–TFR1 complex is clustered into a clathrin-coated vesicle, aided by the adaptor protein complex-2 [70], and gains entry into the cell by endocytosis (Fig. 7.2). Upon internalization, the vesicle loses the clathrin coat to form a smooth vesicle, the sorting endosome. From here, the apotransferrin–TFR1 complex is returned to the plasma membrane, either directly or via the endocytic recycling compartment. Only approximately 1% of the complex enters the late endosomes and is directed to lysosomes [71]. In contrast to the transferrin–TFR1 interaction, transferrin endocytosis is energy- and temperature-dependent [72, 73].

5.1.3 Endosomal Release of Iron from Transferrin

The endosome then undergoes acidification which facilitates the release of iron from transferrin (Fig. 7.2). Acidification is achieved by the entry of H^+ via an ATP-dependent proton pump that reduces the endosomal pH to near 5.5 [74, 75]. This is supported by studies that demonstrated a reduction in cellular TBI uptake due to inhibition of the acidification of endosomes by weak bases, lysosomotropic agents, and inhibitors of H^+-ATPase [75–77]. Iron is then reduced from ferric to ferrous iron by a ferrireductase, probably six-transmembrane epithelial antigen of the prostate 3 (STEAP3). STEAP3 is an NADPH-dependent ferric and cupric reductase which is highly expressed in erythroid cells as well as fetal and adult liver. It is a homodimer with each subunit containing a flavin derivative and a heme moiety as electron acceptors. It has been detected in recycling endosomes co-localizing with transferrin, TFR1, and divalent metal transporter 1 (DMT1), and may form part of a larger complex with these molecules to facilitate iron transport [78, 79]. In addition, *Steap3* deficiency results in low ferrireductase activity in mouse reticulocyte-rich erythrocytes while overexpression of STEAP3 in HEK293 kidney cells exhibits increased ferrireductase activity [78]. These findings indicate that the ferrireductase activity of STEAP3 is important for the efficient delivery of iron to cells by transferrin. Two other members of the STEAP family of proteins, STEAP2 and STEAP4, also exhibit ferric and cupric reductase activity. All three reductases are widely expressed, suggesting the possibility of heterodimer formation, although each is most highly expressed in different tissues [78, 80]. These observations raise the possibility of tissue-specific regulation of metal uptake at least partially based around the activity of the reductases.

5.1.4 Role of Transferrin Receptor 1 in Iron Release from Transferrin

The mechanism of iron release from transferrin following endocytosis and vesicle acidification is poorly understood but there is an accumulation of evidence indicating that the receptor plays an important and active role in the process. It facilitates iron release at endosomal pH [81] and, in contrast to free transferrin, transferrin bound to TFR1 releases iron more readily from the C-lobe than the N-lobe [82]. In addition, the reduction potential of ferric iron co-ordinated by transferrin is increased when the ligand is complexed to TFR1 [83]. The drop in endosomal pH results in a change in the binding footprint of the C-lobe which additionally associates one and maybe two histidine residues of transferrin with a tryptophan and a phenylalanine in the C-terminal tail of TFR1 [84]. TFR1 itself may also undergo a conformational change [85]. The change in the conformation of transferrin may be the trigger for iron release, with changes to the protonation of transferrin (described in Sect. 5.1.5), taking place subsequently [69]. The opening of the C-lobe cleft shifts the structure away from the receptor, possibly allowing other proteins, such as STEAP3, access to the metal atom. Iron release from the N-lobe appears to be directed toward the membrane [40]. Whether there is sufficient room for access by other proteins or whether iron is required to diffuse out from the structure is unknown. The resulting apotransferrin binds to TFR1 with a K_d of approximately 5 nM [69] and is released following exocytosis to the extracellular medium, the rise in pH increasing the K_d approximately 25–35-fold [67, 86].

5.1.5 Transfer of Iron into the Cytosol

The reduced ferrous ion traverses the endosomal membrane into the cytosol mediated by DMT1 (Fig. 7.2). The role of DMT1 in the translocation of iron from the endosome was demonstrated in studies using the Belgrade (*b/b*) rat and microcytic anemic (*mk/mk*) mice which contain a G185R mutation in DMT1 [87–89], resulting in impaired endosomal iron transport. The finding that DMT1 is localized to the plasma and endosomal membranes corroborates its role as an endosomal iron transporter [90]. Cytosolic iron is incorporated into ferritin for storage or into mitochondria for heme protein synthesis.

The apotransferrin–TFR1 complex, still within the endosome, is recycled to the cell surface through exocytic vesicles where apotransferrin dissociates from TFR1 at the extracellular pH of 7.4 [3]. The apotransferrin can be reutilized to bind more circulating iron and another transferrin cell cycle commences. The cycling time of TFR1-mediated endocytosis is cell-type dependent; a cycle is completed within 2–3 min in reticulocytes [91] and in up to 15 min in hepatocytes [92]. Cycling time is increased in reticulocytes of the hemoglobin-deficient (*hbd/hbd*) mouse [93]. This mouse exhibits microcytic anemia caused by a deletion in the *Sec15l* gene [94, 95]. The increase in transferrin cycling time appears to be due to a slowing of exocytosis and may also involve a slowing of endocytosis [93, 96]. Under normal conditions, transferrin protein has an average half-life of approximately 7.5 days while that of TBI is in the range of 1–2.5 h [97], indicating that in its lifetime in the circulation, a transferrin molecule may undergo up to 200 endocytic cycles [98].

5.1.6 Transferrin Receptor 1–HFE Interaction and Cellular Iron Uptake

The physical association between HFE and β2-microglobulin is essential for the cell surface expression of HFE [99] and the HFE-ß2-microglobulin heterodimer can form a ternary complex with TFR1. This interaction was initially reported in human placenta in 1997 and subsequently in other cell types [100–102]. The interaction is pH-dependent [41] with binding occurring at neutral pH but not at pH 6.0. This is similar to the pH-dependency of the TFR1–diferric transferrin interaction as described in Sect. 5.1.1.

TFR1 binds HFE at the same site as it binds transferrin (Fig. 7.1) [41], directly competing with transferrin and causing a decrease in the apparent affinity of the receptor for transferrin [103, 104]. The interaction occurs over an unusually large area, between the α_1 and α_2 domains of HFE and the helical domain of TFR1 [42]. Mutagenesis studies have indicated that the two residues in HFE, which are most important to the interaction, are Val-100 and Trp-103. Mutation of either of these residues resulted in a reduction of affinity of in excess of 4,500 times [105]. Neither Cys-282 nor His-63, mutation of which are associated with iron overload in hereditary hemochromatosis, are directly involved in the interaction: Cys-282 is in the α_3 domain and interacts with ß2-microglobulin [103] and His-63, while positioned in the α_1 domain, does not bind to TFR1 [42, 105]. Several residues in the helical domain of TFR1 participate in binding of HFE and, when mutated, severely reduce binding; tellingly, mutation of these same residues also reduces transferrin binding, confirmation of the overlapping binding sites [106]. Despite the presence of two histidine residues (His-96 and His-172) in the area of interaction of HFE with TFR1 [42], mutation of neither abrogates the pH-dependency of binding; it appears that the pH-dependence is due solely to TFR1 [105].

The interaction of HFE with TFR1 suggested that HFE can modulate iron transport [103, 105, 107]. Perhaps not surprisingly, the interaction of HFE with TFR1 causes a decrease in TBI uptake in hepatocyte-derived cells [108, 109], but, interestingly, appears to increase it in duodenal crypt cells and a Chinese hamster ovary cell model [102, 110], suggesting that the effects of the interaction are cell-type specific. In HFE-overexpressing cells, HFE has been shown to compete with transferrin for TFR1 binding [104, 105], reducing cellular iron uptake from transferrin [101, 111]. HFE and the transferrin–TFR1 complex have been detected in recycling endosomes [112]. However, how HFE impacts on transferrin–TFR1 cycling is controversial. The decrease in TBI uptake has been reported to be accompanied by unaltered TFR1 cycling [101] or a reduction in endocytosis [113] or decreased exocytosis [109]. Cellular iron release does not appear to be affected [109].

5.2 Transferrin Receptor 2-Mediated Iron Uptake

TFR2-mediated TBI uptake has been demonstrated in TFR2 overexpressing Chinese hamster ovary [59, 63] and HeLa [61] cells. TFR2 binds transferrin with an affinity that is up to 30-fold lower than TFR1 [60, 62]. TBI uptake mediated by TFR2 is also pH-dependent. As with TFR1, TFR2 binds diferric transferrin but not apotransferrin at pH 7.4 while at lower pH the converse occurs [60]. This suggests that TBI uptake by TFR2 also occurs by a receptor-mediated endocytic process [63]. In contrast to the widespread expression of TFR1, TFR2 is predominantly expressed by the liver, more specifically in hepatocytes and, indeed, TFR2 has been shown to contribute to TBI uptake by the liver [114]. TFR2 is also involved in the regulation of iron homeostasis as mutations in TFR2 result in iron overload (TFR2-associated hereditary hemochromatosis) [115–117].

Following the identification of TFR2, it was logical to determine whether it interacted with HFE, given the many similarities between TFR1 and TFR2. Nevertheless, initial *in vitro* studies using the soluble extracellular domains of HFE and TFR2 failed to show any interaction between the two fragments [62]. However, TFR2 was shown to co-localize with HFE in duodenal crypt enterocytes by immunohistochemistry [118]. Later, the possibility of an interaction was revisited using overexpressed full-length proteins. These studies have shown that TFR2 and HFE do, indeed, interact, but in a different manner from TFR1 and HFE [119]. The interaction takes place between residues located between amino acids 104 and 250 of TFR2 and in the α_3 domain of HFE (Fig. 7.1). Also, HFE maintains its interaction with TFR2 which contains mutations leading to TFR2-associated hemochromatosis in vivo [119]. Unlike the TFR1–HFE interaction, the interaction between TFR2 and HFE is not dependent on pH between pH 6 and 7.5. As described in Sect. 5.1.6, HFE competes with transferrin for its binding site on TFR1. However, this does not appear to be the case for TFR2, which can bind HFE and transferrin simultaneously [43]. No crystal structure is yet available to confirm the details of the interaction between HFE, TFR2, and transferrin. It remains unclear whether HFE is involved in the regulation of TFR2-mediated TBI transport [108, 120].

6 Regulation of Transferrin and the Transferrin Receptors

6.1 Transferrin

The synthesis of transferrin is regulated by cellular iron levels, hormones such as estrogen and hypoxia [3, 121–123]. Plasma transferrin levels are increased in response to iron deficiency and decreased in iron overload. Elevated estrogen levels are associated with a rise in transferrin levels during pregnancy. Transferrin synthesis is likewise stimulated by hypoxia by a mechanism that involves the binding of hypoxia-inducible factor-1 to the hypoxia response element on the promoter of the transferrin gene [123].

6.2 Transferrin Receptor 1

TFR1-mediated iron uptake is dependent on the expression of TFR1 which is influenced by the stage of development, cellular proliferation, iron status, hypoxia, and inflammation. TFR1 expression and TBI uptake are high in developing erythroid cells and reduced with cellular maturation [124, 125]. Similarly, TFR1 expression is high in the fetal liver [126], with the number of TFR1 decreasing markedly in neonates to relatively low levels in the adult animal [127]. Cells that are actively proliferating take up more TBI due to higher levels of TFR1 expression compared to cells that are quiescent [128, 129]. This is consistent with the high requirements of iron during development. High iron levels are associated with decreased TFR1 expression while iron depletion is associated with increased TFR1 expression [108, 130–132]. The regulation of TFR1 by cellular iron levels is mediated through the iron responsive element–iron regulatory protein (IRE–IRP) post-transcriptional mechanism discussed in Chap. 3. Iron-dependent regulation of TFR1 at the transcriptional level has also been described, although the promoter region responsible remains to be characterized [133]. Hypoxia stimulates TFR1 gene transcription through the activation of the hypoxia-inducible factor-1 [134, 135]. Nitric oxide and hydrogen peroxide [131, 136, 137] as well as cytokines such as tumor necrosis factor-α, interleukin-1β, and interleukin-6 [138, 139] enhance TBI uptake. The effects of nitric oxide and hydrogen peroxide are likely to be mediated by elevation of TFR1 expression through increased RNA-binding activity of IRP1 [131, 136], while the mechanism of action of cytokines is not fully understood.

6.3 *Transferrin Receptor 2*

Like its interaction with HFE, regulation of TFR2 is quite different from that of TFR1. Unlike TFR1, TFR2 mRNA does not contain IREs in its untranslated region and hence is not regulated by iron status [59]. TFR2 protein expression is regulated by transferrin saturation; with higher levels of diferric transferrin increasing TFR2 protein expression during iron overload while lower levels of diferric transferrin in iron deficiency downregulate TFR2 expression as a result of diminished stability of the protein [140, 141]. Like TFR1, TFR2 expression is also regulated by cellular proliferation [129], the cell cycle [60, 142], and cellular differentiation [143]. The regulation of expression of proteins of iron metabolism is discussed in more detail in Chap. 3.

7 Transferrin-Bound Iron Uptake by Mammalian Tissues

The widespread expression of TFR1 indicates that it mediates cellular iron uptake in most types of cells. TBI uptake by TFR1 occurs by a high-affinity receptor-mediated endocytic process which was first described in reticulocytes [144], and thereafter, in a multitude of other cell types such as placental syncytiotrophoblasts, hepatocytes, myocytes, and fibroblasts. Due to the overall similarity of the process of cellular TBI uptake, it will only be described in cells and tissues which play a central role in iron homeostasis or those with specialized functions in iron metabolism such as erythroid cells, duodenum, liver, placenta, brain, and macrophages.

7.1 *Erythroid Cells*

Approximately 70–80% of plasma iron turnover is directed toward the bone marrow for incorporation into developing erythroid cells for hemoglobin synthesis. Erythroid iron is derived exclusively from receptor-mediated endocytosis of transferrin. The rate of TBI uptake corresponds to the stage of maturation of erythroid cells; there are few TFR1 in erythroid progenitor cells while maximal TFR1 expression occurs in intermediate basophilic normoblasts [125]. The number of receptors decreases as the cells mature into reticulocytes, until finally, there is a complete loss of TFR1 as the cells develop into erythrocytes [124, 145].

Most of what we know about TFR1-mediated endocytosis has been accomplished from studies in reticulocytes (see Sect. 5). It is a rapid and efficient process; each endocytic cycle is completed within 3 min [91, 146] with transferrin delivering two atoms of iron to the cells in each cycle [87]. Almost half of the iron taken up is incorporated into heme within 1.5 min, and by 10 min only 12% of the iron is present as non-heme iron [147]. These results indicate that endosomal iron is mainly directed to the mitochondria for heme protein synthesis. Embryos from mice that lack Tfr1 do not survive and suffer from impaired erythropoiesis [148], indicating that functional TFR1 is essential for the supply of iron to developing erythrocytes. The regulation of erythroid iron metabolism is described in more detail in Chap. 10.

7.2 *Duodenum*

The acquisition of iron by duodenal crypt enterocytes is mediated by TFR1-mediated endocytosis of TBI from the circulation. Duodenal iron uptake from plasma transferrin has been shown to be directly proportional to plasma iron concentrations [149]. TFR1 is expressed on the basal membrane of crypt enterocytes and as the cell matures and migrates into the villus, the level of TFR1 expression decreases until it disappears in the absorptive villus enterocyte [150]. This is consistent with the high iron requirement by crypt cells during their proliferative stage. Unlike most cells, the uptake of TBI by duodenal enterocytes does not appear to involve DMT1. Iron uptake from transferrin is not impaired in the Belgrade rat which has a G185R mutation in the DMT1 gene [149], suggesting that DMT1 is not necessary for endosomal iron transport in the duodenum. Furthermore, DMT1 expression is low in crypt enterocytes [89], which provides support for a lack of involvement by DMT1 in the iron uptake process. The mechanism by which endosomal iron is released into the cytosol of crypt cells has not been identified. The iron-free transferrin–TFR1 complex is returned to the basal membrane and the transferrin released back into the plasma.

HFE is expressed in crypt cells and co-localizes with TFR1 [102], implying that HFE regulates duodenal uptake of TBI from the blood. This is evident from an in vivo study in mice which demonstrated that the loss of functional HFE resulted in impaired TBI uptake by the duodenum [151]. The results are consistent with the iron-deficient phenotype of crypt enterocytes reported in subjects with HFE-associated hereditary hemochromatosis [152]. The loss of function of HFE leads to increased expression of iron absorption proteins such as DMT1 and ferroportin [153, 154] and, thus, a dysregulation of non-heme iron absorption. A recent study showed that when Hfe expression was selectively deleted in mouse crypt enterocytes, there was no anomaly in plasma and liver iron concentrations and no change in Dmt1, Dcytb, and ferroportin mRNA expression [155], indicating that duodenal Hfe is not important in systemic iron homeostasis. These findings support the model involving the hepatic peptide, hepcidin described in Chap. 9. Although TFR2 has been detected in crypt enterocytes, co-localizing with HFE [118], its role in duodenal iron metabolism is not understood.

7.3 *Placenta*

The placenta is an ephemeral organ that allows the maternal and fetal circulations to remain separate during pregnancy. Nutrients, oxygen, antibodies, and hormones from the maternal circulation are transferred to the developing fetus by the placenta which also allows waste products to be expelled from the fetal circulation. In humans, the placenta is hemochorial and consists of a single layer of fused cells, the syncytiotrophoblasts. These trophoblasts are in direct contact with maternal blood due to the breakdown of the maternal capillary endothelium.

Iron transport by the syncytiotrophoblasts is unidirectional toward the fetus. The syncytiotrophoblasts are polarized cells with the apical membrane bathed by the maternal circulation and the basal membrane bathed by the fetal circulation. The apical membrane has high levels of TFR1 expression which mediate the uptake of TBI by receptor-mediated endocytosis [156, 157]. Once in the cell, iron is released from the endosomes and the apotransferrin–TFR1 complex is exocytosed back into the maternal circulation. The subsequent transfer of iron across both the endosomal and basal membranes is poorly understood. DMT1 has been detected in the cytoplasm and basal membrane of the syncytiotrophoblasts [158, 159], with some studies reporting little overlap between DMT1 and TFR1 [157, 158] while another demonstrated interaction between TFR1 and HFE [160]. A strong candidate for the basal membrane iron exporter is ferroportin. Ferroportin protein is expressed in abundance on the basal surface of the syncytiotrophoblasts [157, 161, 162]. The loss of functional ferroportin leads to embryonic lethality in mice supporting the notion that ferroportin is essential for maternofetal iron transfer [163]. The presence of copper oxidase activity at the basal placental membrane [164] suggests that a copper oxidase, similar to hephestin in the duodenal enterocyte or ceruloplasmin in hepatic cells, may oxidize the iron released by ferroportin so that it can bind to transferrin in the fetal circulation for delivery of iron to the fetus.

The localization and role of HFE in placental syncytiotrophoblasts is uncertain. Although it has been shown that HFE is present on the apical membrane and co-localizes with TFR1 [100, 160], HFE has also been shown to localize to the basal membrane [157]. Its presence on the apical surface suggests that like in other cell types, HFE may regulate TBI uptake by competing with transferrin for binding to TFR1 [101, 108, 110]. In contrast, the presence of HFE on the basal membrane of syncytiotrophoblasts suggests that it may influence iron export into the fetal circulation. Overexpression of HFE has been shown to inhibit iron export from macrophages and colonic cells [165, 166]. The role of HFE in placental syncytiotrophoblasts remains uncertain.

The rate of iron transfer from the mother to the fetus is greatest in the last trimester during pregnancy and is accompanied by increased TFR1 expression [167]. Iron uptake by placental syncytiotrophoblasts is also regulated by maternal iron levels. The upregulation of the iron transport proteins, TFR1 and DMT1, as well as TBI uptake during maternal iron deficiency [168] may be a protective mechanism to continually provide iron to the developing fetus despite iron depletion in the mother. The involvement of cytokines in placental iron transfer has also been implicated. In iron-deficient rats, placental tumor necrosis factor-α levels are increased while fetal growth is suppressed [169], suggesting a link between iron, cytokine levels and fetal development. Hepcidin, the hepatic regulator of iron homeostasis, when constitutively expressed by the embryo during development results in transcriptional downregulation of placental TFR1 expression that is independent of iron levels and IRE-IRP binding activity [170]. These results suggest that embryonic hepcidin can inhibit iron transfer from the maternal circulation.

7.4 Brain

Although the blood–brain barrier is impervious to plasma proteins, the presence of TFR1 on brain capillary endothelial cells (BCECs) [171, 172] aids in the delivery of iron from plasma transferrin. It is widely accepted that the brain acquires iron by TFR1-mediated endocytosis of diferric transferrin. Transferrin binds to TFR1 on the luminal membrane of brain capillaries and is endocytosed by BCECs. The fate of iron after endocytosis, however, is less clear. Results from an early study suggested that BCECs take up TBI by transcytosis, where transferrin binds to TFR1, the transferrin–TFR1 complex then enters the cell by endocytosis and exits the cell via the abluminal surface of BCEC into the extracellular space [173]. However, the rate of iron accumulation in the brain greatly exceeds that of transferrin which argues for an endocytic–exocytic process where iron dissociates from transferrin in the endosome and the apotransferrin–TFR1 complex is recycled back to the BCEC–plasma interface [174–177]. Cytosolic transfer of iron from the endosome is mediated by DMT1 in other cell types. Whether DMT1 mediates brain endosomal iron transport is uncertain as there is conflicting data on the expression of DMT1 in BCECs [177–180]. Likewise, it is not known how cytosolic iron traverses the abluminal surface of BCEC into the central nervous system. It is thought to involve the iron exporter, ferroportin [181], although there is also evidence against its involvement [182]. Astrocytes in close contact with the abluminal membrane of BCECs have been shown to generate a specialized form of the ferroxidase ceruloplasmin that attaches to membranes with a glycosylphosphatidylinositol anchor [183] which may facilitate iron export via ferroportin.

An alternative model of TBI uptake by BCEC has recently been proposed, one that is independent of DMT1 and which involves astrocytes [184]. In this model, it is proposed that the endosome containing transferrin–TFR1 complex is carried toward the abluminal membrane of BCECs. Iron dissociates from transferrin within the acidic endosome and exits the cell when the endosome fuses with the abluminal membrane. Foot-end processes of astrocytes form close gap junctions with BCECs and the microenvironment at these junctions is likely to be low in pH and rich in ATP, nucleotides, and citrate released by astrocytes [185, 186]. The released iron may bind to citrate, ATP, or transferrin present in brain interstitial fluid [184, 187]. The apotransferrin–TFR1 complex in exosomes is recycled to the luminal surface and released into the circulation. The validity of this model awaits confirmation.

Neurons express both TFR1 and DMT1 [178, 180], indicating that they can acquire TBI by receptor-mediated endocytosis where iron is transported across the endosomal membrane by DMT1. Cytosolic release of iron in the neuron is likely to be mediated by ferroportin [182]. The expression of TFR1 and/or DMT1 in astrocytes, oligodendrocytes, and glial cells is contentious and remains to be ascertained (reviewed in 184).

Iron is required for many brain metabolic processes such as ATP production, myelinogenesis, and neurotransmitter synthesis [177, 184, 188]. The demand for brain iron is dependent on age as well as iron status. In rats, the rate of TBI uptake and TFR1 expression by the BCECs are highest in the developing brain [189, 190]. Under conditions of iron deficiency, TBI transport into the brain is also increased [174]; however, TFR1 expression by BCECs is unaltered. In support of this, Moos and Morgan [191] demonstrated that there was no change in transferrin–TFR1 binding in iron-deficient rats compared to rats with normal iron levels. It is possible that the cycling rate of TFR1 instead is increased.

Despite the regulation of TBI uptake by the brain in response to iron status and the protective role of the blood-brain barrier, the brain can be vulnerable to the harmful effects of iron deficiency and iron excess as seen in neurological and neurodegenerative disorders (see Chap. 23). Like TFR1, HFE is also expressed on brain capillary endothelium [192]. It has been suggested that HFE may be involved in the pathogenesis of brain disorders such as Alzheimer's Disease [193] and Parkinson's Disease [194]. While it is known that brain iron levels are altered in these diseases, the role of HFE is not completely understood, but mutations in the *HFE* gene are thought to impact on brain iron transport, resulting in dysregulated iron accumulation [193].

7.5 Liver

7.5.1 Hepatocytes

Hepatocytes are the major cell type in the liver and also the main site of iron storage in the body. In the liver, iron delivery from plasma transferrin is specifically targeted to hepatocytes [195]. Several pathways of TBI have been characterized in hepatic cells, including the high-affinity low-capacity TFR1-mediated endocytic process and at least three TFR1-independent pathways.

Transferrin Receptor 1-Mediated Endocytosis

Uptake of TBI by hepatocytes via TFR1 is similar to the receptor-mediated endocytic process characterized in reticulocytes (Fig. 7.2). Briefly, transferrin laden with iron binds to TFR1 at the cell surface and is endocytosed. Iron dissociates from transferrin in the endosome and is reduced to the ferrous state by a ferrireductase, possibly STEAP3, and enters the cytosol presumably via DMT1. The iron-deficient transferrin still coupled to TFR1 is transported back to the cell surface by exosomes and released into the circulation where it can bind more iron. In adult hepatocytes, each cycle lasts between 4 and 15 min [92].

Transferrin Receptor 1-Independent Pathways

The procurement of cellular TBI also occurs by TFR1-independent pathways. These mechanisms of TBI uptake have been described in hepatocytes and other cell types including hepatoma cells, melanoma cells, and fibroblasts [126, 196–199]. Since plasma transferrin concentrations are several orders of magnitude greater than that needed to saturate TFR1, TFR1-independent iron transport may account for most of the TBI taken up by hepatocytes.

The first of these TFR1-independent pathways involves the binding of transferrin to low-affinity binding sites at the hepatocyte cell surface. Transferrin is then endocytosed and iron is released from the endosome and is transferred into the cytosol presumably by DMT1. Over time, transferrin uptake reaches a steady state while iron continues to accumulate in the cells [126, 199]. Uptake of transferrin and iron are both temperature-sensitive and energy-dependent. The use of weak bases decreases iron but not transferrin uptake, which is consistent with the inhibition of the acidification process in endosomes [126, 199]. This reaffirms that this process is mediated via a low-affinity binding site which involves endocytosis and that iron release is pH-dependent. When extracellular transferrin concentration is raised, iron uptake by hepatoma and melanoma cells is saturable, demonstrating that uptake is mediated by an iron carrier [198, 199]. In contrast, transferrin binding to the plasma membrane in rat liver was not saturable even at a concentration of 10 μM transferrin, highlighting the low-affinity nature of this process [200].

TFR2 has been postulated as the mediator of this TFR1-independent pathway. Overexpression of TFR2 in Chinese hamster ovary cells confirms that it mediates iron uptake by a receptor-mediated endocytic process [63]. Also, TFR2-overexpressing HeLa cells take up TBI by a mechanism that is comparable to that seen in hepatoma cells [61]. However, results have emerged that suggest TFR2 has a lesser role in hepatic TBI transport than first thought. In these experiments, it was shown that an upregulation of TFR2 protein expression in hepatocytes was not accompanied by an increase in TBI uptake mediated by the TFR1-independent pathway [108]. Similarly, overexpression or underexpression of TFR2 protein in in vitro studies using hepatoma cells elicits moderate changes in iron uptake despite large alterations in protein expression [201]. In addition, in vivo liver iron uptake from plasma transferrin by Tfr2 mutant mice with non-functional Tfr2 was only decreased by approximately 20% compared with wild-type mice with similar iron status [114]. Although these observations suggest that TFR2 does mediate TBI uptake in hepatic cells, they also raise the possibility that another mechanism independent of TFR1 and TFR2 may mediate TBI uptake in hepatocytes. It is hypothesized that TBI uptake via a TFR1- and TFR2-independent pathway is a major contributor to hepatocyte iron loading in disorders of iron overload such as hereditary hemochromatosis.

There is evidence for another TFR1-independent uptake pathway in hepatic cells which does not involve transferrin endocytosis [202]. Instead, iron is released from transferrin at the plasma membrane and enters the cell by a carrier-mediated process [63, 203, 204]. Iron release from transferrin appears to be facilitated by a ferrireductase at the cell surface [205, 206]. Specific ferrous ion chelators inhibit TBI uptake in hepatocytes, suggesting that iron is reduced to the divalent form at the cell surface before internalization [196, 205, 206]. In hepatic cells, TBI uptake is inhibited by NTBI, and similarly, NTBI uptake is inhibited by TBI, suggesting that both TBI and NTBI uptake are mediated by a common transporter [203, 204, 207–209]. NTBI does not affect TBI uptake by a transferrin endocytic process but inhibits the uptake of iron dissociated from transferrin at the plasma membrane. Recently, it was shown that NTBI uptake correlated with TFR2 protein expression in TFR2-overexpressing Chinese hamster ovary cells [63]. Whether TFR2 is involved in this uptake process in other cell types has not been ascertained.

An additional pathway for TBI uptake is fluid-phase endocytosis. Molecules in the fluid phase of the endocytic vesicles are taken up in a non-specific manner. The contents of the vesicles are directed to lysosomes for degradation or exocytosed into the circulation. This process accounts for less than 5–20% of TBI uptake in hepatocytes [196, 210].

7.5.2 Küpffer Cells and Endothelial Cells

TFR1 is expressed and can mediate TBI uptake by non-parenchymal cells of the liver, the Küpffer cells, and endothelial cells, which line the liver sinusoids [195, 211, 212]. TFR1 expression is lower in Küpffer cells [211] and higher in endothelial cells [213] in comparison to hepatocytes.

The high TFR1 expression by endothelial cells led to the suggestion that these cells play an important role in the regulation of liver iron transport, but this has never been confirmed.

Küpffer cells are resident macrophages of the liver and receive most of their iron from erythrophagocytosis, which may explain the lower TFR1 expression. In rats, Tfr1 expression by Küpffer cells is affected by the age as well as iron status of the animals [127]. HFE has also been detected in Küpffer cells [192]. In HFE-associated hereditary hemochromatosis, Küpffer cells, unlike hepatocytes, are relatively spared from iron loading, suggesting that HFE may regulate iron uptake in both cell types using distinct mechanisms. Alternatively, the cells are not as iron loaded due to higher iron export activity by Küpffer cells [214] since ferroportin is highly expressed by macrophages.

7.6 Macrophages

Like Küpffer cells, macrophages in the spleen and bone marrow phagocytose senescent erythroid cells that are at the end of their life span. The presence of TFR1 in macrophages suggests that they can also take up iron from plasma transferrin via TFR1-mediated endocytosis [215–218] although iron uptake by this pathway is likely to be limited in vivo. In contrast to the iron-dependent regulation of TFR1 in other cell types, elevated iron levels enhance TFR1 mRNA and protein expression in macrophages [219]. The presence of HFE increased rather than decreased TBI uptake by these cells [218]. TBI uptake and TFR1 expression by macrophages are downregulated after exposure to lipopolysaccharide and/or interferon-γ despite an increase in IRP1–RNA binding activity [216, 217]. These observations highlight the unconventional manner in which TFR1 expression and TBI uptake are modulated by iron, HFE, and inflammation in macrophages, indicating perhaps the specialized function of these cells of the reticuloendothelial system. Macrophage iron metabolism will be described in more detail in Chap. 11.

Acknowledgments We are grateful to Carly Herbison for assistance with preparation of the figures. The work from this laboratory was supported by research grants from the National Health and Medical Research Council of Australia, Raine Medical Research Foundation, Fremantle Hospital Medical Research Foundation, and the University of Western Australia.

References

1. Charley P, Rosenstein M, Shore E, Saltman P. The role of chelation and binding equilibria in iron metabolism. Arch Biochem Biophys. 1960;88:222–6.
2. Laurell CB. Plasma iron and the transport of iron in the organism. Pharmacol Rev. 1952;4:371–95.
3. Morgan EH. Transferrin biochemistry, physiology and clinical significance. Molec Aspects Med. 1981;4:1–123.
4. Sun H, Li H, Sadler PJ. Transferrin as a metal ion mediator. Chem Rev. 1999;99:2817–42.
5. Taylor DM. The bioinorganic chemistry of actinides in the blood. J Alloys Compd. 1998;271–273:6–10.
6. Hershko C, Graham G, Bates GW, Rachmilewitz EA. Non-specific serum iron in thalassemia: an abnormal serum iron fraction of potential toxicity. Br J Haematol. 1978;40:255–63.
7. Gosriwatana I, Loreal O, Lu S, Brissot P, Porter J, Hider RC. Quantification of non-transferrin-bound iron in the presence of unsaturated transferrin. Anal Biochem. 1999;273:212–20.
8. Loreal O, Gosriwatana I, Guyader D, Porter J, Brissot P, Hider RC. Determination of non-transferrin-bound iron in genetic hemochromatosis using a new HPLC-based method. J Hepatol. 2000;32:727–33.
9. Grootveld M, Bell JD, Halliwell B, Aruoma OI, Bomford A, Sadler PJ. Non-transferrin-bound iron in plasma or serum from patients with idiopathic hemochromatosis. Characterization by high performance liquid chromatography and nuclear magnetic resonance spectroscopy. J Biol Chem. 1989;264:4417–22.
10. Sarkar B. State of iron(III) in normal human serum: low molecular weight and protein ligands besides transferrin. Can J Biochem. 1970;48:1339–50.
11. Breuer W, Ermers MJ, Pootrakul P, Abramov A, Hershko C, Cabantchik ZI. Desferrioxamine-chelatable iron, a component of serum non-transferrin-bound iron, used for assessing chelation therapy. Blood. 2001;97:792–8.

12. Esposito BP, Breuer W, Sirankapracha P, Pootrakul P, Hershko C, Cabantchik ZI. Labile plasma iron in iron overload: redox activity and susceptibility to chelation. Blood. 2003;102:2670–7.
13. Batey RG, Lai Chung Fong P, Shamir S, Sherlock S. A non-transferrin-bound serum iron in idiopathic hemochromatosis. Dig Dis Sci. 1980;25:340–6.
14. Fargion S, Cappellini MD, Sampietro M, Fiorelli G. Non-specific iron in patients with beta-thalassaemia trait and chronic active hepatitis. Scand J Haematol. 1981;26:161–7.
15. Gutteridge JMC, Rowley DA, Griffiths E, Halliwell B. Low-molecular-weight iron complexes and oxygen radical reactions in idiopathic haemochromatosis. Clin Sci. 1985;68:463–7.
16. Durken M, Kohlschutter A, Nielsen P. Non-transferrin bound iron induced by myeloablative therapy. Br J Haematol. 1998;101:393–4.
17. Gafter-Gvili A, Prokocimer M, Breuer W, Cabantchik IZ, Hershko C. Non-transferrin-bound serum iron (NTBI) in megaloblastic anemia: effect of vitamin B12 treatment. Hematol J. 2004;5:32–4.
18. Pootrakul P, Breuer W, Sametband M, Sirankapracha P, Hershko C, Cabantchik ZI. Labile plasma iron (LPI) as an indicator of chelatable plasma redox activity in iron-overloaded beta-thalassemia/HbE patients treated with an oral chelator. Blood. 2004;104:1504–10.
19. Aruoma OI, Bomford A, Polson RJ, Halliwell B. Nontransferrin-bound iron in plasma from hemochromatosis patients: effect of phlebotomy therapy. Blood. 1988;72:1416–9.
20. Jacobs EM, Hendriks JC, van Tits BL, Evans PJ, Breuer W, Liu DY, et al. Results of an international round robin for the quantification of serum non-transferrin-bound iron: need for defining standardization and a clinically relevant isoform. Anal Biochem. 2005;341:241–50.
21. Asaumi A, Ogino T, Akiyama T, Kawabata T, Okada S. Oxidative damages by iron-chelate complexes depend on the interaction with the target molecules. Biochem Mol Biol Int. 1996;39:77–86.
22. Hartwig A, Klyszcz-Nasko H, Schlepegrell R, Beyersmann D. Cellular damage by ferric nitrilotriacetate and ferric citrate in V79 cells: interrelationship between lipid peroxidation, DNA strand breaks and sister chromatid exchanges. Carcinogenesis. 1993;14:107–12.
23. Ogino T, Awai M. Lipid peroxidation and tissue injury by ferric citrate in paraquat-intoxicated mice. Biochim Biophys Acta. 1988;958:388–95.
24. Habel ME, Jung D. Free radicals act as effectors in the growth inhibition and apoptosis of iron-treated Burkitt's lymphoma cells. Free Radic Res. 2006;40:789–97.
25. Inai K, Fujihara M, Yonehara S, Kobuke T. Tumorigenicity study of ferric citrate administered orally to mice. Food Chem Toxicol. 1994;32:493–8.
26. Leanderson P, Tagesson C. Iron bound to the lipophilic chelator, 8-hydroxyquinolone, causes DNA strand breakage in cultured lung cells. Carcinogenesis. 1996;17:545–50.
27. Singh S, Hider RC. Colorimetric detection of the hydroxyl radical: comparison of the hydroxyl-radical-generating ability of various iron complexes. Anal Biochem. 1988;171:47–54.
28. Laurell CB. Studies on the transportation andmetabolism of iron in the body. Acta Physiol Scand. 1947;14(46):1–129.
29. Schade AL, Caroline L. An iron-binding component in human blood plasma. Science. 1946;104:340–1.
30. Wallenius G. A note on serum iron transportation. Scand J Clin Lab Invest. 1952;4:24–6.
31. Bloch B, Popovici T, Levin MJ, Tuil D, Kahn A. Transferrin gene expression visualized in oligodendrocytes of the rat brain by using in situ hybridization and immunohistochemistry. Proc Natl Acad Sci USA. 1985;82:6706–10.
32. Jordan SM, Morgan EH. Plasma protein metabolism during lactation in the rabbit. Am J Physiol. 1970;219:1549–54.
33. Skinner MK, Griswold MD. Sertoli cells synthesize and secrete transferrin-like protein. J Biol Chem. 1980;255:9523–5.
34. Lambert LA, Perri H, Meehan TJ. Evolution of duplications in the transferrin family of proteins. Comp Biochem Physiol B Biochem Mol Biol. 2005;140:11–25.
35. MacGillivray RT, Mendez E, Sinha SK, Sutton MR, Lineback-Zins J, Brew K. The complete amino acid sequence of human serum transferrin. Proc Natl Acad Sci USA. 1982;79:2504–8.
36. Park I, Schaeffer E, Sidoli A, Baralle FE, Cohen GN, Zakin MM. Organization of the human transferrin gene: direct evidence that it originated by gene duplication. Proc Natl Acad Sci USA. 1985;82:3149–53.
37. Jeffrey PD, Bewley MC, MacGillivray RT, Mason AB, Woodworth RC, Baker EN. Ligand-induced conformational change in transferrins: crystal structure of the open form of the N-terminal half-molecule of human transferrin. Biochemistry. 1998;37:13978–86.
38. Bailey S, Evans RW, Garratt RC, Gorinsky B, Hasnain S, Horsburgh C, et al. Molecular structure of serum transferrin at 3.3-A resolution. Biochemistry. 1988;27:5804–12.
39. Anderson BF, Baker HM, Dodson EJ, Norris GE, Rumball SV, Waters JM, et al. Structure of human lactoferrin at 3.2 Å resolution. Proc Natl Acad Sci USA. 1987;84:1769–73.
40. Cheng Y, Zak O, Aisen P, Harrison SC, Walz T. Structure of the human transferrin receptor-transferrin complex. Cell. 2004;116:565–76.

41. Lebrón JA, Bennett MJ, Vaughn DE, Chirino AJ, Snow PM, Mintier GA, et al. Crystal structure of the hemochromatosis protein HFE and characterization of its interaction with transferrin receptor. Cell. 1998;93:111–23.
42. Bennett MJ, Lebron JA, Bjorkman PJ. Crystal structure of the hereditary haemochromatosis protein HFE complexed with transferrin receptor. Nature. 2000;403:46–53.
43. Chen J, Chloupkova M, Gao J, Chapman-Arvedson TL, Enns CA. HFE modulates transferrin receptor 2 levels in hepatoma cells via interactions that differ from transferrin receptor 1/HFE interactions. J Biol Chem. 2007;282:36862–70.
44. Dewan JC, Mikami B, Hirose M, Sacchettini JC. Structural evidence for a pH-sensitive dilysine trigger in the hen ovotransferrin N-lobe: implications for transferrin iron release. Biochemistry. 1993;32:11963–8.
45. Baker HM, Anderson BF, Brodie AM, Shongwe MS, Smith CA, Baker EN. Anion binding by transferrins: importance of second-shell effects revealed by the crystal structure of oxalate-substituted diferric lactoferrin. Biochemistry. 1996;35:9007–13.
46. Pakdaman R, El Hage Chahine JM. A mechanism for iron uptake by transferrin. Eur J Biochem. 1996;236:922–31.
47. MacGillivray RT, Moore SA, Chen J, Anderson BF, Baker H, Luo Y, et al. Two high-resolution crystal structures of the recombinant N-lobe of human transferrin reveal a structural change implicated in iron release. Biochemistry. 1998;37:7919–28.
48. Baker HM, Nurizzo D, Mason AB, Baker EN. Structures of two mutants that probe the role in iron release of the dilysine pair in the N-lobe of human transferrin. Acta Crystallogr D Biol Crystallogr. 2007;63:408–14.
49. Rinaldo D, Field MJ. A computational study of the open and closed forms of the N-lobe human serum transferrin apoprotein. Biophys J. 2003;85:3485–501.
50. He QY, Mason AB, Nguyen V, MacGillivray RT, Woodworth RC. The chloride effect is related to anion binding in determining the rate of iron release from the human transferrin N-lobe. Biochem J. 2000;350:909–15.
51. Wally J, Halbrooks PJ, Vonrhein C, Rould MA, Everse SJ, Mason AB, et al. The crystal structure of iron-free human serum transferrin provides insight into inter-lobe communication and receptor binding. J Biol Chem. 2006;281:24934–44.
52. Lestas AN. The effect of pH upon human transferrin: selective labelling of the two iron-binding sites. Br J Haematol. 1976;32:341–50.
53. Collawn JF, Lai A, Domingo D, Fitch M, Hatton S, Trowbridge IS. YTRF is the conserved internalization signal of the transferrin receptor, and a second YTRF signal at position 31–34 enhances endocytosis. J Biol Chem. 1993;268:21686–92.
54. Fuchs H, Lucken U, Tauber R, Engel A, Gessner R. Structural model of phospholipid-reconstituted human transferrin receptor derived by electron microscopy. Structure. 1998;6:1235–43.
55. Lawrence CM, Ray S, Babyonyshev M, Galluser R, Borhani DW, Harrison SC. Crystal structure of the ectodomain of human transferrin receptor. Science. 1999;286:779–82.
56. Hayes GR, Enns CA, Lucas JJ. Identification of the O-linked glycosylation site of the human transferrin receptor. Glycobiology. 1992;2:355–9.
57. Jing SQ, Trowbridge IS. Identification of the intermolecular disulfide bonds of the human transferrin receptor and its lipid-attachment site. EMBO J. 1987;6:327–31.
58. Schneider C, Sutherland R, Newman R, Greaves M. Structural features of the cell surface receptor for transferrin that is recognized by the monoclonal antibody OKT9. J Biol Chem. 1982;257:8516–22.
59. Kawabata H, Yang R, Hirama T, Vuong PT, Kawano S, Gombart AF, et al. Molecular cloning of transferrin receptor 2. A new member of the transferrin receptor-like family. J Biol Chem. 1999;274:20826–32.
60. Kawabata H, Germain RS, Vuong PT, Nakamaki T, Said JW, Koeffler HP. Transferrin receptor 2-alpha supports cell growth both in iron-chelated cultured cells and in vivo. J Biol Chem. 2000;275:16618–25.
61. Robb AD, Ericsson M, Wessling-Resnick M. Transferrin receptor 2 mediates a biphasic pattern of transferrin uptake associated with ligand delivery to multivesicular bodies. Am J Physiol Cell Physiol. 2004;287:C1769–75.
62. West Jr AP, Bennett MJ, Sellers VM, Andrews NC, Enns CA, Bjorkman PJ. Comparison of the interactions of transferrin receptor and transferrin receptor 2 with transferrin and the hereditary hemochromatosis protein HFE. J Biol Chem. 2000;275:38135–8.
63. Graham RM, Reutens GM, Herbison CE, Delima RD, Chua ACG, Olynyk JK, et al. Transferrin receptor 2 mediates uptake of both transferrin-bound and non-transferrin bound iron. J Hepatol. 2008;48:327–34.
64. Deaglio S, Capobianco A, Cali A, Bellora F, Alberti F, Righi L, et al. Structural, functional, and tissue distribution analysis of human transferrin receptor-2 by murine monoclonal antibodies and a polyclonal antiserum. Blood. 2002;100:3782–9.
65. Jandl JH, Inman JK, Simmons RL, Allen DW. Transfer of iron from serum iron-binding protein to human reticulocytes. J Clin Invest. 1959;38:161–85.
66. Dautry-Varsat A, Ciechanover A, Lodish HF. pH and the recycling of transferrin during receptor-mediated endocytosis. Proc Natl Acad Sci USA. 1983;80:2258–62.

67. Young SP, Bomford A, Williams R. The effect of the iron saturation of transferrin on its binding and uptake by rabbit reticulocytes. Biochem J. 1984;219:505–10.
68. Morgan EH. Effect of pH and iron content of transferrin on its binding to reticulocyte receptors. Biochim Biophys Acta. 1983;762:498–502.
69. Giannetti AM, Snow PM, Zak O, Bjorkman PJ. Mechanism for multiple ligand recognition by the human transferrin receptor. PLoS Biol. 2003;1:E51.
70. Conner SD, Schmid SL. Differential requirements for AP-2 in clathrin-mediated endocytosis. J Cell Biol. 2003;162:773–9.
71. Maxfield FR, McGraw TE. Endocytic recycling. Nat Rev Mol Cell Biol. 2004;5:121–32.
72. Jandl JH, Katz JH. The plasma-to-cell cycle of transferrin. J Clin Invest. 1963;42:314–26.
73. Baker E, Morgan EH. The kinetics of the interaction between rabbit transferrin and reticulocytes. Biochemistry. 1969;8:1133–41.
74. van Renswoude J, Bridges KR, Harford JB, Klausner RD. Receptor-mediated endocytosis of transferrin and the uptake of fe in K562 cells: identification of a nonlysosomal acidic compartment. Proc Natl Acad Sci USA. 1982;79:6186–90.
75. Paterson S, Armstrong NJ, Iacopetta BJ, McArdle HJ, Morgan EH. Intravesicular pH and iron uptake by immature erythroid cells. J Cell Physiol. 1984;120:225–32.
76. Morgan EH. Inhibition of reticulocyte iron uptake by NH_4Cl and CH_3NH_2. Biochim Biophys Acta. 1981;642:119–34.
77. Octave JN, Schneider YJ, Hoffmann P, Trouet A, Crichton RR. Transferrin uptake by cultured rat embryo fibroblasts. The influence of lysosomotropic agents, iron chelators and colchicine on the uptake of iron and transferrin. Eur J Biochem. 1982;123:235–40.
78. Ohgami RS, Campagna DR, Greer EL, Antiochos B, McDonald A, Chen J, et al. Identification of a ferrireductase required for efficient transferrin-dependent iron uptake in erythroid cells. Nat Genet. 2005;37:1264–9.
79. Sendamarai AK, Ohgami RS, Fleming MD, Lawrence CM. Structure of the membrane proximal oxidoreductase domain of human Steap3, the dominant ferrireductase of the erythroid transferrin cycle. Proc Natl Acad Sci USA. 2008;105:7410–5.
80. Ohgami RS, Campagna DR, McDonald A, Fleming MD. The steap proteins are metalloreductases. Blood. 2006;108:1388–94.
81. Bali PK, Zak O, Aisen P. A new role for the transferrin receptor in the release of iron from transferrin. Biochemistry. 1991;30:324–8.
82. Bali PK, Aisen P. Receptor-mediated iron release from transferrin: differential effects on N- and C- terminal sites. Biochemistry. 1991;30:9947–52.
83. Dhungana S, Taboy CH, Zak O, Larvie M, Crumbliss AL, Aisen P. Redox properties of human transferrin bound to its receptor. Biochemistry. 2004;43:205–9.
84. Giannetti AM, Halbrooks PJ, Mason AB, Vogt TM, Enns CA, Bjorkman PJ. The molecular mechanism for receptor-stimulated iron release from the plasma iron transport protein transferrin. Structure. 2005;13:1613–23.
85. Turkewitz AP, Schwartz AL, Harrison SC. A pH-dependent reversible conformational transition of the human transferrin receptor leads to self-association. J Biol Chem. 1988;263:16309–15.
86. Young SP, Aisen P. Transferrin receptors and the uptake and release of iron by isolated hepatocytes. Hepatology. 1981;1:114–9.
87. Bowen BJ, Morgan EH. Anemia of the Belgrade rat: evidence for defective membrane transport of iron. Blood. 1987;70:38–44.
88. Fleming MD, Trenor CC, Su MA, Foernzler D, Beier DR, Dietrich WF, et al. Microcytic anaemia mice have a mutation in Nramp2, a candidate iron transporter gene. Nat Genet. 1997;16:383–6.
89. Fleming MD, Romano MA, Su MA, Garrick LM, Garrick MD, Andrews NC. Nramp2 Is mutated in the anemic Belgrade (b) rat: evidence of a role for Nramp2 in endosomal iron transport. Proc Natl Acad Sci USA. 1998;95:1148–53.
90. Su MA, Trenor CC, Fleming JC, Fleming MD, Andrews NC. The G185R mutation disrupts function of the iron transporter Nramp2. Blood. 1998;92:2157–63.
91. Qian ZM, Morgan EH. Changes in the uptake of transferrin-free and transferrin-bound iron during reticulocyte maturation in vivo and in vitro. Biochim Biophys Acta. 1992;1135:35–43.
92. Morgan EH, Baker E. Iron uptake and metabolism by hepatocytes. Fed Proc. 1986;45:2810–6.
93. Zhang A-S, Sheftel AD, Ponka P. The anemia of "haemoglobin-deficit" (hbd/hbd) mice is caused by a defect in transferrin cycling. Exp Hematol. 2006;34:593–8.
94. Lim JE, Jin O, Bennett C, Morgan K, Wang F, Trenor CC, et al. A mutation in Sec15l1 causes anemia in hemoglobin deficit (hbd) mice. Nat Genet. 2005;37:1270–3.
95. White RA, Boydston LA, Brookshier TR, McNulty SG, Nsumu NN, Brewer BP, et al. Iron metabolism mutant hbd mice have a deletion in Sec15l1, which has homology to a yeast gene for vesicle docking. Genomics. 2005;86:668–73.

96. Garrick MD, Garrick LM. Loss of rapid transferrin receptor recycling due to a mutation in Sec15l1 in hbd mice. Biochim Biophys Acta. 2007;1773:105–8.
97. Katz JH. Iron and protein kinetics studied by means of doubly labeled human crystalline transferrin. J Clin Invest. 1961;40:2143–52.
98. Aisen P. Transferrin receptor 1. Int J Biochem Cell Biol. 2004;36:2137–43.
99. Feder JN, Tsuchihashi Z, Irrinki A, Lee VK, Mapa FA, Morikang E, et al. The hemochromatosis founder mutation in HLA-H disrupts beta2-microglobulin interaction and cell surface expression. J Biol Chem. 1997;272:14025–8.
100. Parkkila S, Waheed A, Britton RS, Bacon BR, Zhou XY, Tomatsu S, et al. Association of the transferrin receptor in human placenta with HFE, the protein defective in hereditary hemochromatosis. Proc Natl Acad Sci USA. 1997;94:13198–202.
101. Roy CN, Penny DM, Feder JN, Enns CA. The hereditary hemochromatosis protein, HFE, specifically regulates transferrin-mediated iron uptake in HeLa cells. J Biol Chem. 1999;274:9022–8.
102. Waheed A, Parkkila S, Saarnio J, Fleming RE, Zhou XY, Tomatsu S, et al. Association of HFE protein with transferrin receptor in crypt enterocytes of human duodenum. Proc Natl Acad Sci USA. 1999;96:1579–84.
103. Feder JN, Penny DM, Irrinki A, Lee VK, Lebron JA, Watson N, et al. The hemochromatosis gene product complexes with the transferrin receptor and lowers its affinity for ligand binding. Proc Natl Acad Sci USA. 1998;95:1472–7.
104. Giannetti AM, Bjorkman PJ. HFE and transferrin directly compete for transferrin receptor in solution and at the cell surface. J Biol Chem. 2004;279:25866–75.
105. Lebrón JA, West Jr AP, Bjorkman PJ. The hemochromatosis protein HFE competes with transferrin for binding to the transferrin receptor. J Mol Biol. 1999;294:239–45.
106. West Jr AP, Giannetti AM, Herr AB, Bennett MJ, Nangiana JS, Pierce JR, et al. Mutational analysis of the transferrin receptor reveals overlapping HFE and transferrin binding sites. J Mol Biol. 2001;313:385–97.
107. Ramalingam TS, West Jr AP, Lebron JA, Nangiana JS, Hogan TH, Enns CA, et al. Binding to the transferrin receptor is required for endocytosis of HFE and regulation of iron homeostasis. Nat Cell Biol. 2000;2:953–7.
108. Chua ACG, Herbison CE, Drake SF, Graham RM, Olynyk JK, Trinder D. The role of Hfe and transferrin receptors 1 and 2 in transferrin-bound iron uptake by hepatocytes. Hepatology. 2008;47:1737–44.
109. Ikuta K, Fujimoto Y, Suzuki Y, Tanaka K, Saito H, Ohhira M, et al. Overexpression of hemochromatosis protein, HFE, alters transferrin recycling process in human hepatoma cells. Biochim Biophys Acta. 2000;1496:221–31.
110. Waheed A, Grubb JH, Zhou XY, Tomatsu S, Fleming RE, Costaldi ME, et al. Regulation of transferrin-mediated iron uptake by HFE, the protein defective in hereditary hemochromatosis. Proc Natl Acad Sci USA. 2002;99:3117–22.
111. Riedel HD, Muckenthaler MU, Gehrke SG, Mohr I, Brennan K, Herrmann T, et al. HFE downregulates iron uptake from transferrin and induces iron-regulatory protein activity in stably transfected cells. Blood. 1999;94:3915–21.
112. Davies PS, Zhang AS, Anderson EL, Roy CN, Lampson MA, McGraw TE, et al. Evidence for the interaction of the hereditary haemochromatosis protein, HFE, with the transferrin receptor in endocytic compartments. Biochem J. 2003;373:145–53.
113. Salter-Cid L, Brunmark A, Li Y, Leturcq D, Peterson PA, Jackson MR, et al. Transferrin receptor is negatively modulated by the hemochromatosis protein HFE: implications for cellular iron homeostasis. Proc Natl Acad Sci USA. 1999;96:5434–9.
114. Chua ACG, Delima RD, Morgan EH, Herbison CE, Tirnitz-Parker JEE, Graham RM, et al. Iron uptake from plasma transferrin by a transferrin receptor 2 mutant mouse model of haemochromatosis. J Hepatol. 2010;52:425–31.
115. Camaschella C, Roetto A, Calì A, De Gobbi M, Garozzo G, Carella M, et al. The gene TFR2 is mutated in a new type of haemochromatosis mapping to 7q22. Nat Genet. 2000;25:14–5.
116. Fleming RE, Ahmann JR, Migas MC, Waheed A, Koeffler HP, Kawabata H, et al. Targeted mutagenesis of the murine transferrin receptor-2 gene produces hemochromatosis. Proc Natl Acad Sci USA. 2002;99:10653–8.
117. Girelli D, Bozzini C, Roetto A, Alberti F, Daraio F, Colombari R, et al. Clinical and pathologic findings in hemochromatosis type 3 due to a novel mutation in transferrin receptor 2 gene. Gastroenterology. 2002;122:1295–302.
118. Griffiths WJ, Cox TM. Co-localization of the mammalian hemochromatosis gene product (HFE) and a newly identified transferrin receptor (TfR2) in intestinal tissue and cells. J Histochem Cytochem. 2003;51:613–24.
119. Goswami T, Andrews NC. Hereditary hemochromatosis protein, HFE, interaction with transferrin receptor 2 suggests a molecular mechanism for mammalian iron sensing. J Biol Chem. 2006;281:28494–8.
120. Waheed A, Britton RS, Grubb JH, Sly WS, Fleming RE. HFE association with transferrin receptor 2 increases cellular uptake of transferrin-bound iron. Arch Biochem Biophys. 2008;474:193–7.
121. McKnight GS, Lee DC, Hemmaplardh D, Finch CA, Palmiter RD. Transferrin gene expression. Effects of nutritional iron deficiency. J Biol Chem. 1980;255:144–7.

122. McKnight GS, Lee DC, Palmiter RD. Transferrin gene expression. Regulation of mRNA transcription in chick liver by steroid hormones and iron deficiency. J Biol Chem. 1980;255:148–53.
123. Rolfs A, Kvietikova I, Gassmann M, Wenger RH. Oxygen-regulated transferrin expression is mediated by hypoxia-inducible factor-1. J Biol Chem. 1997;272:20055–62.
124. Iacopetta BJ, Morgan EH, Yeoh GC. Transferrin receptors and iron uptake during erythroid cell development. Biochim Biophys Acta. 1982;687:204–10.
125. Lesley J, Hyman R, Schulte R, Trotter J. Expression of transferrin receptor on murine hematopoietic progenitors. Cell Immunol. 1984;83:14–25.
126. Trinder D, Morgan E, Baker E. The mechanisms of iron uptake by fetal rat hepatocytes in culture. Hepatology. 1986;6:852–8.
127. Sciot R, Verhoeven G, Van Eyken P, Cailleau J, Desmet VJ. Transferrin receptor expression in rat liver: immunohistochemical and biochemical analysis of the effect of age and iron storage. Hepatology. 1990;11:416–27.
128. Chitambar CR, Massey EJ, Seligman PA. Regulation of transferrin receptor expression on human leukemic cells during proliferation and induction of differentiation. Effects of gallium and dimethylsulfoxide. J Clin Invest. 1983;72:1314–25.
129. Lee AW, Oates PS, Trinder D. Effects of cell proliferation on the uptake of transferrin-bound iron by human hepatoma cells. Hepatology. 2003;38:967–77.
130. Trinder D, Batey RG, Morgan EH, Baker E. Effect of cellular iron concentration on iron uptake by hepatocytes. Am J Physiol. 1990;259:G611–7.
131. Hentze MW, Kuhn LC. Molecular control of vertebrate iron metabolism: mRNA-based regulatory circuits operated by iron, nitric oxide, and oxidative stress. Proc Natl Acad Sci USA. 1996;93:8175–82.
132. Dupic F, Fruchon S, Bensaid M, Loreal O, Brissot P, Borot N, et al. Duodenal mRNA expression of iron related genes in response to iron loading and iron deficiency in four strains of mice. Gut. 2002;51:648–53.
133. Casey JL, Hentze MW, Koeller DM, Caughman SW, Rouault TA, Klausner RD, et al. Iron-responsive elements: regulatory RNA sequences that control mRNA levels and translation. Science. 1988;240:924–8.
134. Lok CN, Ponka P. Identification of a hypoxia response element in the transferrin receptor gene. J Biol Chem. 1999;274:24147–52.
135. Bianchi L, Tacchini L, Cairo G. HIF-1-mediated activation of transferrin receptor gene transcription by iron chelation. Nucleic Acids Res. 1999;27:4223–7.
136. Pantopoulos K, Hentze MW. Activation of iron regulatory protein-1 by oxidative stress in vitro. Proc Natl Acad Sci USA. 1998;95:10559–63.
137. Drapier JC, Hirling H, Wietzerbin J, Kaldy P, Kuhn LC. Biosynthesis of nitric oxide activates iron regulatory factor in macrophages. EMBO J. 1993;12:3643–9.
138. Hirayama M, Kohgo Y, Kondo H, Shintani N, Fujikawa K, Sasaki K, et al. Regulation of iron metabolism in HepG2 cells: a possible role for cytokines in the hepatic deposition of iron. Hepatology. 1993;18:874–80.
139. Kobune M, Kohgo Y, Kato J, Miyazaki E, Niitsu Y. Interleukin-6 enhances hepatic transferrin uptake and ferritin expression in rats. Hepatology. 1994;19:1468–75.
140. Johnson MB, Enns CA. Diferric transferrin regulates transferrin receptor 2 protein stability. Blood. 2004;104:4287–93.
141. Robb A, Wessling-Resnick M. Regulation of transferrin receptor 2 protein levels by transferrin. Blood. 2004;104:4294–9.
142. Warren G, Davoust J, Cockcroft A. Recycling of transferrin receptors in A431 cells is inhibited during mitosis. EMBO J. 1984;3:2217–25.
143. Kawabata H, Germain RS, Ikezoe T, Tong X-J, Green EM, Gombart AF, et al. Regulation of expression of murine transferrin receptor 2. Blood. 2001;98:1949–54.
144. Morgan EH, Appleton TC. Autoradiographic localization of 125-I-labelled transferrin in rabbit reticulocytes. Nature. 1969;223:1371–2.
145. Iacopetta BJ, Morgan EH. Transferrin endocytosis and iron uptake during erythroid cell development. Biomed Biochim Acta. 1983;42:S182–6.
146. Intragumtornchai T, Huebers HA, Finch CA. Transferrin–reticulocyte cycle time in rat reticulocytes. Blut. 1990;60:249–52.
147. Richardson DR, Ponka P, Vyoral D. Distribution of iron in reticulocytes after inhibition of heme synthesis with succinylacetone: examination of the intermediates involved in iron metabolism. Blood. 1996;87:3477–88.
148. Levy JE, Jin O, Fujiwara Y, Kuo F, Andrews NC. Transferrin receptor is necessary for development of erythrocytes and the nervous system. Nat Genet. 1999;21:396–9.
149. Oates PS, Thomas C, Freitas E, Callow MJ, Morgan EH. Gene expression of divalent metal transporter 1 and transferrin receptor in duodenum of Belgrade rats. Am J Physiol Gastrointest Liver Physiol. 2000;278:G930–6.
150. Anderson GJ, Powell LW, Halliday JW. Transferrin receptor distribution and regulation in the rat small intestine. Effect of iron stores and erythropoiesis. Gastroenterology. 1990;98:576–85.

151. Trinder D, Olynyk JK, Sly WS, Morgan EH. Iron uptake from plasma transferrin by the duodenum is impaired in the Hfe knockout mouse. Proc Natl Acad Sci USA. 2002;99:5622–6.
152. Pietrangelo A, Casalgrandi G, Quaglino D, Gualdi R, Conte D, Milani S, et al. Duodenal ferritin synthesis in genetic hemochromatosis. Gastroenterology. 1995;108:208–17.
153. Fleming RE, Migas MC, Zhou X, Jiang J, Britton RS, Brunt EM, et al. Mechanism of increased iron absorption in murine model of hereditary hemochromatosis: increased duodenal expression of the iron transporter DMT1. Proc Natl Acad Sci USA. 1999;96:3143–8.
154. Zoller H, Koch RO, Theurl I, Obrist P, Pietrangelo A, Montosi G, et al. Expression of the duodenal iron transporters divalent-metal transporter 1 and ferroportin 1 in iron deficiency and iron overload. Gastroenterology. 2001;120:1412–9.
155. Vujic Spasic M, Kiss J, Herrmann T, Kessler R, Stolte J, Galy B, et al. Physiologic systemic iron metabolism in mice deficient for duodenal Hfe. Blood. 2007;109:4511–7.
156. Bergamaschi G, Bergamaschi P, Carlevati S, Cazzola M. Transferrin receptor expression in the human placenta. Haematologica. 1990;75:220–3.
157. Bastin J, Drakesmith H, Rees M, Sargent I, Townsend A. Localisation of proteins of iron metabolism in the human placenta and liver. Br J Haematol. 2006;134:532–43.
158. Georgieff MK, Wobken JK, Welle J, Burdo JR, Connor JR. Identification and localization of divalent metal transporter-1 (DMT-1) in term human placenta. Placenta. 2000;21:799–804.
159. Chong WS, Kwan PC, Chan LY, Chiu PY, Cheung TK, Lau TK. Expression of divalent metal transporter 1 (DMT1) isoforms in first trimester human placenta and embryonic tissues. Hum Reprod. 2005;20:3532–8.
160. Gruper Y, Bar J, Bacharach E, Ehrlich R. Transferrin receptor co-localizes and interacts with the hemochromatosis factor (HFE) and the divalent metal transporter-1 (DMT1) in trophoblast cells. J Cell Physiol. 2005;204:901–12.
161. Abboud S, Haile DJ. A novel mammalian iron-regulated protein involved in intracellular iron metabolism. J Biol Chem. 2000;275:19906–12.
162. Donovan A, Brownlie A, Zhou Y, Shepard J, Pratt SJ, Moynihan J, et al. Positional cloning of zebrafish ferroportin1 identifies a conserved vertebrate iron exporter. Nature. 2000;403:776–81.
163. Donovan A, Lima CA, Pinkus JL, Pinkus GS, Zon LI, Robine S, et al. The iron exporter ferroportin/Slc40a1 is essential for iron homeostasis. Cell Metab. 2005;1:191–200.
164. Danzeisen R, Fosset C, Chariana Z, Page K, David S, McArdle HJ. Placental ceruloplasmin homolog is regulated by iron and copper and is implicated in iron metabolism. Am J Physiol Cell Physiol. 2002;282:C472–8.
165. Drakesmith H, Sweetland E, Schimanski L, Edwards J, Cowley D, Ashraf M, et al. The hemochromatosis protein HFE inhibits iron export from macrophages. Proc Natl Acad Sci USA. 2002;99:15602–7.
166. Davies PS, Enns CA. Expression of the hereditary hemochromatosis protein HFE increases ferritin levels by inhibiting iron export in HT29 cells. J Biol Chem. 2004;279:25085–92.
167. McArdle HJ, Morgan EH. Transferrin and iron movements in the rat conceptus during gestation. J Reprod Fertil. 1982;66:529–36.
168. Gambling L, Danzeisen R, Gair S, Lea RG, Charania Z, Solanky N, et al. Effect of iron deficiency on placental transfer of iron and expression of iron transport proteins in vivo and in vitro. Biochem J. 2001;356:883–9.
169. Gambling L, Charania Z, Hannah L, Antipatis C, Lea RG, McArdle HJ. Effect of iron deficiency on placental cytokine expression and fetal growth in the pregnant rat. Biol Reprod. 2002;66:516–23.
170. Martin ME, Nicolas G, Hetet G, Vaulont S, Grandchamp B, Beaumont C. Transferrin receptor 1 mRNA is downregulated in placenta of hepcidin transgenic embryos. FEBS Lett. 2004;574:187–91.
171. Jefferies WA, Brandon MR, Hunt SV, Williams AF, Gatter KC, Mason DY. Transferrin receptor on endothelium of brain capillaries. Nature. 1984;312:162–3.
172. Pardridge WM, Eisenberg J, Yang J. Human blood–brain barrier transferrin receptor. Metabolism. 1987;36:892–5.
173. Fishman JB, Rubin JB, Handrahan JV, Connor JR, Fine RE. Receptor-mediated transcytosis of transferrin across the blood–brain barrier. J Neurosci Res. 1987;18:299–304.
174. Taylor EM, Crowe A, Morgan EH. Transferrin and iron uptake by the brain: effects of altered iron status. J Neurochem. 1991;57:1584–92.
175. Morris CM, Keith AB, Edwardson JA, Pullen RG. Uptake and distribution of iron and transferrin in the adult rat brain. J Neurochem. 1992;59:300–6.
176. Crowe A, Morgan EH. Iron and transferrin uptake by brain and cerebrospinal fluid in the rat. Brain Res. 1992;592:8–16.
177. Moos T, Skjoerringe T, Gosk S, Morgan EH. Brain capillary endothelial cells mediate iron transport into the brain by segregating iron from transferrin without the involvement of divalent metal transporter 1. J Neurochem. 2006;98:1946–58.
178. Burdo JR, Menzies SL, Simpson IA, Garrick LM, Garrick MD, Dolan KG, et al. Distribution of divalent metal transporter 1 and metal transport protein 1 in the normal and Belgrade rat. J Neurosci Res. 2001;66:1198–207.

179. Siddappa AJ, Rao RB, Wobken JD, Leibold EA, Connor JR, Georgieff MK. Developmental changes in the expression of iron regulatory proteins and iron transport proteins in the perinatal rat brain. J Neurosci Res. 2002;68:761–75.
180. Moos T, Morgan EH. The significance of the mutated divalent metal transporter (DMT1) on iron transport into the Belgrade rat brain. J Neurochem. 2004;88:233–45.
181. Wu LJ, Leenders AG, Cooperman S, Meyron-Holtz E, Smith S, Land W, et al. Expression of the iron transporter ferroportin in synaptic vesicles and the blood–brain barrier. Brain Res. 2004;1001:108–17.
182. Moos T, Rosengren Nielsen T. Ferroportin in the postnatal rat brain: implications for axonal transport and neuronal export of iron. Semin Pediatr Neurol. 2006;13:149–57.
183. Jeong SY, David S. Glycosylphosphatidylinositol-anchored ceruloplasmin is required for iron efflux from cells in the central nervous system. J Biol Chem. 2003;278:27144–8.
184. Moos T, Rosengren Nielsen T, Skjorringe T, Morgan EH. Iron trafficking inside the brain. J Neurochem. 2007;103:1730–40.
185. Sonnewald U, Westergaard N, Krane J, Unsgard G, Petersen SB, Schousboe A. First direct demonstration of preferential release of citrate from astrocytes using [^{13}C]NMR spectroscopy of cultured neurons and astrocytes. Neurosci Lett. 1991;128:235–9.
186. Guthrie PB, Knappenberger J, Segal M, Bennett MV, Charles AC, Kater SB. ATP released from astrocytes mediates glial calcium waves. J Neurosci. 1999;19:520–8.
187. Bradbury MW. Transport of iron in the blood–brain-cerebrospinal fluid system. J Neurochem. 1997;69:443–54.
188. Burdo JR, Connor JR. Brain iron uptake and homeostatic mechanisms: an overview. Biometals. 2003;16:63–75.
189. Taylor EM, Morgan EH. Developmental changes in transferrin and iron uptake by the brain in the rat. Brain Res Dev Brain Res. 1990;55:35–42.
190. Moos T, Oates PS, Morgan EH. Expression of the neuronal transferrin receptor is age dependent and susceptible to iron deficiency. J Comp Neurol. 1998;398:420–30.
191. Moos T, Morgan EH. Restricted transport of anti-transferrin receptor antibody (OX26) through the blood–brain barrier in the rat. J Neurochem. 2001;79:119–29.
192. Bastin JM, Jones M, O'Callaghan CA, Schimanski L, Mason DY, Townsend AR. Kupffer cell staining by an HFE-specific monoclonal antibody: implications for hereditary haemochromatosis. Br J Haematol. 1998;103:931–41.
193. Connor JR, Milward EA, Moalem S, Sampietro M, Boyer P, Percy ME, et al. Is hemochromatosis a risk factor for Alzheimer's disease? J Alzheimers Dis. 2001;3:471–7.
194. Dekker MC, Giesbergen PC, Njajou OT, van Swieten JC, Hofman A, Breteler MM, et al. Mutations in the hemochromatosis gene (HFE), Parkinson's disease and parkinsonism. Neurosci Lett. 2003;348:117–9.
195. van Berkel TJ, Dekker CJ, Kruijt JK, van Eijk HG. The interaction in vivo of transferrin and asialotransferrin with liver cells. Biochem J. 1987;243:715–22.
196. Cole ES, Glass J. Transferrin binding and iron uptake in mouse hepatocytes. Biochim Biophys Acta. 1983;762:102–10.
197. Oshiro S, Nakajima H, Markello T, Krasnewich D, Bernardini I, Gahl WA. Redox, transferrin-independent, and receptor-mediated endocytosis iron uptake systems in cultured human fibroblasts. J Biol Chem. 1993;268:21586–91.
198. Richardson DR, Baker E. Two saturable mechanisms of iron uptake from transferrin in human melanoma cells: the effect of transferrin concentration, chelators, and metabolic probes on transferrin and iron uptake. J Cell Physiol. 1994;161:160–8.
199. Trinder D, Zak O, Aisen P. Transferrin receptor-independent uptake of differic transferrin by human hepatoma cells with antisense inhibition of receptor expression. Hepatology. 1996;23:1512–20.
200. Morgan EH, Smith GD, Peters TJ. Uptake and subcellular processing of 59Fe-125I-labelled transferrin by rat liver. Biochem J. 1986;237:163–73.
201. Herbison CE, Thorstensen K, Chua ACG, Graham RM, Leedman P, Olynyk JK, et al. The role of transferrin receptor 1 and 2 in transferrin-bound iron uptake in human hepatoma cells. Am J Physiol. 2009;297:C1567–75.
202. Thorstensen K, Romslo I. The role of transferrin in the mechanism of cellular iron uptake. Biochem J. 1990;271:1–9.
203. Scheiber B, Goldenberg H. Hepatic uptake of iron by receptor-mediated and receptor-independent mechanisms. Z Gastroenterol. 1996;34 Suppl 3:95–8.
204. Trinder D, Morgan E. Inhibition of uptake of transferrin-bound iron by human hepatoma cells by nontransferrin-bound iron. Hepatology. 1997;26:69169–8.
205. Thorstensen K. Hepatocytes and reticulocytes have different mechanisms for the uptake of iron from transferrin. J Biol Chem. 1988;263:16837–41.
206. Thorstensen K, Romslo I. Uptake of iron from transferrin by isolated rat hepatocytes. A redox-mediated plasma membrane process? J Biol Chem. 1988;263:8844–50.

207. Scheiber B, Goldenberg H. The surface of rat hepatocytes can transfer iron from stable chelates to external acceptors. Hepatology. 1998;27:1075–80.
208. Graham RM, Morgan EH, Baker E. Ferric citrate uptake by cultured rat hepatocytes is inhibited in the presence of transferrin. Eur J Biochem. 1998;253:139–45.
209. Chua AC, Olynyk JK, Leedman PJ, Trinder D. Nontransferrin-bound iron uptake by hepatocytes is increased in the Hfe knockout mouse model of hereditary hemochromatosis. Blood. 2004;104:1519–25.
210. Page MA, Baker E, Morgan EH. Transferrin and iron uptake by rat hepatocytes in culture. Am J Physiol. 1984;246:G26–33.
211. Vogel W, Bomford A, Young S, Williams R. Heterogeneous distribution of transferrin receptors on parenchymal and nonparenchymal liver cells: biochemical and morphological evidence. Blood. 1987;69:264–70.
212. Soda R, Tavassoli M. Liver endothelium and not hepatocytes or kupffer cells have transferrin receptors. Blood. 1984;63:270–6.
213. Tavassoli M. The role of liver endothelium in the transfer of iron from transferrin to the hepatocyte. Ann N Y Acad Sci. 1988;526:83–92.
214. Kondo H, Saito K, Grasso JP, Aisen P. Iron metabolism in the erythrophagocytosing kupffer cell. Hepatology. 1988;8:32–8.
215. Oria R, Alvarez-Hernandez X, Liceaga J, Brock JH. Uptake and handling of iron from transferrin, lactoferrin and immune complexes by a macrophage cell line. Biochem J. 1988;252:221–5.
216. Mulero V, Brock JH. Regulation of iron metabolism in murine J774 macrophages: role of nitric oxide-dependent and -independent pathways following activation with gamma interferon and lipopolysaccharide. Blood. 1999;94:2383–9.
217. Wardrop SL, Richardson DR. Interferon-gamma and lipopolysaccharide regulate the expression of Nramp2 and increase the uptake of iron from low relative molecular mass complexes by macrophages. Eur J Biochem. 2000;267:6586–93.
218. Montosi G, Paglia P, Garuti C, Guzman CA, Bastin JM, Colombo MP, et al. Wild-type HFE protein normalizes transferrin iron accumulation in macrophages from subjects with hereditary hemochromatosis. Blood. 2000;96:1125–9.
219. Testa U, Petrini M, Quaranta MT, Pelosi-Testa E, Mastroberardino G, Camagna A, et al. Iron up-modulates the expression of transferrin receptors during monocyte-macrophage maturation. J Biol Chem. 1989;264:13181–7.

Chapter 8
Iron Salvage Pathways

Ann Smith

Keywords Ferritin • Haptoglobin • Heme • Heme oxygenase • Hemoglobin • Hemolysis • Hemopexin • Iron • NTBI • Transferrin

1 Introduction and Overview

Heme catabolism by heme oxygenases (HOs) in macrophages and liver cells allows the heme–iron from red blood cell hemoglobin to be recycled, i.e., to undergo reuse. Mammalian HOs generate Fe(II) in the cytosol from where it is distributed for biochemical and regulatory needs (e.g., heme synthesis, DNA synthesis, and ferritin induction), or stored safely on ferritin, or exported via ferroportin 1 (FPN1) to transferrin for delivery to cells throughout the body. This whole body cycle of iron reclamation is also maintained by several sources of heme in addition to the phagocytosis of effete red blood cells by macrophages. Intravascular hemolysis, whether from the normal wear and tear of circulating erythrocytes or during disease and trauma, provides both hemoglobin–haptoglobin (Hb–Hp) and heme (derived from Hb) in the circulation and within cells. Hb–heme is rapidly oxidized and heme then dissociates. Since heme is redox active, readily accepting and donating electrons, it is important to remove heme from the circulation before it damages cells and circulating molecules. Acting as extracellular antioxidants, hemopexin (HPX) binds heme, dampening its chemical activity, while haptoglobin (Hp) binds hemoglobin (Hb) and transferrin binds iron. The relative amounts of these metal–plasma protein complexes make an impact not only on normal health but also exacerbate a variety of disease states. Heme is removed safely from the circulation by receptor-mediated endocytosis of heme–HPX complexes. The HPX normally recycles intact analogously to transferrin. Most iron and heme–iron, even when bound to extracellular proteins, is in the oxidized ferric (Fe(III)) state. The reduced heme of Hb is one notable exception. Ferro-iron and ferro-heme can be dangerous for cells since they may undergo chemical reactions in the presence of oxygen that produce reactive oxygen species including hydrogen peroxide and superoxide. It is generally accepted that the basis of the cytotoxicity of non-protein bound iron inside cells and non-transferrin bound iron (NTBI) outside cells in iron overload, is when Fe(II) undergoes the Fenton reaction generating the extremely reactive hydroxyl radical.

A. Smith, Ph.D. (✉)
School of Biological Sciences, University of Missouri-K.C., Kansas City, MO 64110, USA
e-mail: smithan@umkc.edu

G.J. Anderson and G. McLaren (eds.), *Iron Physiology and Pathophysiology in Humans*, Nutrition and Health, DOI 10.1007/978-1-60327-485-2_8,

The whole body iron cycle starts with the absorption from the diet of heme by duodenal enterocytes and of iron by all enterocytes. The absorption of heme–iron (i.e., radioactive Hb) is far more effective than that of inorganic iron in humans. More than one third of the body's total daily iron requirement (3 mg) comes from dietary heme–iron (hemoglobin and myoglobin in an average normal diet [1, 2]). Heme is extensively catabolized by HOs in enterocytes [3] or is exported from cells, possibly including enterocytes, via a facilitative transporter, feline leukemia virus subgroup C (FLVCR), which is a member of the major facilitator group of transporters. Recent evidence reinforces the concept that iron supply across the basolateral membrane of enterocytes into the circulation is principally coordinated by systemic signals from the liver with consequences for that organ, for the enterocytes themselves and also for cells of the erythropoietic system. Thus, iron flux across the enterocytes likely responds to the extent of transferrin saturation with iron (normally ~30%) and also, in hemolytic conditions, to the levels of hemoglobin, hemoglobin–haptoglobin [4], heme-HPX, and NTBI. In iron overload conditions, the predominant form of iron in the plasma is NTBI whose uptake via the ion channels DMT1 and ZIP14 into cells, including hepatocytes, is unregulated. FPN1 has been located on the basolateral membrane of enterocytes as well as on the plasma membrane along the sinusoidal border of hepatocytes, where it likely also contributes to the known biliary excretion of iron. Bile flows into the duodenum. Iron is finally removed from the gut as aged enterocytes are "sloughed off" taking their iron with them. This explains why there is no active excretion of iron from the body, and hence why iron reclamation from iron and heme–iron metabolism is so important.

In the context of iron salvage, it is significant that after hepatic uptake of heme–HPX, heme–iron is subsequently incorporated into red blood cells. Heme–HPX can replace iron-transferrin as a growth factor for cultured cells in vitro and may be an iron source for cancer cells in vivo. HPX contributes to iron recycling from heme catabolism and also binds heme in a manner that protects cells and circulating molecules (e.g., HDL [5]) from its oxidizing, chemical reactions. Thus, HPX deficiency states are deleterious since when HPX is low or absent, heme binds to lipids in lipoproteins, cell membranes and induces many events that promote or stimulate inflammation.

Heme–iron for recycling leaves macrophages via ferroportin which is then reutilized by erythroblasts for Hb synthesis. Iron may also leave associated with H- or L-ferritin, which are secreted by macrophages. Ferritin is taken up into certain cells including hepatocytes by receptor-mediated endocytosis followed by catabolism in the lysosomes. Iron is exported from late endosomes and lysosomes into the cytosol via mucolipin and then via FPN1 to transferrin.

Hemoglobin and its globin chains are toxic. Intravascular and extravascular hemolysis releases Hb, and unstable hemoglobins are found in patients with sickle cell disease or thalassemia. In sickle cell disease, HbS will polymerize at low levels of oxygen, sickle erythrocytes generate superoxide and HbS is found deposited in various aggregated and oxidized forms (low-spin ferric denatured HbS) on the cytosolic surface of sickled erythrocyte membranes [6]. Hebbel et al. [7] showed that HbS is inherently unstable and ferro-oxyHbS rapidly loses its heme almost twice as fast as ferro-oxyHbA just like methemoglobin (ferric-Hb). Heme bound to the oxy-form of the α-chains of Hb undergoes auto-oxidation faster than heme bound to the β-chains and like the Hb tetramer, monomeric β-chains bind ferric-heme but less tightly than ferro-heme. After ferric-heme dissociates from globin, the protein itself is cytotoxic and causes vascular damage [8], as shown by in vitro studies with primary bovine aortic endothelial cells. After heme dissociates, a large hydrophobic surface is exposed on globin [9]. Damage by globin to endothelial cells comes not only by absorptive pinocytosis to the plasma membrane but also from membrane insertion of globin as recently shown for neuroglobin [10]. Unlike globin, apo-hemopexin (HPX; at plasma concentrations of 20 μM or higher) is not harmful to cells, e.g., endothelial cells [8] or neurons [11].

The maintenance of whole body iron homeostasis is complex, involving principally the duodenum, liver, and spleen, requiring coordination among several different cell types and proteins. Binding of iron, heme, and Hb by plasma proteins prevents iron loss by the kidneys. Furthermore, copper is needed for normal iron transport across membranes and in the HPX–heme uptake system for coordinated gene regulation (e.g., metallothionein 1 and HO1). The focus here is on the proteins and processes that maintain iron homeostasis. When there are defects in the iron "salvage" pathways, there are serious consequences that can become life threatening. Systemic inflammation-driven pathology, e.g., lipid and lipoprotein oxidation, predominates when heme and iron are present, especially when Hp is low. In such situations, HPX is needed as the last defense against heme toxicity and can become depleted. The importance of transferrin, haptoglobin, and hemopexin as extracellular antioxidants rapidly removing redox-active iron and heme from the circulation but in a manner that safely retains and recycles both heme and its iron is established. Furthermore, iron recycling is important because the body's iron status affects not just iron and heme metabolism but also the functioning of immune system cells. The key and complex relationships between the HPX and Hp systems with macrophages that express CD163 and heme catabolism by heme oxygenases that control whole body heme and iron redistribution are only just being recognized.

2 Hemolytic Anemias, Iron Overload, and Non-Transferrin Bound Iron

2.1 Non-Transferrin Bound Iron (NTBI)

When iron overload develops, transferrin becomes saturated with iron. This can occur in alcoholic cirrhosis, HFE-related hereditary hemochromatosis (HHC), and in certain hemolytic anemias. Clinically, iron overload is defined by more than 75% saturation of transferrin in plasma. As iron levels in the circulation continue to rise, then NTBI is produced whose cellular uptake via ion channel transporters is not regulated. (In contrast, high levels of iron in cells downregulate the levels of transferrin receptors that takes up diferric-transferrin complexes). NTBI is not yet characterized but has been shown to be of relatively small size and was generally assumed to be iron bound to small molecules, e.g., anions such as citrate, or loosely associated with serum albumin. However, Evans et al. [12] concluded that NTBI is not associated with serum albumin. Furthermore, differences must exist between NTBI in mice and humans because in several mouse models of iron overload, mouse NTBI is not detected by the methods used routinely to detect NTBI in humans [12]. For in vitro studies on NTBI, ferric citrate is the predominant model for NTBI Fe(III) uptake. To study Fe(II) uptake, ferric citrate with cell reduction, ferrous sulfate with ascorbate, and some iron chelator complexes have all been employed. Human erythroleukemic K562 cells reduce NTBI by transmembrane ascorbate cycling. Ascorbate dose-dependently stimulates both iron reduction by cells and uptake of iron from ^{55}Fe–ferric citrate [13, 14], and intracellular ascorbate levels rise when cells are incubated with dehydroascorbate. This iron uptake is due to a direct chemical reduction of ascorbate since iron uptake is prevented when ascorbate oxidase is added to the ascorbate-supplemented medium. Importantly, more NTBI enters cells as Fe(II) provided that there is a means to reduce the iron at the cell surface.

The liver is the principal organ for iron storage and, thus, is the main organ affected in iron overload. However, in chronic and/or acute severe iron overload, the cells of the heart and pancreas also succumb to iron toxicity. NTBI uptake takes place via ion channels such as DMT1, where iron is co-transported with protons [15], and also by the zinc transporter, ZIP14 [16], and both depend principally upon iron gradients. Depending upon the needs of hepatocytes and the body's iron status, iron is used for biochemical and metabolic purposes, stored on ferritin or is exported by ferroportin (FPN1) for loading onto transferrin and thus distributed to cells throughout the body, including reticulocytes for heme synthesis (Fig. 8.1). The iron export rate is determined by the number of FPN1 molecules on the plasma membrane, which in turn are regulated by any circulating hepcidin. The classic pathway of iron uptake by transferrin receptor 1 (TfR1) is presumed not important in

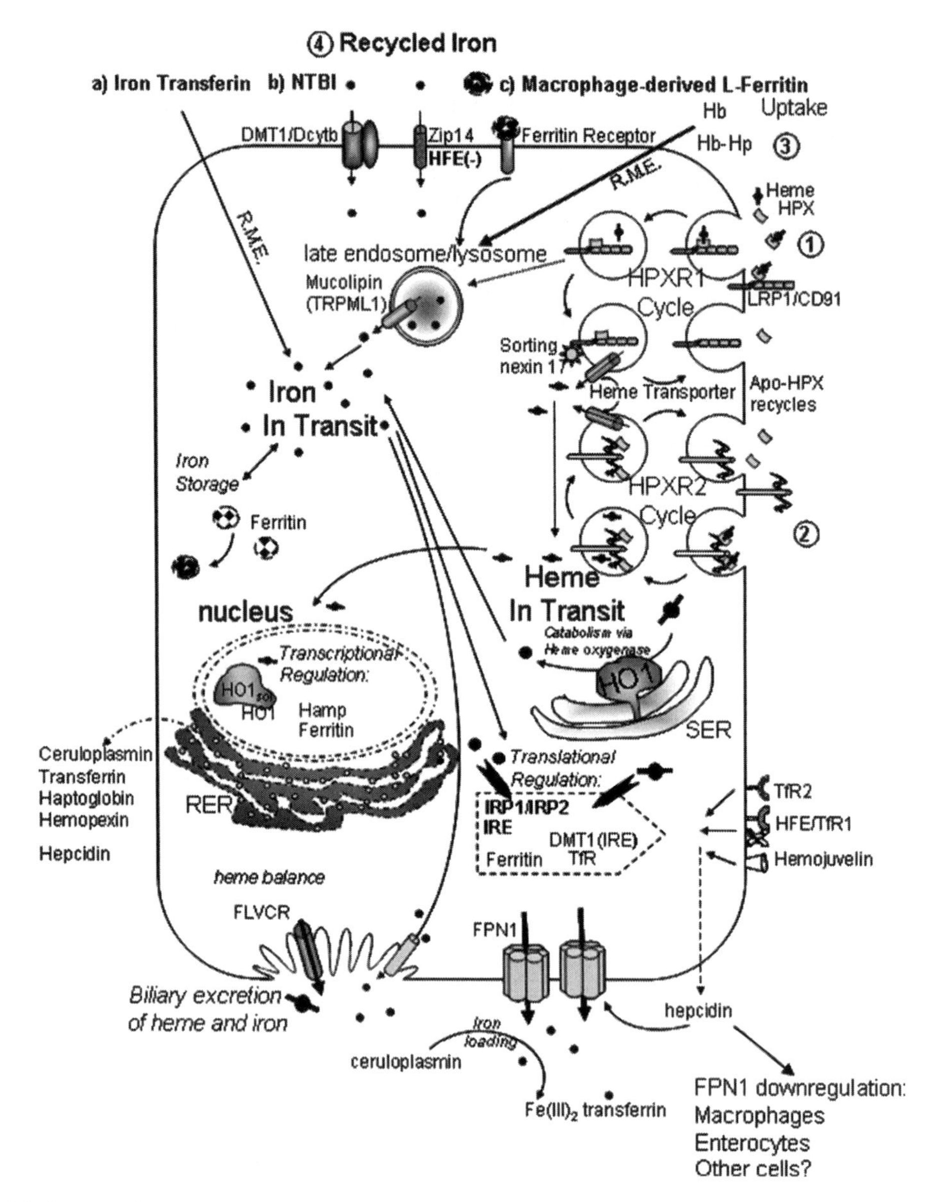

Fig. 8.1 Sources of heme and iron for recycling hemoglobin and its heme–iron via the hepatocyte to maintain heme and iron homeostasis in the whole body. A representative liver parenchymal cell with pathways of iron and heme uptake as well as the intracellular movement of these two molecules is depicted. The secreted proteins or exported iron and heme are exchanged with macrophages (shown in Fig. 8.2) in the spleen and Kupffer cells in the liver, and potentially also in the bone marrow. Uptake of heme–HPX complexes requires a high-affinity, low-capacity receptor HPXR1, the best candidate to date is LRP1/CD91 ①, which is a scavenger receptor with more than 50 ligands, and also by a low-affinity, high-capacity "selective" HPXR2, which may be toll-like receptor 4 ②. Hb uptake via a Hp receptor ③, which appears to differ from CD 163 since it is reported to be expressed only by cells of the monocyte/macrophage lineage; Hb uptake by unknown means. Heme from both Hb–Hp and heme–HPX complexes is degraded by HOs releasing Fe(II). High intracellular iron levels damage cells due to the chemical reactions of non-protein bound intracellular iron, which often referred to as the "labile iron pool (LIP)," but remains controversial [20]. LIP is detected using the fluorescent iron chelators like calcein [21] and LIP is assumed to be the reactive Fe(II) and to increase when cell iron uptake exceeds the storage capacity of iron on cytosolic ferritin. Here, we refer to this iron as "iron in transit" since it is moving from one site in the cell to another (Figs. 8.1 and 8.2). Such free iron has not been incorporated into heme, iron sulfur clusters, or high-affinity mononuclear sites within proteins but is in transit or bound adventitiously to the surface of biomolecules [22]. Biochemical and metabolic purposes for iron include regulation via the IRP/IRE

iron overload due to its inherently low capacity. The importance of the liver for Hb and heme clearance by Hp and by hemopexin (HPX), respectively, as well as for iron recycling is addressed below (and see Fig. 8.1).

What are the possible sources of NTBI in humans? Under normal conditions, iron overload from the diet can be controlled by hepcidin secreted by the liver. As iron levels rise in the liver, hepcidin synthesis is stimulated leading to a downregulation of FPN1, on cells, including enterocytes and macrophages as well as hepatocytes. Thus, iron is retained within these cells. Nonregulated iron uptake across the enterocyte can take place in response to anemia 1 when hepcidin levels are low, e.g., in β-thalassemia [24]. However, if circulating NTBI increases due to increased enterocyte absorption or after a blood transfusion, then NTBI uptake leads to hepatocyte iron overload with anemia because iron is not available to erythroblasts but is retained within the liver and macrophage cells. Urinary hepcidin increases after blood transfusion in β-thalassemia when erythropoiesis is maximally suppressed [208]. Iron administration expands the extramedullary erythropoiesis which improves the anemia in a mouse model of thalassemia intermediary [25]. This suggests that expansion of extramedullary erythropoiesis suppresses hepcidin in β-thalassemic mice.

An increase in intracellular iron from heme catabolism after erythrophagocytosis explains the predominant increase in reticuloendothelial iron seen in type 4 hemochromatosis where there is a missense mutation in the FPN1 gene [26]. Delaby et al. [27] incubated artificially aged murine red blood cells with murine bone marrow-derived macrophages, causing a rapid increase in HO1 and FPN1 RNA and protein as well as ferritin protein. Subsequently, FPN1 levels decreased although HO1 and ferritin levels remained high. The gene expression profile of this iron storage state thus resembled that in inflammation although the pro-inflammatory response of the macrophages was attenuated.

2.2 *Iron Loading of Macrophages by Erythrophagocytosis and in Hemolysis*

Changes in the surface proteins of red blood cells take place as they age. The modified proteins are recognized by specific receptors on macrophages resulting in erythrophagocytosis. After surface binding and engulfment, the heme from hemoglobin is released and degraded by heme oxygenases, thus raising intracellular Fe(II) (Fig. 8.2). It is presumed that, as in hepatocytes, iron is stored, used for regulation and other cellular needs, or is excreted froe macrophages but in this case most likely bound to ferritin rather than loaded onto transferrin. Additional details of reticuloendothelial cell iron metabolism are covered elsewhere (see Chap. 11). It is generally assumed that all of the heme taken up by receptor-mediated endocytosis either as Hb, Hp–Hb, or as heme–HPX is degraded by the macrophage HOs, although this has not yet been shown directly. If any heme avoids breakdown, it may be exported from macrophages by the heme transporter, feline leukemia virus subgroup C receptor (FLVCR; Fig. 8.2), but direct evidence is lacking that this takes place in vivo. Perturbation of the erythrophagocytotic pathway of macrophages in the bone marrow, lung, and liver (Kupffer cells) plays a pathophysiological role in several diseases including HHC, the anemia of chronic

Fig. 8.1 (continued) system or storage on ferritin. Any intracellular iron in excess is presumably exported via FPN1 across the plasma membrane. In addition, several synthetic pathways are shown including those for hepcidin secretion and for the plasma proteins needed to transport redox-active metals: heme, iron, and copper. Heme can also be excreted in the bile [23], likely via FLVCR, as well as iron via DMT1. Iron is recycled via endocytosis of transferrin ④a via the high-affinity, low-capacity TfR1/CD71 and by the low-affinity, high-capacity TfR2; and catabolic non-receptor-mediated transferrin uptake (not shown); by unregulated NTBI uptake via the channels DMT1 and ZIP14 ④b; and by receptor-mediated uptake of ferritin from macrophages ④c

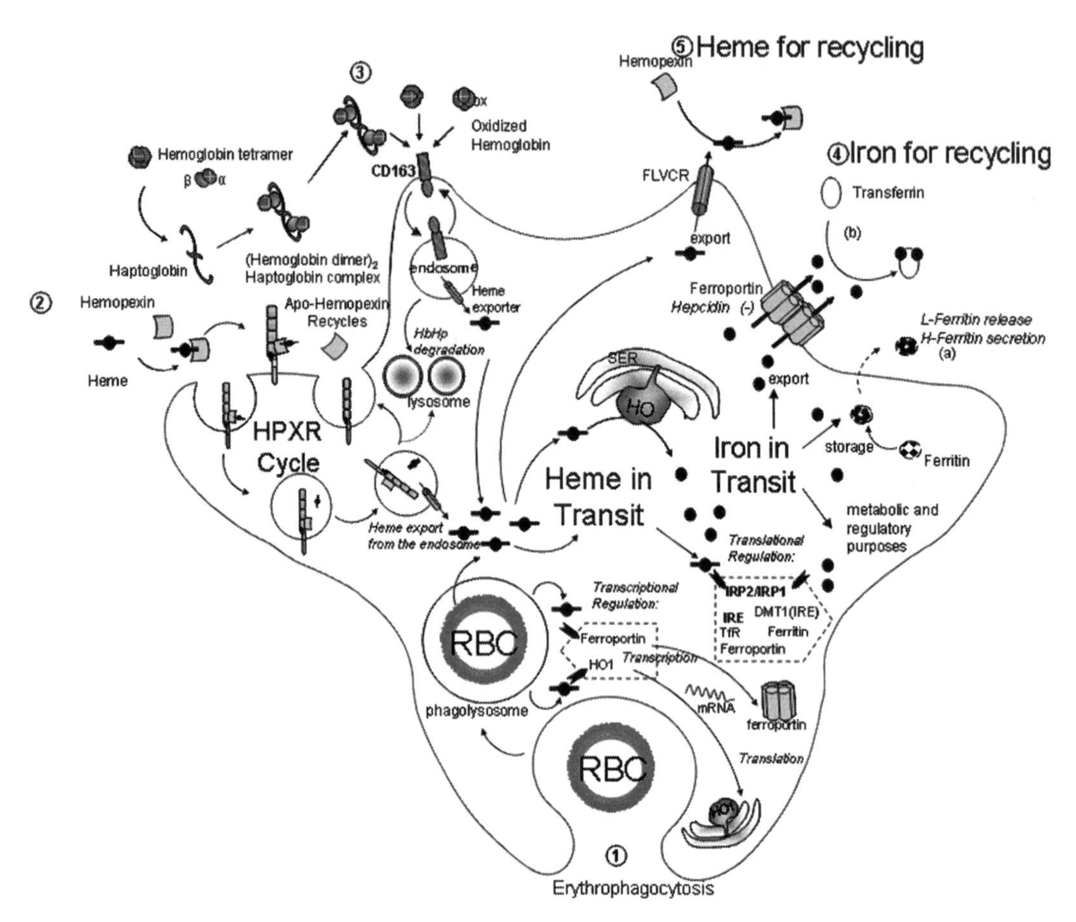

Fig. 8.2 Routes of heme transport in the macrophages for whole body iron recycling. A representative macrophage is depicted with pathways predominantly for heme uptake including phagocytosis of senescent red blood cells (RBC; ①) and low levels of the scavenger receptor, LRP1/CD91 that binds heme-HPX may be present ② and binding of Hb–Hp or Hb to the scavenger receptor CD163 ③ with some extracellular metabolism of Hb by the lipochalin, α1-microglobulin (not shown). Heme may be exported by FLVCR to HPX ⑤ as well as iron export by ferritin ④a and by FPN1 ④b. Limited iron uptake may take place by the TfR1/CD71. The heme exporter in endosomes may be heme carrier protein 1, HCP1, which has been detected in macrophage endosomes together with Hb–Hp [17]. HRG1 is another candidate endosomal heme exporter [18]. Transported heme is degraded by HOs releasing Fe(II). Additional abbreviations used are listed in the legend to Fig. 8.1. Alpha1-microglobulin circulates in blood either free or bound to immunoglobulin A and is proteolytically processed and can be released from IgA in the presence of membranes from ruptured erythrocytes and also by Hb. Whether intact or truncated, it binds heme and degrades it to unknown metabolites with an (as yet uncharacterized) yellow–brown chromophore derived from heme [19]. A truncated α1-microglobulin predominated in the urine of a patient with *extravascular* hemolysis, and was proposed to play a role in extracellular heme catabolism for Hb clearance in hemolytic states. However, whether this protein is involved in iron recycling is currently unknown

disorders as well as in the thalassemias. Loss of the macrophage population expressing the receptor for Hb–Hp (CD163) has dire consequences and is discussed further at the end of this chapter.

Heme–iron recycling in macrophages requires the iron exporter FPN1 as shown by studies with human macrophages and the J774 line of murine macrophages in vitro. Data from type 4 HHC in humans as well as animal models of HHC also support this. Furthermore, the copper status of macrophages affects FPN1 regulation [28] due to the need for the multicopper ferroxidase hephestin for iron export in this cell type. Heme and iron are regulatory molecules, and both are needed to regulate macrophage FPN1 induction, thus influencing release of iron for recycling after hemoglobin catabolism (Fig. 8.2).

After erythrophagocytosis of aged murine or human red blood cells by primary cultures of mouse bone marrow-derived macrophages [29], heme acts to activate transcription first of the HO1 gene and then the FPN1 gene, followed by iron-dependent expression of FPN1. FPN1 mRNA is decreased upon iron depletion by iron chelators and increased with iron loading [30], implicating iron in translational regulation but FPN1 lacks a canonical iron response element like that needed for the translational regulation of ferritin. The iron is presumably derived from the degradation of erythrocytic Hb–heme. Furthermore, transcriptional regulation is supported by the observation that actinomycin D blocked the induction of both FPN1 mRNA and protein after incubating J774 macrophages with senescent erythrocytes. Thus, the iron status of cells expressing FPN1 such as macrophages (and also enterocytes) affects FNP1 in addition to its downregulation by the physical binding of circulating hepcidin, which leads to FPN1 degradation by the proteasome [31]. Three hours after erythrophagocytosis, there was a tenfold increase in HO1, the levels of the iron transporter NRAMP1 had doubled but there was no change in DMT1 protein level. After incubation with ^{59}Fe-labeled rat erythrocytes, iron export rates in J774 macrophages engineered by retroviral transduction to stably express FPN1 were 70% higher than in the control cells. Furthermore, addition of hepcidin to the medium dramatically decreased both FNP1 levels and ^{59}Fe efflux. While non-heme^{59}Fe release was reduced by 50%, there was no change in ^{59}Fe–heme efflux [32], consistent with a specific effect of iron on FPN1. In the context of the whole body, when the liver synthesizes and secretes hepcidin, the predominant cells in which FPN1 levels are decreased are considered to be splenic macrophages and both hepatic parenchymal and Kupffer cells. Cellular iron overload is produced when iron export stops while iron uptake continues, e.g., from NTBI (and iron-transferrin). Heme uptake from Hb, Hb–Hp, and heme-HPX in hemolytic states presumably also contributes to iron overload.

In a related study, erythrophagocytosis increased intracellular heme levels 3.5-fold within 30 min, declining significantly by 3 h but remaining above normal for another 4 h. Heme-arginate (or as the pharmaceutical preparation, Normasang, at 10 or 50 μM) induced FPN1, HO1 and ferritin (FtnH) mRNAs within 4 h. Heme, not iron, is a well-established inducer of HO1 gene transcription [33, 34], and the iron chelator Salicylaldehyde isonicotinoyl hydrazone (SIH) does not decrease HO1 induction. On the other hand, iron is needed for H-Ftn induction since it was prevented by SIH, whereas FPN1 induction was only slightly inhibited. In macrophages and in contrast to the transcriptional regulation of HO1 and FPN1, H-Ftn regulation appeared to be principally at the translational level and iron-dependent. However, FPN1 is regulated transcriptionally by heme in murine Friend erythroleukemia cells [35]. FPN1 and H-Ftn induction by Normosang required heme–iron since Ftn and FPN1 levels were not decreased by SIH when HO1 was inhibited by incubation of the macrophages with tin-PPIX. Consistent with a role for iron, protoporphyrin IX arginate was not an inducer. Thus, FPN1 is regulated by heme at the transcriptional level [36], as previously shown for HO1 regulation in a variety of cell types, including hepatocytes and enterocytes. HO1 is regulated by the transcriptional activator, Nrf2, its binding partner, and a MARE/ARE element [37], and recently similar regulation was reported in murine macrophage line, RAW 264.7 cells incubated with Hb [36]. HO1 is not regulated by iron unless the conditions increase intracellular heme levels, i.e., iron supplementation for extended time periods. Discrepancies in the reported translational regulation of FPN1 by iron are due to multiple transcripts that were first detected in erythroid cells, some of which lacked a 5′IRE [38]. In duodenal and erythroid cells, FPN1B thus evades translational regulation by iron [39]. Heme regulation at the transcriptional level is more important in these two types of cells likely for the coordinate regulation of HO1 and FPN1.

Rapid removal of metHb from the circulation is important to minimize inflammatory responses to the potentially toxic heme and also globin. Hb–Hp complexes are endocytosed by a scavenger receptor, CD163, expressed at high levels on the surface of macrophages [40]. In human macrophages, Hp enhances Hb uptake at low concentrations (e.g., 1 μg/mL), consistent with a high-affinity receptor like CD163, although not at high concentrations (e.g., 100 μg/mL). CD163 is reported to be restricted to cells of the macrophage/monocyte lineage. Hb competes with Hb–Hp for CD163 [41], and therefore likely enters macrophages by this route as well, especially when Hp has been depleted. Uptake of Hb–Hp or Hb leads to both HO1 and ferritin induction [42]. Macrophages play important roles in the immune system and CD163$^+$ macrophages are anti-inflammatory. Dexamethasone, the only documented HO2 inducer, strongly induces CD163 mRNA, resulting in a tenfold increase in these surface receptors. This augments the specific uptake of Hb–Hp complexes [43], which has been proposed to be the basis of a novel anti-inflammatory action of CD163$^+$ macrophages. However, in inflammation when levels of hydrogen peroxide increase, Hb–Hp complexes are oxidized and the heme becomes covalently bound to protein, consequently HO1 is not induced [44].

It is established from patient studies that the binding capacity of Hp is readily exhausted by moderate to severe hemolysis. This is due to the rapid breakdown of Hb–Hp complexes in the lysosomes of hepatic parenchymal cells seen after intravenous injection of radiolabeled Hb–Hp complexes in intact rats (described further below). Presumably, this endocytotic pathway is similar in macrophages. CD163 reportedly undergoes constitutive endocytosis, recycling from early endosomes after ligand-independent internalization [42].

3 Hemoglobin–Haptoglobin (Hb–Hp)

Evidence from both human and animal studies supports that Hp aids in iron recycling of the heme of Hb. Hp binds Hb in a manner that prevents the dangerous oxidizing effects of Hb. Hb is a peroxidase, although not a strong one [45], but is rapidly oxidized in vivo releasing the pro-oxidant heme. Peroxidase cycles of Hb can be activated by H_2O_2 to generate active oxyferryl radicals similar to horseradish peroxidase compounds. When Hp is depleted or low, endotoxin activity catalyzing free radical formation is enhanced as is macrophage activation, platelet adhesion, and even neurotoxicity. In inflammation, nitric oxide (NO) from activated macrophages and other cells binds to the ferroheme of Hb as well as to the thiol of Cysβ93 of globin [46]. This nitrated Hb causes vasoconstriction which leads to ischemia. This NO scavenging of Hb is inhibited by Hp [47].

3.1 Differential Protective Effects of Hp Subtypes

The Hp locus is polymorphic with two common alleles 1 and 2. Thus, Hp exists as three phenotypes: Hp1-1, Hp2-1, or Hp2-2. Homozygous Hp1-1 (β-α1-α1-β) is composed of two identical α1 chains (Mr 9,000 kDa) and Hp2-2 is composed of two identical α2 chains, and Hp2-1 contains one α1 and one α2 chain. The α2 chain has an extra free thiol group, which contributes to the polymerization of Hp2-1 and Hp2-2. Polymers can include up to six or more molecules. Hemoglobin released from erythrocytes during intravascular hemolysis binds immediately to Hp and forms a stable complex. Each Hp molecule binds two αβ Hb dimers (αβHpβα), essentially irreversibly (Kd of 1×10^{-15} mol/L) [48, 49]. Asleh et al. [50] reported a slightly lower value (Kd of 1×10^{-10} mol/L) using surface plasmon resonance. Hp1-1 and Hp2-2 bind Hb dimers equally well but there are differences in function. Significantly, the Hp1-1 phenotype is protective and provides resistance to the development of retinopathy, nephropathy, and cardiovascular disease in diabetes.

In general, Hp1-1–Hb complexes are cleared more rapidly from the circulation than Hp2-2–Hb complexes [51]. Hp2-2 binds Hb with threefold lower affinity than Hp1-1 [50]. Furthermore, Hp2-2 is redox-active and generates free redox iron which leads to, and exacerbates, oxidative stress. In diabetes, Hb is glycated [50] and diabetics with glycated Hp2-2 have greater oxidative tissue injury and vascular disease compared with those expressing Hp1-1, while heterozygotes have an intermediate risk [51]. Glycosylated Hb is bound significantly less tightly (threefold) by both Hp1-1 and Hp2-2.

NTBI is increased in diabetes, and has been proposed to be a better measure of whole body iron than serum Ftn. However, the catalytic iron in these patients differs from NTBI in the plasma of thalassemic patients. CD163 is the receptor responsible for uptake of Hb and Hb–Hp in macrophages and this is downregulated in diabetics. Certainly in the presence of strong oxidants like peroxides, heme can be broken down releasing iron. Fe(III) is probably released, not Fe(II) as from HOs.

One key variable in patient and animal studies that affects iron uptake is the ascorbate (vitamin C) levels in the circulating plasma because reducing systems, particularly ascorbate/dehydroascorbate are needed to generate Fe(II) for uptake across the plasma membrane by divalent metal transporters such as DMT1. The levels of ascorbate in the circulation vary with Hp-type. In men, they are approximately equal in Hp1-1 and Hp2-1 but about 20% less for the Hp2-2 phenotype. In mice, the levels of ascorbate are ~114 μM for the C57Bl/6 strain and, like humans, guinea pigs lack the capacity to synthesize ascorbate de novo and thus are deficient in ascorbate unless receiving a dietary supplement, which clearly impacts studies on iron metabolism [52].

Given the drastic and ongoing increased incidence in obesity and metabolic syndrome in many countries, with the accompanying rise in diabetes (affecting 350 million people worldwide in 2011 and doubled since 1981), glycated Hp2-2 is an additional complicating factor that can generate redox-active iron, which leads to cardiovascular disease [50]. Iron is bound aberrantly by glycated proteins and more loosely than on normal proteins with the potential to increase redox-active iron in the serum and tissues. This was investigated using Hp transgenic mice: the Hp knockout (Hp0) and the same mice expressing human Hp2-2 (Hp2). The amount of redox-active iron in serum, (determined after the addition of 40 μM ascorbate in the presence and absence of iron chelators, e.g., deferiprone), is increased compared with WT in the Hp0 and Hp2 mice. It is further increased by streptozotocin-induced diabetes (after 40 days). The levels of "free" redox-active iron were determined to be ~60–70 nM and were measured in the presence of transferrin whose iron-binding capacity was not saturated.

3.2 *Contribution of Haptoglobin Iron Reclamation to Hepatic Iron Overload in Hereditary Hemochromatosis*

$Hp^{-/-}$ mice develop abnormal iron deposits in the proximal tubules of the kidney as they age but not in the liver or spleen [53]. Iron also accumulated in the proximal tubules after renal ischemia-reperfusion injury or after muscle injury. This provides additional evidence that Hp prevents loss of Hb in the urine and modulates iron loading of the kidney. In HH/HHC, the prevalence of mutations in HFE is high but clinical penetrance of the disease is low. Thus, the hemochromatosis protein HFE is necessary but not a sufficient or sole cause of clinical HHC. Previous studies in humans have shown that the Hp 2-2 phenotype is over presented in Cys282Tyr (C282Y) homozygous HHC patients [54]. Furthermore, iron overload is more pronounced in males (higher serum iron and ferritin levels), suggesting that Hp polymorphisms affects iron metabolism in HHC and that there are gender differences. In men, Hp2-2 has been shown to be associated with an increase in the accumulation of iron by macrophages accompanied by increases in serum ferritin (sFtn). The amount of iron removed by phlebotomy was higher also in patients carrying Hp2-2 [54]. However, in the UK, where 90% patients with HHC are homozygous for HFE C282Y (as are 1 in 150 of the general population), only a minority develop HHC. The Hp2-2 frequencies did not differ and Hp2-2 was, therefore, not considered a risk factor for this population. Blood donors with and without clinical features suggestive of HHC were phenotyped and genotyped but neither transferrin saturation nor sFtn levels differed with Hp type.

The role of Hp as a modifier gene in HHC has been addressed using Hfe knockout mice, as a model of HHC, crossed with mice lacking Hp (i.e., the $Hfe^{-/-}Hp^{-/-}$ double knockout [55]).

In the absence of Hp, significantly less iron was found in the liver than in the $Hfe^{-/-}$ mice. Thus, haptoglobin-mediated heme–iron recovery was proposed to contribute significantly to iron loading in HHC by delivering Hb to liver cells.

3.3 Coordination of Haptoglobin Recovery of Hemoglobin Iron with Heme Reclamation by Hemopexin

The Hp system is coordinately regulated with the hemopexin heme transport system to recycle heme–iron (discussed further below). In HPX null mice, liver Hp mRNA is increased in response to chemically induced hemolysis in HPX null mice [56]. Whether this might lead to the "rebound" in plasma Hp after several transfusions, noted in more than 50 years ago in monkeys [57] and humans [58], is unknown. As a backup system for Hp and for body heme–iron retention, the co-receptors, megalin and cubulin, take up Hb by receptor-mediated endocytosis in kidney proximal tubule cells [59]. This occurs when Hb levels exceed the Hp-binding capacity in plasma or when Hp has been depleted. HPX also prevents loss of heme via the kidney since hemoglobinuria can take place without urinary heme loss [60].

4 Plasma Clearance of Hemoglobin by Haptoglobin and Its Contribution to Iron Recycling

Plasma clearance studies of Hb and Hb–Hp complexes were first undertaken about 40 years ago in man [60–62] and monkeys [57]. Although preformed Hb–Hp complexes were not used, physiologically relevant levels of Hb were employed and these early findings have subsequently been confirmed in rats injected intravenously with doubly radiolabeled Hb (e.g., ^{59}Fe-heme-^{125}I Hb) or Hb–Hp complexes. The early work revealed that Hb is cleared rapidly from the circulation, that Hp plays a role in this process, and that the site of uptake is the liver where both Hb and Hp are degraded. Autoradiography first revealed that after i.v. injection, cyano-metHb was taken up into the parenchymal cells of rabbit liver [63]. More definitive studies with double-radiolabeled Hb provided evidence, over 30 years ago, that hepatic parenchymal cells, not Kupffer cells in the sinusoids, removed Hb intact from the circulation as well as Hb bound to Hp. Thus, heme–iron recovery of ^{59}Fe-Hb by Hp takes place after uptake of intact Hb or of ^{59}Fe-Hb-Hp by the liver [64]. This is intriguing since the scavenger receptor CD 163 for Hb and Hb–Hp is reported to be restricted to cells of the macrophage/monocyte lineage. Thus, it appears that another Hb–Hp receptor may be expressed on hepatic parenchymal cells unless the heme from Hb had been transferred to HPX (see below and Fig. 8.2). Hb appears in the kidney and urine only when Hp is depleted and when plasma Hb levels are extremely high (51 and therein).

To compare the fate of Hb whether bound to Hp or free in plasma, the amount of [^{59}Fe]heme^{125}I-globin injected intravenously is increased relative to the circulating Hp levels. Low amounts of Hb produce Hb–Hp whereas high levels generate free Hb. In either case, 85–95% of [^{59}Fe]Hb was associated with parenchymal cells and less than 15% in sinusoidal Kupffer cells, which constitute only about 5% of the liver volume [65]. In contrast, [^{59}Fe]spherocytic red blood cells were taken up solely by the Kupffer cells. Furthermore, based upon the increased microsomal heme oxygenase (HO) activity, the heme from Hb, Hb–Hp, or from red blood cells was broken down in the same cells into which it had been transported. HO activity in the liver parenchymal cells detectably increased within 4 h after i.v. infusion of soluble Hb. The half-life of Hp-bound Hb was about 20 min compared with 10–15 min for free Hb, i.e., quite rapid and thus consistent with receptor-mediated uptake. Catabolism was also rapid: degraded globin was detected within 15 min after i.v. Hb, with a loss of ^{125}I from the liver. Consequently, about 75% of the Hb was cleared from the circulation within 30 min. When the amount of Hb administered intravenously was within the Hp-binding capacity, liver uptake was about 66% of the dose. In contrast, Hb in excess of Hp was sequestered principally in the kidney, not the liver, as previously reported [66] and some Hb was excreted in the urine. In the liver, non-Hp bound Hb was taken up into parenchymal cells as was Hb–Hp.

Subsequently, Kino and colleagues determined that the clearance rate of preformed [^{59}Fe]Hb–Hp complexes was rapid and similar in human, rats, and cats. The amount of [^{59}Fe]Hb–Hp transported into the liver was saturable (~400 μg Hb–Hp/liver/100 g body weight for 1.5–4 mg Hb–Hp/100 g body weight [67]), and thus indicative of a receptor-mediated process. At a dose of 0.15 mg/100 g body weight, ~66% was recovered in the liver within 30 min with less than 0.5% or 5% in the kidney and spleen, respectively. At the higher concentrations of Hb–Hp, an increasing percentage remained in the blood with a very slight increase in the kidney (overall recoveries ranged from 75% to 84%). They also specifically addressed the relative roles of liver parenchymal cells and Kupffer cells in the uptake of Hb–Hp complexes since this issue remained unresolved [63]. Low-speed centrifugation techniques were used to separate the populations of parenchymal and non-parenchymal cells and after i.v. ^{125}I-Hb–Hp (0.5 mg), the complex was located in the parenchymal cells. Uptake was competed only by unlabeled Hb–Hp, not by asialo-orosomucoid or heme-HPX [67], consistent with distinct and specific binding sites for Hb–Hp on liver parenchymal cells. [^{59}Fe]Hb uptake by rat liver was highest for rat Hp compared with Hb bound to human Hp1-1 and least with Hp2-2. If the hepatic receptor recognized the Hb moiety, then uptake of the heterologous complexes should be similar. Overall, these data support that hepatic parenchymal cells express a Hp receptor, which recognized changes in Hp caused by binding to Hb dimers (see Fig. 8.1). In contrast, the scavenger receptor CD163, reported to bind non-native forms of Hb as well as Hb–Hp complexes [44], appears to preferentially recognize structural determinants on the Hb moiety of Hb–Hp complexes (shown using competitive inhibition [68]).

Significantly, and in contrast to the hemopexin–heme reclamation system, both Hb and Hp are rapidly degraded by the liver [69]. ^{125}I-Hb-Hp passes from organelles of low density (1.05–1.07 g/mL) to those with a higher density (1.07–1.15 g/mL) likely secondary lysosomes [69]. The complex dissociated into two 82 kDa subunits, indicating an initial limited proteolysis, but heme remained bound to the protein. The distribution of radioactivity in various subcellular fractions was consistent with rapid movement of ~40% of the ^{3}H-heme from hemoglobin to both the smooth and rough endoplasmic reticulum within 10 min. However, heme catabolites were not detected until 40–90 min after injection [70]. This is much slower than the heme breakdown following intravenously injected ^{59}Fe-heme-HPX complexes when ^{59}Fe is detected and incorporated into hepatic ferritin within 10 min [71].

Body iron homeostasis is perturbed in $Hp^{-/-}$ mice since these animals have higher than normal iron levels in the kidney proximal tubule cells [4]. Otherwise, the mice are viable but with a small decrease in postnatal viability [72]. These mice are more susceptible than WT mice to the toxic effects of Hb released by phenylhydrazine-induced hemolysis. Phenylhydrazine at 2 mg/10 g body weight is toxic and killed 18% of the WT mice and ~3 times as many $Hp^{-/-}$ mice (55%). In both the WT and $Hp^{-/-}$ mice after 48 h, the hematocrit had decreased to less than 35%, and hemoglobinemia and hemoglobinuria developed that was so severe that both the urine and serum were dark brown in color. Hepatic Hp mRNA was induced in WT mice 4 h after phenylhydrazine. Such an increase would be consistent with the Hp rebound effect after transfusion seen in man [58] and monkeys [57], where plasma Hp levels were increased within 2 h after phenylhydrazine. It is not yet established whether this is due to the effects of heme, iron-induced oxidative stress, or to the ensuing inflammatory response (since Hp is an acute phase reactant). These $Hp^{-/-}$ mice had increased lipid peroxidation in the kidney, but not liver, as shown by elevated lipid peroxidation end products, malonaldehyde content, and 4-hydroxy-2(E)-nonenal. After phenylhydrazine, both WT and the $Hp^{-/-}$ mice had significant amounts of Hb "precipitated" in their renal tubular cells and had similar degrees of hemoglobinuria. This is consistent with acute renal tubular necrosis seen in severe hemolysis or during transfusions with stroma-free Hb, which presumably caused death by renal dysfunction. Even the control mice had compromised renal function. The kidney damage and acute renal failure was due, at least in part, to vasoconstriction since function was restored by administration of vasodilators.

The organ distribution of Hb differs from normal when Hp is lacking. Thus in $Hp^{-/-}$ mice, i.v. ^{125}I-Hb was taken up predominantly in the kidney whereas the liver and spleen are the major sites in WT mice [53]. Also, there was twice as much ^{125}I-Hb in the duodenum and lung compared with WT mice. Tissue iron levels were doubled in the spleen and kidney of $Hp^{-/-}$ but were similar to WT in the liver, duodenum, and serum. The $Hp^{-/-}$ spleen was only half the normal size, although the spleen cell population appeared normal by histology [4]. The acute phase response appeared more robust in the absence of Hp, which is known to be immunosuppressive [73]. Hp is a potent immunosuppressors of lymphocyte function since the levels of alpha1-glycoprotein were significantly higher after a subdermal injection of turpentine in the $Hp^{-/-}$ mice than in WT mice [72]. In their comparison of WT and $Hp^{-/-}$ mice, Lim et al. [72] reported that Hp did not affect the rate of ^{125}I-Hb clearance from the plasma (100 μg ^{125}I-Hb/10 g body wt). However, in these plasma protein clearance studies, the amount of total ^{125}I (i.e., intact and degradation peptides) in plasma was used as an indicator of the remaining Hb, instead of intact ^{125}I-Hb protein solely (e.g., using TCA-precipitable radioactivity). Thus, the total ^{125}I radioactivity includes significant amounts of ^{125}I peptides of Hb destined for excretion. Evidence from several groups shows that Hb is catabolized in lysosomes of both parenchymal cells [69] and of Kupffer cells after uptake by CD163.

Studies with $Hp^{-/-}$ mice have helped reinforce the concept that body iron homeostasis is regulated via systemic signals on cells of the liver, spleen, and duodenum. Based on the premise that the levels of FPN1 control the rate of iron release from enterocytes into the circulation, then circulating levels of hepcidin control absorption of iron from the gut lumen (i.e., diet) by modulating the rate of iron export from the duodenal enterocytes. Iron is also produced from absorbed dietary heme, which at doses designed to mimic normal human meals, is extensively catabolized by enterocytes [3]. Proof of principle studies have demonstrated that enterocytes are the first point for convergence of heme and iron metabolism in the body since only the heme–iron is targeted to transferrin [3] not heme to HPX [3] in the circulation. Whether heme is exported intact across the basal–lateral membrane of enterocytes to HPX under physiological conditions is not known.

Lack of circulating Hp increased iron export from ligated duodenal segments of $Hp^{-/-}$ mice compared with WT but did not alter iron uptake from the lumen. Export was assessed by an indirect method using iron retention in the segment after 5 min of iron uptake followed by a washout [4]. The mRNA levels of DMT1, its reductase duodenal cytochrome b (dCytb), ferritin H and L chains or of duodenal tissue iron were similar in $Hp^{-/-}$ and WT mice. However, FPN1 protein, but not its mRNA, was increased supporting transcriptional regulation of FPN1. The expression of several enzymes of heme biosynthesis, e.g., coproporphyrinogen oxidase, uroporphyrinogen oxidase, protoporphyrinogen oxidase, and uroporphyrin synthase, was decreased in the spleen of $Hp^{-/-}$ mice. The elevated FPN1 in $Hp^{-/-}$ mice was proposed to be a compensation that facilitates iron uptake, allowing more iron into the body. (It is established that FPN1 decreases in mice on an iron-deficient diet and increases in iron overload). Consequently, the $Hp^{-/-}$ liver is presumed to not secrete hepcidin under these circumstances. Based on these observations, Marro et al. [4] proposed that $Hp^{-/-}$ mice mimic the situation where Hp is saturated by Hb, i.e., no circulating Hp. If Hb–Hp is normally cleared from circulation by liver cells (whereas macrophages are presumed crucial for free Hb), then the reason the liver iron is not decreased in $Hp^{-/-}$ mice is because of increased iron flux across the duodenal enterocyte followed by iron uptake into liver. Regulation of FPN1 was perturbed in the $Hp^{-/-}$ macrophages: FPN1 mRNA and HO1 mRNA were increased although this was not reflected at the protein level. However, when RAW264.7 macrophages were incubated with Hb in vitro, a significant increase in FPN1 and HO1 mRNA took place after 4 h and FPN1 protein levels remained high for more than 24 h [4].

5 Plasma Clearance of Heme by Hemopexin and Its Contribution to Heme–Iron Recycling

The transport of heme (iron-protoporphyrin IX) and conservation of body iron stores are part of the overall cyto-protection by the heme-binding plasma protein hemopexin (HPX). HPX links heme and iron metabolism since it delivers heme to liver cells and within minutes, much of this heme is degraded by heme oxygenases releasing the heme–iron. This iron has several fates depending upon the cell type in which it is released and the iron status of the body. It can be used in metabolism including DNA and heme synthesis, and for the regulation of proteins of iron metabolism, or exported or stored on ferritin. The HPX system has a role in iron recycling to erythrocytes. This is strongly supported by published data, but this important activity of HPX is often overlooked. Significantly, the biological function of HPX in iron reclamation has been further substantiated by recent studies in mice that lack HO1, which alters the normal distribution of iron from the liver and spleen to the kidney. This organ then becomes the bastion of protection against iron loss, as discussed later in this section. In the absence of HO1, the metabolism of HPX and Hp is altered as CD163-expressing macrophages die after ingesting erythrocytes.

In this section of the review, we will focus on the role of HPX in iron recycling after describing heme binding by HPX, heme transport, and the biological consequences that are relevant for iron recycling. A comprehensive review of the literature on HPX has recently been published that provides additional details about HPX itself and the HPX-heme transport system [74]. Due to the toxicity of heme that has been well documented, its rapid removal from the circulation by HPX is vital. Lack of HPX increases morbidity in sepsis and contributes to the pathology of sepsis, hemoglobinopathies, malaria, rhabdomyolysis, acute renal failure after hemolysis, tissue injury induced by ischemia/reperfusion [60, 75–78]. When heme and iron levels rise and HPX and Hp are depleted, oxidative stress develops, which contributes to the chronic inflammation observed in some hemolytic diseases [77, 79, 80].

In the brain, free heme from red blood cell hemoglobin or from dying or injured cells, such as neurons, glia, and endothelial cells, has been proposed to substantially contribute to morbidity in cerebral hemorrhage and stroke [81]. Significantly, HPX protects the brain from damage in a mice model of stroke [11], providing the first evidence that heme is toxic to brain cells in stroke. Subsequently, HPX has also been shown to protect the brain in a mice model of intracerebral hemorrhage [82].

5.1 *Heme Toxicity*

HPX is an important extracellular antioxidant [72], which protects all cells from the chemical activity of redox-active heme. Significantly, as recently reviewed [83], HPX is not cytotoxic, nor is it a protease or a hyaluronidase. Furthermore, HPX is difficult to isolate and purify in its native, i.e., properly folded and glycosylated state and, unfortunately, recombinant HPX isolates have not been fully characterized as heme-binding proteins [83]. The toxicity of heme comes from its redox-active iron and the variety of chemical reactions that heme undergoes with oxygen that can destroy essentially all biological molecules. This is seen when HPX levels are reduced by extensive hemolysis. Heme causes lipid peroxidation, a free radical chain reaction, and also affects the function of cells of the immune system, thus contributing to inflammation. Heme triggers the oxidative burst in neutrophils, acts as a mitogen for human peripheral blood mononuclear cells [84, 85], and increases the recruitment of leukocytes to organs [77, 86]. It also activates the toll-like receptor 4 [87], increases the expression of adhesion molecules on endothelial cells [88] and the activity of matrix metalloproteinases contributing to inflammation and autoimmune diseases [89].

HPX is the principal heme-binding protein in essentially all biological fluids including plasma, cerebrospinal fluid [90], amniotic fluid [91], saliva [92], tears [93], and lymph [94]. As described below, heme transfers from albumin to HPX after intravenous heme injection into dogs and kinetic studies in vitro with purified proteins, consistent with the differences in the strength of heme binding by these two proteins. Plasma heme sources for HPX are Hb, myoglobin (Mb), cellular heme–proteins from damaged cells, Hb–Hp complexes, and heme exported by FLVCR to HPX [95]. Other body fluids can contain Hb and Hb–Hp. Plasma HPX is synthesized by hepatocytes whereas other fluids derive HPX from ganglia and photoreceptor cells of the neural retina [96], brain neurons [11], and ependymal cells [97]. When CD 163 expressing macrophage function is compromised, then HPX mRNA increases not only in the liver but also in the spleen and kidney [98].

In contrast to the heme transport function of HPX, all published evidence supports that the abundant albumin, which also binds heme is merely a reservoir for heme as originally proposed in 1971 [99]. Lacking a specific receptor albumin cannot target any of its ligands, including heme, to cells. Albumin does not protect cells from heme toxicity because $HPX^{-/-}$ [56], $Hp^{-/-}$ [72] mice, and the double knockout $HPX^{-/-}Hp^{-/-}$ [100] mice die after chemically induced hemolysis. Human HPX binds heme more tightly (Kd <1 pM; [101]) than human serum albumin (HSA [101–103]) or human globin. HSA binds heme at two sites and relatively weakly (Kds 1 and 10 μM [104]). Heme transfers from HSA to HPX in vitro [103] at physiological molar ratios of the two proteins (ca.70 HSA:1 HPX). Normal adult human plasma HPX concentrations are ~0.6 mg/mL (i.e., ~10 μM) [105–108], ranging from 0.5 to 1.2 mg/mL (~20 μM) in adults. In newborns, levels are ~20% of adults and increase immediately after birth, presumably as the population of hepatocytes increases [109]. In man the heme-binding capacity of HPX would be exceeded by ~95 mg heme/100 mL serum. Intravenous (i.v.) injections of heme (hydroxyhemin) were used to raise heme levels seven times higher than the plasma HPX-heme binding capacity. The concentrations of heme–HPX complexes were initially equal to heme–albumin became tenfold higher within ~2 h [99]. This rapid transfer of heme to HPX was even faster if heme-albumin was injected i.v. instead of heme. This produced twice as much heme bound to HPX than to albumin within 10 min. Heme from [^{59}Fe]-heme- ^{125}I-albumin was taken up by the liver faster than from doubly radiolabeled Hb–Hp complexes, and the induction of microsomal heme oxygenase activity mirrored these heme uptake rates. Overall, these data support that heme dissociation reflected transfer from albumin to HPX before transport to the liver as heme–HPX [64].

A role for HPX in the catabolism of the heme moiety of Hb has been supported by: physical-chemical evidence showing that HPX is the principal heme-binding protein in plasma; autoradiographic studies showing HPX and heme associated with liver parenchymal cells [110]; heme delivery for catabolism in the isolated perfused rat liver; and by studies in animals and in humans [61, 62, 99]. In vivo, after lysis of red blood cells, the released Hb with ferrous heme is rapidly oxidized to metHb (ferric heme) and this heme is then distributed throughout the body by HPX. When equimolar apo-HPX and methemoglobin are incubated together in vitro, 50–70% of hemoglobin heme is bound to HPX at equilibrium [101].

5.2 *Heme Uptake by Receptor-Mediated Endocytosis of Heme–Hemopexin Complexes with Recycling of Intact Hemopexin*

There is strong evidence that hemopexin recycles intact after delivering heme to cells by receptor-mediated endocytosis and co-localizes with transferrin in endosomes. HPX recycling was seen after the uptake of heme from well-defined equimolar [^{59}Fe]-heme-^{125}I-hemopexin complexes both in vivo with intact rats [111] and also after endocytosis is human HepG2 cells [112].

Support for HPX recycling in vivo first came from an analysis of bile pigment formation to assess heme degradation following i.v. heme injection in dogs [99]. Based on a whole body plasma volume of 450 mL and a HPX concentration of 20 μM (0.02 mmol/L), equimolar binding of heme by HPX is equivalent to 5.87 mg heme, which is ~2.45 higher than the amount of heme normally converted to bile pigments (i.e., ~49 mg total and ~2.4 mg/h). Taking into account the finding that heme was cleared from the plasma at a rate of 19.93 mg heme/h, which is very rapid [99], bile pigment production from heme is ~eightfold more than the HPX concentration. Importantly, this is consistent with recycling of HPX.

There is also direct evidence for extensive recycling of ^{125}I-HPX after hepatic uptake of heme-^{125}I-HPX or ^{59}Fe-heme-^{125}I-HPX after i.v. injection in intact rats [111, 113], and from isolated rat hepatocytes [114] and after endocytosis of heme-^{125}I-HPX in human HepG2 hepatoma [112] cells. The in vivo studies clearly revealed that: HPX rapidly targets heme to the liver for catabolism, uptake occurs via a finite number of receptors, and ^{125}I-HPX returns to the circulation intact since it is precipitable from plasma samples with trichloroacetic acid or mono-specific antibodies to HPX and was shown to be the mature size using electrophoresis [111]. Importantly, only a few minutes is needed for the clearance from the circulation of heme-HPX followed by heme catabolism since the heme–iron is detected stored on ferritin within 10 min after i.v. heme-HPX [71]. Iron incorporation into ferritin is sustained for at least 2 h.

Using a tracer dose of 700 pmol of [^{59}Fe]heme-^{125}I-rabbit HPX, the ratio of ^{59}Fe/^{125}I radioactivity in the liver was already 2:1 by 10 min. In addition, there was an inverse relationship between the levels of TCA-precipitable ^{125}I-HPX in liver and serum during the course of heme uptake, consistent with release of intact HPX back to the circulation [113]. The maximal levels of ^{125}I-HPX in the liver occurred 5–10 min after injection and declined by 2 h, while ^{59}Fe-heme uptake accumulated linearly over 2 h. After the i.v. injection of 11 nmol heme-HPX/rat, uptake was saturated at 5 min (~170 pmol ^{125}I-HPX/g liver). HPX delivered heme to the liver and no significant urinary excretion of either ^{125}I or ^{59}Fe was detected and only 1–2% of the dose was found in extra hepatic tissues. In contrast to heme-HPX, only ~3% dose (~3 pmol/gliver) of apo-^{125}I-HPX and ^{125}I-albumin were detected after i.v. injection. All in vivo data show that uptake of heme-HPX and subsequent heme catabolism is faster than uptake of Hb–Hp complexes and Hb degradation.

The receptor-mediated endocytosis of heme-HPX and heme uptake was first revealed by biochemical and morphological studies using human HepG2 and mouse Hepa cells [112]. Furthermore, after endocytosis, HPX returned intact to the medium. Morphological studies using colloidal gold-conjugated heme-HPX and electron microscopy autoradiography of heme-^{125}I-HPX and Hep G2 cells showed HPX in clathrin-coated pits, endosomes, and multivesicular bodies, not lysosomes. Importantly, their orientation in multivesicular bodies relative to the membrane was consistent with that established for ligand-receptor complexes that recycle. HPX was shown to co-localize within vesicles with transferrin by biochemical and morphological techniques: the diaminobenzidine density shift assay with heme-^{125}I-HPX and iron-^{125}I-transferrin and colloidal gold derivatives, respectively. Exposure to the PKC-activating phorbol ester PMA caused a rapid redistribution of HPX receptors from the cell surface that was prevented by a PKC inhibitor, suggesting that this downregulation was due to PKC activation. The receptors were not degraded but recycled back to the cell surface [115]. Thus, HPX and transferrin are the only known recycling metal protein transporters.

The biochemical responses of cells to heme-HPX have been studied in a variety of human cell types including polymorphonuclear leukocytes [116], promyelocytic (HL-60) [117], K562 [118], retinal pigment epithelial (RPE) cells [96], U937 [119], HepG2 [112], placental syncytial BeWo cells [120], and also in rodent cell models including mouse hepatoma cells [121], rat hepatocytes [114], and mouse primary neurons [11]. The number of surface receptors varies slightly with cell type; it is generally similar to transferrin receptors (~40,000 per cell). Internal pools of receptors were detected in mouse Hepa and RPE cells, and while the reported apparent Kd values vary, most are in the nanomolar range.

Two processes of HPX-mediated heme (iron protoporphyrin IX) uptake have been detected in intact rats [111] and isolated rat hepatic parenchymal cells [114]. The "specific" high-affinity uptake has a low capacity whereas the other "selective" uptake has a lower affinity and, interestingly, a high capacity. Both require heme-HPX complexes and have been distinguished from the uptake of non-HPX bound heme by their response to metabolic inhibitors [114]. Thus, there are two types of HPX receptors: one high affinity, low capacity (HPXR1) and one high affinity, high capacity (HPXR2). The specific system in vivo is saturable, has a high affinity (apparent *Km*, approximately 100 nM), and thus exhibits the characteristics of the receptor-mediated system observed in vivo [111]. The cell-associated molar ratio of heme to HPX increased from 1:l with time since heme (1.25 ± 0.25 pmol/10^6 cells in 1 h at 37°C) but not protein (0.51 ± 0.05 pmol/10^8 cells) accumulated. The low-density lipoprotein receptor-related protein (LRP1/CD91) is a high-affinity HPX-binding protein with a reported affinity for heme-HPX of 0.5 nM [122]. LRP1 may be HPXR1 but it is a scavenger cargo receptor that binds a plethora of more than 50 structurally diverse protein ligands [123]. These ligands are usually not native proteins but have either been inactivated or covalently modified sometimes by cleavage (e.g., activated α-2macroglobulin). LRP1 is constitutively endocytosed, targeting some ligands to the lysosomes for degradation, whereas others are efficiently recycled like apolipoprotein E [124]. Sorting nexin 17 is needed for targeting LRP1 to the recycling endosome pathway rather than to lysosomes [125]. In 2005, following some in vitro studies with Chinese hamster ovary cells over expressing LRP1, this scavenger molecule was reported to be the sole receptor for heme-HPX complexes targeting HPX to the lysosomes for degradation [122]. As described here, this is clearly not the normal route. In human promyelocytic HL60 cells, which lack LRP1, heme-HPX induces HO1 [126, 127] and delivers heme to myeloperoxidase [117]. LRP1-negative PEA 13 murine embryonic fibroblasts take up heme-Alex-Fluor-HPX by endocytosis [74]. The multiple examples of evidence for HPX recycling intact from cells after heme delivery from several groups has been summarized above and include data from studies with intact rats [111] and human hepatoma, HepG2 cells [112].

The selective process is needed for the copper-dependent interaction of heme-HPX with the cell growth-associated plasma membrane electron transport pathway in mouse Hepa cells since it is half-saturated at 5 μM complex [128]. Heme-HPX has been identified as a ligand for toll-like receptor 4 [87] and, intriguingly, this binding prevents the release of pro-inflammatory cytokines, independently of HO1 induction. Thus, this may be one way that decreasing HPX levels "opens the door" for pro-inflammatory events to develop.

6 Hemopexin and Iron Salvage

6.1 Plasma Clearance of Heme by Hemopexin in Intra- and Extravascular Hemolysis

Many in vivo studies published in the 1960s and 1970s showed that the liver takes up heme and that HPX is the principal binder and transporter of heme in plasma. The amount of Hb–Hp complexes normally present in plasma from blood collected into anticoagulant is based on the Hb levels that are very low (4–7 μM; 0.04–0.07% of the Hb content of whole blood). Only low protoheme-HPX levels are detectable spectrophotometrically in similarly prepared plasma samples. Any heme-HPX formed from the normal wear and tear of red blood cells in capillary beds will be rapidly removed from the circulation to the liver within 2–3 min. HPX was first characterized in 1971 as a heme complex with a stoichiometry of heme binding of 1:1 [129] in samples of plasma from monkey [130], human [61, 62], and dog [99].

Several features of heme transport by HPX were revealed more than 40 years ago after i.v. injection of ^{14}C-porphyrin-ring labeled heme into dogs [60]. First, HPX is the sole high-affinity heme-binding protein in the plasma. Second, HPX binds both oxidized and reduced heme (ferri- and ferro-protoporphyrin IX, respectively). Third, HPX rapidly clears heme from the circulation mainly to the liver. And, fourth, heme catabolism and heme–iron reutilization starts almost immediately and HPX normally recycles intact from cells. This role for HPX in heme clearance was further supported by studies in humans and primates once again several decades ago. In those days, both heme-HPX and methemalbumin complexes were detected in plasma samples by staining for heme after electrophoresis and quantitation by densitometry. Plasma HPX protein levels were quantitated by immunodiffusion using mono-specific antibodies.

6.2 Enhanced Catabolism of Hemopexin in Severe Hemolysis Depletes Plasma Levels

HPX normally recycles intact after endocytosis and heme delivery but plasma HPX levels are low in chronic and severe hemolytic states [60, 131]. They also decline after intravenous hematin [132–134] used as an experimental model of hemolysis, and after heme infusion (heme-arginate) as therapy for the "heme-deficiency" state in patients with acute intermittent porphyria [135]. "Free" heme, i.e., non-Hb heme, was first found in the plasma of patients with intravascular hemolysis in 1912, detected using a spectrophotometric test now termed the Schumm test after its inventor [136]. Heme bound to HPX and albumin (methemalbumin) was also found in plasma from patients with chronic intravascular hemolysis as first described by Neale [137] and then by Wheby [138]. Notably, in these early studies with hemolytic patients and i.v. hemoglobin, HPX did not completely disappear despite high levels of Hb from hemolysis [62], nor was Hp completely depleted. Based on normal, circulating plasma HPX concentrations, HPX should bind 0.6 mg heme/100 mL (or 16 mg/100 mL if expressed as Hb) and be saturated by 1 mg hematin/kg body weight injected intravenously. At high heme (hematin) levels, HPX is depleted but not at lower levels [61, 62]. Although heme binding to HPX is equimolar, HPX amounts did not decline in molar proportion to the heme dose [132, 134]. Catabolism of HPX leading to lower plasma levels occurs when there is hemoglobinuria and Hp is completely depleted. Also, in the early studies in which the clearance of HPX was determined after injection of heme, it was much slower than that observed for other receptor-mediated uptake processes and for heme-^{125}I-HPX in rats. This is likely due to the transfer of heme from albumin to HPX [103]. The decreases in HPX are due to an increase in the fractional catabolic rate of HPX [131]. HPX levels are depleted when heme is present in the circulation, e.g., when free Hb is present after Hp depletion (both Hb and Hp are degraded in the lysosomes), or when Hp is present but so it non-hemoglobin heme as in hemorrhagic pancreatitis [61] or in some, but not all, children with thalassemia major [139]. Thus, under conditions of unusual heme load, either HPX recycling is not 100%, likely also true for transferrin (Evans Morgan, personal communication), or other mechanisms come into play to account for the enhanced catabolism of HPX. The loss of CD163 expressing macrophages after erythrophagocytosis in HO1$^{-/-}$ mice alters the distribution of iron in the body, requiring the kidney to take over from the liver and spleen as the stronghold for iron reclamation. Certainly, when liver function is compromised or HPX is treated with neuraminidase [133], then the asialo-HPX is rapidly removed via the galactose receptor and degraded [140], as is a chemically modified form of HPX [141].

HPX deficiency states are clearly deleterious in humans and in mice models of i.v. hemolysis. They also contribute to the development of sepsis, where HPX has been shown to be protective [142]. The kidney becomes the organ of last defense against iron loss from the body. When HPX$^{-/-}$ mice are exposed to extensive hemolysis, kidney damage was far more extensive and life threatening than in their WT counterparts [56]. Serum levels of bilirubin, iron, total protein, albumin, WBC, RBC, Hb, HCT, MCV, MCH, RDW, platelet count, PDW, or MPV in HPX$^{-/-}$ mice were the same as WT animals, leading the authors to conclude that HPX does not contribute to iron metabolism or protect against oxidative stress. Importantly, it was later found that as HPX$^{-/-}$ mice mature, the levels of iron increase in the brain accompanied by an increase in malonaldehyde and Cu, Zn superoxide dismutase as parameters of oxidative stress [97], associated with low ferritin expression.

6.3 *Body Iron Stores Regulate Heme–Iron Reutilization by HPX*

Iron reutilization from ^{59}Fe-heme (as hematin) has been compared in normal subjects before and after multiple hematin injections sufficient to deplete HPX and also in patients undergoing intravascular hemolysis. The ^{59}Fe in plasma samples was still heme because it was not removed by dialysis against EDTA, which removes iron from transferrin. Thus, in normal subjects, all of this i.v. ^{59}Fe-hematin was immediately bound to HPX and albumin. One day later, only small amounts of heme-HPX were detected. The plasma clearance rate of heme-HPX was ~7–8 h in three patients and whole body scanning over time showed that heme was first taken up by the liver and its iron rapidly returned to the bone marrow (i.e., sacrum [60]). Notably, this iron was rapidly and extensively reutilized into circulating RBCs (more than half within 48 h, i.e. within one cell life span) and remained for 2–3 months.

Iron deficiency led to a more rapid reutilization of the heme–iron from the liver [60]. When iron overload developed from transfusions in patient with thalassemia, little of the heme–iron injected was incorporated into red blood cells and no radioactivity was detected in the urine. This heme–iron reutilization was slightly slower than for hemoglobin iron [143] or for effete red blood cells [144]. When HPX had been depleted due to sufficiently severe intravascular hemolysis, then the injected heme bound solely to albumin, which produced two components with half-lives averaging 3.9 and 22.2 h in the plasma clearance curve. Some radioactivity was still transported to liver, but the iron reutilization was variable. Similar biphasic clearance curves were seen when a normal person was injected with high heme levels that depleted HPX [60]. In addition, lower amounts of ^{59}Fe-heme did not decrease the endogenous HPX nor increase plasma bilirubin [61].

6.4 *Heme Transport by HPX Is Linked to the Iron Status of Cells*

The effect of changes in iron metabolism on the regulation of heme uptake and the expression of HPX receptors has been studies using a highly differentiated mouse hepatoma cell line (Hepa cells), originally derived from hepatoma BW7756 [145]. After incubation with desferioxamine, iron-deficient Hepa cells express twice the number of high-affinity cell surface HPX receptors (Kd 17 nM; 65,000/cell) and heme uptake increased 60–80% (apparent Km of 160 nM; V_{max} of 7.5 pmol heme/10^6 cells/h) [121]. This change did not require protein synthesis and was due to recruitment from internal pools of HPX receptors. However, when cell iron levels were raised by incubation with ammonium ferric citrate (8.5 and 20 μg/mL for 24 h), heme uptake was only slightly decreased (by 25%), with no discernible effect on the number of surface HPX receptors.

6.5 *The HPX and Hp Systems Are Linked*

HPX is considered the first line of defense against heme-mediated damage to cells during hemolysis, trauma, and ischemia reperfusion injury. A key role for hepatocytes in the metabolism of plasma hemoglobin, in addition to that of macrophages, was first supported by data from rats more than 35 years ago [64]. In mice, HPX prevents endothelial and liver cell damage in chemically induced intravascular hemolysis [56] or an in vitro model for hemolysis that uses high levels of intravascular hematin [146]. When HPX is absent as in the HPX null mice, Hp metabolism changes and compensates (i.e., Hp mRNA in the liver is stabilized [56]). However, when both HPX and Hp are knocked out, lethal inflammation of the liver ensues [100]. Thus, macrophages, which express the CD163 receptor for Hb and Hb–Hp complexes [147] as well as the heme–hemopexin binding proteins, LRP1 and TLR4, are not able to compensate for the loss of both HPX and Hp.

Impairment of CD 163+ macrophages or their loss, as in murine and human HO1 deficiency (described below), is associated with very low HPX but elevated Hp. Transiently impaired Hb scavenging was detected in acute retroviral syndrome (HIV) with Hb–Hp present in the circulation. Early in HIV-1 infection, free Hb in the serum was extremely high (1.68 g/L; normally <0.11 g/L), although there no were other clinical or biochemical signs of hemolysis [148], and the levels of CD163 were only slightly below normal. Overall, these observations suggested that uptake of Hb–Hp by CD163 was somehow defective. This had previously been reported after treatment with gemtuzumab ozogamicin [149], which is a monoclonal antibody used to treat bone marrow cancer (acute myeloid leukemia). This molecule was withdrawn from US markets due to the side effects of hepatotoxicity and liver veno-occlusive disease. In acute syndromes of HIV-1 infection, viral particles compete with Hb–Hp for CD163, which is known to bind porcine reproductive and respiratory syndrome virus and bacteria. In addition, the Hp phenotype might contribute to loss of Hb clearance and affect prognosis in acute viral load. This patient had a Hp2-2 phenotype and Hp2-2 has a higher affinity for CD163 than other Hp phenotypes.

7 Heme Oxygenases Are Linked with Iron Recycling and Iron Overload

Heme oxygenases (HO1 and HO2 isozymes) are the rate-limiting enzymes in the degradation of heme, releasing iron, biliverdin, and carbon monoxide after cleavage of the porphyrin ring [150, 151]. HO1 is highly inducible whereas HO2 is induced ~twofold by dexamethasone [152] and basal HO2 levels are constitutively higher than those of HO1, especially in barrier tissues like testis and brain. The levels of HO1 increase in response to stress [153–155], and conditions that alter iron metabolism, e.g., hypoxia, endocytosis of heme-HPX [126] or of Hb–Hp [42] among others, e.g., inflammation. Overexpression of HO1 prevents cells from dying and provides protection against oxidative stress during organ transplantation and brain neuronal injury [156]. Furthermore, CO exposure often mimics these protective effects by vasodilation [157] and other heme catabolites are also cytoprotective. Biliverdin reductase generates bilirubin, which acts as a free radical scavenger [158]. The Fe(II) released has the potential to be protective due to its regulatory properties via the IRP/IRE system. These include induction of the iron storage protein ferritin, downregulation of iron uptake by TfR1 and DMT1 (IRE). When heme is delivered to cells by HPX, the levels of non-protein bound iron need to be kept low, presumably by promoting storage and export, minimizing iron uptake by TfRs [71]. The heme–iron enters regulatory pools for ferritin and the transferrin receptor 1, which are up- [159] and down- [126] regulated, respectively. HO1 is also induced by heme itself and via Nrf2 (NF-E2 related factor), which is induced by heme-HPX [74]. The genes of the iron exporter FPN1 and HO1 may be coordinately induced by heme, rather than directly by iron. If intracellular Fe(II) levels rise above a certain threshold, then this is potentially toxic to cells (see NTBI section above).

Catabolite protection requires a source of heme and likely at quite high concentrations given the therapeutic levels of CO. Extracellular heme in hemolysis is predominantly in the form of heme-HPX or Hb–Hp, both of which induce HO1. Erythrophagocytosis may become toxic to CD163+ macrophages when intracellular heme levels rise due to inadequate catabolism by HOs and/or diminished export by FLVCR when plasma HPX is depleted. Both HPX and a Albumin accept heme from FLVCR, unless saturated due to hemolysis.

Intriguingly, HO1 and HO2 are cytoprotective even when not enzymatically active. Transfection of catalytically inactive HO1 or HO2 protects U937 and HEK 293 cells, respectively, from peroxide toxicity [158, 160]. Regulated intracellular proteolysis (RIP) generates a soluble form of HO1 ($HO1_{sol}$) that migrates to the nucleus after hepatoma cells are incubated with heme-HPX or non-protein bound heme, and after lung cells are exposed to hypoxia [161, 162]. $HO1_{sol}$ increases nuclear levels of DNA binding proteins and transcription factors, e.g., c-Jun, AP2, CBF and Brn-3, and activates an oxidant-response promoter in *ho1* [161], thus increasing *ho1* transcription when there is oxidative stress [163]. Overexpression of active HO1 in RAW 264.7 macrophage cells reduces NADPH oxidase activity, which is an intracellular source of superoxide [164]. Presumably, this is due in part to competition for the coenzyme NADPH with the obligatory cytochrome-P450 reductase for HOs. HO2 activity is regulated by increasing the affinity for heme at the active site in oxidative stress via two conserved heme regulatory motifs that form a reversible thiol/disulfide redox switch, which is reduced at ambient intracellular redox (range – 170–250 mV) [165] but converted to the disulfide in oxidative stress [166]. This provides a means whereby HO2 integrates heme and carbon monoxide with the redox regulation of metabolism [166].

HO1 is required for normal iron reutilization [167, 168] and hemolytic anemia develops in HO1 deficiency in humans with marked erythrocyte fragmentation and intravascular hemolysis with hematuria but unexpectedly low levels of bilirubin. There is also severe and persistent damage to endothelial cells together with hyperlipidemia and oxidative stress [169]. Although serum iron levels were normal, serum ferritin was elevated and the kidney and liver had extremely high amounts of iron. There were no effects on HO2 expression or on its tissue distribution. In spite of the severe hemolysis, Hp levels were significantly increased whereas HPX was depleted [169]. This is reminiscent of the situation in HPX null mice where Hp and HPX are coordinately regulated after phenylhydrazine-induced hemolysis [56], and perhaps the $CD163^+$ macrophages had been depleted by this treatment.

A principle difference between human HO1 deficiency and young $HO1^{-/-}$ mice is that the mice have splenomegaly and the human patient lacked a spleen (asplenia). In these mice, the lack of HO1 leads to anemia since upon aging there is a loss of CD163-expressing macrophages. HO1 is needed to survive the heme toxicity after erythrophagocytosis [98]. Furthermore, hepatic levels of HPX mRNA and protein are significantly induced even at 7 weeks of age in $HO1^{-/-}$ mice but serum HPX remains low, presumably due to increased catabolism in an effort to keep clearing the heme load in the absence of CD163 expressing macrophages. This loss of the CD163-expressing Kupffer cells in liver, spleen, and also likely in bone marrow, leads to a redistribution of iron reclamation processes in the body. The kidney, an organ that normally plays no role in iron-recycling, now takes over from the liver and spleen. The HPX system is turned on not only in the liver but HPX mRNA is increased in the kidney and spleen as well. The kidney has elevated levels of HPX protein and heme-HPX and heme-albumin may get into the glomerular filtrate and be reabsorbed in proximal tubules of the kidney by nonspecific mechanism such as cubulin and megalin.

Finally, HO1 also regulates iron release from cells and $HO1^{-/-}$ mice and $HO1^{-/-}$ embryonic fibroblasts in vitro are more vulnerable to oxidative stress. In murine $HO1^{-/-}$ fibroblasts, desferioxamine-induced iron efflux was decreased compared with cells from WT mice, whereas iron uptake, either from $FeCl_3$ (in medium containing 10% FBS) or from iron-transferrin, was increased. HEK293 cells overexpressing HO1 together with its obligatory cytochrome p450 reductase [170] had lower iron uptake than controls, although ferritin levels were the same. However, iron efflux (determined after addition of DF to the medium) was twofold higher in the HO1/CPR-293 cells. This iron release was prevented by inhibiting HOs with the heme analog tin-PPIX, supporting that the iron came from heme breakdown. One complicating factor is the presence of high HO2 levels but the HO inhibitor, SnPPIX, also blocked basal levels of iron release. Under conditions of oxidative stress, i.e., selenium deficiency, phenobarbital (PB), which is an inducer of P-450 among other actions, induces HO1 and serum iron levels almost double [171]. The ferrochelatase inhibitor DDC prevented both HO1 induction and the rise in serum iron by PB but not HO1 induction by heme. When oxidative stress was induced by GSH depletion in response to phorone, HO1 was induced and the concomitant rise in serum iron was prevented by the HO1 inhibitor tin-PPIX.

Significantly, ferritin induction is needed for cell survival and forms of ferritin are protective in the cytosol, mitochondria, and nucleus. Ferritin induction requires the iron from heme catabolism, e.g., after endocytosis of heme-HPX since its induction is prevented by simultaneous incubation of heme-HPX with the iron chelator, desferal [159]. The H-ferritin chain [35] is transcriptionally regulated by heme, presumably before regulation by iron from heme catabolism at the translational level. This is an emerging pattern for the regulation of FPN1 too, although it lacks a canonical IRE. Chemical inhibition of HO1 induction prevented ferritin synthesis by exogenous heme [172]. In RAW 264.7 macrophages, heme the oxidant stressor, sodium arsenite, both induced HO1 but only heme increased ferritin synthesis and this was due to iron from heme catabolism. HEK cells overexpressing HO1 had slightly higher ferritin than untransfected cells but were protected from oxidative stress, but without significantly raising ferritin levels. These observations support that heme levels, rather than HO1, limit cellular heme catabolism [173]. A threshold of HO1 expression has been proposed [174], which would be beneficial to cells since it is related to the amount of iron released intracellularly from the active site of HO1. Depending on its rate of release from HO1 and storage on ferritin, this reactive, potentially toxic iron is en route for export by FPN1. $HO1^{-/-}$ animals remain sensitive to hyperoxia-induced injury. These animals had significantly increased levels of hemoproteins and iron but without increased ferritin, suggesting that redox-active iron is accumulating intracellularly. Induced HO1 did not compensate for HO2 loss [175] and this was further supported by disrupting HO1 in the lung implicating iron [176]. Also, iron from heme catabolism by HO1 regulates hyperoxia-dependent induction in human pulmonary endothelial cells [177].

8 Cytoprotection by Hemopexin Requires Heme Oxygenase-1 and Signaling Cascades

The basis for the cytoprotection by the HPX system against heme toxicity comes in part from HO1 induction and ferritin induction but HO1 is one direct link between heme and iron metabolism with iron recycling [11]. Importantly, after endocytosis of heme-HPX, several signaling pathways are activated due to receptor binding that are *not* activated by "free" heme, which is an established inducer of HO1 (and other proteins via the transcription factor, Nrf2). Some of the pathways that come into play in response to receptor binding of heme-HPX, but not heme, activate transcription factors that regulate the expression of proteins that help control copper homeostasis, e.g., metallothioneins that sequester copper and zinc, ferroxidases needed for iron export are copper proteins and copper chaperones like CCS1 for Cu Zn superoxide dismutase (A. Smith; unpublished data). These changes in response to heme-HPX play a key role during oxidative stress in protecting cells from heme and the heme–iron derived from heme catabolism. H-HPX also down regulates the transferrin receptor-1 [126] and decreases synthesis of transferrin (Tf) itself [178], both known iron-regulated proteins. Heme-HPX also induces H-ferritin, a ferroxidase, and to a lesser extent L-ferritin [159]. Ferritin and TfR1 regulation occur principally at the translational level in response to protein binding (IRP1) to iron-responsive elements (IRE) in their mRNA [179], although H-ferritin is regulated by heme. Iron released from the breakdown of heme taken up into cells by HPX will regulate IRP-1/IRE interactions. Unlike heme, heme-HPX regulates metallothioneins [180], stress-activated protein kinase/N-terminal cJun kinase (SAPK/JNK) [181], NFκB [182], PKC [183] and the transcription factor MTF1 [182] for metallothionein synthesis and for the rate-limiting enzyme for GSH synthesis, as well as Nrf2 for quinone oxidoreductases and other protective proteins. Receptor-mediated heme uptake from H-HPX increased transcription of the *ho1* gene [126], thus elevating this enzyme protein level two- to four-fold, and also stimulates RIP to produce a soluble form of HO1 that also activates the *ho1* gene (see section on HOs above).

Few mechanisms for neuroprotection have been established and the neuroprotective effects of HPX via HO1 are important. This was shown using a genetic approach with primary cultures of neurons.

Heme-HPX protects neurons from wild type, but not *ho1*$^{-/-}$ mice, against heme toxicity and chemical-mediated oxidative stress, i.e., the free radical generator, *tert* butyl hydroperoxide [11]. Inflammation accompanies brain injury like stroke and intracerebral hemorrhage, and HPX maintains its structure in an oxidizing extracellular environment due to an extensive disulfide bond network and a lack of free sulfhydryl groups. The heme-HPX complex is stable in the presence of peroxides due to the hindrance of access of hydroperoxides to the bound heme [184] and the heme is prevented from producing radicals. This supports that heme-HPX is able to survive inflammatory conditions in contrast to Hp, which does not protect Hb from peroxide damage. Heme becomes covalently attached to protein in the Hb–Hp complex and cannot reach the nucleus for *ho1* gene activation [44].

9 Iron Recycling via Ferritin

Although ferritin is the principal protein for iron storage and detoxification within cells, it is also considered to help recycle heme–iron after erythrophagocytosis by macrophages. It is not known if hepatic ferritin recycles iron after heme catabolism by the liver and, if so, whether this is part of normal or only pathological conditions. In vitro L-ferritin is secreted from macrophages and H-ferritin from hepatocytes these cells, both ferritins contain iron [185]. The levels of the iron exporter FPN1 play a key role in the erythrocyte Hb-iron cycle by exporting iron for loading onto transferrin (Fig. 8.2). When macrophages depleted of the iron exporter FPN1 by RNAi are incubated in iron-supplemented medium, intracellular iron rises and H-ferritin synthesis is increased. FPN1 is normally downregulated when hepcidin in the circulation binds to it; however, hepcidin is presumed absent in this in vitro system since it is synthesized by the liver. Intracellular heme and iron levels also regulate FPN1 (as described above). Most iron storage takes place within cytosolic ferritin but there are also mitochondrial and nuclear forms that are protective against iron toxicity, particularly in models of oxidative stress in vitro [186, 187].

A dynamic direct role for ferritin in supplying iron for intracellular iron trafficking, e.g., for heme, iron–sulfur center and DNA synthesis, and in iron homeostasis by supplying iron for regulation seems likely but there is little direct evidence. The mechanism for iron release from the ferritin shell is still being characterized and iron chaperones for these processes have not yet been identified. There are two known processes of ferritin degradation. Cationic ferritin was taken up by human fibroblasts and degraded in lysosomes in a chloroquine-inhibitable manner [188]. The iron was proposed to be transported back to cytosol. When FPN1 was overexpressed in HEK293 cells, iron loss from ferritin occurred in the cytosol before mono-ubiquitination of ferritin subunit dimers, which is needed for disassembly of the ferritin nanocages. Ferritin degradation required the proteasome and was unaffected by chloroquine and leupeptin [31].

In iron overload, ferritin containing some iron circulates in plasma and its level is used by physicians to assess the extent of body iron accumulation in patients with inherited or secondary iron overload [189]. This ferritin is the more basic and glycosylated L-subunit rather than the H-subunit, which has ferroxidase activity needed for iron incorporation. One long-held view is that serum ferritin is released when macrophages lyse after extensive erythrophagocytosis. However, more recent evidence suggests active secretion of L-ferritin by hepatocytes [190], although L-ferritin mRNA lacks any obvious sequence that might encode a signal peptide, needed for secretion. Furthermore, ferritin mRNA is found associated with membrane-bound polysomes where proteins destined for secretion are synthesized. Kannengiesser and colleagues [191] explain this apparent anomaly by suggesting that L-ferritin is secreted inefficiently like Plasminogen Activator Inhibitor Type 2, which like ferritin exists in two forms: a non-glycosylated cytosolic form and a glycosylated extracellular form.

A new mutation in ferritin (Thr30Ileu) seems to allow more efficient secretion of ferritin, leading to hyperferritinemia in the absence of iron overload [191].

Recent data support that H-ferritin suppresses the growth of both T- and B-lymphoid cells of the immune system (consistent with the consequences of recombinant ferritin overexpression in HeLa cells observed several years ago [192]). In this process, the secreted H-ferritin also delivers iron to these cells of the immune system [193].

Several lines of evidence support that ferritin is taken up into cells by receptor-mediated endocytosis. The first evidence for ferritin receptors came from classic binding studies using human placenta brush border membranes [194], guinea pig reticulocytes [195], human and porcine [196] and rat [197] liver membranes. Later studies revealed that H- and L-ferritins bind to distinct receptors in transformed human B- and T-lymphoid cells [198] and human T-lymphoid MOLT4 cells [199]. In these studies, the majority of receptors bound H- rather than L-ferritin, with affinities that averaged ~700 nM. The number of sites, but not binding affinity, varied with growth and cell cycle in transformed cells and human erythroid precursors [200]. Maximal binding took place during exponential growth S phase [201] and was also regulated by the iron status of the cell. The fact that no difference in binding affinity was detected in any of these published studies suggests that ferritin receptors are not regulated upon ligand binding by covalent modifications like phosphorylation. Ferritin became pronase-insensitive, supporting internalization via receptor-mediated endocytosis, and this was decreased by chloroquine, which is consistent with a role for lysosomes; however, whether the ferritin receptors are degraded or recycled remains to be established. Like iron uptake by transferrin, ferritin uptake is regulated by cellular iron status. Three iron chelators, desferal, citrate, and diethylene-triamine-pentacetate, all decreased iron uptake from ferritin into rat hepatocytes by 35%, 25%, and 8%, respectively. In contrast, ascorbate increased iron accumulation by 20% [202]. Ferritin binding to microvilli from placental membranes was significantly higher in pregnancy with moderate iron deficiency. Thus, this pathway may help regulate maternal–fetal iron homeostasis [203].

Additional evidence for a role for ferritin in iron recycling has been shown in two types of cells that lack transferrin receptors, which provide evidence that ferritin is potentially the principal nutrient iron source for these cells rather than transferrin. Ferritin-binding sites have been identified in white matter where levels of the transferrin receptor are low [204]. In mouse oligodendrocytes, the T cell immunoglobulin and mucin-domain containing protein Tim 2 is an H-ferritin receptor as shown by binding and antibody blocking studies [205]. These cells require iron to produce myelin [205]. As in macrophages, the number of ferritin-binding sites on oligodendrocytes decreases with iron loading and increases when oligodendrocytes are incubated with iron chelators. The human homolog of Tim2 has not been identified. Serum ferritin levels are three- to eightfold higher in the embryo than in the maternal circulation. Iron is supplied to the stroma and capsule of the developing kidney by Scara-5, a novel ferritin receptor [206]. Thus, ferritin is used instead of transferrin as the iron source for organogenesis. Ferritin can cross endothelial cells in an in vitro model of the blood brain barrier [207]. Thus, ferritin in the systemic circulation likely delivers iron to brain cells in conditions of primary and secondary iron overload.

10 Conclusions

Body iron recycling requires: the plasma proteins transferrin and ferritin which bind iron; hemopexin and haptoglobin, which bind heme and hemoglobin, respectively; heme oxygenases for heme catabolism; as well as the multicopper oxidases including ceruloplasmin and hephestin for iron movement across membranes. The role of these proteins is now recognized as a vital part of the whole process of maintaining body iron, in part via reclamation of heme–iron by CD163-expressing macrophages from the engulfment of effete red blood cells. Hemolytic events occur even in the context of everyday physical exercise like running. Hb is bound by Hp but the catabolism of Hb–Hp complexes after endocytosis means that Hp is readily depleted (e.g., by the lysis of less than 5 mL of blood). Any free Hb is readily oxidized releasing its heme, which is then bound by HPX. Endocytosis of heme-HPX is analogous to that of transferrin and HPX normally recycles intact, the heme is degraded by HOs releasing iron, which can be reutilized by reticulocytes. Thus, a role for HPX in iron recycling is established. This is especially important when Hp levels have declined and to prevent damage to, and iron loss from, the kidney.

Heme does not appear to be effectively reused as an intact molecule and its iron is released by HOs for biochemical and regulatory purposes, for storage, or for export and recycling by transferrin. The levels of these metal-plasma protein complexes in the circulation regulate heme and iron absorption from the gut lumen by changing the expression of molecules including HO1 and FPN1, involved in heme catabolism and iron movement across the basal lateral membrane of the enterocyte. Secreted ferritin is presumed to act in iron recycling from the macrophage to the liver, the organ where most iron is stored. Intact heme delivery from cells by FLVCR to HPX takes place in vitro and may also take place in vivo although it should be noted that some of the cells like macrophages also express surface proteins, including LRP1, that bind heme-HPX complexes. Transferrin receptors are ubiquitously expressed on essentially all cell types unlike those for Hp, HPX, and ferritin. Transferrin is therefore able to distribute iron from heme catabolism to many different tissues and cell types throughout the body. Ferritin replaces transferrin iron in a few cells, e.g., stroma of the developing kidney and in certain brain cells. Iron metabolism in the liver regulates iron recycling via hepcidin. Intracellular iron levels rise when hepcidin levels are increased, since iron is no longer exported from cells via FPN1, which is targeted to the proteasome by hepcidin. Heme activates FPN1 gene expression, as it does HO1 and H-ferritin genes, whereas iron regulates certain FPN isoforms, ferritin, transferrin, and the transferrin receptor1 at the translational level. Much of this information currently comes from studies in rodents. The details of how these events are coordinated in human health and disease, including the respective roles of HPX and Hp, remains to be completely documented. Variations of these mechanisms in barrier tissues also remain to be defined. Such knowledge will likely improve diagnosis and treatment of many hemolytic and neurodegenerative conditions, including the use of hemopexin replacement infusions as therapy.

Acknowledgments The author is grateful to Mr. Taron Davies for his help with the figures, which were based with permission on earlier diagrams of Drs. GJ Anderson and DM Frazer, and to Mr. Peter Hahl for help with the bibliography. Thanks also to both Drs Anderson and McClaren for their editorial support. The author wishes to acknowledge the help of colleagues in both the heme and iron fields, collaborators, technicians, students, and post-doctoral fellows who have contributed to her research on the hemopexin system and to the funding agencies including NIH, AHA, and UMRB that have supported the research.

References

1. Hallberg L, Solvell L. Absorption of hemoglobin iron in man. Acta Med Scand. 1967;181:335–54.
2. Bjorn-Rasmussen E, Hallberg L, Isaksson B, et al. Food iron absorption in man. Applications of the two-pool extrinsic tag method to measure heme and nonheme iron absorption from the whole diet. J Clin Invest. 1974;53:247–55.
3. Smith A. Novel heme–protein interactions: some more radical than others. In: Warren MJ, Smith AG, editors. Tetrapyrroles: birth, life and death. Austin/New York: Landes Bioscience/Springer; 2009. p. 184–207.
4. Marro S, Barisani D, Chiabrando D, et al. Lack of haptoglobin affects iron transport across duodenum by modulating ferroportin expression. Gastroenterology. 2007;133:1261–71.

5. Watanabe J, Grijalva V, Hama S, et al. Hemoglobin and its scavenger protein haptoglobin associate with apoA-1 containing particles and influence the inflammatory properties and function of high density lipoprotein. J Biol Chem. 2009;3:18292–301.
6. Hebbel RP. The sickle erythrocyte in double jeopardy: autoxidation and iron decompartmentalization. Semin Hematol. 1990;27:51–69.
7. Hebbel RP, Morgan WT, Eaton JW, et al. Accelerated autoxidation and heme loss due to instability of sickle hemoglobin. Proc Natl Acad Sci USA. 1988;85:237–41.
8. Tsemakhovich VA, Bamm VV, Shaklai M, et al. Vascular damage by unstable hemoglobins: the role of heme-depleted globin. Arch Biochem Biophys. 2005;436:307–15.
9. Rossi-Fanelli A, Antonini E, Caputo A. Pure native globin from human hemoglobin: preparation and some physico-chemical properties. Biochim Biophys Acta. 1958;28:221.
10. Watanabe S, Wakasugi K. Zebrafish neuroglobin is a cell-membrane-penetrating globin. Biochemistry. 2008;47:5266–70.
11. Li RC, Saleem S, Zhen G, et al. Heme–hemopexin complex attenuates neuronal cell death and stroke damage. J Cereb Blood Flow Metab. 2009;29:953–64.
12. Evans RW, Rafique R, Zarea A, et al. Nature of non-transferrin-bound iron: studies on iron citrate complexes and thalassemic sera. J Biol Inorg Chem. 2008;13:57–74.
13. Lane DJ, Lawen A. Non-transferrin iron reduction and uptake are regulated by transmembrane ascorbate cycling in K562 cells. J Biol Chem. 2008;283:12701–8.
14. Lane DJ, Lawen A. A highly sensitive colorimetric microplate ferrocyanide assay applied to ascorbate-stimulated transplasma membrane ferricyanide reduction and mitochondrial succinate oxidation. Anal Biochem. 2008;373:287–95.
15. MacKenzie B, Takanaga H, Hubert N, Rolfs A, Hediger MA. Functional properties of multiple isoforms of human divalent metal-ion transporter 1 (DMT-1). Biochem J. 2007;403:59–69.
16. Gao J, Zhao N, Knutson MD, et al. The hereditary hemochromatosis protein, HFE, inhibits iron uptake via down-regulation of Zip14 in HepG2 cells. J Biol Chem. 2008;283:21462–8.
17. Schaer CA, Vallelian F, Imhof A, et al. Heme carrier protein (HCP-1) spatially interacts with the CD163 hemoglobin uptake pathway and is a target of inflammatory macrophage activation. J Leukoc Biol. 2008;83:325–33.
18. O'Callaghan KM, Ayllon V, O'Keeffe J, et al. Heme-binding protein HRG-1 is induced by insulin-like growth factor I and associates with the vacuolar H+-ATPase to control endosomal pH and receptor trafficking. J Biol Chem. 2010;285:381–91.
19. Allhorn M, Berggard T, Nordberg J, et al. Processing of the lipocalin alpha(1)-microglobulin by hemoglobin induces heme-binding and heme-degradation properties. Blood. 2002;99:1894–901.
20. Tenopoulou M, Kurz T, Doulias PT, et al. Does the calcein-AM method assay the total cellular 'labile iron pool' or only a fraction of it? Biochem J. 2007;403:261–6.
21. Cabantchik ZI, Glickstein H, Milgram P, et al. A fluorescence assay for assessing chelation of intracellular iron in a membrane model system and in mammalian cells. Anal Biochem. 1996;233:221–7.
22. Imlay JA. Cellular defenses against superoxide and hydrogen peroxide. Annu Rev Biochem. 2008;77:755–76.
23. Petryka ZJ, Pierach CA, Smith A, et al. Billiary excretion of exogenous hematin in rats. Life Sci. 1977;21:1015–20.
24. Papanikolaou G, Tzilianos M, Christakis JI, et al. Hepcidin in iron overload disorders. Blood. 2005;105:4103–5.
25. Ginzburg YZ, Rybicki AC, Suzuka SM, et al. Exogenous iron increases hemoglobin in beta-thalassemic mice. Exp Hematol. 2009;37:172–83.
26. Galli A, Bergamaschi G, Recalde H, et al. Ferroportin gene silencing induces iron retention and enhances ferritin synthesis in human macrophages. Br J Haematol. 2004;127:598–603.
27. Delaby C, Pilard N, Hetet G, et al. A physiological model to study iron recycling in macrophages. Exp Cell Res. 2005;310:43–53.
28. Chung J, Prohaska JR, Wessling-Resnick M. Ferroportin-1 is not upregulated in copper-deficient mice. J Nutr. 2004;134:517–21.
29. Delaby C, Pilard N, Puy H, et al. Sequential regulation of ferroportin expression after erythrophagocytosis in murine macrophages: early mRNA induction by haem, followed by iron-dependent protein expression. Biochem J. 2008;411:123–31.
30. Knutson MD, Vafa MR, Haile DJ, et al. Iron loading and erythrophagocytosis increase ferroportin 1 (FPN1) expression in J774 macrophages. Blood. 2003;102:4191–7.
31. De Domenico I, Vaughn MB, Li L, et al. Ferroportin-mediated mobilization of ferritin iron precedes ferritin degradation by the proteasome. EMBO J. 2006;25:5396–404.
32. Knutson MD, Oukka M, Koss LM, et al. Iron release from macrophages after erythrophagocytosis is up-regulated by ferroportin 1 overexpression and down-regulated by hepcidin. Proc Natl Acad Sci USA. 2005;102:1324–8.

33. Alam J, Shibahara S, Smith A. Transcriptional activation of the heme oxygenase gene by heme and cadmium in mouse hepatoma cells. J Biol Chem. 1989;264:6371–5.
34. Alam J, Cai J, Smith A. Isolation and characterization of the mouse heme oxygenase-1 gene. Distal 5′ sequences are required for induction by heme or heavy metals. J Biol Chem. 1994;269:1001–9.
35. Marziali G, Perrotti E, Ilari R, et al. Transcriptional regulation of the ferritin heavy-chain gene: the activity of the CCAAT binding factor NF-Y is modulated in heme-treated Friend leukemia cells and during monocyte-to-macrophage differentiation. Mol Cell Biol. 1997;17:1387–95.
36. Marro S, Chiabrando D, Messana E, et al. Heme controls ferroportin1 (FPN1) transcription involving Bach1, Nrf2 and a MARE/ARE sequence motif at position −7007 of the FPN1 promoter. Haematologica. 2010; 95:1261–8.
37. Alam J, Stewart D, Touchard C, et al. Nrf2, a Cap'n'Collar transcription factor, regulates induction of the heme oxygenase-1 gene. J Biol Chem. 1999;274:26071–8.
38. Cianetti L, Segnalini P, Calzolari A, et al. Expression of alternative transcripts of ferroportin-1 during human erythroid differentiation. Haematologica. 2005;90:1595–606.
39. Zhang DL, Hughes RM, Ollivierre-Wilson H, et al. A ferroportin transcript that lacks an iron-responsive element enables duodenal and erythroid precursor cells to evade translational repression. Cell Metab. 2009;9:461–73.
40. Madsen M, Moller HJ, Nielsen MJ, et al. Molecular characterization of the haptoglobin.hemoglobin receptor CD163. Ligand binding properties of the scavenger receptor cysteine-rich domain region. J Biol Chem. 2004;279:51561–7.
41. Schaer DJ, Schaer CA, Buehler PW, et al. CD163 is the macrophage scavenger receptor for native and chemically modified hemoglobins in the absence of haptoglobin. Blood. 2006;107:373–80.
42. Schaer CA, Schoedon G, Imhof A, et al. Constitutive endocytosis of CD163 mediates hemoglobin-heme uptake and determines the noninflammatory and protective transcriptional response of macrophages to hemoglobin. Circ Res. 2006;99:943–50.
43. Schaer DJ, Boretti FS, Schoedon G, et al. Induction of the CD163-dependent haemoglobin uptake by macrophages as a novel anti-inflammatory action of glucocorticoids. Br J Haematol. 2002;119:239–43.
44. Buehler PW, Abraham B, Vallelian F, et al. Haptoglobin preserves the CD163 hemoglobin scavenger pathway by shielding hemoglobin from peroxidative modification. Blood. 2009;113:2578–86.
45. Marklund S. Determination of plasma or serum haemoglobin by peroxidase activity employing 2,2′-azino-di-(3-ethyl-benzthiazolinsulphonate-6) as chromogen. Scand J Clin Lab Invest. 1978;38:543–7.
46. Jia L, Bonaventura C, Bonaventura J, et al. S-nitrosohaemoglobin: a dynamic activity of blood involved in vascular control. Nature. 1996;380:221–6.
47. Nakai K, Ohta T, Sakuma I, et al. Inhibition of endothelium-dependent relaxation by hemoglobin in rabbit aortic strips: comparison between acellular hemoglobin derivatives and cellular hemoglobins. J Cardiovasc Pharmacol. 1996;28:115–23.
48. Bowman BH, Kurosky A. Haptoglobin: the evolutionary product of duplication, unequal crossing over, and point mutation. Adv Hum Genet. 1982;12(189–261):453–84.
49. McCormick DJ, Atassi MZ. Hemoglobin binding with haptoglobin: delineation of the haptoglobin binding site on the alpha-chain of human hemoglobin. J Protein Chem. 1990;9:735–42.
50. Asleh R, Guetta J, Kalet-Litman S, et al. Haptoglobin genotype- and diabetes-dependent differences in iron-mediated oxidative stress in vitro and in vivo. Circ Res. 2005;96:435–41.
51. Asleh R, Marsh S, Shilkrut M, et al. Genetically determined heterogeneity in hemoglobin scavenging and susceptibility to diabetic cardiovascular disease. Circ Res. 2003;92:1193–200.
52. Nakagawa K, Asami M. Lack of correlation between lysosomal enzyme activity and ascorbic acid content in brain of lead-treated animals. Toxicol Lett. 1986;30:219–22.
53. Fagoonee S, Gburek J, Hirsch E, et al. Plasma protein haptoglobin modulates renal iron loading. Am J Pathol. 2005;166:973–83.
54. Van Vlierberghe H, Langlois M, Delanghe J, et al. Haptoglobin phenotype 2–2 overrepresentation in Cys282Tyr hemochromatotic patients. J Hepatol. 2001;35:707–11.
55. Tolosano E, Fagoonee S, Garuti C, et al. Haptoglobin modifies the hemochromatosis phenotype in mice. Blood. 2005;105:3353–5.
56. Tolosano E, Hirsch E, Patrucco E, et al. Defective recovery and severe renal damage after acute hemolysis in hemopexin-deficient mice. Blood. 1999;94:3906–14.
57. Sears DA, Huser HJ. Plasma hemoglobin binding and clearance in the rhesus monkey after hemolytic transfusion reactions. Proc Soc Exp Biol Med. 1966;121:116–21.
58. Langley GR, Owen JA, Padanyi R. The effect of blood transfusions on serum haptoglobin. Br J Haematol. 1962;8:392–400.
59. Gburek J, Verroust PJ, Willnow TE, et al. Megalin and cubilin are endocytic receptors involved in renal clearance of hemoglobin. J Am Soc Nephrol. 2002;13:423–30.

60. Sears D. Disposal of plasma heme in normal man and patients with intravascular hemolysis. J Clin Invest. 1970;49:5–14.
61. Sears DA. Plasma heme-binding in patients with hemolytic disorders. J Lab Clin Med. 1968;71:484–94.
62. Sears DA. Depletion of plasma hemopexin in man by hematin injections. Proc Soc Exp Biol Med. 1969;131:371–3.
63. Muller-Eberhard U, Bosman C, Liem HH. Tissue localization of the heme–hemopexin complex in the rabbit and the rat as studied by light microscopy with the use of radioisotopes. J Lab Clin Med. 1970;76:426–31.
64. Bissell DM, Hammaker L, Schmid R. Hemoglobin and erythrocyte catabolism in rat liver: the separate roles of parenchymal and sinusoidal cells. Blood. 1972;40:812–22.
65. Weibel ER, Staubli W, Gnagi HR, et al. Correlated morphometric and biochemical studies on the liver cell. I. Morphometric model, stereologic methods, and normal morphometric data for rat liver. J Cell Biol. 1969;42:68–91.
66. Pimstone NR, Engel P, Tenhunen R, et al. Further studies of microsomal haem oxygenase: mechanism for stimulation of enzyme activity and cellular localization. S Afr Med J. 1971;205:169–74.
67. Kino K, Tsunoo H, Higa Y, et al. Hemoglobin–haptoglobin receptor in rat liver plasma membrane. J Biol Chem. 1980;255:9616–20.
68. Kino K, Tsunoo H, Higa Y, et al. Kinetic aspects of hemoglobin.haptoglobin–receptor interaction in rat liver plasma membranes, isolated liver cells, and liver cells in primary culture. J Biol Chem. 1982;257:4828–33.
69. Higa Y, Oshiro S, Kino K, et al. Catabolism of globin–haptoglobin in liver cells after intravenous administration of hemoglobin–haptoglobin to rats. J Biol Chem. 1981;256:12322–8.
70. Oshiro S, Nakajima H. Intrahepatocellular site of the catabolism of heme and globin moiety of hemoglobin-haptoglobin after intravenous administration to rats. J Biol Chem. 1988;263:16032–8.
71. Davies DM, Smith A, Muller-Eberhard U, et al. Hepatic subcellular metabolism of heme from heme–hemopexin: incorporation of iron into ferritin. Biochem Biophys Res Commun. 1979;91:1504–11.
72. Lim SK, Kim H, Ali A, et al. Increased susceptibility in Hp knockout mice during acute hemolysis. Blood. 1998;92:1870–7.
73. Arredouani M, Matthijs P, Van Hoeyveld E, et al. Haptoglobin directly affects T cells and suppresses T helper cell type 2 cytokine release. Immunology. 2003;108:144–51.
74. Smith A. Mechanisms of cytoprotection by hemopexin. In: Smith KM, Guilard R, Kadish KM, editors. Handbook of porphyrin science biochemistry of tetrapyrroles. Hackensack: World Scientific Publishing Co.; 2011. p. 217–356.
75. Muller-Eberhard U, Javid J, Liem HH, et al. Plasma concentrations of hemopexin, haptoglobin and heme in patients with various hemolytic diseases. Blood. 1968;32:811–15.
76. Comporti M, Signorini C, Buonocore G, et al. Iron release, oxidative stress and erythrocyte ageing. Free Radic Biol Med. 2002;32:568–76.
77. Wagener FA, Volk HD, Willis D, et al. Different faces of the heme-heme oxygenase system in inflammation. Pharmacol Rev. 2003;55:551–71.
78. Kumar S, Bandyopadhyay U. Free heme toxicity and its detoxification systems in human. Toxicol Lett. 2005;157:175–88.
79. Balla J, Vercellotti GM, Nath K, et al. Haem, haem oxygenase and ferritin in vascular endothelial cell injury. Nephrol Dial Transplant. 2003;18 Suppl 5:v8–12.
80. Tracz MJ, Alam J, Nath KA. Physiology and pathophysiology of heme: implications for kidney disease. J Am Soc Nephrol. 2007;18:414–20.
81. Qureshi AI, Tuhrim S, Broderick JP, et al. Spontaneous intracerebral hemorrhage. N Engl J Med. 2001;344:1450–60.
82. Chen L, Zhang X, Chen-Roetling J, et al. Increased striatal injury and behavioral deficits after intracerebral hemorrhage in hemopexin knockout mice. J Neurosurg. 2011;114:1159–67.
83. Mauk MR, Smith A, Grant Mauk A. An alternative view of the proposed alternative activities of hemopexin. Protein Sci. 2011;20:791–805.
84. Graca-Souza AV, Arruda MA, de Freitas MS, et al. Neutrophil activation by heme: implications for inflammatory processes. Blood. 2002;99:4160–5.
85. Arruda MA, Rossi AG, de Freitas MS, et al. Heme inhibits human neutrophil apoptosis: involvement of phosphoinositide 3-kinase, MAPK, and NF-kappaB. J Immunol. 2004;173:2023–30.
86. Wagener FA, Eggert A, Boerman OC, et al. Heme is a potent inducer of inflammation in mice and is counteracted by heme oxygenase. Blood. 2001;98:1802–11.
87. Liang X, Lin T, Sun G, et al. Hemopexin down-regulates LPS-induced proinflammatory cytokines from macrophages. J Leukoc Biol. 2009;86:229–35.
88. Wagener FA, Feldman E, de Witte T, et al. Heme induces the expression of adhesion molecules ICAM-1, VCAM-1, and E selectin in vascular endothelial cells. Proc Soc Exp Biol Med. 1997;216:456–63.
89. Geurts N, Martens E, Van Aelst I, et al. Beta-hematin interaction with the hemopexin domain of gelatinase B/MMP-9 provokes autocatalytic processing of the propeptide, thereby priming activation by MMP-3. Biochemistry. 2008;47:2689–99.

90. Saso L, Leone MG, Mo MY, et al. Differential changes in alpha2-macroglobulin and hemopexin in brain and liver in response to acute inflammation. Biochemistry (Mosc). 1999;64:839–44.
91. Muller-Eberhard U, Bashore R. Assessment of Rh disease by ratios of bilirubin to albumin and hemopexin to albumin in amniotic fluid. N Engl J Med. 1970;282:1163–7.
92. Ramachandran P, Boontheung P, Xie Y, et al. Identification of N-linked glycoproteins in human saliva by glycoprotein capture and mass spectrometry. J Proteome Res. 2006;5:1493–503.
93. Pong JC, Chu CY, Chu KO, et al. Identification of hemopexin in tear film. Anal Biochem. 2011;404:82–5.
94. Leak LV, Liotta LA, Krutzsch H, et al. Proteomic analysis of lymph. Proteomics. 2004;4:753–65.
95. Yang Z, Philips JD, Doty RT, et al. Kinetics and specificity of feline leukemia virus subgroup C receptor (FLVCR) export function and its dependence on hemopexin. J Biol Chem. 2010;285:28874–82.
96. Hunt RC, Hunt DM, Gaur N, et al. Hemopexin in the human retina: protection of the retina against heme-mediated toxicity. J Cell Physiol. 1996;168:71–80.
97. Morello N, Tonoli E, Logrand F, et al. Hemopexin affects iron distribution and ferritin expression in mouse brain. J Cell Mol Med. 2008;13:4192–204.
98. Kovtunovych G, Eckhaus MA, Ghosh MC, et al. Dysfunction of the heme recycling system in heme oxygenase 1-deficient mice: effects on macrophage viability and tissue iron distribution. Blood. 2010;116:6054–62.
99. Drabkin DL. Heme binding and transport – a spectrophotometric study of plasma glycoglobulin hemochromogens. Proc Natl Acad Sci USA. 1971;68:609–13.
100. Tolosano E, Fagoonee S, Hirsch E, et al. Enhanced splenomegaly and severe liver inflammation in haptoglobin/hemopexin double-null mice after acute hemolysis. Blood. 2002;100:4201–8.
101. Hrkal Z, Vodrazka Z, Kalousek I. Transfer of heme from ferrihemoglobin and ferrihemoglobin isolated chains to hemopexin. Eur J Biochem. 1974;43:73–8.
102. Bunn HF, Jandl JH. Exchange of heme among hemoglobins and between hemoglobin and albumin. J Biol Chem. 1968;243:465–75.
103. Morgan WT, Liem HH, Sutor RP, et al. Transfer of heme from heme–albumin to hemopexin. Biochim Biophys Acta. 1976;444:435–45.
104. Beaven GH, Chen S-H, D'Albis A, et al. A spectroscopic study of the haemin–human–serum–albumin system. Eur J Biochem. 1974;41:539–46.
105. Diotallevi P, Balducci E, Canapa A, et al. Plasma level of hemopexin (Hpx) in families with progressive muscular dystrophy (PMD). Boll Soc Ital Biol Sper. 1988;64:531–8.
106. Luft S, Gli ska-Urban D, Brzezi ska B, et al. Serum hemopexin level in rheumatoid arthritis. Reumatologia. 1973;11:279–86.
107. Meiers HG, Lissner R, Mawlawi H, et al. Hemopexin levels of men and women in different age-groups (author's transl). Klin Wochenschr. 1974;52:453–4.
108. Foidart M, Liem HH, Adornato BT, et al. Hemopexin metabolism in patients with altered serum levels. J Lab Clin Med. 1983;102:838–46.
109. Delanghe JR, Langlois MR. Hemopexin: a review of biological aspects and the role in laboratory medicine. Clin Chim Acta. 2001;312:13–23.
110. Liem HH, Tavassoli M, Muller-Eberhard U. Cellular and subcellular localization of heme and hemopexin in the rabbit. Acta Haematol. 1975;53:219–25.
111. Smith A, Morgan WT. Haem transport to the liver by haemopexin. Receptor-mediated uptake with recycling of the protein. Biochem J. 1979;182:47–54.
112. Smith A, Hunt RC. Hemopexin joins transferrin as representative members of a distinct class of receptor-mediated endocytic transport systems. Eur J Cell Biol. 1990;53:234–45.
113. Smith A, Morgan WT. Transport of heme by hemopexin to the liver: evidence for receptor-mediated uptake. Biochem Biophys Res Commun. 1978;84:151–7.
114. Smith A, Morgan WT. Hemopexin-mediated transport of heme into isolated rat hepatocytes. J Biol Chem. 1981;256:10902–9.
115. Smith A, Farooqui SF, Morgan WT. The murine haemopexin receptor. Evidence that the haemopexin-binding site resides on a 20 kDa subunit and that receptor recycling is regulated by protein kinase C. Biochem J. 1991;276:417–25.
116. Okazaki H, Taketani S, Kohno H, et al. The hemopexin receptor on the cell surface of human polymorphonuclear leukocytes. Cell Struct Funct. 1989;14:129–40.
117. Taketani S, Kohno H, Tokunaga R. Cell surface receptor for hemopexin in human leukemia HL60 cells. Specific binding, affinity labeling, and fate of heme. J Biol Chem. 1987;262:4639–43.
118. Taketani S, Kohno H, Tokunaga R. Receptor-mediated heme uptake from hemopexin by human erythroleukemia K562 cells. Biochem Int. 1986;13:307–12.
119. Taketani S, Kohno H, Sawamura T, et al. Hemopexin-dependent down-regulation of expression of the human transferrin receptor. J Biol Chem. 1990;265:13981–5.
120. Van Dijk JP, Kroos MJ, Starreveld JS, et al. Expression of haemopexin receptors by cultured human cytotrophoblast. Biochem J. 1995;307:669–72.

121. Smith A, Ledford BE. Expression of the haemopexin-transport system in cultured mouse hepatoma cells. Links between haemopexin and iron metabolism. Biochem J. 1988;256:941–50.
122. Hvidberg V, Maniecki MB, Jacobsen C, et al. Identification of the receptor scavenging hemopexin–heme complexes. Blood. 2005;106:2572–9.
123. May P, Herz J, Bock HH. Molecular mechanisms of lipoprotein receptor signalling. Cell Mol Life Sci. 2005; 62:2325–38.
124. Heeren J, Grewal T, Jackle S, et al. Recycling of apolipoprotein E and lipoprotein lipase through endosomal compartments in vivo. J Biol Chem. 2001;276:42333–52338.
125. van Kerkhof P, Lee J, McCormick L, et al. Sorting nexin 17 facilitates LRP recycling in the early endosome. EMBO J. 2005;24:2851–61.
126. Alam J, Smith A. Receptor-mediated transport of heme by hemopexin regulates gene expression in mammalian cells. J Biol Chem. 1989;264:17637–40.
127. Collins SJ, Gallo RC, Gallagher RE. Continuous growth and differentiation of human myeloid leukaemic cells in suspension culture. Nature. 1977;270:347–9.
128. Rish KR, Swartzlander R, Sadikot TN, et al. Interaction of heme and heme-hemopexin with an extracellular oxidant system used to measure cell growth-associated plasma membrane electron transport. Biochim Biophys Acta. 2007;1767:1107–17.
129. Heide K, Haupt H, Stoeriko K, et al. On the heme-binding capacity of hemopexin. Clin Chim Acta. 1964;10:460–9.
130. Sears DA, Huser HJ. Plasma hematin-binding and clearance in the rhesus monkey. Proc Soc Exp Biol Med. 1966;121:111–16.
131. Muller-Eberhard U. Hemopexin. N Engl J Med. 1970;283:1090–4.
132. Lane RS, Rangeley DM, Liem HH, et al. Plasma clearance of 125I-labelled haemopexin in normal and haem-loaded rabbits. Br J Haematol. 1973;25:533–40.
133. Conway TP, Morgan WT, Liem HH, et al. Catabolism of photo-oxidized and desialylated hemopexin in the rabbit. J Biol Chem. 1975;250:3067–73.
134. Wochner RD, Spilberg I, Iio A, et al. Hemopexin metabolism in sickle-cell disease, porphyrias and control subjects – effects of heme injection. N Engl J Med. 1974;290:822–6.
135. Muller-Eberhard U, Leim HH, Mathews-Roth M, et al. Plasma levels of hemopexin and albumin in disorders of porphyrin metabolism. Proc Soc Exp Biol Med. 1974;146:694–7.
136. Rosen H, Sears DA, Meisenzahl D. Spectral properties of hemopexin-heme. The Schumm test. J Lab Clin Med. 1969;74:941–5.
137. Neale FC, Aber GM, Northam BE. The demonstration of intravascular haemolysis by means of serum paper electrophoresis and a modification of Schumm's reaction. J Clin Pathol. 1958;11:206–19.
138. Wheby MS, Barrett Jr O, Crosby WH. Serum protein binding of myoglobin, hemoglobin and hematin. Blood. 1960;16:1579–85.
139. Muller-Eberhard U, Cleve H. Immunoelectrophoretic studies of the beta1-haem-binding globulin (haemopexin) in hereditary haemolytic disorders. Nature. 1963;197:602–3.
140. Smith A. Intracellular distribution of haem after uptake by different receptors. Haem–haemopexin and haem-asialo-haemopexin. Biochem J. 1985;231:663–9.
141. Potter D, Chroneos ZC, Baynes JW, et al. In vivo fate of hemopexin and heme-hemopexin complexes in the rat. Arch Biochem Biophys. 1993;300:98–104.
142. Larsen R, Gozzelino R, Jeney V, et al. A central role for free heme in the pathogenesis of severe sepsis. Sci Transl Med. 2010;2:51ra71.
143. Garby L, Noyes WD. J Clin Invest. 1959;38:1479–88.
144. Noyes WD, Bothwell TH, Finch CA. The role of the reticulo-endothelial cell in iron metabolism. Br J Haematol. 1960;6:43–55.
145. Bernhard HP, Darlington GJ, Ruddle FH. Expression of liver phenotypes in cultured mouse hepatoma cells: synthesis and secretion of serum albumin. Dev Biol. 1973;35:83–96.
146. Vinchi F, Gastaldi S, Silengo L, et al. Hemopexin prevents endothelial damage and liver congestion in a mouse model of heme overload. Am J Pathol. 2008;173:289–99.
147. Kristiansen M, Graversen JH, Jacobsen C, et al. Identification of the haemoglobin scavenger receptor. Nature. 2001;409:198–201.
148. Delanghe JR, Philippe J, Moerman F, et al. Impaired hemoglobin scavenging during an acute HIV-1 retroviral syndrome. Clin Chim Acta. 2010;411:521–3.
149. Maniecki MB, Hasle H, Friis-Hansen L, et al. Impaired CD163-mediated hemoglobin-scavenging and severe toxic symptoms in patients treated with gemtuzumab ozogamicin. Blood. 2008;112:1510–14.
150. Morse D, Choi AM. Heme oxygenase-1: the "emerging molecule" has arrived. Am J Respir Cell Mol Biol. 2002;27:8–16.
151. Maines MD. Heme oxygenase: function, multiplicity, regulatory mechanisms, and clinical applications. FASEB J. 1988;2:2557–68.

152. Donnelly LE, Barnes PJ. Expression of heme oxygenase in human airway epithelial cells. Am J Respir Cell Mol Biol. 2001;24:295–303.
153. Ewing JF, Maines MD. Glutathione depletion induces heme oxygenase-1 (HSP32) mRNA and protein in rat brain. J Neurochem. 1993;60:1512–19.
154. Maines MD. Heme oxygenase 1 transgenic mice as a model to study neuroprotection. Methods Enzymol. 2002;353:374–88.
155. Maines MD, Mayer RD, Ewing JF, et al. Induction of kidney heme oxygenase-1 (HSP32) mRNA and protein by ischemia/reperfusion: possible role of heme as both promotor of tissue damage and regulator of HSP32. J Pharmacol Exp Ther. 1993;264:457–62.
156. Panahian N, Yoshiura M, Maines MD. Overexpression of heme oxygenase-1 is neuroprotective in a model of permanent middle cerebral artery occlusion in transgenic mice. J Neurochem. 1999;72:1187–203.
157. Goda N, Suzuki K, Naito M, et al. Distribution of heme oxygenase isoforms in rat liver. Topographic basis for carbon monoxide-mediated microvascular relaxation. J Clin Invest. 1998;101:604–12.
158. Dore S, Takahashi M, Ferris CD, et al. Bilirubin, formed by activation of heme oxygenase-2, protects neurons against oxidative stress injury. Proc Natl Acad Sci USA. 1999;96:2445–50.
159. Sung L, Morales P, Shibata M, et al. Defenses against extracellular heme-mediated oxidative damage: use of iron and copper chelators to investigate the role of redox active iron, copper and heme in the hemopexin heme transport system. In: Badman DG, Bergeron RJ, Brittenham GM, editors. Iron chelators: new development strategies. Sarotoga: Saratoga Publishing Group; 2000. p. 67–86.
160. Hori R, Kashiba M, Toma T, et al. Gene transfection of H25A mutant heme oxygenase-1 protects cells against hydroperoxide-induced cytotoxicity. J Biol Chem. 2002;277:10712–18.
161. Lin Q, Weis S, Yang G, et al. Heme oxygenase-1 protein localizes to the nucleus and activates transcription factors important in oxidative stress. J Biol Chem. 2007;282:20621–33.
162. Suttner DM, Sridhar K, Lee CS, et al. Protective effects of transient HO-1 overexpression on susceptibility to oxygen toxicity in lung cells. Am J Physiol. 1999;276:L443–51.
163. Lin QS, Weis S, Yang G, et al. Catalytic inactive heme oxygenase-1 protein regulates its own expression in oxidative stress. Free Radic Biol Med. 2008;44:847–55.
164. Taille C, El-Benna J, Lanone S, et al. Mitochondrial respiratory chain and NAD(P)H oxidase are targets for the antiproliferative effect of carbon monoxide in human airway smooth muscle. J Biol Chem. 2005;280:25350–60.
165. Jones DP. Redox potential of GSH/GSSG couple: assay and biological significance. Methods Enzymol. 2002; 348:93–112.
166. Yi L, Jenkins PM, Leichert LI, et al. Heme regulatory motifs in heme oxygenase-2 form a thiol/disulfide redox switch that responds to the cellular redox state. J Biol Chem. 2009;284:20556–61.
167. Poss KD, Tonegawa S. Heme oxygenase 1 is required for mammalian iron reutilization. Proc Natl Acad Sci USA. 1997;94:10919–24.
168. Poss KD, Tonegawa S. Reduced stress defense in heme oxygenase 1-deficient cells. Proc Natl Acad Sci USA. 1997;94:10925–30.
169. Yachie A, Niida Y, Wada T, et al. Oxidative stress causes enhanced endothelial cell injury in human heme oxygenase-1 deficiency. J Clin Invest. 1999;103:129–35.
170. Ferris CD, Jaffrey SR, Sawa A, et al. Haem oxygenase-1 prevents cell death by regulating cellular iron. Nat Cell Biol. 1999;1:152–7.
171. Mostert V, Nakayama A, Austin LM, et al. Serum iron increases with acute induction of hepatic heme oxygenase-1 in mice. Drug Metab Rev. 2007;39:619–26.
172. Eisenstein RS, Garcia-Mayol D, Pettingell W, et al. Regulation of ferritin and heme oxygenase synthesis in rat fibroblasts by different forms of iron. Proc Natl Acad Sci USA. 1991;88:688–92.
173. Sheftel AD, Kim SF, Ponka P. Non-heme induction of heme oxygenase-1 does not alter cellular iron metabolism. J Biol Chem. 2007;282:10480–6.
174. Suttner DM, Dennery PA. Reversal of HO-1 related cytoprotection with increased expression is due to reactive iron. FASEB J. 1999;13:1800–9.
175. Dennery PA, Spitz DR, Yang G, et al. Oxygen toxicity and iron accumulation in the lungs of mice lacking heme oxygenase-2. J Clin Invest. 1998;101:1001–11.
176. Dennery PA, Visner G, Weng YH, et al. Resistance to hyperoxia with heme oxygenase-1 disruption: role of iron. Free Radic Biol Med. 2003;34:124–33.
177. Fogg S, Agarwal A, Nick HS, et al. Iron regulates hyperoxia-dependent human heme oxygenase 1 gene expression in pulmonary endothelial cells. Am J Respir Cell Mol Biol. 1999;20:797–804.
178. Smith A. Role of redox-active metals in the regulation of the metallothionein and heme oxygenase gene by heme and hemopexin. In: Ferreira GC, Moura JJG, Franco R, editors. Iron metabolism: inorganic biochemistry and regulatory mechanisms. Weinheim: Wiley-VCH Verlag GmbH; 2008. doi:10.1002/9783527613700.ch05.
179. Casey JL, Hentze MW, Koeller DM, et al. Iron-responsive elements: regulatory RNA sequences that control mRNA levels and translation. Science. 1988;240:924–8.

180. Ren Y, Smith A. Mechanism of metallothionein gene regulation by heme-hemopexin. Roles of protein kinase C, reactive oxygen species, and cis-acting elements. J Biol Chem. 1995;270:23988–95.
181. Eskew JD, Vanacore RM, Sung L, et al. Cellular protection mechanisms against extracellular heme: heme–hemopexin, but not free heme, activates the N-terminal c-Jun kinase. J Biol Chem. 1999;274:638–48.
182. Vanacore R, Eskew J, Morales P, et al. Role for copper in transient oxidation and nuclear translocation of MTF-1, but not of NFκB, by the hemopexin heme transport system. Antioxid Redox Signal. 2000;2:739–52.
183. Smith A, Eskew JD, Borza CM, et al. Role of heme-hemopexin in human T-lymphocyte proliferation. Exp Cell Res. 1997;232:246–54.
184. Timmins GS, Davies MJ, Song DX, et al. EPR studies on the effects of complexation of heme by hemopexin upon its reactions with organic peroxides. Free Radic Res. 1995;23:559–69.
185. Moss D, Fargion S, Fracanzani AL, et al. Functional roles of the ferritin receptors of human liver, hepatoma, lymphoid and erythroid cells. J Inorg Biochem. 1992;47:219–27.
186. Thompson KJ, Fried MG, Ye Z, et al. Regulation, mechanisms and proposed function of ferritin translocation to cell nuclei. J Cell Sci. 2002;115:2165–77.
187. Campanella A, Rovelli E, Santambrogio P, et al. Mitochondrial ferritin limits oxidative damage regulating mitochondrial iron availability: hypothesis for a protective role in Friedreich ataxia. Hum Mol Genet. 2009;18:1–11.
188. Radisky DC, Kaplan J. Iron in cytosolic ferritin can be recycled through lysosomal degradation in human fibroblasts. Biochem J. 1998;336:201–5.
189. Worwood M. Serum ferritin. Crit Rev Clin Lab Sci. 1979;10:171–204.
190. Ghosh S, Hevi S, Chuck SL. Regulated secretion of glycosylated human ferritin from hepatocytes. Blood. 2004;103:2369–76.
191. Kannengiesser C, Jouanolle AM, Hetet G, et al. A new missense mutation in the L ferritin coding sequence associated with elevated levels of glycosylated ferritin in serum and absence of iron overload. Haematologica. 2009;94:335–9.
192. Cozzi A, Corsi B, Levi S, et al. Overexpression of wild type and mutated human ferritin H-chain in HeLa cells: in vivo role of ferritin ferroxidase activity. J Biol Chem. 2000;275:25122–9.
193. Recalcati S, Invernizzi P, Arosio P, et al. New functions for an iron storage protein: the role of ferritin in immunity and autoimmunity. J Autoimmun. 2008;30:84–9.
194. Takami M, Mizumoto K, Kasuya I, et al. Human placental ferritin receptor. Biochim Biophys Acta. 1986;884:31–8.
195. Blight GD, Morgan EH. Transferrin and ferritin endocytosis and recycling in guinea-pig reticulocytes. Biochim Biophys Acta. 1987;929:18–24.
196. Adams PC, Mack U, Powell LW, et al. Isolation of a porcine hepatic ferritin receptor. Comp Biochem Physiol B. 1988;90:837–41.
197. Osterloh K, Aisen P. Pathways in the binding and uptake of ferritin by hepatocytes. Biochim Biophys Acta. 1989;1011:40–5.
198. Anderson GJ, Faulk WP, Arosio P, et al. Identification of H- and L-ferritin subunit binding sites on human T and B lymphoid cells. Br J Haematol. 1989;73:260–4.
199. Moss D, Powell LW, Arosio P, et al. Characterization of the ferritin receptors of human T lymphoid (MOLT-4) cells. J Lab Clin Med. 1992;119:273–9.
200. Gelvan D, Fibach E, Meyron-Holtz EG, et al. Ferritin uptake by human erythroid precursors is a regulated iron uptake pathway. Blood. 1996;88:3200–7.
201. Moss D, Powell LW, Arosio P, et al. Effect of cell proliferation on H-ferritin receptor expression in human T lymphoid (MOLT-4) cells. J Lab Clin Med. 1992;120:239–43.
202. Sibille JC, Kondo H, Aisen P. Uptake of ferritin and iron bound to ferritin by rat hepatocytes: modulation by apotransferrin, iron chelators and chloroquine. Biochim Biophys Acta. 1989;1010:204–9.
203. Liao QK, Kong PA, Gao J, et al. Expression of ferritin receptor in placental microvilli membrane in pregnant women with different iron status at mid-term gestation. Eur J Clin Nutr. 2001;55:651–6.
204. Hulet SW, Hess EJ, Debinski W, et al. Characterization and distribution of ferritin binding sites in the adult mouse brain. J Neurochem. 1999;72:868–74.
205. Todorich B, Zhang X, Slagle-Webb B, et al. Tim-2 is the receptor for H-ferritin on oligodendrocytes. J Neurochem. 2008;107:1495–505.
206. Li JY, Paragas N, Ned RM, et al. Scara5 is a ferritin receptor mediating non-transferrin iron delivery. Dev Cell. 2009;16:35–46.
207. Fisher J, Devraj K, Ingram J, et al. Ferritin: a novel mechanism for delivery of iron to the brain and other organs. Am J Physiol Cell Physiol. 2007;293:C641–9.
208. Kearney SL, Nemeth E, Neufeld EJ, et al. Urinary hepcidin in congenital chronic anemias. Pediatr Blood Cancer. 2007;48:57–63.

Chapter 9
Molecular Regulation of Systemic Iron Metabolism

Tomas Ganz and Sophie Vaulont

Keywords BMP • Hemojuvelin • Hepcidin • HFE • Homeostasis • Iron • SMAD • STAT • TfR2 • TMPRSS6

1 Introduction

In humans, plasma iron concentrations are normally maintained in a relatively narrow range of 10–30 μM with transferrin saturation 20–40%. Prolonged decrease of iron concentrations causes cellular dysfunction and anemia (Chap. 15). Severe and prolonged increase of iron concentrations results in iron deposition in vital organs with consequent tissue injury (Chap. 18). With an average plasma volume of 3 l and iron concentration of 1 mg/l, plasma contains only about 3 mg of iron, a small fraction of the total body iron content of 3–4 g. Assuming free equilibration of iron–transferrin into 15 l of extracellular fluid, extracellular iron amounts to only 15 mg. Under normal circumstances, an average of 25 mg of iron enters this compartment every day, from macrophages recycling the iron of senescent erythrocytes, from hepatocyte storage, and from dietary iron intake. An equal amount of iron exits from the extracellular fluid, largely for hemoglobin synthesis but also for the synthesis of other iron-containing proteins, and to replenish iron stores in hepatocytes. Without regulation, the extracellular fluid compartment would be subject to large changes in iron influx from variable dietary iron content and erythrocyte destruction, and large changes in iron efflux due to variations in erythropoietic and other demand for iron. Mechanisms that adjust iron absorption and recycling to keep extracellular iron concentrations constant also effectively match iron supply to iron demand but would not assure stable iron reserves. Additional circuits must regulate iron absorption to maintain iron stores in the liver that help buffer surges in iron demand. Based on studies of iron absorption in animals and humans, it has long been suspected that a homeostatic system for the regulation of extracellular iron concentrations and iron stores must exist [1]. However, the specific molecular mechanisms, centered on the regulation of the iron efflux channel ferroportin by the hepatic peptide hormone hepcidin (Fig. 9.1), were identified only recently.

T. Ganz, M.D., Ph.D. (✉)
Departments of Medicine and Pathology, David Geffen School of Medicine,
University of California, Los Angeles, CA, USA
e-mail: tganz@mednet.ucla.edu

S. Vaulont, Ph.D.
Institut Cochin, INSERM U567, CNRS, Paris, France
e-mail: vaulont@cochin.inserm.fr

G.J. Anderson and G. McLaren (eds.), *Iron Physiology and Pathophysiology in Humans*, Nutrition and Health, DOI 10.1007/978-1-60327-485-2_9,

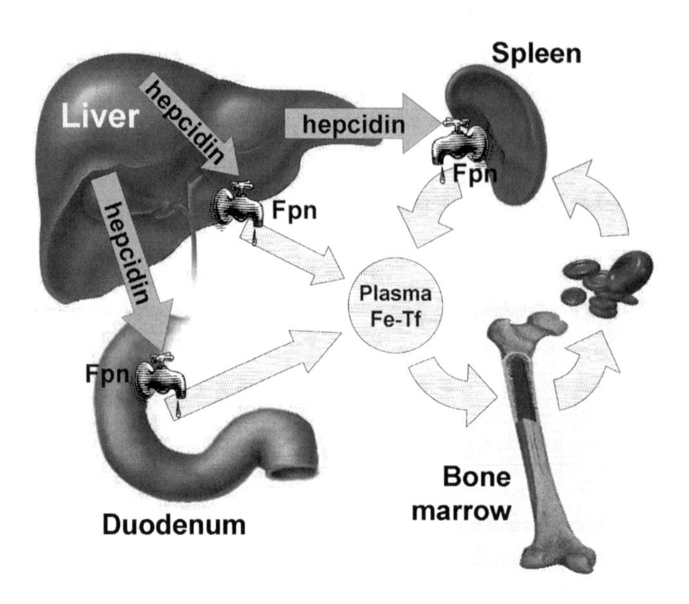

Fig. 9.1 The interaction of hepcidin with ferroportin controls the major flows of iron into extracellular fluid and plasma

2 The Interaction of the Hormone Hepcidin and Its Receptor Ferroportin Regulates Systemic Iron Metabolism

2.1 Hepcidin

Hepcidin is a 25 amino acid (2.7 kD) peptide containing four disulfide bridges [2–4] (Fig. 9.2). It is synthesized in vertebrate hepatocytes as an 84 amino acid prepropeptide that undergoes rapid intracellular processing to mature hepcidin followed by secretion [5]. Hepcidin is an amphipathic cationic peptide that structurally resembles antimicrobial peptides such as defensins and protegrins and displays weak antimicrobial activity in vitro [2, 3]. Although iron- and copper-associated forms of hepcidin have been detected in human urine [6], the biological role (if any) of metallated hepcidin is uncertain.

Hepcidin differs from antimicrobial peptides by greater evolutionary conservation [3] indicative of stricter functional constraints. The involvement of hepcidin in iron metabolism was suggested by its overexpression in the livers of iron-overloaded mice [4], and its essential iron-regulatory role was established by the rapidly progressive iron overload of mice and humans with genetic hepcidin deficiency [7, 8], and the development of severe iron deficiency refractory to oral iron in mice and human overexpressing hepcidin [9, 10]. The administration of synthetic hepcidin peptide to mice produced prolonged hypoferremia [11], demonstrating the in vivo iron-regulatory activity of the 25 amino acid hepcidin peptide.

2.2 Ferroportin

Vertebrate ferroportin [12–14] is also known as solute carrier family 40 (iron-regulated transporter), member 1 (SLC40A1); iron regulated gene 1 (IREG1); solute carrier family 11 (proton-coupled divalent metal ion transporters), member 3 (SLC11A3); and metal transport protein 1 (MTP1). Ferroportin is a 571 amino acid membrane protein with 10 or 12 transmembrane domains and cytoplasmic

human	DTHFPICIFCCGCCHRSKCGMCCKT
chimp	DTHFPICIFCCGCCHRSKCGMCCKT
rhesus	DTHFPICIFCCGCCHRSKCGMCCRT
marmoset	DTHFPICIFCCGCCRQSNCGMCCKT
pig	DTHFPICIFCCGCCRKAICGMCCKT
dog*	DTHFPICIFCCGCCKTPKCGLCCKT
cow	DTHFPICIFCCGCCRKGTCGMCCRT
rat	DTNFPICLFCCKCCKNSSCGLCCIT
mouse	DTNFPICIFCCKCCNNSQCGICCKT
horse	DTHFPICTLCCGCCNKQKCGWCCKT
zebrafish	QSHLSLCRFCCKCCRNKGCGYCCKF
xenopus	QSHLSICVHCCNCCKYKGCGKCCLT

Fig. 9.2 Conservation of hepcidin in vertebrates. *Dark gray shading* denotes the strong conservation of the six N-terminal amino acids that are essential for interaction with ferroportin. *Light shading* denotes the conserved cysteine framework and *the underlined sequence* indicates the highly variable loop region of hepcidin. *Asterisk* multiple dog sequences differing at the C-terminus (…LCCIT, …FCCKT, …LCCKT) are listed in NCBI Protein Database (http://www.ncbi.nlm.nih.gov/entrez/viewer.fcgi?db=protein&id=51095241) and may represent polymorphic variants

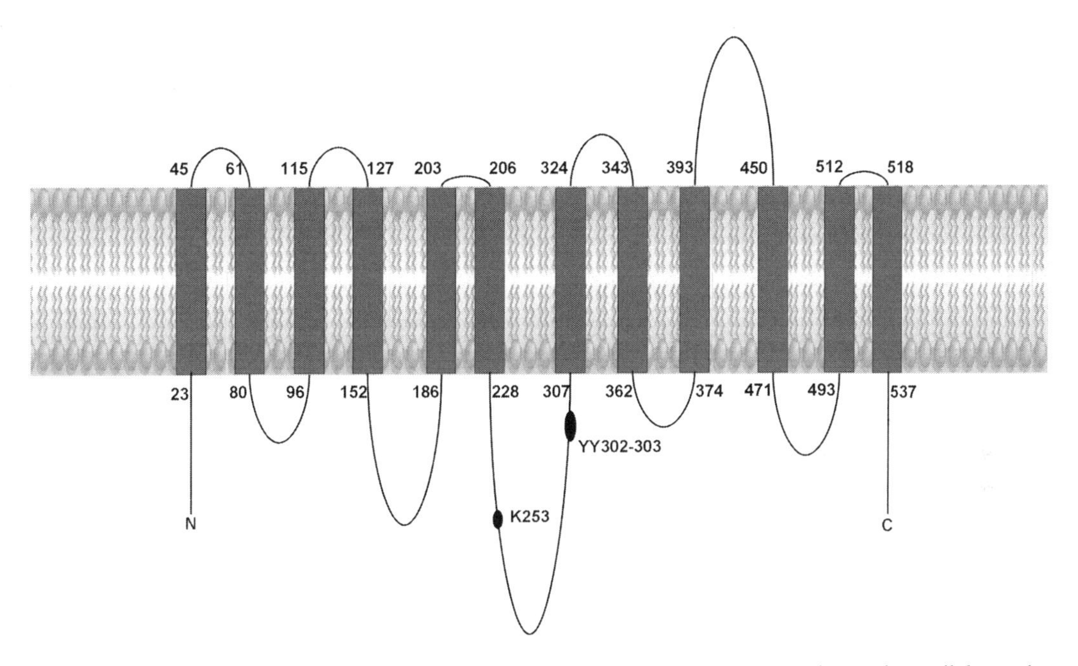

Fig. 9.3 A model of the topology of mammalian ferroportin. Extracellular loops are on the *top*, intracellular on the *bottom*. N- and C-termini and amino acids involved in internalization and degradation are *highlighted*

amino and carboxy termini [15, 16] (Fig. 9.3). Ferroportin constructs expressed in *Xenopus* oocytes or mammalian cells cause iron efflux [12, 13, 17]. Moreover, the mRNA and protein are found in all the cell types that export iron: duodenal enterocytes, placental syncytiotrophoblast, hepatocytes, and macrophages. The iron export function of ferroportin is essential as shown by the embryonic lethal systemic iron deficiency in mice and zebrafish that lack ferroportin [14, 17]. Mice with inactivation of ferroportin in the embryo but not the maternal–fetal interface survive to birth but rapidly become iron deficient and anemic, and manifest abnormal iron accumulation in iron-exporting tissues, including duodenal enterocytes, macrophages and hepatocytes [17]. These findings confirm the essential cellular iron export function of ferroportin.

2.3 *Regulation of Ferroportin by Hepcidin*

Hepcidin regulates cellular iron export by a surprisingly simple mechanism, dependent on hepcidin-induced ferroportin internalization and degradation [18]. This was shown by analyzing the fate of green fluorescent protein (GFP)-tagged ferroportin after exposure to hepcidin in model cell systems [18, 19]. Ferroportin preserves its iron-export function when marked with protein or peptide tags at its carboxy terminus. When expressed in mammalian cell lines, the ferroportin-GFP fusion protein generates membrane-associated fluorescence but upon exposure to 0.1–5 μg/ml hepcidin, the fusion protein is taken up into lysosomes within 1 h and degraded. The molecular mechanism of ferroportin internalization is similar to that of other receptors internalized by their ligands, and involves hepcidin-induced serial phosphorylation and ubiquitination of ferroportin [20]. The large cytoplasmic loop containing residues 229–306 contains the motifs that undergo ligand-induced modification. Tyrosine phosphorylation is required for ferroportin internalization, as revealed by the resistance of Y302F, Y303F double mutants to tyrosine phosphorylation and hepcidin-induced internalization. Subsequent lysine ubiquitination on K253 is required for efficient ferroportin degradation, as the K253A mutant (but not other lysine mutants) is not ubiquitinated and its degradation is very slow. The effect of all these mutations is specific for internalization as they do not impair the iron-exporting function of ferroportin.

In ex vivo macrophages or macrophage-like cell lines, endogenous ferroportin also undergoes internalization and degradation [21, 22]. Conversely, macrophages subjected to iron loading or erythrophagocytosis not only induce hepcidin synthesis but also translocate intracellular ferroportin to the membrane [21]. In duodenal enterocytes, ferroportin is located on basolateral membranes and it is also degraded by a systemic signal, most likely hepcidin [23], as indicated by dramatically increased duodenal ferroportin in states of hepcidin deficiency [24, 25]. Although ferroportin appears to be controlled by hepcidin in both macrophages and enterocytes, the specific mechanisms that determine the subcellular location of ferroportin may differ [22, 23].

2.4 *Genetics of Ferroportin-Related Disorders*

A number of genetically dominant missense (but not nonsense) mutations of ferroportin have been identified. They are manifested either as loss of ferroportin function [26], leading to iron accumulation in macrophages due to decreased cellular iron export, or less commonly, as gain of function [27], leading to hyperabsorption of dietary iron presumably from inappropriately high iron flow through enterocyte ferroportin. In cellular models, loss of function mutations cause defective trafficking of ferroportin to the cell membrane [16, 28], while gain of function mutations cause resistance to hepcidin-induced internalization [16, 28]. A mouse model of heterozygous ferroportin ablation does not manifest disease [17] but a recently identified missense mutation [29] causes iron accumulation in macrophages with iron-restricted erythropoiesis. Based on the genetics of ferroportin-related disease, on biochemical studies, and the dominant-negative effect of clinically significant ferroportin mutations, ferroportin is dimeric or multimeric [30], but this interpretation is not universally accepted [31–33].

2.5 *Structure–Function Analysis of Hepcidin*

Evolutionary analysis of mammalian hepcidin sequences indicates a strong conservation of the disulfide bridge structure and the N-terminal six amino acids (Fig. 9.2). The N-terminus differs in fish and amphibian hepcidins (Fig. 9.2) but the substitutions are quite conservative. Deletion of amino acids from the N-terminus causes progressive loss of activity [34] so that the 20 amino acid form of hepcidin, also naturally found in urine and serum [2, 3], is inactive in cellular ferroportin internalization assays [18, 34] and in vivo [11]. In contrast, the hepcidin structure retains bioactivity in cellular assays when amino acids in the rest of the structure, including the disulfide bonds, are altered [34] although the stability of the molecule may be decreased.

2.6 Hepcidin Catabolism

Fluorescently tagged hepcidin is taken up by ferroportin-expressing cells in culture and colocalizes in lysosomes with GFP-ferroportin (G. Preza et al., in preparation). When radiolabeled hepcidin is given to mice, the tracer is predominantly found in urine but is also taken up by ferroportin-rich tissues [11], indicating that both renal excretion and uptake and degradation in ferroportin-rich tissues could contribute to hepcidin clearance from plasma.

2.7 Cellular Regulation of Ferroportin

Hepcidin is not the only signal that regulates ferroportin. Each macrophage that ingests senescent erythrocytes faces a large load of iron that must be stored or exported, depending on systemic requirements for iron. Whereas the systemic regulation of macrophage iron export is mediated by plasma hepcidin, which internalizes and degrades membrane-associated ferroportin [19], ferroportin is also subject to independent cellular regulation by macrophage heme and iron levels [21, 35, 36]. Cellular iron and heme increase ferroportin mRNA and protein, and induce the translocation of ferroportin from intracellular vesicles to the cellular membrane. The increase in ferroportin is mediated by both transcriptional and translational mechanisms, the latter involving the 5 iron regulatory element (IRE) located in the ferroportin mRNA [37, 38]. The amount of ferroportin on the membrane, and therefore the ability of macrophages to export iron, is thus closely linked to the iron and heme content of each macrophage. In combination, the cellular and systemic regulators deliver iron to extracellular fluid and plasma when iron is required for systemic needs, obtaining it from those macrophages that contain abundant iron and heme.

3 Regulation of Hepcidin Synthesis by Iron

3.1 Hereditary Hemochromatosis Proteins Are Hepcidin Regulators

Analysis of hepcidin expression in patients with hereditary hemochromatosis [8, 39–42] and in mouse models [7, 25, 40, 43–47] revealed that the major forms of juvenile and adult hereditary hemochromatosis are due to deficiency of hepcidin that allows excessive iron absorption and reticuloendothelial iron recycling. The rate of development of iron overload is most severe in the juvenile form of hemochromatosis, which manifest the lowest hepcidin expression, usually caused by homozygous disruption of hepcidin (HAMP) or hemojuvelin (HJV) genes. The adult forms are less hepcidin deficient and are usually caused by homozygous disruption of the genes encoding transferrin receptor 2 (TfR2) or the hemochromatosis gene HFE. Two siblings with phenotypically juvenile form of hereditary hemochromatosis were found to have both homozygous Q317X TfR2 mutations and compound heterozygous C282Y/H63D HFE mutations, suggesting an additive effect of HFE and TfR2 disruption [48]. The simplest explanation of the genotype–phenotype relationships is that HFE, TfR2, and hemojuvelin are regulators of hepcidin, and that HFE and TfR2 are partially redundant and perhaps operating on parallel pathways that converge on hepcidin or hemojuvelin.

3.2 Hemojuvelin

Hemojuvelin (also known as HFE2 and RgmC) was identified as a hepcidin regulator through positional cloning of the gene mutated in most cases of juvenile hemochromatosis [41]. The gene encodes a GPI-linked membrane protein with homology to repulsive guidance molecules (RgmA and RgmB) involved in the development of the central nervous system. Suppression of hemojuvelin by siRNAs proportionally decreased hepcidin mRNA in hepatic cell lines, indicating that hemojuvelin, unlike other Rgm [49], directly regulates hepcidin synthesis and is not principally a developmental mediator. In addition to the membrane-associated GPI-linked form, hemojuvelin also exists as a soluble protein that acts as a suppressor of hepcidin synthesis by hepatocytes in cell culture [49] and in vivo in the mouse [50]. The prohormone convertase furin is responsible for the release of soluble hemojuvelin and may act in the Golgi or on the membrane [51, 52]. The shedding or secretion of hemojuvelin is suppressed by iron [49, 53] through an as yet undefined mechanism and stimulated by hypoxia and iron deficiency in part through increased synthesis of the prohormone convertase furin [51]. Other Rgms act, at least in part, through their interactions with the receptor neogenin, and indeed, such an interaction may modulate the effect of hemojuvelin as well [53, 54], probably through the regulation of hemojuvelin shedding. However, the predominant effect of hemojuvelin on hepcidin synthesis is mediated by its interactions with the BMP pathway [55]. The BMP-dependent effect of hemojuvelin is required for the regulation of hepcidin synthesis by iron-transferrin in primary hepatocytes [56].

3.3 The Bone Morphogenetic Protein (BMP) Pathway in Hepcidin Regulation

With the exception of hepcidin itself, all the genes disrupted in hereditary hemochromatosis encoded proteins whose function was not known. An important insight into how these proteins may fit together came from the phenotype of a liver-specific SMAD4 knockout mouse [57] which manifested systemic iron overload and nearly complete deficiency of hepcidin. SMAD4 is a transcription factor used by the BMP and TGFβ pathways and the phenotype of the SMAD4 knockout implicated both pathways in iron regulation. In unrelated studies [58], RgmB (Dragon) was shown to act as a coreceptor for the BMP receptor and to enhance its signaling, and subsequently, hemojuvelin (RgmC) was also found to act as a coreceptor for the BMP receptor [55] and BMP2, 4 and 9 were shown to be strong inducers of hepcidin synthesis [50, 55, 59]. Based on the comparative potency of their respective ligands, the role of the BMP pathway in hepcidin regulation appears to be much greater that of the TGFβ pathway [50].

The BMP signaling pathway is activated by dimeric ligands that bring together type I and type II receptor serine/threonine kinases on the cell membrane. The constitutively active type II receptor kinase phosphorylates and activates the kinase activity of type I receptor, which in turn phosphorylates the receptor-regulated Smads, Smad 1, 5, and 8. Upon phosphorylation, these Smad proteins form a complex with the common mediator Smad-4. The activated Smad complex translocates into the nucleus and regulates transcription of its target genes. The BMP receptor heterodimers are formed by combining one of three type II receptors (BMPRII, ActRIIA, and ActRIIB) with one of three type I receptors (ALK3, ALK6, and ALK2). Specific combinations of type I and type II receptors are preferentially utilized by different BMP ligands, and additional coreceptors can modify this preference and the intensity of signaling [60]. Multiple BMPs and other potential ligands are expressed in the liver [50] but only a few appear to be involved in the regulation of hepcidin by iron. Although BMP2 and BMP4 interact with hemojuvelin and appear to function in the pathway by which iron regulates hepcidin [56], BMP9 does not interact with hemojuvelin and uses a different BMP receptor heterodimer not involved in iron-related signaling [50, 56]. The dramatic effect of the BMP pathway on hepcidin transcription and the strong phenotype of the hemojuvelin-deficient mice and humans puts them at the center of current models of hepcidin and iron regulation. However, neither hemojuvelin nor the BMPs and their receptors are iron-binding molecules and so they must interact with other molecules that bind iron and can "sense" iron concentrations.

3.4 *Transferrin and Transferrin Receptors 1 and 2*

3.4.1 TfR1

Transferrin receptors 1 and 2 bind holotransferrin (diferric transferrin) as well as monoferric transferrin and both can mediate the cellular uptake of iron (see Chap. 7). The affinity constants for TfR1 and TfR2 binding of holotransferrin are 1.1 and 29 nM, respectively [61], indicating that both receptors would be saturated at physiologic extracellular holotransferrin concentrations which are thousand times higher than the affinity constants. TfR1 is expressed abundantly on erythropoietic precursors and present in most other cell types while TfR2 is hepatocyte-specific. Homozygous ablation of TfR1 is embryonic lethal, producing severe anemia and malformation of the central nervous system [62]. TfR1+/– heterozygotes have iron-deficient erythropoiesis despite iron reserves in macrophages, indicating a defect in iron uptake by erythrocyte precursors [62]. Despite the lack of direct involvement of TfR1 in intestinal iron absorption, iron stores in TfR1 +/– mice are diminished, indicating that the receptor could play a role in iron regulation.

3.4.2 TfR2

The effects of TfR1 deficiency on iron regulation contrast with the effects of TfR2 or transferrin deficiency. Deficiency of TfR2 in mice or humans causes systemic iron overload [63–65] and liver-specific deficiency of TfR2 is sufficient for iron overload, clearly indicating TfR2 involvement in iron regulation [66]. Hepcidin is very low in TfR2-deficient humans [42] and mice [46, 65], indicating that TfR2 defects cause iron overload through the lack of hepcidin.

3.4.3 Holotransferrin

Genetic deficiency of transferrin is associated with a very severe form of iron overload in humans (summarized in [67]) and in mice [68], indicating that transferrin is required for systemic homeostatic regulation of iron. After a test dose of iron, transient increases in transferrin saturation elicit proportional changes in urinary hepcidin concentrations [56]. Holotransferrin, but not elemental iron, induces hepcidin mRNA in freshly isolated hepatocytes [56]. These observations suggest that holotransferrin is an important (although perhaps not the only) form of iron sensed by the systemic homeostatic mechanisms.

3.4.4 Iron Sensing

In the aggregate, genetic studies of transferrin and its receptors suggest that all three are involved in iron regulation, acting by regulating hepcidin synthesis. Based on their reported affinity constants, both transferrin receptors would be saturated with iron-transferrin at physiologic concentrations. Current models of the involvement of TfR1 and TfR2 in iron sensing propose complexes of TfRs with other molecules that effectively lower the affinity of TfRs for holotransferrin so that such complexes could sense changes in holotransferrin concentration in its physiologic range.

3.5 HFE

3.5.1 HFE Regulates Hepcidin

Mutations in the gene HFE are responsible for most cases of hereditary hemochromatosis in patients of European descent. Patients with HFE hemochromatosis carry homozygous or compound heterozygous mutations, and manifest hepcidin mRNA and protein levels that are either lower than normal or normal but inadequate for the high iron load and transferrin saturation [40, 69]. Moreover, patients with HFE hemochromatosis lack the acute hepcidin response to iron ingestion but the chronic response to iron loading is at least partially preserved [69]. Both humans and mice with HFE hemochromatosis are deficient in hepcidin mRNA [40, 43, 45], suggesting decreased hepcidin gene transcription (or less likely, mRNA instability). Transplantation of normal livers into HFE recipients is not followed by reaccumulation of iron, suggesting that HFE expression in the liver is sufficient for iron homeostasis [70, 71] but enterocyte-specific ablation of HFE in mice does not cause an iron disorder [72]. These studies support the idea that HFE acts primarily in the liver by regulating hepcidin. Transplantation of HFE mice with wt bone marrow [73] ameliorated the iron overload and increased hepatic hepcidin mRNA compared to HFE mice transplanted with HFE bone marrow, indicating that HFE in myeloid cells could also contribute to hepcidin regulation.

3.5.2 HFE Interacts with Transferrin Receptors

The HFE gene encodes a membrane protein that forms a heterodimer with β2-microglobulin, and is similar to proteins of the type I major histocompatibility complex. HFE lowers the affinity of TfR1 for holotransferrin [74]. The HFE ectodomain competes with holotransferrin for binding to the TfR1 ectodomain, and the binding sites of HFE and holotransferrin on TfR1 overlap [75, 76]. Moreover, complete TfR1 and holotransferrin compete for HFE in cellular models [77]. Although the TfR2 ectodomain was reported not to bind to the HFE ectodomain, in cellular models with overexpressed whole proteins, TfR2 competed with TfR1 for binding to HFE [78] and TfR2 was stabilized by its interaction with HFE [79]. Unlike the interaction of TfR1 with HFE, the interaction of TfR2 with HFE was not diminished by holotransferrin. In fact, holotransferrin stabilized TfR2 [80, 81], enabling it to compete more effectively for HFE. Based on the phenotypes of mice with a deficiency of transferrin or TfR1 or TfR2, both transferrin receptors could act as sensors for holotransferrin, acting synergistically, and using HFE as a signaling intermediary. Holotransferrin would release HFE from its association with TfR1 and make more HFE available to bind to the holotransferrin-stabilized TfR2. The TfR2–HFE complex would then stimulate hepcidin synthesis.

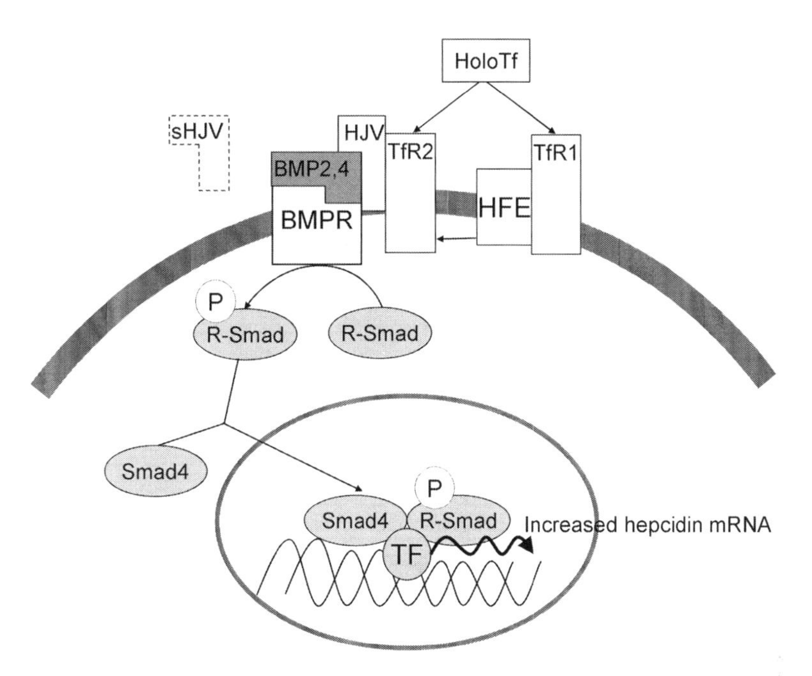

Fig. 9.4 A model of hepcidin regulation by holotransferrin (*holoTf*). Signaling by the receptor complex consisting of BMPR, its ligand BMP2/4, and the coreceptor HJV is stimulated by the binding of holoTf to both TfRs. The binding of holoTf to TfR1 releases HFE and the binding of holoTf to TfR2 stabilizes TfR2, so both HFE and TfR2 can associate with the receptor complex which then phosphorylates R-Smad. R-Smad binds Smad4, they translocate to the nucleus and help form a transcription complex to increase the synthesis of hepcidin mRNA. Soluble HJV (*sHJV*) represses hepcidin expression by selectively inhibiting BMP signaling

3.6 A Model of Hepcidin Regulation

A comprehensive model of hepcidin regulation must account for the effects of known genetic lesions on iron metabolism, and must provide a plausible scheme by which iron is sensed and its concentrations affect the synthesis of the iron-regulatory hormone. A current model of hepcidin regulation (Fig. 9.4) is built around the regulatory complex of hemojuvelin, BMP2/4, and the BMP receptor regulating the transcription of hepcidin via the SMAD pathway. The activity or assembly of this complex is regulated by its association with TfR2 and HFE, with their effects synergistic. The availability of TfR2 and HFE is in turn determined by the concentration of holotransferrin which stabilizes TfR2 and releases HFE from TfR1.

7 Regulation of Systemic Iron Metabolism and Hepcidin Synthesis by Hypoxia-Inducible Transcription Factors

7.1 Gene Regulation by Hypoxia

Hypoxia is a potent regulator of cellular and systemic processes, and has a particularly strong effect on erythropoiesis where it acts as a dominant inducer of the production of erythropoietin. Hypoxia regulates the transcription of erythropoietin and dozens of other hypoxia-regulated genes through heterodimeric hypoxia-inducible transcription factors (HIF) that bind to hypoxia-responsive elements (HRE) in the promoters of target genes [82]. HIF consist of one of three cytoplasmic

HIF1α, HIF2α, or HIF3α that can combine with the constitutive HIF1β subunit. During hypoxia, HIFα subunits accumulate, translocate into the nucleus, and interact with HIF1β and other transcription factors. When oxygen is abundant, HIFα subunits are subjected to hydroxylation on one or two of their prolines, and this modification targets the HIFα for interaction with the von Hippel–Lindau tumor-suppressor protein (VHL) and for degradation. Another oxygen-sensing hydroxylase, FIH-1 (factor inhibiting HIF-1) hydroxylates a specific Asn on HIFα, thereby inhibiting the interaction of HIF with other transcription factors. The hydroxylases contain an essential iron, and their activity is inhibited by iron chelators.

7.2 Iron and Hepcidin Regulation by Hypoxia

Mice and rats subjected to hypoxia respond by increased production of erythropoietin, enhanced erythropoiesis, and increased iron absorption. The increase in iron absorption is, at least in part, independent of the effect of increased erythropoiesis, as revealed by early experiments in which the erythropoietic response is suppressed by nephrectomy or by a combination of irradiation of the bone marrow by radioactive strontium and splenectomy [83, 84]. More recent studies suggest that the increased iron absorption is due to suppression of hepcidin by hypoxia. Mice made hypoxic by exposure to oxygen pressures found at 5,500 m, manifested gradually decreasing hepcidin mRNA but the effect appears to be relatively slow, peaking at 4 days [85], suggesting that the effect on hepcidin included indirect, erythropoiesis-mediated effects of hypoxia. Direct effects of hypoxia on hepatocytes were deduced from hypoxia-exposed hepatocyte cell lines that showed a decrease in hepcidin mRNA within 24–48 h [85, 86]. In the aggregate, these studies suggest that hepcidin is subject to direct regulation by hepatic hypoxia but the relative contribution of direct and indirect effects remains to be demonstrated.

7.3 HIF Involvement in Hepcidin Suppression During Iron Deficiency

Systemic iron deficiency was shown to suppress hepcidin in humans [87, 88]. In mice, the suppression of hepcidin by iron deprivation appears to be partially dependent on HIF1α because mice with ablation of hepatic HIF1α suppress hepcidin mRNA less than do wt mice [89]. Nevertheless, hepcidin suppression still takes place even in HIF1α-deficient mice, indicating that other pathways may also regulate hepcidin during iron deficiency. Although the specific HREs in the hepcidin promoter differ in number, and location between mice and humans, both promoters were found to bind HIF [89]. The HIF-dependent mechanism of hepcidin regulation would be expected to be responsive to hepatocyte iron stores rather than holotransferrin concentration, and thus could complement the effect of the BMP/hemojuvelin/TfR pathway that senses holotransferrin.

8 Regulation of Plasma Iron and of Hepcidin Synthesis by Inflammation

8.1 Hepcidin and the Acute Hypoferremia of Inflammation

Hypoferremia develops within hours of acute infections and persists in states of chronic infection or inflammation (Chaps. 11 and 15). Recent studies indicate that hepcidin is the key mediator of this hypoferremic response. In humans, hepcidin is induced by inflammation within hours and increased hepcidin is followed by hypoferremia a few hours later [90]. The hypoferremic response to turpentine-induced inflammation is lost in hepcidin-deficient mice, indicating that the increased hepcidin concentrations mediate the hypoferremia of inflammation [86]. Injection of hepcidin produces hypoferremia within 1 h [11], in agreement with the time course of the development of hypoferremia in acute infections in humans and in mice. Thus, the role of circulating hepcidin in acute hypoferremia of inflammation is well supported by evidence. Additional mechanisms may contribute to local or systemic hypoferremia. Autocrine secretion of hepcidin by macrophages [91] may act locally to reduce macrophage ferroportin, cause macrophage iron retention, and decrease the local extracellular iron concentrations. In addition, transcriptional suppression of ferroportin by inflammatory stimuli may also contribute to iron retention in macrophages [92, 93].

8.2 Hepcidin and Anemia of Inflammation

Mice and humans chronically overexpressing hepcidin develop not only hypoferremia but also an iron-restricted anemia [9, 10, 94, 95]. Urinary hepcidin is increased in patients with anemia of inflammation [88], suggesting that the overproduction of hepcidin accounts for the defining features of anemia of inflammation: iron-restricted anemia with hypoferremia.

8.3 Regulation of Hepcidin During Infection and Inflammation

The induction of hepcidin by infection or microbial products has been demonstrated in humans [87, 90], in mice [4, 85], and in fish [96]. Infection or microbial products induce hepcidin mRNA directly in primary hepatocytes [4] and in monocytes and macrophages [91, 93, 97–101]. Moreover, media conditioned by lipopolysaccharide-treated blood monocytes induce hepcidin synthesis in isolated hepatocytes and hepatocyte-derived cell lines [87] and this effect is neutralized by anti-IL-6 antibody, indicating that IL-6 is an important macrophage-derived mediator of hepcidin regulation. Unlike wild-type C57Bl6 mice, IL-6-deficient mice injected with turpentine do not acutely increase their hepcidin mRNA, and do not develop hypoferremia, supporting the role of IL-6 in acute hypoferremia of inflammation [101]. Moreover, human volunteers infused with moderate amounts of IL-6 develop increased hepcidin and hypoferremia within hours of infusion [101]. Patients with multicentric Castleman's disease that causes overproduction of IL-6 develop a microcytic anemia with increased serum hepcidin levels but treatment with tocilizumab (anti-IL-6 receptor antibody) decreases hepcidin and reverses the anemia [102]. The transcriptional induction of hepcidin by IL-6 is dependent on the STAT3 pathway [103–105], but may also require the Smad pathway since in liver-specific Smad4 KO mice, IL-6-mediated hepcidin induction is blunted [57]. Other inflammatory mediators and the direct effect of bacterial substances on hepatocytes and macrophages can also induce hepcidin [4, 90, 93, 106, 107] and IL-6-independent pathways may be especially important in the chronic setting. Moreover, the production of increased amounts of hepcidin by macrophages and adipocytes could contribute to hypoferremia in obesity and perhaps other inflammatory disorders [108].

8.4 Regulation of Hemojuvelin by Inflammation

Inflammation not only exerts a stimulatory effect on hepcidin synthesis but also affects the iron-regulatory pathway by suppressing hemojuvelin mRNA [47, 109–111]. Although this remains to be demonstrated experimentally, the suppression of hemojuvelin would be expected to uncouple the iron-regulatory pathway so that the effect of the inflammatory stimuli on hepcidin synthesis would not be outweighed by the opposing effects of iron restriction.

9 Regulation of Hepcidin Synthesis by Erythropoietic Activity

9.1 Erythropoiesis Suppresses Hepcidin Synthesis

It has been known for at least 50 years that increased erythropoietic activity leads to increased intestinal iron absorption [83, 112]. The predicted factor that controls intestinal iron absorption is hepcidin, and indeed hemolytic anemia or hemorrhage both suppress hepcidin synthesis [85, 113, 114]. However, as anticipated by earlier iron absorption studies, anemia does not suppress hepcidin synthesis in the absence of active erythropoiesis [113, 114]. The nature of the factor that signals from the bone marrow to the liver to modulate hepcidin is not yet known.

9.2 Hepcidin Suppression in Expanded but Ineffective Erythropoiesis

β-Thalassemia major and intermedia represent an extreme example of increased erythropoiesis accompanied by premature death of erythroid precursors. Hepcidin is very low in untransfused patients with β-thalassemia intermedia [115, 116] and in the mouse models of β-thalassemia [117–119]. Hepcidin is higher in transfused patients with β-thalassemia but still inappropriately low for the degree of iron overload [115, 116, 120, 121]. A hepcidin-regulating humoral factor present in β-thalassemia was implicated by the observation that sera from patients with β-thalassemia suppressed hepcidin production in hepatocyte cell lines [122]. GDF15, a member of the TGFβ/BMP family of ligands, is produced by erythrocyte precursors and is present at very high concentrations in the plasma of patients with β-thalassemia [123]. At these high concentrations, GDF15 suppressed hepcidin production by primary human hepatocytes and by hepatocyte cell lines and emerged as a strong candidate for bone marrow-derived humoral factor in β-thalassemia. It is not yet clear whether GDF15 contributes to hepcidin regulation in situations where erythroid precursor expansion and apoptosis are less extreme.

10 Summary

Systemic iron homeostasis is mediated predominantly by the interaction of the iron-regulatory hormone hepcidin with the cellular iron efflux channel, ferroportin. In the efferent arm of iron homeostasis, hepcidin binds to ferroportin, causing its internalization and degradation, and thereby inhibiting cellular iron export into extracellular fluid. In the afferent arm of the homeostatic arc, extracellular iron, hepatic iron stores, and inflammation stimulate hepcidin synthesis, and hypoxia and erythropoietic activity suppress it. Direct effects of many of these stimuli on ferroportin synthesis have also been observed and may contribute to iron regulation.

Notes

Since the writing of this article, several important developments updated our understanding of iron homeostasis:

1. The bone morphogenetic protein BMP6 has been shown to be an iron-related ligand of the BMP receptor, necessary for normal hepcidin expression and iron regulation, at least in the mouse [1, 2].
2. The membrane serine protease matriptase 2 (MT-2, also abbreviated TMPRSS6) was found to be a negative regulator of hepcidin [3]. MT-2 acts by cleaving membrane hemojuvelin at an external site [4]. Homozygous or compound heterozygous mutations in MT-2 are a major cause of the rare autosomal recessive disorder iron-refractory iron-deficiency anemia [5] wherein increased circulating hepcidin inhibits iron absorption and recycling without any evidence of inflammation.
3. Accumulating evidence [6, 7] is pointing to two distinct pathways in hepcidin regulation by iron. The first is responsive to extracellular iron, likely sensed as holotransferrin concentration [8]. The extracellular iron pathway modulates signaling by the BMP receptor complex, and requires HFE, TfR2, hemojuvelin and BMP6. The second pathway, historically called the "stores" regulator, responds to intracellular iron and regulates BMP6 concentrations [9] even in the absence of HFE, TfR2 or hemojuvelin. The intracellular regulator exerts its effect on hepcidin even in the absence of BMP6 indicating that other ligands may also be involved.
4. The proposed mechanism of ferroportin internalization by its ligand hepcidin, and the specific roles of hepcidin-induced ferroportin phosphorylation and ubiquitination, have been contested [10] and remain unresolved.
5. Several types of human serum hepcidin assays have been developed and crosscorrelated [11–17] for use in disease-related research and drug development. Assay standardization is underway [14]. Measurements of human serum hepcidin in various disease conditions generally confirmed the regulatory schema presented in this review.

References

1. Bothwell TH, Finch CA. Iron metabolism. Boston: Little, Brown and Company; 1962.
2. Krause A, Neitz S, Magert HJ, Schulz A, Forssmann WG, Schulz-Knappe P, et al. LEAP-1, a novel highly disulfide-bonded human peptide, exhibits antimicrobial activity. FEBS Lett. 2000;480:147–50.
3. Park CH, Valore EV, Waring AJ, Ganz T. Hepcidin, a urinary antimicrobial peptide synthesized in the liver. J Biol Chem. 2001;276:7806–10.
4. Pigeon C, Ilyin G, Courselaud B, Leroyer P, Turlin B, Brissot P, et al. A new mouse liver-specific gene, encoding a protein homologous to human antimicrobial peptide hepcidin, is overexpressed during iron overload. J Biol Chem. 2001;276:7811–19.
5. Valore EV, Ganz T. Posttranslational processing of hepcidin in human hepatocytes is mediated by the prohormone convertase furin. Blood Cells Mol Dis. 2008;40:132–8.
6. Farnaud S, Patel A, Evans R. Modelling of a metal-containing hepcidin. Biometals. 2006;19:527–33.
7. Nicolas G, Bennoun M, Devaux I, Beaumont C, Grandchamp B, Kahn A, et al. Lack of hepcidin gene expression and severe tissue iron overload in upstream stimulatory factor 2 (USF2) knockout mice. Proc Natl Acad Sci USA. 2001;98:8780–5.
8. Roetto A, Papanikolaou G, Politou M, Alberti F, Girelli D, Christakis J, et al. Mutant antimicrobial peptide hepcidin is associated with severe juvenile hemochromatosis. Nat Genet. 2003;33:21–2.
9. Nicolas G, Bennoun M, Porteu A, Mativet S, Beaumont C, Grandchamp B, et al. Severe iron deficiency anemia in transgenic mice expressing liver hepcidin. Proc Natl Acad Sci USA. 2002;99:4596–601.
10. Weinstein DA, Roy CN, Fleming MD, Loda MF, Wolfsdorf JI, Andrews NC. Inappropriate expression of hepcidin is associated with iron refractory anemia: implications for the anemia of chronic disease. Blood. 2002;100:3776–81.

11. Rivera S, Nemeth E, Gabayan V, Lopez MA, Farshidi D, Ganz T. Synthetic hepcidin causes rapid dose-dependent hypoferremia and is concentrated in ferroportin-containing organs. Blood. 2005;106:2196–9.
12. Abboud S, Haile DJ. A novel mammalian iron-regulated protein involved in intracellular iron metabolism. J Biol Chem. 2000;275:19906–12.
13. McKie AT, Marciani P, Rolfs A, Brennan K, Wehr K, Barrow D, et al. A novel duodenal iron-regulated transporter, IREG1, implicated in the basolateral transfer of iron to the circulation. Mol Cell. 2000;5:299–309.
14. Donovan A, Brownlie A, Zhou Y, Shepard J, Pratt SJ, Moynihan J, et al. Positional cloning of zebrafish ferroportin1 identifies a conserved vertebrate iron exporter. Nature. 2000;403:776–81.
15. Liu XB, Yang F, Haile DJ. Functional consequences of ferroportin 1 mutations. Blood Cells Mol Dis. 2005;35:33–46.
16. De Domenico I, Ward DM, Nemeth E, Vaughn MB, Musci G, Ganz T, et al. The molecular basis of ferroportin-linked hemochromatosis. Proc Natl Acad Sci USA. 2005;102:8955–60.
17. Donovan A, Lima CA, Pinkus JL, Pinkus GS, Zon LI, Robine S, et al. The iron exporter ferroportin/Slc40a1 is essential for iron homeostasis. Cell Metab. 2005;1:191–200.
18. Nemeth E, Tuttle MS, Powelson J, Vaughn MB, Donovan A, Ward DM, et al. Hepcidin regulates cellular iron efflux by binding to ferroportin and inducing its internalization. Science. 2004;306:2090–3.
19. Knutson MD, Oukka M, Koss LM, Aydemir F, Wessling-Resnick M. Iron release from macrophages after erythrophagocytosis is up-regulated by ferroportin 1 overexpression and down-regulated by hepcidin. Proc Natl Acad Sci USA. 2005;102:1324–8.
20. De Domenico I, Ward DM, Langelier C, Vaughn MB, Nemeth E, Sundquist WI, et al. The molecular mechanism of hepcidin-mediated ferroportin down-regulation. Mol Biol Cell. 2007;18:2569–78.
21. Delaby C, Pilard N, Goncalves AS, Beaumont C, Canonne-Hergaux F. Presence of the iron exporter ferroportin at the plasma membrane of macrophages is enhanced by iron loading and down-regulated by hepcidin. Blood. 2005;106:3979–84.
22. Chaston T, Chung B, Mascarenhas M, Marks J, Patel B, Srai SK, et al. Evidence for differential effects of hepcidin in macrophages and intestinal epithelial cells. Gut. 2008;57:374–82.
23. Canonne-Hergaux F, Donovan A, Delaby C, Wang HJ, Gros P. Comparative studies of duodenal and macrophage ferroportin proteins. Am J Physiol Gastrointest Liver Physiol. 2006;290:G156–63.
24. Viatte L, Lesbordes-Brion JC, Lou DQ, Bennoun M, Nicolas G, Kahn A, et al. Deregulation of proteins involved in iron metabolism in hepcidin-deficient mice. Blood. 2005;105:4861–4.
25. Huang FW, Pinkus JL, Pinkus GS, Fleming MD, Andrews NC. A mouse model of juvenile hemochromatosis. J Clin Invest. 2005;115:2187–91.
26. Pietrangelo A. The ferroportin disease. Blood Cells Mol Dis. 2004;32:131–8.
27. Sham RL, Phatak PD, West C, Lee P, Andrews C, Beutler E. Autosomal dominant hereditary hemochromatosis associated with a novel ferroportin mutation and unique clinical features. Blood Cells Mol Dis. 2005;34:157–61.
28. Schimanski LM, Drakesmith H, Merryweather-Clarke AT, Viprakasit V, Edwards JP, Sweetland E, et al. In vitro functional analysis of human ferroportin (FPN) and hemochromatosis-associated FPN mutations. Blood. 2005;105:4096–102.
29. Zohn IE, De Domenico I, Pollock A, Ward DM, Goodman JF, Liang X, et al. The flatiron mutation in mouse ferroportin acts as a dominant negative to cause ferroportin disease. Blood. 2007;109:4174–80.
30. De Domenico I, Ward DM, Musci G, Kaplan J. Evidence for the multimeric structure of ferroportin. Blood. 2007;109:2205–9.
31. Goncalves AS, Muzeau F, Blaybel R, Hetet G, Driss F, Delaby C, et al. Wild-type and mutant ferroportins do not form oligomers in transfected cells. Biochem J. 2006;396:265–75.
32. Schimanski LM, Drakesmith H, Talbott C, Horne K, James JR, Davis SJ, et al. Ferroportin: lack of evidence for multimers. Blood Cells Mol Dis. 2008;40:360–9.
33. Pignatti E, Mascheroni L, Sabelli M, Barelli S, Biffo S, Pietrangelo A. Ferroportin is a monomer in vivo in mice. Blood Cells Mol Dis. 2006;36:26–32.
34. Nemeth E, Preza GC, Jung CL, Kaplan J, Waring AJ, Ganz T. The N-terminus of hepcidin is essential for its interaction with ferroportin: structure–function study. Blood. 2006;107:328–33.
35. Knutson M, Wessling-Resnick M. Iron metabolism in the reticuloendothelial system. Crit Rev Biochem Mol Biol. 2003;38:61–88.
36. Delaby C, Pilard N, Puy H, Canonne-Hergaux F. Sequential regulation of ferroportin expression after erythrophagocytosis in murine macrophages: early mRNA induction by heme followed by iron-dependent protein expression. Biochem J. 2008;411:123–31.
37. Liu XB, Hill P, Haile DJ. Role of the ferroportin iron-responsive element in iron and nitric oxide dependent gene regulation. Blood Cells Mol Dis. 2002;29:315–26.
38. Mok H, Jelinek J, Pai S, Cattanach BM, Prchal JT, Youssoufian H, et al. Disruption of ferroportin 1 regulation causes dynamic alterations in iron homeostasis and erythropoiesis in polycythaemia mice. Development. 2004;131:1859–68.

39. Gehrke SG, Kulaksiz H, Herrmann T, Riedel HD, Bents K, Veltkamp C, et al. Expression of hepcidin in hereditary hemochromatosis: evidence for a regulation in response to the serum transferrin saturation and to non-transferrin-bound iron. Blood. 2003;102:371–6.
40. Bridle KR, Frazer DM, Wilkins SJ, Dixon JL, Purdie DM, Crawford DH, et al. Disrupted hepcidin regulation in HFE-associated haemochromatosis and the liver as a regulator of body iron homoeostasis. Lancet. 2003;361:669–73.
41. Papanikolaou G, Samuels ME, Ludwig EH, MacDonald ML, Franchini PL, Dubé MP, et al. Mutations in HFE2 cause iron overload in chromosome 1q-linked juvenile hemochromatosis. Nat Genet. 2004;36:77–82.
42. Nemeth E, Roetto A, Garozzo G, Ganz T, Camaschella C. Hepcidin is decreased in TFR2 hemochromatosis. Blood. 2005;105:1803–6.
43. Ahmad KA, Ahmann JR, Migas MC, Waheed A, Britton RS, Bacon BR, et al. Decreased liver hepcidin expression in the hfe knockout mouse. Blood Cells Mol Dis. 2002;29:361–6.
44. Nicolas G, Viatte L, Lou DQ, Bennoun M, Beaumont C, Kahn A, et al. Constitutive hepcidin expression prevents iron overload in a mouse model of hemochromatosis. Nat Genet. 2003;34:97–101.
45. Muckenthaler M, Roy CN, Custodio AO, Miñana B, de Graaf J, Montross LK, et al. Regulatory defects in liver and intestine implicate abnormal hepcidin and Cybrd1 expression in mouse hemochromatosis. Nat Genet. 2003;34:102–7.
46. Kawabata H, Fleming RE, Gui D, Moon SY, Saitoh T, O'Kelly J, et al. Expression of hepcidin is down-regulated in TfR2 mutant mice manifesting a phenotype of hereditary hemochromatosis. Blood. 2005;105:376–81.
47. Niederkofler V, Salie R, Arber S. Hemojuvelin is essential for dietary iron sensing, and its mutation leads to severe iron overload. J Clin Invest. 2005;115:2180–6.
48. Pietrangelo A, Caleffi A, Henrion J, Ferrara F, Corradini E, Kulaksiz H, et al. Juvenile hemochromatosis associated with pathogenic mutations of adult hemochromatosis genes. Gastroenterology. 2005;128:470–9.
49. Lin L, Goldberg YP, Ganz T. Competitive regulation of hepcidin mRNA by soluble and cell-associated hemojuvelin. Blood. 2005;106:2884–9.
50. Babitt JL, Huang FW, Xia Y, Sidis Y, Andrews NC, Lin HY. Modulation of bone morphogenetic protein signaling in vivo regulates systemic iron balance. J Clin Invest. 2007;117:1933–9.
51. Silvestri L, Pagani A, Camaschella C. Furin mediated release of soluble hemojuvelin: a new link between hypoxia and iron homeostasis. Blood. 2008;111:924–31.
52. Lin L, Nemeth E, Goodnough JB, Thapa DR, Gabayan V, Ganz T. Soluble hemojuvelin is released by proprotein convertase-mediated cleavage at a conserved polybasic RNRR site. Blood Cells Mol Dis. 2008;40:122–31.
53. Zhang AS, Anderson SA, Meyers KR, Hernandez C, Eisenstein RS, Enns CA. Evidence that inhibition of hemojuvelin shedding in response to iron is mediated through neogenin. J Biol Chem. 2007;282:12547–56.
54. Zhang AS, West Jr AP, Wyman AE, Bjorkman PJ, Enns CA. Interaction of hemojuvelin with neogenin results in iron accumulation in human embryonic kidney 293 cells. J Biol Chem. 2005;280:33885–94.
55. Babitt JL, Huang FW, Wrighting DM, Xia Y, Sidis Y, Samad TA, et al. Bone morphogenetic protein signaling by hemojuvelin regulates hepcidin expression. Nat Genet. 2006;38:531–9.
56. Lin L, Valore EV, Nemeth E, Goodnough JB, Gabayan V, Ganz T. Iron transferrin regulates hepcidin synthesis in primary hepatocyte culture through hemojuvelin and BMP2/4. Blood. 2007;110:2182–9.
57. Wang RH, Li C, Xu X, Zheng Y, Xiao C, Zerfas P, et al. A role of SMAD4 in iron metabolism through the positive regulation of hepcidin expression. Cell Metab. 2005;2:399–409.
58. Babitt JL, Zhang Y, Samad TA, Xia Y, Tang J, Campagna JA, et al. Repulsive guidance molecule (RGMa), a DRAGON homologue, is a bone morphogenetic protein co-receptor. J Biol Chem. 2005;280:29820–7.
59. Truksa J, Peng H, Lee P, Beutler E. Bone morphogenetic proteins 2, 4, and 9 stimulate murine hepcidin 1 expression independently of Hfe, transferrin receptor 2 (Tfr2), and IL-6. Proc Natl Acad Sci USA. 2006;103:10289–93.
60. Xia Y, Yu PB, Sidis Y, Beppu H, Bloch KD, Schneyer AL, et al. Repulsive guidance molecule RGMa alters utilization of bone morphogenetic protein (BMP) type II receptors by BMP2 and BMP4. J Biol Chem. 2007;282:18129–40.
61. West Jr AP, Bennett MJ, Sellers VM, Andrews NC, Enns CA, Bjorkman PJ. Comparison of the interactions of transferrin receptor and transferrin receptor 2 with transferrin and the hereditary hemochromatosis protein HFE. J Biol Chem. 2000;275:38135–8.
62. Levy JE, Jin O, Fujiwara Y, Kuo F, Andrews NC. Transferrin receptor is necessary for development of erythrocytes and the nervous system. Nat Genet. 1999;21:396–9.
63. Camaschella C, Roetto A, Cali A, De Gobbi M, Garozzo G, Carella M, et al. The gene TFR2 is mutated in a new type of haemochromatosis mapping to 7q22. Nat Genet. 2000;25:14–5.
64. Fleming RE, Ahmann JR, Migas MC, Waheed A, Koeffler HP, Kawabata H, et al. Targeted mutagenesis of the murine transferrin receptor-2 gene produces hemochromatosis. Proc Natl Acad Sci USA. 2002;99:10653–8.
65. Wallace DF, Summerville L, Lusby PE, Subramaniam VN. First phenotypic description of transferrin receptor 2 knockout mouse, and the role of hepcidin. Gut. 2005;54:980–6.

66. Wallace DF, Summerville L, Subramaniam VN. Targeted disruption of the hepatic transferrin receptor 2 gene in mice leads to iron overload. Gastroenterology. 2007;132:301–10.
67. Knisely AS, Gelbart T, Beutler E. Molecular characterization of a third case of human atransferrinemia. Blood. 2004;104:2607.
68. Trenor III CC, Campagna DR, Sellers VM, Andrews NC, Fleming MD. The molecular defect in hypotransferrinemic mice. Blood. 2000;96:1113–18.
69. Piperno A, Girelli D, Nemeth E, Trombini P, Bozzini C, Poggiali E, et al. Blunted hepcidin response to oral iron challenge in HFE-related hemochromatosis. Blood. 2007;110:4096–100.
70. Crawford DH, Fletcher LM, Hubscher SG, Stuart KA, Gane E, Angus PW, et al. Patient and graft survival after liver transplantation for hereditary hemochromatosis: implications for pathogenesis. Hepatology. 2004;39:1655–62.
71. Bralet MP, Duclos-Vallee JC, Castaing D, Samuel D, Guettier C. No hepatic iron overload 12 years after liver transplantation for hereditary hemochromatosis. Hepatology. 2004;40:762.
72. Spasic MV, Kiss J, Herrmann T, Kessler R, Stolte J, Galy B, et al. Physiologic systemic iron metabolism in mice deficient for duodenal Hfe. Blood. 2007;109:4511–17.
73. Makui H, Soares RJ, Jiang W, Constante M, Santos MM. Contribution of Hfe expression in macrophages to the regulation of hepatic hepcidin levels and iron loading. Blood. 2005;106:2189–95.
74. Feder JN, Penny DM, Irrinki A, Lee VK, Lebrón JA, Watson N, et al. The hemochromatosis gene product complexes with the transferrin receptor and lowers its affinity for ligand binding. Proc Natl Acad Sci USA. 1998;95:1472–7.
75. Lebron JA, West J, Bjorkman PJ. The hemochromatosis protein HFE competes with transferrin for binding to the transferrin receptor. J Mol Biol. 1999;294:239–45.
76. Bennett MJ, Lebron JA, Bjorkman PJ. Crystal structure of the hereditary haemochromatosis protein HFE complexed with transferrin receptor. Nature. 2000;403:46–53.
77. Giannetti AM, Bjorkman PJ. HFE and transferrin directly compete for transferrin receptor in solution and at the cell surface. J Biol Chem. 2004;279:25866–75.
78. Goswami T, Andrews NC. Hereditary hemochromatosis protein, HFE, interaction with transferrin receptor 2 suggests a molecular mechanism for mammalian iron sensing. J Biol Chem. 2006;281:28494–8.
79. Chen J, Chloupkova M, Gao J, Chapman-Arvedson TL, Enns CA. HFE modulates transferrin receptor 2 levels in hepatoma cells via interactions that differ from transferrin receptor 1-HFE interactions. J Biol Chem. 2007;282:36862–70.
80. Johnson MB, Enns CA. Diferric transferrin regulates transferrin receptor 2 protein stability. Blood. 2004;104:4287–93.
81. Robb A, Wessling-Resnick M. Regulation of transferrin receptor 2 protein levels by transferrin. Blood. 2004;104:4294–9.
82. Semenza GL. Hypoxia-inducible factor 1 (HIF-1) pathway. Sci STKE. 2007;2007:cm8.
83. Mendel GA. Studies on iron absorption. I. The relationships between the rate of erythropoiesis, hypoxia and iron absorption. Blood. 1961;18:727–36.
84. Raja KB, Simpson RJ, Pippard MJ, Peters TJ. In vivo studies on the relationship between intestinal iron (Fe3+) absorption, hypoxia and erythropoiesis in the mouse. Br J Haematol. 1988;68:373–8.
85. Nicolas G, Chauvet C, Viatte L, Danan JL, Bigard X, Devaux I, et al. The gene encoding the iron regulatory peptide hepcidin is regulated by anemia, hypoxia, and inflammation. J Clin Invest. 2002;110:1037–44.
86. Leung PS, Srai SK, Mascarenhas M, Churchill LJ, Debnam ES. Increased duodenal iron uptake and transfer in a rat model of chronic hypoxia is accompanied by reduced hepcidin expression. Gut. 2005;54:1391–5.
87. Nemeth E, Valore EV, Territo M, Schiller G, Lichtenstein A, Ganz T. Hepcidin, a putative mediator of anemia of inflammation, is a type II acute-phase protein. Blood. 2003;101:2461–3.
88. Kemna EH, Tjalsma H, Podust VN, Swinkels DW. Mass spectrometry-based hepcidin measurements in serum and urine: analytical aspects and clinical implications. Clin Chem. 2007;53:620–8.
89. Peyssonnaux C, Zinkernagel AS, Schuepbach RA, Rankin E, Vaulont S, Haase VH, et al. Regulation of iron homeostasis by the hypoxia-inducible transcription factors (HIFs). J Clin Invest. 2007;117:1926–32.
90. Kemna E, Pickkers P, Nemeth E, van der Hoeven H, Swinkels D. Time-course analysis of hepcidin, serum iron, and plasma cytokine levels in humans injected with LPS. Blood. 2005;106:1864–6.
91. Theurl I, Theurl M, Seifert M, Mair S, Nairz M, Rumpold H, et al. Autocrine formation of hepcidin induces iron retention in human monocytes. Blood. 2008;111:2392–9.
92. Yang F, Liu XB, Quinones M, Melby PC, Ghio A, Haile DJ. Regulation of reticuloendothelial iron transporter MTP1 (Slc11a3) by inflammation. J Biol Chem. 2002;277:39786–91.
93. Liu XB, Nguyen NB, Marquess KD, Yang F, Haile DJ. Regulation of hepcidin and ferroportin expression by lipopolysaccharide in splenic macrophages. Blood Cells Mol Dis. 2005;35:47–56.
94. Rivera S, Liu L, Nemeth E, Gabayan V, Sorensen OE, Ganz T. Hepcidin excess induces the sequestration of iron and exacerbates tumor-associated anemia. Blood. 2005;105:1797–802.

95. Roy CN, Mak HH, Akpan I, Losyev G, Zurakowski D, Andrews NC. Hepcidin antimicrobial peptide transgenic mice exhibit features of the anemia of inflammation. Blood. 2007;109:4038–44.
96. Shike H, Lauth X, Westerman ME, Ostland VE, Carlberg JM, Van Olst JC, et al. Bass hepcidin is a novel antimicrobial peptide induced by bacterial challenge. Eur J Biochem. 2002;269:2232–7.
97. Peyssonnaux C, Zinkernagel AS, Datta V, Lauth X, Johnson RS, Nizet V. TLR4-dependent hepcidin expression by myeloid cells in response to bacterial pathogens. Blood. 2006;107:3727–32.
98. Nguyen NB, Callaghan KD, Ghio AJ, Haile DJ, Yang F. Hepcidin expression and iron transport in alveolar macrophages. Am J Physiol Lung Cell Mol Physiol. 2006;291:L417–25.
99. Chiou PP, Lin CM, Bols NC, Chen TT. Characterization of virus/double-stranded RNA-dependent induction of antimicrobial peptide hepcidin in trout macrophages. Dev Comp Immunol. 2007;31:1297–309.
100. Sow FB, Florence WC, Satoskar AR, Schlesinger LS, Zwilling BS, Lafuse WP. Expression and localization of hepcidin in macrophages: a role in host defense against tuberculosis. J Leukoc Biol. 2007;82:934–45.
101. Nemeth E, Rivera S, Gabayan V, Keller C, Taudorf S, Pedersen BK, et al. IL-6 mediates hypoferremia of inflammation by inducing the synthesis of the iron regulatory hormone hepcidin. J Clin Invest. 2004;113:1271–6.
102. Kawabata H, Tomosugi N, Kanda J, Tanaka Y, Yoshizaki K, Uchiyama T. Anti-interleukin 6 receptor antibody tocilizumab reduces the level of serum hepcidin in patients with multicentric Castleman's disease. Haematologica. 2007;92:857–8.
103. Wrighting DM, Andrews NC. Interleukin-6 induces hepcidin expression through STAT3. Blood. 2006;108:3204–9.
104. Pietrangelo A, Dierssen U, Valli L, Garuti C, Rump A, Corradini E, et al. STAT3 is required for IL-6-gp130-dependent activation of hepcidin in vivo. Gastroenterology. 2007;132:294–300.
105. Verga Falzacappa MV, Vujic SM, Kessler R, Stolte J, Hentze MW, Muckenthaler MU. STAT3 mediates hepatic hepcidin expression and its inflammatory stimulation. Blood. 2007;109:353–8.
106. Lee P, Peng H, Gelbart T, Beutler E. The IL-6- and lipopolysaccharide-induced transcription of hepcidin in HFE-, transferrin receptor 2-, and beta 2-microglobulin-deficient hepatocytes. Proc Natl Acad Sci USA. 2004;101:9263–5.
107. Rivera S, Gabayan V, Ganz T. In chronic inflammation, there exists an IL-6 independent pathway for the induction of hepcidin. ASH Annu Meet Abstr. 2004;104:3205.
108. Bekri S, Gual P, Anty R, Luciani N, Dahman M, Ramesh B, et al. Increased adipose tissue expression of hepcidin in severe obesity is independent from diabetes and NASH. Gastroenterology. 2006;131:788–96.
109. Krijt J, Vokurka M, Chang KT, Necas E. Expression of Rgmc, the murine ortholog of hemojuvelin gene, is modulated by development and inflammation, but not by iron status or erythropoietin. Blood. 2004;104:4308–10.
110. Constante M, Wang D, Raymond VA, Bilodeau M, Santos MM. Repression of repulsive guidance molecule C during inflammation is independent of Hfe and involves tumor necrosis factor-alpha. Am J Pathol. 2007;170:497–504.
111. Sheikh N, Dudas J, Ramadori G. Changes of gene expression of iron regulatory proteins during turpentine oil-induced acute-phase response in the rat. Lab Invest. 2007;87:713–25.
112. Krantz SB, Goldwasser E, Jacobson LO. Studies on erythropoiesis. XIV. The relationship of humoral stimulation to iron absorption. Blood. 1959;14:654–61.
113. Vokurka M, Krijt J, Sulc K, Necas E. Hepcidin mRNA levels in mouse liver respond to inhibition of erythropoiesis. Physiol Res. 2006;55:667–74.
114. Pak M, Lopez MA, Gabayan V, Ganz T, Rivera S. Suppression of hepcidin during anemia requires erythropoietic activity. Blood. 2006;108:3730–5.
115. Papanikolaou G, Tzilianos M, Christakis JI, Bogdanos D, Tsimirika K, MacFarlane J, et al. Hepcidin in iron overload disorders. Blood. 2005;105:4103–5.
116. Origa R, Galanello R, Ganz T, Giagu N, Maccioni L, Faa G, et al. Liver iron concentrations and urinary hepcidin in beta-thalassemia. Haematologica. 2007;92:583–8.
117. Adamsky K, Weizer O, Amariglio N, Breda L, Harmelin A, Rivella S, et al. Decreased hepcidin mRNA expression in thalassemic mice. Br J Haematol. 2004;124:123–4.
118. Breda L, Gardenghi S, Guy E, Rachmilewitz EA, Weizer-Stern O, Adamsky K, et al. Exploring the role of hepcidin, an antimicrobial and iron regulatory peptide, in increased iron absorption in {beta}-thalassemia. Ann N Y Acad Sci. 2005;1054:417–22.
119. Gardenghi S, Marongiu MF, Ramos P, Guy E, Breda L, Chadburn A, et al. Ineffective erythropoiesis in beta-thalassemia is characterized by increased iron absorption mediated by down-regulation of hepcidin and up-regulation of ferroportin. Blood. 2007;109:5027–35.
120. Kattamis A, Papassotiriou I, Palaiologou D, Apostolakou F, Galani A, Ladis V, et al. The effects of erythropoetic activity and iron burden on hepcidin expression in patients with thalassemia major. Haematologica. 2006;91:809–12.

121. Kearney SL, Nemeth E, Neufeld EJ, Thapa D, Ganz T, Weinstein DA, et al. Urinary hepcidin in congenital chronic anemias. Pediatr Blood Cancer. 2007;48:57–63.
122. Weizer-Stern O, Adamsky K, Amariglio N, Levin C, Koren A, Breuer W, et al. Downregulation of hepcidin and haemojuvelin expression in the hepatocyte cell-line HepG2 induced by thalassaemic sera. Br J Haematol. 2006;135:129–38.
123. Tanno T, Bhanu NV, Oneal PA, Goh SH, Staker P, Lee YT, et al. High levels of GDF15 in thalassemia suppress expression of the iron regulatory protein hepcidin. Nat Med. 2007;13:1096–101.

Supplementary Reference List

1. Meynard D, Kautz L, Darnaud V, Canonne-Hergaux F, Coppin H, Roth MP. Lack of the bone morphogenetic protein BMP6 induces massive iron overload. Nat Genet. 2009;41:478–81.
2. Andriopoulos Jr B, Corradini E, Xia Y, et al. BMP6 is a key endogenous regulator of hepcidin expression and iron metabolism. Nat Genet. 2009;41:482–7.
3. Du X, She E, Gelbart T, et al. The serine protease TMPRSS6 is required to sense iron deficiency. Science. 2008;320:1088–92.
4. Silvestri L, Pagani A, Nai A, De Domenico I, Kaplan J, Camaschella C. The serine protease matriptase-2 (TMPRSS6) inhibits hepcidin activation by cleaving membrane hemojuvelin. Cell Metab. 2008;8:502–11.
5. Finberg KE, Heeney MM, Campagna DR, et al. Mutations in TMPRSS6 cause iron-refractory iron deficiency anemia (IRIDA). Nat Genet. 2008;40:569–71.
6. Ramos E, Kautz L, Rodriguez R, et al. Evidence for distinct pathways of hepcidin regulation by acute and chronic iron loading in mice. Hepatology. 2011;53:1333–41.
7. Corradini E, Meynard D, Wu Q, et al. Serum and liver iron differently regulate the bone morphogenetic protein 6 (BMP6)-SMAD signaling pathway in mice. Hepatology. 2011;54:273–84.
8. Bartnikas TB, Andrews NC, Fleming MD. Transferrin is a major determinant of hepcidin expression in hypotransferrinemic mice. Blood. 2011;117:630–7.
9. Kautz L, Meynard D, Monnier A, et al. Iron regulates phosphorylation of Smad1/5/8 and gene expression of Bmp6, Smad7, Id1, and Atoh8 in the mouse liver. Blood. 2008;112:1503–9.
10. Fourth Congress of the International BioIron Society (IBIS) Biennial World Meeting (BioIron 2011) May 22–26, 2011, Sheraton Vancouver Wall Centre Hotel, Vancouver, BC, Canada. Am J Hematol. 2011;86:E1–E150.
11. Murphy AT, Witcher DR, Luan P, Wroblewski VJ. Quantitation of hepcidin from human and mouse serum using liquid chromatography tandem mass spectrometry. Blood. 2007;110:1048–54.
12. Ganz T, Olbina G, Girelli D, Nemeth E, Westerman M. Immunoassay for human serum hepcidin. Blood. 2008;112:4292–7.
13. Swinkels DW, Girelli D, Laarakkers C, et al. Advances in quantitative hepcidin measurements by time-of-flight mass spectrometry. PLoS One. 2008;3:e2706.
14. Kroot JJ, Kemna EH, Bansal SS, et al. Results of the first international round robin for the quantification of urinary and plasma hepcidin assays: need for standardization. Haematologica. 2009;94:1748–52.
15. Butterfield AM, Luan P, Witcher DR, et al. A dual-monoclonal sandwich ELISA specific for hepcidin-25. Clin Chem. 2010;56:1725–32.
16. Sasu BJ, Li H, Rose MJ, Arvedson TL, Doellgast G, Molineux G. Serum hepcidin but not prohepcidin may be an effective marker for anemia of inflammation (AI). Blood Cells Mol Dis. 2010;45:238–45.
17. Bansal SS, Abbate V, Bomford A, et al. Quantitation of hepcidin in serum using ultra-high-pressure liquid chromatography and a linear ion trap mass spectrometer. Rapid Commun Mass Spectrom. 2010;24:1251–9.

Chapter 10
Erythroid Iron Metabolism

Prem Ponka and Alex D. Sheftel

Keywords Erythrocyte • Erythropoiesis • Globin • Heme • Hemoglobin • Red blood cell • Reticulocyte

1 Introduction

Iron is indispensable for the proper functioning of virtually all cells in the body. However, red blood cells, which contain approximately 80% of organismal iron, have a particularly intimate relationship with this precious metal. It is safe to say that the iron content of erythroid progenitors (e.g., BFU-Es; please see below) is infinitesimal compared to the amount of iron in mature erythrocytes that contain approximately 12×10^8 atoms per cell [1]; hence, the circulating red blood cells hold heme iron in a 20 mM "concentration." Since the developing red cells acquire iron only from diferric transferrin, which carries iron in plasma in about 3 μM concentrations, they have the capacity to increase this concentration 7,000-fold. Based on the value of 2.5 μg non-heme Fe per 100 mL erythrocytes [2], non-heme iron concentrations in erythrocytes are ~40,000-fold lower than those of heme iron. Additionally, the efficacy with which immature red blood cells convert transferrin-borne iron into hemoglobin iron is amazingly high [3, 4]. In the experience of these authors, reticulocytes (immediate progenitors of mature red cells) take up roughly 10 pmol Fe/10^6cells/h from diferric transferrin, corresponding to 6×10^6 atoms Fe/cell/h. Considering the above value of 12×10^8 atoms Fe per erythrocyte, it takes approximately 200 h (or 8.3 days) for iron to accumulate in total erythrocyte hemoglobin. This interval is slightly longer than the average erythroid cell maturation time (~5–6 days) but, since iron uptake by reticulocytes is probably somewhat slower than in bone marrow erythroblasts, the agreement is remarkably close. It needs to be pointed out that the rate with which iron is removed from the circulation by the developing erythroid cells is, under normal conditions, identical to the rate with which iron is released from macrophages following phagocytosis of senescent

P. Ponka, M.D., Ph.D. (✉)
Departments of Physiology and Medicine, Lady Davis Institute for Medical Research, Jewish General Hospital, McGill University, Montreal, QC H3T 1E2, Canada
e-mail: prem.ponka@mcgill.ca

A.D. Sheftel, Ph.D.
University of Ottawa, Ottawa Heart Institute, Ottawa, ON, Canada

G.J. Anderson and G. McLaren (eds.), *Iron Physiology and Pathophysiology in Humans*, Nutrition and Health, DOI 10.1007/978-1-60327-485-2_10,

erythrocytes and hemoglobin catabolism by heme oxygenase 1. This very important aspect of iron metabolism is discussed in Chapter 11.

The fact that all hemoglobin iron is transported from transferrin [5] and that this delivery system operates so efficiently, leaving mature erythrocytes with comparably negligible amounts of non-heme iron, indicates that the iron transport machinery in erythroid cells is part and parcel of the heme biosynthetic pathway. It seems reasonable to propose that the evolutionary forces that led to the development of highly hemoglobinized erythrocytes also dramatically affected numerous aspects of iron metabolism in developing erythroid cells, making them unique in this regard.

The hemoglobin molecule is uniquely suited for the transport of oxygen from the lungs to peripheral tissues without oxidation of its heme[1] (a complex of protoporphyrin IX with ferrous iron) groups and to facilitate the return of carbon dioxide from the tissues back to the lungs [6, 7]. In adult humans, the two primary units of the molecule, the $\alpha\beta$ dimers, associate to form the $\alpha_2\beta_2$ tetramer. Each chain is non-covalently bound to a single heme molecule that sits in a hydrophobic pocket. Since the ferrous iron of each heme group can bind a single oxygen molecule, the hemoglobin tetramer can reversibly bind and transport four molecules of oxygen. In addition to transporting oxygen and carbon dioxide, hemoglobin transports nitric oxide (NO) to tissues where this gaseous molecule plays an important vasodilatory role. Two mechanisms have been proposed to explain this process: (1) oxygen-linked allosteric delivery of NO from *S*-nitrosylated hemoglobin; it has been proposed that NO forms an adduct with cysteine (93) in the β-chain of oxyhemoglobin, forming *S*-nitrosohemoglobin [8], and (2) a nitrite reductase activity of deoxygenated hemoglobin that reduces nitrite to NO and vasodilates blood vessels along the physiological oxygen gradient [9]. Free hemoglobin in the bloodstream is very rapidly catabolized and can be toxic. Hence, one important function of erythrocytes is to prolong the hemoglobin's life span up to 120 days (in humans). Moreover, encasement within erythrocytes allows attainment of a remarkably high hemoglobin concentration of about 5 mM. It is likely that this is the maximal concentration of hemoglobin that, under normal conditions, can be reached in erythrocytes, since "hyperchromic" erythrocytes can be found only in patients with spherocytosis when red blood cells lose their biconcave shape [10].

Hemoglobin synthesis occurs using three independent but stringently coordinated pathways: globin synthesis, which is erythroid specific; heme synthesis that requires protoporphyrin IX synthesis; and the supply of iron from plasma transferrin to mitochondrial ferrochelatase. The two latter ubiquitous pathways are dramatically upregulated in developing red blood cells. One of the goals of this chapter is to convince its readers that in erythroid cells, and only in these cells, the path of iron from transferrin to ferrochelatase and protoporphyrin IX biosynthesis are highly integrated and are, in fact, essential components comprised by one metabolic pathway. Hemoglobin synthesis occurs in the developing red blood cells in the bone marrow in a process known as erythropoiesis that will be briefly discussed below.

2 Erythropoiesis

The average adult's blood contains about 24 trillion (2.4×10^{13}) erythrocytes with a wet weight of approximately 2.4 kg. Red blood cells are produced at a rate of 2.3×10^6 cells/s by a dynamic and exquisitely regulated process that is an integral part of the development of all blood cells, hematopoiesis. In humans, hematopoiesis occurs in the bone marrow of the adult and in the liver of the developing fetus. In addition to the bone marrow, the spleens of mice and rats are also important sites of

[1] Heme is ferroprotoporphyrin IX; hemin is ferric protoporphyrin IX. In this chapter, the term heme is used as a generic expression denoting no particular iron oxidation state.

erythropoiesis. The mature erythrocyte is the product of complex and highly regulated cellular and molecular processes that initiates at the level of the hematopoietic stem cells which have the potential to develop into all morphologically and functionally distinct blood cells. Stem cells, which are present in hematopoietic tissues in very small numbers (<0.01%), are self-renewing, slowly cycling cells that express receptors for stem cell factor (SCF) also known as c-kit receptor (tyrosine-kinase type). Although the regulation of stem cell proliferation and commitment is poorly understood, SCF and some other hematopoietic growth factors seem to be involved in the regulation. The process of commitment is characterized by restriction in the stem cell differentiation capacity, leading to the formation of progenitor cells that differentiate along one lineage [11–13].

Progenitor cells committed toward the erythroid lineage cannot be distinguished by morphologic criteria, but their existence and characteristics can be inferred from their capacity to generate colonies of hemoglobinized cells in vitro [11]. The earliest functionally detectable erythroid precursor is known as the BFU-E (burst-forming unit, erythroid), an early descendant of the hematopoietic stem cell. The BFU-E is detected by its capacity to generate multi-clustered colonies ("erythroid bursts") of hemoglobin-containing cells when marrow is incubated in semisolid medium in the presence of granulocyte macrophage colony-stimulating factor (GM-CSF), interleukin 3 (IL-3), and erythropoietin. BFU-Es are relatively insensitive to erythropoietin both in vitro (requiring a high concentration of the hormone to generate the bursts of erythropoietic colonies) and in vivo.

The BFU-E in turn further develops to yield a class of more mature erythroid precursors, termed CFU-E (colony-forming units, erythroid). These cells are detected by virtue of their capability in cell culture to generate a small cluster of erythroid cells, which mature all the way to erythrocytes. The proliferative capacity of CFU-Es is limited to four or five cell divisions, generating 16–32 progeny red cells. Virtually all CFU-Es are proliferating, and they have an absolute requirement for erythropoietin to maintain viability, undergo cell division and, namely, to differentiate into proerythroblasts.

The first morphologically recognizable erythroid element is the proerythroblast, which is the immediate progeny of a CFU-E. Maturation of the proerythroblast to the circulating red cell involves four to five cell divisions; production of characteristic red cell proteins (hemoglobin, enzymes, and cytoskeletal proteins), surface antigens, and metabolic machinery; loss of replicative capacity and eventually of the nucleus itself; loss of organelles and acquisition of characteristic red cell morphologic features. The proerythroblast stage is succeeded by the basophilic erythroblast. This erythroblast is basophilic because of the high concentration of cytoplasmic ribosomes that accumulate in preparation for the onset of hemoglobin synthesis, which already occurs in these cells at a relatively low rate. The next cell, polychromatophilic erythroblast, displays increasingly deep staining for hemoglobin and a progressive decrease in the concentration of cytoplasmic ribosomes. Cell division continues until the stage of orthochromatic erythroblast in which hemoglobin synthesis continues on relatively stable ribosome-globin mRNA complexes. Extrusion of nuclei from the orthochromatic erythroblasts leads to the formation of reticulocytes. These non-nucleated cells still contain active globin-synthesizing polyribosomes as well as mitochondria that produce heme. At this stage, the reticulocytes are released into the circulation. During the first 24–36 h of circulation in the blood, the reticulocyte is transformed into the mature erythrocyte [14, 15]. The maturation of reticulocytes, which is not fully understood, is characterized by a progressive decrease in the number of polyribosomes and mitochondria, loss of hemoglobin synthetic capacity, loss of transferrin receptor 1 (TfR1), as well as by a decrease in size, and assumption of the biconcave disk shape [14, 15]. During the period of mitochondrial loss, Bcl-X(L), an anti-apoptotic protein that accumulates during erythroblast differentiation and maintains mitochondrial membrane integrity, demonstrated progressive decreases and changes consistent with deamidation [16]. Interestingly, two groups recently reported a role for a Bcl-2 family member, Nix (also called Bnip3L), in the regulation of erythroid maturation through mitochondrial autophagy. $Nix^{-/-}$ mice developed anemia with reduced mature erythrocytes and a compensatory expansion of erythroid precursors. Erythrocytes in the peripheral blood of $Nix^{-/-}$ mice exhibited mitochondrial retention and reduced life span in vivo [17]. Additionally, mitochondria are depolarized in wild type but not Nix-deficient reticulocytes, a feature that appears to be required for the selective incorporation of mitochondria into autophagosomes [18]. Johnstone and her coworkers [19–22] and Blanc et al. [23] showed that reticulocytes lose their TfR1 by "shedding." The loss of TfRs seems to be preceded by the formation of multivesicular bodies containing encapsulated receptors. Fusion of multivesicular bodies with the plasma membrane leads to release of vesicles (exosomes), containing receptors whose extracellular domain is positioned externally, into the circulation. It is unknown how the above processes are triggered, but it is tempting to speculate that reaching a critical concentration of hemoglobin in reticulocytes represents a signal for their activation.

It is remarkable that, although three different and totally distinct pathways are involved in hemoglobin synthesis, virtually no intermediates, i.e., globin chains, intermediates of PPIX synthesis or iron, accumulate in the developing erythroblasts and reticulocytes. This is achieved, at least in part, by a series of negative and positive feedback mechanisms in which heme plays a crucial role. In general, in erythroid cells heme inhibits cellular iron acquisition (reviewed in [5, 24, 25]) and, consequently, heme synthesis, and is essential for the synthesis of globin. The effect of heme on its own synthesis and iron metabolism will be discussed later; here we shall briefly describe the role of heme in globin synthesis. Numerous reports indicate that heme stimulates globin gene transcription and is probably involved in promoting some other aspects of erythroid differentiation. Hemin treatment of erythroid precursors leads to a rapid accumulation of globin mRNA, whereas heme deficiency leads to a decrease in globin mRNA levels [26–30]. These heme-mediated effects likely involve the negative transcriptional regulator Bach1 which functions as a repressor of the Maf recognition elements (MARE, present in the β-globin locus control regions [LCR]) by forming antagonizing heterodimers with small Maf family proteins. Heme positively regulates the β-globin gene expression by blocking the interaction of Bach1 with the MARE in the LCR. This allows the binding of the transcription factor NF-E2p18/Mafk within this region, resulting in β-globin transcription [31, 32].

It has long been known that the translation of globin in intact reticulocytes and their lysates is dependent on the availability of heme [33–37]. Heme deficiency inhibits protein synthesis in part through activation of the heme-regulated inhibitor (HRI). HRI is a cyclic AMP-independent protein kinase which specifically phosphorylates the α-subunit of eukaryotic initiation factor 2 (eIF-2α). Phosphorylation of eIF-2α blocks initiation of protein synthesis. Heme regulates eIF-2α in the other direction by binding to and inhibiting HRI through the formation of disulfide bonds, possibly between two HRI subunits. Disulfide bond formation reverses the inhibition of globin synthesis seen during heme deficiency (reviewed in [37]). The expression of HRI seems to be confined to erythroid cells and, hence, HRI plays an important physiological role in the translation of globin and probably other proteins synthesized in erythroid cells.

In conclusion, in erythroid cells iron is not only the substrate for the synthesis of hemoglobin but also participates in its regulation. The iron protoporphyrin complex appears to enhance globin gene transcription, is essential for globin translation, and supplies the prosthetic group for hemoglobin assembly. Moreover, heme may be involved in the expression (at transcriptional as well as translational levels) of numerous other erythroid-specific proteins.

3 Iron Metabolism and Heme Synthesis in Erythroid Cells

In vertebrates, erythroid cells have by far the greatest need for iron which is used for hemoglobin synthesis with remarkable efficiency and speed [5, 24]. On a per-cell basis, the rate of heme synthesis in the erythron (According to Steadman's Medical Dictionary, Erythron = "the total mass of circulating red blood cells, and that part of the hematopoietic tissue from which they are derived") is at least an order of magnitude higher than in the liver, the second highest heme producer in the organism. Such an exceptionally high capacity of immature erythroid cells to synthesize heme is primarily a result of the unique control of iron metabolism as well as the distinct enzyme of heme biosynthesis, 5-aminolevulinic acid synthase (ALA-S). Because of such an intimate link between iron metabolism and heme synthesis in hemoglobin-synthesizing cells, an overview of this process has to be included in this chapter.

3.1 Overview of Heme Synthesis

Current mechanistic aspects of heme biosynthesis have been thoroughly described in numerous review articles and books [5, 24, 25, 38–40]. It is well established that the synthesis of heme involves eight enzymes, four of which are cytoplasmic and four which are mitochondrial; all of which are encoded by nuclear genes. The first step occurs in the mitochondria and involves condensation of succinyl CoA and glycine to form ALA, a reaction catalyzed by ALA synthase (ALA-S) (Fig. 10.1). The next four biosynthetic steps take place in the cytosol. ALA dehydratase (ALA-D) converts two molecules of ALA to a monopyrrol porphobilinogen (PBG). Two subsequent enzymatic steps convert four molecules of PBG into the cyclic tetrapyrrole uroporphyrinogen III which is then decarboxylated to form coproporphyrinogen III. The final three steps of the biosynthetic pathway, including the insertion of Fe^{2+} into protoporphyrin IX by ferrochelatase, occur in the mitochondria (Fig. 10.1).

All enzymes of the mammalian heme pathway have been cloned and crystallized [5, 24, 38–40]. The genes encoding these enzymes reside on different chromosomes. There are two different genes for the first pathway enzyme, ALA-S. One of these is expressed ubiquitously (ALA-S1, or housekeeping ALA-S) and is encoded on chromosome 3 [42], while the expression of the other is specific to erythroid cells (ALA-S2, or erythroid ALA-S) and is encoded on the X chromosome [43]. These two genes are responsible for the occurrence of ubiquitous and erythroid-specific mRNAs for ALA-S and, consequently, two corresponding isoforms of the enzyme. No tissue-specific isozyme is known for ALA-D but there are subtle differences in 5′ untranslated regions (UTRs) in housekeeping and erythroid ALA-D mRNAs [44]. PBG deaminase (PBG-D) exists in two isoforms, one being present in all cells while the other is expressed only in erythroid cells [45]. However, these isoforms arise from differential splicing of a single gene and from two mRNAs which differ solely in their 5′ ends. There is no evidence that the ubiquitous and the erythroid enzymes would be different in the rest of the pathway. However, variations in mRNAs, caused by the alternative use of the two polyadenylation signals have been reported for ferrochelatase [46]. Interestingly, the preferential utilization of the upstream polyadenylation signal appears to be an erythroid-specific characteristic of ferrochelatase gene expression [47]. Importantly, murine [48] and human [49] ferrochelatase were shown to contain a [2Fe-2S] cluster which seems to be essential for enzyme activity and plays either a redox or regulatory role.

3.2 Overview of Iron Metabolism

All animal cells possess an absolute requirement for iron. However, the very properties of iron that make it indispensable for cells, namely, its ability to donate and accept electrons, also make it potentially hazardous. Iron is virtually insoluble in an aqueous environment under physiological conditions and its participation in one-electron redox reactions produces harmful hydroxyl radicals (also see Chap. 18). Therefore, specialized mechanisms and molecules have evolved for the handling of iron in a soluble, nontoxic form in order that cellular and organismal requirements of this metal can be met [5, 50–57]. In higher organisms, these functions are fulfilled by a number of specialized

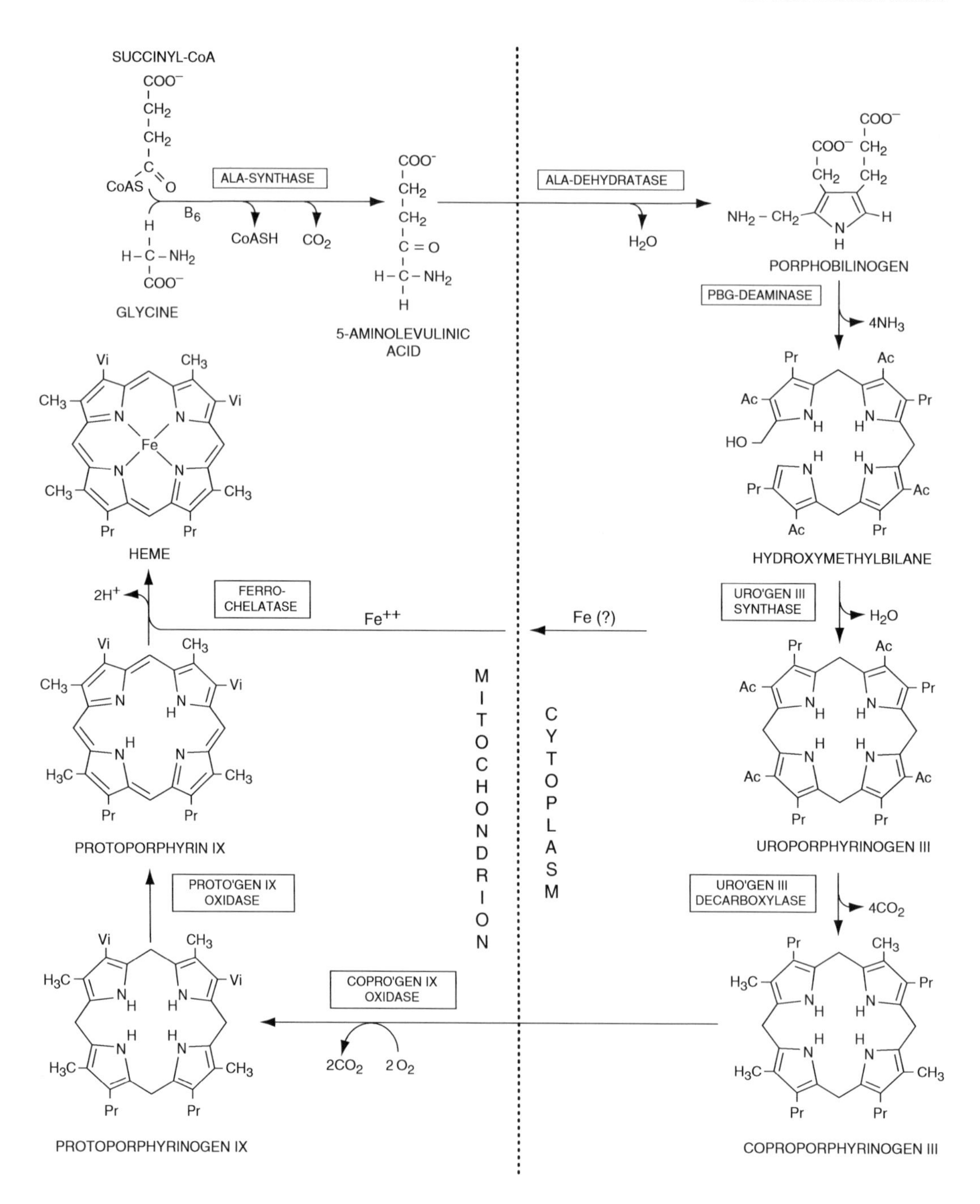

Fig. 10.1 The pathway of heme biosynthesis. *B6* pyridoxal-5′-phosphate, *URO'GEN* uroporphyrinogen, *COPRO'GEN* coproporphyrinogen, *PROTO'GEN* protoporphyrinogen, *Ac* acetate, *Pr* propionate, *Vi* vinyl (Source: Adapted from [41])

proteins, some of which are presented in Table 10.1. Moreover, an elegant regulation system exists that maintains the size of the intracellular pool of "iron-in-transit" at appropriate levels.

Iron is transported between sites of absorption, storage, and utilization by the 80 kDa plasma glycoprotein transferrin which contains two specific high-affinity iron-binding sites with an apparent stability constant for Fe(III) of approximately 10^{23} M^{-1} at neutral pH. Fe(II) does not bind specifically to these sites, and the affinity of transferrin for Fe(III) decreases progressively with decreasing

Table 10.1 Proteins involved in erythroid iron metabolism

Protein	Function	Result of deficiency	Role in erythropoiesis
ABCB7	Required for [Fe–S] on [Fe–S] proteins	XLSA with ataxia	Direct
ABCB10 (ABC-me)	Mitochondrial transport function related to heme synthesis	Unknown	Direct
ALA-S2/eALA-S	First enzyme of heme synthesis; erythroid-specific 5-aminolevulinic acid synthase	X-linked sideroblastic anemia	Direct
Ceruloplasmin (Cp)	Oxidizes exported Fe^{2+}	Neurodegeneration; hypochromic microcytic anemia	Indirect
DMT1/Nramp2	Vesicular and plasma membrane transporter for Fe^{2+}	Hypochromic microcytic anemia in mice. Hypochromic microcytic anemia with iron loading in humans	Direct
Ferritin (H and L)	Prevents Fe toxicity in all cells and during erythropoiesis	H-Ft: embryonic lethality	Indirect
Ferrochelatase	The last enzyme of heme synthesis; Fe^{2+} insertion into protoporphyrin IX	Erythropoietic protoporphyria (EPP)	Direct
Heme oxygenase-1 (HO-1)	Recycling of hemoglobin Fe	Severe anemia and inflammation	Indirect
Huntingtin (Htt) [58]	TfR1 trafficking	Hypochromic anemia in Htt-deficient zebrafish	Probably direct
IRP (1 and 2)	Fe "sensors"; bind to IREs	IRP2: brain Fe overload; microcytic anemia; EPP	Direct (IRP2)
Mitochondrial ferritin	Mitochondrial Fe storage (?)	Unknown; high expression in "ring" sideroblasts	Unknown
Mitoferrin (coded for by *SLC25A37*)	Fe transport to mitochondria	Hypochromic anemia	Direct
Sec15l1	"Vesicle docking"; required for efficient transferrin cycling	"Hemoglobin-deficit" (hbd) mice	Direct
Sideroflexin 1	Mitochondrial transport function related to Fe metabolism	Siderocytic anemia (mice)	Unknown
Steap3	Endosomal ferrireductase	Hypochromic anemia (mice)	Direct
Transferrin (Tf)	Fe(III)-carrier in plasma	Severe anemia (Fe unavailable for erythropoiesis; generalized Fe overload)	Direct
Tf receptor 1 (TfR1)	Membrane receptor for Fe_2-Tf	Embryonic lethality	Direct

pH below neutrality. Physiologically, most cells acquire iron from transferrin by a multistep process involving the specific attachment and internalization of transferrin bound to its cognate receptors (TfR1), followed by release of iron from transferrin by endosomal acidification via the v-ATPase H^+ pump (also see Chap. 7). After iron is released from transferrin, the metal is then translocated to intracellular sites of utilization or storage while the apotransferrin:TfR1 complex is recycled to the cell surface where the apotransferrin is released.

Once iron is released from transferrin within the endosome, the metal is transported across the organellar membrane by a promiscuous, divalent metal transporter, DMT1 (also known as Nramp2 or DCT1 [59, 60]). Since the form of iron bound to transferrin is in the +3 oxidation state, a reduction step, likely catalyzed by Steap3 [61], or another member of the Steap family [62], is required before transport out of the endosome. In erythroid cells, when iron reaches the outer mitochondrial membrane, it is entrapped by an as-yet-unidentified ligand and transferred across the inner membrane to ferrochelatase. The group of Paw has recently demonstrated that mammalian homologs to yeast Mrs3/Mrs4 [63, 64], dubbed "mitoferrins," are responsible for iron import, probably in its Fe^{2+} form, through the mitochondrial inner membrane [65, 66]. Mitoferrin 1 exerts its function primarily in erythroid cells, but mitoferrin 2, which is expressed ubiquitously, cannot support hemoglobinization [66]. Of considerable interest in this context is a recent discovery [67] that mitoferrin 1 physically interacts with ferrochelatase and Abcb10, a mitochondrial inner membrane ATP-binding cassette transporter highly induced during erythroid maturation. The occurrence of a mitoferrin 1-ferrochelatase complex supports the notion that erythroid iron transport consists of a relay of the metal from protein to protein, rather than simply transport of the "free" metal across membranes.

Ferritin is a ubiquitous protein whose only well-defined function is the storage of iron ([50, 51, 68, 69]; Chap. 4). Although ferritin has been postulated to act as an intermediate for heme synthesis in erythroid cells, numerous studies failed to demonstrate that ^{59}Fe from ^{59}Fe-ferritin could be incorporated into hemoglobin [70]. Particularly strong evidence that ferritin is not involved in hemoglobinization has come from a recent study of Kühn and coworkers who demonstrated that the conditional deletion of ferritin heavy chain in adult mice did not cause any decrease in hematocrit or hemoglobin levels [71]. These findings concur with the proposal that the efficient utilization of iron for hemoglobin synthesis requires a direct contact of endosomes with mitochondria [4] and the observations that the intracellular release of iron from ferritin may require its catabolism [72]; all these studies suggest limited availability of ferritin iron for metabolic purposes. These conclusions can be expanded to non-erythroid cells, since a recent report failed to provide any evidence that, in cultivated macrophages, ferritin can make its iron available for heme synthesis [73].

Arosio's laboratory has recently identified a mitochondrial ferritin isoform that can store iron within a shell of homopolymers; however, the function and regulation of this protein is not yet understood [74–76]. Notwithstanding this, it has recently been demonstrated that the overexpression of mitochondrial ferritin causes the redistribution of iron from cytosolic ferritin to mitochondrial ferritin [77] and leads to the inhibition of cancer cells growth [78]. In this context, it should be pointed out that mitochondrial ferritin shows very low expression in all tissues except for testis [74, 76]. Additionally, although mitochondrial ferritin is not expressed in normal erythroblasts, it is expressed in ring sideroblasts of patients with sideroblastic anemia [79].

3.3 Coordinate Regulation of Ferritin and TfR1 Expression

Research conducted on non-erythroid cells cultured in vitro revealed a remarkable regulation system that coordinately regulates the expression of TfR1 and ferritin and, consequently, iron uptake and storage [50–52, 80–86]. A crucial component of this control is that which senses cellular iron levels, carried out by the iron regulatory proteins, IRP-1 (formerly known as IRE-BP [the iron-responsive element-binding protein]) and IRP-2. The coordinate control of TfR1 and ferritin occurs at the posttranscriptional level, and has been mapped to regions known as iron-responsive elements (IRE) that are recognized by IRPs. IREs are nucleotide sequences that form stem-loop structures and are present in the 5′ UTRs of ferritin H- and L-chain mRNAs and in the 3′-UTRs of TfR1 mRNA [87–90]. The IRE is also present in the 5′ UTR of mRNA for erythroid specific ALA-S (ALA-S2) [91–93] (see below). A comprehensive description of this extraordinary regulatory system is beyond the scope of this chapter; however, more intensive details can be found in Chap. 3. Briefly, IRP interaction with IRE controls iron metabolism in non-erythroid cells in the following manner: When cellular iron becomes limiting, IRP-1 is recruited into the high-affinity binding state. The binding of IRP-1 to the IRE in the 5′ UTR of the ferritin mRNA represses the translation of ferritin (and ALA-S2), while an association of IRP-1 with IREs in the

3′ UTR of TfR1 mRNA stabilizes the transcript. On the other hand, the expansion of the "labile iron pool" inactivates IRP-1 and leads to a degradation of IRP-2, resulting in an efficient translation of mRNAs for ferritin and ALA-S2 (occurring in erythroid cells only) and rapid degradation of TfR1 mRNA. However, in spite of this dramatic progress in our understanding of the regulation of proteins involved in iron metabolism, fundamental questions regarding iron transport within the cell remain unanswered.

3.4 *Specific Features of TfR1 Regulation in Erythroid Cells*

Although it is generally assumed that the above mechanism coordinates regulation of iron uptake and storage by all cells, there are some features of erythroid TfR1 regulation that suggest either the existence of erythroid-specific TfRs or at least distinct regulation of their expression: (1) There is evidence from the use of monoclonal antibodies that human erythroid cells may express a unique TfR1 isoform [94]. (2) Murine erythroleukemia (MEL) cells induced to erythroid differentiation respond only slightly to iron chelating agents which stimulate TfR1 expression in proliferating non-erythroid cells. This may be explained by an observation that iron chelators only modestly increase the binding activity of IRPs in differentiating MEL cells [95]. Moreover, in hemoglobin-synthesizing MEL cells, as compared to their undifferentiating counterparts, TfR1 mRNA is virtually unaffected by high concentrations of iron [95]. (3) Heme synthesis inhibitors were shown to strongly inhibit TfR1 expression at both the mRNA and protein [95, 96] levels in nucleated erythroid cells, but had virtually no effect on the expression of TfR1 in cells that did not synthesize hemoglobin [95]. (4) Whereas in non-erythroid cells the transcriptional control of TfR1 expression in response to altered growth rates or iron deprivation does not seem to play a significant role, TfR1 is transcriptionally regulated and "overexpressed" in chick embryo erythroblasts [97] as well as MEL cells induced to synthesize hemoglobin [95]. (5) The recent findings of Schranzhofer et al. suggest that, rather than TfR1 expression being unresponsive to the activity of IRPs, the ability of the IRPs to sense incoming iron decreases, possibly by a more efficient routing of the metal to its site of use [98].

The above discussion would seem to suggest that iron metabolism in hemoglobin-synthesizing cells, in particular those that are in late stages of their maturation stage, may escape the control of the IRE/IRP system. However, two recent reports [99, 100], showing that IRP2$^{-/-}$ mice develop hypochromic microcytic anemia, suggest that IRP2 probably plays at least some role in TfR1 expression in erythroid cells. IRP2$^{-/-}$ animals have increased protoporphyrin IX levels (caused by ALA-S2 hyperexpression in their erythroid precursors) associated with a decrease of TfR1 expression that is a likely cause of anemia. In this context, it is pertinent to mention that the hematopoietic-specific transcription factor Stat5 was recently shown to regulate cellular iron uptake by erythroid cells either by transcriptionally controlling TfR1 [101] or doing so via IRP2 [102].

4 Erythroid-Specific Regulation of Iron Metabolism and Heme Synthesis

Apart from the above-described unique regulation of TfR1 in hemoglobin-synthesizing cells, several other considerations emphasize the idea of erythroid-specific metabolism of iron as well as its critical influence on heme and, consequently, hemoglobin production. As already pointed out, heme synthesis in erythroid cells accounts for about 80% of total body iron turnover and the iron in hemoglobin contains almost 80% of the total iron content of a normal adult. Also, transferrin is the only physiological source of iron for erythroid cell heme synthesis, which is best documented by observations in humans and mice with hereditary atransferrinemia. Both patients and mice with atransferrinemia have severe hypochromic microcytic anemias [5, 50] which can be explained only by the stringent dependency of hemoglobin synthesis on transferrin-bound iron. Furthermore, iron delivery to ferrochelatase, but not a step in protoporphyrin IX synthesis, is rate limiting for heme synthesis in erythroid cells [5]. In other words, either TfR1 levels or a component of the iron transport pathway from Tf-TfR1 association to delivery to the mitochondrial matrix determines the efficiency of heme production in these cells. This conclusion is based on experiments showing that transferrin-independent iron uptake (from iron-salicylaldehyde isonicotinoyl hydrazone complex) in excess of the maximum amount of iron obtained from diferric transferrin, stimulates the synthesis of heme in erythroid cells but is without effect in non-erythroid cells [103–105].

In hemoglobin-synthesizing cells, iron is specifically targeted toward mitochondria which continue to take up the metal with gluttonous appetite even when the synthesis of protoporphyrin IX is suppressed [3, 106–109]. In contrast, in non-erythroid cells, iron in excess of metabolic needs ends up in ferritin [67, 68]. Hence, some specific mechanisms and controls are involved in the transport of iron into mitochondria in erythroid cells, but the nature of these processes, besides the likely role of erythroid-specific mitoferrin 1 [65, 66], is unknown. Based on the fact that transferrin-bound iron is extremely efficiently used for hemoglobin synthesis, that iron is targeted into erythroid mitochondria, and that no cytoplasmic iron transport intermediate can be identified in erythroid cells, an alternative hypothesis of intracellular iron transport has been suggested [3–5]. This model proposes that after iron is released from transferrin in the endosome, it is passed directly from protein to protein until it reaches ferrochelatase in the mitochondrion. Such a transfer would bypass the cytosol, as the transfer of iron between proteins could be mediated by the direct interaction of the endosome with the mitochondrion (Fig. 10.2a). We have recently collected strong experimental evidence, using erythroid cells, supporting this hypothesis that is as follows: (1) iron, delivered to mitochondria via the transferrin-TfR1 pathway, is unavailable to cytoplasmic chelators [4, 119]; (2) transferrin-containing endosomes move to and contact mitochondria [4, 119]; and (3) endosomal movement is required for iron delivery to mitochondria [4, 119]. We have also established that "free" cytoplasmic iron is not efficiently used for heme biosynthesis and that the endosome–mitochondrion interaction increases chelatable mitochondrial iron [119]. Since the majority of cellular iron is processed in the mitochondria of all cells, and not just red ones, it is tempting to speculate that this direct interorganellar iron transport mechanism is ubiquitous. However, Shvartsman et al. have recently documented in a leukemia cell line that the transfer of transferrin-derived iron to mitochondria is blocked by cytosolic chelators [120]. This study quantified compartmental iron levels with the aid of iron-sensitive fluorescent chelators, which are likely to obscure intracellular distribution and may therefore overestimate iron levels.

A further distinction between red-colored cells and the others is that in erythroid cells heme synthesis is controlled by a feedback mechanism in which "uncommitted" heme inhibits iron acquisition from transferrin [121–124]. Although it is still unresolved whether heme inhibits transferrin endocytosis [122] or iron release from transferrin [124], the lack of heme as a negative feedback regulator can help in explaining the aforementioned mitochondrial iron accumulation. This may provide a clue to clinical hematologists as to the pathogenesis of mitochondrial iron accumulation in erythroblasts of patients with sideroblastic anemia. It is essential to point out that this effect of heme is specific for hemoglobin-synthesizing cells, since heme does not inhibit iron uptake in non-erythroid cells [5].

Shortly after the identification of erythroid-specific ALA-S (ALA-S2), it became obvious that most hereditary X-linked sideroblastic anemias (XLSA) cases were caused by mutations in the *ALA-S2* gene [118]. Figure 10.2b provides a schematic representation of mechanisms attributed to XLSA: decreased PPIX formation, slightly increased iron uptake, and substantial accumulation of iron in MtF.

However, there is a certain proportion of patients with hereditary sideroblastic anemia who exhibit autosomal recessive inheritance. Recently, Guernsey et al. [125] described that at least some such patients have a defect in the gene encoding the erythroid-specific mitochondrial carrier protein, SLC25A38. They demonstrated that this transporter is important for the biosynthesis of heme in eukaryotes and conjectured that this protein may be translocating glycine into mitochondria [125]. Needless to say, defects in a putative mitochondrial glycine transporter would be expected to generate a phenotype identical to that seen in patients with defects in ALA-S2 (Fig. 10.2b). It is tempting to speculate that in erythroid cells a common control mechanism, which regulates acquisition of the

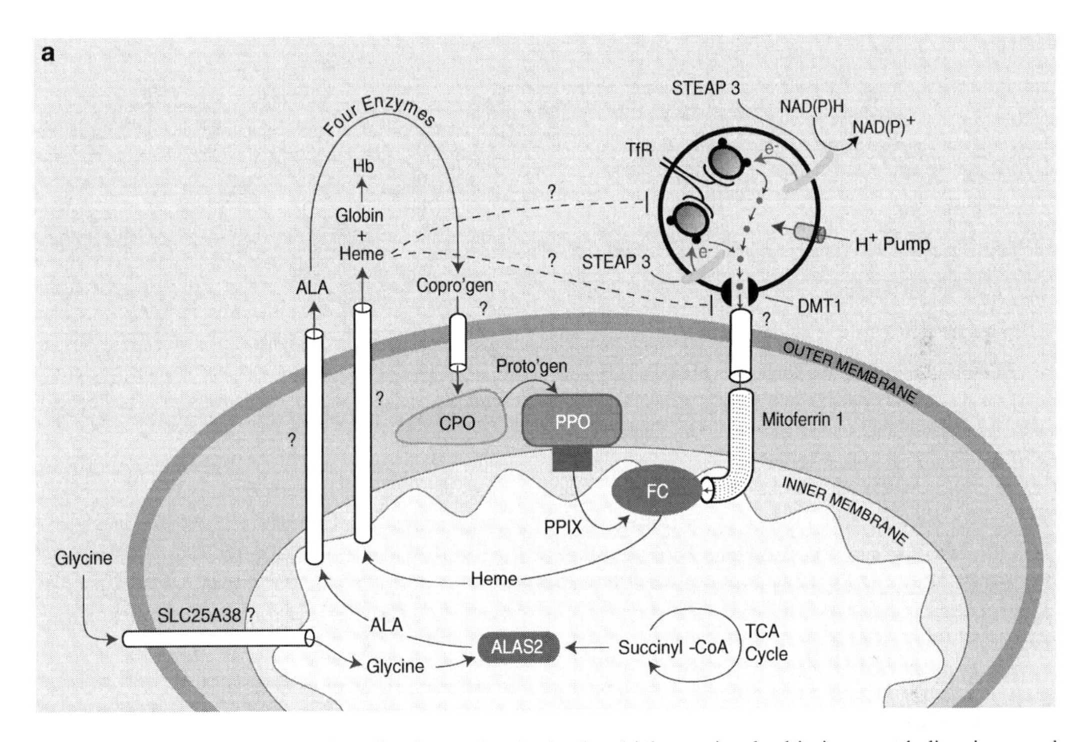

Fig. 10.2 Schematic representation of endosomal and mitochondrial steps involved in iron metabolism in normal erythroid cells (**a**) or those with inhibited heme synthesis (**b**). Iron is released from transferrin within endosomes by a combination of Fe^{3+} reduction by Steap3 (likely when it is still bound to TfR1 [110]) and a decrease in pH (~pH 5.5); following this, Fe^{2+} is transported through the endosomal membrane by DMT1. The post-endosomal path of iron in the developing red blood cells remains elusive or is, at best, controversial. It has been commonly accepted that a low-molecular-weight intermediate chaperones iron in transit from endosomes to mitochondria and other sites of utilization; however, this much sought iron-binding intermediate has never been identified. In erythroid cells, more than 90% of iron must enter mitochondria, since ferrochelatase (*FC*), the enzyme that inserts Fe^{2+} into protoporphyrin IX, resides on the inner leaflet of the inner mitochondrial membrane. Recent research supports the hypothesis that in erythroid cells, a transient mitochondrion–endosome interaction is involved in iron translocation to its final destination. It has been proposed that coproporphyrinogen (Copro'gen; please note that its generation is indicated in Fig. 10.1) is transported into mitochondria by either peripheral-type benzodiazepine receptors [111–113] or ABCB6 [114]. Neither the mechanisms nor the regulation of heme transport from mitochondria to globin polypeptides is known; however, it has been proposed that a carrier protein, heme-binding protein 1 (gene: *HEBP1*), is involved in this process [115–117]. (**b**) Pathological-ringed sideroblasts (iron loaded mitochondria surrounding the nucleus) can arise in patients with defective ALAS2 or SLC25A38 (a putative importer of glycine into erythroid mitochondria) because (**a**) heme, a negative regulator of iron uptake, is deficient; (**b**) iron is specifically targeted to erythroid mitochondria; (**c**) mitochondrial iron cannot be adequately utilized due to lack of PPIX and accumulates in MtF; (**d**) iron normally exits erythroid mitochondria only after being inserted into PPIX [5, 118]. *Hb* hemoglobin, *CPO* coprporphyrinogen oxidase, *PPO* protoporphyrinogen oxidase

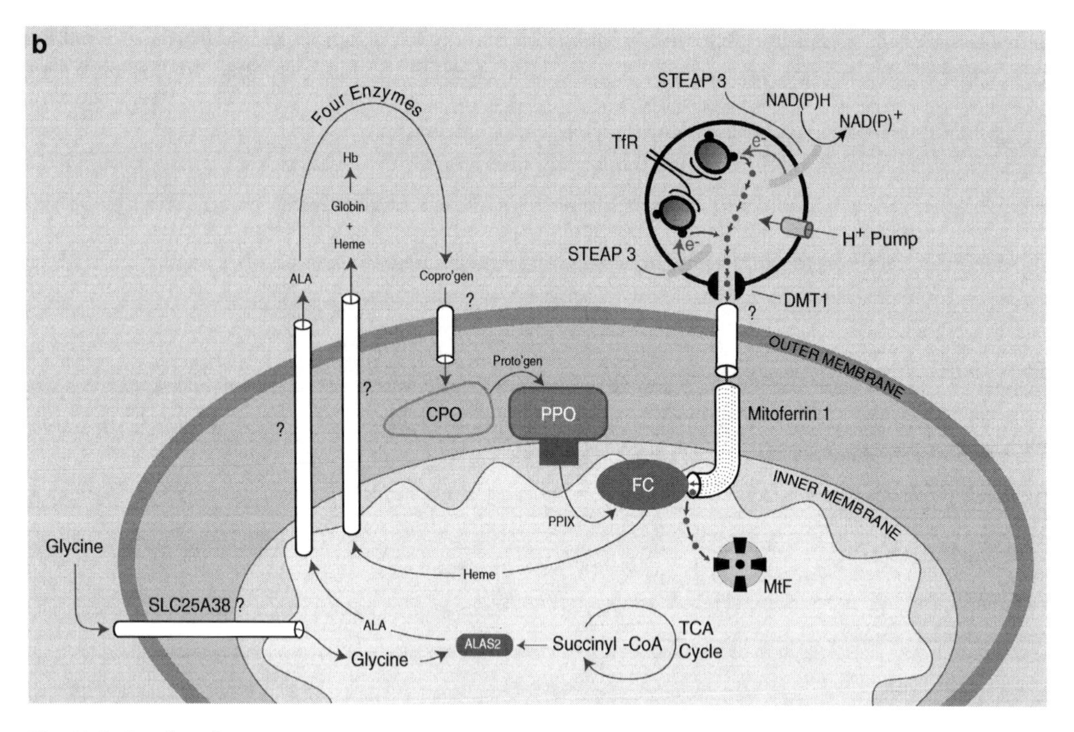

Fig. 10.2 (continued)

two substrates for heme synthesis (iron and glycine), exists. It needs to be pointed out that there are sideroblastic anemias not associated with heme synthesis defects. These conditions, which usually accompany one subtype (RARS) of myelodysplastic syndrome, are outside the scope of this chapter and are discussed elsewhere in this monograph (Chap. 16).

When discussing erythroid-specific ALA-S, there is a need to bring up an interesting and conceptually important development. Until recently, all reported mutations in ALA-S2 were shown to cause XLSA. However, Whatley et al. [126] described several families with ALA-S2 deletions resulting in frameshifts that lead to replacement or deletion of the 19–20 C-terminal residues of the enzyme. Prokaryotic expression studies showed that both mutations markedly increased ALA-S2 activity. These gain-of-function mutations caused a formerly undisclosed form of X-linked dominant protoporphyria, characterized by a high level of zinc-PPIX in erythrocytes; this symptom is reminiscent of erythropoietic protoporphyria caused by ferrochelatase defects in which there is accumulation of free PPIX. The authors explain this finding as indicating that the rate of ALA formation is increased to such an extent that the insertion of Fe^{2+} into PPIX by ferrochelatase becomes rate limiting for heme synthesis. It must be pointed out that this limitation is not ferrochelatase activity, which the authors later point out is in excess of the demands of hemoglobin synthesis, but due to the unavailability of iron for insertion into PPIX. The accumulation of zinc-PPIX is thus caused by a limitation of iron for erythroid heme synthesis, as extensively documented earlier [103–105].

Finally, as already mentioned, erythroid-specific ALA-S is uniquely regulated in erythroid cells. ALA-S2 mRNA contains an IRE in its 5′ UTR that is responsible for the translational induction of ALA-S2 protein by iron [91–93]. This means that in erythroid cells, the rate-limiting and, thus, controlling step in heme synthesis is not the production of ALA but the availability of iron. Moreover, heme has no inhibitory effect on either the activity or synthesis of ALA-S2 [5]. Furthermore, whereas heme inhibits the import of ALA-S1 into mitochondria, it does not inhibit mitochondrial import of erythroid-specific ALA-S [127]. Finally, ALA-S2 enzyme, but not ALA-S1 protein, has been found to associate with succinyl CoA synthetase in mitochondria [128].

5 Integrated View: The Availability of Iron Controls Hemoglobinization

Erythropoiesis is a remarkably complex process that comprises both differentiation of erythroid cells from hematopoietic progenitor cells and induction of hemoglobinization in these cells. During differentiation, the three pathways that lead to the formation of hemoglobin are either transcriptionally induced de novo (globin) or transcriptionally increased (heme synthesis enzymes and TfR1, the gatekeeper for iron entry into the cell). It can be postulated that erythroid differentiation will be associated with a change ("differentiation") in mitochondria that will allow a specific targeting of iron into this organelle; however, it is currently impossible to foresee whether such an alteration is qualitative (induction of new proteins) or simply a quantitative one. Importantly, some changes in mitochondria during erythroid differentiation have already been defined. First, the induction of ALA-S2 is associated with a decrease in the housekeeping ALA-S1 [128]. Second, the erythroid transcription factor GATA-1 has been shown to induce a mitochondrial ABC transporter termed ABCB10 (ABC-me [129, 130]) that localizes to the inner mitochondrial membrane and is postulated to transport (a) yet-to-be-identified substrate(s) from the matrix into the intermembrane space. Importantly, ABCB10 overexpression enhances hemoglobin synthesis in MEL cells [129]. Hence, it seems likely that ABCB10 mediates critical mitochondrial transport functions related to heme synthesis [129]. Notwithstanding the above, recent research has revealed that ABCB10 physically interacts with mitoferrin 1 to enhance its stability and promote mitoferrin 1-dependent mitochondrial heme biosynthesis [131]. Moreover, it can also be assumed that erythroid differentiation is associated with the induction of a heme transporter involved in the export of heme from the mitochondria to the cytosol. Furthermore, a cytosolic heme-binding protein may be needed to safely carry heme from mitochondria to globin chains but, unfortunately, very little is known about this process (Fig. 10.2).

Hence, based on the experimental evidence and above discussions, it can be proposed that one aspect of erythroid differentiation involves an "iron metabolism switch" during which the erythroid-specific pathway and control mechanisms are turned on, leading to their prevalence in erythroblasts and eventually total predominance in reticulocytes. Once all the machinery required for hemoglobin synthesis is induced, its formation is controlled by a series of fine-tuning mechanisms depicted in Fig. 10.3a. In contrast to non-erythroid cells (Fig. 10.3b), heme does not inhibit either the activity or the synthesis of ALA-S, but does inhibit cellular iron acquisition from transferrin in erythroid cells. This negative feedback is likely to explain the mechanism by which the availability of transferrin-derived iron limits the heme synthesis rate, and also clarifies why the system transporting iron to ferrochelatase operates so efficiently, leaving normally mature erythrocytes with negligible amounts of non-heme iron. Since the 5′ UTR of ALA-S2 mRNA contains an IRE, the availability of iron controls ALA-S2 translation, the rate of ALA formation and, consequently, the overall rate of heme synthesis in hemoglobin-synthesizing cells. Because heme is required for globin mRNA translation [37], the overall hemoglobin synthesis rate appears to be controlled by the capacity of erythroid cells to acquire iron from transferrin. Therefore, it is tempting to speculate that erythroid cells with their high requirement for iron, whose biologic availability is so limited, have evolved regulatory mechanisms in which iron controls hemoglobinization.

In conclusion, the regulation of heme synthesis has extensively been studied only in erythroid cells that synthesize approximately 80% of organismal heme, and in the liver, which synthesizes

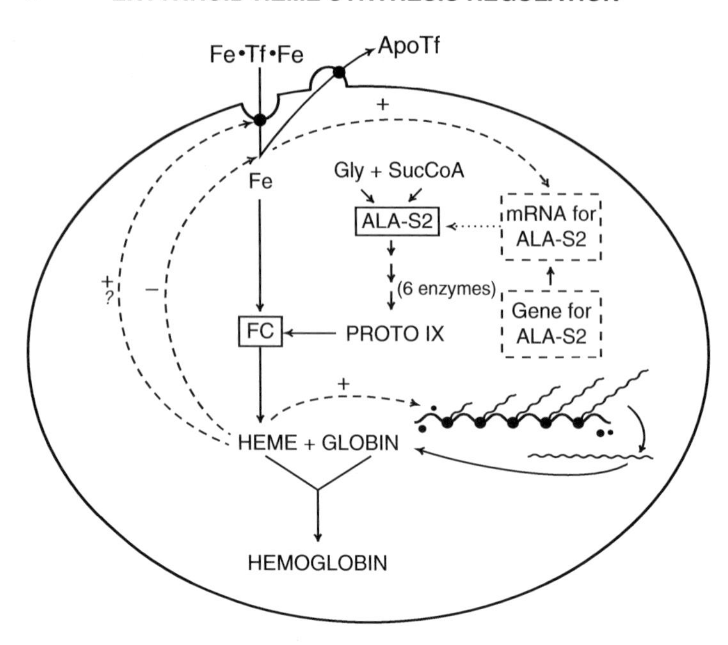

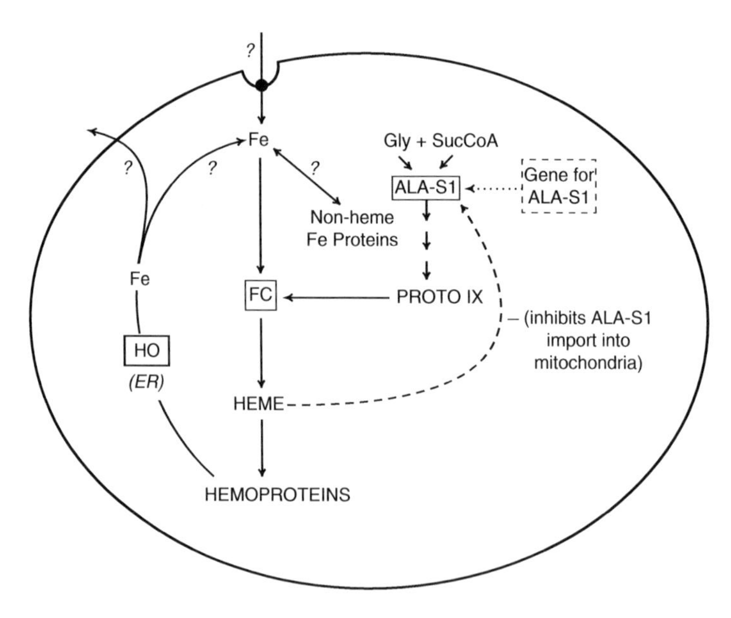

Fig. 10.3 Distinct aspects of heme synthesis regulation in erythroid (**a**) and non-erythroid (**b**) cells. Differences in iron metabolism and in genes for ALA-S likely account for the differences in the rate of heme synthesis and its regulation in erythroid cells as compared to other cells in mammals. (**a**) In erythroid cells, heme inhibits (–) cellular iron acquisition from transferrin (*Tf*) but also serves as a positive feedback regulator (+) that maintains high TfR levels [95, 96]. Heme does not inhibit either the activity or the synthesis of ALA-S2. Because the 5′-UTR of *ALA-S2* mRNA contains an IRE, the availability of iron controls ALA-S2 translation, the rate of ALA formation and, consequently, the overall rate of heme synthesis in hemoglobin-synthesizing cells. Heme is also essential for both globin transcription and translation. In contrast, (**b**) in non-erythroid cells, iron uptake is not regulated by intracellular heme and since the ubiquitous *ALA-S1* mRNA does not contain an IRE, iron availability does not control the overall heme synthesis rate. Additionally, heme represses ALA-S1 by decreasing the half-life of its mRNA [132] and by blocking enzyme's entry into mitochondria [127]. *Gly* glycine, *PROTO IX* protoporphyrin IX, *HO* heme oxygenase, *FC* ferrochelatase, *ER* endoplasmic reticulum (Source: Adapted from [5] and printed with permission)

most of the remaining heme molecules in the human body. One major difference between these two tissues is that the liver synthesizes and degrades heme continuously, whereas erythroid cells generate enormous amounts of heme that stay within the circulating erythrocytes for their life span of 120 days. Hence, the basic principles of the regulation of heme synthesis in the liver and erythroid cells are conceptually totally divergent, but are extremely well tailored for the needs of the respective tissues. Compared to the developing red blood cells, the liver produces heme with much lower rates, but in quantities that satisfy the requirements for the synthesis of hemoproteins. This is achieved by two major factors: the rate-limiting nature of ALA-S1 and the fact that the production of this enzyme is feedback inhibited by heme. In contrast, as extensively discussed above, the synthesis of heme in erythroid cells is comparable to "breaking a dam."

Acknowledgments This work was supported in part by the Canadian Institutes of Health Research. The authors also thank Ms. Rhona Rosenzweig for excellent editorial assistance. This chapter is dedicated to the memory of Herbert M. Schulman.

References

1. Ponka P, Schulman HM, Cox T. Iron metabolism in relation to heme synthesis. In: Dailey HA, editor. Biosynthesis of heme and chlorophylls. New York: McGraw-Hill Publishing Co.; 1990. p. 393–434.
2. Pennell RB. Composition of the normal human red cells. In: Bishop C, Surgenor DM, editors. The red blood cells. New York/London: Academic; 1964. p. 29–69.
3. Richardson DR, Ponka P, Vyoral D. Distribution of iron in reticulocytes after inhibition of heme synthesis with succinylacetone: examination of the intermediates involved in iron metabolism. Blood. 1996;87:3477–88.
4. Zhang AS, Sheftel AD, Ponka P. Intracellular kinetics of iron in reticulocytes: evidence for endosome involvement in iron targeting to mitochondria. Blood. 2005;105:368–75.
5. Ponka P. Tissue-specific regulation of iron metabolism and heme synthesis: distinct control mechanisms in erythroid cells. Blood. 1997;89:1–25.
6. Perutz MF. Molecular anatomy, physiology, and pathology of hemoglobin. In: Stamatoyannopoulos G, Nienhuis AW, et al., editors. The molecular basis of blood disorders. Philadelphia: WB Saunders; 1987. p. 127.
7. Hsia CC. Respiratory function of hemoglobin. N Engl J Med. 1998;338:239–47.
8. Singel DJ, Stamler JS. Chemical physiology of blood flow regulation by red blood cells: the role of nitric oxide and S-nitrosohemoglobin. Annu Rev Physiol. 2005;67:99–145.
9. Gladwin MT. Role of the red blood cell in nitric oxide homeostasis and hypoxic vasodilation. Adv Exp Med Biol. 2006;588:189–205.
10. Kutter D, Coulon N, Stirn F, Thoma M, Janecki J. Demonstration and quantification of "hyperchromic" erythrocytes by haematological analysers: application to screening for hereditary and acquired spherocytosis. Clin Lab. 2002;48:163–70.
11. Koury M, Mahmud M, Rhodes MM. Origin and development of blood cells. In: Greer JP, Foerster J, Rodgers GM, Paraskevas F, Glader B, Arber DA, Means Jr RT, editors. Wintrobe's clinical hematology. 12th ed. Philadelphia/Baltimore/New York: Wolters Kluwer/Lippincott Williams & Wilkins; 2009. p. 79–105.
12. Dessypris EN, Sawyer ST. Erythropoiesis. In: Greer JP, Foerster J, Rodgers GM, Paraskevas F, Glader B, Arber DA, Means Jr RT, editors. Wintrobe's clinical hematology. 12th ed. Philadelphia/Baltimore/New York: Wolters Kluwer/Lippincott Williams & Wilkins; 2009. p. 106–25.
13. Prchal JT. Production of erythrocytes. In: Lichtman MA, Beutler T, Kipps TJ, et al., editors. Williams hematology. 8th ed. New York: McGraw-Hill; 2010. p. 435–47.
14. Rapoport SM. The reticulocyte. Boca Raton: CRC Press; 1986.
15. Houwen B. Reticulocyte maturation. Blood Cells. 1992;18:167–86.
16. Koury MJ, Koury ST, Kopsombut P, Bondurant MC. In vitro maturation of nascent reticulocytes. Blood. 2005;105:2168–74.
17. Sandoval H, Thiagarajan P, Dasgupta SK, et al. Essential role for Nix in autophagic maturation of erythroid cells. Nature. 2008;454:232–5.
18. Zhang J, Ney PA. NIX induces mitochondrial autophagy in reticulocytes. Autophagy. 2008;4:354–6.
19. Pan BT, Johnstone RM. Fate of the transferrin receptor during maturation of sheep reticulocytes in vitro: selective externalization of the receptor. Cell. 1983;33:967–78.

20. Johnstone RM. The Jeanne Manery–Fisher Memorial Lecture 1991. Maturation of reticulocytes: formation of exosomes as a mechanism for shedding membrane proteins. Biochem Cell Biol. 1992;70:179–90.
21. Ahn J, Johnstone RM. Origin of a soluble truncated transferrin receptor. Blood. 1993;81:2442–52.
22. Johnstone RM. Revisiting the road to the discovery of exosomes. Blood Cells Mol Dis. 2005;34:214–9.
23. Blanc L, De Gassart A, Géminard C, Bette-Bobillo P, Vidal M. Exosome release by reticulocytes – an integral part of the red blood cell differentiation system. Blood Cells Mol Dis. 2005;35:21–6.
24. Ponka P. Cell biology of heme. Am J Med Sci. 1999;318:241–56.
25. Ponka P. Iron utilization in erythrocyte formation and hemoglobin synthesis. In: Templeton TM, editor. Molecular and cellular iron transport. New York/Basel: Marcell Dekker, Inc.; 2002. p. 643–77.
26. Ross J, Ikawa Y, Leder P. Globin messenger-RNA induction during erythroid differentiation of cultured leukemia cells. Proc Natl Acad Sci USA. 1972;69:3620–3.
27. Ross J, Sautner D. Induction of globin mRNA accumulation by hemin in cultured erythroleukemia cells. Cell. 1976;8:513–20.
28. Dabney BJ, Beaudet AL. Increase in globin chains and globin mRNA in erythroleukemia cells in response to hemin. Arch Biochem Biophys. 1977;179:106–12.
29. Fuchs O, Ponka P, Borova J, Neuwirt J, Travnicek M. Effect of heme on globin messenger RNA synthesis in spleen erythroid cells. J Supramol Struct Cell Biochem. 1981;15:73–81.
30. Sassa S, Nagai T. The role of heme in gene expression. Int J Hematol. 1996;63:167–78.
31. Igarashi K, Hoshino H, Muto A, et al. Multivalent DNA binding complex generated by small Maf and Bach1 as a possible biochemical basis for beta-globin locus control region complex. J Biol Chem. 1998;273:11783–90.
32. Tahara T, Sun J, Nakanishi K, et al. Heme positively regulated the expression of beta-globin at the locus control region via the transcriptional factor Bach1 in erythroid cells. J Biol Chem. 2004;279:5480–7.
33. Bruns GP, London IM. The effect of hemin on the synthesis of globin. Biochem Biophys Res Commun. 1965;18:236–42.
34. Zucker WV, Schulman HM. Stimulation of globin chain initiation by hemin in the reticulocyte cell-free system. Proc Natl Acad Sci USA. 1968;59:582–9.
35. Crosby JS, Lee K, London IM, Chen J-J. Erythroid expression of the heme-regulated eIF-2α kinase. Mol Cell Biol. 1994;14:3906–14.
36. London IM, Levin DH, Matts RL, Thomas NSB, Petryshyn R, Chen J-J. Regulation of protein synthesis. In: Boyer PD, editor. The enzymes, vol. 18. New York: Academic; 1987. p. 359–80.
37. Chen JJ. Regulation of protein synthesis by the heme-regulated elF2alpha kinase: relevance to anemias. Blood. 2007;109:2693–9.
38. Medlock AE, Dailey HA. Regulation of mammalian heme biosynthesis. In: Warren M-J, Smith AG, editors. Tetrapyrroles: birth, life and death. Austin: Landes Bioscience; 2008. p. 116–27.
39. Ajioka RS, Phillips JD, Kushner JP. Biosynthesis of heme in mammals. Biochim Biophys Acta. 2006;1763:723–36.
40. Heinemann IU, Jahn M, Jahn D. The biochemistry of heme biosynthesis. Arch Biochem Biophys. 2008;474:238–51.
41. Bishop DF, Desnick RJ. Preface. Enzyme. 1982;28:91–3.
42. Cotter PD, Drabkin HA, Varkony T, Smith DI, Bishop DF. Assignment of the human housekeeping delta-aminolevulinate synthase gene (ALAS1) to chromosome band 3p21.1 by PCR analysis of somatic cell hybrids. Cytogenet Cell Genet. 1995;69:207–8.
43. Cotter PD, Willard HF, Gorski JL, Bishop DF. Assignment of human erythroid delta-aminolevulinate synthase (ALAS2) to a distal subregion of band Xp11.21 by PCR analysis of somatic cell hybrids containing X; autosome translocations. Genomics. 1992;13:211–2.
44. Bishop TR, Miller MW, Beall J, Zon LI, Dierks P. Genetic regulation of delta-aminolevulinate dehydratase during erythropoiesis. Nucleic Acids Res. 1996;24:2511–8.
45. Beaumont C, Porcher C, Picat C, Nordmann Y, Grandchamp B. The mouse porphobilinogen deaminase gene. Structural organization, sequence, and transcriptional analysis. J Biol Chem. 1989;264:14829–34.
46. Taketani S, Nakahashi Y, Osumi T, Tokunaga R. Molecular cloning, sequencing, and expression of mouse ferrochelatase. J Biol Chem. 1990;265:19377–80.
47. Chan RY, Schulman HM, Ponka P. Expression of ferrochelatase mRNA in erythroid and non-erythroid cells. Biochem J. 1993;292:343–9.
48. Ferreira GC, Franca R, Lloyd SG, Pereira AS, Moura I, Moura JJ, et al. Mammalian ferrochelatase, a new addition to the metalloenzyme family. J Biol Chem. 1994;269:7062–5.
49. Dailey HA, Finnegan MG, Johnson MK. Human ferrochelatase is an iron–sulfur protein. Biochemistry. 1994;33:403–7.
50. Richardson DR, Ponka P. The molecular mechanisms of the metabolism and transport of iron in normal and neoplastic cells. Biochim Biophys Acta. 1997;1331:1–40.
51. Ponka P, Beaumont C, Richardson DR. Function and regulation of transferrin and ferritin. Semin Hematol. 1998;35:35–54.
52. Ponka P, Lok CN. The transferrin receptor: role in health and disease. Int J Biochem Cell Biol. 1999;31:1111–37.

53. Cairo G, Bernuzzi F, Recalcati S. A precious metal: iron, an essential nutrient for all cells. Genes Nutr. 2006;1:25–39.
54. Andrews NC, Schmidt PJ. Iron homeostasis. Annu Rev Physiol. 2007;69:69–85.
55. Andrews NC. Forging a field: the golden age of iron biology. Blood. 2008;112:219–30.
56. De Domenico I, McVey Ward D, Kaplan J. Regulation of iron acquisition and storage: consequences for iron-linked disorders. Nat Rev Mol Cell Biol. 2008;9:72–81.
57. Hentze MW, Muckenthaler MU, Galy B, Camaschella C. Two to tango: regulation of mammalian iron metabolism. Cell. 2010;142:24–38.
58. Lumsden AL, Henshall TL, Dayan S, Lardelli MT, Richards RI. Huntingtin-deficient zebrafish exhibit defects in iron utilization and development. Hum Mol Genet. 2007;16:1905–20.
59. Fleming MD, Trenor III CC, Su MA, et al. Microcytic anaemia mice have a mutation in Nramp2, a candidate iron transporter gene. Nat Genet. 1997;16:383–6.
60. Fleming MD, Romano MA, Su MA, Garrick LM, Garrick MD, Andrews NC. Nramp2 is mutated in the anemic Belgrade (b) rat: evidence of a role for Nramp2 in endosomal iron transport. Proc Natl Acad Sci USA. 1998;95:1148–53.
61. Ohgami RS, Campagna DR, Greer EL, et al. Identification of a ferrireductase required for efficient transferrin-dependent iron uptake in erythroid cells. Nat Genet. 2005;37:1264–9.
62. Ohgami RS, Campagna DR, McDonald A, Fleming MD. The Steap proteins are metalloreductases. Blood. 2006;108:1388–94.
63. Foury F, Roganti T. Deletion of the mitochondrial carrier genes MRS3 and MRS4 suppresses mitochondrial iron accumulation in a yeast frataxin-deficient strain. J Biol Chem. 2002;277:24475–83.
64. Mühlenhoff U, Stadler JA, Richhardt N, et al. A specific role of the yeast mitochondrial carriers MRS3/4p in mitochondrial iron acquisition under iron-limiting conditions. J Biol Chem. 2003;278:40612–20.
65. Shaw GC, Cope JJ, Li L, et al. Mitoferrin is essential for erythroid iron assimilation. Nature. 2006; 440:96–100.
66. Paradkar PN, Zumbrennen KB, Paw BH, Ward DM, Kaplan J. Regulation of mitochondrial iron import through differential turnover of mitoferrin 1 and mitoferrin 2. Mol Cell Biol. 2009;29:1007–16.
67. Chen W, Dailey HA, Paw BH. Ferrochelatase forms an oligomeric complex with mitoferrin-1 and Abcb10 for erythroid heme biosynthesis. Blood. 2010;116:628–30.
68. Harrison PM, Arosio P. The ferritins: molecular properties, iron storage function and cellular regulation. Biochim Biophys Acta. 1996;1275:161–203.
69. Arosio P, Ingrassia R, Cavadini P. Ferritins: a family of molecules for iron storage, antioxidation and more. Biochim Biophys Acta. 2009;1790:589–99.
70. Ponka P, Richardson DR. Can ferritin provide iron for haemoglobin synthesis? Blood. 1997;89:2611–3.
71. Darshan D, Vanoaica L, Richman L, Beermann F, Kühn LC. Conditional deletion of ferritin H in mice induces loss of iron storage and liver damage. Hepatology. 2009;50:852–60.
72. Kidane TZ, Suable E, Linder MC. Release of iron from ferritin requires lysosomal activity. Am J Physiol Cell Physiol. 2006;291:C445–55.
73. Mikhael M, Sheftel AD, Ponka P. Ferritin does not donate its iron for haem synthesis in macrophages. Biochem J. 2010;429:463–71.
74. Levi S, Corsi B, Bosisio M, et al. A human mitochondrial ferritin encoded by an intronless gene. J Biol Chem. 2001;276:24437–40.
75. Levi S, Arosio P. Mitochondrial ferritin. Int J Biochem Cell Biol. 2004;36:1887–9.
76. Santambrogio P, Biasiotto G, Sanvito F, Olivieri S, Arosio P, Levi S. Mitochondrial ferritin expression in adult mouse tissues. J Histochem Cytochem. 2007;55:1129–37.
77. Nie G, Sheftel AD, Kim SF, Ponka P. Overexpression of mitochondrial ferritin causes cytosolic iron depletion and changes cellular iron homeostasis. Blood. 2005;105:2161–7.
78. Nie G, Chen G, Sheftel AD, Pantopoulos K, Ponka P. In vivo tumor growth is inhibited by cytosolic iron deprivation caused by the expression of mitochondrial ferritin. Blood. 2006;108:2428–34.
79. Cazzola M, Invernizzi R, Bergamaschi G, et al. Mitochondrial ferritin expression in erythroid cells from patients with sideroblastic anemia. Blood. 2003;101:1996–2000.
80. Mikulits W, Schranzhofer M, Beug H, Müllner EW. Post-transcriptional control via iron-responsive elements: the impact of aberrations in hereditary disease. Mutat Res. 1999;437:219–30.
81. Pantopoulos K. Iron metabolism and the IRE/IRP regulatory system: an update. Ann N Y Acad Sci. 2004;1012:1–13.
82. Rouault TA. The role of iron regulatory proteins in mammalian iron homeostasis and disease. Nat Chem Biol. 2006;2:406–14.
83. Leipuviene R, Theil EC. The family of iron responsive RNA structures regulated by changes in cellular iron and oxygen. Cell Mol Life Sci. 2007;64:2945–55.
84. Muckenthaler MU, Galy B, Hentze MW. Systemic iron homeostasis and the iron-responsive element/iron-regulatory protein (IRE/IRP) regulatory network. Annu Rev Nutr. 2008;28:197–213.

85. Leibold EA, Munro HN. Characterization and evolution of the expressed rat ferritin light subunit gene and its pseudogene family. Conservation of sequences within noncoding-regions of ferritin genes. J Biol Chem. 1987;262:7335–41.
86. Hentze MW, Caughman SW, Rouault TA, et al. Identification of the iron-responsive element for the translational regulation of human ferritin mRNA. Science. 1987;238:1570–3.
87. Müllner EW, Kühn LC. A stem-loop in the 3 untranslated region mediates iron-dependent regulation of transferrin receptor mRNA stability in the cytoplasm. Cell. 1988;53:815–25.
88. Rothenberger S, Müllner EW, Kühn LC. The mRNA-binding protein which controls ferritin and transferrin receptor expression is conserved during evolution. Nucleic Acids Res. 1990;18:1175–9.
89. Leibold EA, Laudano A, Yu Y. Structural requirements of iron-responsive elements for binding of the protein involved in both transferrin receptor and ferritin mRNA post-transcriptional regulation. Nucleic Acids Res. 1990;18:1819–24.
90. Barton HA, Eisenstein RS, Bomford A, Munro HN. Determinants of the interaction between the iron-responsive element-binding protein and its binding site in rat L-ferritin mRNA. J Biol Chem. 1990;265:7000–8.
91. Cox TC, Bawden MJ, Martin A, May BK. Human erythroid 5-aminolevulinate synthase: promoter analysis and identification of an iron-responsive element in the mRNA. EMBO J. 1991;10:1891–902.
92. Dandekar T, Stripecke R, Gray NK, et al. Identification of a novel iron-responsive element in murine and human erythroid delta-aminolevulinic acid synthase mRNA. EMBO J. 1991;10:1903–9.
93. Melefors O, Goossen B, Johansson HE, Stripecke R, Gray NK, Hentze MW. Translational control of 5-aminolevulinate syunthase mRNA by iron-responsive elements in erythroid cells. J Biol Chem. 1993;268:5974–8.
94. Cotner T, Gupta AD, Papayannopoulou T, Stamatoyannopoulos G. Characterization of a novel form of transferrin receptor preferentially expressed on normal erythroid progenitors and precursors. Blood. 1989;73:214–21.
95. Chan RY, Seiser C, Schulman HM, Kühn LC, Ponka P. Regulation of transferrin receptor mRNA expression. Distinct regulatory features in erythroid cells. Eur J Biochem. 1994;220:683–92.
96. Hradilek A, Fuchs O, Neuwirt J. Inhibition of heme synthesis decreases transferrin receptor expression in mouse erythroleukemia cells. J Cell Physiol. 1992;150:327–33.
97. Chan LN, Gerhardt EM. Transferrin receptor gene is hyperexpressed and transcriptionally regulated in differentiating erythroid cells. J Biol Chem. 1992;267:8254–9.
98. Schanzhofer M, Schifrer M, Cabrera JA, et al. Remodeling the regulation of iron metabolism during erythroid differentiation to ensure efficient heme biosynthesis. Blood. 2006;107:4159–67.
99. Cooperman SS, Meyron-Holtz EG, Olivierre-Wilson H, Ghosh MC, McConnell JP, Rouault TA. Microcytic anemia, erythropoietic protoporphyria, and neurodegeneration in mice with targeted deletion of iron-regulatory protein 2. Blood. 2005;106:1084–91.
100. Galy B, Ferring D, Minana B, et al. Altered body iron distribution and microcytosis in mice deficient in iron regulatory protein 2 (IRP2). Blood. 2005;106:2580–9.
101. Zhu BM, McLaughlin SK, Na R, et al. Hematopoietic-specific Stat5-null mice display microcytic hypochromic anemia associated with reduced transferrin receptor gene expression. Blood. 2008;112:2071–80.
102. Kerenyi MA, Grebien F, Gehart H, et al. Stat5 regulates cellular iron uptake of erythroid cells via IRP-2 and TfR-1. Blood. 2008;112:3878–88.
103. Ponka P, Schulman HM. Acquisition of iron from transferrin regulates reticulocyte heme synthesis. J Biol Chem. 1985;260:14717–21.
104. Laskey JD, Ponka P, Schulman HM. Control of heme synthesis during Friend cell differentiation: role of iron and transferrin. J Cell Physiol. 1986;129:185–92.
105. Garrick LM, Gniecko K, Hoke JE, al-Nakeeb A, Ponka P, Garrick MD. Ferric-salicylaldehyde isonicotinoyl hydrazone, a synthetic iron chelate, alleviates defective iron utilization by reticulocytes of the Belgrade rat. J Cell Physiol. 1991;146:460–5.
106. Borová J, Ponka P, Neuwirt J. Study of intracellular iron distribution in rabbit reticulocytes with normal and inhibited heme synthesis. Biochim Biophys Acta. 1973;320:143–56.
107. Ponka P, Wilczynska A, Schulman HM. Iron utilization in rabbit reticulocytes. A study using succinylacetone as an inhibitor of heme synthesis. Biochim Biophys Acta. 1982;720:96–105.
108. Adams ML, Ostapiuk I, Grasso JA. The effects of inhibition of heme synthesis on the intracellular localization of iron in rat reticulocytes. Biochim Biophys Acta. 1989;1012:243–53.
109. Morgan EH. Chelator-mediated iron efflux from reticulocytes. Biochim Biophys Acta. 1983;733:39–50.
110. Dhungana S, Taboy CH, Zak O, Larvie M, Crumbliss AL, Aisen P. Redox properties of human transferrin bound to its receptor. Biochemistry. 2004;43:205–9.
111. Verma A, Nye JS, Snyder SH. Porphyrins are endogenous ligands for the mitochondrial (peripheral-type) benzodiazepine receptor. Proc Natl Acad Sci USA. 1987;84:2256–60.
112. Taketani S, Kohno H, Okuda M, Furukawa T, Tokunaga R. Induction of peripheral-type benzodiazepine receptors during differentiation of mouse erythroleukemia cells. A possible involvement of these receptors in heme biosynthesis. J Biol Chem. 1994;269:7527–31.
113. Rampon C, Bouzaffour M, Ostuni MA, et al. Translocator protein (18 kDa) is involved in primitive erythropoiesis in zebrafish. FASEB J. 2009;23:4181–92.

114. Krishnamurthy PC, Du G, Fukuda Y, et al. Identification of a mammalian mitochondrial porphyrin transporter. Nature. 2006;443:586–9.
115. Taketani S, Adachi Y, Kohno H, Ikehara S, Tokunaga R, Ishii T. Molecular characterization of a newly identified heme-binding protein induced during differentiation of murine erythroleukemia cells. J Biol Chem. 1998;273:31388–94.
116. Jacob Blackmon B, Dailey TA, Lianchun X, Dailey HA. Characterization of a human and mouse tetrapyrrole-binding protein. Arch Biochem Biophys. 2002;407:196–201.
117. Welch JJ, Watts JA, Vakoc CR, Yao Y, Wang H, Hardison RC, et al. Global regulation of erythroid gene expression by transcription factor GATA-1. Blood. 2004;04:3136–47.
118. Sheftel AD, Richardson DR, Prchal J, Ponka P. Mitochondrial iron metabolism and sideroblastic anemia. Acta Haematol. 2009;122:120–33.
119. Sheftel AD, Zhang AS, Brown C, Shirihai OS, Ponka P. Direct interorganellar transfer of iron from endosome to mitochondrion. Blood. 2007;110:125–32.
120. Shvartsman M, Fibach E, Cabantchik ZI. Transferrin-iron routing to the cytosol and mitochondria as studied by live and real-time fluorescence. Biochem J. 2010;429:185–93.
121. Ponka P, Neuwirt J. Regulation of iron entry into reticulocytes. I. Feedback inhibitory effect of heme on iron entry into reticulocytes and on heme synthesis. Blood. 1969;33:690–707.
122. Iacopetta B, Morgan E. Heme inhibits transferrin endocytosis in immature erythroid cells. Biochim Biophys Acta. 1984;805:211–6.
123. Ponka P, Schulman HM. Regulation of heme synthesis in erythroid cells: hemin inhibits transferrin iron utilization but not protoporphyrin synthesis. Blood. 1985;65:850–7.
124. Ponka P, Schulman HM, Martinez-Medellin J. Haem inhibits iron uptake subsequent to endocytosis of transferrin in reticulocytes. Biochem J. 1988;251:105–9.
125. Guemsey DL, Jiang H, Campagna DR, et al. Mutations in mitochondrial carrier family gene SLC25A38 cause nonsyndromic autosomal recessive congenital sideroblastic anemia. Nat Genet. 2009;41:651–3.
126. Whatley SD, Ducamp S, Gouya L, et al. C-terminal deletions in the ALAS2 gene lead to gain of function and cause X-linked dominant protoporphyria without anemia or iron overload. Am J Hum Genet. 2008;83:408–14.
127. Munakata H, Sun JY, Yoshida K, et al. Role of the heme regulatory motif in the heme-mediated inhibition of mitochondrial import of 5-aminolevulinate synthase. J Biochem. 2004;136:233–8.
128. Furuyama K, Sassa S. Interaction between succinyl CoA synthetase and the heme-biosynthetic enzyme ALAS-E is disrupted in sideroblastic anemia. J Clin Invest. 2000;105:757–64.
129. Shirhai OS, Gregory T, Yu C, Orkin SH, Weiss MJ. ABE-me: a novel mitochondrial transporter induced by GATA-1 during erythroid differentiation. EMBO J. 2000;19:2492–502.
130. Graf SA, Haigh SE, Corson ED, Shirhai OS. Targeting, import, and dimerization of a mammalian mitochondrial ATP binding cassette (ABC) transporter, ABCB10 (ABC-me). J Biol Chem. 2004;279:42954–63.
131. Chen W, Paradkar PN, Li L, Langer NB, et al. ABCB10 physically interacts with mitoferrin1 (Slc25a37) to enhance its stability and function in the erythroid mitochondria. Proc Natl Acad Sci USA. 2009;106:16263–8.
132. Hamilton JW, Bement WJ, Sinclair PR, Sinclair JF, Alcedo JA, Wetterhahn KE. Heme regulates hepatic 5-aminolevulinate synthase mRNA expression by decreasing mRNA half-life and not by altering its rate of transcription. Arch Biochem Biophys. 1991;289:387–92.

Chapter 11
Iron and the Reticuloendothelial System

Günter Weiss

Keywords Anemia of chronic disease • Erythrophagocytosis • Heme oxygenase • Infection • Inflammation • Interferon-gamma • Interleukins • Macrophages • Monocyte

1 Introduction

Iron is an essential component for all cells and higher eukaryotes due to its central role for oxygen transport, electron transport during mitochondrial respiration, in forming a prosthetic group for central metabolic enzymes, and for the regulation of transcription via its role as the central component of ribonucleotide reductase [1–3]. Moreover, iron catalyzes the formation of hydroxyl radicals, which then modulate the binding affinity of critical transcription factors such as HIF-1 or NF-κB and thus affect the gene expression during inflammation [4]. Therefore, both iron overload and iron deficiency exert subtle effects on essential metabolic pathways and on the growth, proliferation, and differentiation of organisms. The tight control of iron homeostasis is thus a pre-requisite to maintain a sufficient supply of iron for essential metabolic pathways while avoiding the metals' detrimental effects on tissue damage via radical formation. In addition, iron is centrally involved in the regulation of cellular immune function, while on the other hand, it is an essential nutrient for invading microbes and tumor cells. Specifically, microorganisms have evoked multiple strategies to capture and ingest iron, which they need for proliferation, pathogenicity, and defense pathways including biofilm formation [5]. The divergent pathways by which microorganisms can acquire iron have been recently reviewed [6, 7].

While cells of the reticuloendothelial system (RES) play a key role in the control of body iron homeostasis by recycling iron and redistributing the metal to the circulation [8–10], the regulatory network between iron and immune function is of central importance for the pathophysiology and clinical course of diseases such as infections, cancer, or autoimmune disorders. The control over iron homeostasis under these circumstances is one of the most important determinants deciding about the fate of an infectious or malignant disease [11–13].

The close interaction between iron and immunity is underscored by observations that certain immunological proteins do alter cellular iron metabolism, as described for ß2-microglobulin, HFE, a non-classical MHC-I molecule linked to the majority of cases with human hemochromatosis,

G. Weiss, M.D. (✉)
Department of Internal Medicine I, Clinical Immunology and Infectious Diseases, Medical University, A-6020 Innsbruck, Austria
e-mail: guenter.weiss@i-med.ac.at

G.J. Anderson and G. McLaren (eds.), *Iron Physiology and Pathophysiology in Humans*, Nutrition and Health, DOI 10.1007/978-1-60327-485-2_11,

tumor necrosis factor receptor (TNFR), or the natural resistance-associated macrophage protein 1 (NRAMP1). Changes in immune function thus affect iron homeostasis and vice versa [14–18].

In being a central component for all proliferating cells, iron is also a central regulator of immune cell proliferation and function. Lymphocytes are central regulatory cells of specific immunity, which determine the functional activity of cells of the RES. Thus, a sufficient capacity of these cells to proliferate and differentiate is a pre-requisite for normal immune function [19–21]. Iron has turned out to be centrally involved in these processes, and thus, lymphocytes have evoked different mechanisms to acquire iron even under conditions when iron availability is limited. All lymphocyte subsets, which include B- and T-lymphocytes and natural killer (NK) cells, are dependent on transferrin/transferrin receptor (TfR)-mediated iron uptake, while a blockade of this pathway leads to diminished proliferation and differentiation of these cells [22]. Accordingly, mitogenic stimuli, such as phytohemagglutinin, increase TfR surface expression on B and T cells [20]. However, the lymphocyte subsets differ in their dependence on transferrin-mediated iron uptake. Accordingly, the induction of experimental iron overload in rats resulted in a shift in the ratio between T-helper (CD4+) and T-suppressor/cytotoxic T cells (CD8+), with a relative expansion of the latter [13]. Moreover, even T-helper (Th) subset responds differently to iron perturbations [23]. It is well established that there are several subsets of CD4+ T-helper cell that exist in man, termed type 1 (Th1), Th2, Th17, and Treg, each of which produces a typical set of cytokines that regulate different immune effector functions and that cross-react with each other. Th1-derived cytokines such as interferon (IFN)- or tumor necrosis factor (TNF)-ß activate macrophages, thus contributing to the formation of pro-inflammatory cytokines, such as TNF-α, IL-1, or IL-6, and the induction of cytotoxic immune effector mechanisms of macrophages including nitrogen and oxygen radical formation. By contrast, Th2 cells produce IL-4, IL-5, IL-9, and IL-13, which in part exert anti-inflammatory actions via inhibition of various macrophage functions and which activate immune cells involved in allergic reactions (e.g., IgE-secreting B cells). In addition, CD4+ cells with immune-suppressive properties have been described, consisting of T-regulatory $CD25^{+}CD4^{+}$ cells (T_{REG}). Treg inhibit T-cell activation in a cell contact-dependent manner, whereas Th3 cells produce cytokines with immune-deactivating effects such as transforming growth factor (TGF-ß) or IL-10, respectively [24]. In contrast, Th17 cells are major determinants of pro-inflammatory immune effector pathways, thus being centrally involved in many autoimmune diseases [25].

While Th1 clones are very sensitive to treatment with anti-TfR antibodies, resulting in inhibition of their DNA synthesis, Th2 cells are resistant to this procedure. This is partly attributed to the fact that Th2 clones exhibit larger chelatable iron storage pools than Th1 cells. Thus, Th1-mediated immune effector pathways are much more sensitive to changes in iron homeostasis *in vivo* [23]. The latter can partly be referred to a direct regulatory effect of iron on the activity of the central regulatory Th1 cytokine IFN-γ [26].

In contrast, circulating monocytes and tissue macrophages, being the central components of the RES, are differentiating cells and the major regulatory components of iron homeostasis and iron storage within the body.

2 Monocyte/Macrophage Iron Homeostasis

The body's daily demands for iron are estimated between 20 and 30 mg of the metal [1, 27, 28]. While only 10% of this need is compensated by iron absorption from the duodenum, the majority of iron originates from monocytes/macrophages pointing to the essential role of these cells for the recycling of iron from senescent erythrocytes, iron redistribution to the circulation, and thus for the maintenance of body iron homeostasis. In addition, in being cells of the RES monocytes/macrophages play important regulatory roles for iron homeostasis under inflammatory conditions.

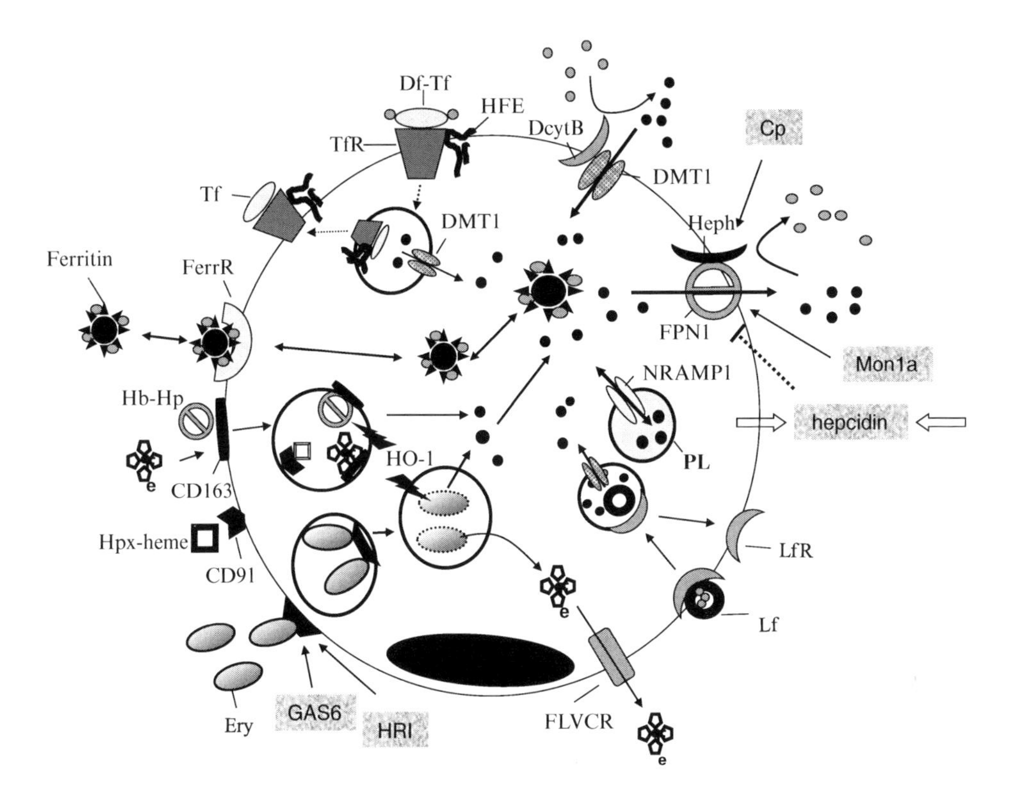

Fig. 11.1 Pathways for iron acquisition and iron release in moncoytes/macrophages and their exogenous modulation. Monocytes/macrophages can acquire iron via transferrin (*Tf*), transferrin receptor (*TfR*)-mediated endocytosis, directly via divalent metal transporter 1 (*DMT1*), by uptake of iron-loaden lactoferrin (*Lf*) via lactoferrin receptors (*LfR*), after binding of hemoglobin–haptoglobin (*Hb–Hp*) complexes or free heme to the CD163 surface receptor, binding of hemopexin–heme (*hpx–heme*) complexes to CD91, both with subsequent endocytosis, respectively, and finally via erythrophagocytosis which requires previous surface binding of erythrocytes and subsequent erythrocytosis. Erythrophagocytosis appears to be positively affected by the growth-arrest-specific gene 6 (*Gas6*) and heme-regulated eIF2alpha kinase (*HRI*), both of which are also produced and released by macrophages. Iron is recycled from erythrocytes and hemoglobin complexes following heme oxygenase-1 (*HO-1*)-mediated degradation of heme. However, heme may be directly released from degraded erythrocytes and then exported by the heme iron exporter, Vlfcr. In addition, the major iron secretory pathway from macrophages is controlled by the protein ferroportin (*FPN1*). The expression and transport capacity of this protein is negatively controlled by the acute-phase peptide hepcidin (from exogenous, liver, and endogenous, macrophage/moncoyte, sources; indicated by arrows) and positively affected by ceruloplasmin (*CP*) and Mon1a. Finally, macrophages express ferritin receptors which may mediate the uptake or release of iron-loaded ferritin from these cells. Ferric iron (*gray*) is reduced on the cell surface by duodenal cytochrome b oxidase (*DcytB*), while ferrous iron (*black*) is oxidized after ferroportin (*FP*)-mediated iron export by the membrane-bound ferroxidase hephaestin (*Heph*)

They are mainly responsible for a diversion of intercellular iron traffic leading to iron retention in the RES and a limited availability of the metal for erythropoiesis, thus leading to the development of anemia of chronic disease, also termed as anemia of inflammation [29–31].

Due to these multiple roles of iron homeostasis in health and disease, monocytes/macrophages have evoked multiple pathways to acquire, store, and recirculate iron (Fig. 11.1) [32, 33]. While the "classical" mammalian iron uptake mechanism via transferrin/TfR-mediated endocytosis is the preferred pathway in lymphocytes and is also used in monocytes/macrophages [34], in addition, the latter have the capacity to acquire the metal by different pathways, some of which are only found in these cells [35].

Specifically, the divalent metal transporter (DMT1) is highly expressed on monocytes and macrophages. DMT1 has initially been identified in rat duodenum where it pumps ferrous iron and other divalent metals by a hydrogen-coupled mechanism across the cell membrane [36]. DMT1 is also of importance for the transfer of iron from the endosome into the cytoplasm [37], and mutations of this transporter are associated with the development of iron deficiency anemia (for a review, see [38]). DMT1 cooperates with a membrane-bound ferric reductase, termed DcytB, which reduces ferric to ferrous iron at the outer membrane which is a pre-requisite to be transported by DMT1[39]. Accordingly, human macrophages take up iron chelates with a higher efficacy than diferric transferrin by a temperature-dependent but pH-independent process [40, 41].

Immune cells also express receptors for H-ferritin [42] which may be involved in the iron turnover and exchange between lymphocytes, hepatocytes, and macrophages [43]. However, the exact functions as well as the regulation of ferritin receptor expression are still elusive. Nonetheless, a recent study identified a novel receptor, Scara5, which mediates the endocytic uptake of ferritin into cells [44]. Opposite, monocytes and macrophages have been shown to act as the major source for serum ferritin [45]. Importantly, different cell types have contrasting preferences for L- or H-chain ferritin [46].

The iron-binding protein, lactoferrin (Lf), is a member of the transferrin family and is able to capture iron while at the same time it exerts distinct effects on immune function by regulating the proliferation and activation of lymphocytes, NK cells, and monocytes [47]. Lf is taken up after binding to specific receptors, Lf receptors (LfR), which are found at the cell surface of macrophages. The Lf/LfR complex is internalized most likely via an endocytotic process [48]. Once taken up, Lf plays regulatory roles within macrophages by modulating on the one hand iron-mediated cytotoxic effector mechanisms against intracellular pathogens via the formation of hydroxyl radicals, while on the other hand, apo-Lf protects macrophages from membrane peroxidation [47]. Evidence for the existence of Lf recirculation in macrophages was provided by experiments, demonstrating that Lf is released from macrophages which have been incubated in Lf-free media [47].

In addition, macrophages can acquire iron via phagocytosis of hemoglobin (Hb)–haptoglobin (Hp) complexes. The CD163 receptor is responsible for this endocytic process leading to removal of Hp–Hb complexes – but not of free Hp or Hb – from the circulation. CD163 is a member of the scavenger receptor cysteine-rich domain family. Interestingly, recent evidence also suggests that CD163 can take up hemoglobin even in the absence of Hp [49]. In addition, monocytes express CD91, the hemopexin receptor, which takes up heme captured by the heme-binding protein, hemopexin, resulting in induction of heme oxygenase-1 (HO-1) with subsequent iron accumulation in monocytes [50]. This receptor has been previously known as the low-density lipoprotein receptor-related protein (LRP)/CD91. Accordingly, endosomal uptake of the heme–hemopexin receptor resulted in lysosomal degradation of hemopexin [50].

Once iron enters the cells, it is either stored within ferritin, utilized upon incorporation into iron-containing enzymes, or exported and transferred to the circulation. An estimate of 10–20% percent remains in the labile iron pool which is important for macrophage effector functions and the regulation of cellular iron homeostasis [33, 51]. The latter is maintained at the posttranscriptional/translational level by interaction of cytoplasmic proteins, so-called iron regulatory proteins (IRP)-1 and 2, with RNA stem-loop structures, iron-responsive elements (IRE). IREs have been identified within the 5 untranslated regions of the mRNAs coding for the central proteins for iron storage (H-chain and L-chain ferritin), iron consumption (erythroid aminolevulinic acid synthase, e-ALAS, the key enzyme in heme biosynthesis), and iron transport (ferroportin), while the mRNA coding for the major iron uptake protein, TfR, bears five IREs within its 3 untranslated region (for a review, see [1, 52, 53]). Iron deficiency in cells stimulates the binding affinity of IRPs to IREs, thus resulting in inhibition of ferritin and e-ALAS expression by blocking the formation of the translation initiation complex [54]. Conversely, binding of IRPs to the IREs within the 3 untranslated region of TfR mRNA increases the expression of this protein by prolonging TfR mRNA half-life and vice versa.

Apart from iron availability, the binding affinities of IRPs are further regulated by NO, hydrogen peroxide, superoxide anion, and hypoxia, conditions and compounds which are found during inflammatory processes [55–60].

Importantly, macrophages/monocytes release iron, which is essential for iron recirculation from degraded erythrocytes. HFE is a non-classical MHC class I molecule which is ubiquitously expressed on cells [61] and which has been found to be mutated in 80% of patients suffering from hereditary hemochromatosis [61–63]. This mutation results in loss of HFE function by disrupting its interaction with ß2-microglobulin. Evidence for the importance of such a condition on iron homeostasis and immune function has been provided earlier by the observation that ß2-microglobulin knockout mice not only develop parenchymal iron overload but also lack CD8+ cells [64, 65]. HFE interacts with transferrin-mediated iron uptake by forming a stoichiometric complex with TfR which lowers the affinity of TfR for iron-loaded transferrin, and thus, HFE affects cellular iron homeostasis [66–69]. Interestingly, HFE also serves as a ligand for the gamma–delta T-cell receptor which may be of importance for enterocyte differentiation [70]. In addition, HFE blocks the iron release from macrophages [71], as transfection of macrophages from hemochromatosis patients carrying the C282Y mutation with wild-type HFE resulted in an increased iron content of these cells [72].

The cellular mechanism underlying these observations may be traced back to modulation of iron release by ferroportin [71, 73]. Ferroportin (also called Ireg1 or SLC11A3) is a transmembrane iron exporter that is implicated in the basolateral transfer of ferrous iron to the circulation. Ferroportin is highly expressed in enterocytes, Kupffer cells, and spleen macrophages [74–76]. Mutations of ferroportin lead to iron overload disorders [77]. After being transported by ferroportin, ferrous iron undergoes oxidation which is maintained by the membrane-bound ferroxidase hephaestin, and ferric iron released from cells is the incorporation into transferrin for subsequent transport within the circulation [78]. Accordingly, monocytes from patients with hemochromatosis and from Hfe–/– mice have been found to be iron depleted [79, 80]. In addition, recent evidence demonstrates that monocytes and macrophages from Hfe–/– mice produce high amounts of the siderophore-capturing peptide lipocalin-2 (Lcn2), leading to macrophage/monocyte iron export [81]. As a consequence, such mice are protected from infection with the intracellular pathogen *Salmonella typhimurium* which has a high need for iron [81].

3 Erythrophagocytosis

Likewise, the major pathway by which monocytes and macrophages acquire iron is via erythrophagocytosis. After a mean half-life of 120 days, senescent erythrocytes express increased quantities of phosphatidylserine residues on their surfaces which are then recognized by macrophage/monocyte surface receptors, leading to attachment of erythrocytes and subsequent phagocytosis. Macrophages have been shown to phagocytose about three times as many erythrocytes as monocytes [82, 83]. Within the macrophage phagolysosome, the erythrocytes are degraded utilizing heme which then undergoes further degradation, a step which is controlled by the enzyme HO-1. This reaction yields iron, biliverdin, and carbon monoxide. Iron can be then shifted into the cytoplasm and incorporated into iron proteins or stored within ferritin [82–84].

Erythrophagocytosis is the most effective iron recycling system in the body, and 90% of the iron needed for erythropoiesis originates from this pathway. As ferroportin is the only known transmembrane iron exporter, the efficacy of iron recycling is linked to the expression of this protein [85]. Overexpression of ferroportin resulted in increased release and export of iron originating from phagocytosed erythrocytes [9]. Accordingly, ferroportin expression appears to be regulated by erythrophagocytosis. During early stages of erythrophagocytosis, an induction of HO-1 and ferroportin expression is observed which is associated with the release of heme into the cytoplasm [86].

At later stages, ferroportin expression is reduced which was linked to iron export and reduction of the cytoplasmic iron pool [8]. This can be also due to several alternative pathways. First, increased systemic iron availability induces the expression of the master iron regulatory peptide hepcidin in the liver [87–89]. Hepcidin is released into the circulation and binds on ferroportin when exposed on the cell surface which results in ferroportin internalization and ubiquitin-mediated degradation of this protein [90, 91]. This results in a blockage of iron export and monocyte/macrophage iron retention. Accordingly, exposure of macrophages to hepcidin reduced the recycling of iron following erythrophagocytosis and significantly decreased the release of non-heme iron from these cells [9, 92]. In addition, both DMT1 and NRAMP1 (see below) are important for iron recycling from senescent erythrocytes by shuttling iron from the phagolysosome to the cytoplasm [10, 93].

Monocytes and macrophages can also release heme via the surface receptor Flvcr (feline leukemia virus subgroup C receptor) [94]. Flvcr appears to be essential for erythropoiesis. In addition, Flvcr is highly expressed in duodenum, the kidney, and also in mononuclear cells and CD34+ progenitor cells. Macrophages, in which *Flvcr* had been deleted neonatally, did not differ from control macrophages in respect to their metabolic response to challenges with iron salts. However, when *Flvcr*-deficient cells were exposed to immunoglobulin-coated red blood cells, they presented with increased intracellular ferritin concentrations. This indicated first, a role of the heme export protein *Flvcr* in erythrophagocytosis, and secondly that heme derived from senescent erythrocytes is not fully degraded within the macrophages. Thus, a certain amount of this molecule is directly released into the circulation via this heme export protein (Fig. 11.1). This could be an important salvage pathway in case of increased erythrocyte degradation as it may occur during hemolytic anemia, malaria, or toxic/inflammatory erythrocyte damage, which exceeds the heme degradation capacity of macrophages. Alternatively, this mechanism could also prevent paralysis of the phagocytosis machinery and innate immune response by an overwhelming erythrophagocytosis and a subsequent drastic increase in intracellular iron concentration. However, heme released by macrophages will be captured by hemopexin in the circulation and redistributed to monocytes/macrophages which take up these complexes via the CD91 pathway. Nonetheless, this data provide evidence for another iron exit pathway from macrophages and monocytes which might be regulated by cytokines under inflammatory condition, thus contributing to macrophage iron retention, hypoferremia, and development of the anemia of chronic disease [29].

Finally, ferroportin expression and thus monocyte iron trafficking are controlled by additional pathways. First, the copper containing ferroxidase ceruloplasmin is not only responsible for the oxidation of ferrous iron but, in doing so, it stabilizes ferroportin [95]. Moreover, recent evidence suggests that a conserved gene, named *Mon1a*, coding for a protein with 556 amino acid residues, is involved in the trafficking of ferroportin within macrophages and thus in iron recycling from these cells [96]. Mice carrying a mutation in *Mon1a* present with increased spleen iron deposition, and accordingly, siRNA-mediated deletion of *Mon1a* resulted in decreased surface expression of ferroportin and macrophage iron retention. This may be referred to the importance of *Mon1a* in membrane trafficking. Accordingly, the expression of several cytokines, such as IL-6 and IL-12, was impaired in LPS-stimulated macrophages in which *Mon1a* expression had been reduced upon siRNA-mediated knockdown. This is of interest in respect to the putative mechanism underlying *Mon1a* action. Of note, two distinct splicing variants of ferroportin have recently been described which differ in their response to iron-mediated regulation [97]. Their tissue specific expression may thus impact on iron recirculation by monocytes/macrophages.

Finally, murine and human monocytes and macrophages produce considerable amounts of hepcidin [98–100]. In contrast to hepdicin expression in the liver, monocyte/macrophage hepcidin expression is not inducible by iron challenge at least in vitro. In contrast, hepcidin expression can by induced upon LPS stimulation which is referred to a TLR4-dependent mechanism [98] and independently from this by IL-6 [100] which results in induction of hepcidin transcription via STAT3-mediated activation [101–103]. Importantly, monocyte/macrophage-derived hepcidin can regulate ferroportin expression in an autocrine fashion, thus resulting in ferroportin internalization and blockage of iron export [100]. Thus, via modulating the expression of cytokine inducers of hepcidin formation in the RES, regulatory molecules, such as Mon1a, may compromise iron homeostasis of these cells [104].

The hepcidin axis is also affected by the heme-regulated eIF2alpha kinase (HRI)[105]. HRI protein is mainly produced in erythroid precursors and is also present in murine macrophages [106]. Hri–/– mice exhibited impaired macrophage maturation and a weaker anti-inflammatory response with reduced cytokine production upon LPS challenge and thus a reduced production of hepcidin. In addition, macrophages from Hri–/– mice presented with an impairment of erythrophagocytosis, providing evidence for the role of HRI in recycling iron from senescent red blood cells [105].

A similar regulatory potential has also been demonstrated for another molecule, growth-arrest-specific gene 6 (Gas6), which is released by murine erythroblasts in response to erythropoietin treatment and which enhances erythropoietin signaling toward target cells [107]. Moreover, Gas6 and its cognate receptors Tyro3, Axl, and Mertk are also expressed by macrophages, and macrophages from Gas6–/– have a reduced capacity for erythrophagocytosis. In addition, loss of Gas6 resulted in increased release of cytokines such as IL-6 or IL-1ß from macrophages [107], cytokines which may also influence the expression of hepcidin, thus affecting monocyte iron homeostasis [41, 75, 108]. This provides another line of evidence that erythropoietic signals have a strong impact on the regulation of body iron homeostasis independent of iron availability [109]. In addition to erythropoietin [110], which downregulates hepcidin expression in the liver, and the putative role of Gas6, the growth differentiation factor-15 (GDF-15), a member of the TGF-ß superfamily which is induced upon erythroblast maturation, has recently been shown to inhibit hepcidin expression, thus contributing to iron overload in patients with thalassemia [111]. It is thus tempting to speculate that erythrophagocytosis may also impact on endogenous macrophage/monocyte expression of hepcidin, thereby ensuring increased ferroportin surface exposure and an efficient iron export and recirculation. However, patients with ACD had no significant differences in circulating GDF-15 levels as compared to controls or subjects with ACD and associated true iron deficiency [112].

4 Regulation of Macrophage/Monocyte Iron Metabolism During Inflammation

Monocytes and macrophage are the conductors that orchestrate iron homeostasis in health and disease and which are at the interface between iron and immunity [11, 33, 113]. This is due to the fact that macrophages need iron to produce highly toxic hydroxyl radicals by the enzyme phagocyte oxidase (phox) [4, 114], while at the same time, macrophages are major storage sites of iron under inflammatory conditions. Cytokines and radicals produced by macrophages as well as acute-phase proteins originating from the liver affect macrophage iron homeostasis by modulating iron uptake and iron release by these cells, leading to increased iron retention within macrophages under inflammatory conditions [34, 41, 115–119]. At the same time, iron modulates macrophage effector pathways by regulating cytokine activities, the induction of the antimicrobial machinery of macrophages, and indirectly via regulating lymphocyte proliferation and activities which then affect macrophage differentiation and activation [11, 21, 120–122]. Since iron is an essential compound for microbial growth and proliferation, the control over iron homeostasis is a central factor in infection. Thus, it is not surprising that phagolysosomal proteins, such as NRAMP1, which are associated with resistance toward infections with intracellular pathogens, also act as iron transporters. NRAMP1 has been identified as an innate immunity gene which was associated with resistance toward infections with intracellular pathogens such as *Leishmania*, *Salmonella*, or *Mycobacteria* species [17, 18]. Ectopic expression of NRAMP1 in COS-1 cells modulated intracellular levels of chelatable iron but did not influence iron uptake which suggested that NRAMP1 may be rather involved in intracellular iron trafficking and mobilization of iron from intracellular vesicles [123, 124]. However, investigations of RAW264.7 macrophage cell line stably transfected with functional or non-functional NRAMP1 demonstrated that macrophages lacking functional NRAMP1 exhibited a significantly higher iron uptake via TfR and, as a consequence of this, an increased iron release mediated via increased ferroportin expression. Accordingly, as a net effect of the altered expression of iron transporters, the overall cellular iron content was lower in macrophages bearing functional NRAMP1 [124]. The attractive hypothesis that NRAMP1 expression may confer resistance toward intracellular pathogens either by limiting the availability of iron to the microbes or by supplying iron for the formation of toxic radicals by the Haber–Weiss reaction is supported by recent findings [125] and by the observation of different immune gene expression patterns along with changes in intracellular iron distribution in cells knocked out for NRAMP1 [126–128]. Moreover, NRAMP1 is able to transport Mn(II), Zn(II), and Fe(II) most likely by a proton gradient-dependent mechanism; however, there is discrepancy as to whether the direction of such a transport is from the cytoplasm to the phagosome or vice versa and if the underlying driving force is pH dependent [129, 130]. Interestingly, NRAMP1 expression appears to be regulated by iron perturbations, with increased NRAMP1 mRNA and protein levels being observed in macrophages loaded with iron [131], which would suggest that NRAMP1 and iron metabolism may regulate each other by a feedback loop.

Therefore, alterations in immune function affect iron homeostasis and vice versa [11, 14–16].

Under inflammatory conditions, iron accumulation and retention by macrophages are controlled by cytokines and acute-phase proteins, which affect the different iron accumulation and release pathways of these cells. These immune regulators act at different stages, thus modulating the expression of critical iron genes at the transcriptional and post-transcriptional levels by IRE/IRP-dependent and independent pathways.

The cause-effective role of cytokines for systemic iron regulation was first confirmed by the observation of sustained hypoferremia in mice injected with TNF-α or IL-1 [132]. Hypoferremia was paralleled by hyperferritinemia which was traced back to transcriptional induction of ferritin expression by cytokines in cells of the RES [133, 134]. In addition, the pro-inflammatory cytokines IL-1 and IL-6 regulate ferritin expression at the translational level by a mechanism being independent from the IRP system, namely, via stimulation of a so-called acute-phase box which is located within the 5 untranslated region of ferritin mRNA [134]. However, only limited information was available on how the induction of ferritin synthesis may lead to hypoferremia and increased iron storage within monocytes/macrophages since these pro-inflammatory cytokines downregulated TfR expression [11, 118]. One possibility was referred to stimulation of erythrophagocytosis by macrophages since TNF-α treatment stimulates phagocytosis of sialidase-treated erythrocytes due to enhanced expression of C3bi (CD11b/CD18) receptors. In addition, the enhanced formation of toxic radicals during inflammatory processes will cause damage of erythrocyte membranes which makes them more susceptible for erythrophagocytosis. Accordingly, the application of sublethal dosages of TNF-α to mice resulted in a shortening of erythrocyte half-life and a faster clearance of these cells from the circulation via erythrophagocytosis [135].

Importantly, pro-inflammatory stimuli can enhance the acquisition of non-transferrin-bound iron by macrophages. IFN-γ, LPS, or TNF-α upregulate DMT1 expression and increase iron influx into activated macrophages [41] (Table 11.1).

The intriguing relationship between immunity and iron homeostasis went into a new dimension upon identification of the acute-phase protein hepcidin [88, 89, 136–138]. The observation that hepcidin deficient mice injected with turpentine did not develop hypoferremia suggested that hepcidin may be involved in the pathogenesis of ACD [139, 140]. The underlying mechanisms appear to be the induction of hepcidin expression by LPS and IL-6 while TNF-α blocks hepcidin expression by hepatocytes in vitro [136, 141]. The cause-effective role of IL-6 and hepcidin for the development of hypoferremia was confirmed by experiments demonstrating that injection of IL-6 into volunteers resulted in increased hepcidin expression and induction of hypoferremia within 24 h. In addition,

Table 11.1 Pathways for the regulation of macrophage/monocyte iron homeostasis by cytokines, acute-phase proteins, and radicals on iron homeostasis (modified from [116])

Factors	Mechanisms
TNF-α	Induces ferritin transcription which promotes iron storage within cells of the RES
	Shortage of erythrocyte half-life (TNF-α) and stimulation of erythrophagocytosis
	Inhibits hepcidin formation
IL-1	Stimulates ferritin transcription and translation, the latter by activating an "acute-phase box" within ferritin mRNA
IL-6	Induces ferritin transcription/translation (see above)
	Stimulates hepcidin formation in monocytes/macrophages
	Stimulates CD163 and increases the uptake of hemoglobin–haptoglobin complexes by macrophages
	Induces heme oxygenase and heme degradation
IFN-γ/LPS	Stimulate DMT1 synthesis and increase uptake of ferrous iron into monocytes
	Downregulate FPN-1 expression, which inhibits iron export from macrophages
	Downregulate TfR via induction of a proximal inhibitory signal
	Induce nitric oxide (NO) formation
IL-4, -10, -13	Increase TfR expression and transferrin-mediated iron uptake into inflammatory macrophages
	Stimulate ferritin translation by inactivating IRP and decreasing NO expression
	IL-10 stimulates CD163 and increases the uptake of hemoglobin–haptoglobin complexes by macrophages
	Il-10 stimulates heme oxygenase expression and heme degradation
NO	Stimulates IRP-1 binding affinity, thus blocking ferritin translation and stabilizing TfR mRNA (feedback regulation with iron by affecting NO formation via modulating iNOS expression)
	Modulates IRP-2 expresison and stability
Oxygen radicals	H_2O_2 when applied extracellularly stimulates IRP-1 activity with blocking of ferritin translation and stabilizing TfR mRNA
	Superoxide anion formed intracellularily inhibits IRP binding affinity
Hepcidin	Formed upon stimulation of mice with LPS, IL-6, TGF-ß, and bone morphogenic proteins
	Blocks iron export from macrophages
	Inhibits duodenal iron absorption
	Exerts autocrine regulation of macrophage iron export
α1-AT	Limits iron uptake by erythroid progenitor cells by interfering with TfR

Abbreviations used: *IL* interleukin, *TNF* tumor necrosis factor, *IFN* interferon, *DMT1* divalent metal transproter-1, *FPN1* ferroportin, *NO* nitric oxide, *H2O2* hydrogen peroxide, *α1-AT* alpha-1 antitrypsin

IL-6 knockout mice which were treated with turpentine in order to induce an inflammatory state did not develop hypoferremia [141]. Part of this may be referred to blockage of iron recirculation from macrophages thanks to the interaction of hepcidin with ferroportin with subsequent reduction of iron export from cells [90, 142, 143]. Accordingly, increased circulating hepcidin concentrations in serum of patients with ACD or a rat model of ACD were associated with decreased ferroportin expression along with reduced duodenal iron absorption and macrophage iron release [143]. However, the induction of hepcidin expression by cytokines is severely impaired in the presence of a concomitant iron deficiency [143–145] pointing to different hierarchies of hepcidin expression by signaling cascades induced by either iron, inflammation, hypoxia, or anemia [146].

In addition, mammalian monocytes and macrophages produce small amounts of hepcidin in response to LPS or IL-6. While the basal expression is relatively low in comparison to the amount of hepcidin produced in the liver, microbial challenges such as group A streptococci and pseudomonas aeruginosa can induce a 20–80 fold increase of hepcidin expression in these cells by a TLR4-dependent pathway [98, 147], while IL-6-mediated induction of hepcidin is mediated via STAT3 activation [101–103]. Interestingly, hepcidin released by macrophages targets ferroportin in an autocrine fashion, thereby promoting macrophage/monocyte iron accumulation during inflammatory processes [100]. This may be a fast-acting defense mechanism of the innate immune system against invading microbes [5, 12, 148]. Thereby, hepcidin targets ferroportin exposed on the cell surface, resulting in immediate blockage of iron release and thus to a reduced availability of the essential microbial nutrient iron in the circulation [5, 12].

However, effects of hepcidin on iron homeostasis appear to occur fast but only for a limited period of time. This has been confirmed by the observation that injection of LPS resulted in induction of hepcidin and development of hypoferremia, which lasted for several hours. Thereafter, serum iron concentrations returned to normal or were even higher than at baseline [149]. Thus, to ensure a sustained modulation of iron homeostasis under inflammatory conditions, a concerted action of different signals exerted by cytokines, acute-phase proteins, and hormones is mandatory [29].

A central regulatory factor which ensures a sustained iron retention in monocytes/macrophages and a reduced expression of ferroportin during inflammation is IFN-γ.

This Th1-derived cytokine IFN-γ not only induces ferritin transcription but also affects ferritin translation, which is based on activation of IRP binding affinity by the cytokine. This is in part due to stimulation of NO formation by IFN-γ [55, 56, 119] which then activates IRP-1 binding to the ferritin IRE, leading to inhibition of ferritin translation [1, 119]. However, NO exerts divergent effects on IRP-2, leading to either stabilization or degradation of this protein [150–152]. This may relate to contrasting effects of positively or negatively charged NO formulations and is determined by the iron status of the cells [153–158]. In addition, NO can also modulate ferritin expression by an IRP-independent mechanism [159]. Moreover, radicals formed during inflammatory processes such as hydrogen peroxide, superoxide anion, as well as hypoxia can modulate the binding affinities of IRPs to target IREs [57, 59, 152]. Specifically, hydrogen peroxide activates IRP-1 by a rapidly inducible process involving kinase/phosphatase signal transduction pathways resulting in post-transcriptional regulation of IRE-regulated target genes such as TfR and ferritin [1, 57, 160]. IFN-γ treatment of monocytes blocks the uptake of transferrin-bound iron via downregulation of TfR expression [11, 41, 118] which is most likely being due to induction of a proximal inhibitory factor by IFN-γ which inhibits TfR transcription. However, IFN-γ induces DMT1 expression and acts synergistically with LPS in this respect. This leads to stimulation of ferrous iron uptake into these cells and promotes their incorporation into ferritin [41]. At the same time, IFN-γ/LPS induce iron retention in macrophages by downregulating the transcriptional expression of ferroportin, thus blocking iron release from these cells [41, 75] which prolongs the blockage of ferroportin-mediated iron release initiated by monocyte/macrophage-derived hepcidin [100]. One might speculate that these two pathways act in a sequential line. Hepcidin mRNA expression in moncoytes/macrophages peaks 3 h after cytokine/LPS stimulation and then returns to baseline levels [100]. Thus, hepcidin may be part of a fast-acting innate immune effector arm aimed to prevent iron export from macrophages which is of relevance in the setting of microbial invasion, thereby reducing circulating iron concentrations and the availability of this nutrient for pathogens [12, 161]. IFN-γ/LPS then block ferroportin transcription, thus ensuring a prolonged blockage of iron export.

While anti-inflammatory cytokines such as IL-4, IL-10, or IL-13 do not affect the suppression of ferroportin mRNA expression by IFN-γ/LPS [41], treatment of murine macrophages with IL-4 and/or IL-13 prior to stimulation with IFN-γ suppresses NO formation and subsequently IRP activation which concomitantly enhances ferritin translation [162]. This has also been found to be true in human monocytic cells, THP-1, which do not express detectable amounts of iNOS [163]. Conversely, TfR mRNA levels increase following pre-treatment of IFN-γ-stimulated macrophages with the anti-inflammatory cytokines. This may be referred to IL-4/IL-13-mediated antagonization of the inhibitory signal which is induced by IFN-γ and which inhibits TfR expression by an IRP-independent pathway [162]. In addition, IL-10 and IL-6 may affect macrophage iron acquisition by stimulating the expression of hemoglobin scavenger receptor, CD163, thus promoting the uptake of hemoglobin–haptoglobin complexes into monocytic cells [164].

The role of Th2-derived cytokines for the development of hyperferritinemia under chronic inflammatory processes was confirmed by a clinical study in patients with Crohn's disease. Patients receiving therapy with human recombinant IL-10 as part of a placebo-controlled, double-blinded study developed a normocytic anemia which was preceded by a significant increase in serum ferritin levels while reticulocyte counts were not affected as compared to placebo treated controls [163]. Both anemia and hyperferritinemia resolved spontaneously within 2–4 weeks after stopping IL-10 therapy. Thus, Th2-derived cytokines may increase iron uptake via induction of TfR and CD163 but will also promote the iron storage within ferritin by activated macrophages. In addition, IL-10 stimulates HO-1 expression and activity, thus promoting iron re-utilization from phagocytosed erythrocytes, hemoglobin–haptoglobin complexes, and hemopexin-bound heme, respectively [165, 166].

In summary, pro- and anti-inflammatory cytokines and, most importantly, acute-phase proteins cooperate at multiple steps in increasing macrophage iron accumulation via stimulation of various iron acquisition pathways of these cells. At the same time, cytokines and hepcidin inhibit iron export from macrophages by downregulation of ferroportin expression, resulting in iron retention within cells of the RES and an iron-restricted erythropoiesis.

As a consequence of these processes, hypoferremia, hyperferritinema, and an iron-restricted anemia develop, termed as anemia of chronic disease (ACD) or anemia of inflammation [29, 31, 167, 168]. The iron restriction to erythroid cells is further aggravated by the action of other acute-phase proteins, such as alpha-1 antitrypsin (α1-AT), which interferes with cellular iron homeostasis in erythroid progenitor cells by competitively blocking the binding of transferrin to TfR, thus reducing TfR-mediated iron uptake [169, 170]. This points to the additional pathophysiological factors playing a role for the development of anemia of chronic disease, namely, a reduced differentiation and proliferation rate of erythroid progenitor cells and an impaired biological activity of erythropoietin. These latter mechanisms relate to the negative effects of cytokines on erythropoietin formation and activity as well as to the induction of toxic or apoptotic pathways in erythroid progenitors by these immune modulators, which are further aggravated by the reduced availability of iron [29, 133, 142, 171–173].

Thus, under conditions of chronic immune activation, the described diversion of iron occurs, resulting in hypoferremia and hyperferritinemia, the main diagnostic hallmarks for the identification of ACD [31, 168, 174, 175]. ACD is the most frequent anemia in hospitalized patients, occurring frequently in subjects suffering from chronic inflammatory disorders, such as autoimmune diseases, chronic infections, or malignancies.

Although the development of anemia is associated with detrimental effects especially in relation to cardiac function, quality of life, growth, and mental development [176], the underlying hypoferremia and the diversion of iron from the circulation may also harbor some potentially positive effects, especially when cancer or infections underlie chronic immune activation.

First, the withdrawal of iron from the circulation and its storage within the RES reduces the availability of this essential nutrient for microorganisms and tumor cells, which need the metal for their growth and proliferation. Thus, limitation of iron availability is a very effective defense strategy of the body to control the growth of pathogens [5, 12]. Moreover, the expression of iron uptake and acquisition systems of microbes or fungi has been linked to their pathogenicity [177, 178]. Accordingly, limitation of iron availability or blockade of iron uptake or recruiting pathways (siderophore systems) affects microbe survival [6, 177, 179–181]. In line with this, macrophages challenged with bacterial pathogens produce and secrete the protein lipocalin-2 which sequesters iron-loaded bacterial siderophores thus limiting their growth [81, 182–184]. Lipocalin-2 (Lcn2, 24p3) captures iron-laden microbial siderophores, thus interfering with the acquisition of siderophore-bound iron by bacteria [182]. Moreover, Lcn2 delivers siderophore-bound iron to mammalian cells, which are able to import the complex via lipocalin-2 receptor (LcnR, 24p3R) [185]. Most interestingly, recent data provide evidence for the existence of mammalian siderophores which are captured by lipocalin-2, thus indicating that lipocalin-2 may be involved in transcellular and transmembrane iron trafficking in mammals [186, 187].

Nonetheless, macrophages challenged with intracellular pathogens, such as *Salmonella* or *Mycobacteria* spp., induce regulatory pathways to limit the availability of iron for these pathogens, which can in part refer to modulation of iron transport by NRAMP1 or ferroportin [123, 125, 181, 188]. Mutations in NRAMP1 have been associated with a reduction of IFN-γ-triggered immune effector pathways such as release of nitrate from macrophages, a mechanism being indicative for endogenous NO formation [189], while overexpression of wild type but not mutant FPN1 reduces the intracellular growth of *S. typhimurium* in J774 macrophages [190], as modulation of ferroportin expression can also control the growth of other bacteria [161, 191].

Accordingly, the development of anemia limits the oxygen transport capacity in general, but rapidly proliferating tissues are more affected since oxygen is an essential compound for energy metabolism and thus for the proliferation of cells.

Third, the reduction of circulating iron strengthens the immune response directed against invading pathogens and tumor cells by stimulating Th1-mediated immune effector pathways of macrophages and by affecting the differentiation of lymphocyte [192].

Specifically, iron loading of monocytes/macrophages results in an inhibition of IFN-γ-mediated pathways such as formation of TNF-α, reduced expression of MHC class II antigens and ICAM-1, decreased formation of neopterin, and impaired tryptophan degradation via IFN-γ-mediated induction of indoleamine 2,3-dioxygenase [26, 115, 122]. As a consequence of this, iron-loaded macrophages have an impaired potential to kill various bacteria, parasites, and fungi (such as *Legionella, Listeria, Ehrlichia, Mycobacteria,* Salmonella, Leishamania, Plasmodia, *Candida*, *Mucor*, and also viruses, *in vitro* and *in vivo)* by IFN-γ-mediated pathways [11, 179, 193–195]. Part of this can be attributed to the reduced formation of NO in the presence of iron since NO is an essential effector molecule of macrophages to fight infectious pathogens and tumor cells [196]. Iron blocks the transcription of inducible NO synthase (iNOS or NOSII), the enzyme being responsible for cytokine-inducible high-output formation of NO by hepatocytes or macrophages [197], and by inhibiting the binding affinity of the transcription factors NF-IL6 and of hypoxia-inducible factor-1 to the iNOS promoter, iron impairs iNOS inducibility by cytokines [120, 198, 199]. According to the regulatory feedback loop, NO produced by activated macrophages activates the IRE-binding function of IRP-1, leading to inhibition of ferritin translation [55, 56], thus linking maintenance of iron homeostasis to NO formation for host defense. In line with this, recent data provided evidence that injection of hepcidin into mice increased their survival following endotoxin injection which was paralleled by reduced formation of cytokines such as TNF-α or IL-6[200]. According to the known interaction of iron with pro-inflammatory immune effector pathways [11, 33, 122, 193, 201], one may speculate that this interesting observation may be due to hepcidin-mediated macrophage iron retention with subsequent inhibition of this pro-inflammatory immune effector pathways.

Via its deactivating effect toward IFN-γ function, iron also affects the Th1/Th2 balance, with Th1 effector functions being weakened while Th2-mediated cytokine production, such as IL-4 activity, is increased, a condition which is a rather unfavorable in case of a tumor disease or an infection [193, 202]. Iron overload also has negative effects on neutrophil function as iron therapy of chronic hemodialysis patients impaired the potential of neutrophils to kill bacteria and reduced their capacity to phagocyte foreign particles [203].

Thus, both iron overload and iron deficiency have unfavorable immunological effects in vivo. Accordingly, mice kept on an iron-rich diet presented with a reduced production of IFN- γ as compared to mice fed with a normal diet, while animals receiving an iron-deficient diet presented with a decreased T-cell proliferation [204]. Both iron-overloaded and iron-deficient mice had an increased mortality when receiving a sublethal dose of LPS as compared to animals with a normal iron status. While a minimum amount of iron is required for the generation of toxic oxygen species by phox [205], macrophage iron overload inhibits the transcription of iNOS and thus the generation of NO [120, 199], the formation of TNF-α, and antigen presentation via MHC II [115, 122], as discussed above.

Thus, investigations of the net effects of disturbances of iron homeostasis on immune function and the course of disease being associated with an activated immune system such as infections, autoimmune disorders, or cancer are of great clinical interest.

Several studies investigated the effects of iron homeostasis on the course or incidence of infections [12]. Interestingly, in one study, iron-deficient children had a reduced incidence of infection as compared to children with a balanced iron status [12, 33]. Accordingly, iron deficiency was associated with a higher percentage of CD8+ cells producing IL-6, a more pronounced expression of T-cell activation markers on lymphocytes, and an increased formation of IFN-γ as compared to Malawian children with a normal iron status [33]. In line with this, oral iron supplementation in children was associated with an increased incidence of malaria in endemic areas and increased odds for a complicated clinical course of the infection [206]. Moreover, children suffering from cerebral malaria due to *Plasmodium falciparum* infection, and receiving iron chelator therapy, desferrioxamine, in addition to a standard antimalarial treatment, presented with an improved clinical course as reflected by a shorter duration of coma and fever and an increased clearance of *Plasmodia* from the circulation [207]. Children receiving desferrioxamine had higher levels of Th1 cytokines and NO, while serum concentration of Th2 cytokines (IL-4) tended to be lower [203, 208] which indicated that withdrawal of iron increases Th1-mediated immune function also in vivo [194]. However, no survival benefit was obtained which may be referred to the poor intracellular penetration of the drug [209].

In Africa, an endemic form of secondary iron overload traced back to the consumption of traditional iron-containing beer linked to a mutation in the ferroportin gene [210] is associated with an increased incidence and mortality from tuberculosis [211]. These data are supported by in vitro findings showing that changes in intramacrophage iron availability stimulate the proliferation of mycobacteria and weaken antimycobacterial defense mechanisms of macrophages [188, 212, 213].

Other infections ranging from bacterial, viral, fungal to parasitic disease where iron overload is associated with a unfavorable course of the infection and/or an impaired immune response have been well summarized in an excellent review [12].

Subsequent studies of macrophage/monocyte iron metabolism under iron-deficient/overload and inflammatory conditions will further extend our knowledge of body iron homeostasis, the impact of erythroid factors on iron recruitment and recirculation, and toward the regulatory pathways in host–pathogen interactions. This may hold the key for future therapeutic developments for the treatment of iron metabolism diseases as well as for anemia of chronic disease. Notably, monocyte/macrophage iron retention seen in inflammation can most effectively be overcome by correcting the underlying disease. However, being aware of the multiple pathways and regulatory factors which control iron homeostasis during inflammation, it is questionable whether modification of one single pathway, e.g., antagonizing of the hepcidin/ferroportin interaction, may have a significant therapeutic effect and whether or not this will improve iron recirculation from macrophages. In addition, we have to acquire new information on adaptive changes of iron homeostasis during therapeutic procedures (e.g., iron supplementation therapy) as well as on the consequences of such interventions on the course of the underlying disease, both of which will be helpful and necessary to optimize therapeutic approaches for correction of disturbances in body iron homeostasis during inflammation.

Acknowledgment Grant support by the Austrian Research Funds-FWF P-19664 is gratefully acknowledged.

References

1. Hentze MW, Muckenthaler MU, Andrews NC. Balancing acts: molecular control of mammalian iron metabolism. Cell. 2004;117:285–97.
2. Nairz M, Weiss G. Molecular and clinical aspects of iron homeostasis: from anemia to hemochromatosis. Wien Klin Wochenschr. 2006;118:442–62.

3. Andrews NC, Schmidt PJ. Iron homeostasis. Annu Rev Physiol. 2007;69:69–85.
4. Rosen GM, Pou S, Ramos CL, Cohen MS, Britigan BE. Free radicals and phagocytic cells. FASEB J. 1995;9:200–9.
5. Schaible UE, Kaufmann SH. Iron and microbial infection. Nat Rev Microbiol. 2004;2:946–53.
6. Hantke K. Iron and metal regulation in bacteria. Curr Opin Microbiol. 2001;4:172–7.
7. Winkelmann G. Microbial siderophore-mediated transport. Biochem Soc Trans. 2002;30:691–6.
8. Delaby C, Pilard N, Puy H, Canonne-Hergaux F. Sequential regulation of ferroportin expression after erythrophagocytosis in murine macrophages: early mRNA induction by haem, followed by iron-dependent protein expression. Biochem J. 2008;411:123–31.
9. Knutson MD, Oukka M, Koss LM, Aydemir F, Wessling-Resnick M. Iron release from macrophages after erythrophagocytosis is up-regulated by ferroportin 1 overexpression and down-regulated by hepcidin. Proc Natl Acad Sci USA. 2005;102:1324–8.
10. Soe-Lin S, Apte SS, Andriopoulos Jr B, Andrews MC, Schranzhofer M, Kahawita T, et al. Nramp1 promotes efficient macrophage recycling of iron following erythrophagocytosis in vivo. Proc Natl Acad Sci USA. 2009;106:5960–5.
11. Weiss G. Iron and immunity: a double-edged sword. Eur J Clin Invest. 2002;32:70–8.
12. Weinberg ED. Iron loading and disease surveillance. Emerg Infect Dis. 1999;5:346–52.
13. de Sousa M, Reimao R, Porto G, Grady RW, Hilgartner MW, Giardina P. Iron and lymphocytes: reciprocal regulatory interactions. Curr Stud Hematol Blood Transfus. 1991;58:171–7.
14. Porto G, Reimao R, Goncalves C, Vicente C, Justica B, de Sousa M. Haemochromatosis as a window into the study of the immunological system: a novel correlation between CD8+ lymphocytes and iron overload. Eur J Haematol. 1994;52:283–90.
15. Meyer PN, Gerhard GS, Yoshida Y, Yoshida M, Chorney KA, Beard J, et al. Hemochromatosis protein (HFE) and tumor necrosis factor receptor 2 (TNFR2) influence tissue iron levels: elements of a common gut pathway? Blood Cells Mol Dis. 2002;29:274–85.
16. Roy CN, Andrews NC. Recent advances in disorders of iron metabolism: mutations, mechanisms and modifiers. Hum Mol Genet. 2001;10:2181–6.
17. Forbes JR, Gros P. Divalent-metal transport by NRAMP proteins at the interface of host-pathogen interactions. Trends Microbiol. 2001;9:397–403.
18. Blackwell JM, Searle S, Goswami T, Miller EN. Understanding the multiple functions of Nramp1. Microbes Infect. 2000;2:317–21.
19. Latunde-Dada GO, Young SP. Iron deficiency and immune responses. Scand J Immunol Suppl. 1992;11:207–9.
20. Brock JH. The effect of iron and transferrin on the response of serum-free cultures of mouse lymphocytes to concanavalin A and lipopolysaccharide. Immunology. 1981;43:387–92.
21. Porto G, De Sousa M. Iron overload and immunity. World J Gastroenterol. 2007;13:4707–15.
22. Seligman PA, Kovar J, Gelfand EW. Lymphocyte proliferation is controlled by both iron availability and regulation of iron uptake pathways. Pathobiology. 1992;60:19–26.
23. Thorson JA, Smith KM, Gomez F, Naumann PW, Kemp JD. Role of iron in T cell activation: TH1 clones differ from TH2 clones in their sensitivity to inhibition of DNA synthesis caused by IgG Mabs against the transferrin receptor and the iron chelator deferoxamine. Cell Immunol. 1991;134:126–37.
24. Farrar JD, Asnagli H, Murphy KM. T helper subset development: roles of instruction, selection, and transcription. J Clin Invest. 2002;109:431–5.
25. Awasthi A, Kuchroo VK. Th17 cells: from precursors to players in inflammation and infection. Int Immunol. 2009;21:489–98.
26. Weiss G, Fuchs D, Hausen A, Reibnegger G, Werner ER, Werner-Felmayer G, et al. Iron modulates interferon-gamma effects in the human myelomonocytic cell line THP-1. Exp Hematol. 1992;20:605–10.
27. Frazer DM, Anderson GJ. The orchestration of body iron intake: how and where do enterocytes receive their cues? Blood Cells Mol Dis. 2003;30:288–97.
28. Brissot P, Troadec MB, Loreal O. The clinical relevance of new insights in iron transport and metabolism. Curr Hematol Rep. 2004;3:107–15.
29. Weiss G, Goodnough LT. Anemia of chronic disease. N Engl J Med. 2005;352:1011–23.
30. Spivak JL. Iron and the anemia of chronic disease. Oncology (Williston Park). 2002;16:25–33.
31. Andrews NC. Anemia of inflammation: the cytokine-hepcidin link. J Clin Invest. 2004;113:1251–3.
32. Weiss G. Iron acquisiton by the reticuloendothelial system. In: Templeton D, editor. Molecular and cellular iron transport. New York: Marcel Dekker Inc.; 2002. p. 467–88.
33. Oppenheimer SJ. Iron and its relation to immunity and infectious disease. J Nutr. 2001;131:616S–35.
34. Fahmy M, Young SP. Modulation of iron metabolism in monocyte cell line U937 by inflammatory cytokines: changes in transferrin uptake, iron handling and ferritin mRNA. Biochem J. 1993;296:175–81.
35. Kaplan J. Mechanisms of cellular iron acquisition: another iron in the fire. Cell. 2002;111:603–6.

36. Gunshin H, Mackenzie B, Berger UV, Gunshin Y, Romero MF, Boron WF, et al. Cloning and characterization of a mammalian proton-coupled metal-ion transporter. Nature. 1997;388:482–8.
37. Fleming MD, Trenor 3rd CC, Su MA, Foernzler D, Beier DR, Dietrich WF, et al. Microcytic anaemia mice have a mutation in Nramp2, a candidate iron transporter gene. Nat Genet. 1997;16:383–6.
38. Andrews NC. The iron transporter DMT1. Int J Biochem Cell Biol. 1999;31:991–4.
39. McKie AT, Barrow D, Latunde-Dada GO, Rolfs A, Sager G, Mudaly E, et al. An iron-regulated ferric reductase associated with the absorption of dietary iron. Science. 2001;291:1755–9.
40. Olakanmi O, Stokes JB, Britigan BE. Acquisition of iron bound to low molecular weight chelates by human monocyte-derived macrophages. J Immunol. 1994;153:2691–703.
41. Ludwiczek S, Aigner E, Theurl I, Weiss G. Cytokine-mediated regulation of iron transport in human monocytic cells. Blood. 2003;101:4148–54.
42. Moss D, Fargion S, Fracanzani AL, Levi S, Cappellini MD, Arosio P, et al. Functional roles of the ferritin receptors of human liver, hepatoma, lymphoid and erythroid cells. J Inorg Biochem. 1992;47:219–27.
43. Ramm GA, Ruddell RG, Subramaniam VN. Identification of ferritin receptors: their role in iron homeostasis, hepatic injury, and inflammation. Gastroenterology. 2009;137:1849–51.
44. Li JY, Paragas N, Ned RM, Qiu A, Viltard M, Leete T, et al. Scara5 is a ferritin receptor mediating non-transferrin iron delivery. Dev Cell. 2009;16:35–46.
45. Cohen LA, Gutierrez L, Weiss A, Leichtmann-Bardoogo Y, Zhang DL, Crooks D, et al. Serum ferritin is derived primarily from macrophages through a non-classical secretory pathway. Blood. 2010;116:1574–84.
46. Fisher J, Devraj K, Ingram J, Slagle-Webb B, Madhankumar AB, Liu X, et al. Ferritin: a novel mechanism for delivery of iron to the brain and other organs. Am J Physiol Cell Physiol. 2007;293:C641–9.
47. Brock JH. The physiology of lactoferrin. Biochem Cell Biol. 2002;80:1–6.
48. Crouch SP, Slater KJ, Fletcher J. Regulation of cytokine release from mononuclear cells by the iron-binding protein lactoferrin. Blood. 1992;80:235–40.
49. Schaer DJ, Schaer CA, Buehler PW, Boykins RA, Schoedon G, Alayash AI, et al. CD163 is the macrophage scavenger receptor for native and chemically modified hemoglobins in the absence of haptoglobin. Blood. 2006;107:373–80.
50. Hvidberg V, Maniecki MB, Jacobsen C, Hojrup P, Moller HJ, Moestrup SK. Identification of the receptor scavenging hemopexin-heme complexes. Blood. 2005;106:2572–9.
51. Kakhlon O, Cabantchik ZI. The labile iron pool: characterization, measurement, and participation in cellular processes(1). Free Radic Biol Med. 2002;33:1037–46.
52. Eisenstein RS, Ross KL. Novel roles for iron regulatory proteins in the adaptive response to iron deficiency. J Nutr. 2003;133:1510S–6.
53. Rouault T, Klausner R. Regulation of iron metabolism in eukaryotes. Curr Top Cell Regul. 1997;35:1–19.
54. Muckenthaler M, Gray NK, Hentze MW. IRP-1 binding to ferritin mRNA prevents the recruitment of the small ribosomal subunit by the cap-binding complex eIF4F. Mol Cell. 1998;2:383–8.
55. Weiss G, Goossen B, Doppler W, Fuchs D, Pantopoulos K, Werner-Felmayer G, et al. Translational regulation via iron-responsive elements by the nitric oxide/NO-synthase pathway. EMBO J. 1993;12:3651–7.
56. Drapier JC, Hirling H, Wietzerbin J, Kaldy P, Kuhn LC. Biosynthesis of nitric oxide activates iron regulatory factor in macrophages. EMBO J. 1993;12:3643–9.
57. Pantopoulos K, Hentze MW. Rapid responses to oxidative stress mediated by iron regulatory protein. EMBO J. 1995;14:2917–24.
58. Schneider BD, Leibold EA. Effects of iron regulatory protein regulation on iron homeostasis during hypoxia. Blood. 2003;102:3404–11.
59. Cairo G, Recalcati S, Pietrangelo A, Minotti G. The iron regulatory proteins: targets and modulators of free radical reactions and oxidative damage. Free Radic Biol Med. 2002;32:1237–43.
60. Leipuviene R, Theil EC. The family of iron responsive RNA structures regulated by changes in cellular iron and oxygen. Cell Mol Life Sci. 2007;64:2945–55.
61. Feder JN, Gnirke A, Thomas W, Tsuchihashi Z, Ruddy DA, Basava A, et al. A novel MHC class I-like gene is mutated in patients with hereditary haemochromatosis. Nat Genet. 1996;13:399–408.
62. Anderson GJ, Powell LW. HFE and non-HFE hemochromatosis. Int J Hematol. 2002;76:203–7.
63. Pietrangelo A. Hereditary hemochromatosis – a new look at an old disease. N Engl J Med. 2004;350:2383–97.
64. Rothenberg BE, Voland JR. beta2 knockout mice develop parenchymal iron overload: a putative role for class I genes of the major histocompatibility complex in iron metabolism. Proc Natl Acad Sci USA. 1996;93:1529–34.
65. Santos M, Schilham MW, Rademakers LH, Marx JJ, de Sousa M, Clevers H. Defective iron homeostasis in beta 2-microglobulin knockout mice recapitulates hereditary hemochromatosis in man. J Exp Med. 1996;184:1975–85.
66. Lebron JA, Bennett MJ, Vaughn DE, Chirino AJ, Snow PM, Mintier GA, et al. Crystal structure of the hemochromatosis protein HFE and characterization of its interaction with transferrin receptor. Cell. 1998;93:111–23.

67. Parkkila S, Waheed A, Britton RS, Bacon BR, Zhou XY, Tomatsu S, et al. Association of the transferrin receptor in human placenta with HFE, the protein defective in hereditary hemochromatosis. Proc Natl Acad Sci USA. 1997;94:13198–202.
68. Ludwiczek S, Theurl I, Artner-Dworzak E, Chorney M, Weiss G. Duodenal HFE expression and hepcidin levels determine body iron homeostasis: modulation by genetic diversity and dietary iron availability. J Mol Med. 2004;82:373–82.
69. Fleming RE, Sly WS. Mechanisms of iron accumulation in hereditary hemochromatosis. Annu Rev Physiol. 2002;64:663–80.
70. Ten Elshof AE, Brittenham GM, Chorney KA, Page MJ, Gerhard G, Cable EE, et al. Gamma delta intraepithelial lymphocytes drive tumor necrosis factor-alpha responsiveness to intestinal iron challenge: relevance to hemochromatosis. Immunol Rev. 1999;167:223–32.
71. Drakesmith H, Sweetland E, Schimanski L, Edwards J, Cowley D, Ashraf M, et al. The hemochromatosis protein HFE inhibits iron export from macrophages. Proc Natl Acad Sci USA. 2002;99:15602–7.
72. Montosi G, Paglia P, Garuti C, Guzman CA, Bastin JM, Colombo MP, et al. Wild-type HFE protein normalizes transferrin iron accumulation in macrophages from subjects with hereditary hemochromatosis. Blood. 2000;96:1125–9.
73. Pietrangelo A. Physiology of iron transport and the hemochromatosis gene. Am J Physiol Gastrointest Liver Physiol. 2002;282:G403–14.
74. McKie AT, Marciani P, Rolfs A, Brennan K, Wehr K, Barrow D, et al. A novel duodenal iron-regulated transporter, IREG1, implicated in the basolateral transfer of iron to the circulation. Mol Cell. 2000;5:299–309.
75. Yang F, Liu XB, Quinones M, Melby PC, Ghio A, Haile DJ. Regulation of reticuloendothelial iron transporter MTP1 (Slc11a3) by inflammation. J Biol Chem. 2002;277:39786–91.
76. Donovan A, Brownlie A, Zhou Y, Shepard J, Pratt SJ, Moynihan J, et al. Positional cloning of zebrafish ferroportin1 identifies a conserved vertebrate iron exporter. Nature. 2000;403:776–81.
77. Pietrangelo A. Hemochromatosis: an endocrine liver disease. Hepatology. 2007;46:1291–301.
78. Vulpe CD, Kuo YM, Murphy TL, Cowley L, Askwith C, Libina N, et al. Hephaestin, a ceruloplasmin homologue implicated in intestinal iron transport, is defective in the sla mouse. Nat Genet. 1999;21:195–9.
79. Cairo G, Recalcati S, Montosi G, Castrusini E, Conte D, Pietrangelo A. Inappropriately high iron regulatory protein activity in monocytes of patients with genetic hemochromatosis. Blood. 1997;89:2546–53.
80. Ludwiczek S, Theurl I, Bahram S, Schumann K, Weiss G. Regulatory networks for the control of body iron homeostasis and their dysregulation in HFE mediated hemochromatosis. J Cell Physiol. 2005;204:489–99.
81. Nairz M, Theurl I, Schroll A, Theurl M, Fritsche G, Lindner E, et al. Absence of functional Hfe protects mice from invasive Salmonella enterica serovar Typhimurium infection via induction of lipocalin-2. Blood. 2009;114:3642–51.
82. Moura E, Noordermeer MA, Verhoeven N, Verheul AF, Marx JJ. Iron release from human monocytes after erythrophagocytosis in vitro: an investigation in normal subjects and hereditary hemochromatosis patients. Blood. 1998;92:2511–9.
83. Kitagawa S, Yuo A, Yagisawa M, Azuma E, Yoshida M, Furukawa Y, et al. Activation of human monocyte functions by tumor necrosis factor: rapid priming for enhanced release of superoxide and erythrophagocytosis, but no direct triggering of superoxide release. Exp Hematol. 1996;24:559–67.
84. Zuckerbraun BS, Billiar TR. Heme oxygenase-1: a cellular Hercules. Hepatology. 2003;37:742–4.
85. Knutson MD, Vafa MR, Haile DJ, Wessling-Resnick M. Iron loading and erythrophagocytosis increase ferroportin 1 (FPN1) expression in J774 macrophages. Blood. 2003;102:4191–7.
86. Delaby C, Pilard N, Hetet G, Driss F, Grandchamp B, Beaumont C, et al. A physiological model to study iron recycling in macrophages. Exp Cell Res. 2005;310:43–53.
87. Ganz T, Nemeth E. Iron imports. IV. Hepcidin and regulation of body iron metabolism. Am J Physiol Gastrointest Liver Physiol. 2006;290:G199–203.
88. Nicolas G, Bennoun M, Porteu A, Mativet S, Beaumont C, Grandchamp B, et al. Severe iron deficiency anemia in transgenic mice expressing liver hepcidin. Proc Natl Acad Sci USA. 2002;99:4596–601.
89. Pigeon C, Ilyin G, Courselaud B, Leroyer P, Turlin B, Brissot P, et al. A new mouse liver-specific gene, encoding a protein homologous to human antimicrobial peptide hepcidin, is overexpressed during iron overload. J Biol Chem. 2001;276:7811–9.
90. Nemeth E, Tuttle MS, Powelson J, Vaughn MB, Donovan A, Ward DM, et al. Hepcidin regulates cellular iron efflux by binding to ferroportin and inducing its internalization. Science. 2004;306:2090–3.
91. De Domenico I, Ward DM, Langelier C, Vaughn MB, Nemeth E, Sundquist WI, et al. The molecular mechanism of hepcidin-mediated ferroportin down-regulation. Mol Biol Cell. 2007;18:2569–78.
92. Delaby C, Pilard N, Goncalves AS, Beaumont C, Canonne-Hergaux F. Presence of the iron exporter ferroportin at the plasma membrane of macrophages is enhanced by iron loading and down-regulated by hepcidin. Blood. 2005;106:3979–84.
93. Soe-Lin S, Apte SS, Mikhael MR, Kayembe LK, Nie G, Ponka P. Both Nramp1 and DMT1 are necessary for efficient macrophage iron recycling. Exp Hematol. 2010;38:609–17.

94. Keel SB, Doty RT, Yang Z, Quigley JG, Chen J, Knoblaugh S, et al. A heme export protein is required for red blood cell differentiation and iron homeostasis. Science. 2008;319:825–8.
95. De Domenico I, Ward DM, di Patti MC, Jeong SY, David S, Musci G, et al. Ferroxidase activity is required for the stability of cell surface ferroportin in cells expressing GPI-ceruloplasmin. EMBO J. 2007;26:2823–31.
96. Wang F, Paradkar PN, Custodio AO, McVey Ward D, Fleming MD, Campagna D, et al. Genetic variation in Mon1a affects protein trafficking and modifies macrophage iron loading in mice. Nat Genet. 2007;39:1025–32.
97. Zhang DL, Hughes RM, Ollivierre-Wilson H, Ghosh MC, Rouault TA. A ferroportin transcript that lacks an iron-responsive element enables duodenal and erythroid precursor cells to evade translational repression. Cell Metab. 2009;9:461–73.
98. Peyssonnaux C, Zinkernagel AS, Datta V, Lauth X, Johnson RS, Nizet V. TLR4-dependent hepcidin expression by myeloid cells in response to bacterial pathogens. Blood. 2006;107:3727–32.
99. Nguyen NB, Callaghan KD, Ghio AJ, Haile DJ, Yang F. Hepcidin expression and iron transport in alveolar macrophages. Am J Physiol Lung Cell Mol Physiol. 2006;291:L417–25.
100. Theurl I, Theurl M, Seifert M, Mair S, Nairz M, Rumpold H, et al. Autocrine formation of hepcidin induces iron retention in human monocytes. Blood. 2008;111:2392–9.
101. Pietrangelo A, Dierssen U, Valli L, Garuti C, Rump A, Corradini E, et al. STAT3 is required for IL-6-gp130-dependent activation of hepcidin in vivo. Gastroenterology. 2007;132:294–300.
102. Verga Falzacappa MV, Vujic Spasic M, Kessler R, Stolte J, Hentze MW, Muckenthaler MU. STAT3 mediates hepatic hepcidin expression and its inflammatory stimulation. Blood. 2007;109:353–8.
103. Wrighting DM, Andrews NC. Interleukin-6 induces hepcidin expression through STAT3. Blood. 2006;108:3204–9.
104. Fraenkel PG, Traver D, Donovan A, Zahrieh D, Zon LI. Ferroportin1 is required for normal iron cycling in zebrafish. J Clin Invest. 2005;115:1532–41.
105. Liu S, Suragani RN, Wang F, Han A, Zhao W, Andrews NC, et al. The function of heme-regulated eIF2alpha kinase in murine iron homeostasis and macrophage maturation. J Clin Invest. 2007;117:3296–305.
106. Chen JJ. Regulation of protein synthesis by the heme-regulated eIF2alpha kinase: relevance to anemias. Blood. 2007;109:2693–9.
107. Angelillo-Scherrer A, Burnier L, Lambrechts D, Fish RJ, Tjwa M, Plaisance S, et al. Role of Gas6 in erythropoiesis and anemia in mice. J Clin Invest. 2008;118:583–96.
108. Nemeth E, Valore EV, Territo M, Schiller G, Lichtenstein A, Ganz T. Hepcidin, a putative mediator of anemia of inflammation, is a type II acute-phase protein. Blood. 2003;101:2461–3.
109. Finch C. Regulators of iron balance in humans. Blood. 1994;84:1697–702.
110. Nicolas G, Viatte L, Bennoun M, Beaumont C, Kahn A, Vaulont S. Hepcidin, a new iron regulatory peptide. Blood Cells Mol Dis. 2002;29:327–35.
111. Tanno T, Bhanu NV, Oneal PA, Goh SH, Staker P, Lee YT, et al. High levels of GDF15 in thalassemia suppress expression of the iron regulatory protein hepcidin. Nat Med. 2007;13:1096–101.
112. Theurl I, Finkenstedt A, Schroll A, Nairz M, Sonnweber T, Bellmann-Weiler R, et al. Growth differentiation factor 15 in anaemia of chronic disease, iron deficiency anaemia and mixed type anaemia. Br J Haematol. 2010;148:449–55.
113. Knutson M, Wessling-Resnick M. Iron metabolism in the reticuloendothelial system. Crit Rev Biochem Mol Biol. 2003;38:61–88.
114. Mastroeni P, Vazquez-Torres A, Fang FC, Xu Y, Khan S, Hormaeche CE, et al. Antimicrobial actions of the NADPH phagocyte oxidase and inducible nitric oxide synthase in experimental salmonellosis. II. Effects on microbial proliferation and host survival in vivo. J Exp Med. 2000;192:237–48.
115. Recalcati S, Pometta R, Levi S, Conte D, Cairo G. Response of monocyte iron regulatory protein activity to inflammation: abnormal behavior in genetic hemochromatosis. Blood. 1998;91:2565–72.
116. Weiss G. Modification of iron regulation by the inflammatory response. Best Pract Res Clin Haematol. 2005;18:183–201.
117. Nairz M, Fritsche G, Brunner P, Talasz H, Hantke K, Weiss G. Interferon-gamma limits the availability of iron for intramacrophage Salmonella typhimurium. Eur J Immunol. 2008;38:1923–36.
118. Byrd TF, Horwitz MA. Regulation of transferrin receptor expression and ferritin content in human mononuclear phagocytes. Coordinate upregulation by iron transferrin and downregulation by interferon gamma. J Clin Invest. 1993;91:969–76.
119. Mulero V, Brock JH. Regulation of iron metabolism in murine J774 macrophages: role of nitric oxide-dependent and -independent pathways following activation with gamma interferon and lipopolysaccharide. Blood. 1999;94:2383–9.
120. Weiss G, Werner-Felmayer G, Werner ER, Grunewald K, Wachter H, Hentze MW. Iron regulates nitric oxide synthase activity by controlling nuclear transcription. J Exp Med. 1994;180:969–76.
121. Recalcati S, Locati M, Marini A, Santambrogio P, Zaninotto F, De Pizzol M, et al. Differential regulation of iron homeostasis during human macrophage polarized activation. Eur J Immunol. 2010;40:824–35.

122. Oexle H, Kaser A, Most J, Bellmann-Weiler R, Werner ER, Werner-Felmayer G, et al. Pathways for the regulation of interferon-gamma-inducible genes by iron in human monocytic cells. J Leukoc Biol. 2003;74:287–94.
123. Kuhn DE, Lafuse WP, Zwilling BS. Iron transport into mycobacterium avium-containing phagosomes from an Nramp1(Gly169)-transfected RAW264.7 macrophage cell line. J Leukoc Biol. 2001;69:43–9.
124. Fritsche G, Nairz M, Theurl I, Mair S, Bellmann-Weiler R, Barton HC, et al. Modulation of macrophage iron transport by Nramp1 (Slc11a1). Immunobiology. 2007;212:751–7.
125. Nairz M, Fritsche G, Crouch ML, Barton HC, Fang FC, Weiss G. Slc11a1 limits intracellular growth of Salmonella enterica sv. Typhimurium by promoting macrophage immune effector functions and impairing bacterial iron acquisition. Cell Microbiol. 2009;11:1365–81.
126. Alter-Koltunoff M, Ehrlich S, Dror N, Azriel A, Eilers M, Hauser H, et al. Nramp1-mediated innate resistance to intraphagosomal pathogens is regulated by IRF-8, PU.1, and Miz-1. J Biol Chem. 2003;278:44025–32.
127. Fritsche G, Dlaska M, Barton H, Theurl I, Garimorth K, Weiss G. Nramp1 functionality increases inducible nitric oxide synthase transcription via stimulation of IFN regulatory factor 1 expression. J Immunol. 2003;171:1994–8.
128. Mulero V, Searle S, Blackwell JM, Brock JH. Solute carrier 11a1 (Slc11a1; formerly Nramp1) regulates metabolism and release of iron acquired by phagocytic, but not transferrin-receptor-mediated, iron uptake. Biochem J. 2002;363:89–94.
129. Canonne-Hergaux F, Gruenheid S, Govoni G, Gros P. The Nramp1 protein and its role in resistance to infection and macrophage function. Proc Assoc Am Physicians. 1999;111:283–9.
130. Jabado N, Jankowski A, Dougaparsad S, Picard V, Grinstein S, Gros P. Natural resistance to intracellular infections: natural resistance-associated macrophage protein 1 (Nramp1) functions as a pH-dependent manganese transporter at the phagosomal membrane. J Exp Med. 2000;192:1237–48.
131. Baker ST, Barton CH, Biggs TE. A negative autoregulatory link between Nramp1 function and expression. J Leukoc Biol. 2000;67:501–7.
132. Alvarez-Hernandez X, Liceaga J, McKay IC, Brock JH. Induction of hypoferremia and modulation of macrophage iron metabolism by tumor necrosis factor. Lab Invest. 1989;61:319–22.
133. Konijn AM, Carmel N, Levy R, Hershko C. Ferritin synthesis in inflammation. II. Mechanism of increased ferritin synthesis. Br J Haematol. 1981;49:361–70.
134. Torti FM, Torti SV. Regulation of ferritin genes and protein. Blood. 2002;99:3505–16.
135. Moldawer LL, Marano MA, Wei H, Fong Y, Silen ML, Kuo G, et al. Cachectin/tumor necrosis factor-alpha alters red blood cell kinetics and induces anemia in vivo. FASEB J. 1989;3:1637–43.
136. Ganz T. Hepcidin, a key regulator of iron metabolism and mediator of anemia of inflammation. Blood. 2003;102:783–8.
137. Loreal O, Brissot P. Hepcidin: small molecule, large future. Rev Med Interne. 2003;24:213–5.
138. Weinstein DA, Roy CN, Fleming MD, Loda MF, Wolfsdorf JI, Andrews NC. Inappropriate expression of hepcidin is associated with iron refractory anemia: implications for the anemia of chronic disease. Blood. 2002;100:3776–81.
139. Nicolas G, Chauvet C, Viatte L, Danan JL, Bigard X, Devaux I, et al. The gene encoding the iron regulatory peptide hepcidin is regulated by anemia, hypoxia, and inflammation. J Clin Invest. 2002;110:1037–44.
140. Fleming RE, Sly WS. Hepcidin: a putative iron-regulatory hormone relevant to hereditary hemochromatosis and the anemia of chronic disease. Proc Natl Acad Sci USA. 2001;98:8160–2.
141. Nemeth E, Rivera S, Gabayan V, Keller C, Taudorf S, Pedersen BK, et al. IL-6 mediates hypoferremia of inflammation by inducing the synthesis of the iron regulatory hormone hepcidin. J Clin Invest. 2004;113:1271–6.
142. Theurl I, Mattle V, Seifert M, Mariani M, Marth C, Weiss G. Dysregulated monocyte iron homeostasis and erythropoietin formation in patients with anemia of chronic disease. Blood. 2006;107:4142–8.
143. Theurl I, Aigner E, Theurl M, Nairz M, Seifert M, Schroll A, et al. Regulation of iron homeostasis in anemia of chronic disease and iron deficiency anemia: diagnostic and therapeutic implications. Blood. 2009;113:5277–86.
144. Darshan D, Frazer DM, Wilkins SJ, Anderson GJ. Severe iron deficiency blunts the response of the iron regulatory gene Hamp and proinflammatory cytokines to lipopolysaccharide. Haematologica. 2010;95:1660–7.
145. Lasocki S, Millot S, Andrieu V, Letteron P, Pilard N, Muzeau F, et al. Phlebotomies or erythropoietin injections allow mobilization of iron stores in a mouse model mimicking intensive care anemia. Crit Care Med. 2008;36:2388–94.
146. Camaschella C, Silvestri L. New and old players in the hepcidin pathway. Haematologica. 2008;93:1441–4.
147. Liu XB, Nguyen NB, Marquess KD, Yang F, Haile DJ. Regulation of hepcidin and ferroportin expression by lipopolysaccharide in splenic macrophages. Blood Cells Mol Dis. 2005;35:47–56.
148. Weiss G. Iron, infection and anemia – a classical triad. Wien Klin Wochenschr. 2002;114:357–67.
149. Constante M, Wang D, Raymond VA, Bilodeau M, Santos MM. Repression of repulsive guidance molecule C during inflammation is independent of Hfe and involves tumor necrosis factor-alpha. Am J Pathol. 2007;170:497–504.
150. Bouton C, Drapier JC. Iron regulatory proteins as NO signal transducers. Sci STKE. 2003;2003:pe17.
151. Bouton C, Oliveira L, Drapier JC. Converse modulation of IRP1 and IRP2 by immunological stimuli in murine RAW 264.7 macrophages. J Biol Chem. 1998;273:9403–8.

152. Hanson ES, Leibold EA. Regulation of the iron regulatory proteins by reactive nitrogen and oxygen species. Gene Expr. 1999;7:367–76.
153. Kim S, Wing SS, Ponka P. S-nitrosylation of IRP2 regulates its stability via the ubiquitin-proteasome pathway. Mol Cell Biol. 2004;24:330–7.
154. Caltagirone A, Weiss G, Pantopoulos K. Modulation of cellular iron metabolism by hydrogen peroxide. Effects of H2O2 on the expression and function of iron-responsive element-containing mRNAs in B6 fibroblasts. J Biol Chem. 2001;276:19738–45.
155. Kim S, Ponka P. Nitric oxide-mediated modulation of iron regulatory proteins: implication for cellular iron homeostasis. Blood Cells Mol Dis. 2002;29:400–10.
156. Hanson ES, Rawlins ML, Leibold EA. Oxygen and iron regulation of iron regulatory protein 2. J Biol Chem. 2003;278:40337–42.
157. Wang J, Chen G, Pantopoulos K. Nitric oxide inhibits the degradation of IRP2. Mol Cell Biol. 2005;25:1347–53.
158. Wang J, Fillebeen C, Chen G, Andriopoulos B, Pantopoulos K. Sodium nitroprusside promotes IRP2 degradation via an increase in intracellular iron and in the absence of S nitrosylation at C178. Mol Cell Biol. 2006;26:1948–54.
159. Mikhael M, Kim SF, Schranzhofer M, Soe-Lin S, Sheftel AD, Mullner EW, et al. Iron regulatory protein-independent regulation of ferritin synthesis by nitrogen monoxide. FEBS J. 2006;273:3828–36.
160. Tacchini L, Gammella E, De Ponti C, Recalcati S, Cairo G. Role of HIF-1 and NF-kappaB transcription factors in the modulation of transferrin receptor by inflammatory and anti-inflammatory signals. J Biol Chem. 2008;283:20674–86.
161. Sow FB, Florence WC, Satoskar AR, Schlesinger LS, Zwilling BS, Lafuse WP. Expression and localization of hepcidin in macrophages: a role in host defense against tuberculosis. J Leukoc Biol. 2007;82:934–45.
162. Weiss G, Bogdan C, Hentze MW. Pathways for the regulation of macrophage iron metabolism by the anti-inflammatory cytokines IL-4 and IL-13. J Immunol. 1997;158:420–5.
163. Tilg H, Ulmer H, Kaser A, Weiss G. Role of IL-10 for induction of anemia during inflammation. J Immunol. 2002;169:2204–9.
164. Graversen JH, Madsen M, Moestrup SK. CD163: a signal receptor scavenging haptoglobin–hemoglobin complexes from plasma. Int J Biochem Cell Biol. 2002;34:309–14.
165. Bach FH. Heme oxygenase-1: a therapeutic amplification funnel. FASEB J. 2005;19:1216–9.
166. Lee TS, Chau LY. Heme oxygenase-1 mediates the anti-inflammatory effect of interleukin-10 in mice. Nat Med. 2002;8:240–6.
167. Cartwright GE. The anemia of chronic disorders. Semin Hematol. 1966;3:351–75.
168. Means Jr RT. Recent developments in the anemia of chronic disease. Curr Hematol Rep. 2003;2:116–21.
169. Graziadei I, Gaggl S, Kaserbacher R, Braunsteiner H, Vogel W. The acute-phase protein alpha 1-antitrypsin inhibits growth and proliferation of human early erythroid progenitor cells (burst-forming units-erythroid) and of human erythroleukemic cells (K562) in vitro by interfering with transferrin iron uptake. Blood. 1994;83:260–8.
170. Weiss G, Graziadel I, Urbanek M, Grunewald K, Vogel W. Divergent effects of alpha 1-antitrypsin on the regulation of iron metabolism in human erythroleukaemic (K562) and myelomonocytic (THP-1) cells. Biochem J. 1996;319:897–902.
171. Jelkmann W. Proinflammatory cytokines lowering erythropoietin production. J Interferon Cytokine Res. 1998;18:555–9.
172. Means Jr RT, Krantz SB. Inhibition of human erythroid colony-forming units by gamma interferon can be corrected by recombinant human erythropoietin. Blood. 1991;78:2564–7.
173. Goodnough LT. Red cell growth factors in patients with chronic anemias. Curr Hematol Rep. 2002;1:119–23.
174. Matzner Y, Levy S, Grossowicz N, Izak G, Hershko C. Prevalence and causes of anemia in elderly hospitalized patients. Gerontology. 1979;25:113–9.
175. Weiss G. Pathogenesis and treatment of anaemia of chronic disease. Blood Rev. 2002;16:87–96.
176. Collins AJ, Ma JZ, Ebben J. Impact of hematocrit on morbidity and mortality. Semin Nephrol. 2000;20:345–9.
177. Schrettl M, Bignell E, Kragl C, Joechl C, Rogers T, Arst Jr HN, et al. Siderophore biosynthesis but not reductive iron assimilation is essential for Aspergillus fumigatus virulence. J Exp Med. 2004;200:1213–9.
178. Boyer E, Bergevin I, Malo D, Gros P, Cellier MF. Acquisition of Mn(II) in addition to Fe(II) is required for full virulence of Salmonella enterica serovar Typhimurium. Infect Immun. 2002;70:6032–42.
179. Kontoghiorghes GJ, Weinberg ED. Iron: mammalian defense systems, mechanisms of disease, and chelation therapy approaches. Blood Rev. 1995;9:33–45.
180. Walter T, Olivares M, Pizarro F, Munoz C. Iron, anemia, and infection. Nutr Rev. 1997;55:111–24.
181. Nairz M, Theurl I, Ludwiczek S, Theurl M, Mair SM, Fritsche G, et al. The co-ordinated regulation of iron homeostasis in murine macrophages limits the availability of iron for intracellular Salmonella typhimurium. Cell Microbiol. 2007;9:2126–40.

182. Flo TH, Smith KD, Sato S, Rodriguez DJ, Holmes MA, Strong RK, et al. Lipocalin 2 mediates an innate immune response to bacterial infection by sequestrating iron. Nature. 2004;432:917–21.
183. Fluckinger M, Haas H, Merschak P, Glasgow BJ, Redl B. Human tear lipocalin exhibits antimicrobial activity by scavenging microbial siderophores. Antimicrob Agents Chemother. 2004;48:3367–72.
184. Berger T, Togawa A, Duncan GS, Elia AJ, You-Ten A, Wakeham A, et al. Lipocalin 2-deficient mice exhibit increased sensitivity to *Escherichia coli* infection but not to ischemia–reperfusion injury. Proc Natl Acad Sci USA. 2006;103:1834–9.
185. Devireddy LR, Gazin C, Zhu X, Green MR. A cell-surface receptor for lipocalin 24p3 selectively mediates apoptosis and iron uptake. Cell. 2005;123:1293–305.
186. Bao G, Clifton M, Hoette TM, Mori K, Deng SX, Qiu A, et al. Iron traffics in circulation bound to a siderocalin (Ngal)-catechol complex. Nat Chem Biol. 2010;6:602–9.
187. Devireddy LR, Hart DO, Goetz DH, Green MR. A mammalian siderophore synthesized by an enzyme with a bacterial homolog involved in enterobactin production. Cell. 2010;141:1006–17.
188. Olakanmi O, Schlesinger LS, Ahmed A, Britigan BE. Intraphagosomal Mycobacterium tuberculosis acquires iron from both extracellular transferrin and intracellular iron pools. Impact of interferon-gamma and hemochromatosis. J Biol Chem. 2002;277:49727–34.
189. Barton CH, Whitehead SH, Blackwell JM. Nramp transfection transfers Ity/Lsh/Bcg-related pleiotropic effects on macrophage activation: influence on oxidative burst and nitric oxide pathways. Mol Med. 1995;1:267–79.
190. Chlosta S, Fishman DS, Harrington L, Johnson EE, Knutson MD, Wessling-Resnick M, et al. The iron efflux protein ferroportin regulates the intracellular growth of Salmonella enterica. Infect Immun. 2006;74:3065–7.
191. Paradkar P, De Domenico I, Durchfort N, Zohn I, Kaplan J, Ward DM. Iron-depletion limits intracellular bacterial growth in macrophages. Blood. 2008;112:866–74.
192. Weiss G, Wachter H, Fuchs D. Linkage of cell-mediated immunity to iron metabolism. Immunol Today. 1995;16:495–500.
193. Mencacci A, Cenci E, Boelaert JR, Bucci P, Mosci P, Fe d'Ostiani C, et al. Iron overload alters innate and T helper cell responses to Candida albicans in mice. J Infect Dis. 1997;175:1467–76.
194. Fritsche G, Larcher C, Schennach H, Weiss G. Regulatory interactions between iron and nitric oxide metabolism for immune defense against *Plasmodium falciparum* infection. J Infect Dis. 2001;183:1388–94.
195. Boelaert JR, Vandecasteele SJ, Appelberg R, Gordeuk VR. The effect of the host's iron status on tuberculosis. J Infect Dis. 2007;195:1745–53.
196. Bogdan C. Nitric oxide and the immune response. Nat Immunol. 2001;2:907–16.
197. MacMicking J, Xie QW, Nathan C. Nitric oxide and macrophage function. Annu Rev Immunol. 1997;15:323–50.
198. Melillo G, Taylor LS, Brooks A, Musso T, Cox GW, Varesio L. Functional requirement of the hypoxia-responsive element in the activation of the inducible nitric oxide synthase promoter by the iron chelator desferrioxamine. J Biol Chem. 1997;272:12236–43.
199. Dlaska M, Weiss G. Central role of transcription factor NF-IL6 for cytokine and iron-mediated regulation of murine inducible nitric oxide synthase expression. J Immunol. 1999;162:6171–7.
200. De Domenico I, Zhang TY, Koening CL, Branch RW, London N, Lo E, et al. Hepcidin mediates transcriptional changes that modulate acute cytokine-induced inflammatory responses in mice. J Clin Invest. 2010;120: 2395–405.
201. Wessling-Resnick M. Iron homeostasis and the inflammatory response. Annu Rev Nutr. 2010;30:105–22.
202. Weiss G, Thuma PE, Mabeza G, Werner ER, Herold M, Gordeuk VR. Modulatory potential of iron chelation therapy on nitric oxide formation in cerebral malaria. J Infect Dis. 1997;175:226–30.
203. Patruta SI, Edlinger R, Sunder-Plassmann G, Horl WH. Neutrophil impairment associated with iron therapy in hemodialysis patients with functional iron deficiency. J Am Soc Nephrol. 1998;9:655–63.
204. Omara FO, Blakley BR. The effects of iron deficiency and iron overload on cell-mediated immunity in the mouse. Br J Nutr. 1994;72:899–909.
205. Collins HL, Kaufmann SH, Schaible UE. Iron chelation via deferoxamine exacerbates experimental salmonellosis via inhibition of the nicotinamide adenine dinucleotide phosphate oxidase-dependent respiratory burst. J Immunol. 2002;168:3458–63.
206. Iannotti LL, Tielsch JM, Black MM, Black RE. Iron supplementation in early childhood: health benefits and risks. Am J Clin Nutr. 2006;84:1261–76.
207. Gordeuk V, Thuma P, Brittenham G, McLaren C, Parry D, Backenstose A, et al. Effect of iron chelation therapy on recovery from deep coma in children with cerebral malaria. N Engl J Med. 1992;327:1473–7.
208. Thuma PE, Weiss G, Herold M, Gordeuk VR. Serum neopterin, interleukin-4, and interleukin-6 concentrations in cerebral malaria patients and the effect of iron chelation therapy. Am J Trop Med Hyg. 1996;54:164–8.
209. Thuma PE, Mabeza GF, Biemba G, Bhat GJ, McLaren CE, Moyo VM, et al. Effect of iron chelation therapy on mortality in Zambian children with cerebral malaria. Trans R Soc Trop Med Hyg. 1998;92:214–8.

210. Gordeuk VR, Caleffi A, Corradini E, Ferrara F, Jones RA, Castro O, et al. Iron overload in Africans and African-Americans and a common mutation in the SCL40A1 (ferroportin 1) gene small star, filled. Blood Cells Mol Dis. 2003;31:299–304.
211. Gordeuk VR. African iron overload. Semin Hematol. 2002;39:263–9.
212. Schnappinger D, Ehrt S, Voskuil MI, Liu Y, Mangan JA, Monahan IM, et al. Transcriptional adaptation of mycobacterium tuberculosis within macrophages: insights into the phagosomal environment. J Exp Med. 2003;198:693–704.
213. Appelberg R. Macrophage nutriprive antimicrobial mechanisms. J Leukoc Biol. 2006;79:1117–28.

Chapter 12
Iron and the Immune System

Hal Drakesmith, Graça Porto, and Maria de Sousa

Keywords HCV • Hemochromatosis • Hepcidin • HIV • Lipocalin-2 • Lymphocytes • Macrophages • Malaria • MHC • TLR4

1 General Introduction

> Whatever concerns health is of real public interest. I take advantage of this to make my address less arduous for you. I shall moreover use the opportunity to show you the practical value of pure research.
>
> Ilya Metchnikoff. Nobel lecture, 1908

Metchnikoff shared the Nobel Prize with Paul Ehrlich 'in recognition of their work in Immunity'. The concept of immunity had preceded by just over 100 years [1], the dim beginning of the realization that some cells could respond to the challenge by foreign bodies clustering round them and phagocytosing them. Macrophages and Ilya Metchnikoff can thus be viewed as pioneers of what we know today to be the immune system. In general, Nobel Prizes in Physiology and Medicine have distinguished immunologists for 'the practical value of pure research', particularly in infection. This chapter will not go against that tradition. Several recent pieces of work, however, point to the fact that the immune system cells are equipped with iron proteins that may have regulatory functions of iron metabolism. The practical value to immunity of such novel functions cannot be disputed. But in a chapter of a book prepared at the beginning of a new century, their possible physiological significance should not be ignored.

Microbes have been shown to be able to leach metals in the inorganic environment [2]. But it was the use of iron by microorganisms that led to the notion that this metal could stand importantly at the frontier between the defenses of living hosts against invading pathogens. With the realization that iron actually existed within red blood cells, those same cells first acknowledged by Metchnikoff of importance to immunity became of growing importance to the understanding of iron recycling in vivo. Macrophages were therefore the first immune system cell to be known to participate in iron

H. Drakesmith, B.A., Ph.D. (✉)
Molecular Immunology Group, Weatherall Institute of Molecular Medicine,
John Radcliffe Hospital, Oxford University, Oxford, OX3 9DS, UK
e-mail: hdrakes@hammer.imm.ox.ac.uk

G. Porto, M.D., Ph.D. • M. de Sousa, M.D., Ph.D., FRCPath
GABBA Program/ICBAS, IBMC, Molecular and Cellular Biology Institute,
University of Porto, 4150-180, Porto, Portugal
e-mail: gporto@ibmc.up.pt; deen112002@yahoo.com

G.J. Anderson and G. McLaren (eds.), *Iron Physiology and Pathophysiology in Humans*, Nutrition and Health, DOI 10.1007/978-1-60327-485-2_12,

metabolism. The novelty in the first decade of the twenty-first century is that all cells of the immune system including lymphocytes may contribute to iron homeostasis. The realization that the full extent of existing subpopulations of macrophages and of lymphocytes is far from complete leads to the conclusion of this chapter with the review of recent work showing how some such subpopulations may behave differently in iron sequestration or release [3] and have different expression in iron overload [4].

In this chapter, we procure to update data showing the effects of iron in immunity. In addition, recent evidence pointing to a reciprocal role of cells of the immune system in iron homeostasis is reviewed. The reader may find additional relevant references in recent reviews of the topic [5].

2 Iron and Innate Immunity: Defending Host Resources

2.1 Introduction

Organisms protect themselves against potentially harmful infection. The network of molecules, cells and organs that perform this defensive and self-preservation function is the immune system. Traditionally the human immune system is divided into two parts, the innate and the adaptive. In the former, pathogens are detected by pattern recognition receptors that bind to structurally conserved components of microbes, and this detection is followed by transcription of genes encoding cytokines that activate other downstream immune mechanisms (including the adaptive immune system). Microbes are killed by the innate system through a variety of methods, for example the complement cascade or following phagocytosis by macrophages. As well as actively destroying pathogens, the innate immune system also denies microbes access to vital host resources and nutrients, including iron. By slowing the growth of invasive organisms, the host gives itself time to mount a specific sterilizing attack – this aspect of the immune response has been termed 'nutritional immunity' [6]. In turn, many pathogens have developed ways of circumventing the host's attempts to withhold iron, in order to ensure their supply. Many virulence genes of pathogens have roles in directly obtaining iron or in manipulating host iron transport, reflecting the requirement for iron to maximize microbial growth and spread. The fight for a crucial nutrient lies at the heart of immunity [7, 8]. The molecular mechanisms of how the host defends its iron resources against pathogenic acquisition, and how the pathogen strikes back, are the subject of the three sections below.

2.2 Iron and Infectious Disease

Iron is utilized in fundamental physiological functions. Iron heme binds oxygen, and iron-sulfur complexes embedded in proteins perform various roles including electron transport and ATP generation. DNA synthesis is also iron-dependent [9–11]. Some bacteria have evolved to use iron in the majority of their proteins and depend upon iron as an energy source [12]. Only two types of organisms are known to science that do not need iron at all – *Borrelia burgdorferi* and Lactobacilli, both of which appear to utilize manganese instead [13, 14]. These exceptions aside, all life forms have a basic requirement for iron to live, thrive and reproduce. Moreover, excess iron is toxic, because of its capacity to catalyze the generation of free radicals. It is probably for these reasons that an increased iron status is generally associated with a poor prognosis in the setting of infection, and current indications suggest high iron predisposes to an unfavorable outcome in some of the world's most common infections: malaria [15, 16], HIV-1 [17, 18], tuberculosis [19] and Hepatitis C virus [20, 21].

During infection, a pathogen must obtain iron from its host or its spread will be stifled. One might expect therefore that specific mechanisms exist to alter host iron transport consequential to pathogen recognition, and that due to the selection pressure for iron acquisition, pathogens have developed methods to manipulate host iron transport for their own benefit. These topics will be considered below.

2.3 Mechanisms of Host Sequestration of Iron: Lipocalin-2 and Hepcidin

Iron is carried around the circulation by the serum protein transferrin, each molecule of which can bind two atoms of iron. However, it is noteworthy that transferrin was discovered not only as an iron-binding protein but also as a bacteriostatic component of human plasma – transferrin was able to halt the growth of the iron-requiring *Shigella dysenteriae* [22]. This seminal paper published in 1946 emphasizes the fundamental intermeshing of iron transport and defense against pathogens. To focus on more recent discoveries regarding iron sequestration as part of an innate immune response, the role of the host protein lipocalin-2 in protecting against bacterial iron acquisition will now be discussed. Iron-carrying siderophores (from the Greek sideros (iron) and phoros (bearing)) are small molecules produced by bacteria whose function is to scavenge iron from their surroundings; during infection, this means from their host. One of the best-studied types of siderophore is the catechol-type enterobactin/enterochelin, made by several types of gram-negative bacteria [23, 24] (Fig. 12.1a). *E. coli* enterobactin has a molecular weight of 669, which exceeds the size-exclusion limit for diffusion across the outer membrane of gram-negative bacteria [25]. Active transport mechanisms therefore exist both to export newly synthesized apo-siderophores and to capture iron-binding enterobactin. The bacterial FepA protein specifically transports Fe-enterobactin for delivery of the metal into the bacterial cytosol [26]. Because of the tremendous affinity of enterobactin for ferric ions, this system facilitates bacterial iron uptake. However, it has been long known that enterobactin is inactive as an iron delivery system in human serum. A human protein, named lipocalin-2 (alternative names are 24p3, siderocalin, NGAL, uterocalin) has been found to bind to Fe-enterobactin with an affinity of 0.11 nM, higher than the affinity of FepA for Fe-enterobactin [27] (Fig. 12.1b). In this way, lipocalin-2 inhibits the enterobactin-mediated pathway of iron acquisition by *E. coli*. Further studies have shown that lipocalin-2 can bind other microbial siderophores such as bacillibactin and carboxymycobactin [28]. Lipocalin-2 is an acute-phase protein, and its expression can be stimulated through the host's pattern-recognition receptor Toll-like receptor-4 (TLR4) [29]. The natural ligand for TLR4 is the ubiquitous bacterial component of gram-negative outer membranes, lipopolysaccharide (LPS). Therefore, the presence of bacteria that use enterobactin is detected because of their obligate co-expression of LPS, and the LPS/TLR4 interaction leads to sequestering of enterobactin through the synthesis of lipocalin-2. The importance of lipocalin-2 in controlling bacterial infections has been revealed using knock-out mice [29]. Lipocalin-2-deleted mice were susceptible to infection with an enterobactin-utilizing strain of *E. coli* whereas the wild-type were able to control the infection. In vitro growth of the same bacterial strain is inhibited by addition to the growth media of lipocalin-2, but this inhibition is counteracted by exogenous equimolar enterobactin. Furthermore, lack of virulence of the enterobactin-utilizing strain of *E. coli* in wild-type mice could be overcome by co-inoculating the bacteria with ferrichrome, a different siderophore that is not bound by lipocalin-2 but can deliver iron to *E.* coli [29]. Interestingly, a vertebrate lipocalin-2 receptor 24p3 has been identified that allows for import into mammalian cells of the iron bound to a bacterial siderophore, removing both the iron and enterobactin from the circulation [30]. Overall, the data suggest that although some strains of bacteria use enterobactin to acquire iron from mammalian hosts, the innate immune response effectively counteracts this through lipocalin-2.

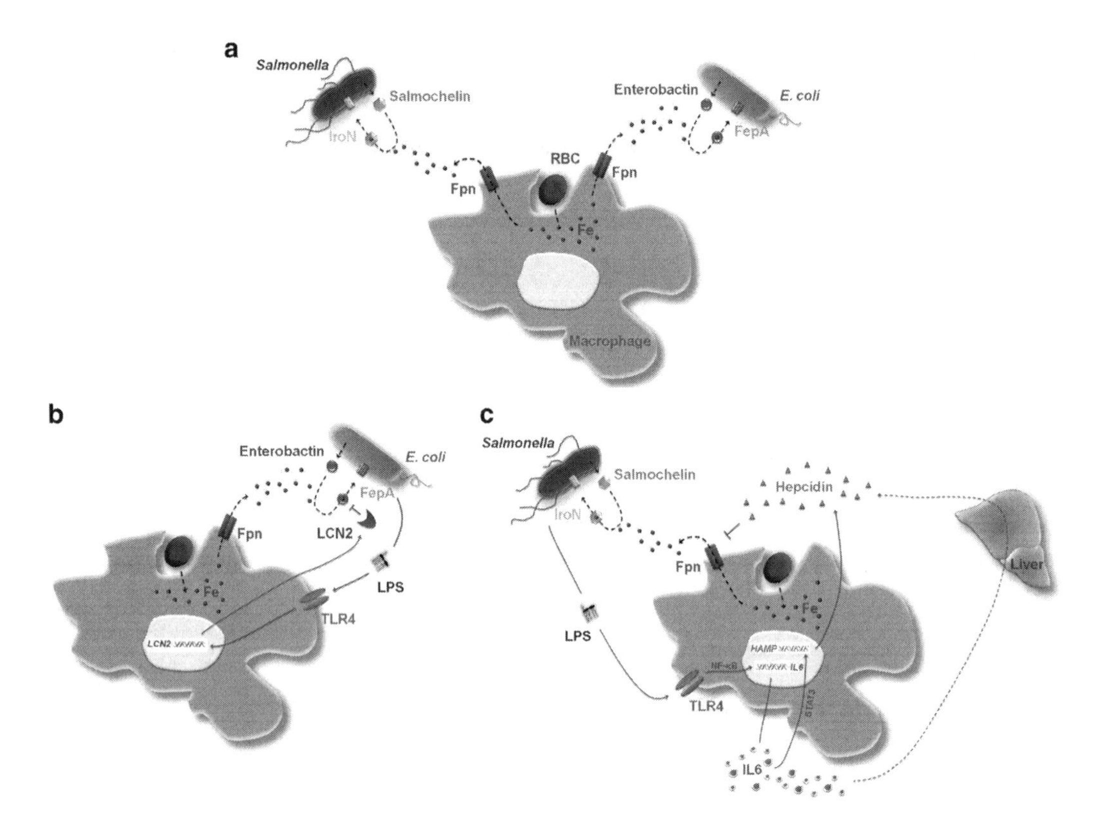

Fig. 12.1 Interactions between microorganisms, the host and iron. (**a**) Macrophages ingest senescent red blood cells and liberate iron from heme, and this iron can be exported back into serum via ferroportin. Iron in serum is a target for scavenging by bacteria – some organisms use the siderophore enterobactin, others may use related but chemically distinct siderophores such as salmochelin. FepA and IroN act as receptors to mediate specific capture of iron-bound siderophores to supply the pathogens with iron, facilitating microbial growth and spread. (**b**) Bacterial components are recognized by host molecules and help initiate anti-microbial responses. In the example shown, bacterial lipopolysaccharide (*LPS*) is bound by the host protein Toll-like receptor 4 (*TLR4*). Innate immune signaling downstream of this recognition event leads to the increased synthesis of lipocalin-2 (*LCN-2*). The bacterial siderophore enterobactin is sequestered by LCN-2, preventing the pathogen from accessing its vital nutrient iron. LCN2-bound to siderophore can be taken up into host cells via 24p3 (not shown). However, some siderophores, for example salmochelin, evade LCN-2 binding and so maintain a supply of iron to the pathogen. (**c**) LPS recognition also leads to the synthesis of hepcidin by both macrophages and liver hepatocytes through the synthesis and action of interleukin-6 (*IL6*). Hepcidin inhibits ferroportin, locking iron in macrophages and reducing serum iron availability. This strategy may deny iron to pathogens that successfully escape LCN-2 restriction. However, it follows that in such circumstances, more iron is present in macrophages, and many types of bacteria are able to successfully colonize this cell type, perhaps utilizing the expanded iron reservoir within

However, this is not the end of the story, and some pathogens have responded by redesigning their siderophores (Fig. 12.1a, b) to evade lipocalin-2 sequestration. Salmonella use siderophores known as salmochelins [31, 32], which are similar to enterobactin but are modified by glucosylation – this alteration increases solubility and stability [33, 34]. In addition, salmochelins are not bound by lipocalin-2 which means salmochelin-synthesizing pathogens escape the mechanisms that restrict the growth of enterobactin-secreting bacteria [35]. However, the glucosylated siderophores also do not bind the bacterial enterobactin importer FepA, meaning an alternative transport system is required for importing salmochelin. In *Salmonella*, the iron-regulated *iroA* gene cluster encodes this machinery [36], along with the enzymes to glucosylate enterobactin. IroB adds glucoses to enterobactin; IroE may linearize the glucosylated siderophore, which is secreted via IroC. IroN then captures and imports iron-bound siderophore through the outer membrane, and IroD releases iron from the siderophore once it is in the cytoplasm [34, 37]. The *iroA* gene cluster is not restricted to *Salmonella*, but is found in a variety of gram-negative bacteria, including the pathogenic varieties of *E. coli.* Fischbasch et al. have found that evasion of lipocalin-2 due to the operation of the *iroA* gene cluster explains the increased virulence of bacterial strains making glusosylated siderophores [35]. Other bacteria also make siderophores that evade lipocalin-2, but use different strategies – for instance *Bacillus anthrax* synthesizes the non-lipocalin-2-binding siderophore petrobactin [38]. It may be that evasion of lipocalin-2 is a necessary step for a bacterial species that is otherwise commensal, to become virulent and pathogenic.

Lipocalin-2, although clearly involved in host defense against bacteria, has not been implicated in modulating host iron transport under normal conditions, although such a role could be possible if a mammalian siderophore could be definitively identified. Instead, mammalian iron homeostasis is maintained by the iron regulatory hormone hepcidin [39] (see Chap. 9), and evidence is accumulating that hepcidin is also involved in the innate immune response to infection (Fig. 12.1c). Hepcidin has some sequence and structural resemblance to the microbicidal beta-defensins, although at present it appears that hepcidin has comparatively weak anti-microbial activity [40–42]. Hepcidin inhibits iron export by binding and causing the degradation of ferroportin [43], in so doing restricting dietary iron absorption through enterocytes and blocking iron recycling from macrophages following erythrophagocytosis [44]. Abrogation of the ferroportin-hepcidin interaction, which occurs with hepcidin-resistant ferroportin mutants such as C326Y, leads to severe systemic iron overload in humans [45]. This finding, along with studies of hepcidin and ferroportin deletion in mice [46, 47], shows that despite the vital importance of iron to physiology, and the necessity of maintaining homeostasis to preserve health, there is a surprising lack of redundancy in the systems tasked with keeping iron in balance. Why should this be? One advantage of such an iron transport 'bottleneck' through ferroportin that is inhibited by only one 'cork' (hepcidin) may be that it allows rapid modulation of serum iron levels. Indeed, infusion of hepcidin can drastically lower serum iron. A 50-μg injection of synthetic hepcidin was enough to reduce serum iron by up to 80% within 1 h [48]. Such a rapid change cannot be accounted for by altering iron absorption, and most likely occurs by locking iron in macrophages through the inhibition of ferroportin. Indeed, injected radiolabelled hepcidin accumulates in ferroportin-rich organs.

A rapid induction of hepcidin expression caused by physiological stimuli could be expected to have similarly potent effects on the geography of iron distribution. As noted above, some bacteria secrete siderophores that obtain iron from their host and avoid the innate immune response strategy of lipocalin-2 secretion. Removing iron from the circulation and locking it in macrophages may be a potent way of denying iron to these pathogens. Several studies have linked hepcidin synthesis to stimulation of the innate immune response by pathogen recognition. Nemeth et al. showed that hepcidin expression during inflammation induced by bacterial LPS is similar to that of an acute phase protein [49]. The pro-inflammatory cytokine interleukin-6 switches on hepcidin expression through the action of the STAT3 transcription factor [50]. IL6 synthesis in turn follows the binding of LPS to TLR4 and the translocation into the nucleus of the transcription factor NF-κB [51]. LPS and TLR4 ligation lead to increased hepcidin expression in both hepatocytes and myeloid cells such as monocytes and neutrophils, and increased serum hepcidin in humans [52–54]. Thus, the detection of LPS initiates the synthesis of host proteins lipocalin-2 (Fig. 12.1b), which prevents bacterial iron acquisition by enterochelin, and hepcidin, which removes iron from extracellular fluids. LPS is not the only TLR agonist that can lead to mammalian hepcidin synthesis – there are indications of other bacterial components such as acylated lipopeptides and flagellin switch on hepcidin too, implicating TLR1, 2, 5 and 6 [55, 56]. In fish, hepcidin synthesis can also be a consequence of exposure to viral nucleic acids [57, 58]. The activation of hepcidin by bacteria can lead to the anemia of infection, for instance following the administration of heat-killed *Brucella abortus* into mice [59]. In this model, the anemia is not responsive to stimulation of erythropoiesis, probably because hepcidin diverts iron away from the bone marrow, reducing its availability for hemoglobin synthesis. Sasu et al. found that suppressing hepcidin's activity using anti-hepcidin neutralizing antibodies allowed the successful treatment of bacteria-induced anemia using erythropoiesis-stimulating agents [59].

These results are particularly interesting given some recent data suggesting that hepcidin induction may contribute to the anemia of malaria [55, 60–63]. Four species of the protozoan parasite *Plasmodium* cause significant human infection, with most fatalities caused by *P. falciparum*-associated malaria. Following an infected mosquito bite, *Plasmodium* sporozoites home to the liver, where they infect hepatocytes and proliferate extensively. Merozoites are then released into blood, where they infect erythrocytes and replicate further. Development of the erythrocyte stage of *Plasmodium* infection is associated with anemia, which is a major contributor to the morbidity of malaria [64, 65]. There are several causes of malarial anemia, including parasite-induced hemolysis, increased uptake of infected and uninfected red cells by macrophages and dyserythropoiesis [65]. An inability to make new red cells could be caused by increased hepcidin synthesis, as appears to be the case in the *Brucella abortus* model of anemia described above. Consistent with this idea, three reports have found increased hepcidin during natural infections [60, 61, 63], and one study of experimental infection of humans also described an increase in serum hepcidin that correlated with anemia [62]. Furthermore, parasitized red blood cells were found to induce hepcidin mRNA expression in co-cultured human leukocytes [55]. If hepcidin induction is shown to have an important role in the pathogenesis of malarial anemia, the development and use of hepcidin antagonists may allow for better treatment of this important disease. Whether the induction of hepcidin following pathogen recognition can control infections has not been determined. It may be that hepcidin and other innate immune defenses such as lipocalin-2 act in concert, so the importance of hepcidin may only be revealed by the use of appropriate multi-knock-out or conditional knock-out mice. It is also not clear whether hepcidin made in the liver or by extra-hepatic sources is likely to be more important during the response to infection. The liver is constantly exposed to bacterial components including LPS derived from the gut flora and delivered via the hepatic portal vein. However, the liver is not in a state of constant inflammation, and is believed to be 'LPS tolerant' compared to other cells of the innate immune response, for example extra-hepatic macrophages [66]. Therefore, although hepatic hepcidin synthesis is undoubtedly crucial in maintaining iron balance, it may be that hepcidin derived from other cell types (monocytes or lymphocytes) contributes to the nutrient deprivation response to infection, particularly at local foci of infection.

Much of the above work has centered on the response to iron acquiring infectious bacterial and eukaryotic pathogens. However, it has become apparent that iron transport is also important in the context of viral infections, as discussed below.

2.4 Viral Manipulation of Iron Metabolism: The Pathogen Strikes Back

Viruses annex the ability of cells to synthesize macromolecules, and utilize this machinery to mass-produce themselves. Cellular factories reprogrammed to actively replicate viruses need raw materials to carry out their new assignment. The generation of ATP, of DNA and of proteins all require iron; many highly conserved enzymes with fundamental roles in cellular physiology are iron-dependent. Depriving infected cells of bioavailable iron, or interrupting crucial iron-dependent processes, can halt viral replication (reviewed in [18]). Iron chelators can inhibit the in vitro growth of Hepatitis B virus (HBV), human cytomegalovirus (HCMV), herpes simplex virus 1, vaccinia virus and human immunodeficiency virus 1 (HIV-1) [67–75]. The life-style of the particular virus determines susceptibility to different types of drug. A recent study on the efficacy of the iron chelator deferiprone and anti-fungal agent ciclopirox illustrates this point [76]. Hoque et al. found that both drugs inhibited HIV-1 replication by preventing the generation of the unusual amino acid hypusine [76]. Hypusine forms part of the host molecule eIF5 [77], a protein which HIV-1 co-opts to promote its own replication [78]. An enzyme that forms hypusine, deoxyhypusine hydroxylase, is iron-dependent [79] and inhibited by the presence of the iron chelator, but is also blocked by the fungicide ciclopirox. Thus, the dependence of HIV-1 on an unusual iron-requiring process can be exploited by well-targeted drugs [78, 80] at least at the cellular level in vitro.

Given the requirement for iron in cellular physiology, one might expect a replication fitness advantage for viruses that targeted iron-acquiring, metabolically active cells. Transferrin receptor-1 (TfR1) is a high-affinity receptor for transferrin-iron, and expression of TfR1 is a marker for rapidly dividing cells. Several viruses in different species have evolved to use TfR1 as a cellular receptor for viral entry: mouse mammary tumor virus [81], the related feline panleukemia and canine parvoviruses [82–85] and the New World hemorrhagic fever-associated clade B arenaviruses of humans [86]. Of these latter viruses, the natural hosts are New World rodents, and in these animals, the cellular protein that binds the viral glycoprotein is also TfR1 [87, 88]. However, the acquisition of human TfR1 binding, which may have occurred as the viral glycoprotein evolved to fit different rodent TfR1, allows zoonotic transmission, with pathogenic consequences [89]. Other clade B arenaviruses can infect humans without using TfR1 as a receptor, but despite being similar to the hemorrhagic-fever associated viruses in other aspects, these arenaviruses are not pathogenic [90]. It is possible that the greater cellular activity of cells expressing high levels of TfR1 may engender a faster rate of viral replication on those viruses that target TfR1, potentially selecting for 'best-fit' variants. Furthermore, binding of viral glycoprotein to TfR1 is not blocked by iron-transferrin, indicating that iron uptake and viral entry could occur concurrently [86]. At present, there are no published studies into the iron-dependency of arenavirus replication, or of whether host iron status influences the outcome of infection.

Changes in body iron have been associated with altered progression of other types of viral infections in humans, although the molecular mechanisms are not always clear. Increased liver iron is frequently observed and is a co-morbidity factor in Hepatitis C virus infection [20, 21, 91]. Excessive iron in the liver can potentiate the formation of free radical species and exacerbate inflammation and fibrosis [92]. Iron depletion therapy of HCV+patients has been found to ameliorate disease and in some cases rescue response to anti-viral therapy (reviewed in [20]). What is the cause of the increased iron that is deleterious in HCV infection? A strong candidate is reduced expression of the iron regulatory hormone hepcidin; HCV is so far unique in being the only pathogen of humans that causes a suppression of hepcidin levels. Several groups have found lower hepcidin (or reduced relatively to serum ferritin compared to uninfected patients) to be a conserved feature of otherwise ethnically and viral-genotypically distinct cohorts of HCV+patients [93–96]. The liver-iron loading observed in hereditary hemochromatosis is generally believed to be the result of relatively reduced hepcidin [97], so by analogy, the iron deposition in the liver in HCV+patients may also be caused by reduced hepcidin. The mechanism by which HCV suppresses hepcidin in vivo is not entirely clear. Reports suggest that reactive oxygen species in virally infected cells or in transgenic mice expressing the HCV polyprotein can act on the hepcidin promoter to reduce transcription [98, 99]. Whether the increased iron concentration in infected hepatocytes as a result of 'viral hemochromatosis' benefits HCV is also a matter of debate. Studies have suggested iron can enhance HCV replication, possibly through promoting translation of viral RNA [100–102], but another group has shown iron can inhibit the viral RNA polymerase [103]. Notwithstanding these issues, the link between HCV and reduced hepcidin is further evidence of the importance of altered iron metabolism in viral infections.

Likewise, an increased iron status, and polymorphisms in the hemoglobin-binding protein haptoglobin, correlates with poor survival in HIV-1 infection [17, 18, 104]. This may be because increased iron availability favors HIV-1 replication [62] or because the iron is advantageous for opportunistic secondary pathogens that colonize the immunodeficient host: One secondary infection particularly associated with HIV-1 is that of Kaposi Herpes Simplex Virus, and intriguingly the incidence of this viral infection has (independently of HIV-1) also been linked to a high-iron environment [105–107]. The importance of iron for HIV-1 replication has been shown by the anti-viral effects of several different iron chelators, which work by different mechanisms [67, 70–72, 74, 75]. In vitro, extra iron can increase synthesis of the viral protein p24 by infected cells [62]. Increased iron levels in bone marrow macrophages also correlates with progression of HIV/AIDS [108]. HIV-1 may deliberately acquire iron for infected cells by manipulation of the hemochromatosis protein HFE [109]. The precise function of HFE remains enigmatic, although it contributes to hepcidin control in hepatocytes [110–112]; it also regulates iron transport in macrophages [113–116]. We found that the Nef protein of HIV-1, known to downregulate HLA-A and HLA-B molecules [117], also downregulates HFE and reroutes it from the cell surface to a trans-golgi-linked compartment [109]. This process leads to iron accumulation in infected macrophages expressing wild-type but not C282Y HFE. This finding has similarities with the earlier discovery that the US2 protein of HCMV targets both HFE, increasing cellular iron levels, and HLA proteins, in order to evade T-cell immunity [118, 119]. The targeting of HLA and HFE by HIV and HCMV viral proteins provides another link between the regulation (and viral manipulation) of the immune system and the control of iron metabolism.

3 Iron and Adaptive Immunity: A New Look into a Classic System

3.1 Interest in the Genetic Control of Lymphocyte Numbers Is Motivated by Immunity but Was First Demonstrated in Hereditary Hemochromatosis Patients

Clinically, interest in abnormal expansion or depletion of particular lymphocyte subsets is generally associated with manifestations of immunity against viral infections specially HIV progression to AIDS. At the systemic level, the importance of lymphocyte numbers is of much greater concern in the immunity literature. As an example, recently Ferreira and co-workers tested 2.3 million variants for association with lymphocyte subsets, including CD4+ and CD8+ T cells, in 2,538 individuals from the general population, trying to identify genetic predictors of lymphocyte levels. Conditional analyses of their results indicated that there are two major independent quantitative trait loci (QTL) in the MHC region that regulate CD4:CD8 ratio: One is located in the class I cluster and influences CD8 levels, whereas the second is located in the class II cluster and regulates CD4 levels [120].

As might have been expected, there is no evidence of interest in possible correlations between genetic predictors of lymphocyte numbers and iron status in the above referred 2,538 individuals analyzed. For historical reasons, as explained in the introduction of this chapter, immunity *not iron homeostasis* is the dominating imprint in the minds of those interested in lymphocytes. But curiously, the first evidence in humans that the numbers of CD8+ T lymphocytes are transmitted in association with genes at the MHC class I region was described some years ago in families of hereditary hemochromatosis patients [121, 122], a study motivated by the consistent observation of abnormalities in the relative and total numbers of peripheral blood CD8+ T lymphocytes in HH patients [123–125].

As reviewed in Chap. 19, hereditary hemochromatosis (HH) is the most common genetic disorder of iron overload. In spite of the fact that more than 80% of patients are homozygous for the C282Y mutation in the *HFE* gene [126], the clinical expression is highly variable. A large proportion of HH patients have low CD8+ T lymphocyte numbers, correlating with a more severe expression of the disease as assessed by high levels of total body iron stores, liver damage and the presence of a larger number of iron overload related symptoms [125, 127]. The reported clinical associations raised the obvious question whether low CD8+ T lymphocyte numbers followed or preceded the development of iron overload. The fact that they were remarkably stable in each individual patient, that they were not corrected by phlebotomy treatment and that they were observed in asymptomatic patients at young ages first favored the hypothesis that they are intrinsic to the genetic defect and not a consequence of the progressive iron overload. This interpretation has now been supported by the demonstration that the CD8+ T lymphocyte numbers are genetically transmitted in association with genes at the MHC-class I region both in HH patients [121, 122] and in normal controls [120, 128]. In HH, this was first demonstrated in family members of patients where CD8+ T-cell numbers were significantly correlated in siblings sharing identical HLA-HFE haplotypes [121]. The question remains if the allele variability in HLA genes in combination with the mutated *HFE* is sufficient to explain the patients' phenotypic heterogeneity or if there is another still unidentified genetic trait in this chromosomal region implicated in the setting of peripheral CD8+ T lymphocyte numbers. The evidence that peripheral blood mononuclear cells from HH patients carrying the C282Y mutation have reduced cell surface expression of MHC class I due to an enhanced endocytosis rate of MHC molecules explained by the triggering of an unfolded protein response [129, 130] supports an interaction between the C282Y mutation and the classical MHC class I route for antigen presentation and lymphocyte activation. Nevertheless, the particular features of the chromosomal region between HLA and *HFE*, namely its remarkable linkage disequilibrium and the high density of genes related to immune responses, make the alternative hypothesis of a novel putative gene/locus involved in the setting of the CD8+ T lymphocyte numbers highly attractive. Work is in progress trying to localize such a putative trait in HH patients and families [131].

3.2 T Lymphocyte Homeostatic Balance Is Compromised in Hereditary Hemochromatosis

One hallmark of T lymphocytes is their capacity of renewal and expansion at the periphery, in a steady-state manner. It is well described that peripheral T lymphocytes are self-renewable cell populations, able to expand in the absence of exogenous antigen stimulation, and tightly regulated by homeostatic mechanisms that control the sizes of their sub compartments, namely the CD4+ and CD8+ T cell pools [132, 133]. It has also been shown that the homeostatic mechanisms controlling the cell renewal and expansion at the periphery are independent for its subpopulations of naïve and memory cells [134, 135]. This kinetic behavior with independent homeostatic regulation of the naïve and memory T cells guarantees the versatility of T-cell repertoires throughout life (persisting after the thymus atrophies at puberty), as well as an extensive modulation of post-thymic selected T-cell specificities for efficient immune responses.

To better address the mechanisms underlying the homeostatic regulation of CD8+ T lymphocytes and its disequilibrium in HH patients, it became necessary to better characterize the distribution of its subpopulations. By using a panel of multiple cell markers previously shown to differentiate CD8+ cell subsets with different functional properties [136], Macedo et al. showed that the low numbers of CD8+ T lymphocytes in HH patients are explained by a defect of the most mature effector cells, lacking the CD27 and CD28 co-receptors, the so-called double negative effector memory cells [4]. It is hoped that by elucidating the networks that down- or upregulate the expression of the subpopulations' related genes one may understand the process of generation, differentiation and self-renewal of these cells.

3.3 How Can Lymphocytes Protect from Iron Toxicity?

The described association in HH patients of a low CD8+ T lymphocyte phenotype with a more severe clinical expression of iron overload [125] supports the notion that these cells may have a role in the protection against iron toxicity, as first proposed by De Sousa in 1978 [137]. The mechanism how lymphocytes could exert this protective role is still not clarified. It is known that lymphocyte activation and expansion depend on the expression of transferrin receptors, required for DNA synthesis and cell division [138], and that both activated and non-activated T lymphocytes synthesize ferritin [139, 140]. More recently, it was shown that lymphocytes express basal hepcidin mRNA levels that increase after T lymphocyte activation and in response to challenge by both holotransferrin (Fe-TF) and ferric citrate in vitro [141]. The same study showed that, like in other cells, lymphocyte hepcidin expression controls intracellular iron levels by regulating the expression of ferroportin, and that inappropriately low expression of hepcidin impairs normal lymphocyte proliferation, therefore establishing hepcidin as a new player in lymphocyte biology [141]. The hypothesis that variations in serum hepcidin may have an impact on T lymphocyte homeostasis is still not tested.

In conclusion, as major circulating blood cell components, lymphocytes may constitute an important 'mobile' and easily 'mobilizable' iron pool with a potential dual function contributing either to protect from iron toxicity through its uptake and retention or as a source of iron through ferroportin mediated export. The latter has been shown recently to occur with a subpopulation of macrophages [3] (see below). The physiological implications of this putative dual behavior are enormous, placing immune system cells in a central position of the complex network not only of regulators of systemic iron balance but also of iron donors to other cells in specific microenvironments. The possibility that a similar phenomenon could occur with some pathogens, to our knowledge, has never been considered.

4 Back to the Future with Macrophages

Although experimental models of spontaneous iron overload developing in lymphocyte deficient mice [142–146] and the more recent finding of the changes in hepcidin mRNA expression in response to challenge by ferric citrate in vitro [141] all point to a role for lymphocytes in iron homeostasis, we wish to conclude the present chapter with another possible 'reciprocal' interaction between immune system cells and iron that may become of exceptional importance in the next decade. This has to do with a recent report from Cairo's group on what they called 'differential regulation of iron homeostasis during human macrophage polarized activation' [3].

By looking at the molecular signature of different types of human macrophages, designated M1 and M2, they observed distinct patterns of iron gene expression in the two types of macrophages. M1 macrophages showed gene expression profiles favoring iron sequestration (ferroportin repression and H ferritin induction), whereas the M2 macrophages had an expression profile that enhanced iron release (ferroportin upregulation and downregulation of ferritin and heme oxygenase). To answer the question whether polarized (M2) macrophages could affect the proliferation of cells present in surrounding tissue microenvironments, they found that after a 24-h incubation of a renal cell carcinoma cell line with conditioned medium of the different macrophage populations had distinct effects. Medium obtained from the M2 population affected the cell line growth by 40%. The proliferation induced by the M2-conditioned medium was reduced in the presence of an iron chelator, HM-DFO [3].

These most elegant experiments stand 102 years from the Nobel lecture of Metchnikoff for his work in immunity. At the beginning of a century where cancer and not infection is a major concern in Western societies, tumor microenvironment begins to be the focus of much attention as unveiling the significance of the presence of macrophages within tumors (TAMs). If macrophages, in addition to doing what Metchnikoff first saw leading him to baptize them phagocytes, and which acquired further public acclaim in immunity in George Bernard Shaw's play 'The Doctor's Dilemma', also control iron availability within tumors, they may actually promote tumor progression (reviewed in [147, 148]) by releasing a critical nutrient in the tumor microenvironment through a mechanism that was only elucidated in the last decade [43].

5 Concluding Remark

We wish to conclude by stating that we felt that there was some danger in accepting to write this chapter. There are enough clues at the beginning of this century telling us that iron and the immune system, as we learnt it last century, was changing as we accepted to write it. The changes, however, will only further sustain Metchnikoff's assertion. Progress in this area will no doubt become one of the best illustrations of the practical value of pure research.

Acknowledgement We gratefully acknowledge SJ Oliveira for the figure depicting the many aspects of the 'iron fight' covered by this chapter.

References

1. Jenner E. An inquiry into the causes and effects of the variolae vaccinae. London: Sampson and Low; 1798.
2. Huchins SR, Davidson MS, Brierley JA, Brierley CI. Microorganisms in reclamation of metals. Ann Rev Microbiol. 1986;40:311–36.
3. Recalcati S, Locati M, Marini A, et al. Differential regulation of iron homeostasis during human macrophage polarized activation. Eur J Immunol. 2010;40:824–35.
4. Macedo F, Porto G, Costa M, Vieira CP, Rocha B, Cruz E. Low numbers of CD8+ T lymphocytesin hereditary hemochromatosis are explained by a decrease of the most mature CD8+ effector memory cells. Clin Exp Immunol. 2010;159:363–71.
5. Porto G, de Sousa M. Iron overload and immunity. World J Gastroenterol. 2007;13:4707–15.
6. Weinberg ED. Nutritional immunity. Host's attempt to withhold iron from microbial invaders. J Am Med Assoc. 1975;231:39–41.
7. Ganz T. Iron in innate immunity: starve the invaders. Curr Opin Immunol. 2009;21:63–7.
8. Schaible UE, Kaufmann SH. Iron and microbial infection. Nat Rev Microbiol. 2004;2:946–53.
9. Ajioka RS, Phillips JD, Kushner JP. Biosynthesis of heme in mammals. Biochim Biophys Acta. 2006;1763:723–36.
10. Hatefi Y. The mitochondrial electron transport and oxidative phosphorylation system. Annu Rev Biochem. 1985;54:1015–69.
11. Jordan A, Reichard P. Ribonucleotide reductases. Annu Rev Biochem. 1998;67:71–98.
12. Ferrer M, Golyshina OV, Beloqui A, Golyshin PN, Timmis KN. The cellular machinery of ferroplasma acidiphilum is iron-protein-dominated. Nature. 2007;445:91–4.
13. Imbert M, Blondeau R. On the iron requirement of lactobacilli grown in chemically defined medium. Curr Microbiol. 1998;37:64–6.
14. Posey JE, Gherardini FC. Lack of a role for iron in the Lyme disease pathogen. Science. 2000;288:1651–3.
15. Prentice AM, Ghattas H, Doherty C, Cox SE. Iron metabolism and malaria. Food Nutr Bull. 2007;28(4 Suppl):S524–39.
16. Sazawal S, Black RE, Ramsan M, et al. Effects of routine prophylactic supplementation with iron and folic acid on admission to hospital and mortality in preschool children in a high malaria transmission setting: community-based, randomised, placebo-controlled trial. Lancet. 2006;367:133–43.
17. McDermid JM, Jaye A, van der Schim Loeff MF, et al. Elevated iron status strongly predicts mortality in West African adults with HIV infection. J Acquir Immune Defic Syndr. 2007;46(4):498–507.
18. Drakesmith H, Prentice A. Viral infection and iron metabolism. Nat Rev Microbiol. 2008;6:6541–52.
19. Boelaert JR, Vandecasteele SJ, Appelberg R, Gordeuk VR. The effect of the host's iron status on tuberculosis. J Infect Dis. 2007;195:1745–53.
20. Franchini M, Targher G, Capra F, Montagnana M, Lippi G. The effect of iron depletion on chronic hepatitis C virus infection. Hepatol Int. 2008;2:335–40.
21. Isom HC, McDevitt EI, Moon MS. Elevated hepatic iron: a confounding factor in chronic hepatitis C. Biochim Biophys Acta. 2009;1790:650–62.
22. Schade AL, Caroline L. An iron-binding component in human blood plasma. Science. 1946;104:340–1.
23. Neilands JB. Siderophores: structure and function of microbial iron transport compounds. J Biol Chem. 1995;270:26723–6.
24. Raymond KN, Dertz EA, Kim SS. Enterobactin: an archetype for microbial iron transport. Proc Natl Acad Sci USA. 2003;100:3584–8.

25. Nikaido H. Porins and specific diffusion channels in bacterial outer membranes. J Biol Chem. 1994;269:3905–8.
26. Annamalai R, Jin B, Cao Z, Newton SM, Klebba PE. Recognition of ferric catecholates by FepA. J Bacteriol. 2004;186:3578–89.
27. Goetz DH, Holmes MA, Borregaard N, Bluhm ME, Raymond KN, Strong RK. The neutrophil lipocalin NGAL is a bacteriostatic agent that interferes with siderophore-mediated iron acquisition. Mol Cell. 2002;10:1033–43.
28. Holmes MA, Paulsene W, Jide X, Ratledge C, Strong RK. Siderocalin (Lcn 2) also binds carboxymycobactins, potentially defending against mycobacterial infections through iron sequestration. Structure. 2005;13:29–41.
29. Flo T, Smith KD, Sato S, et al. Lipocalin 2 mediates an innate immune response to bacterial infection by sequestrating iron. Nature. 2004;432:917–21.
30. Devireddy LR, Gazin C, Zhu X, Green MR. A cell-surface receptor for lipocalin 24p3 selectively mediates apoptosis and iron uptake. Cell. 2005;123:1293–305.
31. Hantke K, Nicholson G, Rabsch W, Winkelmann G. Salmochelins, siderophores of *Salmonella enterica* and uropathogenic *Escherichia coli* strains, are recognized by the outer membrane receptor IroN. Proc Natl Acad Sci USA. 2003;100:3677–82.
32. Muller SI, Valdebenito M, Hantke K. Salmochelin, the long-overlooked catecholate siderophore of Salmonella. Biometals. 2009;22:691–5.
33. Bister B, Bischoff D, Nicholson GJ, et al. The structure of salmochelins: C-glucosylated enterobactins of *Salmonella enterica*. Biometals. 2004;17:471–81.
34. Smith KD. Iron metabolism at the host pathogen interface: lipocalin 2 and the pathogen-associated iroA gene cluster. Int J Biochem Cell Biol. 2007;39:1776–80.
35. Fischbach MA, Lin H, Zhou L, et al. The pathogen-associated iroA gene cluster mediates bacterial evasion of lipocalin 2. Proc Natl Acad Sci USA. 2006;103:16502–7.
36. Baumler AJ, Tsolis RM, van der Velden AW, Stojiljkovic I, Anic S, Heffron F. Identification of a new iron regulated locus of *Salmonella typhi*. Gene. 1996;183:207–13.
37. Fischbach MA, Lin H, Liu DR, Walsh CT. How pathogenic bacteria evade mammalian sabotage in the battle for iron. Nat Chem Biol. 2006;2:132–8.
38. Abergel RJ, Wilson MK, Arceneaux J, et al. Anthrax pathogen evades the mammalian immune system through stealth siderophore production. Proc Natl Acad Sci USA. 2006;103:18499–503.
39. Nemeth E, Ganz T. The role of hepcidin in iron metabolism. Acta Haematol. 2009;122:78–86.
40. Jordan JB, Poppe L, Haniu M, et al. Hepcidin revisited, disulfide connectivity, dynamics, and structure. J Biol Chem. 2009;284:24155–67.
41. Krause A, Neitz S, Magert HJ, et al. LEAP-1, a novel highly disulfide-bonded human peptide, exhibits antimicrobial activity. FEBS Lett. 2000;480:147–50.
42. Park CH, Valore EV, Waring AJ, Ganz T. Hepcidin, a urinary antimicrobial peptide synthesized in the liver. J Biol Chem. 2001;276:7806–10.
43. Nemeth E, Tuttle MS, Powelson J, et al. Hepcidin regulates cellular iron efflux by binding to ferroportin and inducing its internalization. Science. 2004;306:2090–3.
44. Nemeth E, Ganz T. Regulation of iron metabolism by hepcidin. Annu Rev Nutr. 2006;26:323–42.
45. Drakesmith H, Schimanski LM, Ormerod E, et al. Resistance to hepcidin is conferred by hemochromatosis-associated mutations of ferroportin. Blood. 2005;106:1092–7.
46. Donovan A, Lima CA, Pinkus JL, et al. The iron exporter ferroportin/Slc40a is essential for iron homeostasis. Cell Metab. 2005;1:191–200.
47. Lesbordes-Brion JC, Viatte L, Bennoun M, et al. Targeted disruption of the hepcidin 1 gene results in severe hemochromatosis. Blood. 2006;108:1402–5.
48. Rivera S, Nemeth E, Gabayan V, Lopez MA, Farshidi D, Ganz T. Synthetic hepcidin causes rapid dose-dependent hypoferremia and is concentrated in ferroportin-containing organs. Blood. 2005;106:2196–9.
49. Nemeth E, Valore EV, Territo M, Schiller G, Lichtenstein A, Ganz T. Hepcidin, a putative mediator of anemia of inflammation, is a type II acute-phase protein. Blood. 2003;101:2461–3.
50. Wrighting DM, Andrews NC. Interleukin-6 induces hepcidin expression through STAT3. Blood. 2006;108:3204–9.
51. Kumar H, Kawai T, Akira S. Toll-like receptors and innate immunity. Biochem Biophys Res Commun. 2009;388:621–5.
52. Kemna E, Pickkers P, Nemeth E, van der Hoeven H, Swinkels D. Time-course analysis of hepcidin, serum iron, and plasma cytokine levels in humans injected with LPS. Blood. 2005;106:1864–6.
53. Peyssonnaux C, Zinkernagel AS, Datta V, Lauth X, Johnson RS, Nizet V. TLR4-dependent hepcidin expression by myeloid cells in response to bacterial pathogens. Blood. 2006;107:3727–32.
54. Pigeon C, Ilyin G, Courselaud B, et al. A new mouse liver-specific gene, encoding a protein homologous to human antimicrobial peptide hepcidin, is overexpressed during iron overload. J Biol Chem. 2001;276:7811–9.
55. Armitage AE, Pinches R, Eddowes LA, Newbold CI, Drakesmith H. Plasmodium falciparum infected erythrocytes induce hepcidin (HAMP) mRNA synthesis by peripheral blood mononuclear cells. Br J Haematol. 2009;147:769–71.

56. Koening CL, Miller JC, Nelson JM, et al. Toll-like receptors mediate induction of hepcidin in mice infected with *Borrelia burgdorferi*. Blood. 2009;114:1913–8.
57. Zheng W, Liu G, Ao J, Chen X. Expression analysis of immune-relevant genes in the spleen of large yellow croaker (*Pseudosciaena crocea*) stimulated with poly I:C. Fish Shellfish Immunol. 2006;21:414–30.
58. Chiou PP, Lin CM, Bols NC, Chen TT. Characterization of virus/double-stranded RNA-dependent induction of antimicrobial peptide hepcidin in trout macrophages. Dev Comp Immunol. 2007;31:1297–309.
59. Sasu BJ, Cooke KS, Arvedson TL, et al. Anti-hepcidin antibody treatment modulates iron metabolism and is effective in a mouse model of inflammation-induced anemia. Blood. 2010;115:3616–24.
60. de Mast Q, Nadjm B, Reyburn H, et al. Assessment of urinary concentrations of hepcidin provides novel insight into disturbances in iron homeostasis during malarial infection. J Infect Dis. 2009;199:253–62.
61. de Mast Q, Syafruddin D, Keijmel S, et al. Increased serum hepcidin and alterations in blood iron parameters associated with asymptomatic *P. falciparum* and *P. vivax* malaria. Haematologica. 2010;95:1068–74.
62. de Mast Q, van Dongen-Lases EC, Swinkels DW, et al. Mild increases in serum hepcidin and interleukin-6 concentrations impair iron incorporation in haemoglobin during an experimental human malaria infection. Br J Haematol. 2009;145:657–64.
63. Howard CT, McKakpo US, Quakyi IA, et al. Relationship of hepcidin with parasitemia and anemia among patients with uncomplicated *Plasmodium falciparum* malaria in Ghana. Am J Trop Med Hyg. 2007;77:623–6.
64. Haldar K, Mohandas N. Malaria, erythrocytic infection, and anemia. Hematol Am Soc Hematol Educ Program. 2009;87–93.
65. Lamikanra AA, Brown D, Potocnik A, Casals-Pascual C, Langhorne J, Roberts DJ. Malarial anemia: of mice and men. Blood. 2007;110:18–28.
66. Crispe IN. The liver as a lymphoid organ. Annu Rev Immunol. 2009;27:147–63.
67. Traore HN, Meyer D. The effect of iron overload on in vitro HIV-1 infection. J Clin Virol. 2004;31 Suppl 1:S92–8.
68. Chouteau P, Le Seyec J, Saulier-Le Drean B, et al. Inhibition of hepatitis B virus production associated with high levels of intracellular viral DNA intermediates in iron-depleted HepG2.2.15 cells. J Hepatol. 2001;34:108–13.
69. Cinatl Jr J, Cinatl J, Rabenau H, Gumbel HO, Kornhuber B, Doerr HW. In vitro inhibition of human cytomegalovirus replication by desferrioxamine. Antiviral Res. 1994;25:73–7.
70. Georgiou NA, van der Bruggen T, Oudshoorn M, et al. Mechanism of inhibition of the human immunodeficiency virus type 1 by the oxygen radical generating agent bleomycin. Antiviral Res. 2004;63:97–106.
71. Georgiou NA, van der Bruggen T, Oudshoorn M, Hider RC, Marx JJ, van Asbeck BS. Human immunodeficiency virus type 1 replication inhibition by the bidentate iron chelators CP502 and CP511 is caused by proliferation inhibition and the onset of apoptosis. Eur J Clin Invest. 2002;32 Suppl 1:91–6.
72. Georgiou NA, van der Bruggen T, Oudshoorn M, Nottet HS, Marx JJ, van Asbeck BS. Inhibition of human immunodeficiency virus type 1 replication in human mononuclear blood cells by the iron chelators deferoxamine, deferiprone, and bleomycin. J Infect Dis. 2000;181:484–90.
73. Romeo AM, Christen L, Niles EG, Kosman DJ. Intracellular chelation of iron by bipyridyl inhibits DNA virus replication: ribonucleotide reductase maturation as a probe of intracellular iron pools. J Biol Chem. 2001;276:24301–8.
74. Sappey C, Boelaert JR, Legrand-Poels S, Forceille C, Favier A, Piette J. Iron chelation decreases NF-kappa B and HIV type 1 activation due to oxidative stress. AIDS Res Hum Retroviruses. 1995;11:1049–61.
75. Debebe Z, Ammosova T, Jerebtsova M, et al. Iron chelators ICL670 and 311 inhibit HIV-1 transcription. Virology. 2007;367:324–33.
76. Hoque M, Hanauske-Abel HM, Palumbo P, et al. Inhibition of HIV-1 gene expression by Ciclopirox and Deferiprone, drugs that prevent hypusination of eukaryotic initiation factor 5A. Retrovirology. 2009;6:90.
77. Cooper HL, Park MH, Folk JE, Safer B, Braverman R. Identification of the hypusine-containing protein hy+as translation initiation factor eIF-4D. Proc Natl Acad Sci USA. 1983;80:1854–7.
78. Ruhl M, Himmelspach M, Bahr GM, et al. Eukaryotic initiation factor 5A is a cellular target of the human immunodeficiency virus type 1 Rev activation domain mediating trans-activation. J Cell Biol. 1993;123:1309–20.
79. Kim YS, Kang KR, Wolff EC, Bell JK, McPhie P, Park MH. Deoxyhypusine hydroxylase is an Fe(II)-dependent, HEAT-repeat enzyme. Identification of amino acid residues critical for Fe(II) binding and catalysis. J Biol Chem. 2006;281:13217–25.
80. Hauber I, Bevec D, Heukeshoven J, et al. Identification of cellular deoxyhypusine synthase as a novel target for antiretroviral therapy. J Clin Invest. 2005;115:76–85.
81. Ross SR, Schofield J, Farr CJ, Bucan M. Mouse transferrin receptor 1 is the cell entry receptor for mouse mammary tumor virus. Proc Natl Acad Sci USA. 2002;99:12386–90.
82. Hueffer K, Govindasamy L, Agbandje-McKenna M, Parrish CR. Combinations of two capsid regions controlling canine host range determine canine transferrin receptor binding by canine and feline parvoviruses. J Virol. 2003;77:10099–105.
83. Hueffer K, Parker JS, Weichert WS, Geisel RE, Sgro JY, Parrish CR. The natural host range shift and subsequent evolution of canine parvovirus resulted from virus-specific binding to the canine transferrin receptor. J Virol. 2003;77:1718–26.

84. Hueffer K, Parrish CR. Parvovirus host range, cell tropism and evolution. Curr Opin Microbiol. 2003;6:392–8.
85. Parker JS, Murphy WJ, Wang D, O'Brien SJ, Parrish CR. Canine and feline parvoviruses can use human or feline transferrin receptors to bind, enter, and infect cells. J Virol. 2001;75:3896–902.
86. Radoshitzky SR, Abraham J, Spiropoulou CF, et al. Transferrin receptor 1 is a cellular receptor for New World haemorrhagic fever arenaviruses. Nature. 2007;446:92–6.
87. Abraham J, Kwong JA, Albarino CG, et al. Host-species transferrin receptor 1 orthologs are cellular receptors for nonpathogenic new world clade B arenaviruses. PLoS Pathog. 2009;5:e1000358.
88. Radoshitzky SR, Kuhn JH, Spiropoulou CF, et al. Receptor determinants of zoonotic transmission of New World hemorrhagic fever arenaviruses. Proc Natl Acad Sci USA. 2008;105:2664–9.
89. Abraham J, Corbett KD, Farzan M, Choe H, Harrison SC. Structural basis for receptor recognition by New World hemorrhagic fever arenaviruses. Nat Struct Mol Biol. 2010;17:438–44.
90. Flanagan MI, Oldenburg J, Reignier T, et al. New World clade B arenaviruses can use transferrin receptor 1 (TfR1)-dependent and independent entry pathways, and glycoproteins from human pathogenic strains are associated with the use of TfR1. J Virol. 2008;82:938–48.
91. Thursz M. Iron, haemochromatosis and thalassaemia as risk factors for fibrosis in hepatitis C virus infection. Gut. 2007;56:613–4.
92. Kowdley KV. Iron, hemochromatosis, and hepatocellular carcinoma. Gastroenterology. 2004;127(5 Suppl 1): S79–86.
93. Girelli D, Pasino M, Goodnough JB, et al. Reduced serum hepcidin levels in patients with chronic hepatitis C. J Hepatol. 2009;51:845–52.
94. Sugimoto R, Fujita N, Tomosugi N. Impaired regulation of serum hepcidin during phlebotomy in patients with chronic hepatitis C. Hepatol Res. 2009;39:619–24.
95. Fujita N, Sugimoto R, Motonishi S, et al. Patients with chronic hepatitis C achieving a sustained virological response to peginterferon and ribavirin therapy recover from impaired hepcidin secretion. J Hepatol. 2008;49:702–10.
96. Tsochatzis E, Papatheodoridis GV, Koliaraki V, et al. Serum hepcidin levels are related to the severity of liver histological lesions in chronic hepatitis C. J Viral Hepat. 2010;17:800–6.
97. Bridle KR, Frazer DM, Wilkins SJ, et al. Disrupted hepcidin regulation in HFE-associated haemochromatosis and the liver as a regulator of body iron homoeostasis. Lancet. 2003;361:669–73.
98. Miura K, Taura K, Kodama Y, Schnabl B. Brenner DA Hepatitis C virus-induced oxidative stress suppresses hepcidin expression through increased histone deacetylase activity. Hepatology. 2008;48:1420–9.
99. Nishina S, Hino K, Korenaga M, et al. Hepatitis C virus-induced reactive oxygen species raise hepatic iron level in mice by reducing hepcidin transcription. Gastroenterology. 2008;134:226–38.
100. Kakizaki S, Takagi H, Horiguchi N, et al. Iron enhances hepatitis C virus replication in cultured human hepatocytes. Liver. 2000;20:125–8.
101. Cho H, Lee HC, Jang SK, Kim YK. Iron increases translation initiation directed by internal ribosome entry site of hepatitis C virus. Virus Genes. 2008;37:154–60.
102. Theurl I, Zoller H, Obrist P, et al. Iron regulates hepatitis C virus translation via stimulation of expression of translation initiation factor 3. J Infect Dis. 2004;190:819–25.
103. Fillebeen C, Rivas-Estilla AM, Bisaillon M, et al. Iron inactivates the RNA polymerase NS5B and suppresses subgenomic replication of hepatitis C Virus. J Biol Chem. 2005;280:9049–57.
104. Delanghe JR, Langlois MR, Boelaert JR, et al. Haptoglobin polymorphism, iron metabolism and mortality in HIV infection. AIDS. 1998;12:1027–32.
105. Simonart T. Iron: a target for the management of Kaposi's sarcoma? BMC Cancer. 2004;4:1.
106. Simonart T, Noel JC, Andrei G, et al. Iron as a potential co-factor in the pathogenesis of Kaposi's sarcoma? Int J Cancer. 1998;78:720–6.
107. Ziegler JL, Simonart T, Snoeck R. Kaposi's sarcoma, oncogenic viruses, and iron. J Clin Virol. 2001;20:127–30.
108. de Monye C, Karcher DS, Boelaert JR, Gordeuk VR. Bone marrow macrophage iron grade and survival of HIV-seropositive patients. AIDS. 1999;13:375–80.
109. Drakesmith H, Chen N, Ledermann H, Screaton G, Townsend A, Xu XN. HIV-1 Nef down-regulates the hemochromatosis protein HFE, manipulating cellular iron homeostasis. Proc Natl Acad Sci USA. 2005;102:11017–22.
110. Gao J, Chen J, De Domenico I, et al. Hepatocyte-targeted HFE and TFR2 control hepcidin expression in mice. Blood. 2010;115:3374–81.
111. Gao J, Chen J, Kramer M, Tsukamoto H, Zhang AS, Enns CA. Interaction of the hereditary hemochromatosis protein HFE with transferrin receptor 2 is required for transferrin-induced hepcidin expression. Cell Metab. 2009;9:217–27.
112. Vujic Spasic M, Kiss J, Herrmann T, et al. Hfe acts in hepatocytes to prevent hemochromatosis. Cell Metab. 2008;7:173–8.
113. Drakesmith H, Sweetland E, Schimanski L, et al. The hemochromatosis protein HFE inhibits iron export from macrophages. Proc Natl Acad Sci USA. 2002;99:15602–7.

114. Garuti C, Tian Y, Montosi G, et al. Hepcidin expression does not rescue the iron-poor phenotype of Kupffer cells in Hfe-null mice after liver transplantation. Gastroenterology. 2010;139:315–22.
115. Makui H, Soares RJ, Jiang W, Constante M, Santos MM. Contribution of Hfe expression in macrophages to the regulation of hepatic hepcidin levels and iron loading. Blood. 2005;106:2189–95.
116. Montosi G, Paglia P, Garuti C, et al. Wild-type HFE protein normalizes transferrin iron accumulation in macrophages from subjects with hereditary hemochromatosis. Blood. 2000;96:1125–9.
117. Schwartz O, Marechal V, Le Gall S, Lemonnier F, Heard JM. Endocytosis of major histocompatibility complex class I molecules is induced by the HIV-1 Nef protein. Nat Med. 1996;2:338–42.
118. Ben-Arieh SV, Zimerman B, Smorodinsky NI, et al. Human cytomegalovirus protein US2 interferes with the expression of human HFE, a nonclassical class I major histocompatibility complex molecule that regulates iron homeostasis. J Virol. 2001;75:10557–62.
119. Vahdati-Ben Arieh S, Laham N, Schechter C, Yewdell JW, Coligan JE, Ehrlich R. A single viral protein HCMV US2 affects antigen presentation and intracellular iron homeostasis by degradation of classical HLA class I and HFE molecules. Blood. 2003;101:2858–64.
120. Ferreira MA, Mangino M, Brumme CJ, et al. International HIV Controllers Study, Quantitative trait loci for CD4:CD8 lymphocyte ratio are associated with risk of type 1 diabetes and HIV-1 immune control. Am J Hum Genet. 2010;86:88–92.
121. Cruz E, Vieira J, Goncalves R, et al. Involvement of the major histocompatibility complex region in the genetic regulation of circulating CD8 T-cell numbers in humans. Tissue Antigens. 2004;64:25–34.
122. Cruz E, Vieira J, Almeida S, et al. A study of 82 extended HLA haplotypes in HFE-C282Y homozygous hemochromatosis subjects: relationship to the genetic control of CD8+ T-lymphocyte numbers and severity of iron overload. BMC Med Genet. 2006;7:16.
123. Porto G, Reimao R, Goncalves C, Vicente C, Justiça B, De Sousa M. Haemochromatosis as a window into the study of the immunological system: a novel correlation between CD8+ lymphocytes and iron overload. Eur J Haematol. 1994;52:283–90.
124. Porto G, Vicente C, Teixeira MA, et al. Relative impact of HLA and CD4/CD8 ratios on the clinical expression of hemochromatosis. Hepatology. 1997;25:397–402.
125. Cruz E, Melo G, Lacerda R, Almeida S, Porto G. The CD8+ T-lymphocyte profile as a modifier of iron overload in HFE hemochromatosis: an update of clinical and immunological data from 70 C282Y homozygous subjects. Blood Cells Mol Dis. 2006;37:33–9.
126. Feder JN, Gnirke A, Thomas W, et al. A novel MHC class I like gene is mutated in patients with hereditary haemochromatosis. Nat Genet. 1996;13:399–406.
127. Cardoso EMP, Hagen K, De Sousa M, Hulcrantz R. Hepatic damage in C282Y homozygotes relates to low numbers of CD8+ cells in the liver lobuli. Eur J Clin Invest. 2001;31:45–53.
128. Vieira J, Cardoso C, Pinto J, et al. A putative gene located at the MHC class I region around the D6S105 marker contributes to the setting of CD8+ T-lymphocyte numbers in humans. Int J Immunogenet. 2007;34:359–67.
129. De Almeida SF, Carvalho IF, Cardoso CS, et al. HFE crosstalks with the MHC class I antigen presentation pathway. Blood. 2005;106:971–7.
130. De Almeida SF, Fleming JV, Azevedo J, Carmo-Fonseca M, De Sousa M. Stimulation of an unfolded protein response impairs MHC class I expression. J Immunol. 2007;178:3612–9.
131. Cruz E, Whittington C, Krikler SH, et al. A new 500 kb haplotype associated with high CD8+ T-lymphocyte numbers predicts a less severe expression of hereditary hemochromatosis. BMC Med Genet. 2008;9:97.
132. Rocha B, Dautigny N, Pereira P. Peripheral T lymphocytes: expansion potential and homeostatic regulation of pool sizes and CD4/CD8 ratios in vivo. Eur J Immunol. 1989;19:905–11.
133. Freitas AA, Rocha B. Population biology of lymphocytes: the flight for survival. Annu Rev Immunol. 2000;18:83–111.
134. Tanchot C, Fernandes HV, Rocha B. The organization of mature T-cell pools. Philos Trans R Soc Lond B Biol Sci. 2000;355:323–8.
135. Almeida AR, Rocha B, Freitas AA, Tanchot C. Homeostasis of T cell numbers: from thymus production to peripheral compartmentalization and the indexation of regulatory T cells. Semin Immunol. 2005;17:239–49.
136. Monteiro M, Evaristo C, Legrand A, Nicoletti A, Rocha B. Cartography of gene expression in CD8 single cells: novel CCR7- subsets suggest differentiation independent of CD45RA expression. Blood. 2007;109:2863–70.
137. De Sousa M. Lymphoid cell positioning: a new proposal for the mechanism of control of lymphoid cell migration. Symp Soc Exp Biol. 1978;32:393–410.
138. Neckers LM, Cossman J. Transferrin receptor induction in mitogen-stimulated human T lymphocytes is required for DNA synthesis and cell division and is regulated by interleukin 2. Proc Natl Acad Sci USA. 1983;80:3494–8.
139. Dörner MH, Silverstone A, Nishiya K, de Sostoa A, Munn G, de Sousa M. Ferritin synthesis by human T lymphocytes. Science. 1980;209:1019–21.
140. Vezzoni P, Levi S, Gabri E, Pozzi MR, Spinazze S, Arosio P. Ferritins in malignant and non-malignant lymphoid cells. Br J Haematol. 1986;62:105–10.

141. Pinto JP, Dias V, Zoller H, et al. Hepcidin Messenger RNA expression in human lymphocytes. Immunology. 2010;130:217–30.
142. de Sousa M, Reimão R, Lacerda R, Hugo P, Kaufmann SH, Porto G. Iron overload in beta 2-microglobulin-deficient mice. Immunol Lett. 1994;39:105–11.
143. Santos M, Schilham MW, Rademakers LH, Marx JJ, de Sousa M, Clevers H. Defective iron homeostasis in beta 2-microglobulin knockout mice recapitulates hereditary hemochromatosis in man. J Exp Med. 1996;184:1975–85.
144. Santos MM, de Sousa M, Rademakers LH, Clevers H, Marx JJ, Schilham MW. Iron overload and heart fibrosis in mice deficient for both beta2-microglobulin and Rag1. Am J Pathol. 2000;157:1883–92.
145. Cardoso EM, Macedo MG, Rohrlich P, et al. Increased hepatic iron in mice lacking classical MHC class I molecules. Blood. 2002;100:4235–41.
146. Muckenthaler MU, Rodrigues P, Macedo MG, et al. Molecular analysis of iron overload in beta2-microglobulin-deficient mice. Blood Cells Mol Dis. 2004;33:125–31.
147. Mantovani A, Sica A. Macrophages, innate immunity and cancer: balance, tolerance, and diversity. Curr Opin Immunol. 2010;22:231–7.
148. Cairo G, Recalcati S, Mantovani A, Locati M. Iron trafficking and metabolism in macrophages: contribution to the polarized phenotype. Trends Immunol. 2011;32:241–7.

Section III
Disorders of Iron Homeostasis: Anemias

Chapter 13
Iron Deficiency

Barry Skikne and Chaim Hershko

Keywords Anemia • Autoimmune gastritis • *Helicobacter pylori* • Hemoglobin • Iron absorption • Iron deficiency • Iron fortification • Oral iron therapy • Pregnancy • Soluble transferrin receptor

1 Introduction

Iron deficiency is one of the most frequent hematological disorders encountered in the clinical setting. Iron is not only an element necessary for hemoglobin production but is also an important component of at least 200 cellular enzymes that are essential for normal cellular functions. The manifestations of iron deficiency vary from those related to the anemia of iron deficiency and to those related to tissue iron deficiency, not related to anemia. These include negative effects on work capacity [1] and endurance, low birth weight and preterm delivery, and effects on motor and mental development in infants, children, and adolescents [2–4]. These changes may lead to adverse socioeconomic and socioemotional [5] effects. Manifestations of anemia and tissue iron depletion often overlap and coexist.

The causes of iron deficiency vary significantly during different stages of life and according to gender and socioeconomic circumstances. Dietary iron intake, as well as other dietary constituents that influence food iron absorption, are also important. Iron deficiency anemia may be the presenting clinical feature of occult gastrointestinal bleeding and may herald underlying malignancy [6].

The development of erythropoietin therapy for various clinical causes of anemia has lead to an evolving concept of functional or relative iron deficiency [7–9], also termed iron-restricted erythropoiesis. Administration of erythropoietin results in expansion of erythroid precursors in the bone marrow as well as significantly accelerated erythropoiesis. Under these circumstances, the rate and amount of iron mobilization from existing iron stores may lag behind the rate of hemoglobin production. This leads to decreased iron incorporation into hemoglobin, with an effect on erythropoiesis similar to that seen in absolute iron deficiency, where iron stores are absent.

During the past decade, significant strides have been made in the understanding of different aspects of iron metabolism, most of which are covered in other chapters. Most of these have not yet

B. Skikne, M.D. (✉)
Celgene Corporation, Overland Park, KS, USA
e-mail: bskikne@celgene.com

C. Hershko, M.D.
Department of Hematology, Shaare Zedek Medical Center and Hebrew University of Jerusalem, Jerusalem, Israel
e-mail: hershko@szmc.org.il

G.J. Anderson and G. McLaren (eds.), *Iron Physiology and Pathophysiology in Humans*, Nutrition and Health, DOI 10.1007/978-1-60327-485-2_13,

been applied at the clinical level. It is likely that some of these parameters will be brought to the clinical arena, once their clinical applications are understood and assays developed that can be implemented in clinical laboratories.

2 Diagnosis of Iron Deficiency

In most instances, uncomplicated iron deficiency anemia is not difficult to diagnose, even though no single laboratory measurement accurately defines this disorder. The diagnosis of iron deficiency requires multiple laboratory assays [9]. Measurements of body iron need to reflect the complete spectrum of iron status from iron overload to severe iron deficiency. The laboratory measurements listed in the following discussion allow determination of iron status, distinguishing normal iron stores from depleted iron stores, and negative iron status where iron deficit is present producing an overall debit of iron in tissue and cellular components. Serum ferritin has been used as the main marker to indicate depleted iron stores. The development of negative iron status prior to progression to anemia has been determined by serum iron, total iron binding capacity and transferrin saturation and/or red blood cell protoporphyrin levels, and more recently the circulating transferrin receptor level. More advanced stages of iron deficiency lead to anemia, and the severity of the anemia reflects the level of iron deficit.

The anemia of chronic disease, caused by inflammation, infection, or neoplasia, alters laboratory studies used to define iron status and is often a confounding factor in the diagnosis of iron deficiency. This difficulty arises especially in the earlier stages of anemia of chronic disease, and when both disorders occur concurrently. The most useful tests to help distinguish these disorders will be discussed and are listed in Table 13.1.

2.1 *Hemoglobin/Hematocrit*

Red blood cells produced under iron-restricted conditions become hypochromic and microcytic. This is an evolving process that may take months to become clearly apparent since only 1% of the circulating red cell population is replaced each day. If concomitant pathological conditions are present, and the erythropoietin drive is blunted for any reason, less than 1% of the red cell pool may be replaced each day, further delaying the peripheral blood changes of iron-deficient erythropoiesis. When more than 10% of the red cell population is hypochromic, automated counters may clearly identify the effects of iron-restricted erythropoiesis.

The hemoglobin value itself is a poor indicator of the presence of iron deficiency anemia, as shown in both clinical and population studies. There is a significant overlap in hemoglobin levels between normal subjects and patients with iron deficiency [10, 11]. Furthermore, significant differences in hemoglobin reference ranges are seen in different races or populations [12, 13]. Iron deficiency is not the most frequent cause of anemia in some populations, especially in developing countries where anemia of chronic inflammation, infections such as malaria [14, 15], vitamin B12 or folate deficiency, malnutrition, and other factors related to poverty may play a role. Considerable overlap in hemoglobin levels and indices occur in all of the aforementioned disorders. In studies from the Ivory Coast, only 20% of anemias in adult males were due to iron deficiency, and only in preschool children was iron deficiency the major cause of anemia. In school-aged children and women, 50% of the anemias could be attributed to iron deficiency [14]. A drop in hemoglobin concentration is frequently the last measurement to become abnormal in iron deficiency and signifies advanced iron deficiency. When active bleeding is the cause of iron deficiency, anemia may be primarily due to blood loss, rather than limitation of erythropoiesis by iron deficiency.

Table 13.1 Laboratory markers for evaluation of body iron status and iron deficiency

Test	Advantages	Limitations	Range in ID[a]
Hemoglobin	Widely available	Poor specificity	Usually normal in early ID
		Slow evolution	<13 g/dL males[b]
		Late marker of IDA	<12 g/dL females
			<11 g/dL pregnancy and children
MCV	Marker of iron-deficient erythropoiesis	Poor specificity, overlap with ACD, slow evolution	≤80 fl
RDW			>14.2%
Reticulocyte hemoglobin content	Early indicator of iron-deficient erythropoiesis	Requires sophisticated automated counters	<27.5 pg
		Cannot store sample	
Ferritin	Reflects iron stores	Poor specificity in presence of inflammation	<12–15 ng/mL
	Marker of depleted iron stores		
Fe/TIBC	Specific in uncomplicated iron-deficient erythropoiesis	Poor specificity in inflammation	<50 ug/dL iron
		Oral contraceptives and pregnancy raise TIBC	>350 μg/dL TIBC
Protoporphyrin (Zinc)	Iron-deficient erythropoiesis	Poor delineation of IDA and ACD	>80 μg/dL
		Raised in lead poisoning	
sTfR	Iron-deficient erythropoiesis	Raised levels with increased erythropoiesis, including EPO therapy	Varies by kit manufacturer
sTfR/ferritin	Estimates whole range of body iron	Confounded by inflammation	

[a]ID = iron deficiency
[b]WHO criteria for anemia

2.2 *Reticulocyte Hemoglobin Content*

Reticulocytes are the earliest red blood cells to enter the circulation after their release from the bone marrow. They provide real-time assessment of the functional state of the bone marrow, in contrast to standard red blood cell indices, which reflect erythropoiesis over the prior 2–3 months. Newer automated cell counters have the ability to measure hemoglobin content within reticulocytes, reticulocyte cell volume (MCVr), and mean cellular hemoglobin content of reticulocytes (CHr on the ADVIA, Bayer Diagnostics, and Ret He on the Sysmex XE-2100, Sysmex Corp [7]). These measurements are early sensitive indices of iron-deficient erythropoiesis, reflecting iron available for production of new red blood cells [16]. CHr levels decline significantly in iron deficiency [16, 17, 18] and do not decline in patients with anemia of chronic inflammation [17]. An important advantage of CHr is that it directly reflects iron incorporation into erythrocyte hemoglobin and thus indirectly reflects functional availability of iron in the bone marrow, indicating early iron deficiency, prior to changes in some of the traditional biochemical measurements and prior to development of anemia [19]. In a study in healthy 9–12-month-old infants, CHr level <27.5 pg accurately indicated iron deficiency compared to hemoglobin levels, and when abnormal, there was an increased risk of developing anemia in the following year (risk ratio 9:1) [20].

CHr has equivalent sensitivity to serum transferrin receptor (TfR) measurement in detecting iron deficiency anemia [17]. Similar to serum TfR, CHr may differentiate concurrent iron deficiency occurring in combination with anemia of chronic inflammation [17]. CHr has high sensitivity and specificity in dialysis patients and more accurately predicts a response to iron therapy than serum ferritin, transferrin saturation, or percent hypochromic red blood cells [21]. The major disadvantage related to these measurements is that the required laboratory instruments are not universally available.

2.3 Serum Ferritin

Serum ferritin levels reflect iron stores (iron stores are proportional to the logarithm of ferritin). A serum ferritin level below 12–15 μg/L indicates depleted iron stores. An important shortcoming of the serum ferritin measurement is that it is increased by inflammation, infection, hyperthyroidism, malignancies, and liver disease; thus a normal ferritin level may occur in the presence of iron deficiency. In population studies where inflammation or infection is prevalent, threshold levels indicating depleted iron stores are raised to 30–40 μg/L [22]. Serum ferritin levels correlate positively with CRP in populations with high rates of infection, including malaria [22, 23]. In renal patients on chronic hemodialysis, ferritin levels less than 100–200 μg/L alone, or less than 400 μg/L together with a transferrin saturation of $<20\%$, indicate that response to erythropoietin administration is unlikely to occur because of reduced storage iron and the need to administer intravenous iron.

An innovative measurement of iron status that is not confounded by the commonly occurring acute inflammatory response of serum ferritin measurement is serum ferritin iron. The normal serum ferritin iron range is 10–35 ng/mL, while iron deficiency values are less than 10 ng/mL. Most patients with inflammation have normal to raised serum ferritin iron levels reflecting their adequate iron stores. Further information can be gained by calculating the ratio of serum ferritin iron to total serum ferritin (iron/protein) [24]. The current assay requires multiple steps, making it time-consuming and not cost effective.

2.4 Serum Iron, Total Iron Binding Capacity, and Transferrin

Serum iron, total iron binding capacity (TIBC), and transferrin saturation measurements are widely used, but their specificity is limited to uncomplicated iron deficiency. Serum iron levels are affected by a number of factors. Serum iron should always be drawn after an overnight fast because iron levels may vary with the type and content of iron in the prior meal. Iron absorbed from a meal typically clears from the serum within 6–8 h after absorption. Serum iron levels also have a diurnal variation, and day-to-day variations may be seen [25]. Morning iron levels tend to be higher than afternoon levels; however, this is not always consistent, and the opposite may occur. Hypoferremia occurs in both iron deficiency and anemia of chronic inflammation, where iron stores are adequate. In chronic inflammation, cytokines lead to a decrease in serum iron, with hepcidin playing an important role in moderating these events [26–30].

TIBC is an indirect measure of serum transferrin. Most modern clinical laboratories measure the transferrin level, which is then converted to TIBC. The transferrin level decreases in response to inflammation. In iron deficiency, transferrin rises late in the development of a negative iron balance; this occurs slightly earlier than the intrinsic changes in red blood cell measurements. Transferrin levels rise during pregnancy and on taking estrogen.

2.5 Zinc Protoporphyrin

Zinc protoporphyrin (ZP) levels have been used as a laboratory marker of iron deficiency. When this assay is performed in the clinical setting, red blood cells should undergo washing to remove possible plasma constituents that may interfere with the fluorescence readings. This measurement has been used as one of three laboratory markers of iron deficiency [15]. Zinc protoporphyrin levels rise in anemia of chronic inflammation as well as iron deficiency, and levels may also rise in lead toxicity. In a study in the Ivory Coast, the high prevalence of malaria and inflammatory disorders complicated the detection of iron deficiency using the ZP measurement [15], and there was a significant correlation between ZP and CRP in preschool children, the group with the highest prevalence of inflammation. Based on these results, ZP may overestimate the prevalence of iron deficiency anemia in population studies where infection/inflammation may be prevalent. In patients with renal failure, the RBC ZP level does not adequately detect iron deficiency in patients on erythropoietin replacement [31].

2.6 Circulating Transferrin Receptor

Erythropoiesis is highly dependent on a continuous supply of iron from the circulation. This iron, bound to transferrin, is taken up by transferrin receptors, transmembrane proteins predominantly present on the external surface of normoblasts in the bone marrow. Soluble transferrin receptor (sTfR) is a truncated form of erythroid precursor surface transferrin receptor [32]. The sTfR level is an indirect quantitative measurement of TfR. A decrease in iron supply from the circulation results in upregulation of TfR on the normoblast surface, via a mechanism that involves stabilization of the TfR mRNA (see Chap. 3).

Inadequate iron supply for hemoglobin synthesis results in iron-deficient erythropoiesis. This state has been defined as a transferrin saturation below 18%. Iron-deficient erythropoiesis may occur when there is markedly increased iron requirement in the presence of normal transferrin saturation, for example, in patients with thalassemia major. Iron-deficient erythropoiesis may also occur in iron-replete patients who have enhanced erythropoiesis secondary to erythropoietin administration. In iron deficiency, surface TfR numbers increase significantly on erythroid precursors, accompanied by elevated sTfR levels [33]. The enhanced erythropoietic activity that occurs in hemolytic anemias, megaloblastic anemias, myelodysplastic syndromes, and erythropoietin administration also give rise to elevated sTfR levels.

Serum ferritin and sTfR levels reflect different stages of iron status. As iron stores decrease, serum ferritin declines until iron stores are fully depleted, when the ferritin level is <12–15 μg/L. Once iron stores are depleted and further iron loss occurs, sTfR begins to rise as iron-deficient erythropoiesis progressively develops. The sTfR becomes abnormal before other laboratory markers of iron-deficient erythropoiesis become abnormal such as transferrin saturation, MCV, erythrocyte protoporphyrin, and finally hemoglobin [34].

The sTfR does not rise in inflammatory states and can be used to diagnose iron deficiency in patients with concomitant anemia of chronic disease [15, 18, 35, 36, 37]. In populations where inflammation and infections are highly prevalent, no correlation is seen between CRP and sTfR [22, 37, 38, 39]. In a study in the Ivory Coast, sTfR was the most reliable indicator of iron deficiency [15], and there was no association between malarial infection (which can cause hemolysis) and sTfR. The combination of hemoglobin and sTfR may be adequate in some population studies for detection of iron deficiency since sTfR is not affected by inflammation or infection. In patients with either uncomplicated iron deficiency or clear-cut anemia of chronic inflammation, TIBC measurement is as discerning as sTfR in distinguishing between the two disorders [40, 41]. In situations where iron deficiency and anemia of chronic inflammation coexist, ferritin levels may be normal or raised, and elevation of sTfR is helpful in identifying the presence of iron deficiency [41]. In anemia of chronic inflammation with raised sTfR level, the bone marrow iron stain may not always show depleted iron stores [37]. In a study of 130 patients with anemia of chronic disease, 54% had normal or low sTfR levels, while 46% had raised sTfR levels. Other classic indices of iron deficiency such as MVC and transferrin saturation were significantly lower in those with raised sTfR levels, compared with those with normal sTfR levels. Not all patients with raised sTfR levels had absent iron stores, suggesting that functional iron deficiency may be present in a proportion of patients with anemia of chronic inflammation, with stainable iron detectable in the bone marrow [37]. From a clinical standpoint, iron status markers are assayed in a sequential manner, sTfR after the serum ferritin and transferrin saturation [42]. If the transferrin saturation is less than 18% and serum ferritin is between 100 and 200 ng/mL, then the sTfR may be helpful. If sTfR is raised, iron deficiency is present in addition to anemia of chronic disease. If the ferritin is below 100 ng/mL, then iron deficiency is likely to be present, while a patient with a ferritin >200 ng/mL is unlikely to have associated iron deficiency. STfR measurement is unlikely to help in these circumstances. Sequential measurements of sTfR during treatment of populations with iron deficiency can provide a valuable marker of response, with decreasing levels as iron-deficient erythropoiesis is alleviated [43].

A drawback of the universal use of sTfR assay is the variability of reported ranges with different manufacturers. These differences may relate to differences in sTfR standard reagents. Placental-derived sTfR standard reagents may give higher sTfR levels than do standards isolated from serum [44], possibly due to higher immunologic activity of the latter standards. These differences between assays will be eliminated when reference materials are produced and utilized to standardize different assay systems.

2.7 *Transferrin Receptor/Ferritin Ratio*

The sTfR/ferritin ratio is a valuable measure of iron deficiency since sTfR rises with tissue iron deficiency while ferritin decreases as iron stores decline. The sTfR/ferritin ratio was first used as a measure of body iron content in a phlebotomy study in normal subjects [34]. Subjects underwent weekly phlebotomy of 150 mL until hemoglobin levels dropped by 2 g/dL from baseline and remained at the new level, without rising over the following 3 weeks. Failure of hemoglobin to rise indicated that iron stores were depleted and insufficient to supply iron for the production of new hemoglobin. The total amount of iron removed with each phlebotomy was calculated, based on the iron content of the hemoglobin removed. Total body iron was then calculated retrospectively at each phlebotomy time point and showed significant correlation with the sTfR/ferritin ratios at each time point [34]. Correction for iron absorption was also considered in the calculations. The body iron measurement is also corrected for body weight, which may be especially important when studying children with different weights. However, there are no definitive validation studies in young age groups or in pregnancy. The use of this ratio to determine iron deficiency has been validated by others [45]. The index was significantly different in pure iron deficiency, compared with anemia of chronic inflammation or combined iron deficiency with inflammation. However, the diagnostic performance of the index was not superior to sTfR or CHr [17].

A significant advantage of this ratio to measure iron status is that the assays can be done on small capillary blood samples, which makes the method highly suitable for use in population studies, especially when only small blood volumes can be obtained. These measurements have also been adapted to dried blood spots, which are easily collected in epidemiologic studies especially in infants and young children [46].

The ratio can be applied to estimate body iron in individual subjects and in population studies. Subsets can easily be evaluated especially when performing intervention studies to improve iron nutrition, and limited interim surveys can be performed. The relationship between sTfR/ferritin and body iron may not be equivalent with the use of different sTfR assays. With one assay method using the same reagents as described [33], body iron can be calculated as follows [47]:

$$\text{Body Iron (mg/kg)} = -[\log(\text{TfR/SF}) - 2.8229] / -0.1207.$$

Both TfR and SF are expressed in µg/L to obtain this TfR/SF ratio. This calculation can be useful in measuring responses to iron interventions. In an iron fortification study of fish sauce in Vietnam using NaFeEDTA, a mean iron increment of 201 mg was measured, equivalent to the absorption of about 12% of fortified iron on a daily basis, while a mean increment of only 26 mg occurred in the control group [43].

The sTfR/ferritin ratio is limited by infections, inflammation, and liver disease which influence ferritin levels independent of iron status. This effect on ferritin value necessitates the use of a marker such as C-reactive protein to detect the presence of inflammation. When inflammation is present, ferritin levels are regarded as inaccurate, and if inflammation is confirmed with a C-reactive protein measurement, the ratio may be considered inaccurate. There remains, however, a significant difference between anemia secondary to iron deficiency and anemia of chronic disease. The sTfR/log ferritin will invariably be >2 in iron deficiency and combined iron deficiency with chronic disease, and <1 in anemia of chronic disease [41]. The sTfR is not influenced by the presence of inflammation and can be used to detect iron deficiency when inflammation is present [40].

Another disadvantage of the sTfR/ferritin ratio as a measure of body iron status is that it has only been validated with one of the available assay systems. Unfortunately, variable ranges have been reported for sTfR, depending on the source of the assay.

Tissue iron deficiency may develop in the absence of anemia. In a study of pregnant Jamaican women, as many as 30% had tissue iron deficiency without anemia [48]. Iron deficiency during pregnancy or infancy can have deleterious effects on intellect and learning capabilities. The use of body iron measurements based on the sTfR/ferritin ratio allows study of the effects of body iron status and tissue iron deficiency on various parameters of daily activity. Measurement of iron status using the ratio may allow early detection of tissue iron deficiency, permitting early intervention strategies to combat and correct iron deficiency.

A further application of these measurements includes iron fortification studies, allowing results to be obtained soon after their implementation. In the past, using older measures, interventions had to be studied over long periods to obtain meaningful results. The utility of this method is illustrated in a study of anemic Vietnamese women, one group of whom received a meal fortified with 10 mg iron as NaFeEDTA 6 days per week, while a control group received no additional iron [43]. Significant changes in body iron could be identified within 3 months using this method. This approach allows early decisions to be made concerning the need to continue with a given strategy.

2.8 Bone Marrow Iron Content

Iron staining of the bone marrow is regarded as the gold standard for the quantitation of body iron content. The amount of visualized iron correlates with total body iron. Absent stainable iron is regarded as definitive iron deficiency. There are, however, some pitfalls with this approach. Although stainable iron may not be visualized, small amounts of iron may be present in the marrow since ferritin iron does not stain with the Perl's stain. This residual iron contributes significantly to the iron supply for erythropoiesis.

There are several drawbacks to the direct quantification of bone marrow iron. Bone marrows are invasive, painful, and costly procedures; therefore, surrogate blood testing of iron status is clearly desirable. Marrow iron distribution is not uniform, thus variances in visual quantification do occur, and variability in observer quantification is also an issue. New automated scanning procedures of bone marrow slides stained for iron may overcome these drawbacks [49].

3 Causes of Iron Deficiency

Although recent evidence suggests that the iron status of developed populations is improving and the incidence of iron deficiency anemia is declining, the worldwide prevalence of iron deficiency continues to be a significant problem. Populations residing in underdeveloped countries are especially vulnerable. Even within developed countries, certain population subgroups are at risk for developing iron deficiency due to heightened physiological requirements. These include infants, growing children, adolescents during the growth spurt, and menstruating and pregnant women. Besides these physiological situations, there are a number of pathological disorders that necessitate iron replacement. The causes of iron deficiency are noted in Table 13.2.

Iron deficiency may be caused by a single disorder; however, in many cases, multiple causative factors interact to produce iron deficiency. Furthermore, a number of additional causes of anemia may contribute to the development of anemia in iron deficiency, especially when iron deficiency is encountered in hospitalized patients.

3.1 Inadequate Dietary Iron Intake

The typical western diet contains approximately 6 mg/1,000 kCal. If caloric intake is restricted in any way, such as in individuals restricting food intake, or in food faddism, with diet containing reduced iron content, it is likely that iron depletion will develop, especially in conditions of concurrent increased iron demands such as menstruation, rapid growth spurt in children and adolescents, and during pregnancy. To achieve an adequate iron intake, an individual may require ingestion of greater than 2,000 kCal in a day. Ingestion of 2,000 kCal may approximate ingestion of 12 mg of iron.

Table 13.2 Causes of iron deficiency

Inadequate dietary iron intake
Single-food diets in infancy
Dieting, fasting, malnutrition
Diet containing inhibitors of iron absorption
Accelerated iron requirements
Growth spurts in childhood/adolescence
Menstruation
Pregnancy
Erythropoietin therapy
Increased iron losses
Bleeding from gastrointestinal, genitourinary tracts
Hemosiderinuria due to intravascular hemolysis
Parasitic infestations
Exercise related
Blood donation
Decreased absorption of iron
Diseases of stomach or proximal small bowel
Celiac disease
Helicobacter pylori gastritis
Autoimmune atrophic gastritis
Chronic inflammation
Iron-refractory iron deficiency anemia

If the dietary intake contains few inhibitors and approximately 15% of the iron is absorbed, this would be equivalent to absorption of 1.8 mg iron. However, should the diet contain inhibitors of iron absorption, and the amount of iron absorbed decline by about 66%, then less than 1 mg will be absorbed, and a negative iron balance will ensue. Therefore, the dietary content of inhibitors and enhancers plays a more important role than does the iron content of the diet [50].

3.2 Diet Containing Inhibitors of Iron Absorption

Differences in iron status occurring in different parts of the world relate in part to differences in dietary constituents. Many dietary constituents affect nonheme iron absorption. Populations consuming diets rich in meat and ascorbic acid, both facilitators of iron absorption, tend to have less iron deficiency [50] than populations consuming diets rich in inhibitors of iron absorption such as phytates and polyphenols. Diets high in fiber and/or calcium [51–53] have a negative effect on iron absorption, but to a lesser extent than those rich in phytates and polyphenols. Diets containing lower calcium content, taken with food that enhances absorption, do not have an inhibitory effect on either nonheme or heme iron absorption [54], compared to high calcium-containing diets.

3.3 Accelerated Iron Requirements

3.3.1 Growth Spurt and Iron Requirements

A sizeable growth spurt occurs in adolescent males and females, resulting in increased iron requirements, secondary to expansion of the blood volume, increase in lean body mass, and onset of menstruation in females [55]. The increase in total blood volume raises the requirements for iron by an additional 0.14 mg iron per day in females and 0.18 mg per day in males. This additional iron is utilized not only to expand the total red cell mass but also to increase the Hb concentration from a mean of 130 g/L to 133 g/L in females and 141 g/L in males. The increase in lean body mass requires an additional 0.33 mg iron per day in females and 0.55 mg per day in males. Apart from the above requirements, females require additional iron to replace blood lost with the onset of menstruation, amounting to an average of 0.56 mg per day (range 0.17–1.08 mg) [55, 56].

3.3.2 Pregnancy and Iron Requirements

Pregnancy creates a significantly increased demand for iron secondary to the physiological expansion of maternal red cell mass, fetal iron requirements, placental growth, and delivery-associated iron loss. Iron requirements during pregnancy amount to approximately 500–700 mg, or an additional 2.5 mg per day over the 1 mg basal daily requirement. Women with multiple pregnancies are especially prone to develop iron deficiency anemia because of the cumulative increased iron demands from each pregnancy. Iron deficiency anemia in pregnancy is associated with increased fetal loss due to prematurity and increased prevalence of low birth weight and perinatal mortality. Storage iron depletion itself may not be detrimental; however, it is important to avoid tissue iron depletion.

Unless dietary iron intake is sufficient and taken in a bioavailable form, it is likely that most women with adequate iron stores before pregnancy (serum ferritin > 60 μg/L) will develop depleted iron stores, and those with lower iron stores at the start of pregnancy (ferritin < 50 μg/L) will develop iron-deficient erythropoiesis, if not iron deficiency anemia. Even with daily ingestion of iron supplements, stores are likely to decline during pregnancy. In a study of 176 pregnant women evaluated during the third trimester, the majority of whom were taking iron supplements, 30% had depleted iron stores at the start of the third trimester (mean serum ferritin 15 μg/L) and 51% had depleted iron stores during the last month of the third trimester (mean serum ferritin 13 μg/L) [57]. Similarly, in a double-blind placebo-controlled study, iron stores declined significantly during pregnancy even in women taking 66 mg of ferrous fumarate per day. However, women taking ferrous fumarate showed a less severe decline in ferritin levels and transferrin saturation, and higher hemoglobin levels, compared with placebo [58]. Studies in pregnant women in Jamaica showed similar results. Patients receiving placebo showed a decline in iron stores and hemoglobin concentration compared with patients given iron supplements [48]. It is estimated that an additional daily iron intake of 22–36 mg [59] would be required to prevent the development of iron deficiency anemia during pregnancy; however, it is difficult for most pregnant women to achieve this level of iron intake from diet alone. An iron supplement containing 20–30 mg iron in a bioavailable form should be sufficient to achieve this level of iron requirement. This amount of iron supplementation is unlikely to cause significant gastrointestinal side effects. The dietary components play an important role in moderating the amount of iron that will be absorbed, unless iron is taken on an empty stomach. If the diet contains inhibitors of iron absorption, the aforementioned dose may be inadequate. The best time to take iron supplements is on retiring at night.

The postpartum period is another phase during which iron deficiency is frequently encountered. It is likely that patients who are iron deficient at delivery will remain iron deficient in the postpartum period. Women treated with iron during pregnancy tend to have improved postpartum iron status compared to those not receiving iron [59].

3.3.3 Erythropoietin Therapy

Patients with anemia secondary to chronic renal failure are frequently treated with erythropoietin (EPO), especially when they are on dialysis. Their body iron stores and whole body iron status commonly decline despite ingestion of oral iron [31]. Under normal circumstances, iron requirement for ongoing erythropoiesis is met by a combination of iron derived from breakdown of senescent red cells in the reticuloendothelial system, dietary absorption, and iron stores. During basal erythropoiesis, iron recovered from red cell breakdown is the main source of iron for new red cell production. When erythropoiesis is accelerated by administration of EPO, iron supply from body stores and from absorption become increasingly important, while iron supply from red cell catabolism remains stable. When patients are anemic, the contribution of iron from breakdown of senescent RBC is limited. When iron stores are ample, much of the heightened iron requirement can be met from stores, although the iron mobilization from stores may lag behind the accelerated iron requirement of the bone marrow. In this situation, the availability of additional iron for erythropoiesis becomes dependent on the amount of iron that can be absorbed from the gastrointestinal tract. The extent to which iron absorption can compensate for increased demands determines the severity of iron-deficient erythropoiesis that may develop following expansion of erythropoiesis. Iron absorption does increase significantly after EPO administration. In a study in normal subjects, nonheme iron absorption from a standard meal increased fivefold from 6% to 32% after administration of EPO. Absorption of heme iron (which is absorbed through a different pathway than nonheme iron) also increased modestly from 47% to 59%. Absorption of supplemental iron taken with food was approximately one third of absorption of iron taken alone. When 50 mg ferrous sulfate was taken alone, baseline absorption after EPO administration increased more than threefold, from 7% to 25%. When this dose was taken with food, absorption rose from 2% to 18% following EPO administration [60]. The increased iron absorption occurring after EPO administration can be ascribed both to a decline in iron stores secondary to the expanding erythroid mass, and to enhanced erythropoiesis. Because EPO administration results in increased iron utilization, a response or lack of response to EPO may be predicted based on serum TfR and ferritin levels at baseline. A TfR>8 mg/L and a ferritin level<50 μg/L at baseline indicate iron deficiency and the need to ensure adequate iron replacement during EPO therapy, while a serum TfR<6 mg/L at baseline predicts an adequate response [31].

In patients on maintenance EPO therapy, iron status declines even when oral iron is taken. Patients with adequate iron stores have steeper declines in iron status because of lower iron absorption. If iron stores are depleted, indicated by a serum ferritin <50 μg/L, iron absorption is unlikely to meet the increased iron requirements, and therefore intravenous iron replacement is recommended. For patients with ferritin levels in the intermediate range (50–100 μg/L), decreasing hemoglobin or serum ferritin levels indicate that oral iron is not meeting the increased demands, indicating the need for intravenous iron administration. When ferritin levels are raised greater than 100 μg/L, iron stores should be adequate for hemoglobin synthesis. Oral iron replacement may be adequate in these patients; however, intravenous iron is indicated if ferritin level declines. For most patients, overall iron status will decline, necessitating intravenous iron replacement [31, 61].

3.4 *Increased Iron Losses*

3.4.1 Gastrointestinal Tract Bleeding as the Cause of Iron Deficiency Anemia

Blood loss is the most common cause of iron deficiency in adults, and the various causes are well described. It is always essential to exclude pathological disorders, especially of the gastrointestinal (GI) tract, in patients without obvious causes for iron deficiency. Ingestion of aspirin and nonsteroidal anti-inflammatory drugs should not be overlooked as a cause because even low doses of aspirin taken to prevent atherosclerotic complications may cause significant GI bleeding.

In adults over 50 years of age presenting with iron deficiency anemia, underlying malignancies should always be considered and excluded. In a recent study in the United Kingdom of patients presenting with iron deficiency anemia with no obvious cause, colon cancer accounted for 6.3% of the cases [62]. Only 1.2% were female, while 14% were male. Cancer of the upper or lower gastrointestinal tract accounted for only 7% of the cases. Other studies reported that 2–14% of patients presenting with iron deficiency anemia had colon cancer [63]. Eighty-nine percent of the patients had cancer involving the right side of the colon, and the average age was 70 [58–82] years [62]. Most patients with right-sided colon cancer have no symptoms other than those related to iron deficiency anemia. When the cancer is significantly advanced, symptoms may include local discomfort or a mass. It is therefore imperative that all patients over 50 years of age presenting with iron deficiency anemia should undergo colonoscopy with or without upper endoscopy.

Most causes of unexplained iron deficiency involve benign disorders of the upper gastrointestinal tract (77%) versus the lower gastrointestinal tract (11%) [62]. The diagnoses include gastritis (46%, including 32% taking nonsteroidal medications), duodenitis (23%, including 13% with *Helicobacter pylori*, discussed below), hiatal hernia 4%, gastric ulcer (<1%), duodenal ulcer (1%), and esophageal cancer (<1%). Disorders of the lower intestinal tract include celiac disease (<1%), benign colonic polyps (4%), hemorrhoids (3%), and diverticular disease (4%). No cause of iron deficiency could be found in 5% of patients. The causes of blood loss from the gastrointestinal tract may vary between differing geographical areas, where intestinal parasites may play an important role. In a study in Vietnam, 46% of anemic women were infected with intestinal parasites, including *Ascaris lumbricoides* (24%), *Trichuris trichuria* (32%), and hookworm (9%) [43]. Of these infestations, only hookworm is known to have a significant effect on gastrointestinal blood losses.

3.4.2 Excess Iron Losses in Athletes

Athletes undergoing endurance training, especially adolescent and young adult females, are prone to develop iron deficiency, with or without anemia. Iron status declines because of expanding red cell mass and muscle mass, and additional iron loss may occur from GI tract bleeding, especially when anti-inflammatory drugs are regularly used. In addition, minimal iron loss may occur from traumatic (foot-strike) hemolysis.

3.4.3 Hemolysis as a Cause of Iron Deficiency

Chronic intravascular hemolysis is an infrequent cause of iron deficiency. Hemoglobin in plasma exceeding the binding capacity of haptoglobin is filtered through the glomeruli, after which a small amount of hemoglobin is reabsorbed by the renal tubular cells. Within these cells, iron is released from the hemoglobin molecule by the heme oxidase enzyme and taken up by ferritin. The ferritin molecules subsequently form hemosiderin, and this iron is lost into the urine when these tubular cells are sloughed off at the end of their lifespan. Hemosiderin in urine can be identified by staining of urine sediment with Prussian Blue stain. Hemoglobin not reabsorbed by the tubular cells passes into the urine and can be detected by a dipstick or visually if there is frank hemoglobinuria. Classical causes of chronic intravascular hemolysis include paroxysmal nocturnal hemoglobinuria, malaria, intravascular damage of red blood cells on artificial mechanical heart valves or due to microvascular diseases, sickle-cell disease, and glucose-6-phosphate dehydrogenase deficiency.

3.5 Decreased Absorption of Iron

Decreased dietary iron absorption may be secondary to defective extraction of iron from food, failure to present this iron in a suitable form for absorption by proximal small bowel, or malabsorption of iron presented in a suitable form because of abnormal gastrointestinal tract mucosa as in celiac disease [64].

3.5.1 Role of *Helicobacter pylori* and Autoimmune Gastritis in Obscure or Refractory Iron Deficiency Anemia

Conventional endoscopic and radiographic methods fail to identify a source of gastrointestinal blood loss in up to one-third of males and postmenopausal females, and in most young women with iron deficiency anemia [65–67]. Referral for hematological evaluation is likely to occur when iron deficiency anemia persists despite a negative gastrointestinal workup or when anemia is unresponsive to standard oral iron treatment.

In recent years, there has been increasing recognition of subtle, nonbleeding gastrointestinal conditions that may result in abnormal iron absorption leading to iron deficiency anemia in the absence of gastrointestinal symptoms. The most prominent disorders are celiac disease [68], autoimmune gastritis [69, 70], and *Helicobacter pylori* gastritis [71, 72]. The availability of convenient, noninvasive screening methods for identifying celiac disease (endomysial and gliadin antibodies), autoimmune atrophic gastritis (serum gastrin, parietal cell antibodies), and *H. pylori* infection (antibody screening and urease breath test) greatly facilitates the recognition of patients with these entities and their possible role in causing iron deficiency anemia.

In a recent prospective observational study, 300 consecutive patients referred for hematologic evaluation of obscure or refractory IDA have been investigated employing the above methods for identifying nonbleeding gastrointestinal conditions responsible for the anemia [73–75]. The mean age of subjects was 39 ± 18 y, and 251 of 300 (84%) were women. A likely cause of IDA was identified in 93% of patients. As expected in females of reproductive age, only 10% had a source of gastrointestinal bleeding identified. A history of menorrhagia was present in 32% of patients. The second most common abnormality was *autoimmune atrophic gastritis* documented in 77 IDA patients (26%) of whom 39 had coexistent *H. pylori* infection. *H. pylori* infection was the only positive finding in 57 patients (19%). There were 13 new cases of *adult celiac disease* (4%) manifested in IDA only. Refractoriness to oral iron treatment was found in 100% of patients with celiac disease, 69% with autoimmune atrophic gastritis, 68% with *H. pylori* infection, but in only 10% of subjects with no underlying abnormality. Celiac disease is an uncommon immunologically mediated disorder associated with development of abnormal small bowel mucosal cells. A common clinical manifestation of the disease is gluten intolerance. The incidence of iron deficiency at presentation of celiac disease varies according to sex and age; in patients presenting at greater than 14 years of age, iron deficiency anemia is found in 52% of females versus 39% in males, whereas at 2–14 years of age, it is present in 23% of females and 32% in males [64].

The following section focuses on the role of *H. pylori* infection and autoimmune gastritis, two entities which are not widely recognized as conditions commonly associated with refractory or obscure IDA.

3.5.2 Significance of *Helicobacter pylori* Gastritis in Explaining Iron Deficiency

The role of *H. pylori* in causing iron deficiency anemia is unsettled, as *H. pylori* infection is common in the normal population. Population surveys involving thousands of subjects [76] conducted over diverse geographic areas indicate that *H. pylori* is associated with a slight decrease in ferritin levels implying diminished iron stores, but there was no evidence of a high prevalence of iron deficiency anemia associated with *H. pylori* seropositivity in these populations.

A cause-and-effect relation between *H. pylori* and serious gastrointestinal pathology, including duodenal ulcer, atrophy of the gastric body predisposing to gastric ulcer, and cancer, or mucosa-associated lymphoid tissue (MALT) lymphoma, is well established and strongly supported by the beneficial effects of *H. pylori* eradication in these conditions [77]. Consequently, in a search for evidence supporting a cause-and-effect relation between *H. pylori* and iron deficiency anemia, it is necessary to focus on possible beneficial effects of *H. pylori* eradication on refractory iron deficiency anemia. Indeed studies indicate that failure to respond to oral iron treatment in *H. pylori*-positive patients was more than twice as common as in *H. pylori*-negative subjects, and successful *H. pylori* eradication resulted in an increase in hemoglobin indistinguishable from that in previously responsive iron deficiency anemia patients [73–75]. These observations agree with a number of previous studies [72, 78, 79] conducted in young females refractory to oral iron treatment in whom improvement occurred following *H. pylori* eradication even in the absence of continued iron administration.

Because menstrual blood loss is a compounding factor in evaluating the role of *H. pylori* in the pathogenesis of IDA in young females, studies in males with negative gastrointestinal workup and poor initial response to oral iron treatment would be more useful for assessing the relation between *H. pylori* and unexplained IDA. In a recent study involving 25 males with unexplained IDA and *H. pylori* [75], all previously refractory patients achieved normal hemoglobin levels after *H. pylori* eradication with follow-up periods of 4–69 months. This was accompanied by a significant decrease in *H. pylori* IgG antibodies and serum gastrin levels. Sixteen patients discontinued iron treatment, maintaining normal hemoglobin and ferritin, and may be considered cured. Remarkably, 4 of the 16 achieved normal hemoglobin without receiving oral iron after *H. pylori* eradication.

A number of mechanisms may explain the relation between *H. pylori* gastritis and iron deficiency anemia, including occult gastrointestinal bleeding and competition for dietary iron by the bacteria. However, the most likely explanation is the effect of *H. pylori* on the composition of gastric juice. Studies by Annibale et al. show that gastric acidity and ascorbate content, both critical for normal iron absorption, are adversely affected by *H. pylori* infection. Conversely, H. *pylori* eradication results in normalization of gastric pH and ascorbate content restoring normal iron absorption [80].

3.5.3 Significance of Autoimmune Atrophic Gastritis in Explaining Iron Deficiency

Screening for autoimmune gastritis relies on the coexistence of increased serum gastrin and autoantibodies to gastric parietal cells. In most such patients, gastric mucosal histology shows chronic gastritis and atrophic gastritis [74]. Increased serum gastrin is the consequence of increased secretion in response to achlorhydria by G-cells in the gastric antrum and duodenum which are characteristically spared by autoimmune gastritis involving only the proximal two-thirds of the stomach. This combination of abnormalities is typical of pernicious anemia but is largely unrecognized in the context of iron deficiency anemia.

In pernicious anemia, gastric atrophy involving the proximal two-thirds of the stomach but sparing the antrum was first documented by Faber and Bloch in 1900 [81]. Abnormal gastric secretion associated with pernicious anemia was designated "achylia gastrica" [82]. Subsequently, Faber et al. described 59 patients with achylia gastrica and anemia, but only 15 of these had pernicious anemia. The remaining 37 patients had hypochromic anemia. They were mostly women, responding only to large doses of iron but tending to relapse [83, 84]. Cumulative experience up to 1933 with hypochromic anemia associated with achlorhydria was summarized in a landmark study by Wintrobe and Beebe involving 498 patients [85]. By comparison with pernicious anemia, patients with hypochromic anemia and achylia gastrica were 35–50 years old or about 10 years younger; 96% were females compared with a roughly equal gender in pernicious anemia. They had no neurological complications, and the anemia was microcytic instead of macrocytic. Free hydrochloric acid in gastric juice was absent in the vast majority of patients in both groups. The most important difference was that a fatal course was almost universal in untreated pernicious anemia, whereas only one of the 498 patients with achylia gastrica and hypochromic anemia died.

Despite these differences between pernicious anemia and hypochromic anemia associated with achylia gastrica, certain similarities were recognized by Wintrobe and Beebe [85]. In hypochromic anemia and achlorhydria, there was an increased prevalence of pernicious anemia among family members, and progression of hypochromic anemia to pernicious anemia was repeatedly observed. The frequent association of thyroid disease with both types of anemia was also recognized. In both types of anemia, it was noted that achlorhydria may precede development of anemia by many years. Based on the marked difference in gender and younger age of hypochromic anemia patients, the authors concluded that an added factor must be the increased physiologic needs associated with menstruation and pregnancy. In view of failure to respond to conventional doses of oral iron treatment, it was concluded that iron absorption in this condition is abnormal and lack of free hydrochloric acid may be the fundamental disorder responsible for "idiopathic hypochromic anemia."

Unfortunately, the concept of gastric atrophy as a common cause of iron deficiency anemia has been largely forgotten and ignored in subsequent surveys of gastrointestinal causes of iron deficiency anemia [86]. It is possible that the discovery of intrinsic factor, of cobalamin, and the profound change in management and prognosis of pernicious anemia resulted in decreased interest in iron deficiency, a less exotic consequence of achylia gastrica, despite the fact that this type of anemia was more common in achylia gastrica than megaloblastic anemia. Although the advent of gastroscopic methodology confirmed the coexistence of iron deficiency anemia and gastric mucosal atrophy, there was no consensus regarding the role of achlorhydria in the pathogenesis of iron deficiency [87–91]. It was even suggested that gastric atrophy may be the result and not the cause of chronic iron deficiency.

Following the demonstration of antibodies to gastric parietal cells in pernicious anemia, it was also shown that sera in over 20% of patients with iron deficiency anemia are positive for the same antibodies [92]. Increased incidence of iron deficiency anemia only occurred in patients with histamine-fast achlorhydria who also had biopsy evidence of atrophic gastritis. Likewise, in a more recent study [69] employing gastric mucosal biopsies and serologic screening, autoimmune achlorhydric gastric atrophy has been implicated in 20% of subjects with iron deficiency anemia without evidence of gastrointestinal blood loss. These observations have been confirmed and extended in a series of studies [70] where 27% of patients with refractory iron deficiency anemia without gastrointestinal symptoms were found to have atrophic gastritis, a percentage almost identical with the proportion of subjects with autoimmune atrophic body gastritis found in subsequent studies. Impaired iron absorption in pernicious anemia is corrected by normal, but not by neutralized gastric juice, indicating that lack of gastric acidity is the key factor in abnormal iron absorption [93]. Other studies have also shown that iron absorption is heavily dependent on normal gastric secretion and acidity for dissolving and reducing dietary iron [94, 95]. Although atrophic gastritis may impair both cobalamin and iron absorption simultaneously, in young women in whom menstruation and pregnancy represent an added strain on iron requirements, iron deficiency will develop years before depletion of cobalamin stores.

3.5.4 Possible Role of *H. pylori* in the Pathogenesis of Autoimmune Gastritis

In order to define the relation between iron deficiency anemia, pernicious anemia, and *H. pylori* infection, 160 patients with autoimmune gastritis were studied of whom 83 presented with microcytic anemia, 48 with normocytic, and 29 with macrocytic anemia [74].

The mean age of patients with microcytic anemia was 41 ± 15 y, 18 years younger than the mean age of the other groups. Low serum cobalamin was found in 100% of the macrocytic, 92% of the normocytic, and 46% of the microcytic groups. Iron deficiency was found in all patients with microcytic anemia, but also in 50% of the normocytic and 10% of the macrocytic patients. Thus, a considerable proportion of patients had combined iron and cobalamin deficiency. Endoscopic studies were available in 87 patients and gastric mucosal histology in 69. Histology was defined as atrophic gastritis in 50%, chronic gastritis (chronic inflammation) in 42%, MALT lymphoma in 3%, gastric polyp in 3%, and adenocarcinoma of the stomach in 1 patient. In an additional 18 cases, the gastric mucosa was described as normal macroscopically, but no biopsies were taken. The proportion of patients with atrophic gastritis was 9/13 (69%) in patients with macrocytic anemia and 13/32 (41%) in microcytic anemia. Conversely, the proportion of patients with chronic inflammation in the macrocytic group was 2/13 (15%) compared with 18/32 (56%) in microcytic anemia. Stratification by age cohorts of autoimmune gastritis from <20 to >60 y showed coexistent *H. pylori* infection in 87.5% at age <20 y, 47% at 20–40 y, 37.5% at 41–60 y, and 12.5% at age >60y. With ages increasing from <20 to >60 y, there was a progressive increase in serum ferritin from 4 ± 2 to 37 ± 41 μg/L and serum gastrin from 349 ± 247 to 800 ± 627 u/mL, and decrease in cobalamin from 392 ± 179 to 108 ± 65 pg/mL.

The high prevalence of *H. pylori* in young patients with autoimmune gastritis and its almost total absence in elderly patients with pernicious anemia implies that *H. pylori* infection in autoimmune gastritis may represent an early phase of disease in which an infectious process is gradually replaced by an autoimmune disease terminating in burned-out infection and irreversible destruction of gastric body mucosa. The relation between *H. pylori* and pathogenesis of pernicious anemia is still unsettled [96]. *H. pylori*-infected subjects have circulating IgG antibodies directed against epitopes on gastric mucosal cells. Of these, the most likely target of an autoimmune mechanism triggered by *H. pylori* and directed against gastric parietal cells by means of antigenic mimicry [97–104] is H + K+-ATPase, a protein that is the most common autoantigen in pernicious anemia. Conversely, *H. pylori* eradication in patients with autoimmune atrophic gastritis is followed by improved gastric acid and ascorbate secretion in many and complete remission of atrophic gastritis in a variable proportion of patients [105–107]. Failure to achieve remission by *H. pylori* eradication in many patients does not argue against the role of *H. pylori* in the pathogenesis of autoimmune gastritis but more likely indicates that a point of no return may be reached beyond which the autoimmune process may no longer require the continued presence of the inducing pathogen.

In view of the above considerations, initial testing for celiac disease (anti-endomysial antibodies), autoimmune type A atrophic gastritis (gastrin, antiparietal antibodies), and *H. pylori* (IgG antibodies followed by urease breath test) provides high-sensitivity screening and an effective starting point for further investigation. This is recommended in all patients with obscure iron deficiency anemia and in those refractory to oral iron treatment. Interpretation of positive serology for *H. pylori* confirmed by positive urease breath test requires clinical judgment as 20–50% of the healthy population in industrialized countries will have such findings. In such patients, refractoriness to oral iron treatment may justify a "test-and-treat" approach of *H. pylori* eradication as currently advocated in the management of dyspeptic patients [108]. Cure of previously refractory iron deficiency anemia by *H. pylori* eradication may be regarded as evidence supporting a cause-and-effect relation. The recently reported disorder, iron-refractory iron deficiency anemia due to mutations of the TMPRSS6 gene which encodes matriptase-2, should also be considered when other causes of iron refractoriness have been excluded [109] (see Chap. 26).

4 Prevalence of Iron Deficiency

Historically, iron deficiency has been estimated to affect approximately 30% of the world population [110]. Prevalence of iron deficiency can be evaluated on the basis of age, sex, race, socioeconomic status, and regional variances, including altitude. Several studies in the past have utilized anemia as a surrogate indicator of iron deficiency. More recent data refutes the use of hemoglobin as the sole indicator of iron deficiency since the hemoglobin level is influenced by other factors affecting surveyed populations, including socioeconomic factors, infections, other inflammatory conditions, and altitude. In view of the availability of specific laboratory tests covering several aspects of iron status, the use of hemoglobin as the sole indicator of iron deficiency should be abandoned. Newer measurements to diagnose iron deficiency in population studies have included, in addition to hemoglobin levels, serum ferritin, transferrin saturation, free erythrocyte protoporphyrin, and C-reactive protein as an indicator of inflammation. Iron deficiency is present when at least two of the following three measurements are abnormal: low serum ferritin, low transferrin saturation with a raised or high normal TIBC, or a raised free erythrocyte protoporphyrin. A low ferritin by itself may indicate that anemia is secondary to iron deficiency; however, this only reflects depleted stores and it is possible that tissue iron deficiency is not occurring and some other cause is responsible for the anemia. A second abnormal measure of iron status would confirm that iron deficiency is the probable cause of the anemia [111].

The serum TfR/ferritin ratio provides a significantly improved quantitative measure of iron status, independent of hemoglobin level [13, 47, 112]. However, when infection or inflammation is present, body iron measurement becomes unreliable because ferritin behaves as an acute phase reactant. A number of population studies have used only hemoglobin levels, some with high incidences of anemia; however, specific iron studies were not obtained [113]. Such reports are not included in this review.

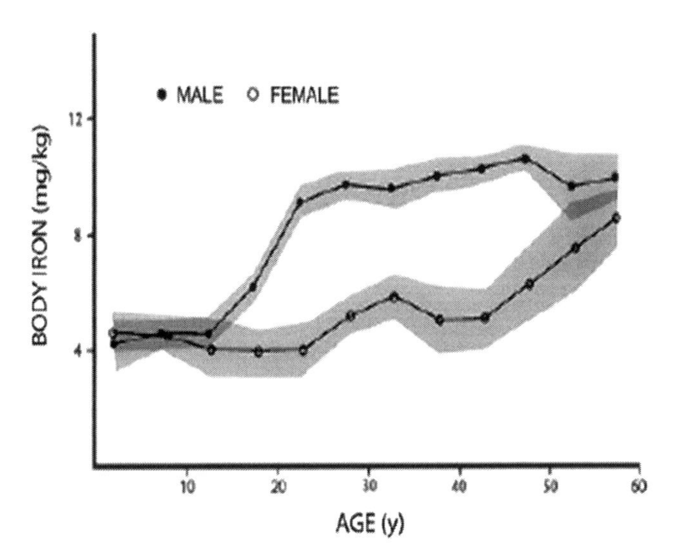

Fig. 13.1 Effect of age and sex on body iron based on blood specimens collected in the NHANES III. *Shaded* areas represent ±SEM for each 5-year interval (From [47])

The effects of age, sex, and infections and the need to utilize a spectrum of tests and not rely solely on hemoglobin levels are illustrated by a study performed in the Ivory Coast in West Africa. The prevalence of iron deficiency was 41–63% in women and children and 13% in men. Iron deficiency anemia was present in 30–66% of the iron-deficient women and children, and 30% of iron-deficient men. Overall, iron deficiency accounted for about 50% of cases of anemia in this population where malaria, other infections, and hemoglobinopathies were also prevalent [15].

4.1 *Effect of Age, Growth, and Sex*

Studies measuring whole body iron in a population sample from NHANES III [114] indicate a significant effect of age and sex on iron status (Fig. 13.1) [47]. Body iron status remains stable until late adolescence in both sexes. An abrupt rise occurs in late teenage years in males. In females, body iron remains on a plateau due to menstruation and childbearing, but begins to slowly rise after the childbearing years, and menopause begins. Thereafter, iron status increases continuously, eventually reaching levels equivalent to males after 50 years of age. In males, iron stores continue to rise from adolescence to the third decade, after which iron stores plateau, but rise slowly over the next three decades. The incidences of iron deficiency in various parts of the world are noted in Table 13.3. This table does not reflect all studies that have been completed. These studies rely on specific markers of iron deficiency and do not include the incidences of iron deficiency anemia.

4.2 *Toddlers (Age 12–35 Months) and Preschool Children*

In the USA, iron deficiency occurs in approximately 2.4 million children, and iron deficiency anemia occurs in approximately 490,000 children [110, 114]. During the first year of life, approximately 50% of infants have tissue iron deficiency. A further decline in iron status occurs during the second year of life, after which body iron status improves steadily over the next 2 years, despite a rapid growth spurt. The incidence of iron deficiency varies with race and ethnicity in the USA. In the

Table 13.3 Prevalence of iron deficiency in developing and developed countries

	Developing countries	Developed countries
Toddlers (1–3 years old)	63% [15]	31% [120]
		7–9% [115]
Children (5–16 years old)	47% [15]	1–5% [120]
	15% [128]	8–10% girls
		<1% boys
Menstruating women	41% [15]	9–16% [120][a]
		7% [13]
		15% [112]
		36% [146]
Pregnancy	30% [48]	30% [144]
	56% [55]	20% [145]
		10% [57]
Men	13% [15]	1–5% [121]
		6% [146][b]
Elderly	–	3–7% [121]
		3–4% males
		6–7% females

[a]White 8–10%, Black 15–19%, Hispanic 19–22%
[b]Recreational athletes

NHANES IV study (conducted 1999–2002), 8% of toddlers were iron deficient. Hispanic children had the highest incidence of iron deficiency (12%), versus 6% in white toddlers and 6% in black toddlers [115]. Iron deficiency was highest (20%) in overweight toddlers, versus 7% for normal weight toddlers. The incidence of iron deficiency was also influenced by proficiency of the mothers in speaking and understanding English (7% among those whose mothers did, versus 14% among those whose mothers did not speak or understand English). Attendance at day care also played a role; the incidence was half that of those that did not attend day care (5% vs. 10%) [115]. In this survey, Hispanic children were more likely to be overweight and less likely to be in day care. An association between overweight children and iron deficiency was also seen previously in children 2–16 years of age [116, 117]. Several factors may play a role in these findings, including inadequate iron content of the diet, especially diets high in calories, with poor micronutrient levels, for example, excessive ingestion of juices and milk.

In a study in Bolivia evaluating body iron measurements in children and their mothers, hemoglobin levels rose from 99 g/L and 100 g/L in the first and second years of life to 120 g/L at 4 years of age. Mean body iron content rose from a deficient state at 1 year to reach 3.85 mg/kg by 4 years of age, which was a similar iron value to that seen in their mothers [112]. An interesting observation in this study was the significant correlation between body iron content in the children and their mothers. Iron-replete mothers tended to have iron-replete infants, while iron-deficient mothers had iron-deficient infants. However, in a study from Australia, iron status of 6-month-old children did not show any difference whether or not their mothers were given iron supplements during pregnancy, and whether or not the mothers were iron deficient at the time of childbirth [118]. The children also did not show differences in iron status at 4 years of age related to their mothers' iron status at the time of childbirth. These contrasting observations are related to the influence of diet and its iron content and availability, which is the likely common factor between each household in underdeveloped populations. In developed countries, where the population is well nourished and a variety of food sources are available, children may have different iron status from their mothers. An additional factor is the relationship of iron status in the mother during gestation and its influence on iron status of the infant [119].

In the Ivory Coast study, iron deficiency was present in 63% of children aged 2–5 years. Iron deficiency anemia occurred in about two-thirds of these with an overall incidence of 39% [15].

4.3 *School-Age Children (Age 6–15 Years)*

It is estimated that 46% of the world's children have anemia, the majority of these living in underdeveloped areas [56]. Whether these children have iron deficiency alone, anemia of chronic infection, or other causes of anemia, such as vitamin B12 or folate deficiency, is unclear. These estimates are easily corroborated by the study from Ivory Coast, where 47% of children had iron deficiency, of which about one half (25%) were anemic [15].

4.4 *Pregnancy*

Hemoglobin levels normally decline during pregnancy. Under normal physiological conditions, expansion of the red cell mass occurs, provided adequate iron stores are present. There are two causes for the decline in hemoglobin concentration, the first being the physiological expansion of plasma volume leading to dilution of hemoglobin, the second being the propensity to develop iron deficiency. Increased iron required by the fetus, placenta, and umbilical cord leads to a significant decline in iron stores during pregnancy, reflected by changes in serum ferritin as well as sTfR.

It is estimated that 48% of pregnant women worldwide have anemia, and in underdeveloped countries, the incidence is as high as 56% [57]. In Bolivia, pregnant women had a mean serum ferritin of 15 ug/L versus a mean of 29 ug/L in nonpregnant women; however, tissue iron deficiency was not evident in pregnancy as measured by serum TfR itself. Body iron content calculated for each individual averaged 1.31 ± 3.67 mg/kg in pregnant women and 3.99 ± 4.3 mg/kg in nonpregnant women [112]. In a study of anemic pregnant women in Jamaica, the mean ferritin level was 11 µg (range 4–32 µg/L), mean sTfR was 7.9 ± 3.4 mg/L, and mean sTfR/ferritin ratio was 650 (range 187–2,258). Mean body iron was 0.085 ± 4.5 mg/kg, and half the women had tissue iron deficiency.

Iron supplementation somewhat prevents iron depletion during pregnancy. In an Australian study comparing 20 mg iron versus placebo administered from 20 weeks of gestation, significant differences in Hb and ferritin concentrations were observed in the two groups at delivery (128 g/L versus 121 g/L and 16.1 µg/L versus 11.1 µg/L, respectively) [118]. In general, because iron stores are frequently depleted during pregnancy, serum ferritin has poor specificity for iron deficiency, while serum TfR has greater specificity.

4.5 *Menstruating Women*

Studies in the USA indicate a low incidence of iron deficiency in menstruating women, utilizing older criteria to detect iron deficiency, including serum ferritin, transferrin saturation, and free erythrocyte protoporphyrin, and iron deficiency anemia by addition of hemoglobin. However, differences in incidence were noted within different population groups. Iron deficiency occurred in 11% and 12% of the population in the NHANES III and NHANES 1999–2000 survey, while iron deficiency anemia occurred in 4% and 3%, respectively [121]. In white non-Hispanics, iron deficiency incidence was 8–10%, in blacks, 15–19%, and in Mexican Americans, 19–22% in these two study time periods [121]. Body iron measurements have recently been employed to examine the prevalence of iron deficiency in the USA. Mean ferritin was 34 ug/L (range 12–94 ug/L), mean serum TfR was 6.3±2.6 mg/L, mean sTfR/ferritin ratio was 172 (range 54–544), and body iron was 4.9±4.1 mg/kg [47]. The frequency distribution of this population was not linear in the lower portion of the curve, in keeping with a minor population of iron-deficient women. Mixed distribution analyses allowed differentiation of these populations. The normal population had a mean body iron of 5.5 mg/kg, while 7% of the population had iron deficiency with a mean whole body iron deficit of –3.9 mg/kg.

In a study in Bolivia, examining the influence of high altitude on body iron, a similar frequency distribution of body iron status occurred in mothers and their children, except that the children's iron status was shifted toward the lower end of the spectrum. Iron deficiency occurred in 15% of the women [112], which was half the incidence in children living in the same household (31%). Iron deficiency severe enough to cause anemia (iron deficit greater than 4 mg/kg) occurred in approximately 6% of mothers and 12% of their offspring. Anemia occurred in about one-third of all women with absent iron stores (defined by body iron<0 mg/kg). Similar to the USA figures mentioned above, 83% of Bolivian women had a mean body iron of 5.3 mg/kg, while 17% iron-deficient women had a mean body iron deficit of –2.3 mg/kg [112].

The incidence of iron deficiency and iron deficiency anemia varies significantly in different parts of the world, and when populations have concurrent infections, as demonstrated in studies in Ivory Coast [15], the prevalence can be difficult to define clearly. As demonstrated in this study, iron deficiency occurred in 41% of the women and iron deficiency anemia occurred in approximately half of these (20%).

4.6 Males Aged 20–65 Years

In a subsample from the NHANES III study in men between 20 and 65 years of age, mean ferritin concentration was 109 µg/L (range 66–285 µg/L), mean sTfR was 6.1±2.7 mg/L, and the geometric mean TfR/Ferritin ratio was 42 (range 19–93), equivalent to body iron stores of 9.89±2.82 mg/kg, consistent with a single normal distribution.

In men from Ivory Coast, mean serum ferritin concentration was 65 µg/L and mean sTfR was 7.2 mg/L, not dissimilar to the values reported in the USA study noted above [15]. Iron depletion was present in 13% of the men, and 30% of these (4% overall) had iron deficiency anemia.

4.7 Elderly (Over 65 Years of Age)

The incidence of anemia in the elderly rises from approximately 8% in the 65–74 year age group to 13% in the 75–84 year age group to 24% in the 85 year and older age group [121]. Data from the NHANES III study (1988–1994) in noninstitutionalized subjects 65 yrs and older indicated that 20% of anemic subjects had iron deficiency. Approximately 16% of the iron-deficient population had iron deficiency combined with folate or vitamin B12 deficiency [121]. In a number of previous population studies, anemia was presumed to be due to iron deficiency. However the NHANES III study clearly established that nutritional deficiencies account for only one-third of all causes of anemia in this age group. In subjects 70 years and older, iron deficiency was present in 4% and 7% of males and females, respectively, and in 3% and 6% of males and females in a more recent NHANES study in 1999–2000. Iron deficiency anemia occurred in 2% of the females in the NHANES III study and 1% of females in the more recent NHANES study [120].

4.8 *Effect of Altitude*

Diminished oxygen tension at high altitude leads to increased hemoglobin levels, mediated by increased erythropoietin production. Expansion of hemoglobin mass requires increased iron mobilization from stores as well as increased iron absorption from the diet. There is evidence, based on animal models, that hypoxia has a direct stimulating effect on iron absorption, possibly mediated by downregulation of hepcidin [122]. A rise in hemoglobin of 10 g/L requires an additional 33.8 mg of iron/L of blood. Thus a 60-kg woman with an average blood volume of 67 mL/kg, or total blood volume of 4.02 L, will require an additional 135 mg of iron to produce a rise in hemoglobin of 10 g/L (or 1 g/dL). Although this amount appears trivial, it may be difficult for some women to accomplish based on poor dietary iron intake, excess menstrual losses, and further pregnancies.

As noted previously, studies relying on hemoglobin measurements as markers of iron deficiency tend to overestimate its prevalence. In a study at high altitude in Bolivia, the prevalence of iron deficiency was estimated to be between 27% and 52%. When more specific measurements were introduced, the level of iron deficiency was <10% [123]. In another study of menstruating women in Bolivia, rising altitude at 1,000 m intervals had no effect on body iron status in children younger than 5 years of age; however, diminished iron status occurred in mothers living at altitudes greater than 3,000 m [112]. Serum ferritins in mothers at altitudes below and above 3,000 m were 30 μg/L and 23 μg/L, respectively, mean serum TfR values were 6.61 mg/L and 7.97 mg/L, respectively, and mean body iron was 30% lower at the higher altitude (4.32 mg/kg and 2.77 mg/kg, respectively) [112]. When only hemoglobin levels were used in this study, anemia prevalence was 27% in women of menstruating age; however, body iron measurements indicated that only 5.7% had tissue iron depletion severe enough to produce anemia (which requires a tissue iron deficit greater than −4 mg/kg). Similar findings were noted in children, of whom 45% were anemic, but only 12% had tissue iron deficiency that could cause anemia. The discrepancy between the prevalence of anemia and the prevalence of tissue iron depletion severe enough to cause anemia can be explained by the fact that iron deficiency is not the only cause of anemia in such populations. Furthermore, in this study, hemoglobin may have been erroneously corrected for differences in altitude.

5 Therapy for Iron Deficiency Anemia

When iron deficiency is identified, whether in an individual patient or a population, it is always necessary to investigate and establish causes, evaluate the clinical consequences of the iron deficiency, and establish a plan to correct the deficiency. Different strategies are required for the management of iron deficiency, depending on the population undergoing therapy. Iron depletion may require correction of iron balance in whole population segments where fortification of the diet may be required, or iron supplementation may be directed toward specific members of a population. Iron fortification may not always be the desired strategy since it may be harmful to certain population members, for example, where the gene for hemochromatosis is prevalent.

Diets containing inadequate amounts of iron or those that contain excess inhibitors of iron absorption are important causes of iron deficiency, especially in situations of coexistent increased iron demand. These causative factors often coexist, for example, during the 4th–12th month of infancy, when there is increased iron requirement due to expansion of body tissues and red blood cell mass. Approximately 0.9 mg of iron is required per day during this time. Milk contains only about 0.2 mg of iron per deciliter, or about 1.5 mg per 100 Kcal. If cow's milk (which has a lower iron bioavailability than human breast milk) is ingested, the amount of iron absorbed may be insufficient to meet the growing child's iron requirement and additional iron fortification or supplementation of the diet are necessary to avoid a negative iron balance. A similar circumstance occurs during menstruation or pregnancy, when there is enhanced iron requirement. Under these circumstances, if there is insufficient dietary intake, for example, due to food faddism and/or a diet containing increased inhibitors of iron absorption, iron deficiency is likely to develop. On the other hand, ingestion of a diet rich in vitamin C, meat, or other animal proteins is protective against iron deficiency by enhancing iron absorption. This partly explains the lower incidence of iron deficiency in developed countries. Population studies have shown an inverse correlation between meat ingestion and prevalence of iron deficiency.

5.1 Dietary Iron Fortification

Various strategies have been devised to prevent iron deficiency. In most developed countries, it has been the practice to fortify the diet with iron. Iron is routinely added to flour in 49 countries. Fortification can be large scale or localized to certain population sectors. Specific iron fortification programs directed at populations with higher iron requirements (such as children, adolescents, and pregnant women) would be beneficial and should perhaps replace nationwide fortification programs.

There are a number of pitfalls associated with large-scale fortification. If the prevalence of the iron-loading gene for genetic hemochromatosis is high in a population, this segment may experience severe complications. Besides this, the dietary vehicle may contain inhibitors that interact with the particular iron fortificant, and iron compounds may have different absorption properties depending on the specific food vehicle. Commonly studied iron fortificants include NaFeEDTA [124–127], ferrous fumarate, and electrolytic iron. NaFeEDTA does not have unacceptable organoleptic properties on the fortificant, and it is bioavailable and water soluble. In Africa, fortification of staple cereals has been common. In a recent study in Kenyan schoolchildren [128], NaFeEDTA at two different doses, or electrolytic iron, was compared to no supplementary iron, added to whole grain maize flower. NaFeEDTA at 56 mg/kg was superior in correcting iron deficiency anemia compared to a lower dose (28 mg/kg) of NaFeEDTA and to electrolytic iron, which had no beneficial effect. The lower NaFeEDTA dose diminished the prevalence of iron deficiency but not the incidence of iron deficiency anemia [128]. In contrast, others report that electrolytic iron is the elemental iron that should be used in cereal flours. These differences may relate to the type of cereal used. Whole grain flour has a higher phytate content than low-extraction flour. When phytate content is high, EDTA chelates iron, preventing its binding to phytate, thus making it more likely to be absorbed. On the other hand, meals containing less phytate may promote absorption of electrolytic iron over NaFeEDTA. Various food vehicles have been utilized in different populations. In a study in Vietnam, fish sauce, consumed by more than 80% of the population, was fortified with 10 mg iron as NaFeEDTA. This was added to the diet daily for 6 days each week over a 6-month period and compared with a control group. This intervention led to higher hemoglobin and ferritin levels and lower sTfR levels in the iron-fortified group. The incidence of iron deficiency anemia declined from 58% to 20%, and the incidence of iron deficiency dropped from 62% in the control group to 33% in the treatment group [43].

Because iron compounds such as ferrous sulfate that are readily soluble in water promote fat oxidation and cause unacceptable organoleptic changes in food, alternative iron compounds for targeted fortification have been evaluated. These include ferrous fumarate, which produces no significant organoleptic effect. Studies comparing absorption from ferrous fumarate to ferrous sulfate added to infant cereals show no differences in iron absorption. Absorption from ferrous fumarate and ferrous sulfate contained in a rice cereal was 2.58% from each compound or 0.2 mg of a 7.5 mg dose. Further studies of a chocolate drink powder designed for targeted fortification in children and containing 5 mg iron per serving showed similar results of 3.31% absorption from ferrous fumarate and 2.28% from ferrous sulfate [129]. Processing of the drink ingredients after addition of the iron salts significantly improved absorption of ferrous fumarate to 5.3% compared with 2.6% from ferrous sulfate. These studies suggest that when ferrous compounds are taken in the diet, iron enters a common pool in the gastrointestinal tract, where it comes under the influence of inhibitory ligands contained in the diet, such as phytates and polyphenols. In the study mentioned above however, processing during manufacture of the chocolate drink appeared to alter assimilation from this common iron pool.

When instituting iron fortification strategies, it is important to evaluate response because initial positive results obtained under well-controlled circumstances in pilot studies may not reflect outcomes under realistic conditions when large fortification programs are implemented.

5.2 *Oral Iron Therapy*

The majority of patients with iron deficiency anemia respond readily to oral iron replacement. Although a number of iron compounds exist for oral use, significant differences in iron bioavailability occur between the various compounds. Ferrous iron salts have superior bioavailability compared to ferric iron salts. Furthermore, a single iron compound may vary in bioavailability depending on the manner in which it is coated during manufacture. Some iron tablets may be almost totally unavailable for absorption because the tablet coating is resistant to dissolution in the stomach. Tablets may pass whole or only partly dissolved through the gastrointestinal tract. Each iron compound form may be manufactured by a number of different companies. In the USA, there are at least 15 brands of ferrous sulfate, at least 7 brands of ferrous fumarate, 3 brands of ferrous gluconate, and 5 brands containing polysaccharide iron. In addition, there is at least one brand containing two iron compounds.

Because of relatively low cost and reasonable bioavailability, ferrous sulfate is the iron compound used most often for oral iron therapy. It is also commonly used as a standard for comparison. Ferrous sulfate is, however, associated with a number of gastrointestinal side effects that often lead to poor compliance or discontinuation of therapy. A number of alternative iron compounds have been manufactured in an attempt to lessen side effects and thereby enhance acceptability, with the hope of having equal, if not improved, bioavailability. Apart from the compounds mentioned below, very few iron preparations exist with bioavailability equivalent to ferrous sulfate while at the same time having decreasing side effects. Ferrous fumarate, ferrous lactate, ferrous succinate, and ferrous glutamate have similar bioavailability to ferrous sulfate, based on studies using double radioisotopic labeling techniques [130].

A number of preparations with slow iron-release properties have been designed, but for the most part, bioavailability does not equal that of standard ferrous sulfate tablets, although there are some exceptions. One of these is ferrous sulfate suspended in a gastric delivery system which is retained in the stomach for 5–12 h [48]; however, this preparation is not commercially available.

An important determinant of efficacy of iron therapy pertains to the side effects induced by the iron preparation. This is the single most important cause of noncompliance with iron therapy. A number of side effects have been described, almost exclusively involving the gastrointestinal tract. Common side effects include constipation, nausea, heartburn, intestinal gas, diarrhea, and loss of appetite. Side effects may necessitate a dose reduction or change in the manner or form in which iron is taken. Side effects are directly related to the dose of iron and frequency of ingestion, although the latter is less important. Iron is customarily prescribed to be taken three times per day; however, this dosing schedule is probably unnecessary for most patients, unless they have significantly accelerated iron loss or iron requirements. This may occur as a result of chronic bleeding, during pregnancy or in situations where there is markedly enhanced erythropoiesis such as with erythropoietin therapy [60]. At lower doses of iron, it is difficult to demonstrate significantly increased side effects compared to placebo [59]; however, higher doses of iron are associated with increased side effects. One study compared 222 mg iron, given as either ferrous fumarate or ferrous sulfate, with placebo; subjects taking placebo had a 14% incidence of side effects, while in those taking ferrous sulfate and ferrous fumarate, the incidence of side effects was significantly higher at 28% and 26%, respectively. There were no differences in incidence and type of side effects between ferrous sulfate and ferrous fumarate. One percent of the placebo group discontinued taking tablets because of side effects, compared to 10% of the group taking ferrous sulfate and 6% of those taking ferrous fumarate [129].

The dose of iron or frequency of iron intake can be reduced to once or twice per day for most patients who do not have excessive requirements. Furthermore, high doses are not necessarily required during times of major iron requirement such as pregnancy. This was shown in an iron supplement study of pregnant women in Australia, using low-dose ferrous sulfate at 20 mg per day versus a placebo control group. Most previous studies in pregnancy utilized 100 mg iron per day, a dose which is approximately threefold higher than required. At the end of pregnancy, 3% of the treatment group had iron deficiency anemia versus 11% in the placebo group, the rate of iron deficiency without anemia was reduced to 35% compared with 58% in the placebo group, and hemoglobin levels were higher in the iron-supplemented group at week 28 and at delivery. At 6 months postpartum, 16% of the women in the iron-supplemented group were iron deficient versus 29% in the control group [59]. At this low dose, no intolerance to iron was encountered compared with the control group.

Reducing the frequency of iron ingestion from once daily to once or twice weekly may decrease the incidence of side effects and lead to proportionately higher iron absorption from each intermittent dose of iron, compared to that with daily intake. This is based on the theory that iron taken daily or more frequently may result in diminished luminal iron uptake by the mucosal cell and diminished transport from the cell into the portal circulation because iron taken up from the previous day's dose may still be present in the mucosal cell and may block further iron uptake from the bowel lumen. However, a study has shown no advantage to administering iron less than once a day [131]. It was reported that absorption from weekly administration would likely fall short of the amount of iron required in most situations where iron supplementation is used, such as pregnancy. Iron absorption from a daily dose was a nonsignificant 3% lower compared to weekly iron administration, regardless of whether iron was taken alone or with food. Absorption amounted to 4.2 mg from daily iron administration compared with 4.8 mg from a weekly dose [131]. Extrapolation of the data indicates a sixfold higher total iron assimilation when iron is taken daily rather than weekly. Furthermore, reducing administration to less than once per day may not diminish side effects appreciably because the majority of side effects originate in the upper gastrointestinal tract. These symptoms often occur soon after iron ingestion and are caused by the effects of released iron on the gastrointestinal tract mucosa. The only advantage to less frequent ingestion is less frequent symptoms.

A number of strategies may be used to diminish side effects of iron. If a single daily dose on an empty stomach fails to alleviate symptoms, iron should be taken with food; however, this significantly reduces iron absorption. Ingestion of vitamin C with the meal may help improve iron assimilation in this situation. Taking ferrous iron solution may help occasionally if iron tablets are intolerable, but usually, this results in similar side effects. In general, an erythropoietic response to iron therapy should be seen within 4–6 weeks of iron replacement therapy. When a response does not occur, reasons for a lack of response should be actively pursued.

A concern has been raised that ingestion of iron supplements may interfere with zinc absorption. When pregnant women ingested 20 mg of ferrous sulfate daily, no differences in serum zinc concentrations were observed at delivery or 6 months postpartum. At delivery, 51% of the iron-supplemented group versus 59% of the placebo group were zinc deficient (zinc levels $<9.8\ \mu$mol/L), while 7% of the iron-supplemented group and 10% of the placebo group were zinc deficient at 6 months postpartum [59].

Under most circumstances when iron deficiency anemia is treated, the hematological response is prompt, with a discernable change in laboratory markers of hematopoiesis within 14 days. In general, hemoglobin levels rise by approximately 1 g/L per day after starting iron therapy. Lack of response to iron therapy may be due to poor compliance, or concurrent disorders of the bone marrow, the most common of which is anemia of chronic disease. The use of poorly bioavailable iron preparations or concurrent ongoing blood loss may also result in lack of response. The latter problem can be identified by testing the feces for occult blood. If the hemoglobin level fails to rise, a hematological response may be evidenced by a raised reticulocyte count. Reticulocyte hemoglobin content (CHr) is an early, sensitive indicator of a favorable response to iron administration [17, 18, 19]. Iron malabsorption may occur with disorders involving the small bowel or gastric mucosa (see above). Performing an iron tolerance test with an iron preparation known to be well absorbed will be helpful in identifying this possibility. The iron tolerance test may not accurately reflect total absorption, especially from iron compounds designed to dissolve as delayed-release formulations. For the most part, however, this method can be used to measure relative iron absorption from a particular preparation or "brand" of iron. This method is also useful in the clinical arena, when patients on oral iron therapy fail to respond. This may be due to iron malabsorption related to an underlying gastrointestinal disease. Alternatively, poor absorption may occur because of poor iron bioavailability from the iron tablet. If there is suspicion that a particular brand of iron is poorly absorbed in a patient and this is confirmed in an iron tolerance test, the test should be repeated using a ferrous sulfate solution. If absorption from this solution is still abnormal, iron malabsorption is the likely cause. If absorption from ferrous sulfate solution is normal, then the problem lies with the iron compound that the patient was taking, in some cases due to thick enteric coating that does not dissolve in the stomach. It is important to use a brand of oral iron with proven efficacy, rather than to randomly purchase any over-the-counter preparations.

Although ferrous sulfate has been the traditional iron salt used for replacement, other ferrous salts, including ferrous fumarate and ferrous gluconate, have equivalent efficacy and can be used for initial therapy. These iron compounds should be tried when ferrous sulfate induces intolerable side effects. The concomitant administration of ascorbic acid enhances iron absorption from these preparations, and some oral iron preparations contain added vitamin C. Vitamin C may also improve iron mobilization from iron stores, and administration of vitamin C may improve hematological indices in hemodialysis patients [23].

5.3 *Oral Iron Therapy During Erythropoietin Administration*

Therapy with erythropoiesis-stimulating agents (ESA) has been used primarily for patients with anemia of chronic renal failure. Other indications for erythropoietin therapy include anemia of chronic inflammation, anemia with HIV infection, myelodysplastic syndromes, and patients receiving chemotherapy, although the latter has come to be considered inadvisable for a number of malignancies. ESA therapy necessitates increased iron delivery to the erythroid bone marrow to produce hemoglobin. In most situations, iron mobilization from iron stores meets this enhanced requirement; however, a number of studies report subtle changes of iron-deficient erythropoiesis under these circumstances. Some studies used normal volunteer subjects whose erythroid response may exceed that in patients with complex diseases. Furthermore, the form of oral iron replacement used in some studies may have less than adequate efficacy. With ESA treatment, the rate of iron mobilization from stores may be unable to match iron requirements of an expanding red cell mass. Consequently, to obtain optimal response from a given dose of ESA, additional iron replacement is often necessary. It has been suggested that iron absorbed from oral iron supplements is inadequate to meet the enhanced requirements of ESA therapy. This presumption may not be correct in all cases, and significant controversy exists concerning the optimal route of iron replacement. Intravenous iron dosing is advocated by most authorities to obtain optimal response to ESAs. Intravenous iron preparations must be catabolized in macrophages to release iron, in order for iron to become available for use by the erythroid marrow. The difference in rate and magnitude of the erythropoietic response to administered intravenous iron or oral iron may be negligible.

5.4 *Intravenous Iron Therapy*

Intravenous iron replacement is indicated in limited clinical situations. It should be reserved for patients who are intolerant to oral iron therapy, have iron malabsorption, or have iron losses that cannot be adequately replenished to keep up with the rate of bleeding. Intravenous iron therapy may also be used during ESA administration, especially in anemia of chronic renal disease, where oral iron replacement is usually inadequate to replenish or maintain adequate iron status. Iron deficiency is the most common cause of erythropoietin hyporesponsiveness. Because patients on hemodialysis are unable to maintain a stable iron balance, oral iron administration often fails to maintain adequate iron stores, especially if they are treated with ESAs. Intravenous iron therapy is frequently administered to maximize the efficacy of ESAs [132]. However, the National Kidney Foundation Kidney Disease Outcomes Quality Initiative anemia guidelines caution against the regular administration of intravenous iron when ferritin levels exceed 500 μg/L [133]. Autologous blood donation is another situation where intravenous iron may be useful.

There are four parenteral iron preparations currently available for use in the United States. These preparations have a carbohydrate ligand and ferric hydroxide or paramagnetic ferric oxide iron cores. The iron core particles differ in size, and there are differences in affinity of the bond between the core iron and the carbohydrate moiety. There are two main risks associated with the administration of these preparations – anaphylaxis-type reactions and bioactive iron reactions. Anaphylactic reactions are usually related to the carbohydrate ligand, which may cause immune responses predominantly occurring with dextran. The bond between the carbohydrate and iron core influences the rate of iron release from the carbohydrate ligand in the reticuloendothelial system, predominantly in the bone marrow, spleen, and liver. Bioactive iron reactions occur when iron is released in intracellular or extracellular spaces and precipitate adverse reactions, including hypotension, abdomen, flank or chest pain, myalgias, arthralgias, nausea, vomiting, or diarrhea.

Iron dextran, which has been available the longest, has been associated with adverse side effects, including hypotension, bronchospasm, anaphylaxis, and death. The rate of intolerance has been reported to be 2.5%, including a 0.7% rate of life-threatening anaphylactoid reactions [134]. Three alternative preparations now available include ferric gluconate (Ferrlecit®), which has an intolerance rate of 0.44–1.7% [135, 136]; iron sucrose (Venofer®) [137], a drug available in Europe for over 50 years; and ferumoxytol (Feraheme®) [138]. In a study of 144 hemodialysis patients with sensitivity to iron dextran, treated with ferric gluconate, 88% had no adverse reaction [134]. In another study of 130 patients with intolerance to iron dextran, neither ferric gluconate nor iron sucrose was associated with any serious adverse events. There were 14 nonserious adverse events in eight patients attributed to iron sucrose, none of which resulted in discontinuation of therapy [137]. Initial studies with ferumoxytol have shown anaphylaxis/anaphylactoid reactions of 0.2% and other reactions that can be associated with hypersensitivity in 3.7% [138].

These preparations can be used for the treatment of iron deficiency or the maintenance of iron stores. An advantage of iron dextran is that doses up to 1,000 mg can be administered in a single infusion, while only 125 mg of ferric gluconate can be safely given at a time. In a study of iron sucrose in hemodialysis patients [137], up to 200 mg of iron sucrose was administered intravenously undiluted over 2–5 min, or diluted in normal saline over 15–30 min. Doses of the latter two intravenous iron preparations can be repeated more frequently than weekly, but it is preferable to give them weekly, unless there is a compelling reason to obtain a faster correction of the iron deficit. Ferumoxytol is given on days 1 and 5, each at a dose of 510 mg as a rapid intravenous injection. Few patients have been tested with additional doses, and possible increased adverse reactions to repeat doses need to be followed. Approximately 170 mg of iron is required to obtain a 10 g/L rise in hemoglobin in a 70-kg male, based on a total blood volume of 4.9 L.

Although intravenous iron has beneficial effects in treating iron deficiency or functional iron deficiency in patients treated with ESAs, excess intravenous iron administration generates oxidative stress, inflammation, endothelial dysfunction, and renal injury [133, 139, 140]. Nondextran iron preparations may increase this propensity. Differences exist between iron sucrose and ferric gluconate in their ability to donate iron directly to transferrin (gluconate > sucrose > iron dextran) [141], indicating that a labile iron fraction may develop with these intravenous iron preparations, especially if serum UIBC is low [141]. This may cause proteinuria and increased plasma levels of lipid peroxidation products [133]. The long-term effects of excess intravenous iron preparations on vascular function [142], systemic inflammatory responses, atherogenesis, and rate of renal disease progression [143] require careful study, especially since cardiovascular disease is the primary cause of death in patients with end-stage renal disease.

The iron status of patients taking iron therapy, whether oral or intravenous, should be monitored intermittently, to establish whether iron stores are adequately replenished, and to avoid iron overload that may occur with unmonitored long-term iron replacement.

References

1. Haas JD, Brownlie T. Iron deficiency and reduced work capacity: a critical review of the research to determine a causal relationship. J Nutr. 2001;131:676S–88.
2. Halterman JS, Kaczorowski JM, Aligne CA, Auinger P, Szilagyi PG. Iron deficiency and cognitive achievement among school-aged children and adolescents in the United States. Pediatrics. 2001;107:1381–6.
3. Algarin C, Peirano P, Garrido M, Pizarro F, Lozoff B. Iron deficiency anemia in infancy: long- lasting effects on auditory and visual system functioning. Pediatr Res. 2003;53:217–23.
4. Verdon F, Burnand B, Stubi CL, et al. Iron supplementation for unexplained fatigue in non-anemic women: double blind randomized placebo controlled trial. BMJ. 2003;326:1124–7.
5. Carter RC, Jacobson JL, Burden MJ, et al. Iron deficiency anemia and cognitive function in infancy. Pediatrics. 2010;126:e427–34.
6. Willoughby JMT, Laitner SM. Audit of the investigation of iron deficiency anemia in a district general hospital, with sample guidelines for future practice. Postgrad Med J. 2000;76:218–22.
7. Brugnara C, Schiller B, Moran J. Reticulocyte hemoglobin equivalent (Ret He) and assessment of iron-deficient states. Clin Lab Haematol. 2006;28:303–8.
8. Macdougall IC, Cavill I, Hulme B, et al. Detection of functional iron-deficiency during erythropoietin treatment: a new approach. BMJ. 1992;304:225–6.
9. Macdougall IC, Horl WH, Jacobs C, et al. European best practice guidelines 6–8: assessing and optimizing iron stores. Nephrol Dial Transplant. 2000;15:20–32.
10. Goodnough LT, Skikne B, Brugnara C. Erythropoietin, iron, and erythropoiesis. Blood. 2000;96(3):823–33.
11. Cook JD, Alvarado J, Gutniskey A, et al. Nutritional deficiency and anemia in Latin America: a collaborative study. Blood. 1971;38:591–603.
12. Cohen JH, Haas JD. The comparison of mixed distribution analysis with a three-criteria model as a method for estimating the prevalence of iron deficiency anemia in Costa Rican children aged 12–23 months. Int J Epidemiol. 1999;28:82–9.
13. Frith-Terhune Al, Cogswell ME, Khan LK, Will JC, Ramakrishnan U. Iron deficiency anemia: higher prevalence in Mexican American than in non-Hispanic white females in the third National Health and Nutrition Examination Survey. Am J Clin Nutr. 2000;72:963–8.
14. Milman N, Byg KE, Mulvad G, Pedersen HS, Bjerregaard P. Haemoglobin concentrations appear to be lower in indigenous Greenlanders than in Danes: assessment of haemoglobin in 234 Greenlanders and in 2804 Danes. Eur J Haematol. 2001;67:23–9.

15. Asobayire FS, Adou P, Davidsson L, Cook JD, Hurrell RF. Prevalence of iron deficiency with and without concurrent anemia in population groups with high prevalences of malaria and other infections: a study in cote d'Ivoire. Am J Clin Nutr. 2001;74:776–82.
16. Kitua AY, Smith TA, Alonso PL, et al. The role of low level plasmodium falciparum parasitemia in anemia among infants living in an area of intense and perennial transmission. Trop Med Int Health. 1997;2:325–39.
17. Mast AE, Blinder MA, Lu Q, Flax S, Dietzen DJ. Clinical utility of the reticulocyte hemoglobin content in the diagnosis of iron deficiency. Blood. 2002;99:1489–92.
18. Markovic M, Majkic-Singh N, Ignjatovic S, Singh S. Reticulocyte haemoglobin content vs. soluble transferrin receptor and ferritin index in iron deficiency anemia accompanied with inflammation. Int J of Lab Haematol. 2007;29:341–6.
19. Brugnara C, Zurakowski D, DiGnzio J, Boyd T, Platt O. Reticulocyte haemoglobin content to diagnose iron deficiency in children. JAMA. 1999;281:2225–30.
20. Ullrich C, Wu A, Armsby C, et al. Screening healthy infants for iron deficiency using reticulocyte hemoglobin content. JAMA. 2005;294:924–30.
21. Fishbane S, Galgano C, Langley Jr RC, Canfield W, Maesaka JK. Reticulocyte hemoglobin content in the evaluation of iron status of hemodialysis patients. Kidney Int. 1997;52:217–22.
22. Kuvibidila S, Yu LC, Ode DL, Warrier RP, Mbefe V. Assessment of iron status of Zairian women of childbearing age by serum transferrin receptor. Am J Clin Nutr. 1994;60:603–9.
23. Tarng DC, Huang TP, Chen TW, Yang WC. Erythropoietin hyporesponsiveness: from iron deficiency to iron overload. Kidney Int Soc Nephrol. 1995;69:S107–18.
24. Herbert V, Jayatilleke E, Shaw S, et al. Serum ferritin iron, a new test, measures human body iron stores uncompounded by inflammation. Stem Cells. 1997;15:291–6.
25. Dale JC, Burritt MF, Zinsmeister AR. Diurnal variation of serum iron, iron-binding capacity, transferrin saturation, and ferritin levels. Am J Clin Pathol. 2002;117:802–8.
26. Pak M, Lopez MA, Gabayan V, Ganz T, Rivera S. suppression of hepcidin during anemia requires erythropoietic activity. Blood. 2006;108:3730–5.
27. Detivaud L, Nemeth E, Boudjema K, et al. Hepcidin levels in humans are correlated with hepatic iron stores, hemoglobin levels, and hepatic function. Blood. 2005;106:746–8.
28. Nemeth E, Valore EV, Territo M, Schiller G, Lichtenstein A, Ganz T. Hepcidin, a putative mediator of anemia of inflammation, is a type II acute-phase protein. Blood. 2003;101:2461–3.
29. Weinstein DA, Roy CN, Fleming MD, Loda MF, Wolfsdorf JI, Andrews NC. Inappropriate expression of hepcidin is associated with iron refractory anemia: implications for the anemia of chronic disease. Blood. 2002;100:3776–81.
30. Kemna E, Tjalsma H, Laarakkers C, Nemeth E, Willems H, Swinkels D. Novel urine hepcidin assay by mass spectrometry. Blood. 2005;106:3268–70.
31. Ahluwalia N, Skikne BS, Savin V, Chonko A. Markers of masked iron deficiency and effectiveness of EPO therapy in chronic renal failure. Am J Kidney Dis. 1997;30(4):532–41.
32. Shih YJ, Baynes RD, Hudson BG, Flowers CH, Skikne BS, Cook JD. Serum transferrin receptor is a truncated form of tissue receptor. J Biol Chem. 1990;265:19077–81.
33. Cook JD, Skikne BS, Baynes RD. Serum transferrin receptor. Annu Rev Med. 1993;44:63–74.
34. Skikne BS, Flowers CH, Cook JD. Serum transferrin receptor: a quantitative measure of tissue iron deficiency. Blood. 1990;75:1870–6.
35. Ferguson BJ, Skikne BS, Simpson KM, Baynes RD, Cook JD. Serum transferrin receptor distinguishes the anemia of chronic disease from iron deficiency anemia. J Lab Clin Med. 1992;119:385–90.
36. Ahuwalia N, Lammi-Keefe CJ, Bendel RB. Iron deficiency and anemia of chronic disease in elderly women: a discriminant-analysis approach for differentiation. Am J Clin Nutr. 1995;61:590–6.
37. Suominen P, Punnonen K, Rajamaki A, Irjala K. Evaluation of new immunoenzymometric assay for measuring soluble transferrin receptor to detect iron deficiency in anemic patients. Clin Chem. 1997;43:1641–6.
38. Nielsen OJ, Andersen LS, Hansen NE, Hansen TM. Serum transferrin receptor levels in anemic patients with rheumatoid arthritis. Scand J Clin Lab Invest. 1994;54:75–82.
39. Siebert S, Williams BD, Henley R, Ellis R, Cavill I, Worwood M. Single value of serum transferrin receptor is not diagnostic for the absence of iron stores in anemic patients with rheumatoid arthritis. Clin Lab Haematol. 2003;25:155–60.
40. Wians Jr FH, Urban JE, Keffer JH, Kroft SH. Discriminating between iron deficiency anemia and anemia of chronic disease using traditional indices of iron status vs transferrin receptor concentration. Am J Clin Pathol. 2001;115:112–8.
41. Punnonen K, Irjala K, Rajamaki A. Serum transferrin receptor and its ratio to serum ferritin in the diagnosis of iron deficiency. Blood. 1997;89:1052–7.
42. Weiss G, Goodnough LT. Anemia of chronic disease. N Engl J Med. 2005;352:1011–23.

43. Thuy PV, Berger J, Davidsson L, et al. Regular consumption of NaFeEDTA-Fortified Fish Sauce improves iron status and reduces the prevalence of anemia in anemic Vietnamese women. Am J Clin Nutr. 2003;78:284–90.
44. Kogan AE, Filatov VL, Kara AN, Levina AA, Katrukha AG. Comparison of soluble and placental transferrin receptors as standards for the determination of soluble transferrin receptor in humans. Int J Lab Hematol. 2007;29:335–40.
45. Souminen P, Punnonen K, Rajamaki A, Irjala K. Serum transferrin receptor and transferrin receptor-ferritin index identify healthy subject with sub-clinical iron deficits. Blood. 1998;92:934–9.
46. Cook JD, Flowers CH, Skikne BS. An assessment of dried blood-spot technology for identifying iron deficiency. Blood. 1998;92:1807–13.
47. Cook JD, Flowers CH, Skikne BS. The quantitative assessment of body iron. Blood. 2003;9:3359–64.
48. Simmons WK, Cook JD, Bingham KC, et al. Evaluation of gastric delivery system for iron supplementation in pregnancy. Am J Clin Nutr. 1993;58:622–6.
49. Tawfik O, O'Neal MF, Davis M, Cunningham MT, Skikne B, Chapman KD. A newly proposed iron stain quantitation method in bone marrow smears using an automated cellular imaging system. Am J Clin Pathol. 2006;126:643–4.
50. Fleming DJ, Jacques PF, Dallal GE, Tucker KL, Wilson PWF, Wood RJ. Dietary determinants of iron stores in a free-living elderly population. The Framingham heart study. Am J Clin Nutr. 1998;67:722–33.
51. Cook JD, Dassenko SA, Whittaker P. Calcium supplementation: effect on iron absorption. Am J Clin Nutr. 1991;53:106–11.
52. Hallberg L, Rossander-Hulten L, Brune M, Gleerup A. Calcium and iron absorption: mechanism of action and nutritional importance. Eur J Clin Nutr. 1992;46:317–27.
53. Hallberg L, Brune M, Erlandsson M, Snadberg AS, Rossander-Hulten L. Calcium: effect of different amounts on nonheme – and heme-iron absorption in humans. Am J Clin Nutr. 1991;53:112–9.
54. Roughead ZK, Zito CA, Hunt JR. Initial uptake and absorption of nonheme iron and absorption of heme iron in humans are unaffected by the addition of calcium as cheese to a meal with high iron bioavailability. Am J Clin Nutr. 2002;76:419–25.
55. Beard JL. Iron requirements in adolescent females. J Nutr. 2000;130:440S–2.
56. Hallberg L. Iron requirements, iron balance and iron deficiency in menstruating and pregnant women. In: Hallberg L, Asp NG, editors. Iron nutrition in health and disease. London: John Libbey & Co; 1996. p. 165–82.
57. Carriaga MT, Skikne BS, Finley B, Cutler B, Cook JD. Serum transferrin receptor for the detiction of iron deficiency in pregnancy. Am J Clin Nutr. 1991;54:1077–81.
58. Milman N, Agger AO, Nielsen OJ. Iron supplementation during pregnancy. Dan Med Bull. 1991;38:471–6.
59. Makrides M, Crowther CA, Gibson RA, Gibson RS, Skeaff CM. Efficacy and tolerability of low-dose iron supplements during pregnancy: a randomized controlled trial. Am J Clin Nutr. 2003;78:145–53.
60. Skikne BS, Cook JD. Effect of enhanced eryrhropoiesis on iron absorption. J Lab Clin Med. 1992;20:746–54.
61. Skikne BS, Ahluwalia N, Fergusson B, Chonko A, Cook JD. Effects of erythropoietin therapy on iron absorption in chronic renal failure. J Lab Clin Med. 2000;135:452–8.
62. Raje D, Mukhtar H, Oshowo A, Ingham Clark C, Chir M. What proportion of patients referred to secondary care with iron deficiency anemia have colon cancer? Dis Colon Rectum. 2007;50:1211–4.
63. Acher PL, Al-Mishlab T, Rahman M, Bates T. Iron deficiency anemia and delay in the diagnosis of colorectal cancer. Colorectal Dis. 2003;5:145–8.
64. Bardella MT, Fredella C, Saladino V, et al. Gluten intolerance. Gender and age-related differences in symptoms. Scand J Gastroenterol. 2005;40:15–9.
65. Rockey DC, Cello JP. Evaluation of the gastrointestinal tract in patients with iron-deficiency anemia. N Engl J Med. 1993;329:1691–5.
66. McIntyre AS, Long RG. Prospective survey of investigations in outpatients referred with iron deficiency anemia. Gut. 1993;34:1102–7.
67. Bini EJ, Micale PL, Weinshel EH. Evaluation of the gastrointestinal tract in pre-menopausal women with iron deficiency anemia. Am J Med. 1998;105:281–6.
68. Dickey W, Hughes D. Prevalence of celiac disease and its endoscopic markers among patients having routine upper gastrointestinal endoscopy. Am J Gastroenterol. 1999;94:2182–6.
69. Dickey W, Kenny BD, McMillan SA, Porter KG, McConnell JB. Gastric as well as duodenal biopsies may be useful in the investigation of iron deficiency anemia. Scand J Gastroenterol. 1997;32:469–72.
70. Annibale B, Capurso G, Chistolini A, et al. Gastrointestinal causes of refractory iron deficiency anemia in patients without gastrointestinal symptoms. Am J Med. 2001;111:439–45.
71. Choe YH, Kwon YS, Jung MK, et al. Helicobacter pylori-associated iron-deficiency anemia in adolescent female athletes. J Pediatr. 2001;139:100–4.
72. Annibale B, Marignani M, Monarca B, et al. Reversal of iron deficiency anemia after Helicobacter pylori eradication in patients with asymptomatic gastritis. Annu Int Med. 1999;131:668–72.

73. Hershko C, Hoffbrand AV, Keret D, et al. Role of autoimmune gastritis, Helicobacter pylori and celiac disease in refractory or unexplained iron deficiency anemia. Haematologica. 2005;90:585–95.
74. Hershko C, Ronson A, Souroujon M, et al. Variable hematologic presentation of autoimmune gastritis: age-related progression from iron deficiency to cobalamin depletion. Blood. 2006;107:1673–9.
75. Hershko C, Ianculovich M, Souroujon M. A hematologist's view of unexplained iron deficiency anemia in males: impact of Helicobacter pylori eradication. Blood Cells Mol Dis. 2007;38:45–53.
76. Milman N, Rosenstock S, Andersen L, et al. Serum ferritin, hemoglobin, and Helicobacter pylori infection: a seroepidemiologic survey comprising 2794 Danish adults. Gastroenterology. 1998;115:268–74.
77. Suerbaum S, Michetti P. Helicobacter pylori infection. N Engl J Med. 2002;347:1175–86.
78. Choe YH, Kim SK, Son BK, et al. Randomized placebo-controlled trial of Helicobacter pylori eradication for iron-deficiency anemia in preadolescent children and adolescents. Helicobacter. 1999;4:135–9.
79. Choe YH, Lee JE, Kim SK. Effect of helicobacter pylori eradication on sideropenic refractory anaemia in adolescent girls with Helicobacter pylori infection. Acta Paediatr. 2000;89:154–7.
80. Annibale B, Capurso G, Lahner E, et al. Concomitant alterations in intragastric pH and ascorbic acid concentration in patients with Helicobacter pylori gastritis and associated iron deficiency anaemia. Gut. 2003;52:496–501.
81. Faber K, Bloch CE. Über die pathologischen Veränderungen am digestion-stractus bei der perniciösen anämie und über die sogenannte darm atrophie. Zeitschrift Klin Med. 1900;40:98.
82. Faber K. Achylia gastrica mit Anämie. Medizinishe Klinik. 1909;5:1310–25.
83. Faber K. Anämische Zustände bei der chronischen Achylia Gastrica. Klin Echnschr. 1913;50:958.
84. Faber K, Gram HC. Relations between achylia gastrica and simple and pernicious anemia. Arch Intern Med. 1924;34:658–68.
85. Wintrobe MM, Beebe RT. Idiopathic hypochromic anemia. Medicine. 1933;12:187–243.
86. Hershko C, Patz J, Ronson A. The anemia of achylia gastrica revisited. Blood Cells Mol Dis. 2007;39:178–83.
87. Beutler E, Fairbanks VF, Fahey JL. Clinical disorders of iron metabolism. New York: Grune& Stratton; 1963. p. 80–3.
88. Davidson WMB, Markson JL. The gastric mucosa in iron deficiency anaemia. Lancet. 1955;269:639–43.
89. Badenoch J, Evans JR, Richards WCD. The stomach in hypochromic anemia. Brit J Haematol. 1957;3:175–85.
90. Lees F, Rosenthal FD. Gastric mucosal lesions before and after treatment in iron-deficiency anemia. Quart J Med. 1958;27:19–26.
91. Editorial. Achlorhydria and anaemia. Lancet. 1960;2:27–8.
92. Dagg JH, Goldberg A, Gibbs WN, Anderson JR. Detection of latent pernicious anemia in iron -deficiency anemia. Brit Med J. 1966;2:619–21.
93. Cook JD, Brown GM, Valberg LS. The effect of achylia gastrica on iron absorption. J Clin Invest. 1964;43:1185–91.
94. Schade SG, Cohen RJ, Conrad ME. The effect of hydrochloric acid on iron absorption. N Engl J Med. 1968;279:621–4.
95. Bezwoda W, Charlton R, Bothwell T, et al. The importance of gastric hydrochloric acid in the absorption of nonheme food iron. J Lab Clin Med. 1978;92:108–16.
96. Stopeck A. Links between Helicobacter pylori infection, cobalamin deficiency, and pernicious anemia. Arch Intern Med. 2000;160:1229–30.
97. Appelmelk BJ, Simoons-Smit I, Negrini R, et al. Potential role of molecular mimicry between Helicobacter pylori lipopolysaccharide and host Lewis blood group antigens in autoimmunity. Infect Immun. 1996;64:2031–40.
98. Negrini R, Savio A, Appelmelk BJ. Autoantibodies to gastric mucosa in Helicobacter pylori infection. [review]. Helicobacter. 1997;2:S13–6.
99. Ma JY, Borch K, Sjostrand SE, et al. Positive corrélation between H, K-adenosine triphosphatase autoantibodies and Helicobacter pylori antibodies in patients with pernicious anemia. Scand J Gastroenterol. 1994;29:961–5.
100. Claeys D, Faller G, Appelmelk BJ, et al. The gastric H+, K+-ATPase is a major autoantigen in chronic Helicobacter pylori gastritis with body mucosa atrophy. Gastroenterology. 1998;115:340–7.
101. Negrini R, Savio A, Poiesi C, et al. Antigenic mimicry between Helicobacter pylori and gastric mucosa in the pathogenesis of body atrophic gastritis. Gastroenterology. 1996;111:655–65.
102. Jassel SV, Ardill JE, Fillmore D, et al. The rise in circulating gastrin with age is due to increases in gastric autoimmunity and Helicobacter pylori infection. QJM. 1999;92:373–7.
103. Appelmelk BJ, Negrini R, Moran AP, Kuipers EJ. Molecular mimicry between Helicobacter pylori and the host. Trends Microbiol. 1997;5:70–3.
104. Rad R, Schmid RM, Prinz C. Helicobacter pylori, iron deficiency, and gastric autoimmunity. Blood. 2006;107:4969–70.
105. Annibale B, Di Giulio E, Caruana P, et al. The long-term effects of cure of *Helicobacter pylori* infection on patients with atrophic body gastritis. Aliment Pharmacol Ther. 2002;16:1723–31.

106. Kaptan K, Beyan C, Ural AU, et al. *Helicobacter pylori*: is it a novel causative agent in vitamin B12 deficiency? Arch Intern Med. 2000;160:1349–53.
107. Haruma K, Mihara M, Okamoto E, et al. Eradication of *Helicobacter pylori* increases gastric acidity in patients with atrophic gastritis of the corpus-evaluation of 24-h pH monitoring. Aliment Pharmacol Ther. 1999;13:155–62.
108. McColl KEL, Murray LS, Gillen D, et al. Randomized trial of endoscopy with testing for *Helicobacter pylori* compared with non-invasive H pylori testing alone in the management of dyspepsia. BMJ. 2002;324:999–1002.
109. Finberg KE. Iron-refractory iron deficiency anemia. Semin Hematol. 2009;46:378–86.
110. DeMaeyer EM, Adiels-Tegman M. The prevalence of anemia in the world. World Health Stat Q. 1985;38:302–16.
111. Looker AC, Dallman PR, Carroll MD, Gunter EW, Johnson CL. Prevalence of iron deficiency in the United States. JAMA. 1997;227:973–6.
112. Cook JD, Boy E, Flowers C, del Carmen Daroca M. The influence of high-altitude living on body iron. Blood. 2005;106:1441–6.
113. Rahimova S, Perry GS, Sarbanescu F, et al. Prevalence of anemia among displaced and nondisplaced mothers and children – Azerbaijan, 2001. MMWR Morb Mortal Wkly Rep. 2004;53:610–4.
114. National Center for Health Statistics. Plan and Operation of the Third National Health and Nutrition Examination Survey (NHANES III), 1988–1994. Hyattsville: National Center for Health Statistics; 1994.
115. Brotanek JM, Gosz J, Weitzman M, Flores G. Iron deficiency in early childhood in the United States: risk factors and racial/ethnic disparities. Pediatrics. 2007;120:568–75.
116. Nead KG, Halterman JS, Kaczorowski JM, Auinger P, Weitzman M. Overweight children and adolescents: a risk group for iron deficiency. Pediatrics. 2004;114:104–8.
117. Pinhas-Hamiel O, Newfield RS, Koren I, Agmon A, Lilos P, Phillip M. Greater prevalence of iron II deficiency in overweight and obese children and adolescents. Int J Obes Relat Metab Disord. 2003;27:416–8.
118. Zhou SJ, Gibson RA, Makrides M. Rôutine iron supplementation in pregnancy has no effect on iron status of children at six months and four years of age. J Pediatr. 2007;151:438–40.
119. DePee S, Bloem MW, Sari M, Kiess L, Yip R, Kosen S. The high prevalence of low hemoglobin concentration among Indonisian infants aged 3–5 months is related to maternal anemia. J Nutr. 2002;132:2215–21.
120. Looker AC, Cogswell ME, Gunter EW. Iron deficiency – United States: 1999-2000. MMWR Weekly. 2002;51:897–9.
121. Guralnik JM, Eisenstaedt RS, Ferrucci L, Klein HG, Woodman RC. Prevalence of anemia in persons 65 years and older in the United States: evidence for a high rate of unexplained anemia. Blood. 2004;104:22263–8.
122. Nicolas G, Chauvet C, Viatte L, et al. The gene encoding the iron regulatory peptide hepcidin is regulated by anemia, hypoxia, and inflammation. J Clin Invest. 2002;110:1037–44.
123. Berger J, Aguayo VM, Tellez W, Lujan C, Traissac P, San Miguel JL. Weekly iron supplementation is as effective as 5 day per week iron supplementation in Bolivian school children living at high altitude. Eur J Clin Nutr. 1997;51:381–6.
124. Hurrell RF. Fortification: overcoming technical and practical barriers. J Nutr. 2002;132(Suppl):806S–12.
125. Garby L, Areekul S. Iron supplementation in the Thai Fish sauce. Ann Trop Med Parasitol. 1974;68:467–76.
126. Viteri FE, Alvarez E, Batres R, et al. Fortification of sugar with iron sodium ethylenediaminotetraacetate (FeNaEDTA) improves iron status in semirural Guatemalan populations. Am J Clin Nutr. 1995;61:1153–63.
127. Ballot DE, MacPhail TH, Bothwell M, Gillooly M. Fortification of curry powder with NaFe(III)EDTA in an iron-deficient population. Am J Clin Nutr. 1989;49:162–9.
128. Andang'o PEA, Osendarp SJM, Ayah R, West CE, et al. Efficacy of iron-fortified whole maize flour on iron status of school children in Kenya: a randomized controlled trial. Lancet. 2007;369:1799–806.
129. Hurrell RF, Reddy MB, Dassenko SA, Cook JD, Shepherd D. Ferrous fumarate fortification of a chocolate drink powder. Brit J Nutr. 1991;65:271–83.
130. Brise H, Hallberg L. Absorbability of different iron compounds. Acta Med Scand Suppl. 1962;17:23–37.
131. Cook JD, Reddy MB. Efficacy of weekly compared with daily iron supplementation. Am J Clin Nutr. 1995;62:117–20.
132. Besarab A. More than a decade of experience and still no consensus: controversies in iron therapy. Clin J Am Soc Nephrol. 2006;1(Suppl 1):S1–3.
133. KDOQI Clinical practice guidelines and clinical practice recommendations for anemia in chronic kidney disease: update 2006. Am J Kidney Dis 2006; 47(Suppl 3):S11–145.
134. Fishbane S, Ungureanu VD, Maesaka JK, Kaupke CJ, Lim V, Wish J. The safety of intravenous iron dextan in hemodialysis patients. Am J Kidney Dis. 1996;28:529–34.
135. Michael B, Coyne DW, Fishbane S, et al. Sodium ferric gluconate complex in hemodialysis patients: adverse reactions compared to placebo and iron dextran. Kidney Int. 2002;61:1830–9.

136. Miller HJ, Hu J, Valentine JK, Gable PS. Efficacy and tolerability of intravenous ferric gluconate in the treatment of iron deficiency anemia in patients without kidney disease. Arch Intern Med. 2007;167:1327–8.
137. Charytan C, Schwenk MH, Al-Saloum MM, Spinowitz BS. Safety of iron sucrose in hemodialysis patients intolerant to other potential iron products. Nephron Clin Pract. 2004;96:C63–6.
138. Lu M, Cohen MH, Rieves D, Pazdur R. FDA report: ferumoxytol for intravenous iron therapy in adult patients with chronic kidney disease. Am J Hematol. 2010;85:315–9.
139. Drueke T, Witko-Sarsat V, Massy Z, et al. Iron therapy, advanced oxidation protein products, and carotid artery intima-media thickness in end-stage renal disease. Circulation. 2002;106:2212–7.
140. Reis KA, Guz G, Ozdemir H, et al. Intravenous iron therapy as a possible risk factor for atherosclerosis in end-stage renal disease. Int Heart J. 2005;46:255–64.
141. Van Wyck D, Anderson J, Johnson K. Labile iron in parenteral iron formulations: a quantitative and comparative study. Nephrol Dial Transplant. 2004;19:561–5.
142. Rooyakkers TM, Stroes ES, Kooistra MP, et al. Ferric saccharate induces oxygen radical stress and endothelial dysfunction in vivo. Eur J Clin Invest. 2002;32(Suppl 1):9–16.
143. Zager RA. Parenteral iron compounds potent oxidents but mainstays of anemia management in chronic renal disease. Clin J Am Soc Nephrol. 2006;1(Suppl 1):S24–31.
144. Krafft A, Perewusnyk G, Hanseler E, Quack K, Huch R, Breymann C. Effect of postpartum iron supplementation on red cell and iron parameters in non-anemic iron-deficient women: a randomized placebo- controlled study. BJOG. 2005;112:445–50.
145. Akesson A, Bjellerup P, Berglund M, Bremme K, Vahter M. Serum transferrin receptor;a specific marker of iron deficiency in pregnancy. Am J Clin Nutr. 1998;68:1241–6.
146. Sinclair LM, Hinton PS. Prevalence of iron deficiency with and without anemia in recreationally active men and women. J Am Diet Assoc. 2005;105:975–8.

Chapter 14
The Liabilities of Iron Deficiency

John L. Beard and Carrie Durward

Keywords Anemia • Brain • Development • Fetus • Iron deficiency • Liabilities • Neuronal function • Physical performance • Pregnancy • Thermoregulation

1 General Clinical Manifestations

The overt physical manifestations of iron deficiency include the generic symptoms of anemia, which are tiredness, lassitude, and general feelings of lack of energy [1, 2]. Clinical manifestations of iron deficiency are glossitis, angular stomatitis, koilonychia (spoon nails), blue sclera, esophageal webbing (Plummer-Vinson Syndrome), and microcytic hypochromic anemia. Behavioral disturbances such as pica, which is characterized by abnormal consumption of nonfood items such as dirt (geophagia) and ice (pagophagia), are often present in iron deficiency, but clear biological explanations for these abnormalities are lacking. More recently, restless legs syndrome (RLS) has been described as being causally related to iron deficiency anemia [3]. This aphasic involuntary muscle contraction appears related to altered movement of iron to and within motor-control centers in the brain and is treatable in most cases with either iron or levodopa [4]. Neuro-maturational delays have been described by many research groups and will be discussed in detail in a later section. Physiological manifestations of iron deficiency have also been noted in immune function, thermoregulatory performance, energy metabolism, and exercise or work performance [2]. The current understanding of the iron biology underlying deficits in the neurobiology, muscle and energy metabolism, and consequences specific to pregnancy outcomes will be discussed in the remaining sections of this chapter.

2 Conceptual Relationship between Severity of Iron Deficiency and Sequelae

The conceptual relationship between functional consequences of iron deficiency and specific outcomes goes back to research from 30 years ago when research groups were looking at exercise performance and temperature regulation [5–9]. Those research groups clearly established that few

J.L. Beard • C. Durward (✉)
Department of Nutritional Sciences, Pennsylvania State University, University Park, PA, USA
e-mail: carrie.durward@gmail.com

G.J. Anderson and G. McLaren (eds.), *Iron Physiology and Pathophysiology in Humans*, Nutrition and Health, DOI 10.1007/978-1-60327-485-2_14,

consequences of iron deficiency occurred in the absence of anemia. Exchange transfusion studies and other approaches showed biochemical and hormonal signaling of metabolism were sensitive to increasing severity of iron deficiency, with biologically meaningful changes frequently observed at about the same severity of iron deficiency as when anemia became present. This, however, is largely an academic question because tissue iron deficits occur simultaneously with deficits in oxygen transport in naturally occurring iron deficiency anemia. Good examples are the 50% decreases in muscle myoglobin content, cytochrome oxidase activity and electron transport capacity in skeletal muscle with iron deficiency at the same time, and the subjects have a 50% decreased oxygen transport capacity due to anemia [8]. Individual cell types within organs may have their own specific iron requirements, and compete with other cells for available iron delivered by transferrin or other transport proteins. The adaptive strategies for acquisition of iron and intracellular metabolism, or export, are described elsewhere in this text. It is not likely, however, that all cell types have the same iron requirements and ability to retain cellular iron when availability from extracellular sources becomes limiting. Application of new genomic, proteomic, and metabolomic approaches will likely provide new evidence as to the different approaches that immune cells, myocytes, hepatocytes, and neurons may all employ to prevent cellular depletion of iron contents [8]. The most accurate approach to the human studies regarding consequences of iron deficiency is to consider individuals along a continuum of iron nutriture with different functional consequences arising at different stages of severity [6, 10].

3 Neuronal Function and Iron Deficiency

Out of necessity, a number of the studies cited below rely on animal studies to identify the brain biology that is altered by dietary iron deficiency. The early autopsy studies of Hallgren established the large heterogeneity of iron distribution in the human brain [11]. There is evidence from both human infant development studies [12] and studies of older humans with certain neurological disorders such as restless legs syndrome [13, 14] that are consistent with depletion of brain iron when there is systemic iron status depletion. In RLS, there is a strong inverse correlation between serum ferritin levels and RLS symptoms and neuroleptic-induced akathisia [3, 15]. There is a lower CSF ferritin in these patients, and MRI analysis also shows a significantly lower brain iron concentration [16, 17]. These patients have a strong urge to move their legs at rest, and this urge is relieved with movement. Importantly, correction of the brain iron status of these patients will frequently improve symptoms [18]. Other neuropathologies associated with likely abnormalities of brain iron metabolism include amyotrophic lateral sclerosis in which there is an association between H63D mutations in HFE and the clinical pathology [19–23].

3.1 Acquisition, Location, and Function of Iron

The brain primarily obtains iron via transferrin receptors expressed on endothelial cells on the brain microvasculature, though recent evidence also indicates that non-transferrin bound iron also fluxes across the blood-brain barrier [24–26]. The rate of iron uptake into the brain is increased when the iron status of the subject is low and is decreased when the iron status is higher [27]. The choroid plexus is a rich source of transferrin mRNA, and transferrin secreted by this organ presumably is used for the distribution of iron to glia and neurons for use or storage [28]. While plasma transferrin (Tf) can move across the blood-brain barrier and become part of the circulating pool of transferrin in cerebrospinal fluid, brain-produced Tf has a slightly different structure than systemic Tf and may play a distinct role [27, 29, 30]. H-ferritin has been documented as binding to neurons as well as cells of the blood-brain barrier and may function as an iron transport protein in addition to its well-described role in intracellular iron storage [31, 32]. Brain iron is located primarily in microglia and oligodendrocytes where it is involved in numerous metabolic activities that are related to the functioning of the particular cells of interest.

Dietary iron deficiency results in a heterogeneous depletion of iron in different regions of the brain [30, 33] with corresponding changes in the gene expression for transferrin [28], transferrin receptor [28, 34], and DMT-1 [27, 35]. In addition, ferroportin is present in the blood-brain barrier and its functioning is likely related to the presence of astrocyte projections in close proximity to the epithelial cells of the barrier [36, 37]. While there is a great scarcity of data in humans, autopsy analyses of RLS brains that have a low brain iron diagnosed by MRI also have this general profile of iron management proteins [38, 39]. Iron deficiency during periods of early development results in functional deficits consistent with declines in brain iron in the hippocampus, striatum, and prefrontal cortex [40].

3.2 Iron Functioning in the Brain and Sensitivity to Iron Deficiency

Alterations in CNS functioning have been broken into morphological changes, bioenergetics, hypo-myelination, and alterations in neurochemistry, based on the available literature in animal models. There is substantial evidence that nerve cells are structurally different in iron-deficient animals [41, 42], but analogous data are missing in human infants. There are morphological changes in hippocampus where dendritic arborization is decreased when iron deficiency occurs during the perinatal period [41, 42]. This is likely related to altered electrical activity in hippocampal nerve fibers [43–45].

Neurochemical studies using high-energy proton nuclear magnetic resonance show that energy metabolism in the hippocampus is also dramatically altered by early life iron deficiency [46]. The relative sorting of iron to preserve intracellular iron-dependent processes apparently fails to preserve sufficient iron for mitochondrial functioning in these brain regions as ratios of creatinine to phosphocreatine are consistent with limitations in electron transfer reactions.

One of the earliest described consequences of iron deficiency in animal models was hypo-myelination of nerve cells [47], which persists despite later iron repletion [48]. Oligodendrocytes need abundant amounts of iron for production of myelin lipids and proteins [49–51]. Such compositional changes resulting from disrupted iron homeostasis in the early stages of growth may contribute to the abnormal behavior that has been observed in developmental testing of auditory and visual evoked potentials.

3.3 Development and Brain Iron Location

Regions of the brain rich in iron in adulthood – substantia nigra, globus pallidus, nucleus accumbens – are not the regions that have a high iron content in early life and are far less affected by dietary iron deficiency than are other regions [30, 52]. Iron concentrations in CSF are approximately 15–25 μg/L in humans, 14 μg/L in monkeys, and 5–20 μg/L in mice [53], but the developmental dependency of these levels is unknown. In RLS, CSF iron levels may be normal despite lower CSF ferritin concentrations, and this has been related to brain iron deficiency in these patients [14, 18, 54]. The role of the cerebrospinal fluid in the delivery of iron to various brain cells is not well understood [55], although recent data suggest that H ferritin may play a role [16]. In rat and human brains, most ferritin is found in microglia and oligodendrocytes, whereas in mice, most is in astrocytes. Ferritin levels correlate with brain iron content and are highest at birth and decline thereafter in the newborn rat [56]. Moreover, the concentration can be directly affected by the body iron burden [57]. Studies in postnatal iron deficiency involving ferritin ratios (H:L) in brain reveal a dramatic effect of iron deficiency and the expression of these two subunits of the ferritin molecule [32, 58–60]. The developmental roles of the two subunits relative to iron storage or use and detoxification are unknown, although accumulation of iron in certain brain regions is believed to play a role in a number of neuropathologies [59].

3.4 *Iron Deficiency Effects During Development*

Dallman [61, 62] demonstrated two decades ago that young rats deprived of iron in early postnatal life have significantly lower (27%) whole-brain iron content than do controls 28 days postnatally and were quite resistant to restoration of their normal complement of brain iron (still 20% lower) despite aggressive dietary repletion for 45 days. Although these studies were landmark investigations at the time, they were usually misinterpreted to indicate that brain iron content was very static and not at all sensitive to dietary iron deficiency. The last decade of research shows animal models are quite sensitive to iron depletion and refeeding [12, 33]. There are few human MRI data in iron deficiency, although there is evidence from weighted T2 relaxation times that systemic iron deficiency is associated with depleted striatal and nigra iron contents [13]. In contrast, genetic alterations that lead to iron accumulation in the brain, such as pantothenate kinase 2 deficiency, are easily identified via MRI [63].

Iron is required for proper myelination of the spinal cord and white matter of cerebellar folds [64]. Oligodendrocytes are responsible for the synthesis of fatty acids [50] and cholesterol for myelin, and both of these metabolic processes require iron [65]. In iron deficiency, oligodendrocytes appear immature [48] and this could be causally related to delayed motor maturation and perhaps behavioral alterations in young humans [66–68]. These investigators demonstrated a slowed nerve conduction velocity during an auditory evoked potential test. The reversibility of this finding is still being investigated, but current data suggest the alteration in nerve conduction velocity persists for many years [12, 69].

3.5 *Neurotransmitters*

The role of intraneuronal iron in metabolism is varied and involves the incorporation of iron into enzymes of oxidation-reduction or electron transport, synthesis and packaging of neurotransmitters, uptake and degradation of the neurotransmitters, and iron incorporation into other proteins that may directly or indirectly alter brain function through peroxide reduction, amino acid metabolism, and fat desaturation.

3.5.1 Oxidation-Reduction

Mackler demonstrated that cytochrome concentrations in mitochondria from the brain of iron-deficient animals were not different from those of controls whereas muscle metabolism was significantly changed [70]. More recent studies with proton NMR, however, have demonstrated clear alterations in bioenergetic profiles in vivo [46, 71].

3.5.2 Synthesis and Degradation

Iron is a cofactor for a number of enzymes related to neurotransmitter synthesis and degradation [72]. Nutritional iron deficiency would be expected to lead to decreased activities of these enzymes, but this has not been consistently observed. When brain iron levels were reduced by as much as 40% with dietary restriction in postweanling rats, there was no change in the activity of tyrosine hydroxylase, tryptophan hydroxylase, monoamine oxidase, succinate hydroxylase, or cytochrome C oxidase [73]. Aminobutyric acid transaminase and glutamate decarboxylase activities were decreased, and subsequent studies demonstrated functional changes in glutamate and glutamine metabolism [59, 74, 75]. The turnover of norepinephrine, dopamine, and serotonin in brain homogenates was also unaffected by iron deficiency [76], but more sophisticated approaches have not be used in recent years. Monoamine oxidase and aldehyde dehydrogenase are critical in the catabolism of neurotransmitters in the dopaminergic, serotoninergic, and noradrenergic systems of the brain, but appear to be unaffected by dietary iron deficiency [70].

3.5.3 γ-Aminobutyric Acid

There is a similarity in brain iron distribution and the brain regions that receive input from γ-aminobutyric acid (GABA) [77]. Because GABA release will modulate the activity of dopaminergic neurons, it is important to determine if GABA metabolism is altered by iron deficiency. Iron deficiency in utero and postweaning are associated with significant decreases in glutamate decarboxylase, glutamate dehydrogenase, and GABA transaminase activities [74, 78]. These latter two enzymes are shunt enzymes responsible for the synthesis and degradation of GABA and the findings are consistent with the proton-NMR imaging of striatum and hippocampus [71].

3.5.4 Dopamine

The dopaminergic system has been shown to be sensitive to experimental changes in iron status [79]. As whole-brain iron content drops 15% below normal, biological and behavioral alterations occur that may result from changes in the dopaminergic system [80–83]. Striatum dopamine D_1 and D_2 receptor densities and the dopamine transporter are significantly lower (25–35%) in postweaning iron-deficient rats, and the dopamine transporter is also significantly lower in density in several brain regions [80, 84].

Recent in vivo animal data demonstrate that extracellular dopamine is elevated in the striatum of postweaning iron-deficient rats and returns to normal levels when brain iron content and iron status return to normal [83]. Attentional processing of environmental information is highly dependent on appropriate rates of dopamine clearance from the interstitial space, which suggests that iron status may affect behavior through effects on dopamine metabolism [40]. A number of the alterations in functioning in iron-deficient human infants and monkeys may be attributed to changes in dopamine metabolism in the mesolimbic and the nigrostriatal tracts [85, 86].

3.5.5 Serotonin and Norepinephrine

As part of their initial survey of neurotransmitter systems that may be affected by iron deficiency, Youdim and colleagues measured the concentrations of serotonin, norepinephrine, and their primary metabolites 5-hydroxy indole acetic acid and normetanephrine [87, 88]. They observed no significant alterations in concentrations of these neurotransmitters or metabolites in the striatum of rats.

Other groups have also failed to observe consistent alterations in their concentrations in extracellular fluid in the brain [83]. However, ligand binding studies demonstrated significantly lower densities of the serotonin transporter in striatum of iron-deficient mice [89] as well as other regions of the brain in iron-deficient rats [90]. These observations have significance because the dopamine, norepinephrine, and serotonin transporters have a high degree of homology as well as a similar trafficking [91, 92]. The observations of a consistent decrease in dopamine transporter density in the striatum of iron-deficient rats, in combination with the one study of serotonin transporter, suggest a more general role of iron in the removal of neurotransmitters from the synaptic cleft [84].

3.6 Developmental Models

In a series of studies, investigators demonstrated a prompt recovery of brain iron in nearly all brain regions with feeding of a high-iron diet after experiencing iron deficiency in utero or during early lactation [40]. In contrast, human infants may have persistent effects of early life iron deficiency that extend into adulthood [93]. Thus, it is possible that despite brain iron repletion, important biological switches for the acquisition of brain iron in early development may be irreversibly altered. The recent findings from rodent models which used variable time points of iron repletion support this concept of persistent effects of transient periods of brain iron deficiency [94, 95].

4 Thermoregulation

Iron-deficient humans and lab animals are not able to effectively thermoregulate when exposed to cold [96]. Correction of iron status improves or corrects this deficit in functioning [97–99]. This alteration in homeostasis has usually been attributed to alterations in the neuroendocrine system that controls thermoregulation, specifically changes in norepinephrine (NE) and thyroid hormone metabolism. Support for this concept comes from animal studies in which iron-deficient rats had increased plasma NE and decreased thyroid hormone [99–101]. Other associated changes that have not yet been examined in this context include bioenergetic capabilities to generate heat and the roles of other neuropeptides and neurotransmitters in these processes [71]. In the earliest human study, Martinez-Torres et al. found that iron-deficient anemic subjects had a significantly lower oral temperature after 60 min of exposure cold water bath of 28°C [102]. Beard et al. found that after a 100-min cold water bath of 28°C that women with iron deficiency anemia (IDA) had significantly lower rectal temperatures than the control group [5, 103, 104]. A dietary depletion and repletion study by Lukaski et al. found that iron-deficient women had lower skin and rectal temperatures during cold air exposure (16°C) and that iron therapy restored temperature regulation [98].

4.1 Human Studies

One of the first studies of the neuroendocrine liabilities of iron deficiency was the study of Oski in iron-deficient infants [105] where he observed that iron-deficient infants had significant elevations of urinary NE and its metabolites. Intramuscular iron treatment reduced the urinary NE and its metabolite MHPG (3-methoxy-4-hydroxyphenylglycol) levels to normal within 1 week indicating that sympathetic nervous system (SNS) metabolism of monoamines is strongly affected by iron status. Martinez-Torres and colleagues observed that iron-deficient and IDA subjects had baseline plasma NE values almost double those of the control subjects; this difference was further exaggerated with cold exposure [102]. The apparent increased activation of SNS activity with increased NE spillover into plasma and urine was confirmed in the study by Lukaski when they showed that iron-deficient nonanemic women had significantly higher NE concentration during cold air exposure at baseline [98]. A third human study of iron status and thermoregulation failed to reproduce these finding when subjects were matched for body fat and day of the menstrual cycle [5].

4.2 Animal Studies

The section on brain monoamines and iron deficiency noted that both animal studies and cell culture studies demonstrated that neuronal iron deficiency is associated with alterations in the synthesis of NE and its reuptake through the NE transporter [106]. Studies with a focus on SNS activity are consistent with the concept that iron deficiency alters the reuptake, catabolism, and clearance of NE. IDA is associated with increased plasma and urinary NE [99, 100], decreased NE content in tissues such as heart, liver, and brown adipose tissue [107], and increased fractional turnover in such tissues [96, 108]. The observations that T4 and T3 replacement therapy did not alter NE metabolism in iron-deficient rats suggests independent effects of iron deficiency on NE and thyroid metabolism [108].

4.3 Thyroid Hormone Human Studies

The identification of slightly lower (5–10%) T3 levels in IDA women in the original cold stress studies [102] was confirmed in the second study conducted with cold air stress [98], but these studies suffered from inappropriate body size and menstrual cycle controls. When female subjects were matched for body fat and day of the menstrual cycle, IDA women had lower plasma thyroxine (T4) and triiodothyronine (T3) than control women both at baseline and after cold exposure [109]. Modestly iron-deficient women without anemia were similar to control subjects. Iron supplementation (79 mg elemental iron/day for 12 weeks) corrected thermoregulation and plasma thyroid hormone levels in iron-deficient and anemic women [5].

In a recent study of IDA children without a cold stress, thyroid function was not found to be abnormal and there was no significant change in thyroid hormone levels with correction of anemia [110]. However, in response to TRH injections, IDA children tended to reach peak TSH concentration more slowly ($p=0.08$) than control subjects and did not have a significantly lower total TSH response or peak TSH value.

In another recent study of iron-deficient, nonanemic adolescent girls, there was a significant correlation between T4 concentration and ferritin ($r=0.52$) and between TSH and ferritin ($r=-0.3$), indicating that the severity of the iron deficiency may affect the severity of thyroid hormone metabolism alterations [111]. They also had higher reverse triiodothyronine (rT3) concentrations, indicating that a larger than normal portion of the T4 pool was metabolized to the physiologically inactive metabolite. Overall, iron-deficient girls were not found to have a functional deficiency of thyroid hormone.

4.4 Thyroid Hormone Animal Studies

In animal studies, IDA results in decreased T3 and T4 levels [109, 112] and changes in plasma kinetics. These alterations are reversed by iron repletion [99] or by exchange transfusion [97, 101, 113].

Several steps in thyroid metabolism have been investigated in animal models as possible causes of decreased thyroid hormone in iron deficiency. IDA animals fail to increase circulating TSH when exposed to cold [97]. In addition, despite lower baseline TSH levels, IDA rats have a blunted TSH response to TRH injection [101]. Thyroid peroxidase (TPO) is the first enzyme in thyroid hormone synthesis and is iron-dependent and heme-containing. In a recent study, thyroid peroxidase activity was decreased in iron-deficient animals when compared to pair fed controls [112]. The decrease in activity was more substantial in more severely anemic animals. Once thyroxin has been released, it is converted to the active form T3 via a selenium-dependent 5′-deiodinase enzyme (5′DI). The early studies of Dillman showed that injected T3 was effective in preventing hypothermia in iron deficient, thyroidectomized rats, whereas T4 was not [99]. Subsequent studies showed that liver 5′DI activity was decreased in IDA [108].

4.5 Related Clinical Issues

An intriguing connection between thyroid function and iron deficiency is the connection between iron and iodine status. There is a high prevalence of iron deficiency and anemia in areas of endemic goiter which may reduce the effectiveness of iodine fortification programs [114, 115]. Indeed, IDA has been shown to decrease the effectiveness of iodine supplementation [116]. Similarly, in children with IDA, iron supplementation has been shown to increase the efficacy of iodized salt or oil supplementation. Dual fortification of salt with iron and iodine to reduce anemia also increases the efficacy of the iodine fortification [116].

Anemic dialysis patients have been found to have a decreased TSH response to TRH in comparison to control patients [117]. This abnormality was corrected after the correction of anemia via EPO therapy (and parental iron for 4/5 subjects). The anemic patients were also found to have decreased fT4, fT3, and total T4 in response to TRH administration as compared to controls. However, correction of anemia did not return thyroid hormone levels to control levels, though fT3 was significantly increased. These responses of the thyroid system in human patients as well as the transfusion experiments in rodents suggest that this segment of the thyroid abnormality in iron deficiency anemia is related to anemia per se.

Regulation of metabolic rate and heat loss rates have only been superficially examined in animal models of iron deficiency anemia [99, 113], but neither study was able to remove the confounding role of decreased body fat in iron deficiency. In the two human studies that controlled for body fat between groups during cold exposure, O_2 consumption (VO_2) was lower in iron deficiency [5, 98]. Depletion of essential pools of iron for bioenergetic production of ATP could be limiting to the metabolic response just as it may be limiting to exercise performance or brain cell functioning.

5 Physical Performance

There is strong evidence that iron deficiency anemia [118] impairs physical performance, resulting in reduced aerobic capacity, reduced endurance capacity, increased exercise heart rate, and increased blood lactate with exercise [119–125]. These impairments are proportional to the severity of the anemia [122, 125] and are corrected through improvement of hemoglobin [126] by transfusion or iron treatment [119–121, 123]. Although iron deficiency without anemia does not impact aerobic capacity [127–130], it affects physical performance in other ways. Iron deficiency results in tissue iron deficiency before it progresses to full-fledged anemia, and there is evidence that muscle iron deficiency in the absence of anemia may result in impaired endurance, reduced energetic efficiency, and decreased ability to benefit from training.

A classic animal study by Davies et al. separated the effects of decreased oxygen transport and decreased muscle iron enzyme activity on physical performance [131]. They measured two iron markers, hematocrit (a marker of oxygen transport) and muscle pyruvate oxidase (a marker of muscle functional iron content), and two measures of physical performance, VO_2 max and endurance capacity, over 7 days of iron repletion. They found that the recovery pattern of hematocrit paralleled the recovery of VO_2 max and the recovery pattern of muscle pyruvate oxidase followed that of endurance [131]. A follow-up study, which used exchange transfusion to equalize the Hb of the control and anemic rats, found that VO_2 max was corrected to within 15% of the control values, while endurance was not changed, further supporting the idea that the reduced aerobic capacity of anemia results primarily from reduced oxygen transport while the effect on endurance is primarily caused by decreased muscle functional iron content [8].

Animal studies have clearly shown that iron deficiency and IDA impair endurance and have provided further evidence that this deficit is due to reduced oxidative capacity of the tissues rather than anemia [132–134]. However, laboratory studies have in general been unable to link iron deficiency to endurance in humans [127, 130, 135]. The negative findings may be due to many factors including the small sample sizes, failure to prove tissue iron deficiency, variations in the work level during the endurance test, and the difficulty in testing physical endurance capabilities in humans due to issues of motivation [136]. However, one recent study by Brutsaert et al. used a dynamic knee extension test that measures progressive muscle fatigue during submaximal exercise while largely removing the effect of motivation [137]. After iron supplementation, iron-deficient subjects had decreased muscle fatigue, as measured by the force of maximal voluntary static contractions at the end of the test, while there was no difference in the placebo group [137].

Iron deficiency has also been shown to impair the ability of subjects to benefit from athletic training, both in endurance and aerobic measures [129, 138–140]. The strongest evidence for the negative effect of iron deficiency on adaptation to training comes from a 15-km time trial study of previously untrained women with iron deficiency [140]. They found that after training, the supplemented group had significantly greater improvements both in endurance time and VO_2 max than the placebo group [138, 140]. Further analysis of the data from this study showed that these changes were driven by a subset of women who had elevated serum transferrin receptor (sTfR) at baseline [138, 139]. In addition, in the less depleted subset (with lower sTfR levels), iron treatment did not have significant effects on endurance trial time or VO_2 max [139]. These findings indicate that iron depletion without tissue level iron deficiency (as indicated by in increased sTfR) does not have an effect on endurance or aerobic adaptation to training. These results have serious implications for earlier studies of physical functioning in nonanemic iron deficiency that did not measure sTfR and indicate the importance of establishing a functional deficiency in the tissue of interest. Although not all studies of physical training on iron-deficient subjects have shown a deficit [127, 141], these negative results may be due to small sample sizes, or as discussed above, failure to show functional tissue iron deficiency [139].

Iron deficiency may also have a negative effect on physical performance by decreasing energetic efficiency. Although an early cross-sectional study by Zhu and Haas found no difference in δ-efficiency between a sample of iron-deficient women and controls [142], a follow-up experimental study found that iron treatment significantly increased the energetic efficiency of iron-deficient women during a 15-km time trial [130]. When compared to the placebo group, the iron-treated women had 2.0 kJ/min lower energy expenditure and 5.1% lower VO_2 max [130]. A recent study of recreationally active iron-deficient men and women found that iron supplementation resulted in significantly increased gross energetic efficiency during endurance exercise when compared to the placebo group [143]. In a field study done by Li et al. on female cotton mill workers, supplementation of iron-deficient and IDA women significantly decreased mean heart rate and increased energetic efficiency at work by 467 kJ/day [144]. In addition, despite limitations to increased production imposed by the speed of the machines the women worked on, they were able to show that both production (Yuan/day) and production efficiency (in Yuan/mJ of energy expenditure) were significantly increased in the iron-treated group [144]. These findings begin to show us the extensive consequences of impaired physical performance due to iron deficiency.

Several other studies have examined the economic impacts of impaired physical performance due to iron status [144–146]. The strongest evidence is from a study of IDA in rubber tree tappers in Indonesia [145]. This study found that at baseline, anemic subjects collected about 18.7% less rubber than the nonanemic control group. After treatment, the IDA workers who had received iron supplements collected a similar amount of rubber as the nonanemic group and 14.5% more rubber than the placebo group [145]. A study of iron-deficient tea pickers in Sri Lanka found that iron supplementation resulted in a significant increase in tea picked of 0.3 kg/d [146]. Although this is a small change, it is impressive considering the initial mean Hb concentration of the workers was relatively high, only 11 g/dL. In contrast, those subjects whose initial Hb was <9 g/dl increased their output by nearly 2 kg tea/day after supplementation. In a subset that wore activity monitors, iron supplementation was found to cause very significant increases in daily physical activity outside of work [146]. This change was also found in the previously mentioned study of cotton mill workers [144]. In the cotton mill study, the iron-supplemented group had a statistically significant increase in energy expended during leisure when compared to the placebo group, as calculated from heart rate data. Analysis of activity diaries showed that the supplemented workers spent about 30 min more per day working in the kitchen or shopping [144]. This connection between iron deficiency anemia and voluntary activity is well supported by the animal literature [132, 147, 148].

This decrease in voluntary activity and leisure time activities shows us that the impact that iron deficiency and IDA have on physical performance has far-reaching consequences beyond athletic performance and economic productivity. Such deficits may affect an individual's ability to fulfill their social responsibilities such as childcare and household chores such as cooking, with obvious consequences for child development, nutrition, and overall quality of life. Although the evidence for iron deficiency impairing physical performance is sometimes equivocal, this area of research has broad impacts due to the prevalence of iron deficiency worldwide.

6 Liabilities in Pregnancy

Iron requirements increase quite dramatically during pregnancy for expansion of the maternal blood volume, placental growth, and fetal growth. Quantitatively, these requirements change from <1 mg Fe/day in a reproductive age female to a median requirement of 4.6 mg Fe/day and a 90th percentile requirement of nearly 6.75 mg Fe/day by the third trimester [149]. The sinks for iron during an entire pregnancy include an expansion of the red cell mass (450 mg), needs for fetal and placental iron (370 mg), and blood losses during and after delivery (150–250 mg). Thus the total estimated additional needs are 1,040–1,240 mg of iron. Of course, these requirements are not equal in all trimesters: In the first trimester, iron for the fetus (25 mg) and the umbilicus and placenta (5 mg) totals 30 mg of iron. Much of the expansion of the red cell mass occurs in the second trimester, while most of the fetal deposition of iron occurs in the third trimester.

6.1 Iron for the Maternal Red Cell Mass and Anemia

The red cell mass in pregnancy is not static and can be affected by the amount of iron supplementation that has occurred during the pregnancy [150]. For example, when supplemental iron was provided to a group of women, the expansion of the red cell mass was approximately 570 mg of iron, whereas when no supplementation was provided, the expansion was only 260 mg of iron. It has been suggested that for every 10 g/L increase in maternal Hb desired, there is a need for an additional 175 mg of absorbed iron [151]. The World Health Organization recommends iron supplements of between 30 and 60 mg/d if the woman has low iron stores (e.g., ferritin <30 ug/L). It is easy to assume that more iron and higher Hb are better, but there are data that demonstrate a negative outcome to an overly elevated Hb concentration [152]. Consumption of large doses of iron supplements have been related to oxidative damage, and the gastrointestinal side effects may be related to the poor compliance in many populations of pregnant women [153, 154]. This alternative approach of non-daily low-dose iron supplementation appears to be effective in some situations of only modest iron deficits.

6.2 Iron Supplementation and Maternal Red Cell Responses

The decline in Hb in the first trimester is now seen as a normal physiological event and is the result of expansion of the plasma volume. Overzealous supplementation to prevent this physiological anemia has been associated with risk of poor fetal outcomes in at least one study [155]. The normal nadir of Hb is between 24 and 32 weeks of gestation after which the Hb concentration again rises to levels similar to that seen in the first trimester. The extent of this Hb readjustment may be affected by iron reserves as the large expansion of the red cell mass in the second trimester and early third trimester usually depletes all iron reserves and physiological anemia may now be replaced with nutritional anemia.

Maternal Hb concentration and infant outcomes have a U-shaped curve with an increased risk for poor outcomes at each end of the distribution [156]. High Hb likely reflects an improper expansion of the plasma volume, as in preeclampsia, with increased infant mortality and morbidity [157]. The variation in the amount of hemodilution is considerable and makes the relatively simple Hb measurement quite unreliable with regard to diagnosis of iron deficiency anemia. Current target Hb concentrations in each trimester are based on supplementation trials which suggest that Hb > 110 g/L in the first and third trimesters and 105 g/L in the second trimester represent reasonable clinical expectations of lower normal levels [149].

6.3 Iron Absorption

Maternal iron stores are usually limited in women, and the capacity to increase the efficiency of absorption of dietary iron appears to maximize at around 40–60% for non-heme iron in the second trimester [158–160]. The adaptive responses in placental transfer of iron with severe iron deficiency includes upregulation of placental ferritin receptors and presumably an increase in placental-fetal transfer of iron [161, 162]. These attempts to maximize iron delivery to the fetus often have limited success as there is still a smaller-than-normal endowment of iron for the newborn and subsequent postnatal infant iron deficiency results (see sections below) [163].

6.4 Consequences of a Negative Iron Balance

The consequences of depletion of the essential body pools of iron include anemia, altered hormone metabolism, altered energy metabolism, depressed immune functioning, and changes in behavior and cognition [164, 165]. The impacts of each of these consequences on maternal and fetal survival, fetal growth, and postnatal development are still being examined and include direct and indirect effects of anemic hypoxia, placental delivery of iron, and alterations in hormonal control of pregnancy due to alterations in the stress-hypothalamic-pituitary-adrenal axis system [163]. Maternal anemia has been related to maternal mortality, fetal mortality, fetal growth retardation, pregnancy complications, and to a small amount infant growth [166–169]. The vast majority of the studies on anemia and pregnancy outcome have not separated the effects of iron deficiency from the effects of anemia.

6.4.1 Anemia and Birth Weight, Gestational Age, and Infant Mortality

Most reviewers of the scientific literature will agree that there is a U-shaped curve relationship between the maternal hemoglobin concentration and the proportion of low birth weight (LBW) infants [169]. The cause of the elevation in prevalence of LBW infants at the upper end of the distribution of Hb is believed to be improper expansion of the maternal plasma volume [170], while insufficient erythropoiesis and poor volume expansion may be associated with the low Hb concentrations at the other end of the distribution curve. The optimal maternal Hb for minimal incidence of LBW in the published literature varies. The hemoglobin concentration and the definition of "anemia" are trimester-dependent with a clear nadir of concentration in mid gestation. Since many of these studies did not use finite times of sampling, the variations may well reflect the timing of sampling and not true discrepancies in the relationship of data to outcomes [171].

The severity of anemia is an additional factor associated with an increased risk of LBW and prematurity, even though the exact causes of the anemia are not known [171, 172]. There is a median relative risk (RR) of 4.9 for severe anemia, with moderate anemia having a median risk of approximately 2.0. In a study of pregnancy outcome where malaria is endemic, Verhoeff et al. [173] reported an RR of 1.6 for intrauterine growth retardation in a study of 1,423 live-born singleton births in rural Malawi if maternal Hb was <80 g/L in the first trimester, compared to no effect of moderate anemia at delivery. Iron-folate administration during pregnancy reduced the prevalence of prematurity, while malaria intervention was effective in promoting fetal growth.

Several research groups have computed relative risks for the impact of iron deficiency anemia on pregnancy complications while controlling for other causes of anemia [169, 174]. In a study in the USA, Scholl and colleagues [175] showed that iron deficiency anemia in the first trimester was more strongly related to prematurity and LBW (RR = 3.1) than anemia of any cause later in pregnancy. They concluded from this that iron deficiency in the first trimester was important but anemia at other times had little effect. In Chinese mothers in early pregnancy (<8 weeks), moderate iron deficiency anemia conferred an RR of 2.96 for prematurity and LBW [176]. This suggests that iron deficiency anemia has an impact on fetal growth and development similar to anemia in general.

6.4.2 Maternal Anemia and Mortality

Maternal mortality is correlated with the severity of anemia in pregnancy [177]. In his review of reports from 1950 to 1999, Rush examined the relationship of maternal anemia, usually at delivery, with both antepartum and postpartum death. He concluded that severe anemia (Hb <6–7 g/L) is associated with an increased rate of maternal death. In very severe anemia, the death rate may be as high as 20% greater than a comparison group. When the Hb is this low, compensatory mechanisms begin to fail, lactic acid levels rise, and cardiac failure may occur. While no direct causal relationships between iron deficiency anemia and mortality are usually demonstrated, it is reasonable to expect that it is contributory to death rates.

6.5 Maternal Iron Deficiency and Fetal Outcomes

Plasma ferritin is not a sensitive indicator of iron status by the middle of the second trimester and, as a result, has little sensitivity as a predictor of poor fetal outcomes [178]. There is a significant relationship of elevated ferritin with preterm birth, LBW, and also preeclampsia [175, 179], suggesting possible relationships of ferritin as an acute phase marker and not an iron status biomarker [180]. Higher ferritin concentrations may be more an indication of upper genital tract infection and a subsequent development of spontaneous preterm delivery than an indication that higher iron status is detrimental for fetal growth and development. Lao et al. [181] reported on an analysis of birth outcomes for 488 nonanemic women. They observed a significant inverse relationship between maternal ferritin quartiles and infant birth weight with an increased risk of prematurity and neonatal asphyxia in those mothers with the highest quartile of ferritin. In an analysis of the Preterm Prediction Study of the National Institute of Child Health and Human Development Maternal-Fetal Medicine Units network conducted from 1992 to 1996, there was a similar relationship [179, 182]. Regardless of the gestational age at sampling (19, 26, or 36 weeks), ferritin in the highest quartile was associated with the lower mean birth weights than those in the other three quartiles of ferritin. The adjusted odds ratio was significant, however, only in the 26-week sample with an odds ratio of 2.0 for premature delivery and 2.7 for small birth weight (<1,500 g). In the 2002 follow-up analysis, utilizing cervical ferritin concentrations at 22–24 weeks of gestation, the adjusted odds ratio of very premature delivery (<32 weeks) was as high as 6.3. There was also a strong correlation with other markers of inflammation from cervical fluid. These studies suggest that elevations of ferritin in mid gestation increase the risk for pregnancy complications. Iron supplementation trials can answer the question of whether prevention of the decrease in iron status can improve birth outcomes.

Prophylactic iron supplementation during the first trimester of pregnancy in poor women improved birth weight, lowered the incidence of prematurity, but did not alter the incidence of small for gestational age deliveries [183]. The timing and dose of supplementation, as well as the frequency of supplementation, are important considerations in interventions during pregnancy [153, 184].

6.5.1 Maternal Iron Status and Subsequent Infant Development

Despite the concept that the fetus is an effective parasite for iron, the previously discussed information indicates that fetal development is compromised when maternal iron status is compromised. One dimension now receiving attention vis-à-vis iron status is neurodevelopment of the infant [40]. In an important study several years ago, Tamura and colleagues noted a relationship between newborn cord ferritin levels and cognition and behavior at 5 years of age [185]. The children were compared by their cord blood ferritin in the two median ferritin quartiles, and those in the lowest quartile scored lower on a number of tests including language ability, fine motor skills, and tractability. Since cord blood ferritin is correlated with maternal iron status, these data suggest that poor iron status at birth is related to later infant development. The intervention study of Presozio et al. [186] reached a similar conclusion regarding the benefit of iron supplementation in pregnancy on infant scores in tests of motor and mental development at 12 months of age. More recently, a study in South Africa [187, 188] showed that infants of iron-deficient anemic mothers had lower developmental scores, assessed with the Griffith scale at 9 months of age, than infants of mothers who were not anemic. All infants in this study were of full gestational age and weight; thus intrauterine growth failure and severe maternal anemia (<85 g/L) were excluded. These anemic mothers had increased amounts of depression and altered mother-child interactions compared to iron-supplemented mothers. Indeed, maternal postpartum depression related to Hb concentration in the months after delivery of the infant may contribute to changes in infant development. This is not to suggest that iron supplementation will lead to smarter children. A recent study showed that very modest iron supplementation (20 mg/d) of mothers in New Zealand had no effect on the IQ of the infants at 4 years of age despite a reduction in prevalence of IDA from 11% to 1% during pregnancy [189]. The authors did show that behaviors of the infants were affected by the iron intervention in pregnancy, but they could not separate direct biological effects of the iron on fetal growth and development from the indirect effect that would be expected through the improved iron status of the mother during and after the pregnancy. Mother-child interactions can be quite sensitive to the nutritional status of the infant and the mother.

6.5.2 Maternal Iron Deficiency and Infant Iron Status

The relationship between moderately anemic mothers and infant hematology has been reviewed [167, 190]. There is a general correlation between maternal Hb in the third trimester with the infant Hb at 9 months of age [191]. However, this relationship is not observed when the overall prevalence rates of anemia are so high as to remove the possibility that there are "normal" Hb concentrations in both mothers and infants [192]. In a number of other studies reviewed by Allen, Milman, and Scholl, there is a reoccurring theme that maternal anemia may be related to infant anemia in early life on some occasions, but more commonly the relationship is more strongly expressed at 9–12 months of age when infant iron stores have been exhausted [167, 169, 190]. Thus, there is the concept that iron-depleted and moderately anemic mothers provide sufficient delivery of iron for infant growth and erythropoiesis in utero, but fail to provide sufficient iron for normal growth and development over the next 12 months of life.

7 Conclusions

The liabilities of iron deficiency on human functioning are diverse and likely involve the effects of deficits on essential tissue essential iron pools as well as to deficits in oxygen transport to the tissues. Importantly, the impact of these deficits on functioning can have persistent, and perhaps lifelong, effects if the deficiency occurs during periods of organogenesis. The epigenesis of effects of early life iron deficiency will be the challenge of the next decade as well as understanding the complexity of the contribution of genetic variability to iron biology in humans.

References

1. Bothwell TH. Overview and mechanisms of iron regulation. Nutr Rev. 1995;53:237–45.
2. Beard JL. Iron biology in immune function, muscle metabolism and neuronal functioning. J Nutr. 2001;131:568S–80.
3. Allen RP, Earley CJ. The role of iron in restless legs syndrome. Mov Disord. 2007;22(S18):S440–8.
4. Gamaldo CE, Benbrook AR, Allen RP, Oguntimein O, Earley CJ. A further evaluation of the cognitive deficits associated with restless legs syndrome (RLS). Sleep Med. 2008;9:500–5.
5. Beard JL, Borel MJ, Derr J. Impaired thermoregulation and thyroid function in iron-deficiency anemia. Am J Clin Nutr. 1990;52:813–9.
6. Beard J, Finch CA, Mackler B. Deleterious effects of iron deficiency. Prog Clin Biol Res. 1981;77:305–10.
7. Woodson RD. Hemoglobin concentration and exercise capacity. Am Rev Respir Dis. 1984;129:S72–5.
8. Davies KJ, Donovan CM, Refino CJ, Brooks GA, Packer L, Dallman PR. Distinguishing effects of anemia and muscle iron deficiency on exercise bioenergetics in the rat. Am J Physiol. 1984;246:E535–43.
9. Finch CA, Huebers H. Perspectives in iron metabolism. N Engl J Med. 1982;306:1520–8.
10. Dallman PR. Biochemical basis for the manifestations of iron deficiency. Annu Rev Nutr. 1986;6:13–40.
11. Hallgren B, Sourander P. The effect of age on the non-haemin iron in the human brain. J Neurochem. 1958;3:41–51.
12. Lozoff B, Georgieff MK. Iron deficiency and brain development. Semin Pediatr Neurol. 2006;13:158–65.

13. Earley CJ, Barker PB, Horska A, Allen RP. MRI-determined regional brain iron concentrations in early- and late-onset restless legs syndrome. Sleep Med. 2006;7:458–61.
14. Earley CJ, Connor JR, Beard JL, Malecki EA, Epstein DK, Allen RP. Abnormalities in CSF concentrations of ferritin and transferrin in restless legs syndrome. Neurology. 2000;54:1698–700.
15. O'Keeffe ST. Iron deficiency with normal ferritin levels in restless legs syndrome. Sleep Med. 2005;6:281–2.
16. Clardy SL, Earley CJ, Allen RP, Beard JL, Connor JR. Ferritin subunits in CSF are decreased in restless legs syndrome. J Lab Clin Med. 2006;147:67–73.
17. Mizuno S, Mihara T, Miyaoka T, Inagaki T, Horiguchi J. CSF iron, ferritin and transferrin levels in restless legs syndrome. J Sleep Res. 2005;14:43–7.
18. Earley CJ, Heckler D, Allen RP. The treatment of restless legs syndrome with intravenous iron dextran. Sleep Med. 2004;5:231–5.
19. Wang XS, Lee S, Simmons Z, et al. Increased incidence of the Hfe mutation in amyotrophic lateral sclerosis and related cellular consequences. J Neurol Sci. 2004;227:27–33.
20. Wang XS, Simmons Z, Liu W, Boyer PJ, Connor JR. Differential expression of genes in amyotrophic lateral sclerosis revealed by profiling the post mortem cortex. Amyotroph Lateral Scler. 2006;7:201–10.
21. Goodall EF, Greenway MJ, van Marion I, Carroll CB, Hardiman O, Morrison KE. Association of the H63D polymorphism in the hemochromatosis gene with sporadic ALS. Neurology. 2005;65:934–7.
22. Levenson CW. Trace metal regulation of neuronal apoptosis: from genes to behavior. Physiol Behav. 2005;86:399–406.
23. Sutedja NA, Sinke RJ, Van Vught PW, et al. The association between H63D mutations in HFE and amyotrophic lateral sclerosis in a Dutch population. Arch Neurol. 2007;64:63–7.
24. Burdo JR, Antonetti DA, Wolpert EB, Connor JR. Mechanisms and regulation of transferrin and iron transport in a model blood-brain barrier system. Neuroscience. 2003;121:883–90.
25. Burdo JR, Connor JR. Brain iron uptake and homeostatic mechanisms: an overview. Biometals. 2003;16:63–75.
26. Burdo JR, Simpson IA, Menzies S, Beard J, Connor JR. Regulation of the profile of iron-management proteins in brain microvasculature. J Cereb Blood Flow Metab. 2004;24:67–74.
27. Moos T, Skjoerringe T, Gosk S, Morgan EH. Brain capillary endothelial cells mediate iron transport into the brain by segregating iron from transferrin without the involvement of divalent metal transporter 1. J Neurochem. 2006;98:1946–58.
28. Han J, Day JR, Connor JR, Beard JL. Gene expression of transferrin and transferrin receptor in brains of control vs. iron-deficient rats. Nutr Neurosci. 2003;6:1–10.
29. Moos T, Morgan EH. Transferrin and transferrin receptor function in brain barrier systems. Cell Mol Neurobiol. 2000;20:77–95.
30. Moos T, Rosengren Nielsen T, Skjorringe T, Morgan EH. Iron trafficking inside the brain. J Neurochem. 2007;103:1730–40.
31. Surguladze N, Thompson KM, Beard JL, Connor JR, Fried MG. Interactions and reactions of ferritin with DNA. J Biol Chem. 2004;279:14694–702.
32. Fisher J, Devraj K, Ingram J, et al. Ferritin: a novel mechanism for delivery of iron to the brain and other organs. Am J Physiol Cell Physiol. 2007;293:C641–9.
33. Erikson KM, Pinero DJ, Connor JR, Beard JL. Regional brain iron, ferritin and transferrin concentrations during iron deficiency and iron repletion in developing rats. J Nutr. 1997;127:2030–8.
34. Siddappa AJ, Rao RB, Wobken JD, et al. Iron deficiency alters iron regulatory protein and iron transport protein expression in the perinatal rat brain. Pediatr Res. 2003;53:800–7.
35. Burdo JR, Menzies SL, Simpson IA, et al. Distribution of divalent metal transporter 1 and metal transport protein 1 in the normal and Belgrade rat. J Neurosci Res. 2001;66:1198–207.
36. Dringen R, Bishop GM, Koeppe M, Dang TN, Robinson SR. The pivotal role of astrocytes in the metabolism of iron in the brain. Neurochem Res. 2007;32:1884–90.
37. Wu LJ, Leenders AG, Cooperman S, et al. Expression of the iron transporter ferroportin in synaptic vesicles and the blood-brain barrier. Brain Res. 2004;1001:108–17.
38. Earley CJ, Connor JR, Beard JL, Clardy SL, Allen RP. Ferritin levels in the cerebrospinal fluid and restless legs syndrome: effects of different clinical phenotypes. Sleep. 2005;28:1069–75.
39. Wang X, Wiesinger J, Beard J, et al. Thy1 expression in the brain is affected by iron and is decreased in restless legs syndrome. J Neurol Sci. 2004;220:59–66.
40. Lozoff B, Beard J, Connor J, Barbara F, Georgieff M, Schallert T. Long-lasting neural and behavioral effects of iron deficiency in infancy. Nutr Rev. 2006;64:S34–43. S72–S91.
41. Jorgenson LA, Sun M, O'Connor M, Georgieff MK. Fetal iron deficiency disrupts the maturation of synaptic function and efficacy in area CA1 of the developing rat hippocampus. Hippocampus. 2005;15:1094–102.
42. Jorgenson LA, Wobken JD, Georgieff MK. Perinatal iron deficiency alters apical dendritic growth in hippocampal CA1 pyramidal neurons. Dev Neurosci. 2003;25:412–20.

43. McEchron MD, Alexander DN, Gilmartin MR, Paronish MD. Perinatal nutritional iron deficiency impairs hippocampus-dependent trace eyeblink conditioning in rats. Dev Neurosci. 2008;30:243–54.
44. McEchron MD, Cheng AY, Liu H, Connor JR, Gilmartin MR. Perinatal nutritional iron deficiency permanently impairs hippocampus-dependent trace fear conditioning in rats. Nutr Neurosci. 2005;8:195–206.
45. McEchron MD, Paronish MD. Perinatal nutritional iron deficiency reduces hippocampal synaptic transmission but does not impair short- or long-term synaptic plasticity. Nutr Neurosci. 2005;8:277–85.
46. Rao R, Tkac I, Townsend EL, Gruetter R, Georgieff MK. Perinatal iron deficiency alters the neurochemical profile of the developing rat hippocampus. J Nutr. 2003;133:3215–21.
47. Yu GS, Steinkirchner TM, Rao GA, Larkin EC. Effect of prenatal iron deficiency on myelination in rat pups. Am J Pathol. 1986;125:620–4.
48. Beard JL, Wiesinger JA, Connor JR. Pre- and postweaning iron deficiency alters myelination in Sprague-Dawley rats. Dev Neurosci. 2003;25:308–15.
49. Morath DJ, Mayer-Proschel M. Iron deficiency during embryogenesis and consequences for oligodendrocyte generation in vivo. Dev Neurosci. 2002;24:197–207.
50. Ortiz E, Pasquini JM, Thompson K, et al. Effect of manipulation of iron storage, transport, or availability on myelin composition and brain iron content in three different animal models. J Neurosci Res. 2004;77:681–9.
51. Connor JR, Menzies SL. Relationship of iron to oligodendrocytes and myelination. Glia. 1996;17:83–93.
52. Pinero DJ, Li NQ, Connor JR, Beard JL. Variations in dietary iron alter brain iron metabolism in developing rats. J Nutr. 2000;130:254–63.
53. Bradbury MW. Transport of iron in the blood-brain-cerebrospinal fluid system. J Neurochem. 1997;69:443–54.
54. Bartzokis G, Tishler TA, Shin IS, Lu PH, Cummings JL. Brain ferritin iron as a risk factor for age at onset in neurodegenerative diseases. Ann NY Acad Sci. 2004;1012:224–36.
55. Dwork AJ. Effects of diet and development upon the uptake and distribution of cerebral iron. J Neurol Sci. 1995;134(Suppl):45–51.
56. Miller MW, Roskams AJ, Connor JR. Iron regulation in the developing rat brain: effect of in utero ethanol exposure. J Neurochem. 1995;65:373–80.
57. Chen Q, Connor JR, Beard JL. Brain iron, transferrin and ferritin concentrations are altered in developing iron-deficient rats. J Nutr. 1995;125:1529–35.
58. Han J, Day JR, Connor JR, Beard JL. H and L ferritin subunit mRNA expression differs in brains of control and iron-deficient rats. J Nutr. 2002;132:2769–74.
59. Iii AM, Mitchell TR, Neely EB, Connor JR. Metabolic analysis of mouse brains that have compromised iron storage. Metab Brain Dis. 2006;21:77–87.
60. Zhang X, Surguladze N, Slagle-Webb B, Cozzi A, Connor JR. Cellular iron status influences the functional relationship between microglia and oligodendrocytes. Glia. 2006;54:795–804.
61. Dallman PR, Spirito RA. Brain iron in the rat: extremely slow turnover in normal rats may explain long-lasting effects of early iron deficiency. J Nutr. 1977;107:1075–81.
62. Dallman PR, Siimes MA, Manies EC. Brain iron: persistent deficiency following short-term iron deprivation in the young rat. Br J Haematol. 1975;31:209–15.
63. Rao C, Murthy V, Hegde R, Asha, Vishwanath. Hallervorden Spatz disease. Indian J Pediatr. 2003;70:513–514.
64. Rice D, Barone Jr S. Critical periods of vulnerability for the developing nervous system: evidence from humans and animal models. Environ Health Perspect. 2000;108(Suppl 3):511–33.
65. Morath DJ, Mayer-Proschel M. Iron modulates the differentiation of a distinct population of glial precursor cells into oligodendrocytes. Dev Biol. 2001;237:232–43.
66. Roncagliolo M, Garrido M, Walter T, Peirano P, Lozoff B. Evidence of altered central nervous system development in infants with iron deficiency anemia at 6 mo: delayed maturation of auditory brainstem responses. Am J Clin Nutr. 1998;68:683–90.
67. Burden MJ, Westerlund AJ, Armony-Sivan R, et al. An event-related potential study of attention and recognition memory in infants with iron-deficiency anemia. Pediatrics. 2007;120:e336–45.
68. Peirano P, Algarin C, Garrido M, Algarin D, Lozoff B. Iron-deficiency anemia is associated with altered characteristics of sleep spindles in NREM sleep in infancy. Neurochem Res. 2007;32:1665–72.
69. Lozoff B, Jimenez E, Hagen J, Mollen E, Wolf AW. Poorer behavioral and developmental outcome more than 10 years after treatment for iron deficiency in infancy. Pediatrics. 2000;105:E51.
70. Mackler B, Person R, Miller LR, Finch CA. Iron deficiency in the rat: effects on phenylalanine metabolism. Pediatr Res. 1979;13:1010–1.
71. Ward KL, Tkac I, Jing Y, et al. Gestational and lactational iron deficiency alters the developing striatal metabolome and associated behaviors in young rats. J Nutr. 2007;137:1043–9.
72. Beard J. Iron deficiency alters brain development and functioning. J Nutr. 2003;133:1468S–72.
73. Ashkenazi R, Ben-Shachar D, Youdim MB. Nutritional iron and dopamine binding sites in the rat brain. Pharmacol Biochem Behav. 1982;17(Suppl 1):43–7.

74. Li D. Effects of iron deficiency on iron distribution and gamma-aminobutyric acid (GABA) metabolism in young rat brain tissues. Hokkaido Igaku Zasshi. 1998;73:215–25.
75. Erikson KM, Shihabi ZK, Aschner JL, Aschner M. Manganese accumulates in iron-deficient rat brain regions in a heterogeneous fashion and is associated with neurochemical alterations. Biol Trace Elem Res. 2002;87:143–56.
76. Yehuda S, Youdim MB. Brain iron: a lesson from animal models. Am J Clin Nutr. 1989;50:618–29.
77. Hill JM. Iron concentration reduced in ventral pallidum, globus pallidus, and substantia nigra by GABA-transaminase inhibitor, gamma-vinyl GABA. Brain Res. 1985;342:18–25.
78. Taneja V, Mishra KP, Agarwal KN. Effect of maternal iron deficiency on GABA shunt pathway of developing rat brain. Indian J Exp Biol. 1990;28:466–9.
79. Beard JL, Connor JR. Iron status and neural functioning. Annu Rev Nutr. 2003;23:41–58.
80. Erikson KM, Jones BC, Beard JL. Iron deficiency alters dopamine transporter functioning in rat striatum. J Nutr. 2000;130:2831–7.
81. Erikson KM, Jones BC, Hess EJ, Zhang Q, Beard JL. Iron deficiency decreases dopamine D1 and D2 receptors in rat brain. Pharmacol Biochem Behav. 2001;69:409–18.
82. Youdim MB, Ben-Shachar D, Ashkenazi R, Yehuda S. Brain iron and dopamine receptor function. Adv Biochem Psychopharmacol. 1983;37:309–21.
83. Nelson C, Erikson K, Pinero DJ, Beard JL. In vivo dopamine metabolism is altered in iron-deficient anemic rats. J Nutr. 1997;127:2282–8.
84. Wiesinger JA, Buwen JP, Cifelli CJ, Unger EL, Jones BC, Beard JL. Down-regulation of dopamine transporter by iron chelation in vitro is mediated by altered trafficking, not synthesis. J Neurochem. 2007;100:167–79.
85. Lubach GR, Coe CL. Preconception maternal iron status is a risk factor for iron deficiency in infant rhesus monkeys (Macaca mulatta). J Nutr. 2006;136:2345–9.
86. Golub MS, Hogrefe CE, Germann SL, Capitanio JP, Lozoff B. Behavioral consequences of developmental iron deficiency in infant rhesus monkeys. Neurotoxicol Teratol. 2006;28:3–17.
87. Youdim MB, Green AR. Biogenic monoamine metabolism and functional activity in iron-deficient rats: behavioural correlates. Ciba Found Symp. 1976;51:201–25.
88. Youdim MB, Green AR. Iron deficiency and neurotransmitter synthesis and function. Proc Nutr Soc. 1978;37:173–9.
89. Morse AC, Beard JL, Jones BC. A genetic developmental model of iron deficiency: biological aspects. Proc Soc Exp Biol Med. 1999;220:147–52.
90. Burhans MS, Dailey C, Beard Z, et al. Iron deficiency: differential effects on monoamine transporters. Nutr Neurosci. 2005;8:31–8.
91. Miranda M, Sorkin A. Regulation of receptors and transporters by ubiquitination: new insights into surprisingly similar mechanisms. Mol Interv. 2007;7:157–67.
92. Melikian HE. Neurotransmitter transporter trafficking: endocytosis, recycling, and regulation. Pharmacol Ther. 2004;104:17–27.
93. Lozoff B, Kaciroti N, Walter T. Iron deficiency in infancy: applying a physiologic framework for prediction. Am J Clin Nutr. 2006;84:1412–21.
94. Beard JL, Unger EL, Bianco LE, Paul T, Rundle SE, Jones BC. Early postnatal iron repletion overcomes lasting effects of gestational iron deficiency in rats. J Nutr. 2007;137:1176–82.
95. Unger EL, Paul T, Murray-Kolb LE, Felt B, Jones BC, Beard JL. Early iron deficiency alters sensorimotor development and brain monoamines in rats. J Nutr. 2007;137:118–24.
96. Brigham D, Beard J. Iron and thermoregulation: a review. Crit Rev Food Sci Nutr. 1996;36:747–63.
97. Beard J, Green W, Miller L, Finch C. Effect of iron-deficiency anemia on hormone levels and thermoregulation during cold exposure. Am J Physiol. 1984;247:R114–9.
98. Lukaski HC, Hall CB, Nielsen FH. Thermogenesis and thermoregulatory function of iron-deficient women without anemia. Aviat Space Environ Med. 1990;61:913–20.
99. Dillman E, Gale C, Green W, Johnson DG, Mackler B, Finch C. Hypothermia in iron deficiency due to altered triiodothyronine metabolism. Am J Physiol. 1980;239:R377–81.
100. Beard J, Tobin B, Smith SM. Norepinephrine turnover in iron deficiency at three environmental temperatures. Am J Physiol. 1988;255:R90–6.
101. Beard J, Tobin B, Green W. Evidence for thyroid hormone deficiency in iron-deficient anemic rats. J Nutr. 1989;119:772–8.
102. Martinez-Torres C, Cubeddu L, Dillmann E, et al. Effect of exposure to low temperature on normal and iron-deficient subjects. Am J Physiol. 1984;246:R380–3.
103. Borel MJ, Beard JL, Farrell PA. Hepatic glucose production and insulin sensitivity and responsiveness in iron-deficient anemic rats. Am J Physiol. 1993;264:E380–90.
104. Borel MJ, Smith SH, Brigham DE, Beard JL. The impact of varying degrees of iron nutriture on several functional consequences of iron deficiency in rats. J Nutr. 1991;121:729–36.

105. Voorhess ML, Stuart MJ, Stockman JA, Oski FA. Iron deficiency anemia and increased urinary norepinephrine excretion. J Pediatr. 1975;86:542–7.
106. Beard JL, Wiesinger JA, Jones BC. Iron chelation decreases norepinephrine transporter concentrations in PC12 cells and iron deficient rat brain. Brain Res. 2006;1092:47–58.
107. Beard JL. Neuroendocrine alterations in iron deficiency. Prog Food Nutr Sci. 1990;14:45–82.
108. Brigham DE, Beard JL. Effect of thyroid hormone replacement in iron-deficient rats. Am J Physiol. 1995;269:R1140–7.
109. Beard JL, Brigham DE, Kelley SK, Green MH. Plasma thyroid hormone kinetics are altered in iron-deficient rats. J Nutr. 1998;128:1401–8.
110. Tienboon P, Unachak K. Iron deficiency anaemia in childhood and thyroid function. Asia Pac J Clin Nutr. 2003;12:198–202.
111. Eftekhari MH, Keshavarz SA, Jalali M, Elguero E, Eshraghian MR, Simondon KB. The relationship between iron status and thyroid hormone concentration in iron-deficient adolescent Iranian girls. Asia Pac J Clin Nutr. 2006;15:50–5.
112. Hess SY, Zimmermann MB, Arnold M, Langhans W, Hurrell RF. Iron deficiency anemia reduces thyroid peroxidase activity in rats. J Nutr. 2002;132:1951–5.
113. Beard J. Feed efficiency and norepinephrine turnover in iron deficiency. Proc Soc Exp Biol Med. 1987;184:337–44.
114. Wegmuller R, Camara F, Zimmermann MB, Adou P, Hurrell RF. Salt dual-fortified with iodine and micronized ground ferric pyrophosphate affects iron status but not hemoglobin in children in Cote d'Ivoire. J Nutr. 2006;136:1814–20.
115. Zimmermann MB. The influence of iron status on iodine utilization and thyroid function. Annu Rev Nutr. 2006;26:367–89.
116. Zimmermann M, Adou P, Torresani T, Zeder C, Hurrell R. Persistence of goiter despite oral iodine supplementation in goitrous children with iron deficiency anemia in Cote d'Ivoire. Am J Clin Nutr. 2000;71:88–93.
117. Ramirez G, Bittle PA, Sanders H, Bercu BB. Hypothalamo-hypophyseal thyroid and gonadal function before and after erythropoietin therapy in dialysis patients. J Clin Endocrinol Metab. 1992;74:517–24.
118. Schmidauer C, Sojer M, Seppi K, et al. Transcranial ultrasound shows nigral hypoechogenicity in restless legs syndrome. Ann Neurol. 2005;58:630–4.
119. Celsing F, Blomstrand E, Werner B, Pihlstedt P, Ekblom B. Effects of iron deficiency on endurance and muscle enzyme activity in man. Med Sci Sports Exerc. 1986;18:156–61.
120. Edgerton VR, Ohira Y, Hettiarachchi J, Senewiratne B, Gardner GW, Barnard RJ. Elevation of hemoglobin and work tolerance in iron-deficient subjects. J Nutr Sci Vitaminol (Tokyo). 1981;27:77–86.
121. Gardner GW, Edgerton VR, Barnard RJ, Bernauer EM. Cardiorespiratory, hematological and physical performance responses of anemic subjects to iron treatment. Am J Clin Nutr. 1975;28:982–8.
122. Gardner GW, Edgerton VR, Senewiratne B, Barnard RJ, Ohira Y. Physical work capacity and metabolic stress in subjects with iron deficiency anemia. Am J Clin Nutr. 1977;30:910–7.
123. Ohira Y, Edgerton VR, Gardner GW, Senewiratne B, Barnard RJ, Simpson DR. Work capacity, heart rate and blood lactate responses to iron treatment. Br J Haematol. 1979;41:365–72.
124. Tufts DA, Haas JD, Beard JL, Spielvogel H. Distribution of hemoglobin and functional consequences of anemia in adult males at high altitude. Am J Clin Nutr. 1985;42:1–11.
125. Woodson RD, Wills RE, Lenfant C. Effect of acute and established anemia on O2 transport at rest, submaximal and maximal work. J Appl Physiol. 1978;44:36–43.
126. Finch CA, Deubelbeiss K, Cook JD, et al. Ferrokinetics in man. Medicine (Baltimore). 1970;49:17–53.
127. Klingshirn LA, Pate RR, Bourque SP, Davis JM, Sargent RG. Effect of iron supplementation on endurance capacity in iron-depleted female runners. Med Sci Sports Exerc. 1992;24:819–24.
128. Newhouse IJ, Clement DB, Taunton JE, McKenzie DC. The effects of prelatent/latent iron deficiency on physical work capacity. Med Sci Sports Exerc. 1989;21:263–8.
129. Rowland TW, Deisroth MB, Green GM, Kelleher JF. The effect of iron therapy on the exercise capacity of nonanemic iron-deficient adolescent runners. Am J Dis Child. 1988;142:165–9.
130. Zhu YI, Haas JD. Altered metabolic response of iron-depleted nonanemic women during a 15-km time trial. J Appl Physiol. 1998;84:1768–75.
131. Davies KJ, Maguire JJ, Brooks GA, Dallman PR, Packer L. Muscle mitochondrial bioenergetics, oxygen supply, and work capacity during dietary iron deficiency and repletion. Am J Physiol. 1982;242:E418–27.
132. Edgerton VR, Bryant SL, Gillespie CA, Gardner GW. Iron deficiency anemia and physical performance and activity of rats. J Nutr. 1972;102:381–99.
133. Perkkio MV, Jansson LT, Henderson S, Refino C, Brooks GA, Dallman PR. Work performance in the iron-deficient rat: improved endurance with exercise training. Am J Physiol. 1985;249:E306–11.
134. Finch CA, Miller LR, Inamdar AR, Person R, Seiler K, Mackler B. Iron deficiency in the rat. Physiological and biochemical studies of muscle dysfunction. J Clin Invest. 1976;58:447–53.

135. LaManca JJ, Haymes EM. Effects of iron repletion on VO2max, endurance, and blood lactate in women. Med Sci Sports Exerc. 1993;25:1386–92.
136. Haas JD, Brownlie T. Iron deficiency and reduced work capacity: a critical review of the research to determine a causal relationship. J Nutr. 2001;131:676S–90.
137. Brutsaert TD, Hernandez-Cordero S, Rivera J, Viola T, Hughes G, Haas JD. Iron supplementation improves progressive fatigue resistance during dynamic knee extensor exercise in iron-depleted, nonanemic women. Am J Clin Nutr. 2003;77:441–8.
138. Brownlie T, Utermohlen V, Hinton PS, Giordano C, Haas JD. Marginal iron deficiency without anemia impairs aerobic adaptation among previously untrained women. Am J Clin Nutr. 2002;75:734–42.
139. Brownlie T, Utermohlen V, Hinton PS, Haas JD. Tissue iron deficiency without anemia impairs adaptation in endurance capacity after aerobic training in previously untrained women. Am J Clin Nutr. 2004;79:437–43.
140. Hinton PS, Giordano C, Brownlie T, Haas JD. Iron supplementation improves endurance after training in iron-depleted, nonanemic women. J Appl Physiol. 2000;88:1103–11.
141. Jensen CA, Weaver CM, Sedlock DA. Iron supplementation and iron status in exercising young women. J Nutr Biochem. 1991;2:368–73.
142. Zhu YI, Haas JD. Iron depletion without anemia and physical performance in young women. Am J Clin Nutr. 1997;66:334–41.
143. Hinton PS, Sinclair LM. Iron supplementation maintains ventilatory threshold and improves energetic efficiency in iron-deficient nonanemic athletes. Eur J Clin Nutr. 2007;61:30–9.
144. Li R, Chen X, Yan H, Deurenberg P, Garby L, Hautvast JG. Functional consequences of iron supplementation in iron-deficient female cotton mill workers in Beijing, China. Am J Clin Nutr. 1994;59:908–13.
145. Basta SS, Soekirman DS, Karyadi D, Scrimshaw NS. Iron deficiency anemia and the productivity of adult males in Indonesia. Am J Clin Nutr. 1979;32:916–25.
146. Edgerton VR, Gardner GW, Ohira Y, Gunawardena KA, Senewiratne B. Iron-deficiency anaemia and its effect on worker productivity and activity patterns. Br Med J. 1979;2:1546–9.
147. Edgerton VR, Diamond LB, Olson J. Voluntary activity, cardiovascular and muscular responses to anemia in rats. J Nutr. 1977;107:1595–601.
148. Hunt JR, Zito CA, Erjavec J, Johnson LK. Severe or marginal iron deficiency affects spontaneous physical activity in rats. Am J Clin Nutr. 1994;59:413–8.
149. Food and Nutrition Board. Dietary reference intakes for vitamin A, vitamin K, arsenic, boron, chromium, copper, iodine, iron, manganese, molybdenum, nickel, silicon, vanadium, and zinc. Washington, DC: National Academy Press; 2001. http://www.iom.edu/Reports.aspx?Search=Dietary%20Reference%20Intakes%20for%20Micronutrients&Date=1/1/2001 t1/12/2001.
150. De Leeuw NK, Lowenstein L, Hsieh YS. Iron deficiency and hydremia in normal pregnancy. Medicine (Baltimore). 1966;45:291–315.
151. Beaton GH. Iron needs during pregnancy: do we need to rethink our targets? Am J Clin Nutr. 2000;72:265S–71.
152. Milman N. Iron prophylaxis in pregnancy-general or individual and in which dose? Ann Hematol. 2006;85:821–8.
153. Casanueva E, Viteri FE, Mares-Galindo M, et al. Weekly iron as a safe alternative to daily supplementation for nonanemic pregnant women. Arch Med Res. 2006;37:674–82.
154. Pena-Rosas JP, Nesheim MC, Garcia-Casal MN, et al. Intermittent iron supplementation regimens are able to maintain safe maternal hemoglobin concentrations during pregnancy in Venezuela. J Nutr. 2004;134:1099–104.
155. Allen LH. Pregnancy and iron deficiency: unresolved issues. Nutr Rev. 1997;55:91–101.
156. Murphy JF, O'Riordan J, Newcombe RG, Coles EC, Pearson JF. Relation of haemoglobin levels in first and second trimesters to outcome of pregnancy. Lancet. 1986;1:992–5.
157. Steer P, Alam MA, Wadsworth J, Welch A. Relation between maternal haemoglobin concentration and birth weight in different ethnic groups. BMJ. 1995;310:489–91.
158. Barrett JF, Whittaker PG, Williams JG, Lind T. Absorption of non-haem iron from food during normal pregnancy. BMJ. 1994;309:79–82.
159. O'Brien KO. Regulation of mineral metabolism from fetus to infant: metabolic studies. Acta Paediatr Suppl. 1999;88:88–91.
160. O'Brien KO, Zavaleta N, Caulfield LE, Yang DX, Abrams SA. Influence of prenatal iron and zinc supplements on supplemental iron absorption, red blood cell iron incorporation, and iron status in pregnant Peruvian women. Am J Clin Nutr. 1999;69:509–15.
161. Gambling L, Charania Z, Hannah L, Antipatis C, Lea RG, McArdle HJ. Effect of iron deficiency on placental cytokine expression and fetal growth in the pregnant rat. Biol Reprod. 2002;66:516–23.
162. Hindmarsh PC, Geary MP, Rodeck CH, Jackson MR, Kingdom JC. Effect of early maternal iron stores on placental weight and structure. Lancet. 2000;356:719–23.
163. Allen LH. Biological mechanisms that might underlie iron's effects on fetal growth and preterm birth. J Nutr. 2001;131:581S–9.

164. Jones BC, Reed CL, Hitzemann R, et al. Quantitative genetic analysis of ventral midbrain and liver iron in BXD recombinant inbred mice. Nutr Neurosci. 2003;6:369–77.
165. Beard J. Iron. In: Bowman BA, Russell RM, editors. Present knowledge in nutrition. 9th ed. Washington, DC: International Life Sciences Press; 2006.
166. Allen LH. Anemia and iron deficiency: effects on pregnancy outcome. Am J Clin Nutr. 2000;71:1280S–4.
167. Allen LH. Multiple micronutrients in pregnancy and lactation: an overview. Am J Clin Nutr. 2005;81:1206S–12.
168. Brabin BJ, Hakimi M, Pelletier D. An analysis of anemia and pregnancy-related maternal mortality. J Nutr. 2001;131:604S–15.
169. Scholl TO. Iron status during pregnancy: setting the stage for mother and infant. Am J Clin Nutr. 2005;81:1218S–22.
170. Yip R. Significance of an abnormally low or high hemoglobin concentration during pregnancy: special consideration of iron nutrition. Am J Clin Nutr. 2000;72:272S–9.
171. Rasmussen K. Is there a causal relationship between iron deficiency or iron-deficiency anemia and weight at birth, length of gestation and perinatal mortality? J Nutr. 2001;131:590S–603.
172. Rasmussen KM, Stoltzfus RJ. New evidence that iron supplementation during pregnancy improves birth weight: new scientific questions. Am J Clin Nutr. 2003;78:673–4.
173. Verhoeff FH, Brabin BJ, van Buuren S, et al. An analysis of intra-uterine growth retardation in rural Malawi. Eur J Clin Nutr. 2001;55:682–9.
174. Brabin BJ, Premji Z, Verhoeff F. An analysis of anemia and child mortality. J Nutr. 2001;131:636S–48.
175. Scholl TO, Reilly T. Anemia, iron and pregnancy outcome. J Nutr. 2000;130:443S–7.
176. Zhou LM, Yang WW, Hua JZ, Deng CQ, Tao X, Stoltzfus RJ. Relation of hemoglobin measured at different times in pregnancy to preterm birth and low birth weight in Shanghai, China. Am J Epidemiol. 1998;148:998–1006.
177. Rush D. Nutrition and maternal mortality in the developing world. Am J Clin Nutr. 2000;72:212S–40.
178. Goldenberg RL, Tamura T. Prepregnancy weight and pregnancy outcome. J Am Med Assoc. 1996;275:1127–8.
179. Tamura T, Goldenberg RL, Johnston KE, Cliver SP, Hickey CA. Serum ferritin: a predictor of early spontaneous preterm delivery. Obstet Gynecol. 1996;87:360–5.
180. Beard JL, Murray-Kolb LE, Rosales FJ, Solomons NW, Angelilli ML. Interpretation of serum ferritin concentrations as indicators of total-body iron stores in survey populations: the role of biomarkers for the acute phase response. Am J Clin Nutr. 2006;84:1498–505.
181. Lao TT, Tam KF, Chan LY. Third trimester iron status and pregnancy outcome in non-anaemic women; pregnancy unfavourably affected by maternal iron excess. Hum Reprod. 2000;15:1843–8.
182. Ramsey PS, Tamura T, Goldenberg RL, et al. The preterm prediction study: elevated cervical ferritin levels at 22 to 24 weeks of gestation are associated with spontaneous preterm delivery in asymptomatic women. Am J Obstet Gynecol. 2002;186:458–63.
183. Siega-Riz AM, Hartzema AG, Turnbull C, Thorp J, McDonald T, Cogswell ME. The effects of prophylactic iron given in prenatal supplements on iron status and birth outcomes: a randomized controlled trial. Am J Obstet Gynecol. 2006;194:512–9.
184. Milman N, Byg KE, Bergholt T, Eriksen L. Side effects of oral iron prophylaxis in pregnancy–myth or reality? Acta Haematol. 2006;115:53–7.
185. Tamura T, Goldenberg RL, Hou J, et al. Cord serum ferritin concentrations and mental and psychomotor development of children at five years of age. J Pediatr. 2002;140:165–70.
186. Preziosi P, Prual A, Galan P, Daouda H, Boureima H, Hercberg S. Effect of iron supplementation on the iron status of pregnant women: consequences for newborns. Am J Clin Nutr. 1997;66:1178–82.
187. Beard JL, Hendricks MK, Perez EM, et al. Maternal iron deficiency anemia affects postpartum emotions and cognition. J Nutr. 2005;135:267–72.
188. Perez EM, Hendricks MK, Beard JL, et al. Mother-infant interactions and infant development are altered by maternal iron deficiency anemia. J Nutr. 2005;135:850–5.
189. Zhou SJ, Gibson RA, Crowther CA, Baghurst P, Makrides M. Effect of iron supplementation during pregnancy on the intelligence quotient and behavior of children at 4 y of age: long-term follow-up of a randomized controlled trial. Am J Clin Nutr. 2006;83:1112–7.
190. Milman N. Iron and pregnancy-a delicate balance. Ann Hematol. 2006;85:559–65.
191. Savoie N, Rioux FM. Impact of maternal anemia on the infant's iron status at 9 months of age. Can J Public Health. 2002;93:203–7.
192. Kilbride J, Baker TG, Parapia LA, Khoury SA, Shuqaidef SW, Jerwood D. Anaemia during pregnancy as a risk factor for iron-deficiency anaemia in infancy: a case-control study in Jordan. Int J Epidemiol. 1999;28:461–8.

Chapter 15
The Anemia of Inflammation and Chronic Disease

Cindy N. Roy

Keywords Anemia • Chronic disease • Erythropoiesis • Erythropoietin • Ferritin • Infection • Inflammation • Macrophage • Reticuloendothelial • Transferrin receptor

Abbreviations

AICD	Anemia associated with inflammation and chronic disease
BFU-E	Erythroid blast forming units
CD71	Transferrin receptor
CD91	Hemopexin receptor
CFU-E	Erythroid colony-forming units
CKD	Chronic kidney disease
Cp	Ceruloplasmin
Epo	Erythropoietin
EpoR	Erythropoietin receptor
FLVCR	Feline leukemia virus subgroup C, receptor
Fpn	Ferroportin
Ft	Ferritin
GATA	Binding protein 2
HF	Heart failure
HNF	Hepatocyte nuclear factor
HO-1	Heme oxygenase 1
IBD	Inflammatory bowel disease
IFN	Interferon
IL	Interleukin
LRP	Low density lipoprotein receptor-related protein
NFκb	Nuclear factor κb
NSAIDS	Nonsteroidal anti-inflammatory drugs
PS	Phosphatidyl serine
RA	Rheumatoid arthritis
SLE	Systemic lupus erythematosus

C.N. Roy, PhD (✉)
Division of Geriatric Medicine and Gerontology, Johns Hopkins University, Baltimore, MD, USA
e-mail: croy6@jhmi.edu

G.J. Anderson and G. McLaren (eds.), *Iron Physiology and Pathophysiology in Humans*, Nutrition and Health, DOI 10.1007/978-1-60327-485-2_15,

sTfR Soluble/serum transferrin receptor
Tf Transferrin
TfR Transferrin receptor
TIBC Total iron binding capacity
TNF Tumor necrosis factor.

1 Prevalence

Anemia associated with inflammation and chronic disease (AICD) is a commonly observed anemia, second only to iron deficiency anemia in its prevalence in developed countries. It is a mild, normocytic, normochromic anemia that is characterized by adequate or increased iron in macrophages and low serum iron, a blunted response of erythroid precursors to erythropoietin (Epo), and decreased erythrocyte survival. Such an anemia is associated with bacterial, viral, or parasitic infections, but as antibiotics have become widely available, the incidence of long-lasting suppurative infections has decreased. AICD is classically associated with chronic disease states that generate systemic inflammatory mediators [1], including autoimmune disorders – like rheumatoid arthritis (RA), systemic lupus erythematosus (SLE) [2], or inflammatory bowel disease (IBD) – and cancer. More recently, anemia has been recognized as a significant risk multiplier or comorbid factor in the context of severe trauma [3], heart failure (HF) [4], chronic kidney disease (CKD) [5], aging [6], and frailty [7, 8]. Finally, the anemia associated with inflammation or infection is increasingly recognized as a cause of anemia in the developing world apart from nutritional deficiencies [9]. While the incidence of anemia related to nutritional deficiencies, Epo deficiency, and blood loss overlaps with AICD in many patients, inflammation is clearly involved in the pathogenesis of anemia in these complex disease states.

Estimates of the prevalence of AICD vary widely among study groups depending upon the laboratory criteria for inclusion, the underlying disorder, and the demographics of the subjects involved. Table 15.1 highlights a few representative studies from a number of diseases associated with AICD. While most studies report only the incidence of anemia within the particular disease group, some used additional criteria to diagnose AICD.

Table 15.1 Incidence of anemia in disease groups associated with AICD

Disorder	Subgroup	Anemia (all causes)	AICD (% total)	Reference
Infection	Tuberculosis	20%	NR	[10]
	HIV/AIDS	12–37%	NR	[11]
Trauma	Heart transplant	72%	NR	[12]
	Intensive care	~40%	NR	[3]
Autoimmune	RA	16%	NR	[13]
	SLE	16%	NR	[14]
		34%	NR	[15]
	IBD	9–74%	NR	[16]
		41%	24%	[17]
Cancer	Palliative care	>50%	NR	[18]
		39%	NR	[19]
		41%	NR	[20]
		68–77%	36–52%	[21]
CKD		40%	NR	[22]
HF		32%	NR	[23]
Aging	>65 years	10–11%	~2%	[24]
		21%	~6%	[25]
		8.5%	NR	[26]

NR not reported

2 Review of the Erythropoiesis Cycle

As we review the physiology and molecular pathology associated with AICD, it is important to highlight several key features of erythropoiesis that have already been discussed in Chap. 10. Erythropoiesis begins in the bone marrow (Fig. 15.1a). Maturation of erythroid precursors occurs in "erythroid" or "blood islands." Here, erythroid precursors develop in association with a central macrophage, which supports their development and assists with the extrusion of the erythroblast nucleus [27, 28]. Epo [29] promotes survival and allows proliferation of erythroid precursors [erythroid colony-forming units (CFU-E) and erythroblasts] that express the Epo receptor (EpoR) [30]. Survival of erythroid precursors is closely linked to their ability to successfully hemoglobinize. To furnish the iron for hemoglobin, early precursors, the erythroblasts, express abundant transferrin receptor 1 (TfR1/CD71) [31–34] to acquire iron from the serum protein, transferrin (Tf) [35, 36]. Much of erythropoiesis is ineffective, as many precursors do not complete full development, but instead undergo apoptosis [30]. Upon maturation, reticulocytes shed TfR into the serum (sTfR), which negatively correlates with the amount of iron available to developing erythrocytes [37]. Reticulocytes that successfully mature are released from their bone marrow niche where they continue to mature in the circulation (Fig. 15.1b). For a more detailed discussion of erythroid iron handling, please see Chap. 10.

Mature red cells circulate approximately 120 days in humans and approximately 50 days in mice; after which, they senesce and express phosphatidyl serine (PS) on the outer membrane leaflet [38]. These senescent [39] red cells are phagocytosed by tissue macrophages [38] (Fig. 15.1c). Little is known concerning the specific macrophages responsible for erythrocyte turnover. Many are present in the splenic red pulp and are differentiated from other splenic macrophages by the expression of F4/80 [40]. These macrophages recognize PS and phagocytose senescent red cells. Various components of the aged erythrocyte are then recycled.

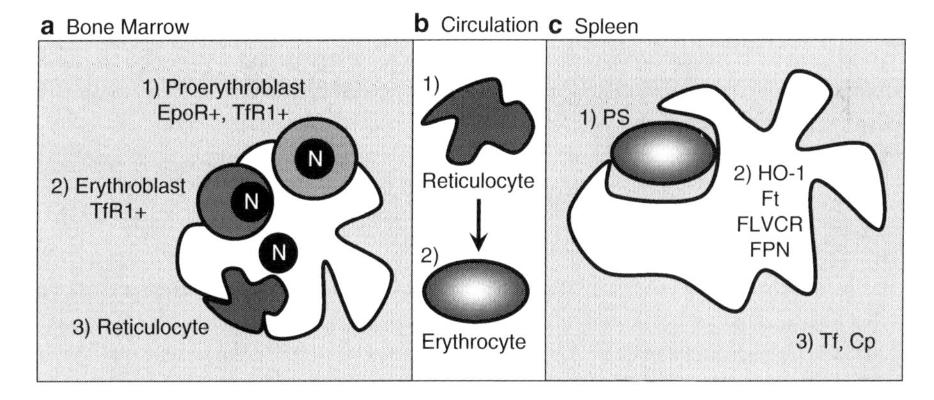

Fig. 15.1 Cycle of erythropoiesis. Erythroid cells develop in the bone marrow (**a**) in a specific environment or "niche" called erythroid islands, or erythroblastic islets. Here, erythrocyte progenitors maintain physical contact with central macrophages as they develop. Proliferation of proerythroblasts is dependent upon Epo and TfR1. Epo receptor (*EpoR*) is downregulated at the erythroblast stage, but TfR1 is required for hemoglobinization. Upon maturation to reticulocytes, TfR1 is shed and the erythroblast nucleus (*N*) is extruded and phagocytosed by the central macrophage. Reticulocytes continue to mature in circulation to erythrocytes (**b**). Senescent erythrocytes express phosphatidyl serine (*PS*) and are phagocytosed by macrophages of the spleen (**c**). Heme is returned to the serum by the feline leukemia virus, subgroup C, receptor (*FLVCR*). Heme oxygenase-1 (*HO-1*) degrades some heme. The iron recycled from heme is returned to transferrin (*Tf*) in the serum by ferroportin (*FPN*). Ceruloplasmin (*Cp*) converts Fe^{2+} transported by FPN to Fe^{3+} for binding to Tf. See text for references. Figure courtesy of the author

The feline leukemia virus, subgroup C, receptor (FLVCR) has recently emerged as an intriguing point of control for reticuloendothelial iron homeostasis. This channel is capable of releasing heme from macrophages [40, 41]. It has been hypothesized that this function allows the macrophage to avoid accumulation of damaging heme. The heme is likely bound by hemopexin, then returned to macrophages and hepatocytes via the hemopexin receptor, CD91/low density lipoprotein–related protein (LRP), which undergoes endocytosis. Heme and hemopexin are then degraded in the lysosome [42] (see also Chap. 8).

Alternatively, or in addition, heme oxygenase-1 (HO-1) [43] catabolizes heme from senescent red cells and allows for recycling of elemental iron, though the exact machinery required for phagosomal iron export is unclear [44–47]. Ferroportin (FPN), which is expressed in these macrophages, is a critical control point for the regulation of elemental iron egress [48, 49]. It is the only transporter known to facilitate cellular release of elemental iron. Some iron is stored within the macrophage in a complex with ferritin (Ft) [50–53], while some is released to the circulation. Virtually, nothing is known concerning the signals that dictate whether heme or elemental iron is released from the macrophage. Likewise, very little is known of the regulators that control whether iron is stored in Ft or released from the macrophage. Ferrous iron released from macrophages is oxidized to ferric iron, then loaded onto Tf in a process that involves the serum copper oxidase, Ceruloplasmin (Cp) [54–56]. Thus, Tf closes the loop between erythrocyte production and turnover. For a more detailed discussion of reticuloendothelial iron handling, please see Chap. 11.

3 Diagnosis and Treatment

Traditionally, AICD has been considered a diagnosis of exclusion in patients with unexplained anemia accompanying another illness. The anemia can be normochromic and normocytic or, if accompanied by iron deficiency, it can be hypochromic and microcytic. At present there is no definitive diagnostic test; rather, a diagnosis of AICD is made considering the overall clinical picture and laboratory findings, which typically include low serum iron, low total iron-binding capacity (TIBC, an indirect measure of Tf), and normal or elevated serum Ft (sFt) [57]. When examined after Perls' staining, bone marrow macrophages typically show retained iron in spite of iron-restricted erythropoiesis [58, 59]. Levels of C-reactive protein and the erythroid sedimentation rate may be elevated, indicative of an inflammatory process [60]. Soluble transferrin receptor (sTfR) levels are only increased if iron deficiency is also present. An index based on measurements of sTfR and sFt has been proposed to differentiate AICD from iron deficiency anemia [61, 62], but it is not widely used. Cytokine measurements, particularly measurement of interleukin (IL)-6 might, theoretically, be helpful [63], but they are not used routinely in medical practice. Measurement of hepcidin antimicrobial peptide levels may be of use in the diagnosis of AICD associated with some chronic diseases [64, 65], but it is not yet clear whether hepcidin will be a universal predictor of anemia in all cases. The putative role of hepcidin in the pathogenesis of AICD will be discussed in more detail later in this chapter.

Unfortunately, there is often little urgency associated with the treatment of AICD. In the context of short-term conditions, AICD should resolve when the underlying disease is abated. When a chronic disease underlies AICD, the gradual development of anemia, possibly without obvious symptoms, can easily be ignored. However, even mild anemia is increasingly recognized as an important independent contributor to adverse health outcomes such as disability, frailty, and mortality, especially in older adults [7, 66–69]. Since many chronic diseases such as HF, CKD, and cancer cannot yet be cured, only managed, early diagnosis and treatment of anemia in the context of chronic disease is likely to substantially increase quality of life for many patients with chronic disease [70–72] and to reduce the economic burden associated with treatment of the underlying condition [73, 74].

Treatment options for patients with AICD must be carefully weighed based on the severity of the anemia, the specific disease underlying AICD, and whether other causes of anemia are contributing [57]. Since AICD is derived from the innate immune response to infection, there is little support for the use of exogenous iron or erythroid-stimulating agents in the course of anemia due to infection. However, in the case of autoimmune disorders or end-stage renal disease, iron treatment in conjunction with erythroid-stimulating agents can be effective [70, 75–77]. Since AICD, alone, is a mild anemia, transfusions are only warranted in life-threatening situations that usually involve another anemia due to other pathologies. When treating such patients, the target hemoglobin level that should be achieved will depend upon their age, sex, and race and is a hotly debated topic that will not be reviewed here [78].

4 Features of AICD

The severity of the systemic reaction to infection or disease seems a better prognostic marker for anemia than the actual time course of the disease. Very active disease (associated with joint pain and tenderness, fever, accelerated erythrocyte sedimentation rate, and weight loss) was shown to correlate with the most severe anemia in RA patients. In contrast, the severity of the anemia did not correlate with the number of years patients had endured RA [79]. Likewise, in the context of infection, the onset of anemia is relatively rapid (within 6 weeks) but subsequently stabilizes despite the duration of the infection for many months [80]. This stabilization suggests the establishment of a new equilibrium for erythropoiesis that is likely dependent upon both the intensity of cytokine expression and the portfolio of cytokines involved. The anemia associated with inflammation likely results from pleiotropic effects of cytokines at the various stages of erythropoiesis and turnover (Fig. 15.2) which were described above. The major features of AICD include:

1. Low serum iron and iron sequestration in reticuloendothelial cells
2. Hypoproliferative erythroid precursors
3. A modest decrease in erythrocyte survival

We will use examples from specific disease states to highlight these common "endophenotypes" of AICD.

4.1 Low Serum Iron (Hyposideremia/Hypoferremia) and Reticuloendothelial Iron Sequestration

4.1.1 Cytokines and Reticuloendothelial Iron Cycling

Because many infections are resolved quickly by the immune system, hyposideremia may be the only feature of AICD that actually manifests during an infection. Hyposideremia (which is low serum iron, also called "hypoferremia") is associated with bacterial [81, 82], viral [83–86], and parasitic [87] infections.

It has been clear for some time that the low serum iron levels observed during inflammation result from impaired iron release by the reticuloendothelial system [82, 88–90]. Tumor necrosis factor (TNF)α [91, 92], IL-1α [91, 92], and IL-6 [93, 94] are each associated with hyposideremia, but whether their effects are direct or indirect in relation to reticuloendothelial iron cycling remains somewhat unclear. The recent discovery of Hepc certainly argues for molecular mediators between cytokine production and regulation of the reticuloendothelial system.

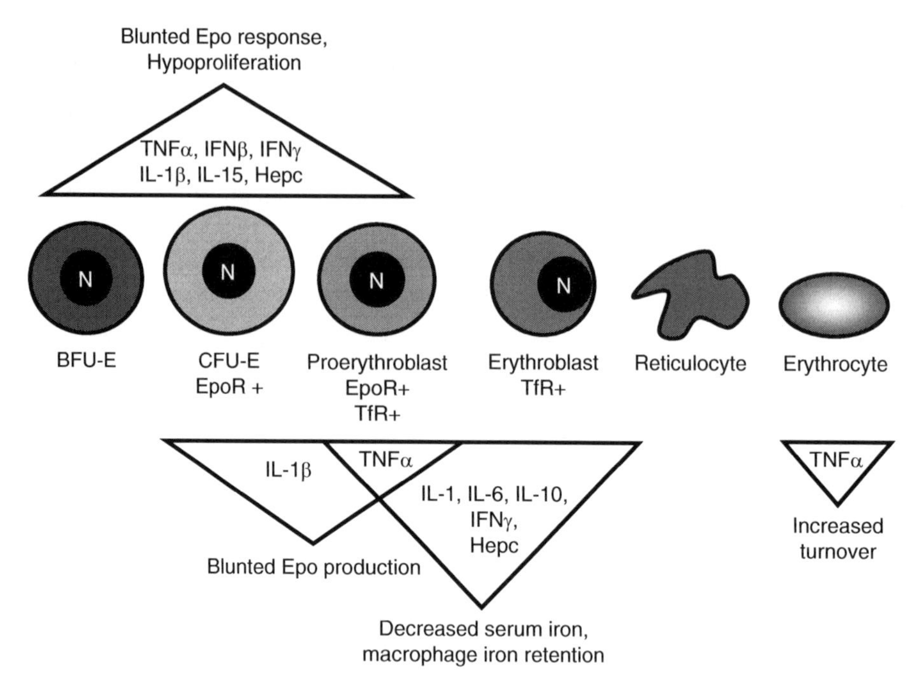

Fig. 15.2 Cytokine regulation of erythropoiesis. The anemia associated with inflammation and chronic disease (*AICD*) inhibits erythropoiesis along the development continuum. Various cytokines (enclosed in triangles) inhibit proliferation of early erythroid precursors by acting directly on early precursors and by reducing Epo production. Cytokines also prevent iron release from macrophages, resulting in hypoferremia and decreased proliferation and differentiation of later erythroblasts. Finally, cytokines reduce erythrocyte survival. See text for references. Figure courtesy of the author

4.1.2 IL-6 and Hepcidin

IL-6 is the primary cytokine that induces hepcidin expression [64]. Though IL-1α is also capable of inducing hepcidin after 24 h, this induction occurs through the elaboration of IL-6 in response to IL-1α [64]. IL-6 has been shown to correlate with the incidence or severity of anemia in a number of diseases associated with AICD including RA [95], ovarian cancer [96], SLE [97], and the morbidity associated with aging [8, 98]. While we would expect hepcidin levels to be increased in these patients, those data are not yet available. The small size and unique structure of hepcidin has made it exceedingly difficult to assay in serum and urine, so very few studies have assessed hepcidin expression in patients. However, hepcidin has been shown to be elevated in patients with iron refractory anemia and liver adenomas [99], in patients with elevated sFt and anemia [64], and in humans injected with LPS [100]. Antibiotic treatment of one patient with epididymitis and sepsis returned urinary hepcidin levels to normal [64], suggesting treatment of the underlying disorder may resolve hepcidin overexpression.

Hepcidin was first identified for its similarity to defensin-like cationic peptides involved in host defense [101, 102]. While it does have some antimicrobial activity, it is not a very strong agent. The primary antimicrobial role of hepcidin is likely to be in the sequestration of iron from pathogens. Hepcidin induces hypoferremia by inhibiting reticuloendothelial iron egress through FPN [103, 104]. Injection of hepcidin peptide [105] or overexpression of hepcidin in mice [106, 107] results in low serum iron concentrations as expected. Monocytes from AICD patients have decreased FPN, decreased iron regulatory protein (IRP) activity, and increased Ft [108], consistent with hepcidin-dependent sequestration of iron, though serum or urinary hepcidin were not determined in this study.

Table 15.2 Molecular mechanisms to reduce serum iron

Mediator	Target(s)	Remarks	References
TNFα	Ft	None	[111, 112]
IFNγ	IRP2, Ft, DMT1, FPN	Ft, DMT1, and FPN all have putative binding/regulatory sites for IRP2	[116–118]
Prostaglandins	Ft	None	[119]
Hepcidin	FPN	Induces internalization and degradation	[103, 104]
Cp	Fe^{2+}	Converts to Fe^{3+} to load onto Tf	[124, 125]

Hepcidin also reduces intestinal iron absorption [109] by reducing FPN expression at the enterocyte basolateral surface. However, because most of the iron required for erythropoiesis in adults is recycled from senescent erythrocytes, this regulatory step has little initial impact in the setting of AICD. For more discussion of the molecular basis of hepcidin action, see Chap. 9.

4.1.3 Hepcidin-Independent Mechanisms of Iron Sequestration

TNFα fails to induce hepcidin expression [110], yet expression of TNFα results in low serum iron [111, 112] and anemia [113, 114]. This suggests hepcidin-independent mechanisms exist which may regulate other proteins involved in cellular iron handling and result in reticuloendothelial iron sequestration. Ft is a likely target within the macrophage for such regulation. TNFα treatment of the human monocytic cell line U937 resulted in increased transcription of Ft. TNFα treatment also increased the relative amount of radiolabeled iron sequestered in Ft [115].

Studies in human U937 [115] and in murine J774 [116] and RAW264.7 [117] macrophage cell lines implicated IFNγ in iron regulatory protein-2-mediated accumulation of Ft. IFNγ, in combination with lipopolysaccharide, was shown to increase expression of divalent metal-ion transporter 1 (DMT1) and to downregulate expression of FPN in the human monocytic cell lines U937 and THP-1 [118]. Both of these studies are consistent with iron sequestration. Cyclopentenone prostaglandins have also been shown to target Ft accumulation in human monocytes [119]. For a summary of cytokines effects on serum iron, see Table 15.2.

Patients with IBD treated with IL-10 may become anemic [120]. Higher doses of IL-10 were shown to correlate with increased sFt and sTfR. IL-10 was also shown to increase Ft transcription and translation in human monocytic THP-1 cells [121], yet IL-10 does not seem to induce transcription of hepcidin [122].

The drawback to most of these in vitro studies is their use of monocytes or monocytic cell lines that are not fully differentiated and lack potential signals from interacting erythrocytes. More studies in coculture systems and whole animal models are needed to validate the findings in primary monocytes or cultured cell lines.

4.1.4 Additional Regulatory Changes

In addition to the blockade of reticuloendothelial iron egress, the concentration of Tf in the serum (assayed by TIBC) is decreased [123]. Since this increases the relative ratio of diferric Tf to monoferric forms, it might encourage more efficient iron uptake by reticulocytes in the face of decreasing serum iron [59]. Additionally, Cp levels can be elevated during infection [124, 125]. Cp promotes the oxidation of FeII to FeIII for loading on Tf and sequestration of FeII from various pathogens. Despite these changes in favor of Tf uptake in erythroid precursors, alpha-1 antitrypsin, an acute phase protein, has been shown to compete with Tf for binding to the TfR and may thus inhibit erythropoiesis by reducing erythroid iron acquisition from Tf [126, 127].

4.2 Hypoproliferation of Erythroid Precursors and the "Blunted Epo" Phenomenon

Despite the inhibitory effects of iron restriction on erythropoiesis, AICD is also characterized by disturbances in Epo-dependent regulation of the erythron. This disturbance is usually described as a "blunted Epo response." Understanding the biological mechanisms behind this pathophysiological response has been exceedingly difficult due to the number of events that modulate Epo responsiveness of erythroid precursors. The regulatory block in the Epo axis differs among studies and patient groups – sometimes even among patients with essentially the same underlying disease. These seeming contradictions are likely the result of an insufficient understanding of the disease process and the inherent problems associated with sampling patients during the course of their treatment, when regulatory systems are in flux.

4.2.1 Blunted Epo Production

Whatever the cause of anemia, decreased circulating hemoglobin reduces tissue oxygen tension and induces production of Epo in the peritubular fibroblast-like interstitial cells of the kidney [128]. As the anemia becomes more severe, Epo levels should increase to stimulate proliferation and differentiation of CFU-E and proerythroblasts.

The blunted Epo response is sometimes synonymous with insufficient Epo production. A comparison of Epo production in patients with infection and malignancy to patients with anemia due to iron deficiency and primary hematopoietic disorders [129] found no correlation between Epo and anemia in patients with infection or malignancy. Furthermore, these levels were lower than those in the patients with anemia from other etiologies. Similar observations of blunted Epo production have been made in AICD patients when compared to patients with hereditary spherocytosis [108].

Zucker et al. demonstrated blunted Epo production in a cohort of patients with infections and RA [130]. Patients with infection and inflammation had normal to elevated Epo, but the increase was not in keeping with the amount of Epo produced in patients with equally severe anemia due to iron or folate deficiency [130]. In the same study, addition of exogenous Epo to cultured bone marrow induced appropriate heme synthesis in these patients.

Blunted Epo production has been described in the context of RA [131–136], AIDS [137], cancer [138], trauma [139], tuberculosis [140], malaria [141], and aging [142–144]. A "pre-anemic" state of increased Epo levels and normal hemoglobin has been described in individuals with inflammation [145], suggesting prolonged inflammation diminishes the sensitivity of the Epo response. Recombinant human Epo has been shown to be effective for improving hemoglobin in RA patients [146], though it does not improve measures of RA disease activity itself.

Cytokines are likely involved in the regulation of Epo production in response to oxygen tension [147]. IL-1β has also been shown to dampen the response of Epo to hypoxia through inactivation of hepatocyte nuclear factor 4α [148]. Both IL-1β and TNFα promote recruitment of GATA-binding protein 2 and nuclear factor κb to suppress transcription of Epo [149]. In contrast, IL-6 and IFNγ do not regulate Epo production [150, 151]. This suggests that the cytokine profile associated with a particular disease is important with respect to the features of AICD that may arise [152] and should be used to develop more sensitive diagnostics or individualized treatments for AICD.

The anemia associated with systemic lupus erythematosus (SLE) stems from various pathologies, including aplasia, iron deficiency, autoimmune hemolysis, cyclophosphamide-induced myelotoxicity, and chronic renal insufficiency [2]. But SLE has provided some added insight into the problem of blunted Epo production in AICD. Close to half (46%) of SLE patients in one study had autoantibodies against Epo [153]. Whether these antibodies participate in clearance of Epo from the system or might interfere with Epo detection is not yet clear. However, the patients with anti-Epo antibodies did not have more severe anemia than their SLE counterparts lacking anti-Epo antibodies, suggesting the anti-Epo antibodies are not the cause of anemia in these patients. Even SLE patients without anti-Epo antibodies had lower Epo levels than expected, which suggests blunted Epo production consistent with AICD [154].

As is the case for SLE, the anemia associated with chronic kidney disease is a complex entity [5]. Epo deficiency secondary to kidney failure is clearly involved in the pathogenesis of the anemia in these patients, but treatment with Epo and exogenous iron does not fully resolve this anemia, indicating other pathogenic factors are at work. Patients with chronic kidney disease also have significant inflammation [60]. For this reason, AICD is a common complication of patients with CKD and end-stage renal disease.

4.2.2 Blunted Erythron Response to Epo

In contrast to the Epo deficiency described above, sometimes the blunted Epo response refers to a failure of the erythron to respond to available Epo. Zucker et al. contrasted their findings in patients with infection and inflammation (described above) with patients with malignancy [130]. Epo levels were increased in patients with malignancy (a finding consistent with decreased hemoglobin). However, heme synthesis was not sufficiently increased in response to exogenous Epo in bone marrow cultures of these patients. This seems to be a relatively common feature in the anemia associated with cancer [155] (see also Chap. 24). At least two other groups have described RA patients with elevated circulating Epo, but hypoproliferative erythroid precursors [156, 157]. Hepcidin overexpressing transgenic mice also have circulating Epo levels greater than phlebotomized controls with identical hemoglobin concentration, yet the erythron of hepcidin transgenic mice fails to increase reticulocyte production in response to this available Epo [107]. Both blunted Epo production and the blunted erythron response to Epo have been observed in patients with lung cancer [158].

4.2.3 Pleiotropic Effects of Individual Cytokines

Early efforts to investigate how cytokines modulate proliferation of erythroid progenitors in inflammatory states studied precursors cultured from murine spleen and human and murine bone marrow [159, 160]. The earliest precursors were designated blast-forming units (BFU-E) and more mature precursors, colony-forming units (CFU-E). Only CFU-E require Epo, as BFU-E proliferation and survival occur without expression of EpoR [30] (Fig. 15.2). Emerging data suggest that individual cytokines regulate particular erythroid targets. However, the effects of combinations of cytokines are unclear, and this underscores the importance of continued research toward understanding how the full complement of cytokines expressed in an individual may contribute to the pathogenesis of AICD.

TNFα

TNFα is closely associated with disease activity and anemia in RA patients [161]. TNFα is capable of suppressing erythroid development from CFU-E and BFU-E [95, 162]. Similarly, chronic treatment of mice with TNFα resulted in an erythropoietic block in CFU-E in bone marrow and spleen [113, 163]. Since these cultures initially contain accessory cells that may produce secondary signaling molecules, Means and colleagues depleted the accessory cells and then found no TNFα-mediated colony inhibition [164]. They went on to show the hypothesized secondary signaling molecule was

IFNβ [165] (see below). In contrast, Roodman and colleagues tested several hematopoietic cell lines and found proliferation of these lines was inhibited by TNFα alone. However, the effect seemed to be specific to a particular subset of cells that could not be clearly defined [166].

Davis and colleagues applied these findings to patient care and demonstrated that anti-TNFα antibodies relieved the blockade of erythropoiesis, increasing hemoglobin while decreasing Epo and IL-6 in RA patients [167]. BFU-E also increased in the bone marrow of RA patients treated with anti-TNFα antibody [168].

IL-1β

IL-1β is increased in anemic RA patients relative to non-anemic RA patients and inhibits erythroid colony formation of normal bone marrow [95, 169]. The inhibitory effect on bone marrow cultures is probably mediated through IFNγ (see below) [170]. However IL-1β, alone, inhibits proliferation of human erythroleukemia cell lines [171], suggesting that this cytokine can act directly on some erythroid precursors.

IFN

IFNγ inhibits proliferation and differentiation of early erythroid precursors, BFU-E and CFU-E [172, 173]. Secondary signals [174], such as nitric oxide [175] or IL-15 [176], elaborated from accessory cells are likely to be involved. IFNγ inhibits proliferation and differentiation of precursors by decreasing expression of stem cell factor and EpoR [177]. These regulatory targets are specific, as expression of insulin-like growth factor receptor is unchanged. In addition to preventing proliferation and maturation of erythroid precursors, IFNγ may also induce apoptosis, as it increases expression of Fas in erythroid progenitors [178, 179].

IFNβ has also been shown to inhibit erythropoiesis in erythroid islands [180]. This effect requires expression of the type I interferon receptor, but the signaling pathways that result in anemia are not yet understood.

Hepcidin

Over production of hepcidin attenuates erythropoiesis in vivo despite sufficient Epo production [107]. Whether this is due to a direct effect of hepcidin on the erythron [181] or the iron-restricted erythropoiesis that results from sequestration of iron in the reticuloendothelial system [102] is not yet clear.

4.3 Erythrocyte Survival

The modest decrease in erythropoietic capacity in the bone marrow is exacerbated in AICD by decreased survival of circulating erythrocytes. In the classical contexts of AICD, this is not related to hemolysis. However, in the settings of SLE and CKD, autoimmune hemolysis [2] and the effects of membrane dialysis [60] can confound and contribute to the severity of AICD.

Early attempts to quantitate survival of peripheral erythrocytes relied on Ashby differential red cell agglutination techniques and chromium labeling. Labeled erythrocytes from normal donors have decreased survival times in patients with disease without regard to the techniques used to label the cells [182–185]. Labeled erythrocytes from donors with inflammation have normal survival times in healthy recipients. The most likely explanation for these results would be an increase in the rate of erythrocyte turnover by the reticuloendothelial system of patients with inflammation, rather than a deficiency intrinsic to the red cell [186, 187]. It is likely that inflammatory cytokines play an additional role in the regulation of macrophage "surveillance" of circulating red cells, reducing their tolerance of erythrocyte anomalies that must increase as erythrocytes age.

No specific cytokine has been closely tied to this phenomenon, but TNFα and IL-1 are, again, important mediators. A comparison of the effects of recombinant TNFα or recombinant IL-1α on red cell survival [91] showed this feature was most apparent in TNFα-treated rats, though detectable in IL-1α-treated rats. A study in RA patients reported anemic patients had higher serum IL-1α levels and decreased erythrocyte survival, as measured by red cell–bound immunoglobulins [188]. Overexpression of hepcidin in transgenic mice does not alter erythrocyte survival [107].

The decreased red cell survival in AICD is consistent with an activated inflammatory state. Faster turnover of erythrocytes without iron recycling would also contribute to elevated iron stores in macrophages of patients with AICD. It does seem important, however, to consider the potential contribution of intestinal blood loss or enteropathy, especially in the context of RA. The majority of patients with RA take nonsteroidal anti-inflammatory drugs (NSAIDs) [189], and their use increases with age [190]. NSAIDs contribute to inflammation of the intestine and enteropathy [191], making these important study groups especially susceptible to gastrointestinal bleeding. Hemoglobin, serum iron, and sFt levels were found to be similar in anemic rheumatology patients without regard to the presence of gastrointestinal lesions or fecal occult blood [192]. Thus, until enteropathy can be ruled out in individuals with decreased erythrocyte survival, it may be an important confounder.

5 Conclusions

AICD is best defined as anemia in the context of adequate iron stores. Functional iron deficiency results from an inability to access or utilize iron sequestered in the reticuloendothelial system. Hypoproliferation of erythroid precursors results in failed attempts to offset losses associated with increased erythrocyte turnover. The specific disease underlying AICD critically impacts the presentation of anemia. The relative expression of pro-inflammatory cytokines, serum hepcidin, and other signaling molecules in various disease states must be investigated further to improve treatment options for individuals.

Acknowledgments My thanks to my mentor, Dr. Nancy Andrews, for her guidance in the preparation of this chapter and for so much more beyond it.

References

1. Cartwright GE. The anemia of chronic disorders. Semin Hematol. 1966;3:351–75.
2. Giannouli S, Voulgarelis M, Ziakas PD, Tzioufas AG. Anaemia in systemic lupus erythematosus: from pathophysiology to clinical assessment. Ann Rheum Dis. 2006;65:144–8.
3. Robinson Y, Hostmann A, Matenov A, Ertel W, Oberholzer A. Erythropoiesis in multiply injured patients. J Trauma. 2006;61:1285–91.
4. Anand I, McMurray JJ, Whitmore J, et al. Anemia and its relationship to clinical outcome in heart failure. Circulation. 2004;110:149–54.
5. van der Putten K, Braam B, Jie KE, Gaillard CA. Mechanisms of disease: erythropoietin resistance in patients with both heart and kidney failure. Nat Clin Pract Nephrol. 2008;4:47–57.
6. Ershler WB. Biological interactions of aging and anemia: a focus on cytokines. J Am Geriatr Soc. 2003;51(3 Suppl):S18–21.

7. Chaves PH, Xue QL, Guralnik JM, Ferrucci L, Volpato S, Fried LP. What constitutes normal hemoglobin concentration in community-dwelling disabled older women? J Am Geriatr Soc. 2004;52:1811–6.
8. Leng S, Chaves P, Koenig K, Walston J. Serum interleukin-6 and hemoglobin as physiological correlates in the geriatric syndrome of frailty: a pilot study. J Am Geriatr Soc. 2002;50:1268–71.
9. Calis JC, Phiri KS, Faragher EB, et al. Severe anemia in Malawian children. N Engl J Med. 2008;358:888–99.
10. Cartwright GE, Lauritsen MA, Jones PJ, Merrill IM, Wintrobe MM. The anemia of infection. I. Hypoferremia, hypercupremia, and alterations in porphyrin metabolism in patients. J Clin Invest. 1946;25:65–80.
11. Sullivan PS, Hanson DL, Chu SY, Jones JL, Ward JW. Epidemiology of anemia in human immunodeficiency virus (HIV)-infected persons: results from the multistate adult and adolescent spectrum of HIV disease surveillance project. Blood. 1998;91:301–8.
12. Muller HM, Horina JH, Kniepeiss D, et al. Characteristics and clinical relevance of chronic anemia in adult heart transplant recipients. Clin Transpl. 2001;15:343–8.
13. Young A, Koduri G. Extra-articular manifestations and complications of rheumatoid arthritis. Best Pract Res Clin Rheumatol. 2007;21:907–27.
14. Burling F, Ng J, Thein H, Ly J, Marshall MR, Gow P. Ethnic, clinical and immunological factors in systemic lupus erythematosus and the development of lupus nephritis: results from a multi-ethnic New Zealand cohort. Lupus. 2007;16:830–7.
15. AlSaleh J, Jassim V, ElSayed M, Saleh N, Harb D. Clinical and immunological manifestations in 151 SLE patients living in Dubai. Lupus. 2008;17:62–6.
16. Wilson A, Reyes E, Ofman J. Prevalence and outcomes of anemia in inflammatory bowel disease: a systematic review of the literature. Am J Med. 2004;116(Suppl. 7A):44S–9.
17. Revel-Vilk S, Tamary H, Broide E, et al. Serum transferrin receptor in children and adolescents with inflammatory bowel disease. Eur J Pediat. 2000;159:585–9.
18. Bron D, Meuleman N, Mascaux C. Biological basis of anemia. Semin Oncol. 2001;28(2 Suppl. 8):1–6.
19. Birgegard G, Aapro MS, Bokemeyer C, et al. Cancer-related anemia: pathogenesis, prevalence and treatment. Oncology. 2005;68(Suppl. 1):3–11.
20. Harrison L, Shasha D, Shiaova L, White C, Ramdeen B, Portenoy R. Prevalence of anemia in cancer patients undergoing radiation therapy. Semin Oncol. 2001;28(2 Suppl. 8):54–9.
21. Dunn A, Carter J, Carter H. Anemia at the end of life: prevalence, significance, and causes in patients receiving palliative care. J Pain Sympt Manag. 2003;26:1132–9.
22. Agarwal AK. Practical approach to the diagnosis and treatment of anemia associated with CKD in elderly. J Am Med Direct Assoc. 2006;7(9 Suppl):S7–12.
23. de Silva R, Rigby AS, Witte KK, et al. Anemia, renal dysfunction, and their interaction in patients with chronic heart failure. Am J Cardiol. 2006;98:391–8.
24. Guralnik JM, Eisenstaedt RS, Ferrucci L, Klein HG, Woodman RC. Prevalence of anemia in persons 65 years and older in the United States: evidence for a high rate of unexplained anemia. Blood. 2004;104:2263–8.
25. Semba RD, Ricks MO, Ferrucci L, et al. Types of anemia and mortality among older disabled women living in the community: the women's health and aging study I. Aging Clin Exp Res. 2007;19:259–64.
26. Zakai NA, Katz R, Hirsch C, et al. A prospective study of anemia status, hemoglobin concentration, and mortality in an elderly cohort: the cardiovascular health study. Arch Intern Med. 2005;165:2214–20.
27. Chasis JA. Erythroblastic islands: specialized microenvironmental niches for erythropoiesis. Curr Opin Hematol. 2006;13:137–41.
28. Kawane K, Fukuyama H, Kondoh G, et al. Requirement of DNase II for definitive erythropoiesis in the mouse fetal liver. Science. 2001;292:1546–9.
29. Graber SE, Krantz SB. Erythropoietin and the control of red cell production. Annu Rev Med. 1978;29:51–66.
30. Koury MJ, Sawyer ST, Brandt SJ. New insights into erythropoiesis. Curr Opin Hematol. 2002;9:93–100.
31. Iacopetta BJ, Morgan EH, Yeoh GC. Transferrin receptors and iron uptake during erythroid cell development. Biochim Biophys Acta. 1982;687:204–10.
32. Horton MA. Expression of transferrin receptors during erythroid maturation. Exp Cell Res. 1983;144:361–6.
33. Levy JE, Jin O, Fujiwara Y, Kuo F, Andrews NC. Transferrin receptor is necessary for development of erythrocytes and the nervous system. Nat Genet. 1999;21:396–9.
34. Ponka P, Lok CN. The transferrin receptor: role in health and disease. Int J Biochem Cell Biol. 1999;31:1111–37.
35. Jandl JH. Transfer of iron from serum iron-binding protein to human reticylocytes. J Clin Invest. 1959;38:161–85.
36. Bernstein SE. Hereditary hypotransferrinemia with hemosiderosis, a murine disorder resembling human atransferrinemia. J Lab Clin Med. 1987;110:690–705.
37. Beguin Y. Soluble transferrin receptor for the evaluation of erythropoiesis and iron status. Clin Chim Acta. 2003;329:9–22.
38. Bratosin D, Mazurier J, Tissier JP, et al. Cellular and molecular mechanisms of senescent erythrocyte phagocytosis by macrophages. A review. Biochimie. 1998;80:173–95.

39. Schroit AJ, Madsen JW, Tanaka Y. In vivo recognition and clearance of red blood cells containing phosphatidylserine in their plasma membranes. J Biol Chem. 1985;260:5131–8.
40. Taylor PR, Martinez-Pomares L, Stacey M, Lin HH, Brown GD, Gordon S. Macrophage receptors and immune recognition. Annu Rev Immunol. 2005;23:901–44.
41. Keel SB, Doty RT, Yang Z, et al. A heme export protein is required for red blood cell differentiation and iron homeostasis. Science. 2008;319:825–8.
42. Hvidberg V, Maniecki MB, Jacobsen C, Hojrup P, Moller HJ, Moestrup SK. Identification of the receptor scavenging hemopexin-heme complexes. Blood. 2005;106:2572–9.
43. Poss KD, Tonegawa S. Heme oxygenase 1 is required for mammalian iron reutilization. Proc Natl Acad Sci USA. 1997;94:10919–24.
44. Baranano DE, Wolosker H, Bae BI, Barrow RK, Snyder SH, Ferris CD. A mammalian iron ATPase induced by iron. J Biol Chem. 2000;275:15166–73.
45. Gomes MS, Appelberg R. Evidence for a link between iron metabolism and Nramp1 gene function in innate resistance against *Mycobacterium avium*. Immunology. 1998;95:165–8.
46. Canonne-Hergaux F, Gruenheid S, Govoni G, Gros P. The Nramp1 protein and its role in resistance to infection and macrophage function. Proc Assoc Am Physicians. 1999;111:283–9.
47. Jabado N, Canonne-Hergaux F, Gruenheid S, Picard V, Gros P. Iron transporter Nramp2/DMT-1 is associated with the membrane of phagosomes in macrophages and Sertoli cells. Blood. 2002;100:2617–22.
48. Donovan A, Lima CA, Pinkus JL, et al. The iron exporter ferroportin/Slc40a1 is essential for iron homeostasis. Cell Metab. 2005;1:191–200.
49. Knutson MD, Oukka M, Koss LM, Aydemir F, Wessling-Resnick M. Iron release from macrophages after erythrophagocytosis is up-regulated by ferroportin 1 overexpression and down-regulated by hepcidin. Proc Natl Acad Sci USA. 2005;10:1324–8.
50. Custer G, Balcerzak S, Rinehart J. Human macrophage hemoglobin–iron metabolism in vitro. Am J Hematol. 1982;13:23–36.
51. Galli A, Bergamaschi G, Recalde H, et al. Ferroportin gene silencing induces iron retention and enhances ferritin synthesis in human macrophages. Br J Haematol. 2004;127:598–603.
52. Bornman L, Baladi S, Richard MJ, Tyrrell RM, Polla BS. Differential regulation and expression of stress proteins and ferritin in human monocytes. J Cell Physiol. 1999;178:1–8.
53. Theurl I, Ludwiczek S, Eller P, et al. Pathways for the regulation of body iron homeostasis in response to experimental iron overload. J Hepatol. 2005;43:711–9.
54. Sarkar J, Seshadri V, Tripoulas NA, Ketterer ME, Fox PL. Role of ceruloplasmin in macrophage iron efflux during hypoxia. J Biol Chem. 2003;278:44018–24.
55. Harris ZL, Durley AP, Man TK, Gitlin JD. Targeted gene disruption reveals an essential role for ceruloplasmin in cellular iron efflux. Proc Natl Acad Sci USA. 1999;96:10812–7.
56. Cartwright GE, Wintrobe MM. The question of copper deficiency in man. Am J Clin Nutr. 1964;15:94–110.
57. Weiss G, Goodnough LT. Anemia of chronic disease. N Engl J Med. 2005;352:1011–23.
58. Song JS, Park W, Bae SK, et al. The usefulness of serum transferrin receptor and ferritin for assessing anemia in rheumatoid arthritis: comparison with bone marrow iron study. Rheumatol Int. 2001;21:24–9.
59. Erslev AJ. Williams hematology. 6th ed. New York: McGraw-Hill; 2001.
60. Kaysen GA. The microinflammatory state in uremia: causes and potential consequences. J Am Soc Nephrol. 2001;12:1549–57.
61. Punnonen K, Irjala K, Rajamaki A. Serum transferrin receptor and its ratio to serum ferritin in the diagnosis of iron deficiency. Blood. 1997;89:1052–7.
62. Brugnara C. Iron deficiency and erythropoiesis: new diagnostic approaches. Clin Chem. 2003;49:1573–8.
63. Raj DS. Role of interleukin-6 in the anemia of chronic disease. Sem Arthrit Rheumat. 2009;38:382–8.
64. Nemeth E, Valore EV, Territo M, Schiller G, Lichtenstein A, Ganz T. Hepcidin, a putative mediator of anemia of inflammation, is a type II acute-phase protein. Blood. 2003;101:2461–3.
65. Ganz T, Olbina G, Girelli D, Nemeth E, Westerman M. Immunoassay for human serum hepcidin. Blood. 2008;112:4292–7.
66. Sibley JT, Blocka KL, Haga M, Martin WA, Murray LM. Clinical course and predictors of length of stay in hospitalized patients with rheumatoid arthritis. J Rheumatol. 1990;17:1623–7.
67. Penninx BW, Guralnik JM, Onder G, Ferrucci L, Wallace RB, Pahor M. Anemia and decline in physical performance among older persons. Am J Med. 2003;115:104–10.
68. Mishra TK, Mishra SK, Mohanty NK, Rath PK. Prevalence, prognostic importance and therapeutic implications of anemia in heart failure. Indian Heart J. 2005;57:670–4.
69. Han C, Rahman MU, Doyle MK, et al. Association of anemia and physical disability among patients with rheumatoid arthritis. J Rheumatol. 2007;34:2177–82.
70. Kaltwasser JP, Kessler U, Gottschalk R, Stucki G, Moller B. Effect of recombinant human erythropoietin and intravenous iron on anemia and disease activity in rheumatoid arthritis. J Rheumatol. 2001;28:2430–6.

71. Silverberg DS, Wexler D, Iaina A, Schwartz D. The interaction between heart failure and other heart diseases, renal failure, and anemia. Semin Nephrol. 2006;26:296–306.
72. Crawford J, Cella D, Cleeland CS, et al. Relationship between changes in hemoglobin level and quality of life during chemotherapy in anemic cancer patients receiving epoetin alfa therapy. Cancer. 2002;95:888–95.
73. Nissenson AR, Wade S, Goodnough T, Knight K, Dubois RW. Economic burden of anemia in an insured population. J Manag Care Pharm. 2005;11:565–74.
74. Ershler WB, Chen K, Reyes EB, Dubois R. Economic burden of patients with anemia in selected diseases. Value Health. 2005;8:629–38.
75. Weiss G, Meusburger E, Radacher G, Garimorth K, Neyer U, Mayer G. Effect of iron treatment on circulating cytokine levels in ESRD patients receiving recombinant human erythropoietin. Kidney Int. 2003;64:572–8.
76. Gasche C, Lomer MC, Cavill I, Weiss G. Iron, anaemia, and inflammatory bowel diseases. Gut. 2004;53:1190–7.
77. Goodnough LT, Skikne B, Brugnara C. Erythropoietin, iron, and erythropoiesis. Blood. 2000;96:823–33.
78. Singh AK, Fishbane S. The optimal hemoglobin in dialysis patients – a critical review. Semin Dial. 2008;21:1–6.
79. Jeffrey MR. Some observations on anemia in rheumatoid arthritis. Blood. 1953;8:502–18.
80. Cartwright GE, Wintrobe MM. The anemia of infection. XVII. A review. Adv Int Med. 1952;5:165–226.
81. Elin RJ, Wolff SM, Finch CA. Effect of induced fever on serum iron and ferritin concentrations in man. Blood. 1977;49:147–53.
82. Letendre ED, Holbein BE. Mechanism of impaired iron release by the reticuloendothelial system during the hypoferremic phase of experimental Neisseria meningitidis infection in mice. Infect Immun. 1984;44:320–5.
83. Olivares M, Walter T, Osorio M, Chadud P, Schlesinger L. Anemia of a mild viral infection: the measles vaccine as a model. Pediatrics. 1989;84:851–5.
84. Fuchs D, Zangerle R, Artner-Dworzak E, et al. Association between immune activation, changes of iron metabolism and anaemia in patients with HIV infection. Eur J Haematol. 1993;50:90–4.
85. Cemeroglu AP, Ozsoylu S. Haematologic consequences of viral infections including serum iron status. Eur J Pediatr. 1994;153:171–3.
86. Spada C, Treitinger A, Hoshikawa-Fujimura AY. HIV influence on hematopoiesis at the initial stage of infection. Eur J Haematol. 1998;61:255–60.
87. Lalonde RG, Holbein BE. Role of iron in *Trypanosoma cruzi* infection of mice. J Clin Invest. 1984;73:470–6.
88. Freireich EJ, Miller A, Emerson CP, Ross JF. The effect of inflammation on the utilization of erythrocyte and transferrin bound radioiron for red cell production. Blood. 1957;12:972–83.
89. Noyes WD, Bothwell TH, Finch CA. The role of the reticulo-endothelial cell in iron metabolism. Br J Haematol. 1960;6:43–55.
90. Haurani FI, Young K, Tocantins LM. Reutilization of iron in anemia complicating malignant neoplasma. Blood. 1963;22:73–81.
91. Moldawer LL, Marano MA, Wei H, et al. Cachectin/tumor necrosis factor-alpha alters red blood cell kinetics and induces anemia in vivo. FASEB J. 1989;3:1637–43.
92. Alvarez-Hernandez X, Liceaga J, McKay IC, Brock JH. Induction of hypoferremia and modulation of macrophage iron metabolism by tumor necrosis factor. Lab Invest. 1989;61:319–22.
93. Kobune M, Kohgo Y, Kato J, Miyazaki E, Niitsu Y. Interleukin-6 enhances hepatic transferrin uptake and ferritin expression in rats. Hepatology. 1994;19:1468–75.
94. Nieken J, Mulder NH, Buter J, et al. Recombinant human interleukin-6 induces a rapid and reversible anemia in cancer patients. Blood. 1995;86:900–5.
95. Voulgari PV, Kolios G, Papadopoulos GK, Katsaraki A, Seferiadis K, Drosos AA. Role of cytokines in the pathogenesis of anemia of chronic disease in rheumatoid arthritis. Clin Immunol. 1999;92:153–60.
96. Maccio A, Madeddu C, Massa D, et al. Hemoglobin levels correlate with interleukin-6 levels in patients with advanced untreated epithelial ovarian cancer: role of inflammation in cancer-related anemia. Blood. 2005;106:362–7.
97. Ripley BJ, Goncalves B, Isenberg DA, Latchman DS, Rahman A. Raised levels of interleukin 6 in systemic lupus erythematosus correlate with anaemia. Ann Rheum Dis. 2005;64:849–53.
98. Maggio M, Guralnik JM, Longo DL, Ferrucci L. Interleukin-6 in aging and chronic disease: a magnificent pathway. J Gerontol A Biol Sci Med Sci. 2006;61:575–84.
99. Weinstein DA, Roy CN, Fleming MD, Loda MF, Wolfsdorf JI, Andrews NC. Inappropriate expression of hepcidin is associated with iron refractory anemia: implications for the anemia of chronic disease. Blood. 2002;100:3776–81.
100. Kemna E, Pickkers P, Nemeth E, van der Hoeven H, Swinkels D. Time-course analysis of hepcidin, serum iron, and plasma cytokine levels in humans injected with LPS. Blood. 2005;106:1864–6.
101. Park CH, Valore EV, Waring AJ, Ganz T. Hepcidin, a urinary antimicrobial peptide synthesized in the liver. J Biol Chem. 2001;276:7806–10.
102. Krause A, Neitz S, Magert HJ, et al. LEAP-1, a novel highly disulfide-bonded human peptide, exhibits antimicrobial activity. FEBS Lett. 2000;480:147–50.

103. Nemeth E, Tuttle MS, Powelson J, et al. Hepcidin regulates cellular iron efflux by binding to ferroportin and inducing its internalization. Science. 2004;306:2090–3.
104. De Domenico I, Ward DM, Langelier C, et al. The molecular mechanism of hepcidin-mediated ferroportin down-regulation. Mol Biol Cell. 2007;18:2569–78.
105. Rivera S, Nemeth E, Gabayan V, Lopez MA, Farshidi D, Ganz T. Synthetic hepcidin causes rapid dose-dependent hypoferremia and is concentrated in ferroportin-containing organs. Blood. 2005;106:2196–9.
106. Nicolas G, Bennoun M, Porteu A, et al. Severe iron deficiency anemia in transgenic mice expressing liver hepcidin. Proc Natl Acad Sci USA. 2002;99:4596–601.
107. Roy CN, Mak HH, Akpan I, Losyev G, Zurakowski D, Andrews NC. Hepcidin antimicrobial peptide transgenic mice exhibit features of the anemia of inflammation. Blood. 2007;109:4038–44.
108. Theurl I, Mattle V, Seifert M, Mariani M, Marth C, Weiss G. Dysregulated monocyte iron homeostasis and erythropoietin formation in patients with anemia of chronic disease. Blood. 2006;107:4142–8.
109. Laftah AH, Ramesh B, Simpson RJ, et al. Effect of hepcidin on intestinal iron absorption in mice. Blood. 2004;103:3940–4.
110. Nemeth E, Rivera S, Gabayan V, et al. IL-6 mediates hypoferremia of inflammation by inducing the synthesis of the iron regulatory hormone hepcidin. J Clin Invest. 2004;113:1271–6.
111. Feelders RA, Vreugdenhil G, Eggermont AM, Kuiper-Kramer PA, van Eijk HG, Swaak AJ. Regulation of iron metabolism in the acute-phase response: interferon gamma and tumour necrosis factor alpha induce hypoferraemia, ferritin production and a decrease in circulating transferrin receptors in cancer patients. Eur J Clin Invest. 1998;28:520–7.
112. Laftah AH, Sharma N, Brookes MJ, et al. Tumour necrosis factor-alpha causes hypoferraemia and reduced intestinal iron absorption in mice. Biochem J. 2006;397:61–7.
113. Johnson RA, Waddelow TA, Caro J, Oliff A, Roodman GD. Chronic exposure to tumor necrosis factor in vivo preferentially inhibits erythropoiesis in nude mice. Blood. 1989;74:130–8.
114. Capocasale RJ, Makropoulos DA, Achuthanandam R, et al. Myelodysplasia and anemia of chronic disease in human tumor necrosis factor-alpha transgenic mice. Cytometry A. 2008;73:148–59.
115. Fahmy M, Young SP. Modulation of iron metabolism in monocyte cell line U937 by inflammatory cytokines: changes in transferrin uptake, iron handling and ferritin mRNA. Biochem J. 1993;296:175–81.
116. Recalcati S, Taramelli D, Conte D, Cairo G. Nitric oxide-mediated induction of ferritin synthesis in J774 macrophages by inflammatory cytokines: role of selective iron regulatory protein-2 downregulation. Blood. 1998;91:1059–66.
117. Kim S, Ponka P. Effects of interferon gamma and lipopolysaccharide on macrophage iron metabolism are mediated by nitric oxide-induced degradation of iron regulatory protein 2. J Biol Chem. 2000;275:6220–6.
118. Ludwiczek S, Aigner E, Theurl I, Weiss G. Cytokine-mediated regulation of iron transport in human monocytic cells. Blood. 2003;101:4148–54.
119. Elia G, Polla B, Rossi A, Santoro MG. Induction of ferritin and heat shock proteins by prostaglandin A1 in human monocytes. Evidence for transcriptional and posttranscriptional regulation. Eur J Biochem. 1999;264:736–45.
120. Fedorak RN, Gangl A, Elson CO, et al. Recombinant human interleukin 10 in the treatment of patients with mild to moderately active Crohn's disease. The Interleukin 10 Inflammatory Bowel Disease Cooperative Study Group. Gastroenterology. 2000;119:1473–82.
121. Tilg H, Ulmer H, Kaser A, Weiss G. Role of IL-10 for induction of anemia during inflammation. J Immunol. 2002;169:2204–9.
122. Lee P, Peng H, Gelbart T, Wang L, Beutler E. Regulation of hepcidin transcription by interleukin-1 and interleukin-6. Proc Natl Acad Sci USA. 2005;102:1906–10.
123. Jarnum S, Lassen NA. Albumin and transferrin metabolism in infectious and toxic diseases. Scand J Clin Lab Invest. 1961;13:357–68.
124. Markowitz H, Gubler CJ, Mahoney JP, Cartwright GE, Wintrobe MM. Studies on copper metabolism. XIV. Copper, ceruloplasmin and oxidase activity in sera of normal human subjects, pregnant women, and patients with infection, hepatolenticular degeneration and the nephrotic syndrome. J Clin Invest. 1955;34:1498–508.
125. Beaumier DL, Caldwell MA, Holbein BE. Inflammation triggers hypoferremia and de novo synthesis of serum transferrin and ceruloplasmin in mice. Infect Immun. 1984;46:489–94.
126. Graziadei I, Kaserbacher R, Braunsteiner H, Vogel W. The hepatic acute-phase proteins alpha 1-antitrypsin and alpha 2-macroglobulin inhibit binding of transferrin to its receptor. Biochem J. 1993;290:109–13.
127. Graziadei I, Gaggl S, Kaserbacher R, Braunsteiner H, Vogel W. The acute-phase protein alpha 1-antitrypsin inhibits growth and proliferation of human early erythroid progenitor cells (burst-forming units-erythroid) and of human erythroleukemic cells (K562) in vitro by interfering with transferrin iron uptake. Blood. 1994;83:260–8.
128. Nangaku M, Eckardt KU. Hypoxia and the HIF system in kidney disease. J Mol Med. 2007;85:1325–30.
129. Ward HP, Kurnick JE, Pisarczyk MJ. Serum level of erythropoietin in anemias associated with chronic infection, malignancy, and primary hematopoietic disease. J Clin Invest. 1971;50:332–5.

130. Zucker S, Friedman S, Lysik RM. Bone marrow erythropoiesis in the anemia of infection, inflammation, and malignancy. J Clin Invest. 1974;53:1132–8.
131. Pavlovic-Kentera V, Ruvidic R, Milenkovic P, Marinkovic D. Erythropoietin in patients with anaemia in rheumatoid arthritis. Scand J Haematol. 1979;23:141–5.
132. Baer AN, Dessypris EN, Goldwasser E, Krantz SB. Blunted erythropoietin response to anaemia in rheumatoid arthritis. Br J Haematol. 1987;66:559–64.
133. Hochberg MC, Arnold CM, Hogans BB, Spivak JL. Serum immunoreactive erythropoietin in rheumatoid arthritis: impaired response to anemia. Arthritis Rheum. 1988;31:1318–21.
134. Boyd HK, Lappin TR, Bell AL. Evidence for impaired erythropoietin response to anaemia in rheumatoid disease. Br J Rheumatol. 1991;30:255–9.
135. Remacha AF, la SA Rodriguez-de, Garcia-Die F, Geli C, Diaz C, Gimferrer E. Erythroid abnormalities in rheumatoid arthritis: the role of erythropoietin. J Rheumatol. 1992;19:1687–91.
136. Kendall R, Wasti A, Harvey A, et al. The relationship of haemoglobin to serum erythropoietin concentrations in the anaemia of rheumatoid arthritis: the effect of oral prednisolone. Br J Rheumatol. 1993;32:204–8.
137. Spivak JL, Barnes DC, Fuchs E, Quinn TC. Serum immunoreactive erythropoietin in HIV-infected patients. J Am Med Assoc. 1989;261:3104–7.
138. Miller CB, Jones RJ, Piantadosi S, Abeloff MD, Spivak JL. Decreased erythropoietin response in patients with the anemia of cancer. N Engl J Med. 1990;322:1689–92.
139. Hobisch-Hagen P, Wiedermann F, Mayr A, et al. Blunted erythropoietic response to anemia in multiply traumatized patients. Crit Care Med. 2001;29:743–7.
140. Ebrahim O, Folb PI, Robson SC, Jacobs P. Blunted erythropoietin response to anaemia in tuberculosis. Eur J Haematol. 1995;55:251–4.
141. el Hassan AM, Saeed AM, Fandrey J, Jelkmann W. Decreased erythropoietin response in *Plasmodium falciparum* malaria-associated anaemia. Eur J Haematol. 1997;59:299–304.
142. Ferrucci L, Guralnik JM, Bandinelli S, et al. Unexplained anaemia in older persons is characterised by low erythropoietin and low levels of pro-inflammatory markers. Br J Haematol. 2007;136:849–55.
143. Ershler WB, Sheng S, McKelvey J, et al. Serum erythropoietin and aging: a longitudinal analysis. J Am Geriatr Soc. 2005;53:1360–5.
144. Carpenter MA, Kendall RG, O'Brien AE, et al. Reduced erythropoietin response to anaemia in elderly patients with normocytic anaemia. Eur J Haematol. 1992;49:119–21.
145. Ferrucci L, Guralnik JM, Woodman RC, et al. Proinflammatory state and circulating erythropoietin in persons with and without anemia. Am J Med. 2005;118:1288.
146. Pincus T, Olsen NJ, Russell IJ, et al. Multicenter study of recombinant human erythropoietin in correction of anemia in rheumatoid arthritis. Am J Med. 1990;89:161–8.
147. Faquin WC, Schneider TJ, Goldberg MA. Effect of inflammatory cytokines on hypoxia-induced erythropoietin production. Blood. 1992;79:1987–94.
148. Krajewski J, Batmunkh C, Jelkmann W, Hellwig-Burgel T. Interleukin-1beta inhibits the hypoxic inducibility of the erythropoietin enhancer by suppressing hepatocyte nuclear factor-4alpha. Cell Mol Life Sci. 2007;64:989–98.
149. La Ferla K, Reimann C, Jelkmann W, Hellwig-Burgel T. Inhibition of erythropoietin gene expression signaling involves the transcription factors GATA-2 and NF-kappaB. FASEB J. 2002;16:1811–3.
150. Jelkmann W, Pagel H, Wolff M, Fandrey J. Monokines inhibiting erythropoietin production in human hepatoma cultures and in isolated perfused rat kidneys. Life Sci. 1992;50:301–8.
151. Frede S, Fandrey J, Pagel H, Hellwig T, Jelkmann W. Erythropoietin gene expression is suppressed after lipopolysaccharide or interleukin-1 beta injections in rats. Am J Physiol. 1997;273:R1067–71.
152. Cazzola M, Ponchio L, de Benedetti F, et al. Defective iron supply for erythropoiesis and adequate endogenous erythropoietin production in the anemia associated with systemic-onset juvenile chronic arthritis. Blood. 1996;87:4824–30.
153. Schett G, Firbas U, Fureder W, et al. Decreased serum erythropoietin and its relation to anti-erythropoietin antibodies in anaemia of systemic lupus erythematosus. Rheumatology. 2001;40:424–31.
154. Voulgarelis M, Kokori SI, Ioannidis JP, Tzioufas AG, Kyriaki D, Moutsopoulos HM. Anaemia in systemic lupus erythematosus: aetiological profile and the role of erythropoietin. Ann Rheum Dis. 2000;59:217–22.
155. Corazza F, Beguin Y, Bergmann P, et al. Anemia in children with cancer is associated with decreased erythropoietic activity and not with inadequate erythropoietin production. Blood. 1998;92:1793–8.
156. Birgegard G, Hallgren R, Caro J. Serum erythropoietin in rheumatoid arthritis and other inflammatory arthritides: relationship to anaemia and the effect of anti-inflammatory treatment. Br J Haematol. 1987;65:479–83.
157. Nielsen OJ, Andersen LS, Ludwigsen E, et al. Anaemia of rheumatoid arthritis: serum erythropoietin concentrations and red cell distribution width in relation to iron status. Ann Rheum Dis. 1990;49:349–53.
158. Dowlati A, R'Zik S, Fillet G, Beguin Y. Anaemia of lung cancer is due to impaired erythroid marrow response to erythropoietin stimulation as well as relative inadequacy of erythropoietin production. Br J Haematol. 1997;97:297–9.

159. Means Jr RT, Krantz SB. Progress in understanding the pathogenesis of the anemia of chronic disease. Blood. 1992;80:1639–47.
160. Smith MA, Knight SM, Maddison PJ, Smith JG. Anaemia of chronic disease in rheumatoid arthritis: effect of the blunted response to erythropoietin and of interleukin 1 production by marrow macrophages. Ann Rheum Dis. 1992;51:753–7.
161. Vreugdenhil G, Lowenberg B, Van Eijk HG, Swaak AJ. Tumor necrosis factor-alpha is associated with disease activity and the degree of anemia in patients with rheumatoid arthritis. Eur J Clin Invest. 1992;22:488–93.
162. Akahane K, Hosoi T, Urabe A, Kawakami M, Takaku F. Effects of recombinant human tumor necrosis factor (rhTNF) on normal human and mouse hemopoietic progenitor cells. Int J Cell Cloning. 1987;5:16–26.
163. Johnson CS, Chang MJ, Furmanski P. In vivo hematopoietic effects of tumor necrosis factor-alpha in normal and erythroleukemic mice: characterization and therapeutic applications. Blood. 1988;72:1875–83.
164. Means Jr RT, Dessypris EN, Krantz SB. Inhibition of human colony-forming-unit erythroid by tumor necrosis factor requires accessory cells. J Clin Invest. 1990;86:538–41.
165. Means Jr RT, Krantz SB. Inhibition of human erythroid colony-forming units by tumor necrosis factor requires beta interferon. J Clin Invest. 1993;91:416–9.
166. Roodman GD, Bird A, Hutzler D, Montgomery W. Tumor necrosis factor-alpha and hematopoietic progenitors: effects of tumor necrosis factor on the growth of erythroid progenitors CFU-E and BFU-E and the hematopoietic cell lines K562, HL60, and HEL cells. Exp Hematol. 1987;15:928–35.
167. Davis D, Charles PJ, Potter A, Feldmann M, Maini RN, Elliott MJ. Anaemia of chronic disease in rheumatoid arthritis: in vivo effects of tumour necrosis factor alpha blockade. Br J Rheumatol. 1997;36:950–6.
168. Papadaki HA, Kritikos HD, Valatas V, Boumpas DT, Eliopoulos GD. Anemia of chronic disease in rheumatoid arthritis is associated with increased apoptosis of bone marrow erythroid cells: improvement following anti-tumor necrosis factor-alpha antibody therapy. Blood. 2002;100:474–82.
169. Schooley JC, Kullgren B, Allison AC. Inhibition by interleukin-1 of the action of erythropoietin on erythroid precursors and its possible role in the pathogenesis of hypoplastic anaemias. Br J Haematol. 1987;67:11–7.
170. Means Jr RT, Dessypris EN, Krantz SB. Inhibition of human erythroid colony-forming units by interleukin-1 is mediated by gamma interferon. J Cell Physiol. 1992;150:59–64.
171. Maury CP, Andersson LC, Teppo AM, Partanen S, Juvonen E. Mechanism of anaemia in rheumatoid arthritis: demonstration of raised interleukin 1 beta concentrations in anaemic patients and of interleukin 1 mediated suppression of normal erythropoiesis and proliferation of human erythroleukaemia (HEL) cells in vitro. Ann Rheum Dis. 1988;47:972–8.
172. Raefsky EL, Platanias LC, Zoumbos NC, Young NS. Studies of interferon as a regulator of hematopoietic cell proliferation. J Immunol. 1985;135(4):2507–12.
173. Wang CQ, Udupa KB, Lipschitz DA. Interferon-gamma exerts its negative regulatory effect primarily on the earliest stages of murine erythroid progenitor cell development. J Cell Physiol. 1995;162:134–8.
174. Mamus SW, Beck-Schroeder S, Zanjani ED. Suppression of normal human erythropoiesis by gamma interferon in vitro. Role of monocytes and T lymphocytes. J Clin Invest. 1985;75:1496–503.
175. Maciejewski JP, Selleri C, Sato T, et al. Nitric oxide suppression of human hematopoiesis in vitro. Contribution to inhibitory action of interferon-gamma and tumor necrosis factor-alpha. J Clin Invest. 1995;96:1085–92.
176. Mullarky IK, Szaba FM, Kummer LW, et al. Gamma interferon suppresses erythropoiesis via interleukin-15. Infect Immun. 2007;75:2630–3.
177. Taniguchi S, Dai CH, Price JO, Krantz SB. Interferon gamma downregulates stem cell factor and erythropoietin receptors but not insulin-like growth factor-I receptors in human erythroid colony-forming cells. Blood. 1997;90:2244–52.
178. Dai C, Krantz SB. Interferon gamma induces upregulation and activation of caspases 1, 3, and 8 to produce apoptosis in human erythroid progenitor cells. Blood. 1999;93:3309–16.
179. Dai CH, Price JO, Brunner T, Krantz SB. Fas ligand is present in human erythroid colony-forming cells and interacts with Fas induced by interferon gamma to produce erythroid cell apoptosis. Blood. 1998;91:1235–42.
180. Yoshida H, Okabe Y, Kawane K, Fukuyama H, Nagata S. Lethal anemia caused by interferon beta produced in mouse embryos carrying undigested DNA. Nat Immunol. 2005;6:49–56.
181. Dallalio G, Law E, Means Jr RT. Hepcidin inhibits in vitro erythroid colony formation at reduced erythropoietin concentrations. Blood. 2006;107:2702–4.
182. Hyman GA, Gellhorn A, Harvey JL. Studies on the anemia of disseminated malignant neoplastic disease. II. Study of the life span of the erythrocyte. Blood. 1956;11:618–31.
183. Alexander WR, Richmond J, Roy LM, Duthie JJ. Nature of anaemia in rheumatoid arthritis. II. Survival of transfused erythrocytes in patients with rheumatoid arthritis. Ann Rheum Dis. 1956;15:12–20.
184. Freireich EJ, Ross JF, Bayles TB, Emerson CP, Finch SC. Radioactive iron metabolism and erythrocyte survival studies of the mechanism of the anemia associated with rheumatoid arthritis. J Clin Invest. 1957;36:1043–58.
185. Hollingsworth JW, Hollingsworth DR. Study of total red cell volume and erythrocyte survival using radioactive chromium in patients with advanced pulmonary tuberculosis. Ann Intern Med. 1955;42:810–5.

186. Richmond J, Alexander WR, Potter JL, Duthie JJ. The nature of anaemia in rheumatoid arthritis. V. Red cell survival measured by radioactive chromium. Ann Rheum Dis. 1961;20:133–7.
187. Dinant HJ, de Maat CE. Erythropoiesis and mean red-cell lifespan in normal subjects and in patients with the anaemia of active rheumatoid arthritis. Br J Haematol. 1978;39:437–44.
188. Salvarani C, Casali B, Salvo D, et al. The role of interleukin 1, erythropoietin and red cell-bound immunoglobulins in the anaemia of rheumatoid arthritis. Clin Exp Rheumatol. 1991;9:241–6.
189. Varma J. Do nonsteroidal anti-inflammatory drugs cause lower gastrointestinal bleeding? A brief review. J Am Board Fam Pract. 1989;2:119–22.
190. Hirschowitz BI. Nonsteroidal antiinflammatory drugs and the gastrointestinal tract. Gastroenterologist. 1994;2:207–23.
191. Davies NM, Jamali F, Skeith KJ. Nonsteroidal antiinflammatory drug-induced enteropathy and severe chronic anemia in a patient with rheumatoid arthritis. Arthritis Rheum. 1996;39:321–4.
192. Doube A, Collins AJ. Anaemia in patients with arthritis: are simple investigations helpful? Br J Rheumatol. 1988;27:303–5.

Chapter 16
Disorders of Red Cell Production and the Iron-Loading Anemias

Stefano Rivella

Keywords Anemia • Erythropoietin • Hepcidin • Hypoproliferative • Ineffective erythropoiesis • Iron overload • Jak2 • Normal • Stress erythropoiesis • Thalassemia

1 Introduction

Anemias are a numerous and diverse group of disorders, ranging from limited erythroid precursor production to premature senescence of RBCs. In many cases, anemia is associated with hypoproliferative erythropoiesis (HE), while in other forms, with ineffective erythropoiesis (IE). HE leads to a reduction of the erythron and consequent anemia by absent or limited proliferation of the erythroid precursors. In contrast, the anemia in IE occurs despite expansion of the erythron. In some cases, IE is triggered by impaired maturation of the erythroid precursors while, in others, by hemolysis and/or premature senescence of RBCs. In some forms of hypoproliferative anemia, administration of iron and an erythropoiesis-stimulating agent (ESA), such as recombinant human erythropoietin (rhEPO), might be required. In aplastic and IE-associated anemias, blood transfusion and iron chelation may be necessary as supportive therapies.

2 Hypoproliferative Erythropoiesis-Associated Anemias

Hypoproliferative erythropoiesis (HE)-associated anemias are a large and diverse group of disorders. In a proportion of HE-associated anemias, the erythroid precursors have the potential to sustain a normal erythropoiesis under optimal conditions of iron and erythropoietin (EPO) administration, such as in many forms of chronic kidney disease (CKD). In other cases, the anemia is caused by limited or impaired production of erythroid progenitor cells, as in aplastic anemia (AA) or pure red cell aplasia. CKD and AA will be discussed as examples of different forms of HE-associated anemia (Table 16.1).

S. Rivella, Ph.D. (✉)
Department of Pediatric Hematology–Oncology, Children's Cancer and Blood Foundation Laboratories, Weill Medical College of Cornell University, New York, NY, USA
e-mail: str2010@med.cornell.edu

G.J. Anderson and G. McLaren (eds.), *Iron Physiology and Pathophysiology in Humans*, Nutrition and Health, DOI 10.1007/978-1-60327-485-2_16,

Table 16.1 Main features associated with anemias resulting from hypoproliferative or ineffective erythropoiesis

Hypoproliferative erythropoiesis				
Cause[a]	Kidney failure EPO/iron ↑	Tumor infection Hamp/IL6 ↑	Toxic agents	Inherited mutations
Leading to	CDK	Anemia of inflammation	Aplastic anemia	Aplastic anemia
It may require	Administration of EPO and iron	Transfusion and chelation	Transfusion and chelation/BMT	Transfusion and chelation/BMT
Ineffective erythropoiesis				
Cause[a]	Toxic agents or limited folate/B12	Toxic agents or mutations in ALAS2 ↓	Mutations in red cell PGK ↓	Mutations in beta-globin ↓
Leading to	Megaloblastic anemia	SA	PKD	Beta-thalassemia SCD
It may require	Administration of folate/B12	Phlebotomy, transfusion, and chelation/BMT	Transfusion and chelation/BMT	Transfusion and chelation/BMT

[a] Only some of the many potential causes that can lead to hypoproliferative or ineffective erythropoiesis are listed. Similarly, only a partial inventory of therapeutic approaches is presented, limited to iron and EPO administration or transfusion and iron chelation. The descending arrow might indicate reduction of mRNA or protein synthesis, limited enzymatic activity, or alteration of the protein properties

2.1 *Chronic Kidney Disease*

Chronic kidney disease, also referred to as chronic renal failure, encompasses a spectrum of diseases with mild renal impairment at one end and end-stage renal disease (ESRD) at the other, the latter requiring hemodialysis for survival. Anemia develops during the early stages of CKD, and is common in patients with ESRD as a result of diminished production of EPO. In general, the marrow erythroid lineages appear normal. However, the bone marrow is abnormal in the context of the anemia and expected increased erythroid activity. In cases of acute renal failure, erythroid hypoplasia has also been observed [1]. In anemic patients, hypoxia is one of the common factors responsible for CKD progression. CKD also plays an important role in the morbidity and mortality associated with cardiovascular disease, infection, and related side effects [2–4]. Correction of anemia by rhEPO has been shown to improve the quality of life and survival of patients affected by CDK [3–5].

In CDK patients, detection of both absolute and functional iron deficiency is important because these are the most common causes of hyporesponsiveness to rhEPO. Absolute iron deficiency may be due to inadequate iron intake, reduced bioavailability of dietary iron, increased utilization of iron, or chronic blood loss. The percent saturation of transferrin and serum ferritin concentration cutoff levels for absolute iron deficiency in CKD patients are <20% and <100 μg/L, respectively. The serum ferritin cutoff in CDK patients is determined by the observation that chronic inflammation increases serum ferritin levels approximately threefold compared to that of normal individuals [6].

Functional iron deficiency is the most common cause of a poor response to rhEPO therapy. It is a condition in which there is a failure to release iron rapidly enough to keep pace with the demands of erythropoiesis. However, it may be more difficult to diagnose since iron-related parameters may indicate adequate iron stores. In these cases, ferritin levels may be normal or high, even though the supply of iron to the erythron is limited. The Kidney Disease Outcomes Quality Initiative (K/DOQI) of the National Kidney Foundation recommends maintaining transferrin saturation levels above 20% and a lower limit of serum ferritin equal to 200 μg/L and 100 μg/L for CKD patients who do and do not require the hemodialysis, respectively. In general, iron deficiency is accompanied by reductions in the serum iron concentration and transferrin saturation and by elevations in the red cell distribution width, free erythrocyte protoporphyrin concentration, total iron binding capacity (TIBC), percentage of hypochromic red blood cells, and circulating transferrin receptor levels [7]. Serum soluble transferrin receptor levels, however, reflect ongoing erythropoiesis but not iron availability in rhEPO-treated chronic dialysis patients [8, 9]. Reticulocyte Hb content (CHr) represents a snapshot of the immediate availability of bone marrow iron and therefore may represent a useful test for guiding iron therapy [10–13]. Unfortunately, these parameters can be influenced by factors other than iron status, most notably inflammation, malnutrition, and infection.

CDK patients might be affected by uremia, which is associated with a chronic inflammatory state [14, 15]. Even in the absence of overt infection or inflammation, many ESRD patients show increased levels of acute-phase proteins, such as C-reactive protein (CRP), and cytokines such as interleukin (IL)-1, IL-6, IL-10, IL-13, interferon (IFN)-γ, and tumor necrosis factors TNF-alpha and TNF-gamma [16, 17]. Hepcidin might also exert a role in this disorder [18, 19], since hepcidin is also induced during inflammation. Under such conditions, hepcidin transcription is likely to be activated by IL-6 and its receptor through STAT-3 [20–22]. It has also been demonstrated that p53 binds the hepcidin promoter activating its expression, suggesting that upregulation of hepcidin by p53 is part of a defense mechanism against cancer through iron deprivation, and that hepcidin induction by p53 might be involved in the pathogenesis of the anemia accompanying cancer [23]. An additional factor that might play a role in the anemia of inflammation is the product of the growth arrest–specific gene 6 (*Gas6*), which enhances Epo receptor signaling by activating the serine-threonine kinase Akt in erythroid cells [24]. In the absence of *Gas6*, it has been shown that erythroid progenitors are hyporesponsive to Epo and fail to restore hematocrit levels in response to anemia, while in a mouse model hypomorphic for Epo production, Gas6 synergized with Epo in restoring hematocrit levels. It has been suggested that Gas6 influences erythropoiesis via a paracrine erythroblast-independent mechanism. In addition, the activity of Gas6 on erythroid cells may involve macrophages. The role of macrophages in the anemia of inflammation has been proposed by several groups based on the observation that macrophages may be able to produce hepcidin or inflammatory cytokines [24–27]. In particular, proinflammatory cytokines may antagonize the action of EPO by exerting an inhibitory effect on erythroid progenitor cells, while high hepcidin levels may interfere with ferroportin-mediated iron release, thus explaining why CKD patients have high ferritin levels, poor intestinal iron absorption, and disturbed iron release from the reticuloendothelial system [19, 28].

In clinical practice, functional iron deficiency is confirmed by the erythropoietic response to a course of parenteral iron and is excluded by the failure of the erythroid response to intravenous iron administration [29]. However, supplying intravenous iron may be associated with acute adverse events and should be carefully monitored [4, 6, 30]. For monitoring the response to rhEPO, hemoglobin (Hb) levels should be determined after 4 weeks of therapy. If the Hb level increases by less than 1 g/dL, iron status should be reevaluated and iron supplementation considered [31–33]. If no response is achieved after 8 weeks as an optimal dose in the absence of iron deficiency, a patient is considered non-responsive to erythropoietic agents. Two main mechanisms could explain resistance to endogenous and exogenous EPO. First, as mentioned previously, EPO resistance might be caused by inflammation [34]. Second, patients treated with rhEPO may develop neutralizing antibodies to recombinant and endogenous EPO, causing pure red cell aplasia. The incidence of this adverse effect peaked in 2002 [35, 36], and it has now abated, although very rarely patients may still develop anti-EPO antibodies [37, 38] and became transfusion dependent [35–37, 39].

2.2 *Aplastic Anemia*

Aplastic anemia (AA) is a rare, potentially life-threatening hematopoietic stem-cell disorder that results in pancytopenia and a hypocellular bone marrow. Often fatty replacement occurs in the marrow with a near absence of hematopoietic stem cells. Although most of AA cases are acquired, there are unusual forms due to inherited bone marrow failure syndromes, e.g., Fanconi's anemia, dyskeratosis congenita, amegakaryocytic thrombocytopenia, and Shwachman-Diamond syndrome [40]. Failure to diagnose an inherited form may lead to inappropriate supportive therapy, immunosuppressive treatment, and conditioning for bone marrow transplantation [41].

A large number of studies support apoptosis of hematopoietic stem cells as the underlying defect in AAs. For instance, Fanconi's anemia is triggered by mutations in genes that modulate DNA stability, the resulting pancytopenia being associated with and marked by increased rate of bone marrow apoptosis [42, 43]. In addition, TNF-alpha and TNF-gamma may be overexpressed in the marrow of these patients [44], leading to suppression of erythropoiesis [45, 46]. Similarly, acquired aplastic anemias are likely to result from the death of hematopoietic stem cells by an autoimmune mechanism. In aplastic anemia, autoreactive lymphocytes might target $CD34^+$ cells, CD34 being a surrogate marker that identifies, mainly hematopoietic stem cells. It has been shown that a significant proportion of $CD34^+$ cells in aplastic anemia patients exhibit an increased expression of Fas and become the targets of T lymphocytes which, in the same patients, overexpress FasL [42, 47, 48]. In addition, many patients affected by AA show a positive clinical response to immunosuppressive agents [40, 41, 49]. Environmental exposure to drugs, viruses, and toxins is thought to trigger the aberrant immune response in some patients, but most cases are classified as idiopathic. Similar to other autoimmune diseases, aplastic anemia has a varied clinical course; some patients have mild symptoms that necessitate little or no therapy, whereas others present with life-threatening pancytopenia constituting a medical emergency [41, 49]. Paroxysmal nocturnal hemoglobinuria and myelodysplastic syndrome commonly arise in patients with aplastic anemia, showing a pathophysiological link between these disorders [50, 51].

Management of aplastic anemia consists of supportive therapy and treatment aimed at restoring normal bone-marrow activity. Some forms of inherited and acquired aplastic anemia can be effectively treated by allogeneic bone-marrow transplantation. In some cases of acquired aplastic anemia, immunosuppression, using antithymocyte and antilymphocyte globulin, ciclosporin and high-dose cyclophosphamide can be effective [41, 52, 53]. In all forms of AA, supportive therapy involves red cell and platelet transfusions, and, in cases of long-term use of transfusion therapy, iron chelation [54, 55].

3 Ineffective Erythropoiesis and the Iron-Loading Anemias

Ineffective erythropoiesis is associated with all those conditions in which erythroid progenitor precursors either fail to mature, die in the process of becoming erythrocytes, or develop into erythrocytes that are abnormal and die prematurely despite all the necessary factors in the bone marrow to support erythropoiesis. Although the erythron is expanded in IE, this results in only a limited number of erythrocytes being produced, far fewer than the pool of erythroid progenitor cells. This includes conditions ranging from megaloblastic anemia (MA), where early erythroid progenitor precursors die prematurely, to red cell pyruvate kinase deficiency (PDK), where it is mostly hemolysis of mature erythroid cells that triggers IE. In beta-thalassemia, IE is characterized by a combination of premature death of nucleated erythroid cells and a shorter life span of RBCs. In addition, new observations point to a role for limited erythroid cell differentiation in the development of IE in this disorder [56]. Alternatively, IE can be defined by ferrokinetic parameters as described originally by Huff and collaborators [57, 58] and further elaborated on by Finch and colleagues [59–63]. Ferrokinetic studies were performed by the injection of ^{59}Fe into normal and anemic individuals. Red cell iron turnover was then estimated with consideration paid to the clearance time of ^{59}Fe after administration, the plasma iron turnover, and the subsequent rate of incorporation of ^{59}Fe in RBCs [57]. Based on these measurements, it was determined that the iron uptake by RBCs was equal to 80–90% of the injected ^{59}Fe 10–14 days post administration in normal individuals. In patients affected by IE, such as those with beta-thalassemia major, this percentage was reduced to 10–30%

during the same time period [59]. These and subsequent ferrokinetic studies introduced the notion that intravascular erythroid cell death was responsible for IE in thalassemia [64, 65].

As examples of IE-associated anemia, MA, sideroblastic anemia, red cell PKD, and some hemoglobinopathies will be discussed (Table 16.1). In particular, beta-thalassemia will be utilized to further discuss the relationship between IE, iron metabolism, and iron overload.

3.1 Megaloblastic Anemias

MA is caused most commonly by a deficiency of folate or cobalamin (vitamin B12), thus affecting DNA synthesis. Folate, in the form of tetrahydrofolate (THF) coenzymes, is required for the synthesis of thymidylate and purines and is indirectly involved in the methylation of cytosines in DNA [66], while cobalamin deficiency limits the intracellular supply of THF coenzymes [67]. In these conditions, DNA synthesis is affected in all hematopoietic lineages. The bone marrow is cellular and shows remarkable features, especially in the erythroid lineage, where there are increased numbers of large immature-appearing erythroblasts and myeloblasts (i.e., megaloblasts). In addition, cytogenetic studies have shown increased chromosomal breakage. MA is characterized by macrocytic erythrocytes, hypersegmented neutrophilic granulocytes, and reticulocytopenia. The differentiation of erythroid cells is ineffective, resulting in anemia due to an inability of erythroid colony forming units (CFU-E) and proerythroblasts to form reticulocytes. Failure to produce new erythrocytes stimulates EPO production, which, in turn, increases the proportion of erythroid cells at the CFU-E and proerythroblast stages of development [68, 69]. When erythroblasts derived from a murine model of MA were grown in folate-rich medium, they survived, proliferated, and underwent terminal maturation [69]. IE is observed in MA patients based on the increased ratio of erythroid precursors to reticulocytes. Elevated plasma iron turnover, increased lactate dehydrogenase and bilirubin levels in the plasma, and extramedullary hemolysis also support IE and hemolysis in MA [70–75].

Studies in patients with anemia due to folate or vitamin B12 deficiency have shown that impaired DNA synthesis increases hematopoietic cell death. In particular, the high rate of proliferation of their erythroid progenitors likely makes these cells more susceptible than others to impaired DNA synthesis. In vitro and in vivo models of folate deficiency were used to study the relationship between S-phase accumulation of the progenitors and apoptosis in MA [68, 69, 75, 76]. The results indicate that folate-deficient cells accumulate in S-phase where they undergo apoptosis [66, 68, 77–79]. Addition of thymidine to the folate-free medium inhibited apoptosis and rescued the cells, thus suggesting that folate deficiency leads to a defect in thymidine synthesis with consequent uracil misincorporation into DNA. This misincorporation of uracil into DNA may induce double-stranded breakage of the DNA with consequent induction of an apoptotic process [66, 68, 69, 76, 78]. However, studies in folate and vitamin B12-deficient patients [80, 81] did not find increased incorporation of uracil in the DNA of their blood cells [82]. Treatment of MA consists of folate or cobalamin administration. Occasionally, transfusions are required when the hematocrit is less than 15% or when the patient is debilitated, infected, or in heart failure.

3.2 Pyruvate Kinase Deficiency

Among glycolytic defects causing chronic non-spherocytic hemolytic anemia, red cell pyruvate kinase deficiency (PKD) is the most common, with heterozygote frequencies ranging from 0.24% to 3.1% [83–86]. Red cell PKD is transmitted as an autosomal recessive trait and is a genetically heterogeneous disorder, with different mutations causing different kinetics and electrophoretic changes in the corresponding enzyme. The erythrocyte PK mRNA is synthesized from the corresponding erythroid-specific promoter of the gene called PK-LR located on chromosome 1. To date, more than 150 different mutations in the PK-LR gene have been associated with PKD. Most patients with hereditary non-spherocytic hemolytic anemia manifest only symptoms of chronic hemolysis, only a few having minimal RBCs in their circulation due to very severe PKD. Other potential complications associated with red cell PKD are iron overload [87], severe jaundice, and cholecystolithiasis [88].

No specific therapy is available. Treatment of this disease is, therefore, based on supportive measures [83, 84]. Dietary supplementation of folic acid and other B vitamins is recommended to prevent deficiencies of these factors due to increased erythrocyte production. Red cell transfusions may be required in severely anemic cases, particularly in the first years of life. Splenectomy usually results in an increase in Hb of 1–3 g/dL and reduces or even eliminates the need for transfusion support [83]. This therapeutic option, however, must be weighed carefully, since in some patients, it may not be beneficial, and it may increase the likelihood of sepsis in children and thromboembolic events in adults [89]. Iron chelation may be required since iron overload has been documented in PKD, even in non-transfused patients [90, 91]. In the latter patients, iron overload was demonstrated by observing that their serum ferritin level was higher than that in matched controls, and some were affected by liver siderosis, fibrosis, and cirrhosis. These studies underlined the importance of evaluating the iron status of all PKD patients in order to prevent the clinical consequences of iron overload. Although no studies have been carried out so far to assess the mechanism that leads to iron overload in red cell PKD, increased intestinal iron absorption, triggered by enhanced erythropoiesis due to chronic hemolysis, is likely to be the cause, these conditions having been documented in red cell PKD. Morphologic abnormalities are not a prominent finding, but polychromatophilia, anisocytosis, poikilocytosis, and nucleated red blood cells can be observed. Erythrocyte life span is moderately to severely reduced, depending on the severity of the anemia and the level of splenic congestion, reticuloendothelial hyperplasia, and erythrophagocytosis. In addition, pathologic and histologic findings suggest IE, since normoblastic erythroid hyperplasia of the bone marrow and extramedullary hematopoiesis can be observed in patients affected by this disease.

Since red cell PKD is a monogenic disorder with no definitive cure, potential therapeutic approaches involve gene addition strategies similar to those that have been evaluated in hemoglobinopathies [92, 93]. The rationale for this approach is based on studies involving gene transfer techniques and murine models of red cell PKD. The feasibility of gene therapy in PKD was first demonstrated by Tani and colleagues [94], who introduced the human liver-specific PK-RL cDNA into mouse bone marrow cells using a retroviral vector. They demonstrated prolonged expression of human liver PK-RL mRNA in both the peripheral blood and hematopoietic organs of normal mouse with long-term bone marrow chimeras. Additional studies were performed using two murine transgenic models expressing low (hRPK-lo) or high (hRPK-hi) levels of the human-specific cDNA of the PK-RL gene under control of the human erythroid PK-RL promoter and a cassette containing elements of the beta-globin locus control region (uLCR) [95]. This approach was designed to test the tissue specificity, level of expression, and therapeutic potential of a cassette harboring human erythroid PK-RL cDNA that potentially could be introduced into viral vectors and utilized for gene transfer into bone marrow cells. The hRPK-lo and hRPK-hi mouse lines were crossed with a red cell PKD mouse model to evaluate whether expression of human erythroid PK-RL reduced the pathophysiological features associated with this disorder. hRPK-lo mice showed RBC PK activity at the same level of normal littermates, with mean Hb levels of 13.0 g/dL and reduced reticulocytosis, while hRPK-hi mice had PK activity double that of controls with no hemolytic anemia, with Hb levels of about 15.1 g/dL and almost normal reticulocyte counts. However, even with a high level of expression of the transgene, splenomegaly was still present. Interestingly, the authors observed an inverse correlation between human PK activity and the number of apoptotic erythroid progenitors in the spleen. These data provided direct evidence that the metabolic alteration responsible for PK deficiency not only leads to hemolysis of RBCs but also affects erythroid progenitor maturation, further contributing to IE [96].

3.3 Sideroblastic Anemias

Acquired or inherited sideroblastic anemias (SA) are a heterogeneous group of disorders that have in common the presence of large numbers of ringed sideroblasts in the marrow. Sideroblasts are erythroblasts containing large amounts of non-heme iron aggregates deposited within the cristae of the mitochondria. They are visible under light microscopy as Prussian blue positive granules surrounding the nucleus. Disorders associated with the formation of sideroblasts might exhibit impaired hematopoiesis as a primary defect, in particular erythropoiesis, or a series of defects affecting multiple organs, including the bone marrow. The former group of disorders can be classified as primary acquired SAs, a subset of myelodysplastic manifestations, or secondary acquired SAs, resulting from ingestion of drugs, alcohol or other toxins, or inherited SAs, as in the case of X-linked SA or XLSA.

In the case of primary and secondary SAs, the primary defects have not been elucidated, although alteration of mitochondria function may have a role in the initiation or progression of these disorders [97–99]. Compromised mitochondrial function could be related to mitochondrial genome mutations, alterations in mitochondrial iron metabolism, or exacerbation of physiological pathways involving caspases, leading to the activation of the mitochondrial pathway to apoptotic cell death [99–101]. In secondary SA, discontinuation of the offending insult drug usually restores normal erythropoiesis [102–105]. In primary SA, if patients require chronic blood transfusions, iron chelation might be required [55, 106]. However, even in a subset of non-transfused patients, IE may be elevated [107–109] and iron absorption increased [110].

XLSA is the most common form of congenital sideroblastic anemia associated with molecular defects of the erythroid-specific 5-aminolevulinate synthase isoenzyme (ALAS2), which is involved in the biosynthesis of heme. In most cases, a mutation in the ALAS2 gene appears to affect the affinity of the enzyme for its cofactor, pyridoxal 5-phosphate [111, 112]. In fact, many of XLSA patients are, to some extent, responsive to pyridoxine, which is metabolized to pyridoxal 5-phosphate. In other circumstances, the ALAS2 gene mutation either decreases the enzymatic activity of the gene product [113] or abrogates its interaction with protein partners [114], thus rendering patients resistant to pyridoxine supplementation [115]. While an ALAS-E-deficient mouse has been generated [116, 117], experimental production of ringed sideroblasts has not been observed and the mice died by E11.5. The life span of the embryos was extended to E19.0 by crossing the ALAS-E-deficient mice with animals expressing the human ALAS-E gene at a level lower than the wt gene [118]. In these hypomorphic embryos, most of the primitive erythroid cells were transformed into ringed sideroblasts. Definitive ringed sideroblasts were also observed, and the majority of the circulating definitive erythroid cells exhibited enucleated erythrocytes containing iron deposits. Interestingly, these iron-overloaded cells suffered from an alpha/beta-globin chain imbalance. Unfortunately, analysis of the iron distribution and IE in adult mice was prevented by embryonic lethality. These results suggest that limiting the heme supply provokes ringed sideroblast formation. This conclusion is supported by studies in the zebrafish mutant *shiraz*, which exhibits severe anemia and is embryonically lethal due to deletion of the gene glutaredoxin 5 (*GRLX5*). The absence of *GRLX5* expression leads to insufficient biogenesis of mitochondrial iron-sulfur (Fe/S) clusters and deregulated iron regulatory protein 1 (IRP1) activity. Reduced IRP1 activity, in turn, leads to the stabilization of transferrin receptor 1 mRNA, and repression of ferritin and ALA-synthase 2 (*ALAS2*) translation with impaired heme synthesis. The iron-sensing protein IRP2 has no role in *shiraz* [119]; however, being regulated by proteasomal degradation through iron and heme binding [120], it has increased activity in a low-heme environment. A patient carrying a homozygous mutation in *GRLX5* has been described. This mutation alters the correct splicing of *GRLX5,* severely limiting its synthesis. The patient showed iron overload and a low number of ringed sideroblasts, mimicking the observations in zebrafish [121]. Moreover, the anemia was worsened by blood transfusions but partially reversed by iron chelation. It was suggested that IRP2, less degraded by low heme, further contributed to repressed synthesis of ferritin and ALAS2 in erythroblasts, thereby increasing mitochondrial iron. Iron chelation probably reduced the IRP2 excess, leading to improved heme synthesis and decreased anemia.

In SA patients, the rate of cell destruction is usually normal or only moderately increased to levels easily compensated by bone marrow. IE has been documented in SA mainly by ferrokinetic studies. The half-life of intravenously injected tracer doses of radioactive iron is less than in normal individuals (25–40 min versus 90 min, respectively). The plasma iron turnover, however, is generally increased (1.5–5.9 mg/dL versus 0.30–0.70 mg/dL), and incorporation of radioactive iron into heme and its delivery to the blood as newly synthesized Hb are depressed (15–30% versus 70–90%). The RBC life span varies from 40 to 120 days. As in other kinds of anemia characterized by IE, the total fecal stercobilin excreted per day may be greater than can be accounted for by the catabolism of circulating Hb. Iron overloading regularly accompanies this disorder and may be the cause of death. Iron storage might be enhanced if mutations in the *Hfe* gene are co-inherited [122, 123]. If the anemia is not too severe or if it can be partially corrected by the administration of pyridoxine, phlebotomy may be used to diminish the iron burden. However, in other cases, the use of iron chelators is preferred [55, 106].

3.4 Hemoglobinopathies

Sickle cell disease (SCD) and beta-thalassemia represent the most common hemoglobinopathies caused, respectively, by the alteration of structural features and deficient production of the beta chain of the Hb molecule. SCD and the thalassemias are quite common in Asian, African, African-American, and Mediterranean populations [124]. It has been estimated that approximately 7% of the world population are carriers of such disorders, and that 300,000–400,000 children with severe forms of these diseases are born each year [125].

A single mutation leads to SCD, causing an adenine (A) to thymidine (T) substitution in codon 6 (GAG-GTG), which leads to insertion of valine in place of glutamic acid in the beta-globin chain. The resulting Hb (HbS) has the unique property of polymerizing when deoxygenated [124]. When the polymer becomes abundant, the red cells "sickle," stiff rods form that stretch and distort the red cells. These distorted cells can obstruct blood flow through the small vessels, affecting many organs and tissues. The restricted oxygen delivery to the tissues damages cells, injures organs, and produces pain.

In contrast, the thalassemias are a group of disorders due to a large number of heterogeneous mutations causing abnormal globin gene expression resulting in the total absence or quantitative reduction of globin chain synthesis [124]. Patients affected by Cooley's anemia require chronic blood transfusions to sustain life and chelation therapy to prevent iron overload. Those affected by beta-thalassemia intermedia, a milder form of the disease, do not require chronic blood transfusions, but eventually develop elevated body iron loads as well due to increased gastrointestinal iron absorption [126].

Many SCD patients require blood transfusions to prevent deleterious and painful vaso-occlusive crises and iron chelation to alleviate complications due to iron overload. Non-transfused patients also become iron overloaded and, in the absence of chelation therapy, exhibit elevated serum transferrin saturations and ferritin levels. Iron overload is responsible for the most damaging effects of SCD and the thalassemias, making iron chelation a major focus of the management of these diseases. In conditions of increased iron absorption, iron accumulates in parenchymal tissues, where it can cause significant toxicity as compared to that within reticuloendothelial cells [127]. As loading continues, the capacity of transferrin, the main transport protein of iron, to bind and detoxify this essential metal may be exceeded. The resulting non-transferrin-bound iron (NTBI) fraction within plasma may promote generation of free radicals, propagators of oxygen-related damage [127–130].

Excess iron and NTBI are deposited in liver parenchymal cells as well as other organs. The heart and endocrine tissues are particularly susceptible. The identity of the hepatocyte NTBI uptake molecules has not yet been clarified. DMT1 is a potential candidate in view of the fact that NTBI uptake is increased in cells where DMT1 mRNA and protein expression has been upregulated [131, 132]. A few additional candidates have been proposed, such as *ZIP14*, originally described as a zinc transporter [133, 134], and neutrophil gelatinase–associated lipocalin (*NGAL*), which is elevated in beta-thalassemia [135] and has been shown to be a siderophore iron-binding protein as well as a growth factor [136, 137]. However, in the case of all these potential NTBI transporters, information is still inadequate to draw firm conclusions.

The progressive accumulation of iron may lead to dysfunction of the liver, endocrine glands, and heart [138, 139]. Iron-induced liver disease is a common cause of death in transfused patients [140]. Within 2 years transfusions, collagen formation and portal fibrosis are observed, and in the absence of chelation therapy, cirrhosis may develop [141]. Iron-induced liver disease may be complicated by transfusion-related hepatitis [142]. Chronic iron deposition also damages the thyroid, parathyroid, adrenal glands, and exocrine pancreas. Iron loading within the anterior pituitary may cause disturbances in sexual maturation. Iron-induced myocardial dysfunction may be the most important factor determining the survival of patients with beta-thalassemia. Extensive iron deposits in the heart are associated with cardiac hypertrophy and dilatation, myocardial fiber degeneration, and, occasionally, fibrosis. In unchelated patients, symptomatic cardiac disease is observed after about 10 years of transfusion therapy and may be aggravated by pulmonary hypertension [143, 144]. Therefore, even if the goal of transfusion therapy is the correction of anemia, efforts need to be undertaken in order to limit the damage due to iron overload [145].

Definitive cures for thalassemia are presently available (e.g., bone marrow transplantation) or are in development (e.g., beta-globin gene transfer using hematopoietic stem cells) [93, 146]. Proof of concept that additive gene transfer could cure beta-thalassemia and other forms of hemoglobinopathy was achieved with a mouse model of beta-thalassemia intermedia (*th3/+*). *Th3/+* mice harbor a deletion that eliminates both the *minor* and *major* beta-globin genes in heterozygosity [147, 148]. The *th3/+* mice show Hb levels in the range of 9–10 g/dL. Adult *th3/+* mice have a degree of disease severity (hepatosplenomegaly, anemia, aberrant erythrocyte morphology) comparable to that of patients affected by beta-thalassemia intermedia. Efficient transfer of the human beta-globin gene together with large segments (3.2 kb) of its locus control region (LCR) into murine hematopoietic stem cells was achieved using recombinant lentiviruses. Transplantation of these cells into *th3/+*mice resulted in sufficient levels of human beta-globin expression to markedly reduce anemia in BM chimeras [93, 149–153]. Thalassemia major mice, (*th3/th3*) were not used in these studies because they do not survive fetal life since the switch from embryonic to adult Hb production in mice occurs at 14–15 days of gestation [93]. Fetal liver cells removed from live *th3/th3* embryos were transplanted into lethally irradiated animals, thus generating the first adult mice affected by thalassemia major [93]. Transplantation of *th3/th3* fetal liver cells transduced with a lentiviral vector carrying the human beta-globin gene rescued the mice from lethal anemia and reduced the severity of the splenomegaly, extramedullary hematopoiesis, and hepatic iron overload that characterizes this model [93]. Generation of *th3/+* and *th3/th3* was central to investigating the relation between IE and iron metabolism [56, 154], as we will describe in the next section.

3.5 *Ineffective Erythropoiesis and Iron Overload*

In beta- and alpha-thalassemia major, as well as in Hb-H disease, IE is evidenced by ferrokinetic studies, as well as increased plasma levels of EPO and soluble transferrin receptor [59, 64, 155, 156]. Iron absorption studies in subjects affected by beta-thalassemia intermedia show that the rate of iron loading from the gastrointestinal tract is approximately three to four times greater than normal [126, 139, 157–161]. In non-transfused patients with severe thalassemia, abnormal dietary iron absorption results in an increased body iron burden between 2 and 5 g per year depending on the severity of erythroid expansion [162]. Regular transfusions double this rate of iron accumulation. Increased iron absorption also plays a role in beta-thalassemia major, where its importance is inversely related to Hb levels [61, 163]. Erlandson et al. [163] documented increased iron absorption in three non-transfused SCD patients with Hb levels of 6.5–8.7 g/dL. Increased reticulocytosis was observed together with anemia, which suggests that IE also occurs in such patients. In the same study, patients affected by beta-thalassemia major were compared before and after transfusion therapy. The results clearly showed that iron absorption was elevated in the absence of transfusion therapy, whereas it was decreased after transfusion. Moreover, in the presence of transfusions, endogenous erythropoiesis was suppressed [163]. Thus, it is likely that increased iron absorption is a feature of all hemoglobinopathies associated with IE. This study and previous investigations led to the conclusion that iron absorption in humans is regulated by the combined influences of hypoxia, the body's iron stores [164–166], and the erythropoietic demand for iron [154, 167].

The mechanisms that control iron homeostasis predict signaling through iron-absorbing duodenal cells, iron-storing hepatocytes, and iron-recycling macrophages by regulators, historically defined as the "store" and "erythroid" regulators [168]. To date, the only candidate for the storage regulator is hepcidin, a circulating peptide hormone [165, 169] (Fig. 16.1a) (see also Chap. 9). Fluctuating levels of hepcidin affect iron absorption as well as the concentration of iron in macrophages [170–172]. Circulating iron is derived mainly from recovery of iron from senescent erythrocytes, through phagocytosis by tissue macrophages, particularly in the spleen. The Hb is catabolized in the macrophages, the iron being liberated from heme by heme oxygenase. Ferroportin is critical for export of the iron. Therefore, fluctuating hepcidin levels can change the ratio between stored and released iron. In the presence of IE, iron absorption and the amount of iron released from macrophages are expected to increase. In a study by Kattamis, liver hepcidin mRNA levels correlated with Hb concentrations and inversely related to with serum transferrin receptor, EPO, and NTBI levels [173]. In beta-thalassemic patients, urinary hepcidin levels were suppressed in relation to the iron burden, whereas transfusion led to its increase. In other studies, the hepcidin to ferritin ratio was used to correlate hepcidin expression with the degree of iron burden. In SCD patients, urinary hepcidin was suppressed and inversely associated with erythropoietic drive [174–176].

The function of the putative erythroid regulator is to maintain the production of erythrocytes irrespective of the body's iron balance. While increased amounts of the erythroid regulator are extremely helpful in resolving transient blood loss, in hemoglobinopathies, its continued overexpression will result in iron overload due to the inadequacy of IE in addressing anemia. After phlebotomy, hemolysis, or EPO administration, hepcidin production is decreased [167, 177, 178], indicating that the erythroid regulator exerts its activity, at least in part, by suppressing production of this peptide. Two major lines of thought identify the erythroid regulator as either a diffusible factor or an intrinsic cellular process, both of which repress hepcidin expression. Increased erythropoiesis, through secretion of soluble mediators, could directly influence hepcidin production. Erythropoiesis also causes a decrease in tissue and serum iron levels, which could downregulate hepcidin. Alternatively, anemia could cause hypoxia, triggering EPO expression or activation of transcription factors that repress hepcidin synthesis.

Pak et al. [179] administered inhibitors of erythropoiesis after phlebotomy to disassociate the effects of anemia, hypoxia, and Epo from those of increased erythropoiesis and iron use. Phlebotomized mice developed anemia, tissue hypoxia, increased Epo levels, increased erythropoiesis, and decreased serum iron and hepatic hepcidin mRNA levels. When erythropoietic inhibitors were administered, serum and tissue iron together with hepcidin mRNA rose dramatically, even though the mice were anemic. These results suggest that the dominant regulators of hepcidin during increased erythropoiesis include a signal arising from erythropoietic activity (also in the spleen) or

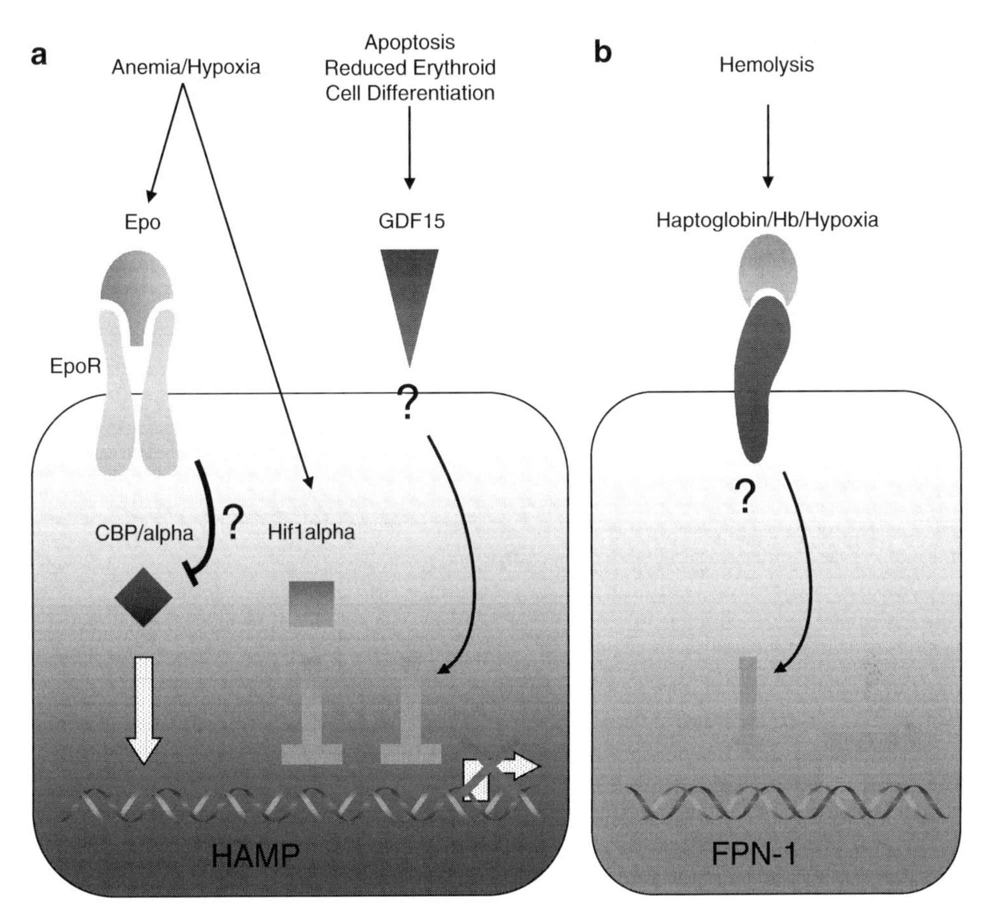

Fig. 16.1 Putative proteins involved in increased iron absorption under conditions of ineffective erythropoiesis. The main factors and pathways regulating hepcidin in the liver (**a**) and ferroportin in the duodenum (**b**) are described in the text. The question marks indicate that the pathway and potential protein partners have not yet been characterized

the effects of increased iron use on plasma or tissue iron. The existence of an erythroid factor is also supported by studies in which the sera of patients affected by beta-thalassemia or hereditary hemochromatosis associated with mutations in the *Hfe* gene were compared in terms of their ability to induce the expression of hepcidin and other factors related to iron metabolism. Sera from beta-thalassemia major and intermedia patients downregulated hepcidin expression in the HepG2 cell line. In contrast, the majority of sera from hereditary hemochromatosis patients induced an increase in hepcidin expression, which correlated with transferrin saturation [180]. A candidate for the erythroid regulator has been proposed called *GDF15* (Fig. 16.1a). Compared to controls, GDF15 is elevated in the serum of beta-thalassemic patients and suppresses hepcidin expression in vitro [181]. *GDF15* is a member of the TGF-beta superfamily of proteins, which are known to control cell proliferation, differentiation, and apoptosis in numerous cell types. Interestingly, *GDF15*, also called *MIC-1*, can be modulated by p53. Conditioned medium from cells expressing this protein can suppress the growth of certain tumor cells provided they express *TGF-beta* receptors and *SMAD4* [182–184]. However, the mechanism of action and efficacy of *GDF15* in repressing hepcidin expression still needs to be elucidated.

Alternatively, studies by Yoon et al. and Peyssonnaux et al. [185, 186] emphasize the role of the hypoxia factor Hif1alpha (and potentially Hif2alpha) in controlling iron absorption and erythropoiesis

(Fig. 16.1a). Using several conditional transgenic lines to modify expression of the hypoxic response, they demonstrated that the hypoxia-inducible transcription factor Hif1alpha binds the hepcidin promoter, downregulating its expression under hypoxic conditions. Their studies also suggest a more general role for the hypoxia pathway in coordinating iron metabolism and oxygen transport by the simultaneous coordinated expression of hepcidin, ferroportin, and *EPO*.

These studies might also indicate that several factors act synergistically leading to hepcidin downregulation when both increased erythropoiesis and hypoxia exist. This model recognizes the individual role of soluble erythroid factors, hypoxia, and iron levels, although their separate effect on hepcidin synthesis would be of a lower magnitude. This was illustrated by using several mouse models of beta-thalassemia. However, these mouse models need to be carefully compared to beta-thalassemia patients before any conclusion can be extended to humans [187]. For instance, thalassemia intermedia mice exhibit approximately 9–10 g/dL of Hb. With these Hb levels, IE may be less severe than in patients affected by thalassemia intermedia whose Hb levels can be significantly lower than 9 g/dL [176]. Small differences in Hb levels likely affect hypoxia, hepcidin synthesis, and iron distribution to a larger extent. In contrast, mice affected by thalassemia major are not transfused. Therefore, IE is more severe, and synthesis of hepcidin lower than that is found in thalassemia major patients who are chronically transfused [174, 176].

Keeping these differences in mind, much important information can be obtained by studying thalassemic mice. These studies were the first to indicate that mice affected by beta-thalassemia major (*th3/th3*) and intermedia (*th3/+* and *th1/th1*) had low or relatively low hepcidin expression compared to that seen in iron overload [188–191]. Further, gene expression analysis indicated that the mRNA levels of *Hfe* and *Cebpα* were reduced in the liver of thalassemic animals that expressed low hepcidin [154]. Since *Cebpα*-KO and *Hfe*-KO mice showed low hepcidin expression [192], these factors might be involved in the low hepcidin expression observed in thalassemia. In particular, *Cebpα* decreased in *th3/th3* mice that showed the lowest level of hepcidin expression. Therefore, *Hfe* could play a direct role in hepcidin regulation in beta-thalassemia, while low *Cebpα* levels might further decrease hepcidin expression in conditions of extreme IE. In contrast, in transfused mice, hepcidin, *Hfe*, and *Cebpα* expressions are probably augmented due to the combined effects of reduced anemia, increased iron content, and suppression of erythropoiesis [154]. In particular, a potential link between *Cebpα* and hepcidin was suggested by a recent study in which it was shown that Epo, through EpoR signaling, inversely mediates hepcidin expression in a dose-related fashion in freshly isolated mouse hepatocytes and in HepG2 cells [184] (Fig. 16.1a). Interestingly, chromatin immunoprecipitation experiments showed a significant decrease of *Cebpα* binding to the hepcidin promoter after Epo supplementation, suggesting the involvement of this transcription factor in the response of hepcidin to Epo [193].

It is also possible that genes which do not control hepcidin synthesis might be influenced by the erythroid demand, further increasing the rate of iron absorption. Quite interestingly, analysis of 1-year-old *th3/+* mice indicated that hepcidin expression was similar to or greater than that of control mice, and that it was upregulation of ferroportin in the duodenum rather than hepcidin that caused iron overload [154]. As previously noted [185, 186], increasing levels of hypoxia can trigger upregulation of ferroportin in the duodenum (Fig. 16.1b), although the same has not been observed in *th3/th3* mice. It has been shown that *th3/th3* erythroid cells differentiate less and contain less alpha-globin mRNA than *th3/+* cells [56]. This supports the notion that the severity of the thalassemic mutation is proportional to IE and the amount of iron absorbed, but inversely proportional to the level of Hb synthesized. In contrast, *th3/+* mice, that produce definitive erythroid cells, could increase free Hb and reduce haptoglobin serum levels over time. This may cause an increase of ferroportin in the duodenum based on the observation that *haptoglobin*-KO mice transport significantly more iron from the duodenal mucosa to the plasma than to control mice [194]. In the same study, it was also suggested that increased free Hb levels might activate ferroportin expression.

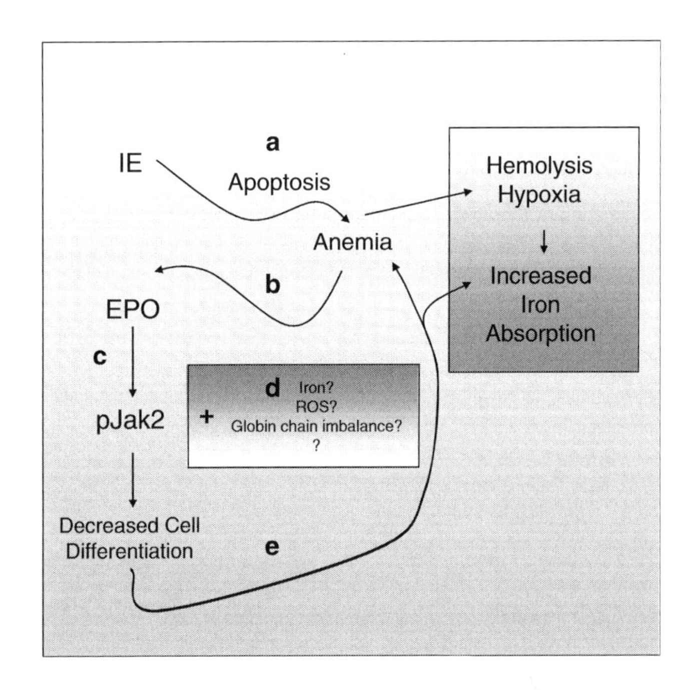

Fig. 16.2 Potential correlation between Jak2, ineffective erythropoiesis, and iron absorption. During the early stage of beta-thalassemia, genetic defect and cell death lead to, anemia (**a**), triggering Epo synthesis (**b**). Increased Epo production prompts proliferation of more erythroid progenitor cells through Jak2 signaling (**c**). However, additional intrinsic and extrinsic factors likely limit erythroid cell differentiation in association with the phosphorylated and active form of Jak2, pJak2 (**d**). In turn, pJak2 and these yet uncharacterized factors exacerbate anemia, leading to even higher Epo levels and increasing levels of IE (**e**)

IE seems to be one of the primary mechanisms leading to iron overload; however, the relationship between IE, iron absorption, and iron deposition needs further explanation in light of some previous as well as more recent observations. Past observations indicate that iron deficiency is very common among non-transfused patients with sickle cell anemia [195, 196], while more recent observations challenge the notion of IE in SCA [56]. Although premature destruction or elimination of abnormal non-nucleated erythroid cells (e.g., hemolytic anemia and phagocytosis) [197] and death of erythroid precursors by apoptosis have normally been considered almost exclusively the causes that lead to IE, new studies indicate that limited erythroid cell differentiation may also contribute [56].

Ferrokinetic studies led to the introduction of the concept of IE. According to this model of IE, iron is rapidly absorbed by the bone marrow in patients affected by the disease, but is then slowly released into the circulation due to death of the erythroid cells in this organ. In beta-thalassemia patients, measurements predict that 80% of the erythroid precursors would die in the bone marrow [65]. However, subsequent studies have indicated that the percentage of apoptotic cells is much lower than the value predicted, although apoptosis is increased compared to normal individuals [198]. Mice affected by beta-thalassemia also exhibit a relatively small increase in apoptosis of their erythroid cells compared to normal mice. This was attributed to a greater than normal percentage of erythroid cells in S-phase, exhibiting an erythroblast-like morphology. Thalassemic cells were associated with the expression of cell cycle–promoting genes such as EpoR, Jak2, Cyclin-A, Cdk2, Ki-67, and the anti-apoptotic protein Bcl-X_L. They also differentiated less than normal cells in vitro. Jak2 was partially responsible for limited cell differentiation, since administration of a Jak2 inhibitor to thalassemic mice decreased spleen size with limited effect on anemia. While these data do not exclude a role for apoptosis in IE, it has been proposed that expansion of the erythroid pool followed by limited cell differentiation exacerbates IE in thalassemia (Fig. 16.2). Apart from the message that Jak2 inhibitors have the potential to limit splenomegaly and hence the necessity for splenectomy in this disorder, this study indicates that the percentage of expected cell death in bone marrow may be less than anticipated.

If this scenario is correct, depending on the level of IE, a certain proportion of the absorbed iron in thalassemia would not be utilized for erythropoiesis, but rather diverted directly toward storage in

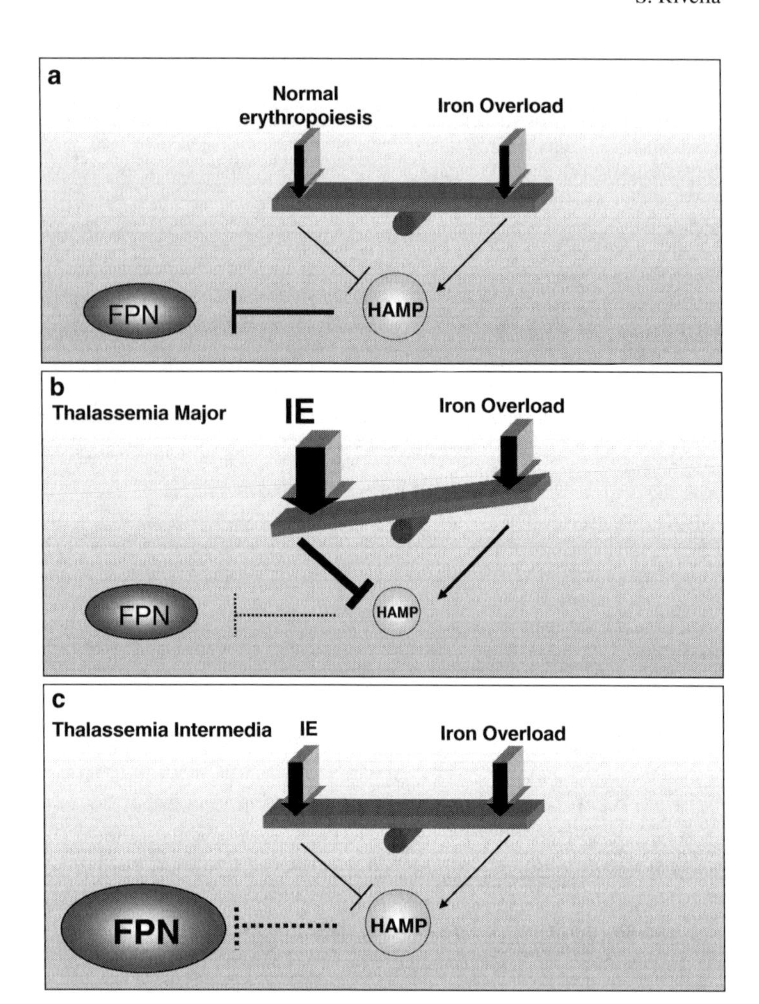

Fig. 16.3 Schematic representation of iron absorption in beta-thalassemia intermedia and major. Under normal conditions, hepcidin controls the amount of ferroportin in the duodenum so as to maintain iron balance (**a**). In mice affected by thalassemia, iron homeostasis is mediated by the relative amount of hepcidin mRNA synthesized in the liver and ferroportin produced in the duodenum. In conditions of severe IE, such as in beta-thalassemia major, the levels of hepcidin are extremely low (**b**). In beta-thalassemia intermedia the amount of hepcidin is similar to that observed in normal mice. However, the amount of ferroportin is increased in the duodenum (**c**). The dotted line indicates that no correlation has been investigated between the levels of hepcidin mRNA in the liver and the protein secreted into the bloodstream, which may be reduced in conditions of IE

the liver [154]. In particular, *th3/th3* mice exhibited extremely high levels of transferrin saturation (>95%), total serum iron, and non-transferrin bound iron (5 and 6 times higher than control animals). They also have more iron in the parenchymal cells of their livers and much less in Kupffer cells and their spleens compared to animals with lower levels of anemia. Low levels of iron were observed in the BM of both *th3/+* and *th3/th3* mice. These observations suggest that the iron absorbed in response to IE might exceed the amount required for erythropoiesis and be transported directly into the liver for storage. Therefore, an alternative explanation for the original ferrokinetic studies could be that a portion of the iron administered to patients affected by IE would be taken up by liver parenchymal cells rather than be utilized by erythroid cells. As a consequence, in the ferrokinetic studies, the iron "missing" from the circulation would not necessarily translate into apoptosis of the red cells. This scenario does not negate the role of apoptosis in IE, but rather introduces the notion that reduced erythroid differentiation also limits the production of mature red cells in beta-thalassemia.

Another consequence of this scenario is that while the iron levels observed in *th3/th3* mice would trigger an elevated production of hepcidin under normal conditions (Fig. 16.3b), the extreme level of IE in these animals prevents hepcidin from sensing the iron burden and keeps its expression very low. In *th3/+* mice, which have a lower erythropoietic drive than *th3/th3* mice, hepcidin expression is likely to be determined by the relative ratio between anemia and iron overload, which varies with age and the relative synthesis of ferroportin in the duodenum (Fig. 16.3c).

4 Summary

Future studies should address whether abnormal iron absorption could be prevented by administration of hepcidin. Mouse models of beta-thalassemia and SCD could be utilized as a first step. In addition, the use of Jak2 inhibitors may be of value in limiting IE and, consequently, abnormal iron absorption. Anemia and iron metabolism will need to be carefully monitored. However, the decreased levels of hepcidin observed in the urine of thalassemic patients [175] and the lack of alternatives to splenectomy indicate that such therapeutic approaches are worth investigating for their potential to reduce iron overload and IE in thalassemia and other hemoglobinopathies.

References

1. Pasternack A, Wahlberg P. Bone marrow in acute renal failure. Acta Med Scand. 1967;181:505–11.
2. Iseki K, Kohagura K. Anemia as a risk factor for chronic kidney disease. Kidney Int Suppl. 2007;72:S4–9.
3. Horl WH. Clinical aspects of iron use in the anemia of kidney disease. J Am Soc Nephrol. 2007;18:382–93.
4. Horl WH. Iron therapy for renal anemia: how much needed, how much harmful? Pediatr Nephrol. 2007;22:480–9.
5. Evans RW, Rader B, Manninen DL. The quality of life of hemodialysis recipients treated with recombinant human erythropoietin. Cooperative multicenter EPO clinical trial group. J Am Med Assoc. 1990;263:825–30.
6. Locatelli F, Aljama P, Barany P, et al. Revised European best practice guidelines for the management of anaemia in patients with chronic renal failure. Nephrol Dial Transplant. 2004;19 Suppl 2:ii1–47.
7. Brugnara C. Iron deficiency and erythropoiesis: new diagnostic approaches. Clin Chem. 2003;49:1573–8.
8. Chiang WC, Tsai TJ, Chen YM, Lin SL, Hsieh BS. Serum soluble transferrin receptor reflects erythropoiesis but not iron availability in erythropoietin-treated chronic hemodialysis patients. Clin Nephrol. 2002;58:363–9.
9. Macdougall IC, Cavill I, Hulme B, et al. Detection of functional iron deficiency during erythropoietin treatment: a new approach. Br Med J. 1992;304:225–6.
10. Bovy C, Gothot A, Delanaye P, Warling X, Krzesinski JM, Beguin Y. Mature erythrocyte parameters as new markers of functional iron deficiency in haemodialysis: sensitivity and specificity. Nephrol Dial Transplant. 2007;22:1156–62.
11. Chuang CL, Liu RS, Wei YH, Huang TP, Tarng DC. Early prediction of response to intravenous iron supplementation by reticulocyte haemoglobin content and high-fluorescence reticulocyte count in haemodialysis patients. Nephrol Dial Transplant. 2003;18:370–7.
12. Brugnara C, Schiller B, Moran J. Reticulocyte hemoglobin equivalent (Ret He) and assessment of iron-deficient states. Clin Lab Haematol. 2006;28:303–8.
13. Kim JM, Ihm CH, Kim HJ. Evaluation of reticulocyte haemoglobin content as marker of iron deficiency and predictor of response to intravenous iron in haemodialysis patients. Int J Lab Hematol. 2008;30:46–52.
14. Kimmel PL, Phillips TM, Simmens SJ, et al. Immunologic function and survival in hemodialysis patients. Kidney Int. 1998;54:236–44.
15. Bergstrom J, Lindholm B, Lacson Jr E, et al. What are the causes and consequences of the chronic inflammatory state in chronic dialysis patients? Semin Dial. 2000;13:163–75.
16. Kaysen GA. The microinflammatory state in uremia: causes and potential consequences. J Am Soc Nephrol. 2001;12:1549–57.
17. Macdougall IC, Cooper AC. Hyporesponsiveness to erythropoietic therapy due to chronic inflammation. Eur J Clin Invest. 2005;35 Suppl 3:32–5.
18. Roy CN, Andrews NC. Anemia of inflammation: the hepcidin link. Curr Opin Hematol. 2005;12:107–11.
19. Roy CN, Mak HH, Akpan I, Losyev G, Zurakowski D, Andrews NC. Hepcidin antimicrobial peptide transgenic mice exhibit features of the anemia of inflammation. Blood. 2007;109:4038–44.
20. Wrighting DM, Andrews NC. Interleukin-6 induces hepcidin expression through STAT3. Blood. 2006;108:3204–9.
21. Pietrangelo A, Dierssen U, Valli L, et al. STAT3 is required for IL-6-gp130-dependent activation of hepcidin in vivo. Gastroenterology. 2007;132:294–300.
22. Verga Falzacappa MV, Vujic Spasic M, Kessler R, Stolte J, Hentze MW, Muckenthaler MU. STAT3 mediates hepatic hepcidin expression and its inflammatory stimulation. Blood. 2007;109:353–8.
23. Weizer-Stern O, Adamsky K, Margalit O, et al. Hepcidin, a key regulator of iron metabolism, is transcriptionally activated by p53. Br J Haematol. 2007;138:253–62.

24. Angelillo-Scherrer A, Burnier L, Lambrechts D, et al. Role of Gas6 in erythropoiesis and anemia in mice. J Clin Invest. 2008;118:583–96.
25. Theurl I, Mattle V, Seifert M, Mariani M, Marth C, Weiss G. Dysregulated monocyte iron homeostasis and erythropoietin formation in patients with anemia of chronic disease. Blood. 2006;107:4142–8.
26. Theurl I, Theurl M, Seifert M, et al. Autocrine formation of hepcidin induces iron retention in human monocytes. Blood. 2008;111:2392–9.
27. Dallalio G, Law E, Means Jr RT. Hepcidin inhibits in vitro erythroid colony formation at reduced erythropoietin concentrations. Blood. 2006;107:2702–4.
28. Deicher R, Horl WH. Hepcidin: a molecular link between inflammation and anaemia. Nephrol Dial Transplant. 2004;19:521–4.
29. Besarab A. Evaluating iron sufficiency: a clearer view. Kidney Int. 2001;60:2412–4.
30. KDOQI clinical practice guidelines and clinical practice recommendations for anemia in chronic kidney disease. Am J Kidney Dis 2006;47:S11–145.
31. Weiss G, Goodnough LT. Anemia of chronic disease. N Engl J Med. 2005;352:1011–23.
32. Winn RJ. The NCCN guidelines development process and infrastructure. Oncology. 2000;14:26–30.
33. Rizzo JD, Lichtin AE, Woolf SH, et al. Use of epoetin in patients with cancer: evidence-based clinical practice guidelines of the American Society of Clinical Oncology and the American Society of Hematology. Blood. 2002;100:2303–20.
34. van der Putten K, Braam B, Jie KE, Gaillard CA. Mechanisms of disease: erythropoietin resistance in patients with both heart and kidney failure. Nat Clin Pract Nephrol. 2008;4:47–57.
35. Casadevall N, Nataf J, Viron B, et al. Pure red-cell aplasia and antierythropoietin antibodies in patients treated with recombinant erythropoietin. N Engl J Med. 2002;346:469–75.
36. Bunn HF. Drug-induced autoimmune red-cell aplasia. N Engl J Med. 2002;346:522–3.
37. Macdougall IC. Adverse event issue management: what have we learnt from pure red cell aplasia (PRCA)? Nephrol Dial Transplant. 2005;20 Suppl 8:viii18–21.
38. Macdougall IC. Antibody-mediated pure red cell aplasia (PRCA): epidemiology, immunogenicity and risks. Nephrol Dial Transplant. 2005;20 Suppl 4:iv9–15.
39. Pollock C, Johnson DW, Horl WH, et al. Pure red cell aplasia induced by erythropoiesis-stimulating agents. Clin J Am Soc Nephrol. 2008;3:193–9.
40. Brodsky RA, Jones RJ. Aplastic anaemia. Lancet. 2005;365:1647–56.
41. Marsh J. Making therapeutic decisions in adults with aplastic anemia. Hematology Am Soc Hematol Educ Program 2006:78–85.
42. Testa U. Apoptotic mechanisms in the control of erythropoiesis. Leukemia. 2004;18:1176–99.
43. Li X, Le Beau MM, Ciccone S, et al. Ex vivo culture of Fancc–/– stem/progenitor cells predisposes cells to undergo apoptosis, and surviving stem/progenitor cells display cytogenetic abnormalities and an increased risk of malignancy. Blood. 2005;105:3465–71.
44. Dufour C, Corcione A, Svahn J, et al. TNF-alpha and IFN-gamma are overexpressed in the bone marrow of Fanconi anemia patients and TNF-alpha suppresses erythropoiesis in vitro. Blood. 2003;102:2053–9.
45. Li J, Sejas DP, Zhang X, et al. TNF-alpha induces leukemic clonal evolution ex vivo in Fanconi anemia group C murine stem cells. J Clin Invest. 2007;117:3283–95.
46. Bijangi-Vishehsaraei K, Saadatzadeh MR, Werne A, et al. Enhanced TNF-alpha-induced apoptosis in Fanconi anemia type C-deficient cells is dependent on apoptosis signal-regulating kinase 1. Blood. 2005;106:4124–30.
47. Killick SB, Cox CV, Marsh JC, Gordon-Smith EC, Gibson FM. Mechanisms of bone marrow progenitor cell apoptosis in aplastic anaemia and the effect of anti-thymocyte globulin: examination of the role of the Fas-Fas-L interaction. Br J Haematol. 2000;111:1164–9.
48. Killick SB, Marsh JC. Aplastic anaemia: management. Blood Rev. 2000;14:157–71.
49. Alter BP. Diagnosis, genetics, and management of inherited bone marrow failure syndromes. Hematology (Am Soc Hematol Educ Program). 2007;2007:29–39.
50. Ohara A, Kojima S, Hamajima N, et al. Myelodysplastic syndrome and acute myelogenous leukemia as a late clonal complication in children with acquired aplastic anemia. Blood. 1997;90:1009–13.
51. Araten DJ, Nafa K, Pakdeesuwan K, Luzzatto L. Clonal populations of hematopoietic cells with paroxysmal nocturnal hemoglobinuria genotype and phenotype are present in normal individuals. Proc Natl Acad Sci USA. 1999;96:5209–14.
52. Young NS, Scheinberg P, Calado RT. Aplastic anemia. Curr Opin Hematol. 2008;15:162–8.
53. Young NS, Calado RT, Scheinberg P. Current concepts in the pathophysiology and treatment of aplastic anemia. Blood. 2006;108:2509–19.
54. Vichinsky E, Pakbaz Z, Onyekwere O, et al. Patient-reported outcomes of deferasirox (Exjade(R), ICL670) versus deferoxamine in sickle cell disease patients with transfusional hemosiderosis. Substudy of a randomized open-label phase II trial. Acta Haematol. 2008;119:133–41.

55. Porter J, Galanello R, Saglio G, et al. Relative response of patients with myelodysplastic syndromes and other transfusion-dependent anaemias to deferasirox (ICL670): a 1-yr prospective study. Eur J Haematol. 2008;80:168–76.
56. Libani IV, Guy EC, Melchiori L, et al. Decreased differentiation of erythroid cells exacerbates ineffective erythropoiesis in beta-thalassemia. Blood. 2008;112:875–85.
57. Huff RL, Hennessy TG, Austin RE, Garcia JF, Roberts BM, Lawrence JH. Plasma and red cell iron turnover in normal subjects and in patients having various hematopoietic disorders. J Clin Invest. 1950;29:1041–52.
58. Huff RL, Elmlinger PJ, Garcia JF, Oda JM, Cockrell MC, Lawrence JH. Ferrokinetics in normal persons and in patients having various erythropoietic disorders. J Clin Invest. 1951;30:1512–26.
59. Finch CA, Sturgeon P. Erythrokinetics in Cooley's anemia. Blood. 1957;12:64–73.
60. Cazzola M, Finch CA. Evaluation of erythroid marrow function in anemic patients. Haematologica. 1987;72:195–200.
61. Cazzola M, Pootrakul P, Huebers HA, Eng M, Eschbach J, Finch CA. Erythroid marrow function in anemic patients. Blood. 1987;69:296–301.
62. Pootrakul P, Huebers HA, Finch CA, Pippard MJ, Cazzola M. Iron metabolism in thalassemia. Birth Defects Orig Artic Ser. 1988;23:3–8.
63. Cazzola M, Finch CA. Iron balance in thalassemia. Prog Clin Biol Res. 1989;309:93–100.
64. Pootrakul P, Kitcharoen K, Yansukon P, et al. The effect of erythroid hyperplasia on iron balance. Blood. 1988;71:1124–9.
65. Finch CA, Deubelbeiss K, Cook JD, et al. Ferrokinetics in man. Medicine. 1970;49:17–53.
66. Koury MJ, Price JO, Hicks GG. Apoptosis in megaloblastic anemia occurs during DNA synthesis by a p53-independent, nucleoside-reversible mechanism. Blood. 2000;96:3249–55.
67. Herbert V, Zalusky R. Interrelations of vitamin B12 and folic acid metabolism: folic acid clearance studies. J Clin Invest. 1962;41:1263–76.
68. Koury MJ, Horne DW. Apoptosis mediates and thymidine prevents erythroblast destruction in folate deficiency anemia. Proc Natl Acad Sci USA. 1994;91:4067–71.
69. Koury MJ, Horne DW, Brown ZA, et al. Apoptosis of late-stage erythroblasts in megaloblastic anemia: association with DNA damage and macrocyte production. Blood. 1997;89:4617–23.
70. Hamilton HE, Sheets RF, De GE, Dahlin RE. Studies with inagglutinable erythrocyte counts; analysis of mechanism of Cooley's anemia. J Clin Invest. 1950;29:714–22.
71. Heller P, Weinstein HG, West M, Zimmerman HJ. Enzymes in anemia: a study of abnormalities of several enzymes of carbohvdrate metabolism in the plasma and erythrocytes in patients with anemia, with preliminary observations of bone marrow enzymes. Ann Intern Med. 1960;53:898–913.
72. Lindahl J. Quantification of ineffective erythropoiesis in megaloblastic anaemia by determination of endogenous production of 14CO after administration of glycine-2-14C. Scand J Haematol. 1980;24:281–91.
73. Dudley 3rd GM, Coltman Jr CA. Resolution of ineffective erythropoiesis of pernicious anemia and "strongly suggestive" folate lack in response to folic acid. Am J Clin Nutr. 1970;23:147–55.
74. Emerson PM, Wilkinson JH. Lactate dehydrogenase in the diagnosis and assessment of response to treatment of megaloblastic anaemia. Br J Haematol. 1966;12:678–88.
75. Bills ND, Koury MJ, Clifford AJ, Dessypris EN. Ineffective hematopoiesis in folate-deficient mice. Blood. 1992;79:2273–80.
76. Kelley LL, Green WF, Hicks GG, Bondurant MC, Koury MJ, Ruley HE. Apoptosis in erythroid progenitors deprived of erythropoietin occurs during the G1 and S phases of the cell cycle without growth arrest or stabilization of wild-type p53. Mol Cell Biol. 1994;14:4183–92.
77. Lin HL, Chen CJ, Tsai WC, Yen JH, Liu HW. In vitro folate deficiency induces apoptosis by a p53, Fas (Apo-1, CD95) independent, bcl-2 related mechanism in phytohaemagglutinin-stimulated human peripheral blood lymphocytes. Br J Nutr. 2006;95:870–8.
78. Stenman UH, Simons K, Grasbeck R. Vitamin B 12-binding proteins in normal and leukemic human leukocytes and sera. Scand J Clin Lab Invest. 1968;21:202–10.
79. Alperin JB, Hutchinson HT, Levin WC. Studies of folic acid requirements in megaloblastic anemia of pregnancy. Arch Intern Med. 1966;117:681–8.
80. Ramsahoye BH, Burnett AK, Taylor C. Nucleic acid composition of bone marrow mononuclear cells in cobalamin deficiency. Blood. 1996;87:2065–70.
81. Ren J, Ulvik A, Refsum H, Ueland PM. Uracil in human DNA from subjects with normal and impaired folate status as determined by high-performance liquid chromatography–tandem mass spectrometry. Anal Chem. 2002;74:295–9.
82. Koury MJ, Ponka P. New insights into erythropoiesis: the roles of folate, vitamin B12, and iron. Annu Rev Nutr. 2004;24:105–31.
83. Garcia SC, Moragon AC, Lopez-Fernandez ME. Frequency of glutathione reductase, pyruvate kinase and glucose-6-phosphate dehydrogenase deficiency in a Spanish population. Hum Hered. 1979;29:310–3.

84. Abu-Melha AM, Ahmed MA, Knox-Macaulay H, Al-Sowayan SA, el-Yahia A. Erythrocyte pyruvate kinase deficiency in newborns of eastern Saudi Arabia. Acta Haematol. 1991;85:192–4.
85. Mohrenweiser HW, Fielek S. Elevated frequency of carriers for triosephosphate isomerase deficiency in newborn infants. Pediatr Res. 1982;16:960–3.
86. Mohrenweiser HW. Functional hemizygosity in the human genome: direct estimate from twelve erythrocyte enzyme loci. Hum Genet. 1987;77:241–5.
87. Salem HH, Van Der Weyden MB, Firkin BG. Iron overload in congenital erythrocyte pyruvate kinase deficiency. Med J Aust. 1980;1:531–2.
88. Zanella A, Fermo E, Bianchi P, Valentini G. Red cell pyruvate kinase deficiency: molecular and clinical aspects. Br J Haematol. 2005;130:11–25.
89. Chou R, DeLoughery TG. Recurrent thromboembolic disease following splenectomy for pyruvate kinase deficiency. Am J Hematol. 2001;67:197–9.
90. Andersen FD, d'Amore F, Nielsen FC, van Solinge W, Jensen F, Jensen PD. Unexpectedly high but still asymptomatic iron overload in a patient with pyruvate kinase deficiency. Hematol J. 2004;5:543–5.
91. Zanella A, Berzuini A, Colombo MB, et al. Iron status in red cell pyruvate kinase deficiency: study of Italian cases. Br J Haematol. 1993;83:485–90.
92. Pawliuk R, Westerman KA, Fabry ME, et al. Correction of sickle cell disease in transgenic mouse models by gene therapy. Science. 2001;294:2368–71.
93. Rivella S, May C, Chadburn A, Riviere I, Sadelain M. A novel murine model of Cooley anemia and its rescue by lentiviral-mediated human beta-globin gene transfer. Blood. 2003;101:2932–9.
94. Tani K, Yoshikubo T, Ikebuchi K, et al. Retrovirus-mediated gene transfer of human pyruvate kinase (PK) cDNA into murine hematopoietic cells: implications for gene therapy of human PK deficiency. Blood. 1994;83:2305–10.
95. Kanno H, Utsugisawa T, Aizawa S, et al. Transgenic rescue of hemolytic anemia due to red blood cell pyruvate kinase deficiency. Haematologica. 2007;92:731–7.
96. Kanno H, Fujii H, Wei DC, et al. Frame shift mutation, exon skipping, and a two-codon deletion caused by splice site mutations account for pyruvate kinase deficiency. Blood. 1997;89:4213–8.
97. Napier I, Ponka P, Richardson DR. Iron trafficking in the mitochondrion: novel pathways revealed by disease. Blood. 2005;105:1867–74.
98. Bottomley SS. Congenital sideroblastic anemias. Curr Hematol Rep. 2006;5:41–9.
99. Fontenay M, Cathelin S, Amiot M, Gyan E, Solary E. Mitochondria in hematopoiesis and hematological diseases. Oncogene. 2006;25:4757–67.
100. Zermati Y, Garrido C, Amsellem S, et al. Caspase activation is required for terminal erythroid differentiation. J Exp Med. 2001;193:247–54.
101. Kolbus A, Pilat S, Husak Z, et al. Raf-1 antagonizes erythroid differentiation by restraining caspase activation. J Exp Med. 2002;196:1347–53.
102. Sharp RA, Lowe JG, Johnston RN. Anti-tuberculous drugs and sideroblastic anaemia. Br J Clin Pract. 1990;44:706–7.
103. Hines JD, Grasso JA. The sideroblastic anemias. Semin Hematol. 1970;7:86–106.
104. Harriss EB, Macgibbon BH, Mollin DL. Experimental sideroblastic anaemia. Br J Haematol. 1965;11:99–106.
105. Verwilghen R, Reybrouck G, Callens L, Cosemans J. Antituberculous drugs and sideroblastic anaemia. Br J Haematol. 1965;11:92–8.
106. Wells RA, Leber B, Buckstein R, et al. Iron overload in myelodysplastic syndromes: a Canadian consensus guideline. Leuk Res. 2008;32:1338–53.
107. Ghoti H, Amer J, Winder A, Rachmilewitz E, Fibach E. Oxidative stress in red blood cells, platelets and polymorphonuclear leukocytes from patients with myelodysplastic syndrome. Eur J Haematol. 2007;79:463–7.
108. Metzgeroth G, Rosee PL, Kuhn C, et al. The soluble transferrin receptor in dysplastic erythropoiesis in myelodysplastic syndrome. Eur J Haematol. 2007;79:8–16.
109. Mahesh S, Ginzburg Y, Verma A. Iron overload in myelodysplastic syndromes. Leuk Lymphoma. 2008;49:427–38.
110. Winder A, Lefkowitz R, Ghoti H, et al. Urinary hepcidin excretion in patients with myelodysplastic syndrome and myelofibrosis. Br J Haematol. 2008;142:669–71.
111. Cox TC, Bottomley SS, Wiley JS, Bawden MJ, Matthews CS, May BK. X-linked pyridoxine-responsive sideroblastic anemia due to a Thr388-to-Ser substitution in erythroid 5-aminolevulinate synthase. N Engl J Med. 1994;330:675–9.
112. Cotter PD, May A, Li L, et al. Four new mutations in the erythroid-specific 5-aminolevulinate synthase (ALAS2) gene causing X-linked sideroblastic anemia: increased pyridoxine responsiveness after removal of iron overload by phlebotomy and coinheritance of hereditary hemochromatosis. Blood. 1999;93:1757–69.
113. Furuyama K, Fujita H, Nagai T, et al. Pyridoxine refractory X-linked sideroblastic anemia caused by a point mutation in the erythroid 5-aminolevulinate synthase gene. Blood. 1997;90:822–30.
114. Furuyama K, Sassa S. Interaction between succinyl CoA synthetase and the heme-biosynthetic enzyme ALAS-E is disrupted in sideroblastic anemia. J Clin Invest. 2000;105:757–64.

115. Astner I, Schulze JO, van den Heuvel J, Jahn D, Schubert WD, Heinz DW. Crystal structure of 5-aminolevulinate synthase, the first enzyme of heme biosynthesis, and its link to XLSA in humans. EMBO J. 2005;24:3166–77.
116. Nakajima O, Takahashi S, Harigae H, et al. Heme deficiency in erythroid lineage causes differentiation arrest and cytoplasmic iron overload. EMBO J. 1999;18:6282–9.
117. Yamamoto M, Nakajima O. Animal models for X-linked sideroblastic anemia. Int J Hematol. 2000;72:157–64.
118. Nakajima O, Okano S, Harada H, et al. Transgenic rescue of erythroid 5-aminolevulinate synthase-deficient mice results in the formation of ring sideroblasts and siderocytes. Genes Cells. 2006;11:685–700.
119. Wingert RA, Galloway JL, Barut B, et al. Deficiency of glutaredoxin 5 reveals Fe-S clusters are required for vertebrate haem synthesis. Nature. 2005;436:1035–9.
120. Hentze MW, Kuhn LC. Molecular control of vertebrate iron metabolism: mRNA-based regulatory circuits operated by iron, nitric oxide, and oxidative stress. Proc Natl Acad Sci USA. 1996;93:8175–82.
121. Camaschella C, Campanella A, De Falco L, et al. The human counterpart of zebrafish shiraz shows sideroblastic-like microcytic anemia and iron overload. Blood. 2007;110:1353–8.
122. Peto TE, Pippard MJ, Weatherall DJ. Iron overload in mild sideroblastic anaemias. Lancet. 1983;1:375–8.
123. Nearman ZP, Szpurka H, Serio B, et al. Hemochromatosis-associated gene mutations in patients with myelodysplastic syndromes with refractory anemia with ringed sideroblasts. Am J Hematol. 2007;82:1076–9.
124. Steinberg MH, Forget BG, Higgs DR, Nagel RL. Disorders of hemoglobin: genetics, pathophysiology and clinical management. Cambridge: Cambridge University Press; 2001.
125. Weatherall DJ, Clegg JB. Inherited haemoglobin disorders: an increasing global health problem. Bull World Health Organ. 2001;79:704–12.
126. Pippard MJ, Callender ST, Warner GT, Weatherall DJ. Iron absorption and loading in beta-thalassaemia intermedia. Lancet. 1979;2:819–21.
127. Pippard MJ, Callender ST, Finch CA. Ferrioxamine excretion in iron-loaded man. Blood. 1982;60:288–94.
128. Rachmilewitz EA, Weizer-Stern O, Adamsky K, et al. Role of iron in inducing oxidative stress in thalassemia: can it be prevented by inhibition of absorption and by antioxidants? Ann N Y Acad Sci. 2005;1054:118–23.
129. Esposito BP, Breuer W, Sirankapracha P, Pootrakul P, Hershko C, Cabantchik ZI. Labile plasma iron in iron overload: redox activity and susceptibility to chelation. Blood. 2003;102:2670–7.
130. Pootrakul P, Breuer W, Sametband M, Sirankapracha P, Hershko C, Cabantchik ZI. Labile plasma iron (LPI) as an indicator of chelatable plasma redox activity in iron-overloaded beta-thalassemia/HbE patients treated with an oral chelator. Blood. 2004;104:1504–10.
131. Chua AC, Olynyk JK, Leedman PJ, Trinder D. Nontransferrin-bound iron uptake by hepatocytes is increased in the Hfe knockout mouse model of hereditary hemochromatosis. Blood. 2004;104:1519–25.
132. Baker E, Baker SM, Morgan EH. Characterisation of non-transferrin-bound iron (ferric citrate) uptake by rat hepatocytes in culture. Biochim Biophys Acta. 1998;1380:21–30.
133. Liuzzi JP, Lichten LA, Rivera S, et al. Interleukin-6 regulates the zinc transporter Zip14 in liver and contributes to the hypozincemia of the acute-phase response. Proc Natl Acad Sci USA. 2005;102:6843–8.
134. Liuzzi JP, Aydemir F, Nam H, Knutson MD, Cousins RJ. Zip14 (Slc39a14) mediates non-transferrin-bound iron uptake into cells. Proc Natl Acad Sci USA. 2006;103:13612–7.
135. Roudkenar MH, Halabian R, Oodi A, et al. Upregulation of neutrophil gelatinase-associated lipocalin, NGAL/Lcn2, in beta-thalassemia patients. Arch Med Res. 2008;39:402–7.
136. Schmidt-Ott KM, Mori K, Li JY, et al. Dual action of neutrophil gelatinase-associated lipocalin. J Am Soc Nephrol. 2007;18:407–13.
137. Oudit GY, Sun H, Trivieri MG, et al. L-type Ca2+ channels provide a major pathway for iron entry into cardiomyocytes in iron-overload cardiomyopathy. Nat Med. 2003;9:1187–94.
138. Olivieri NF. Progression of iron overload in sickle cell disease. Semin Hematol. 2001;38:57–62.
139. Olivieri NF, Weatherall DJ. Clinical aspects of beta-thalassemia. In: Steinberg MH, Forget BG, Higgs DR, Nagel RL, editors. Disorders of hemoglobin: genetics, pathophysiology and clinical management. Cambridge: Cambridge University Press; 2001. p. 277–341.
140. Propper RD, Cooper B, Rufo RR, et al. Continuous subcutaeneous administration of deferoxamine in patients with iron overload. N Engl J Med. 1977;297:418–23.
141. Berdoukas V, Bohane T, Tobias V, et al. Liver iron concentration and fibrosis in a cohort of transfusion-dependent patients on long-term desferrioxamine therapy. Hematol J. 2005;5:572–8.
142. Thursz M. Iron, haemochromatosis and thalassaemia as risk factors for fibrosis in hepatitis C virus infection. Gut. 2007;56:613–4.
143. Taher A, Aoun E, Sharara AI, et al. Five-year trial of deferiprone chelation therapy in thalassaemia major patients. Acta Haematol. 2004;112:179–83.
144. Taher A. Iron overload in thalassemia and sickle cell disease. Semin Hematol. 2005;42:S5–9.
145. Vichinsky E, Butensky E, Fung E, et al. Comparison of organ dysfunction in transfused patients with SCD or beta thalassemia. Am J Hematol. 2005;80:70–4.

146. Rivella S, Sadelain M. Therapeutic globin gene delivery using lentiviral vectors. Curr Opin Mol Ther. 2002;4:505–14.
147. Ciavatta DJ, Ryan TM, Farmer SC, Townes TM. Mouse model of human beta zero thalassemia: targeted deletion of the mouse beta maj- and beta min-globin genes in embryonic stem cells. Proc Natl Acad Sci USA. 1995;92:9259–63.
148. Yang B, Kirby S, Lewis J, Detloff PJ, Maeda N, Smithies O. A mouse model for beta 0-thalassemia. Proc Natl Acad Sci USA. 1995;92:11608–12.
149. Imren S, Payen E, Westerman KA, et al. Permanent and panerythroid correction of murine beta thalassemia by multiple lentiviral integration in hematopoietic stem cells. Proc Natl Acad Sci USA. 2002;99:14380–5.
150. Persons DA, Allay ER, Sawai N, et al. Successful treatment of murine beta-thalassemia using in vivo selection of genetically-modified, drug-resistant hematopoietic stem cells. Blood. 2003;102:506–13.
151. Hanawa H, Persons DA, Nienhuis AW. High-level erythroid lineage-directed gene expression using globin gene regulatory elements after lentiviral vector-mediated gene transfer into primitive human and murine hematopoietic cells. Hum Gene Ther. 2002;13:2007–16.
152. Samakoglu S, Lisowski L, Budak-Alpdogan T, et al. A genetic strategy to treat sickle cell anemia by coregulating globin transgene expression and RNA interference. Nat Biotechnol. 2006;24:89–94.
153. Puthenveetil G, Scholes J, Carbonell D, et al. Successful correction of the human beta-thalassemia major phenotype using a lentiviral vector. Blood. 2004;104:3445–53.
154. Gardenghi S, Marongiu MF, Ramos P, et al. Ineffective erythropoiesis in beta-thalassemia is characterized by increased iron absorption mediated by down-regulation of hepcidin and up-regulation of ferroportin. Blood. 2007;109:5027–35.
155. Rees DC, Williams TN, Maitland K, Clegg JB, Weatherall DJ. Alpha thalassaemia is associated with increased soluble transferrin receptor levels. Br J Haematol. 1998;103:365–9.
156. Sohan K, Billington M, Pamphilon D, Goulden N, Kyle P. Normal growth and development following in utero diagnosis and treatment of homozygous alpha-thalassaemia. Br J Obstet Gynecol. 2002;109:1308–10.
157. Celada A. Iron overload in a non-transfused patient with thalassaemia intermedia. Scand J Haematol. 1982;28:169–74.
158. Bannerman RM, Keusch G, Kreimer-Birnbaum M, Vance VK, Vaughan S. Thalassemia intermedia, with iron overload, cardiac failure, diabetes mellitus, hypopituitarism and porphyrinuria. Am J Med. 1967;42:476–86.
159. Cossu P, Toccafondi C, Vardeu F, et al. Iron overload and desferrioxamine chelation therapy in beta-thalassemia intermedia. Eur J Pediatr. 1981;137:267–71.
160. Fiorelli G, Fargion S, Piperno A, Battafarano N, Cappellini MD. Iron metabolism in thalassemia intermedia. Haematologica. 1990;75:89–95.
161. Piperno A, Mariani R, Arosio C, et al. Haemochromatosis in patients with beta-thalassaemia trait. Br J Haematol. 2000;111:908–14.
162. Hershko C, Rachmilewitz EA. Mechanism of desferrioxamine-induced iron excretion in thalassaemia. Br J Haematol. 1979;42:125–32.
163. Erlandson ME, Walden B, Stern G, Hilgartner MW, Wehman J, Smith CH. Studies on congenital hemolytic syndromes, IV. Gastrointestinal absorption of iron. Blood. 1962;19:359–78.
164. Fleming RE, Sly WS. Hepcidin: a putative iron-regulatory hormone relevant to hereditary hemochromatosis and the anemia of chronic disease. Proc Natl Acad Sci USA. 2001;98:8160–2.
165. Nicolas G, Bennoun M, Devaux I, et al. Lack of hepcidin gene expression and severe tissue iron overload in upstream stimulatory factor 2 (USF2) knockout mice. Proc Natl Acad Sci USA. 2001;98:8780–5.
166. Pigeon C, Ilyin G, Courselaud B, et al. A new mouse liver-specific gene, encoding a protein homologous to human antimicrobial peptide hepcidin, is overexpressed during iron overload. J Biol Chem. 2001;276:7811–9.
167. Nicolas G, Chauvet C, Viatte L, et al. The gene encoding the iron regulatory peptide hepcidin is regulated by anemia, hypoxia, and inflammation. J Clin Invest. 2002;110:1037–44.
168. Finch C. Regulators of iron balance in humans. Blood. 1994;84:1697–702.
169. Ganz T. Hepcidin – a peptide hormone at the interface of innate immunity and iron metabolism. Curr Top Microbiol Immunol. 2006;306:183–98.
170. De Domenico I, Ward DM, Langelier C, et al. The molecular mechanism of hepcidin-mediated ferroportin down-regulation. Mol Biol Cell. 2007;18:2569–78.
171. Nemeth E, Preza GC, Jung CL, Kaplan J, Waring AJ, Ganz T. The N-terminus of hepcidin is essential for its interaction with ferroportin: structure–function study. Blood. 2006;107:328–33.
172. Paradkar P, De Domenico I, Durchfort N, Zohn I, Kaplan J, Ward DM. Iron-depletion limits intracellular bacterial growth in macrophages. Blood. 2008;112:866–74.
173. Kattamis A, Papassotiriou I, Palaiologou D, et al. The effects of erythropoetic activity and iron burden on hepcidin expression in patients with thalassemia major. Haematologica. 2006;91:809–12.
174. Kearney SL, Nemeth E, Neufeld EJ, et al. Urinary hepcidin in congenital chronic anemias. Pediatr Blood Cancer. 2007;48:57–63.

175. Papanikolaou G, Tzilianos M, Christakis JI, et al. Hepcidin in iron overload disorders. Blood. 2005;105:4103–5.
176. Origa R, Galanello R, Ganz T, et al. Liver iron concentrations and urinary hepcidin in beta-thalassemia. Haematologica. 2007;92:583–8.
177. Nicolas G, Viatte L, Bennoun M, Beaumont C, Kahn A, Vaulont S. Hepcidin, a new iron regulatory peptide. Blood Cells Mol Dis. 2002;29:327–35.
178. Vokurka M, Necas E. Hepcidin – a peptide regulating the quantity and distribution of iron in the body in healthy and disease states. Cas Lek Cesk. 2003;142:465–9.
179. Pak M, Lopez MA, Gabayan V, Ganz T, Rivera S. Suppression of hepcidin during anemia requires erythropoietic activity. Blood. 2006;108:3730–5.
180. Weizer-Stern O, Adamsky K, Amariglio N, et al. Downregulation of hepcidin and haemojuvelin expression in the hepatocyte cell-line HepG2 induced by thalassaemic sera. Br J Haematol. 2006;135:129–38.
181. Tanno T, Bhanu NV, Oneal PA, et al. High levels of GDF15 in thalassemia suppress expression of the iron regulatory protein hepcidin. Nat Med. 2007;13:1096–101.
182. Kannan K, Amariglio N, Rechavi G, Givol D. Profile of gene expression regulated by induced p53: connection to the TGF-beta family. FEBS Lett. 2000;470:77–82.
183. Kannan K, Amariglio N, Rechavi G, et al. DNA microarrays identification of primary and secondary target genes regulated by p53. Oncogene. 2001;20:2225–34.
184. Tan M, Wang Y, Guan K, Sun Y. PTGF-beta, a type beta transforming growth factor (TGF-beta) superfamily member, is a p53 target gene that inhibits tumor cell growth via TGF-beta signaling pathway. Proc Natl Acad Sci USA. 2000;97:109–14.
185. Yoon D, Pastore YD, Divoky V, et al. Hypoxia-inducible factor-1 deficiency results in dysregulated erythropoiesis signaling and iron homeostasis in mouse development. J Biol Chem. 2006;281:25703–11.
186. Peyssonnaux C, Zinkernagel AS, Schuepbach RA, et al. Regulation of iron homeostasis by the hypoxia-inducible transcription factors (HIFs). J Clin Invest. 2007;117:1926–32.
187. Van Wyck DB, Tancer ME, Popp RA. Iron homeostasis in beta-thalassemic mice. Blood. 1987;70:1462–5.
188. Adamsky K, Weizer O, Amariglio N, et al. Decreased hepcidin mRNA expression in thalassemic mice. Br J Haematol. 2004;124:123–4.
189. Weizer O, Adamsky K, Breda L, et al. Hepcidin expression in cultured liver cells responds differently to iron overloaded sera derived from patients with thalassemia and hemochromatosis. The American Society of Hematology 46th Annual Meeting. San Diego. Blood 2004;104:873A.
190. De Franceschi L, Daraio F, Filippini A, et al. Liver expression of hepcidin and other iron genes in two mouse models of beta-thalassemia. Haematologica. 2006;91:1336–42.
191. Weizer-Stern O, Adamsky K, Amariglio N, et al. mRNA expression of iron regulatory genes in beta-thalassemia intermedia and beta-thalassemia major mouse models. Am J Hematol. 2006;81:479–83.
192. Courselaud B, Pigeon C, Inoue Y, et al. C/EBPalpha regulates hepatic transcription of hepcidin, an antimicrobial peptide and regulator of iron metabolism. Cross-talk between C/EBP pathway and iron metabolism. J Biol Chem. 2002;277:41163–70.
193. Pinto JP, Ribeiro S, Pontes H, et al. Erythropoietin mediates hepcidin expression in hepatocytes through EPOR signalling and regulation of C/EBPalpha. Blood. 2008;111:5727–33.
194. Morra S, Barisani D, Chiabrando D, et al. Lack of haptoglobin affects iron transport across duodenum modulating ferroportin expression. Gastroenterology. 2007;133:1261–71.
195. Rao KR, Patel AR, McGinnis P, Patel MK. Iron stores in adults with sickle cell anemia. J Lab Clin Med. 1984;103:792–7.
196. Vichinsky E, Kleman K, Embury S, Lubin B. The diagnosis of iron deficiency anemia in sickle cell disease. Blood. 1981;58:963–8.
197. Angelucci E, Bai H, Centis F, et al. Enhanced macrophagic attack on beta-thalassemia major erythroid precursors. Haematologica. 2002;87:578–83.
198. Centis F, Tabellini L, Lucarelli G, et al. The importance of erythroid expansion in determining the extent of apoptosis in erythroid precursors in patients with beta-thalassemia major. Blood. 2000;96:3624–9.

Section IV
Disorders of Iron Homeostasis: Iron Overload and Related Conditions

Chapter 17
The Pathology of Hepatic Iron Overload

Yves Deugnier and Bruno Turlin

Keywords Cirrhosis • Ferritin • Fibrosis • Hemosiderin • Hepatocellular carcinoma • Iron overload • Liver • Perls' Prussian blue

1 Introduction

Since the discovery of the *HFE* gene in 1996 [1], tremendous advances have been made both in our understanding of normal and abnormal iron metabolism and in the noninvasive assessment of iron overload. Currently, hepatic iron excess can be reliably diagnosed using MRI and most genetic iron overload syndromes can be identified by laboratory tests [2]. This has resulted in restricting the place of liver pathology in the management of iron-overloaded patients to the assessment of associated lesions, especially fibrosis, and to the diagnosis of iron overload that remains unclassified by genetic molecular markers.

2 A Semiological Approach to Hepatic Iron Overload

The pathologist identifies iron overload, describes its cellular and lobular distribution, assesses its amount semiquantitatively, and reports associated lesions, especially fibrosis. In doing so, he/she participates in the assessment of prognosis and may usefully direct clinical investigation toward a specific cause.

2.1 Identification of Iron Overload

Iron deposits are difficult to identify with the usual stains unless they are abundant. Therefore, routine histochemical stains must include an iron stain, together with hematoxylin and eosin (H&E), and a connective tissue stain [3]. Perls' stain is the most widely used [4]. It allows for the identification of

Y. Deugnier, M.D. (✉)
Liver Unit and CIC INSERM 0203, Pontchaillou University Hospital, Rennes 35033, France
e-mail: yves.deugnier@univ-rennes1.fr

B. Turlin, M.D.
Department of Pathology, Pontchaillou University Hospital, Rennes 35033, France

G.J. Anderson and G. McLaren (eds.), *Iron Physiology and Pathophysiology in Humans*, Nutrition and Health, DOI 10.1007/978-1-60327-485-2_17,

membrane-bound lysosomal hemosiderin that consists of Fe^{2+}. The combined assessment of both Fe^{2+} and Fe^{3+} requires the use of the related Prussian blue stain (also known as Perls' Prussian blue). Within the normal range of hepatic iron concentration, iron is usually undetectable even when using specific stains [5, 6].

2.2 *Characterization of Iron Overload*

Parenchymal cells (hepatocytes and bile duct cells) as well as mesenchymal cells (endothelial cells from the portal circulation, central veins, and sinusoids, macrophages within portal tracts and fibrous septa, and Kupffer and fat-storing cells from sinusoids) may be affected by iron deposition. The abundance and cellular distribution of iron deposits often differ from one acinar zone to another and from one lobule to another. Therefore, the pathologist's report must include a descriptive and semiquantitative assessment of iron excess according to its cellular, lobular, and organ distribution.

2.2.1 Distribution

Assessing the cellular and lobular distribution of iron deposits allows three types of hepatic iron overload to be distinguished (a) *Parenchymal iron overload* is characterized by iron deposition within hepatocytes. Iron usually accumulates as fine granules predominating at the biliary pole of cells. It is distributed throughout the lobule according to a decreasing gradient, from periportal to centrilobular areas. Mesenchymal iron deposits may be found, but at a later stage when hepatocytic iron is high enough to induce cell necrosis. (b) *Mesenchymal iron overload* corresponds to iron deposition within sinusoidal cells – chiefly Kupffer cells – and/or portal macrophages. Iron-loaded cells are either isolated or grouped together with no lobular systematization. When associated, hepatocytic iron deposits are rough, sparse, and usually located close to iron-loaded macrophages. (c) *Mixed iron overload* presents with the histological characteristics of the previous two types and corresponds usually to complex conditions or to massive iron loading. Assessing the homogeneous or heterogeneous pattern of iron distribution from one lobule (nodule) to another is also necessary, especially with respect to etiology and in the case of a cirrhotic patient.

2.2.2 Quantitation

Semiquantitative Grading by Light Microscopy

The semiquantitative grading of hepatic iron by light microscopy is a reliable option for quantifying hepatic iron excess. Scheuer et al. [7] introduced the concept of "grading" iron deposition in liver biopsies. Since then, numerous grading methods have been proposed [3]. Both the original and modified Scheuer's scoring systems are based on the percentage of iron-overloaded hepatocytes. Although they were not satisfactorily validated, they remain widely used in routine practice because of their simplicity. The system proposed by the authors (Table 17.1) has been well validated in both hemochromatotic [9, 10] and nonhemochromatotic [11] iron overload disorders, but, as it is a form of computerized morphometric semiquantitation [12, 13], it remains mainly used for research purposes.

Hepatic Iron Concentration (HIC)

The biochemical determination of HIC on a liver sample is considered as the "iron" standard [5], whatever the method used (colorimetry or atomic absorption spectrometry). In normal subjects, HIC ranges from 10 to 35 μmol/g of dry weight [5]. Iron excess is considered as mild up to 150 μmol/g,

Table 17.1 Histological grading of iron storage. From Deugnier and Turlin [8]8

Hepatocytic iron	0, 3, 6, 9, or 12	HIS
	According to granule size in each Rappaport area	0–36
Sinusoidal iron	0, 1, 2, 3, or 4	SIS
	According to granule size in each Rappaport area	0–12
Portal iron	0, 1, 2, 3, or 4	PIS
	According to % of iron-overloaded macrophages, biliary cells, and vascular walls	0–12
Total iron score		0–60

HIS hepatocytic iron score, *SIS* sinusoidal iron score, *PIS* portal iron score

moderate between 150 and 300 μmol/g, and important above 300 μmol/g. Cases with HIC greater than 1000 μmol/g are exceptional. Results obtained from fresh tissue and from deparaffinized blocks are equivalent [14]. The determination of HIC on deparaffinized tissue must be advocated because it allows for histological control, which is especially relevant when iron distribution is heterogeneous as in the cirrhotic liver [15–17]. The paramagnetic properties of iron have been exploited to detect and quantify iron by MRI. When using a well-calibrated 1.5 T device, there exists an excellent inverse correlation between biochemical HIC and the MRI signal, allowing for an accurate detection of hepatic iron excess within the range 50–350 μmol/g [18]. In addition, MRI may help to identify the heterogeneous distribution of iron within the liver and, by studying other organs, to differentiate parenchymal (normal splenic signal and low hepatic, pancreatic, and cardiac signals) from mesenchymal (decreased splenic signal) iron overload [19]. For these reasons and because it is a noninvasive procedure, MRI tends to replace liver biopsy and biochemistry for the identification of iron overload and for the determination of HIC.

2.3 Associated Lesions

One of the most important goals of the pathologist is to make an inventory of associated lesions in order to assess the prognosis (especially with respect to fibrosis) and, when necessary, to guide toward the right etiology of iron excess.

3 Diagnosis of Hepatic Iron Overload According to Its Cause

The types of iron overload and the spectrum of associated lesions vary between different types of disease.

3.1 Genetic Iron Overload

3.1.1 Genetic Hemochromatosis

Genetic hemochromatosis or, merely, hemochromatosis, refers to four main autosomal recessive disorders, two of late onset (adult type: HFE hemochromatosis and iron overload related to mutation on the transferrin receptor 2 gene) and two of early onset (juvenile type: related to mutations in the *hemojuvelin* or *HAMP* (hepcidin) genes). These disorders share a common pathophysiology consisting in an impairment of hepcidin production or activity. Therefore, they exhibit similar histological features. By far, the most common is HFE hemochromatosis.

HFE Hemochromatosis

In early HFE hemochromatosis, iron remains located at the biliary pole of hepatocytes. It is distributed according to a decreasing gradient from periportal to centrilobular areas. This results in a typical parenchymal iron overload pattern. However, as emphasized by Brunt et al. [20, 21], while predominantly Kupffer cell iron staining may serve as a strong negative predictor of HFE hemochromatosis, the reverse (with predominantly parenchymal cell loading) is not necessarily true. As cellular iron load increases, sideronecrosis occurs. This is a key event corresponding to acidophilic or lytic necrosis of hepatocytes due to iron excess. It leads to the redistribution of iron toward nonparenchymal cells and then to heavily iron-laden Kupffer cell aggregates close to necrotic hepatocytes. Mild chronic inflammation is commonly found [9]. Necroinflammatory changes precede the development of portal and periportal fibrosis, portal–portal bridging fibrosis, and then cirrhosis [9]. Cirrhosis related to HFE hemochromatosis resembles biliary cirrhosis. It consists of large fibrous septa, but the vascular architecture of the liver is retained for a long time as disease progresses. This likely explains why portal hypertension and hepatic failure are rare features in HFE hemochromatosis [22]. According to one study, 25–50% of hemochromatosis patients are still diagnosed at the cirrhotic stage. In the absence of other causes of chronic liver disease, cirrhosis develops when the hepatic iron concentration exceeds 300 μmol/g. Whether fibrosis was able to regress or not following venesection therapy was addressed by Falize et al. [23] in 36 C282Y homozygotes presenting with severe fibrosis on their initial liver biopsy. These authors demonstrated that fibrosis regressed in 69% of patients with initial bridging fibrosis and in 35% of patients with initial cirrhosis. In addition, they proposed a predictive index for fibrosis regression based upon gamma globulins, platelet count, and prothrombin activity.

It is mandatory to assess whether, at the time of diagnosis, the patient's liver is cirrhotic or not in order to define follow-up policy, especially regarding cancer screening. Liver biopsy is no longer necessary for diagnosing C282Y homozygosity, but it remains the reference means for assessing fibrosis. Guyader et al. [24] demonstrated that when the liver was not clinically enlarged and serum ferritin level was lower than 1000 ng/ml and serum AST level was normal, there was never a significant liver fibrosis (i.e., grade 3 or 4 fibrosis according to the METAVIR scoring system). On the contrary, when one, two, or all these conditions were not met, there was a significant risk of fibrosis, calculated as 1/(1+exp[−(−6.7620+3.2934 AST (iu/l)+0.0013 ferritin (ng/ml)+2.5317 hepatomegaly (0:1))]). Other equations of prediction of (non)fibrosis have been proposed based upon age and serum ferritin levels, or serum ferritin levels, serum AST levels, and platelet count, but either they are not extensively validated or they were not as simple for clinical use as Guyader's algorithm [25, 26]. Currently, there is a global consensus to perform liver biopsy for fibrosis evaluation in C282Y homozygotes with either increased liver size, serum ferritin levels higher than 1000 ng/ml, or abnormal serum AST levels, except when the diagnosis of cirrhosis is clinically obvious or when the predictive equation gives a risk close to 100%. It is likely that when noninvasive measurement of hepatic fibrosis by biochemical tests and/or elastometry is validated in hemochromatosis, the indication for liver biopsy will become exceptional in C282Y homozygotes. It is important to stress that Guyader's algorithm does not apply to HFE genotypes other than C282Y homozygosity and to non-HFE causes of iron overload.

Primary liver cancer (PLC) accounts for 27.5–45% of deaths in hemochromatosis patients [27]. The relative risk for a patient with hemochromatosis to develop PLC has been calculated as greater than 200 [28–30]. The main risk factors are male sex, age over 50 years, cirrhosis, and associated (co)carcinogenic factors such as chronic alcoholism, tobacco smoking, and HBV and HCV infections [28–31]. Most cases correspond to classic hepatocellular carcinoma (HCC) which has developed in a cirrhotic liver [31, 32]. However, attention has to be paid to some specific features. First, PLC may develop whether the patient has been treated or not. Second, about 20% of PLC are diagnosed in the absence of cirrhosis [31, 32]. Third, as demonstrated by Morcos et al. [32], cholangiocarcinoma or HCC with biliary differentiation may account for one third of PLC cases in C282Y homozygotes. Fourth, two types of preneoplastic lesions – iron-free foci (IFF) [9, 33] and Von Meyenburg complexes [33] – have been reported. Iron-free foci consist of sublobular nodular clusters of hepatocytes devoid of iron or with low iron content within an otherwise iron-overloaded liver [9]. Most often, they exhibit a proliferative pattern, with either large or small cell dysplasia in 50% of cases. More than half of the patients with IFF on their initial liver biopsy have been reported to further develop PLC compared to less than 10% with no IFF at initial biopsy [33]. Von Meyenburg complexes have also been reported as abnormally numerous in the surrounding liver of patients with hemochromatosis complicated with either HCC or cholangiocarcinoma [32, 34].

Non-HFE Hemochromatosis

The histological presentation of iron overload related to non-HFE hemochromatosis [35] is identical to that of HFE hemochromatosis. TfR2 hemochromatosis is responsible for mild to moderate parenchymal iron excess that leads rarely to cirrhosis in the absence of comorbid factors such as chronic excessive alcohol consumption. Juvenile hemochromatosis is responsible for marked iron overload of mixed pattern with parenchymal predominance. Cirrhosis is the rule at diagnosis.

3.1.2 Other Genetic Iron Overload Syndromes

Ferroportin Disease

Ferroportin disease [35] is a dominant hereditary iron overload disorder characterized by phenotypic variability. In the majority of cases, it results in Kupffer cell iron loading, predominantly in acinar zone 1 (mesenchymal type), with no significant fibrosis even when HIC exceeds 300 μmol/g. This corresponds to the classic asymptomatic form with elevated hyperferritinemia contrasting with normal or mildly increased transferrin saturation (type A). However, one case of ferroportin A disease complicated with HCC in the absence of significant fibrosis has been reported [36], which suggests that this type of iron overload may also be deleterious on the long term. Rarely, iron is predominantly located within parenchymal cells and the histological picture is similar to that of HFE hemochromatosis with, in some cases, either severe fibrosis or cirrhosis (type B). Then, transferrin saturation is usually markedly elevated. Autosomal dominant parenchymal iron overload reported in families from the Solomon Islands is likely to be related to ferroportin disease [37].

Other Hereditary Iron Overload Syndromes

Such syndromes are exceptional. In hereditary aceruloplasminemia [38] or hypoceruloplasminemia [39], a disease transmitted as a recessive trait, iron is found predominantly in parenchymal cells. No case of liver cirrhosis has been described even in the most heavily iron-loaded cases. In autosomal recessive genetic atransferrinemia [40], iron overload is related to both increased duodenal absorption and transfusions. It is characterized by a mixed pattern associating parenchymal and mesenchymal iron deposition. Finally, African iron overload [41], originally termed "Bantu siderosis," is also characterized by a mixed pattern and complicated with cirrhosis in up to 90% of cases [42]. It is related to excessive iron intake and likely furthered by non-HFE genetic factors.

3.2 *Nongenetic Iron Overload*

3.2.1 Excessive Iron Supply

When administered parenterally (i.e., through multiple transfusions), iron is initially localized within Kupffer cells and portal macrophages. With time, it is redistributed toward surrounding parenchymal cells, which results in a mixed and heterogeneous pattern. In cases of excessive chronic iron intake, parenchymal or mixed hepatic iron overload may develop, as reported in elite road cyclists [43].

3.2.2 Inflammatory Syndromes

Inflammatory conditions are a frequent cause of mesenchymal hepatic siderosis related to a defect of iron release from Kupffer cells due to increased production of hepcidin. Iron deposits are usually sparse and distributed throughout the lobule.

3.2.3 Chronic Liver Diseases

Noncirrhotic Chronic Liver Disease

Granular iron deposition in hepatocytes and/or mesenchymal cells may be found in every type of chronic noncirrhotic liver disease regardless of its cause. Iron excess is commonly slight or mild (HIC <100 μmol/g dry weight) and distributed heterogeneously with a trend for parenchymal iron to predominate in acinar zone 1 and for mesenchymal iron to be panacinar. The cause(s) of such "siderosis" remain(s) unknown. It is likely that various nonspecific factors (inflammation, cell necrosis, etc.) are involved, together with polymorphisms in iron-related genes and specific interactions between iron metabolism and the etiological agent of liver disease. Whether this type of iron excess is clinically relevant with respect to fibrosis and cancer risk is still debated [2].

Alcoholic Liver Disease

Mesenchymal or mixed mild hepatic siderosis is found in up to 57% of chronic alcoholics [44], even in the absence of cirrhosis. A direct effect of alcohol on hepcidin production could be involved [45]. It was for the distinction between alcoholic siderosis and genetic hemochromatosis that Bassett et al. [46] proposed the hepatic iron index consisting of the ratio of HIC (as μmol/g dry weight) to age. A threshold of 1.9–2 was found to distinguish the two conditions accurately.

Nonalcoholic Fatty Liver Disease (NAFLD) and Dysmetabolic Iron Overload Syndrome (DIOS)

Early descriptions of nonalcoholic steatohepatitis in Australian and American patients reported iron deposition in 10–95% of cases [47]. This wide range was likely due to differences in the methods used for iron assessment and to the high variability in case definition, since some series consisted of overweight patients while others consisted of morbidly obese individuals. At the same time, our group reported that most cases of unexplained hepatic iron excess were associated with metabolic abnormalities, especially increased body mass index, and were characterized by high serum ferritin levels with normal or subnormal transferrin saturation [48, 49]. We therefore proposed the concept of DIOS, also known as "insulin resistance–associated hepatic iron overload" [48]. The histological pattern of DIOS is typically mixed [50]. HIC reaches a ceiling of 100 μmol/g dry weight, but in 30% of cases, the hepatic iron index exceeds 2. Either steatosis or steatohepatitis is present in 50% of cases [50]. Bridging fibrosis or cirrhosis is found in 12% of cases [50]. The concept of DIOS encompasses siderosis associated with NAFLD and extends to unexplained hepatic iron overload with normal histology in subjects with metabolic abnormalities. Whether iron may be involved in the development of fibrosis in DIOS patients and whether its removal may be beneficial remains debated.

Viral Hepatitis

In acute viral hepatitis, iron is often found as punctate inclusions in endothelial cells and, in the resolving phase, in PAS-diastase-resistant granules within Kupffer cells and portal tract macrophages. In chronic hepatitis, hepatic iron deposition is found in 35–56% of cases [51]. This was especially demonstrated in patients with chronic hepatitis related to the hepatitis C virus (HCV). The histological pattern is usually mesenchymal, with frequent iron deposits in endothelial cells. An "endothelial pattern" of iron deposition was even reported as associated with fibrosis progression and lack of response to interferon [52]. Iron excess has been shown to correlate with necroinflammatory changes and to decrease after interferon therapy [53]. Moreover, iron removal before or at the time of interferon therapy could result in histological improvement, even in nonresponders [54]. Recently, a negative effect of HCV infection on hepatic hepcidin production was shown, which may explain, at least partly, abnormalities of iron metabolism found in patients with chronic hepatitis C [55].

Wilson Disease

Mixed iron overload is frequently found in the liver of patients with Wilson disease [56]. Its mechanism is likely multifactorial and involves low serum ceruloplasmin levels, hemolysis, necroinflammatory changes, and cirrhosis.

Porphyria Cutanea Tarda (PCT)

Both moderate to marked hepatocellular and mesenchymal iron accumulation are often found in the liver of patients with PCT regardless of the presence of HFE mutations [57]. Careful examination may allow for a correct diagnosis when identifying porphyrin crystals in tissue sections.

Cirrhosis

Regardless of the cause of cirrhosis, significant liver siderosis is found in 35–78% of patients with end-stage liver disease [16–18, 58]. Iron deposition presents with a parenchymal pattern and predominates in the remaining periportal areas. It has a heterogeneous distribution from one nodule to another, and the absence of iron within fibrous septa, biliary cells, and vascular walls allows for the correct diagnosis of "iron overload secondary to cirrhosis" instead of that of hemochromatosis [16]. Thus, in case of cirrhosis, HIC should be interpreted according to histological findings. It is likely that non-transferrin-bound iron (NTBI) plays a key role in the development of this type of iron overload. Indeed, in severe cirrhosis, serum transferrin levels are low due to hepatic failure, which results in increased saturation of transferrin and, then, in the appearance of NTBI, a special form of iron that is avidly taken up by hepatocytes [59]. In addition, decreased hepcidin production has been reported in patients with cirrhosis [60], which may result in increased intestinal iron absorption and iron release from macrophages.

3.2.4 Hepatocellular Carcinoma (HCC)

HCC tissue is commonly iron poor, and the expression of hepcidin mRNA is markedly suppressed in cancerous, but not in noncancerous, human HCC tissues, irrespective of ferroportin or transferrin receptor 2 expression [61]. This possibly reflects an increased demand for bioavailable iron and a high iron turnover in neoplastic cells. Conversely, parenchymal or mixed iron overload has been reported in the nontumorous part of the liver in more than 80% of patients with HCC, which has developed on a noncirrhotic liver [62, 63]. Nahon et al. [64] showed that liver iron overload was associated, independently from the carriage of the C282Y mutation, with a higher risk of HCC in patients with alcoholic but not HCV-related cirrhosis. These data support the idea that iron may be both a negative marker of neoplastic transformation and a (co)carcinogenic factor [8].

3.2.5 Blood Disorders

In well-compensated anemias with ineffective erythropoiesis (thalassemias, multifactorial sidero-blastic anemias, congenital dyserythropoietic syndromes, etc.), intestinal iron absorption is increased secondary to the impairment of iron incorporation into red cell precursors. With time, severe hepatic iron overload resembling hemochromatosis may develop, even in the absence of blood transfusions. Once transfusions are required, iron accumulates in both parenchymal and mesenchymal cells [65].

In hemolytic anemias with normal erythropoiesis, iron deposition predominates in macrophages as punctuate granules in the early stages. Large Kupffer cell aggregates (siderotic nodules) develop in more advanced disease, requiring regular blood transfusions. When macrophage iron storage capacity is exceeded, iron is secondarily redistributed toward hepatocytes. In the absence of iron removal, portal fibrosis may occur [65].

4 Liver Histology in the Management of Iron Overload Syndromes

Liver biopsy is no longer necessary to ascertain iron overload, and MRI, together with the level of transferrin saturation, may identify the correct etiology, especially with respect to the choice of geno-typing tests. Assessment of associated lesions, especially fibrosis, will remain the major goal of liver biopsy until noninvasive tests for fibrosis are validated in patients with iron overload syndromes.

In the presence of a hemochromatosis phenotype (i.e., increased transferrin saturation with paren-chymal iron deposition), performing liver biopsy depends on HFE genotyping. In C282Y homozy-gotes, Guyader's algorithm can be used to decide whether to perform liver biopsy or not. For C282Y-H63D compound heterozygotes, the situation is more complex. In a subject presenting with mild increases in transferrin saturation (usually between 45% and 60%) and serum ferritin (usually <500 ng/ml) and with no biochemical abnormalities or clinical liver symptoms, it can be reasonably assumed that the HFE genotype is responsible for the abnormalities in iron metabolism and that the patient is free of risk of fibrosis. In such cases, liver biopsy is not necessary. However, when faced with more pronounced abnormalities of iron metabolism and/or abnormal liver tests, a codamaging factor is suggested [66]. Other HFE genotypes do not result in clinically relevant abnormalities of iron metabolism.

Liver biopsy remains suitable to diagnose any additional cause of either iron overload or chronic liver disease. In these cases, the most frequent finding is heterogeneous parenchymal iron overload complicating alcoholic or viral liver disease. Much more rarely, liver biopsy discovers marked iron overload, suggesting an associated mutation on another gene involved in iron metabolism. Then, the precise description of iron deposition and associated lesions may help in identifying the cause of the disease: mesenchymal or mixed iron deposition with no significant fibrosis is suggestive of ferroportin disease (which sometimes presents with TS >60%), while parenchymal iron overload suggests a diagnosis of juvenile hemochromatosis (mutations in *hemojuvelin* or *HAMP*) in a young adult with severe fibrosis, or transferrin receptor 2–related hemochromatosis in an adult with or without fibrosis.

In the absence of hemochromatosis phenotype (i.e., low, normal, or slightly elevated transferrin saturation), the question is whether increased serum ferritin levels are related to iron overload or not. MRI can replace liver biopsy to answer this question, and histological examination of the liver can be limited to patients with significant iron deposition at MRI (i.e., hepatic iron concentration >100 μmol/g dry weight) and/or elevated serum transaminase levels and/or abnormal noninvasive predictive tests of fibrosis. The most frequent finding is of mild and mixed iron overload with either metabolic or alcoholic steatohepatitis, chronic hepatitis C, or porphyria cutanea tarda. Rarely, histological examination reveals marked iron overload with no significant fibrosis corresponding to either ferroportin disease (mesenchymal type – normal or slightly increased transferrin saturation) or to hereditary aceruloplasminemia (parenchymal type – low transferrin saturation).

Finally, in routine practice, hepatic iron is frequently found in liver biopsies performed in the absence of clinical suspicion of iron excess. This always should be indicated in the pathologist's report since iron excess, even when mild, is suspected to be involved as a codamaging factor in various conditions including insulin-resistance syndrome and diabetes, cardiovascular complications, and cancer.

References

1. Feder JN. The hereditary hemochromatosis gene (HFE): a MHC class I-like gene that functions in the regulation of iron homeostasis. Immunol Res. 1999;20:175–85.
2. Deugnier Y, Brissot P, Loréal O. Iron and the liver: update 2008. J Hepatol. 2008;48:S113–23.
3. Turlin B, Deugnier Y. Evaluation and interpretation of iron in the liver. Sem Diag Pathol. 1998;15:237–45.
4. Turlin B, Loreal O, Moirand R, Brissot P, Deugnier Y, Ramee MP. Histochemical detection of hepatic iron. A comparative study of four Stains. Ann Pathol. 1992;12:371–3.
5. Brissot P, Bourel M, Herry D, et al. Assessment of liver iron content in 271 patients: a reevaluation of direct and indirect methods. Gastroenterology. 1981;80:557–65.
6. Imbert-Bismut F, Charlotte F, Turlin B, et al. Low hepatic iron concentration: evaluation of two complementary methods, colorimetric assay and iron histological scoring. J Clin Pathol. 1999;52:430–4.
7. Scheuer P, Williams R, Muir A. Hepatic pathology in relatives of patients with haemochromatosis. J Pathol Bacteriol. 1962;84:53–64.
8. Deugnier Y, Turlin B. Iron and hepatocellular carcinoma. J Gastroenterol Hepatol. 2001;16:491–4.
9. Deugnier YM, Loreal O, Turlin B, et al. Liver pathology in genetic hemochromatosis: a review of 135 homozygous cases and their bioclinical correlations. Gastroenterology. 1992;102:2050–9.
10. Deugnier YM, Turlin B, Powell LW, et al. Differentiation between heterozygotes and homozygotes in genetic hemochromatosis by means of a histological hepatic iron index: a study of 192 cases. Hepatology. 1993;17:30–4.
11. Turlin B, Deugnier Y. Histological assessment of liver siderosis. J Clin Pathol. 1997;50:971.
12. Deugnier Y, Margules S, Brissot P, et al. Comparative study between biochemical and histological methods and image analysis in liver iron overload. J Clin Pathol. 1982;35:45–51.
13. Olynyk J, Hall P, Sallie R, Reed W, Shilkin K, Mackinnon M. Computerized measurement of iron in liver biopsies: a comparison with biochemical iron measurement. Hepatology. 1990;12:26–30.
14. Olynyk JK, O'Neill R, Britton RS, Bacon BR. Determination of hepatic iron concentration in fresh and paraffin-embedded tissue: diagnostic implications. Gastroenterology. 1994;106:674–7.
15. Deugnier Y, Turlin B, le Quilleuc D, et al. A reappraisal of hepatic siderosis in patients with end-stage cirrhosis: practical implications for the diagnosis of hemochromatosis. Am J Surg Pathol. 1997;21:669–75.
16. Ludwig J, Hashimoto E, Porayko MK, Moyer TP, Baldus WP. Hemosiderosis in cirrhosis: a study of 447 native livers. Gastroenterology. 1997;112:882–8.
17. Villeneuve JP, Bilodeau M, Lepage R, Cote J, Lefebvre M. Variability in hepatic iron concentration measurement from needle-biopsy specimens. J Hepatol. 1996;25:172–7.

18. Gandon Y, Olivie D, Guyader D, et al. Non-invasive assessment of hepatic iron stores by MRI. Lancet. 2004;363:357–62.
19. Pietrangelo A. Non-invasive assessment of hepatic iron overload: are we finally there? J Hepatol. 2005;42:153–4.
20. Brunt EM, Olynyk JK, Britton RS, Janney CG, Di Bisceglie AM, Bacon BR. Histological evaluation of iron in liver biopsies: relationship to HFE mutations. Am J Gastroenterol. 2000;95:1788–93.
21. Brunt EM. Pathology of hepatic iron overload. Semin Liver Dis. 2005;25:392–401.
22. Fracanzani AL, Fargion S, Romano R, et al. Portal hypertension and iron depletion in patients with genetic hemochromatosis. Hepatology. 1995;22:1127–31.
23. Falize L, Guillygomarc'h A, Perrin M, et al. Reversibility of hepatic fibrosis in treated genetic hemochromatosis: a study of 36 cases. Hepatology. 2006;44:472–7.
24. Guyader D, Jacquelinet C, Moirand R, et al. Noninvasive prediction of fibrosis in C282Y homozygous hemochromatosis. Gastroenterology. 1998;115:929–36.
25. Beaton M, Guyader D, Deugnier Y, Moirand R, Chakrabarti S, Adams P. Noninvasive prediction of cirrhosis in C282Y-linked hemochromatosis. Hepatology. 2002;36:673–8.
26. Morrison ED, Brandhagen DJ, Phatak PD, et al. Serum ferritin level predicts advanced hepatic fibrosis among U.S. Patients with phenotypic hemochromatosis. Ann Intern Med. 2003;138:627–33.
27. Kowdley KV. Iron, hemochromatosis, and hepatocellular carcinoma. Gastroenterology. 2004;127(5 Suppl 1):S79–86.
28. Bradbear RA, Bain C, Siskind V, et al. Cohort study of internal malignancy in genetic hemochromatosis and other chronic nonalcoholic liver diseases. J Nat Cancer Inst. 1985;75:81–4.
29. Fracanzani AL, Conte D, Fraquelli M, et al. Increased cancer risk in a cohort of 230 patients with hereditary hemochromatosis in comparison to matched control patients with non-iron-related chronic liver disease. Hepatology. 2001;33:647–51.
30. Niederau C, Fischer R, Sonnenberg A, Stremmel W, Trampisch HJ, Strohmeyer G. Survival and causes of death in cirrhotic and in noncirrhotic patients with primary hemochromatosis. N Engl J Med. 1985;313:1256–62.
31. Deugnier YM, Guyader D, Crantock L, et al. Primary liver cancer in genetic hemochromatosis: a clinical, pathological, and pathogenetic study of 54 cases. Gastroenterology. 1993;104:228–34.
32. Morcos M, Dubois S, Bralet MP, Belghiti J, Degott C, Terris B. Primary liver carcinoma in genetic hemochromatosis reveals a broad histologic spectrum. Am J Clin Pathol. 2001;116:738–43.
33. Deugnier YM, Charalambous P, Le Quilleuc D, et al. Preneoplastic significance of hepatic iron-free foci in genetic hemochromatosis: a study of 185 patients. Hepatology. 1993;18:1363–9.
34. Blanc JF, Bernard PH, Carles J, Le Bail B, Balabaud C, Bioulac-Sage P. Cholangiocarcinoma arising in Von meyenburg complex associated with hepatocellular carcinoma in genetic haemochromatosis. Eur J Gastroenterol Hepatol. 2000;12:233–7.
35. Pietrangelo A. The ferroportin disease. Blood Cells Mol Dis. 2004;32:131–8.
36. Rosmorduc O, Wendum D, Arrive L, et al. Phenotypic expression of ferroportin disease in a family with the N144H mutation. Gastroenterol Clin Biol. 2008;32:321–7.
37. Arden KE, Wallace DF, Dixon JL, et al. A novel mutation in ferroportin1 is associated with haemochromatosis in a Solomon islands patient. Gut. 2003;52:1215–7.
38. Miyajima H, Takahashi Y, Kono S. Aceruloplasminemia, an inherited disorder of iron metabolism. Biometals. 2003;16:205–13.
39. Kono S, Suzuki H, Takahashi K, et al. Hepatic iron overload associated with a decreased serum ceruloplasmin level in a novel clinical type of aceruloplasminemia. Gastroenterology. 2006;131:240–5.
40. Beutler E, Gelbart T, Lee P, Trevino R, Fernandez MA, Fairbanks VF. Molecular characterization of a case of atransferrinemia. Blood. 2000;96:4071–4.
41. Gordeuk VR. African iron overload. Semin Hematol. 2002;39:263–9.
42. Gordeuk V, Mukiibi J, Hasstedt SJ, et al. Iron overload in Africa. Interaction between a gene and dietary iron content. N Engl J Med. 1992;326:95–100.
43. Deugnier Y, Loreal O, Carre F, et al. Increased body iron stores in elite road cyclists. Med Sci Sports Exerc. 2002;34:876–80.
44. Jakobovits AW, Morgan MY, Sherlock S. Hepatic siderosis in alcoholics. Dig Dis Sc. 1979;24:305–10.
45. Harrison-Findik DD. Role of alcohol in the regulation of iron metabolism. World J Gastroenterol. 2007;13:4925–30.
46. Bassett ML, Halliday JW, Powell LW. Value of hepatic iron measurements in early hemochromatosis and determination of the critical iron level associated with fibrosis. Hepatology. 1986;6:24–9.
47. Brunt EM. Pathology of nonalcoholic steatohepatitis. Hepatol Res. 2005;33:68–71.
48. Mendler MH, Turlin B, Moirand R, et al. Insulin resistance-associated hepatic iron overload. Gastroenterology. 1999;117:1155–63.
49. Moirand R, Mortaji AM, Loreal O, Paillard F, Brissot P, Deugnier Y. A new syndrome of liver iron overload with normal transferrin saturation. Lancet. 1997;349:95–7.

50. Turlin B, Mendler MH, Moirand R, Guyader D, Guillygomarc'h A, Deugnier Y. Histologic features of the liver in insulin resistance-associated iron overload. A study of 139 patients. Am J Clin Pathol. 2001;116:263–70.
51. Bonkovsky HL, Lambrecht RW, Shan Y. Iron as a co-morbid factor in nonhemochromatotic liver disease. Alcohol. 2003;30:137–44.
52. Kaji K, Nakanuma Y, Sasaki M, Unoura M, Kobayashi K, Nonomura A. Hemosiderin deposition in portal endothelial cells: a novel hepatic hemosiderosis frequent in chronic viral hepatitis B and C. Hum Pathol. 1995;26:1080–5.
53. Boucher E, Bourienne A, Adams P, Turlin B, Brissot P, Deugnier Y. Liver iron concentration and distribution in chronic hepatitis C before and after interferon treatment. Gut. 1997;41:115–20.
54. Fontana RJ, Israel J, LeClair P, et al. Iron reduction before and during interferon therapy of chronic hepatitis C: results of a multicenter, randomized, controlled trial. Hepatology. 2000;31:730–6.
55. Fujita N, Sugimoto R, Takeo M, et al. Hepcidin expression in the liver: relatively low level in patients with chronic hepatitis C. Mol Med. 2007;13:97–104.
56. Hayashi H, Yano M, Fujita Y, Wakusawa S. Compound overload of copper and iron in patients with Wilson's disease. Med Mol Morph. 2006;39:121–6.
57. Alla V, Bonkovsky HL. Iron in nonhemochromatotic liver disorders. Sem Liver Dis. 2005;25:461–72.
58. Cotler SJ, Bronner MP, Press RD, et al. End-stage liver disease without hemochromatosis associated with elevated hepatic iron index. J Hepatol. 1998;29:257–62.
59. Brissot P, Wright TL, Ma WL, Weisiger RA. Efficient clearance of non-transferrin-bound iron by rat liver. Implications for hepatic iron loading in iron overload states. J Clin Invest. 1985;76:1463–70.
60. Detivaud L, Nemeth E, Boudjema K, et al. Hepcidin levels in humans are correlated with hepatic iron stores, hemoglobin levels, and hepatic function. Blood. 2005;106:746–8.
61. Kijima H, Sawada T, Tomosugi N, Kubota K. Expression of hepcidin mRNA is uniformly suppressed in hepatocellular carcinoma. BMC Cancer. 2008;8:167.
62. Turlin B, Juguet F, Moirand R, et al. Increased liver iron stores in patients with hepatocellular carcinoma developed on a noncirrhotic liver. Hepatology. 1995;22:446–50.
63. Ko C, Siddaiah N, Berger J, et al. Prevalence of hepatic iron overload and association with hepatocellular cancer in end-stage liver disease: results from the national hemochromatosis transplant registry. Liver Int. 2007;27:1394–401.
64. Nahon P, Sutton A, Rufat P, et al. Liver iron, HFE gene mutations, and hepatocellular carcinoma occurrence in patients with cirrhosis. Gastroenterology. 2008;134:102–10.
65. Bottomley SS. Secondary iron overload disorders. Semin Hematol. 1998;35:77–86.
66. Walsh A, Dixon JL, Ramm GA, et al. The clinical relevance of compound heterozygosity for the C282Y and H63D substitutions in hemochromatosis. Clin Gastroenterol Hepatol. 2006;4:1403–10.

Chapter 18
Hepatic Pathobiology of Iron Overload

Richard G. Ruddell and Grant A. Ramm

Keywords Cirrhosis • Fibrosis • Free radical • Heart • Hepatocellular carcinoma • Ischemic heart disease • Liver • Pancreas • Reactive oxygen species

Abbreviations

4-HNE	4-Hydroxynonenal
AP-1	Activator protein 1
ATP	Adenosine triphosphate
CYP	Cytochrome P450
ECM	Extracellular matrix
GSH	Glutathione
HCC	Hepatocellular carcinoma
ICAM-1	Intracellular adhesion molecule-1
IL	Interleukin
MDA	Malondialdehyde
MMPs	Matrix metalloproteinases
MPTP	Mitochondrial permeability transition pore
NFκB	Nuclear factor κB
PKC-ζ	Protein kinase C-ζ
PPARγ	Peroxisome proliferator-activated receptor-γ
ROS	Reactive oxygen species
TBA	Thiobarbituric acid
TGF-β	Transforming growth factor-β
Tim-2	T cell immunoglobulin and mucin domain-2
TIMPs	Tissue inhibitors of metalloproteinases
TNFα	Tumor necrosis factor-α
αSMA	α-Smooth muscle actin (αSMA)
IHD	Ischemic heart disease

R.G. Ruddell, Ph.D. • G.A. Ramm, Ph.D. (✉)
Hepatic Fibrosis Group, Queensland Institute of Medical Research, Brisbane, QLD, Australia
e-mail: Grant.Ramm@qimr.edu.au

G.J. Anderson and G. McLaren (eds.), *Iron Physiology and Pathophysiology in Humans*, Nutrition and Health, DOI 10.1007/978-1-60327-485-2_18,

1 Iron and Oxidative Stress

1.1 Introduction

Iron is an essential nutrient and plays an important role as a cofactor in a number of physiologically crucial processes. Intestinal absorption is tightly regulated as the human body has no dedicated iron excretory pathway. In excess, iron is toxic to the cell thanks to its catalytic properties, which leads to the generation of reactive and damaging oxygen radicals. This chapter will outline the mechanisms by which iron in excess leads to cellular damage and the relationship of iron to the initiation of hepatic fibrosis, the development of cirrhosis and hepatocellular carcinoma (HCC) and its role in ischemic heart disease and diabetes linked to iron overload.

1.2 Iron-Mediated Generation of Reactive Oxygen Species

Iron has an intrinsic ability to catalyze reactions that lead to the generation of the labile hydroxyl radical ($OH^{\cdot}$), and it is thought to be through this mechanism that iron negatively impacts cellular function and viability. The hydroxyl radical is generated through the Fenton and Haber–Weiss reactions where iron is reduced by the superoxide radical (O_2^{-}) to ferrous iron, which reacts with hydrogen peroxide (H_2O_2) to produce $OH^{\cdot}$. This reaction can occur anywhere iron is present and is normally under tight cellular regulation due to the potential damage $OH^{\cdot}$ can inflict on the cell. The reactive oxygen species (ROS) O_2^{-} and H_2O_2 are the by-products of aerobic respiration reactions by cytochrome P450 (CYP) 2E1 and are also produced by the membrane-bound NADPH oxidase complex [1] (see Fig. 18.1). Iron is also able to catalyse the production of NO_2^{+} from peroxynitrite ($ONOO^{-}$).

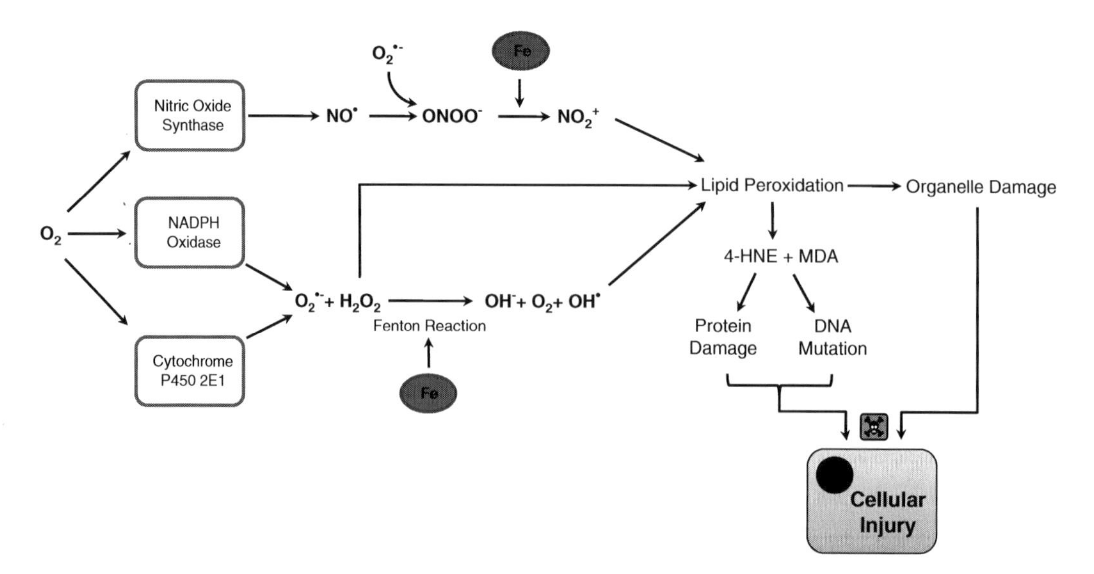

Fig. 18.1 Iron-mediated generation of reactive oxygen species. Acting as a catalyst in the Fenton reaction, iron promotes the generation of the hydroxyl (*OH*$^{\cdot}$) radical from the superoxide radical O_2^{-} and hydrogen peroxide (*H2O2*). Iron is also able to catalyse the formation of the nitronium anion NO_2^{+} from the peroxynitrite radical $ONOO^{-}$. Both processes require the presence of the superoxide radical O_2^{-}, which is itself generated as a by-product of aerobic respiration. Both $OH^{\cdot}$ and $ONOO^{-}$ are then able to take part in lipid peroxidation of polyunsaturated fatty acids, yielding conjugated dienes which can then further react leading to the eventual production of 4-hydroxynonenal (*4-HNE*) and malondialdehyde (*MDA*). Lipid peroxidation leads to organelle dysfunction and eventually damage to DNA and cellular proteins (adapted from Philippe et al. [44])

Peroxynitrite is formed during times of elevated O_2^- and also requires the presence of the radical NO· produced by nitric oxide synthase. Peroxynitrite also reacts with iron to produce the reactive NO_2^+ species (Fig. 18.1) [2, 3].

Both OH· and NO_2^+ are highly reactive and are central to the development of lipid peroxidation and damage to both proteins and DNA. Microsomal membranes and organelles such as peroxisomes and mitochondria usually produce high levels of ROS under normal physiological conditions. In order to keep this potential source of damaging reactive species in check, enzymes such as catalase, superoxide dismutase and glutathione peroxidase catalyse the breakdown of reactive oxygen species to non-toxic by-products [4]. In addition, antioxidants provide a more passive form of protection against ROS-induced damage. For example, glutathione (GSH) can neutralise free radicals and ROS directly via a chemical reaction or in combination with enzymatic reactions involving glutathione reductase or glutathione peroxidase [5]. Antioxidant agents such as vitamin A, C and E also limit ROS damage by breaking the chain reaction that leads to lipid peroxidation. Other antioxidants, such as diallylsulfide, can act as inhibitors of CYP2E1 thereby reducing the availability of superoxide radical (O_2^-) that is transformed to OH· by iron [3]. During times of iron overload (e.g. in hemochromatosis), the burden of cellular iron can overwhelm these antioxidant mechanisms and ROS reacts with polyunsaturated phospholipids within organelles and other cell membranes. In this setting, oxidation of amino acids leads to the formation of protein adducts, DNA strand breaks and protein fragmentation, with clear consequences for altered cellular integrity and metabolic function [6].

1.3 Lipid Peroxidation

The OH· formed by iron-catalysed reactions is second only to elemental fluorine in terms of its reactivity. OH· is able to catalyse the transfer of electrons from lipids of the cell membrane back to the free radical resulting in lipid peroxidation. This process affects polyunsaturated fatty acids as they contain multiple double bonds between which lie methylene (CH_2) groups that are especially susceptible to peroxidation. Intramolecular rearrangement of double bonds within these radicals yields conjugated dienes, and in the presence of oxygen, lipid radicals form lipid peroxyl radicals [7]. These lipid peroxyl radicals can self-perpetuate by reacting with more fatty acids and also form lipid hydroperoxide, which is susceptible to cleavage by ferrous and ferric iron chelates with decomposition to alkoxyl and peroxyl free radicals, respectively. Lipid hydroperoxides undergo intramolecular cyclization and decomposition to generate thiobarbituric acid (TBA)-reactants and the breakdown by-products malondialdehyde (MDA), 4-hydroxynonenal (4-HNE), ketones, alcohol, ethane and pentane [7, 8]. In turn, MDA and 4-HNE are frequently used as markers of oxidative stress as they are readily localized using specific antibodies. Lipid peroxidation of membranes throughout the cell results in membrane fragility and can lead to dysfunction of a number of different organelles which compromises cell function (Fig. 18.1) [9]. These organelles include lysosomes, which store excess iron, mitochondria and endoplasmic reticulum, leading to problems with energy and protein production [9].

1.4 Iron-Mediated Intracellular Damage

1.4.1 Lysosomal Fragility

Iron accumulation within lysosomes is frequently observed in patients with iron overload [10]. Intracellular iron requirements are typically met by turnover and recycling of iron already present in the cell. In dividing cells, access to iron is gained through the internalisation of transferrin-bound iron with subsequent iron liberation achieved in late endosomes. During iron overload, autophagocytosis of macromolecules such as ferritin and hemosiderin containing substantial amounts of iron is thought to result in lysosomes becoming iron loaded [11]. Labile iron can readily generate ROS as outlined in the previous sections (Fig. 18.1), and sequestration in the lysosome is believed to represent one of many protective mechanisms that exist within the cell. Excessive lysosomal iron is thought to lead to lysosomal fragility and dysfunction through lipid peroxidation [12]. The loss of lysosomal integrity has important ramifications when one considers that the iron is then released into the cytoplasm along with a number of hydrolytic enzymes [7, 13]. Evidence of lysosomal fragility is seen in patients with hemochromatosis where elevated levels of the lysosomal enzymes N-acetyl-β glucosaminidase and acid phosphatase are seen in liver tissue [13, 14]. Lysosomal enzyme levels returned to near normal after repeated phlebotomy [14]. Animal models of iron overload have also demonstrated the presence of lysosomal fragility as evidenced by elevated lysosomal enzyme activity [15, 16].

1.4.2 Mitochondrial Abnormalities

As mentioned previously, mitochondrial dysfunction is also a consequence of iron overload. In a rat model of iron overload and in isolated normal rat mitochondria, iron has been found to be deleterious to the mitochondrial electron transport chain [17, 18]. While this is principally due to an iron-induced decrease in cytochrome C oxidase activity, it is unclear if iron mediates changes in the enzyme or in functionally dependent phospholipids. Lysosomal enzymes have also been shown to induce cytochrome C release and oxidant production [19]. Although this study did not look specifically at the role of iron, it does suggest that lysosomal fragility may be implicated in disrupted mitochondrial function. The hydroxyl radical is also known to be formed by the iron-dependent Fenton reaction in the mitochondria during times of oxidant stress [20]. Given the propensity for lipid peroxidation by $OH^{\cdot}$, this may represent an important source of ROS during iron overload. Acute iron overload in the rat has been shown to lead to iron loading of the mitochondria with an accompanying rise in lipid peroxidation and glutathione oxidation. Mitochondrial uncoupling was also observed, but this did not alter phosphorylation efficiency or the cellular adenosine triphosphate (ATP) levels. These data suggest that mitochondrial uncoupling may represent a protective mechanism limiting the damage caused by acute iron overload [21].

Opening of the mitochondrial permeability transition pore (MPTP) is another important mechanism by which mitochondrial stress can lead to apoptosis. Induction of the MPTP results in rapid mitochondrial depolarization, uncoupling of oxidative phosphorylation and osmotic swelling of the inner membrane-matrix compartment. The subsequent release of cytochrome c is known to activate various caspase enzymes, resulting ultimately in apoptosis [22]. Studies using isolated rat hepatocytes have shown that free chelatable iron is able to open the MPTP leading to mitochondrial DNA release and hepatocyte apoptosis [23]. Mitochondrial dysfunction in hepatic iron overload is also caused by decreased Ca^{2+} sequestration [24], increased Ca^{2+} release [25] and mitochondrial DNA damage and release [26, 27]. The release of Ca^{2+} from mitochondria suggests a permeability problem in iron overload, which may explain the decreased sequestration.

Interestingly, a recent study examined the role of glucosylxanthone derived from *Mangifera indica* in the prevention of iron-mediated mitochondrial damage [28]. This study suggested that the antioxidant activity of mangiferin is due its iron-chelating properties, suggesting that it could be a potential candidate for chelation therapy in diseases related to abnormal iron overload [28].

1.4.3 Protein and DNA Damage

Another consequence of lipid peroxidation is the damage to DNA and proteins, as lipid peroxidation products such as 4-HNE and MDA can react with DNA bases [29] and the ε-NH_2 group of lysine and histidine residues [30]. Acetaldehyde, derived from ethanol oxidation, is also known to bind MDA in a synergistic manner, generating new hybrid adducts called MDA-acetaldehyde adducts [31]. These adducts may play a role in disease development. For example, MDA-acetaldehyde adducts have been shown to play a role in progression of liver fibrosis as they have been linked to the secretion of several cytokines and chemokines by liver endothelial cells and hepatic stellate cells [32–34].

A considerable volume of evidence indicates that excess iron can induce DNA damage in both animal models of iron overload and in vitro in hepatocyte culture [7]. DNA damage is of particular significance in patients with hemochromatosis, a disease which shows a high incidence of HCC linked to DNA mutation/damage. Several studies show increased levels of etheno-DNA adducts derived from lipid peroxidation of DNA in hemochromatosis liver [35]. Etheno-DNA adducts are generated by 4-HNE when it contacts DNA [35]. Mutation of the p53 tumor suppressor gene, which regulates cell cycle progression and DNA repair, is a common finding in patients with hemochromatosis-linked HCC [36]. Iron is also known to directly associate with DNA in a manner that is not entirely random [37]. For example, iron-mediated Fenton oxidants of DNA occur preferentially at the following sites – R***T***GT TA***T***TY CT***T***R ***NGG***G – leading to cleavage at the site of the bold, underlined nucleotides [37].

1.5 *Summary*

The toxicity associated with excessive iron in the main can be attributed to its catalytic role in the generation of various ROS including OH˙. The ROS then partake in a number of self-perpetuation reactions that lead to lipid peroxidation, protein adduct formation and DNA mutation. At physiological concentrations of iron, cells and organs are well equipped to deal with these unwanted effects of iron. However at pathological concentrations, protective mechanisms can be overwhelmed, leading to cell apoptosis and necrosis, ultimately leading to organ failure. The following sections will highlight the pathological role of iron in liver disease, ischemic heart disease and the diabetic pancreas.

2 Genesis of Hepatic Fibrosis and Development of Cirrhosis

2.1 *Introduction*

Injury to any organ will result in a wound healing response [38]. If the injury is severe enough and or sustained, scar tissue will form at the site of injury. Chronic injury of the liver is no exception and gives rise to a wound healing response typically associated with fibrosis, and if the injury is prolonged, cirrhosis [39–41]. Cirrhosis is characterized by widespread fibrosis in addition to the appearance of nodules of regenerating hepatocytes. The nodules of hepatocytes are circular areas surrounded by scar tissue. The size and architecture of the nodes of hepatocytes, in turn, defines the type of cirrhosis which can be termed either macronodular or micronodular. Those nodes centered on a hepatic vein are termed macronodular, whereas nodes that lack lobular organisation are micronodular. Cirrhosis of the liver is normally accompanied by a number of life-threatening sequelae including portal hypertension caused by hepatic vein compression, leading to ascites and esophageal varices, jaundice, hepatocellular carcinoma and hepatic encephalopathy. In the normal liver the extracellular matrix (ECM) forms the framework of the liver and a fine balance is struck between deposition and degradation. During chronic liver injury the balance between deposition and degradation of components of the ECM becomes perturbed. This is accomplished by the transition of the hepatic stellate cell from a fat-storing phenotype to that typically associated with a myofibroblast. The myofibroblastic or activated hepatic stellate cell expresses a variety of scar tissue ECM components, namely fibrillary collagens type I and III in addition to collagen type IV, fibronectin, elastin and laminin [42]. In addition, activated hepatic stellate cells also express various tissue inhibitors of metalloproteinases (TIMPs) that prevent the breakdown of the scar ECM, thereby ensuring the perpetuation of the fibrotic tissue [42]. At present the only way to successfully resolve liver fibrosis is to treat the underlying cause of the liver injury. In patients suffering from hemochromatosis, this is typically achieved by phlebotomy [43]. Cirrhosis is known to be more resistant to resolution and can persist long after the injurious agent has been removed. The following sections will discuss in detail the iron-mediated processes that permit the development of fibrosis and cirrhosis.

2.2 *Initiation of Fibrosis*

The normal liver exhibits a tremendous capacity to tolerate injury and regenerate, even in the continued presence of an injurious stimulus. This can be demonstrated by the fact that clinical liver disease caused by excessive alcohol intake, hemochromatosis and viral hepatitis can often take many years to present [42]. Iron has been implicated as either the main cause or as an aggravating factor in a number of different types of liver disease that lead to cirrhosis [44]. Under normal physiological conditions, intestinal iron absorption is tightly regulated by the peptide hepcidin [45]. In the human body there is no dedicated iron excretion process and dysregulation of the iron uptake process leads to iron overload. Under normal physiological conditions, most uptake of iron by hepatocytes occurs via the internalisation of transferrin-bound iron [46]. Indeed internalisation of iron by hepatocytes also represents one of the few iron excretory pathways where it is excreted via the biliary system [16].

During times of iron overload, i.e. hemochromatosis, iron loading occurs in hepatocytes proximal to the portal tract (acinar zone 1) [43]. It also appears that there is a hepatic iron threshold of 60 μmol/g over which early evidence of hepatic fibrogenesis, in the form of hepatic stellate cell activation, is seen [43]. When the hepatic iron concentration reaches levels between 250 and 400 μmol/g, liver cirrhosis is often present [47–49]. Kupffer cells are the resident macrophage of the liver and normally reside in the hepatic sinusoid. They are also known to play an important part in iron metabolism and, in the latter stages of hemochromatosis, can store considerable amounts of iron [50]. It is excessive iron loading of hepatocytes and eventually Kupffer cells in hemochromatosis that is believed to be an initiating event that causes the transition of the liver from healthy to fibrotic. The role of iron in cirrhosis is somewhat clouded by the fact that another source of injury seems to be required for clinically relevant liver disease to become apparent [51]. The prevalence of cirrhosis in male C282Y homozygous patients is approximately 4–6% [51]. These results are at odds with the findings that as many as 100% of male C282Y homozygous subjects display biochemical evidence of iron loading [51]. Taken together, these findings clearly suggest that other factors are important in determining if an iron-loaded patient goes on to develop cirrhosis. It has been proposed that a second injurious insult is required for homozygous C282Y patients to develop clinically relevant liver disease, and to date, excessive alcohol consumption, viral hepatitis and obesity are the most frequently encountered cofactors [44]. The following sections will cover the role iron plays in initiating the cellular changes that lead ultimately to cirrhosis.

2.2.1 The Role of the Hepatocyte

Injury to the parenchymal cells of the liver is generally required for cirrhosis to develop. Hepatocytes perform numerous critical roles including iron storage, bile secretion and detoxification. In the course of performing these roles, hepatocytes are frequently exposed to numerous injurious stimuli. As the hepatic parenchyma is one of the principal sites of iron storage, this renders the hepatocyte susceptible to the oxidant stress generated by iron. Numerous pathways and mechanisms exist that protect cells from oxidant stress, but iron in excess can overrun these mechanisms resulting in cell injury and/or cell death.

Iron has been shown to initiate both apoptosis [52] and necrosis [53] of hepatocytes. In both cases hepatocyte death is thought to be due to oxidant stress with the degree of hepatocyte apoptosis being directly proportional to the hepatic iron concentration [52]. Hepatocyte apoptosis is mainly observed in the pericentral regions or acinar zone 3 which, interestingly, is also the area associated with the activated hepatic stellate cell phenotype yet distal to the site of early iron loading [43]. Key indicators of oxidant stress in hepatocytes are the presence of the aldehydes MDA and 4-HNE [54]. These aldehydes are known to form protein adducts which can interfere with cell function causing apoptosis/necrosis [44]. Both can exert their effects away from their source of origin, and this may represent a mechanism by which hepatocyte apoptosis occurs distal to the regions of iron loading [43]. Transforming growth factor-β (TGF-β) is known to be synthesised by hepatocytes in the livers of patients with iron overload due to the C282Y mutation in HFE [55]. Many studies have demonstrated the importance of TGF-β as a profibrogenic cytokine [42], although it should be noted that TGF-β expression is not exclusive to hepatocytes in livers with excess iron [56]. Experimental iron loading of isolated hepatocytes has also been shown to induce the expression of interleukin (IL)-6 through the transcription factor activator protein 1 (AP-1) [57]. In addition, iron also renders cultured hepatocytes insensitive to the protection from oxidant stress elicited by tumor necrosis factor-α (TNFα) [58]. As the ECM around the hepatocytes changes to that associated with fibrosis, hepatocytes become more susceptible to oxidant stress making them more likely to undergo apoptosis or necrosis [59]. Iron has also been shown to facilitate CYP2E1-induced hepatocyte damage by enhancing oxidant stress within the cell [60]. This finding is of particular relevance to alcoholic liver disease or in patients with hemochromatosis who consume excess alcohol, where the combination of iron and alcohol results in increased oxidative stress within hepatocytes.

2.2.2 The Role of the Kupffer Cell

Along with the hepatocyte, the Kupffer cell (resident hepatic macrophage) plays a major role in iron metabolism. As part of the reticuloendothelial system, these cells are responsible (in part) for the phagocytosis of senescent red blood cells and recycling heme-bound iron back to the plasma [46]; Kupffer cells have also been shown to phagocytose sideronecrotic hepatocytes [50]. During times of iron overload, Kupffer cells, especially late in the disease, can contain relatively high concentrations of iron [50] and this is particularly apparent in hemochromatosis associated with mutations in ferroportin [61]. Expression of ferroportin at the cell surface is under the regulation of hepcidin, and mutations in ferroportin are thought to prevent release of iron from the Kupffer cell [61].

Ferrous iron has been shown to directly regulate the activity of the transcription factor nuclear factor κB (NFκB) in cultured rat Kupffer cells, enhancing the expression of TNFα [62, 63]. It is also apparent that iron may be a cofactor, enhancing the expression of NFκB-dependent genes (TNFα and IL-6) in a rat model of cholestasis [64] and alcoholic liver disease [63]. It has been postulated that oxidant stress within the Kupffer cell, leading to the release of IL-6 and TNFα, is a key mechanism that leads to activation of the hepatic stellate cell leading to its transformation to a profibrogenic myofibroblast [65]. IL-6 and TNFα are known in other forms of liver disease to be key regulators of the events leading to liver fibrosis and cirrhosis [42]. Interestingly IL-6 has also been shown to enhance hepatic iron uptake through transferrin, and it also upregulates the expression of serum ferritin [66] possibly worsening the oxidant stress already present within the liver. In hemochromatosis, iron loading of Kupffer cells has also been shown to induce the expression of intracellular adhesion molecule-1 (ICAM-1) by adjacent hepatocytes [50]. The exact mechanism by which this occurs is unresolved, but ICAM-1 expression in the liver is sensitive to the presence TNFα [67]. ICAM-1 is known to mediate the binding and adhesion of leukocytes to cells and has been shown to be a crucial component in liver regeneration following injury [68].

Kupffer cells are known to phagocytose iron-loaded hepatocytes that are undergoing apoptosis [52]. Previous studies have shown that phagocytosis of apoptotic hepatocytes by Kupffer cells leads to their activation, enhancing their pro-inflammatory and profibrogenic role [69]. Activated Kupffer cells and activated hepatic stellate cells are also often found in close proximity in hereditary hemochromatosis; thus Kupffer cell activation has been suggested as an important event leading to fibrosis and cirrhosis [50]. Evidence also suggests that iron in combination with other factors such as alcohol leads to the activation of Kupffer cells in other liver diseases not related to iron overload [65, 70, 71].

2.2.3 The Role of Other Cell Types

The Hepatic Sinusoidal Endothelial Cell

Hepatic sinusoidal endothelial cells separate hepatocytes and hepatic stellate cells from the blood and form the lining of the hepatic sinusoid. They play an important role in regulating hepatic microcirculation, and together with Kupffer cells, they play a role in the reticuloendothelial system, representing the most powerful scavenger pathway in the body. In the cirrhotic liver, sinusoidal endothelial cells lose their fenestrations and become pseudo-capillarized, thus greatly affecting the flow of nutrient and oxygen across the space of Dissé to the hepatic stellate cell and hepatocyte. The role that sinusoidal endothelial cells play in iron metabolism is relatively unexplored, and subsequently their role in the development of cirrhosis linked to iron is even less well known. It is known that endothelial cells express mRNAs for a number of proteins involved in iron homeostasis (i.e. transferrin receptors 1 and 2, divalent metal transporter-1, ferroportin and hephaestin), but currently their role in iron metabolism remains to be clarified [72]. Feeding a carbonyl iron diet to rats has been shown to induce acinar zone 1 loading of endothelial cells, as well as hepatocytes and Kupffer cells. This leads to the co-localization of hepatic iron with collagen α1(I) transcripts, MDA protein adducts and TGF-β1 expression in hepatocytes and hepatic stellate cells, accompanied by minor necrosis and inflammation [73]. In addition, colloidal iron is known to induce rapid defenestration and thickening of endothelial cells, but it is not known if the observed changes are due to the direct toxic effects of iron or due to the subsequent increases in oxidative stress. Experimentally induced hemolytic anemia leading to iron overload of the spleen, kidney and liver does not alter the iron content of the resident endothelial cells [74]. It therefore seems likely that iron during periods of overload may affect endothelial cell function and induce defenestration. The consequences of this, i.e. decreased sinusoidal blood flow and portal hypertension, are clearly important pathological factors associated with cirrhosis.

Cells of the Immune System

Unlike liver diseases such as viral hepatitis, alcoholic liver disease and non-alcoholic steatohepatitis, fibrosis and cirrhosis linked to hemochromatosis develops with very little evidence of inflammation [9]. Mild inflammation [75] and necrosis (sideronecrosis) [76] have been observed in periportal areas of the liver associated with extreme iron loading. Infiltration of the liver by CD3-positive T lymphocytes has been observed and correlated with hepatic iron concentration [75]; however, the consequences of these observations remain unknown. A clear decrease in cytotoxic CD8-positive T lymphocytes has been well characterized in patients with hemochromatosis and is particularly apparent in patients with cirrhosis [77, 78]. Cytotoxic T cells play an important role in the removal of infected cells, tumor cells and damaged or dysfunctional cells. The exact role that CD8-positive T lymphocytes play in iron-induced cirrhosis remains somewhat of an enigma.

Liver Progenitor Cells

Liver progenitor cells are responsible for liver regeneration during times of liver injury when hepatocyte division is inhibited. Progenitor cell proliferation has been shown to occur in conditions such as alcoholic liver disease, viral hepatitis, non-alcoholic fatty liver disease and hereditary hemochromatosis [79, 80]. Experimental iron loading of rat livers using carbonyl iron leads to the appearance of liver progenitor cells in the periportal region and, with continued iron loading, also in the pericentral region of the acinus. These cells were found to be free of iron and also negative for transferrin, indicating that progenitor cell expansion was a consequence of iron overload and is not directly causative [80]. It has recently been shown that progenitor cells acting through lymphotoxin-β are able to induce signaling events in hepatic stellate cells that are thought to contribute to the regenerative and fibrogenic response of the liver to injury [79]. Therefore, while iron does not appear to directly contribute to liver progenitor cell-mediated fibrogenic processes, progenitor cell expansion is implicated as mediating the response of the hepatic stellate cell to injury.

2.3 Iron and the Hepatic Stellate Cell

The hepatic stellate cell is primarily responsible for the qualitative and quantitative ECM changes associated with liver fibrosis and cirrhosis. In the normal healthy liver, hepatic stellate cells exist in the space of Dissé in close proximity to the sinusoidal endothelial cells and Kupffer cells on one side and the hepatocytes on the other. This close proximity makes them a key mediator in the transport of soluble factors from the circulation to the hepatic parenchyma. They also store considerable amounts of vitamin A in intracellular vesicles, with the amount dependent on their location within the liver [81]. Typically hepatic stellate cells located in areas near the portal tract (periportal) have been shown to contain significantly more vitamin A than those near the central vein of the hepatic lobule (pericentral) [82]. The hepatic stellate cell is highly sensitive to various stimuli that trigger transdifferentiation of the cell to a myofibroblast associated with proliferation, chemotaxis, fibrogenesis, contractility and leukocyte chemoattraction [83]. The number of receptors expressed by the hepatic stellate cell is considerable, and they are known to respond to chemokines (chemokine C-C ligands (CCL) 2 and 5), cytokines (interleukins 1β, 6, 8, 10, interferonγ and TNFα), growth factors (platelet-derived growth factor-BB, insulin-like growth factor-1, TGFβ and epidermal growth factor) and neuroendocrine agents (serotonin [84], angiotensin and endothelin) [42]. When in their quiescent stage, hepatic stellate cells also express the mRNAs for a number of genes known to be important in iron homeostasis (e.g. hepcidin, ferroportin 1, ceruloplasmin and transferrin receptors 1 and 2) [72]. In addition, the hepatic stellate cell is the only resident liver cell known to express bone morphogenetic protein 6 [85], which has recently been shown to be a key regulator of hepcidin expression [86, 87]. These findings alone suggest that hepatic stellate cells may be important in iron sensing or, alternatively, iron may facilitate hepatic stellate cell activation. The dazzling array of events that lead to the activation of the hepatic stellate cell is complex and still being deciphered. What is clear is that the myofibroblastic hepatic stellate cell is directly responsible for the scar matrix seen in the fibrotic liver which is the main event in the development of liver cirrhosis. Scar tissue of the cirrhotic liver is readily identified in histochemical sections using the collagen stain Sirius red, and similarly, myofibroblastic hepatic stellate cells can be identified using antibodies to α-smooth muscle actin (αSMA) [88] The following sections will outline those events mediated directly by iron, by oxidant stress as a result of iron and iron-associated/binding proteins that result in hepatic stellate cell activation.

2.3.1 Patterns of Hepatic Stellate Cell Activation and Matrix Remodeling as a Result of Iron Overload

In the early stages of iron overload when hepatic iron concentrations are around 60 μmol/g dry weight, αSMA-positive or activated hepatic stellate cells are located in regions close to the central vein [43]. This is distal to the site of iron loading which usually occurs in regions close to the portal tract. As iron loading progresses, activated hepatic stellate cells appear in areas close to and eventually in areas near to the portal tract [43]. While this would appear to be counterintuitive, as in hereditary hemochromatosis injury occurring initially in periportal areas, it has also been observed in another liver disease state (hepatitis C) where activated hepatic stellate cells appear in apparently healthy liver tissue [89]. The reason for this observation is unclear, but it would seem that soluble factors are able to influence hepatic stellate cells distal to their source. A number of animal models have also been used to model iron overload, but contrary to results seen in human hereditary hemochromatosis, activated hepatic stellate cells were found close to siderotic hepatocytes. Feeding the carbonyl iron diet to rats has been shown to induce acinar zone 1 loading of hepatocytes, Kupffer cells and sinusoidal endothelial cells. This led to the co-localization of hepatic iron with collagen α1(I) transcripts, MDA protein adducts and TGFβ1 expression in hepatocytes and hepatic stellate cells [73]. Similar results were observed in male gerbils subcutaneously dosed with iron dextran [56]. Iron loading of the liver induced the expression of collagen by hepatic stellate cells around the iron foci (periportal areas) with animals going on to develop micronodular cirrhosis after 4 months of iron dextran injections. Marked proliferation of hepatic stellate cells around the regions of regenerating hepatocyte nodules was also observed [56].

Matrix remodeling, regulated by TIMPs and matrix metalloproteinases (MMPs), is also known to occur in patients with iron overload, and this is thought to contribute directly to the progression of hepatic fibrosis [90]. TIMP1 is known to be elevated during times of cirrhosis, is expressed by activated hepatic stellate cells and plays a key role in preventing scar tissue breakdown [91]. In addition to the upregulated expression of TIMP1 by hepatic stellate cells, the other arm of matrix remodeling, namely MMP expression, remains relatively unchanged in hemochromatosis patients [90]. This study did not, however, go on to describe the distribution of TIMP1 and MMPs in the cirrhotic liver.

2.3.2 Direct Effects of Iron on Hepatic Stellate Cell Activation

During iron overload, the hepatic stellate cell is not the principal site of iron storage. However, hepatic stellate cells undoubtedly have the ability to sequester iron [92, 93], thus presenting a possible mechanism by which iron and iron-related oxidant stress may influence hepatic stellate cell biology. Both iron ascorbate and ferric nitrilotriacetate have been shown to directly enhance the exchange of Na^+/H^+ leading to accelerated hepatic stellate cell proliferation and collagen type 1 expression in vitro [94]. Gardi et al. were also able to show that ferric iron was able to modestly enhance collagen synthesis and, at higher doses, induce the proliferation of hepatic stellate cells and the activity of MMP-2 [95]. In culture, iron aldehydes and other pro-oxidants were found to induce heme oxygenase expression within activated hepatic stellate cells but were not able to induce the expression of collagen mRNA. Heme oxygenase is known to have an important role in protecting cells from oxidant stress [96]. In addition, other fibroblastic cell types have been shown to respond to iron overload in a fibrogenic manner, with enhanced expression of TGFβ1 and collagen type 1 being observed after iron loading in vitro [97].

Role of Iron-Binding Proteins in Hepatic Stellate Cell Activation

A number of proteins that interact with iron have been shown to be important in hepatic stellate cell activation, including the iron-storage protein ferritin. Normally ferritin acts to store iron within the cell in an inert but biologically available form. During times of iron overload and inflammation, serum ferritin becomes markedly elevated. The precise reasons why serum ferritin is elevated are unknown, but it has been postulated that ferritin may have additional roles other than simply iron storage. In iron overload conditions, ferritin released from damaged hepatocytes and/or Kupffer cells may contribute significantly to the local hepatic ferritin concentration. A number of studies have identified specific receptors for both H- and L-ferritin subunits which appear to be involved in ferritin endocytosis [93, 98–100]. T-cell immunoglobulin and mucin domain-2 (Tim-2) and transferrin receptor 1 have been identified as H-ferritin endocytic receptors [98, 100, 101] whereas Scara5 internalises L-ferritin [99]. The physiological relevance of these findings is unknown as much of this work was conducted in cell lines. Hepatic stellate cells express Tim-2 [102], although it is unclear whether this is the receptor responsible for ferritin endocytosis in these cells [93]. Ferritin has been shown to act as a pro-inflammatory cytokine in hepatic stellate cell biology, by inducing a protein kinase C-ζ (PKC-ζ)-dependent signaling event, elicited via an as yet unknown receptor, which results in the upregulation of NFκB-regulated inflammatory genes (IL-1β, inducible nitric oxide synthase, ICAM-1, CCL5) associated with the profibrogenic phenotype of hepatic stellate cells [102]. Of interest, these signaling pathways appear to be entirely independent of iron, as iron-free apoferritin and recombinant H- and L-ferritins all had similar effects on gene expression [102]. Activated hepatic stellate cells also express both transferrin receptors, which mediates the enhanced expression of αSMA and collagen α_1(I) [92]. These two proteins may represent important profibrogenic factors associated with iron overload and hemochromatosis.

Cytoglobin is an iron-binding protein that has been shown to protect the hepatic stellate cell against oxidative stress and has been investigated as a potential suppressor of hepatic stellate cell activation. Cytoglobin was first identified in activated hepatic stellate cells [103] and has now been described in many splanchnic fibroblast cells. It is a new member of the hexacoordinate globin superfamily [104]. The precise role of cytoglobin is unclear, but it has been shown to scavenge toxic radicals such as nitric oxide, peroxynitrite and hydrogen peroxide, thereby protecting cells from oxidant stress [105].

2.3.3 Role of Iron-Mediated Oxidant Stress in Hepatic Stellate Cell Activation

The general consensus is that hepatic stellate cells in vivo are not directly subject to iron-induced oxidant stress due to iron uptake. Rather, hepatic stellate cell activation during iron overload is a result of the release of ROS, protein adducts and various cytokines and chemokines from hepatocytes and Kupffer cells. Early studies performed by Parola et al. showed lipid peroxidation (induced by iron and ascorbic acid) and 4-HNE can directly influence procollagen gene expression and synthesis in hepatic stellate cells [106]. Using the iron-dextran model of iron overload in the gerbil, Montosi and colleagues [96] were unable to find evidence of ferritin accumulation (suggesting no iron uptake), or the presence of MDA-protein adducts in activated hepatic stellate cells surrounding iron-laden hepatocytes. In culture, however, iron, aldehydes and other pro-oxidants were able to induce the expression of heme oxygenase but not collagen mRNA [96]. This is work was further supported by in vitro studies using hepatocyte-conditioned medium from cells treated with ferric nitrilotriacetate to induce hepatocyte oxidant stress. The conditioned medium was able to stimulate enhanced hepatic stellate cell proliferation and also the activity of Na^+/H^+ exchanger, a protein known to regulate cell proliferation [107]. MDA and 4-HNE have also been shown by others to induce procollagen expression in hepatic stellate cells and fibroblast cells [108]. ROS derived from hepatocytes expressing CYP2E1 was observed to increase the rate of hepatic stellate cell proliferation and the levels of αSMA and collagen expression in culture, effects enhanced by the presence of ferric nitrilotriacetate [109]. Conversely, other in vitro studies using conditioned medium from iron-loaded hepatocytes have shown the opposite effects, where proliferation of activated hepatic stellate cells was inhibited through a TGFβ1-dependent mechanism [110]. Other studies were also unable to show any effects of 4-HNE and MDA on the activation of hepatic stellate cells as assessed by the expression of αSMA protein [111]. Thus the role of these lipid peroxidation by-products on hepatic stellate cell activation remains controversial.

2.4 *Fibrosis/Cirrhosis Therapies*

Phlebotomy is frequently used to treat patients with hereditary hemochromatosis presenting with iron overload, and in general this is a highly effective therapy at reducing both iron levels and fibrosis [43, 49]. As iron is also implicated in a number of other diseases that lead to cirrhosis, including viral hepatitis [112], alcoholic liver disease [113] and non-alcoholic fatty liver disease [114], phlebotomy has been trialed as a therapy for these diseases with varying degrees of success. Antioxidants have also been investigated as potential therapeutics in iron-associated liver fibrosis. Vitamin E (α-tocopherol) has been shown to completely inhibit iron overload-induced fibrosis in the gerbil [56], with others showing this possibly occurs through the inhibition of the formation of aldehyde adducts [115]. However, no thorough studies have been performed using vitamin E as a therapy for iron-induced fibrosis in human subjects due to the efficacy of phlebotomy therapy.

2.5 *Summary*

In summary, hepatic cirrhosis is a life-threatening consequence of iron overload. Cirrhosis is the abnormal deposition of scar tissue within the liver and is usually the result of prolonged iron overload within the liver. Iron loading occurs primarily in the hepatocytes in the periportal regions of the liver, gradually extending to regions closer to the central vein with time. As iron loading reaches extreme levels, Kupffer cells also exhibit significant levels of iron. It is the iron loading of these cells and the concomitant oxidative stress that lead to cellular necrosis and apoptosis. As hepatocytes and Kupffer cells undergo necrosis and apoptosis, they release a number of different mediators that contribute to the activation of the hepatic stellate cell. The activated hepatic stellate cell then begins the process of scar matrix deposition associated with fibrosis. As the injury due to iron continues, the activated hepatic stellate cell will continue to deposit scar tissue until the liver becomes cirrhotic. The cellular interactions and major cytokines and growth factors that are believed to play a role in the genesis of hepatic cirrhosis are summarised in Fig. 18.2. The damage caused to hepatocytes and Kupffer cells by excess iron deposition, combined with the abnormal liver architecture due to scar tissue deposition, leads to the morbidity and mortality associated with hepatic iron overload. If diagnosed early, phlebotomy is highly effective at reducing iron burden and simultaneously the liver can return to a normal architecture.

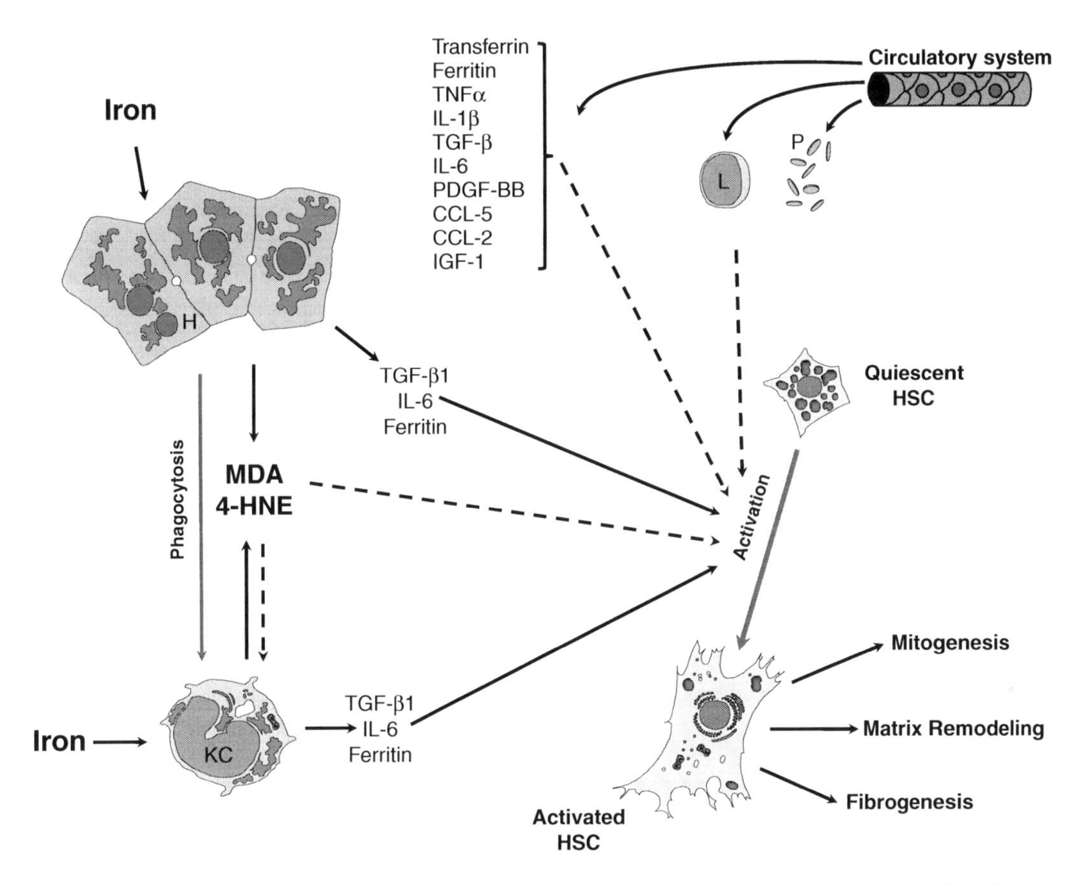

Fig. 18.2 Cellular interactions and mechanisms leading to wound healing in hepatic iron overload. Iron deposition in hepatocytes (*H*) and Kupffer cells (*KC*) subsequent to increased intestinal iron absorption leads to lipid peroxidation, cellular damage and eventually apoptosis and necrosis. Lipid peroxidation by-products 4-hydroxynonenal (*4-HNE*) and malondialdehyde (*MDA*), as well as transforming growth factor-β (*TGF*-β) and interleukin 6 (*IL-6*) and the iron-storage protein ferritin released by dying cells, are then postulated to play a role in the phenotypic transformation of the hepatic stellate cell (*HSC*) to a myofibroblast. The transformed HSC is then primarily responsible for matrix remodeling and scar tissue deposition in the livers of hemochromatotic patients. The role that lymphocytes (*L*), platelets (*P*) and the immune system in general play in the development of fibrosis/cirrhosis is not fully understood. An array of other factors known to play a role in the development of cirrhosis associated with other types of liver injury have also been postulated to influence cirrhosis linked to hemochromatosis. Dashed arrows represent potential pathways requiring further investigation. CCL-5, chemokine (*C-C motif*) ligand-5; CCL-2, chemokine (*C-C motif*) ligand-2; IGF-1, insulin-like growth factor-1; IL-1β, interleukin 1β; PDGF-BB, platelet-derived growth factor-BB; TNFα, tumor necrosis factor-α (adapted from Ramm and Ruddell [9])

3 Iron and the Pancreas

The pancreas is an organ that exhibits both endocrine and exocrine functions. During pathological iron overload, areas of the pancreas including β-cells and acini [116] show evidence of iron loading and this phenomenon is thought to be responsible for the diabetes observed in patients suffering from extreme iron overload. The exocrine function of the pancreas also appears to be affected in patients with iron overload as a consequence of frequent chronic blood transfusion [117]. Studies performed using rats indicate that β-cells express higher levels of transferrin receptor than α-cells, and that with progressive iron loading, β-cells demonstrate elevated intracellular ferritin levels and eventually stainable iron [118]. Studies on the mammalian pancreas have shown that β-cells also express a number of proteins involved in iron homeostasis, and these include hepcidin, ferroportin and DMT-1 [119]. Restriction of iron in the Otsuka Long-Evans Tokushima fatty rat model of type 2 diabetes resulted in decreased oxidative stress in the pancreas as indicated by markers of lipid peroxidation; furthermore, peroxisome proliferator-activated receptor-δ (PPARδ) and insulin expression were found to increase [120]. PPARδ is known to play a role lipid accumulation, and the PPARδ agonist GW-501516 has been used experimentally to treat pathologies associated with the metabolic syndrome in obese men [121]. Iron chelation or phlebotomy may represent mechanisms to treat the pathologies associated with type 2 diabetes. It is apparent that the β-cell is particularly ill-equipped to deal with oxidant stress due to low expression levels of superoxide dismutase and glutathione peroxidase [122]. Given that β-cell iron loading is seen in patients with β-thalassemia and hemochromatosis and the ability of iron to catalyse the formation of ROS, it is not unreasonable to hypothesise that the observed diabetes maybe due to the presence of iron in the β-cell. A separate study found that while mutations in *HFE* are linked to diabetes mellitus, they were not linked with pancreatitis and pancreatic adenocarcinoma [123]. This would suggest that damage sustained by the iron-loaded pancreas is not widespread and may be limited to β-cells. Damage to β-cells can also be mediated by cytokines such as TNFα and IL-1β, resulting in decreased insulin production [124]. In patients with β-thalassemia that received frequent blood transfusion, this was found not to be the case as levels of these cytokines were not elevated [125]. It has also been suggested that diabetes associated with iron overload may be more the result of hepatic insulin resistance leading to diabetes rather than a lack of insulin production [126, 127]. In addition, Suvarna and colleagues found in chronically transfused β-thalassemia patients a correlation between hyper-insulinemia and indicators of iron overload before the onset of frank diabetes mellitus [126].

In summary, iron accumulation occurs within the parenchyma of the pancreas in diseases such as hemochromatosis and in chronically transfused β-thalassemia patients. Iron is associated with decreased insulin signaling; whether this is due to decreased insulin production by β-cells or is due to decreased hepatic insulin sensitivity remains to be definitively proven.

4 Hepatocellular Carcinoma

4.1 Introduction

HCC is a common primary malignancy of the liver [128] that usually occurs secondary to liver diseases with diverse etiologies. Afflictions of the liver that cause cirrhosis are generally a prerequisite for the development of HCC, and in patients with compensated cirrhosis, HCC is the number one cause of mortality [129]. One such disease is hereditary hemochromatosis. Patients suffering with hemochromatosis have an estimated overall rate of HCC of approximately 6–10% [130, 131]. This translates to an approximate 20–200-fold increased risk of developing HCC [132], leading to 25–45% of all premature deaths associated with hemochromatosis [133–135]. Other risk factors that are also known to increase the chances of a patient with hemochromatosis developing HCC include viral infection (hepatitis B and C), male gender, excessive alcohol consumption and non-alcoholic fatty liver disease [136]. The exact role of the various cells and processes thought to be involved are still being dissected. However, chronic liver injury typically results in the impaired function and proliferation of hepatocytes, invoking a coordinated mobilisation of the liver progenitor cell compartment. Liver progenitor cells are readily transformed in vivo and have high rates of proliferation [137]. A number of studies have now implicated liver progenitor cells in the progression of HCC [138, 139].

4.2 Mechanism of Iron-Induced Hepatocellular Carcinoma

Iron loading of the liver, whether it is due to hemochromatosis, high dietary intake or β-thalassemia, has been linked directly to the increased risk of developing HCC [130, 140, 141]. Iron loading of the liver also occurs in other forms of chronic liver disease [44], and the role that this iron plays in the progression from cirrhosis to HCC remains unclear. Iron is an essential nutrient known to be crucial in normal cell function; however, in excess, iron and the resultant oxidant stress induced by iron have a demonstrated capacity to induce carcinogenic changes [36]. Iron has also been shown to stimulate the proliferation of both normal hepatocytes and hepatoma cell lines [142–144]. The early stages of HCC are characterized by iron-free foci within the livers of patients with hemochromatosis which are thought to be areas of rapidly dividing hepatocytes or stem cells [136]. As the tumor increases in size, angiogenesis and tumor encapsulation become important factors regulating tumor size and spread. The following sections will discuss the role iron plays in the development HCC in the context of iron overload.

4.2.1 Iron and DNA Damage

The transcription factor p53 regulates the progression of the cell cycle and is intimately linked to the suppression of tumor growth. It is activated by a number of different stress factors, including DNA damage, reactive oxygen species and osmotic shock. The resulting cellular effects of p53 activation include the activation of DNA repair genes, arrest of the cell cycle at the G_1/S checkpoint and the initiation of apoptosis. Mutations that alter or inhibit the functionality of p53 have been linked directly to carcinogenesis. The oxidative stress associated with iron loading in the livers of patients with hemochromatosis has been shown to cause mutations in the p53 gene predisposing them to HCC. Three studies have identified a number of mutations within the p53 gene [36, 145, 146]. Each of these studies identified different hotspots within the gene, for example, codon 220 [146], codons 249 and 250 [36] and codons 273 and 298 [145]. The difference in the mutational hotspots identified by these studies were attributed to possible differences in the prevalence of other contributing factors such as viral hepatitis and alcoholic liver disease [145]. Iron-mediated ROS generation via the Fenton reaction is thought to lead to point mutations in DNA. Iron is known to directly associate with DNA, and it is thought that the location of this iron binding may determine the substrate and nature of the damage [37]. For example, iron-mediated oxidative damage to DNA occurs preferentially at the following sites – R***T***GT, TA***T***TY, CT***T***R and ***NGG***G – leading to cleavage at the site of the bold underlined nucleotide [37]. Extensive mechanisms exist to 'repair' damaged DNA; however, these mechanisms may be overwhelmed during times of iron loading, resulting in base-pair transversion [37]. At present the presence of other mutations associated with HCC is relatively underreported.

4.2.2 Iron and Proliferation

Given that iron is an essential component of many cellular functions, it is logical that its availability would be an important factor in regulating cell proliferation. Iron has been shown to promote the proliferation of a number of cells of hepatocyte lineage in vitro [143, 144], and it has also been shown to stimulate hepatocyte growth and hepatomegaly in a rodent model of iron overload [142]. Several studies have shown that iron-chelating agents are able to inhibit hepatocyte growth, suggesting that they have a potential role as anti-tumor agents [144, 147]. The exact mechanism that underlies the increased rate of hepatocyte proliferation in response to iron remains largely unexplored; however, some evidence indicates a direct effect of iron on cyclin D1 expression [142]. Cyclin D1 is known to regulate cell cycle progression. Iron overload in rat liver has been shown to significantly increase cyclin D1 expression in the hepatocyte, resulting in elevated rates of hepatocyte proliferation [142]. Chronic iron overload in rats has also been shown to induce the proliferation of the liver stem cell compartment [80]. Similarities between the choline-deficient, ethionine-supplemented diet (also carcinogenic) and the carbonyl-iron-supplemented diet were observed, except that stem cells induced by carbonyl iron were negative for transferrin [80].

4.2.3 Iron and Non-parenchymal Cells

As mentioned previously, HCC is generally preceded by cirrhosis [131, 136], and the one cell type known to be primarily responsible for scar matrix deposition in the cirrhotic liver is the hepatic stellate cell [9]. A growing body of evidence suggests that the hepatic stellate cell is an important mediator in the processes that are involved in the development of HCC [148–150]. While hepatic stellate cells are not a major site of iron storage, they are recognised as a potential mediator of the effects of iron in fibrosis and they are activated in response to hepatic iron loading [43, 92, 93, 102, 151]. The iron-binding protein transferrin and the iron-storage protein ferritin have both been shown to elicit profibrogenic changes in hepatic stellate cells [92, 102]. Hepatic stellate cells may also play a role in mediating angiogenesis of the solid tumor being able to promote endothelial proliferation in response to soluble factors released by a hepatoma cell line [149]. Hepatic stellate cells, or more specifically activated myofibroblasts, also play a role in host defense, encapsulating the tumor and influencing local hepatic invasion [152, 153].

4.2.4 Iron and the Immune System

The immune system plays an important role in regulating the growth of tumors in a number of organs and HCC is no exception [154]. Iron is also a recognised mediator of immune function and vice versa [155], and during times of iron overload, it is plausible that altered immune function due to iron may alter the progression of HCC. While the interactions between iron and immunity and the immune response to HCC have been extensively investigated, the impact of iron overload on the immune response to HCC remains somewhat of an enigma. The local HCC tumor microenvironment is known to be immunosuppressive [156], and immune cells from patients with HCC exhibit a significant decrease in the numbers of CD16+ NK cells [157]. The mechanisms behind this decreased NK activity in patients with HCC are unknown; however, low counts of NK cells are seen in patients with hemochromatosis, and thus the two may be related [158]. Non-transferrin-bound iron is known to inhibit CD4+ T-lymphocyte proliferation [159], and this may in part be responsible for the reduced CD4+ cells seen in patients with β-thalassemia and hemochromatosis [136]. Iron-laden ferritin is also known to regulate T-lymphocyte proliferation and function [160] possibly through a newly described H-ferritin receptor [98]. Iron is also known to inhibit the tumoricidal activity of peritoneal macrophages [161].

4.3 HCC Therapies

The prognosis for a patient suffering with HCC is poor often because of the advanced stages of the cancer at the time of diagnosis, preventing liver transplantation [132]. When diagnosed early, treatment modalities include resection, transplantation and percutaneous ablation. The most widely used percutaneous ablation methods include ethanol injection and radiofrequency ablation. Other methods also trialed include acetic acid injection, boiling saline injection and cryotherapy to name but a few [162]. Success of these methods is dependent upon tumor size with smaller tumors (less than 2 cm) being treated with almost 100% success rates [162]. Phlebotomy is frequently used to treat patients with hemochromatosis and is very effective at lowering iron levels and preventing transition to cirrhosis which is frequently accompanied by HCC [132]. Once cirrhosis (whatever the cause) has developed, patients are still at an elevated risk of developing HCC; however, improved management of the tumor and complications of cirrhosis have significantly prolonged the life expectancy of patients [129]. Investigations into the therapeutic value of iron chelation have shown the ability of agents such as deferoxamine and ICL670 to inhibit the growth of hepatoma cell lines [144, 147], but the effects of these agents in vivo remain unproven.

4.4 Summary

HCC is a very common primary malignancy of the liver. It occurs in cirrhotic patients, and for those suffering with hemochromatosis, it is the number one cause of premature death. Iron is known to play a key role in the transition of the healthy liver to cirrhosis. It can also mutate DNA leading to dysregulation of the tumor suppressor gene p53. Iron is a vital component of many cellular reactions, and chelation of iron has been shown to significantly decrease the proliferation of cells derived from HCC. Iron also induces the proliferation of the stem cell compartment which has been shown to be an important step in the progression to HCC. Relatively little is known about the effects of high iron levels on the immune system and how this impacts the progression of HCC. It is known that high iron levels negatively impact upon CD4+ T-cell numbers, macrophage function and NK cell counts. Treatment for HCC can be effective if the disease is diagnosed in its early stages, and this can be achieved by regular monitoring of those patients with chronic liver disease. Advances in the detection methods used to determine the transition from cirrhosis to HCC currently represent the best way to minimise the impact of HCC on patient health.

5 Iron and Ischemic Heart Disease

5.1 Introduction

Ischemic heart disease (IHD) can be defined as the acute or chronic loss of oxygenated blood supply to the heart muscle leading to reduced heart function. IHD can be a stable condition (angina) apparent during times of mild to moderate physical exertion, or it can be unstable, deteriorating with time resulting in myocardial infarction and death. The cause of the decrease in cardiac blood flow is often associated with smoking, hypertension, a diet high in saturated fats and cholesterol, and type 2 diabetes mellitus. The net effect of these factors is the partial occlusion and decreased elasticity of the coronary artery leading to reduced cardiac muscle blood supply. The commonest cause of coronary artery occlusion is atherosclerosis, a process whereby fatty acids, cholesterol, calcium, fibrous tissue and macrophages are deposited to form an atheroma on the lumen of the artery wall. With time, the atheroma will usually get bigger and can result in the total blockade of the coronary artery leading to death. Reduced oxygenated blood flow to the cardiac muscle leads to hypoxia and the rapid development of necrosis in those tissues affected.

Recent scientific advances suggest that hypoxia-linked necrosis in the heart is a coordinated event involving a number of signaling pathways. ATP depletion is an initiating factor in ischemia-induced necrotic cell death with calcium and ROS also playing a role. During necrosis, elevated cytosolic calcium levels and ROS lead to mitochondrial dysfunction, loss of ATP production and activation of proteases and phospholipases. The necrosing cell also releases immunomodulatory factors that mediate inflammation and engulfment by phagocytes.

5.2 Identification of Iron as a Potential Mediator of Ischemic Heart Disease

The role of iron in ischemic heart disease is controversial and has been the source of much debate, with some studies indicating a correlation [163, 164] and others no correlation [165, 166]. The contentious hypothesis is that sustained or mild iron deficiency is protective against ischemic heart disease. How, why and if iron depletion is protective against IHD will be covered in the following section. A possible link between iron and IHD was first identified in 1981 [163] when it was observed that premenopausal women exhibit rates of heart disease lower than three in 1,000 per year. One factor common to almost all premenopausal women under the age of 45 is the low levels of stored iron and median serum ferritin levels of 25 ng/ml [163]. The levels of serum ferritin (an indicator of body iron stores) in women correlate with the incidence of IHD, and in older women with higher levels of serum ferritin, there is an observed increase in death due to IHD [167]. In this study the observed correlation did not specify how or why iron status may affect the prevalence or severity of IHD.

Although the work of Sullivan proposed a role for iron in IHD, several other studies have failed to demonstrate such a link [166, 168, 169]. Most recently, a prospective study of a healthy population in France found no major role for iron status in the development of IHD [165]. Interestingly, the correlation between iron and IHD prevalence is also dependent upon ethnicity [170]. Black South African men have far lower rates of IHD and, due to the practice of preparing food in iron cooking vessels, can have levels of hepatic iron approaching 2% dry weight [171]. Conversely men and women of Indian origin with low iron stores have a far higher rate of IHD, comparable or greater than the local white population [172]. While the iron status of a person may or may not correlate with likelihood of developing IHD or its severity, a role for iron in the pathologies associated with IHD has been widely reported.

5.3 Mechanisms of Iron-Induced Injury in the Ischemic Heart

Given the well-described catalytic role of iron in the generation of ROS, perhaps the most plausible explanation for the negative role of iron in IHD can be linked to this function. Indeed, data do exist demonstrating a role for iron in catalysing the formation of the hydroxyl radical in the aging rat heart following ischemia and reperfusion [173]. These effects were not observed in younger rat hearts and may represent a mechanism contributing to the increased sensitivity of the myocardium to hydrogen peroxide [173]. Iron has also been shown to mediate changes in myocardial membrane turnover and integrity, with the iron-chelating agent deferoxamine reducing lactate dehydrogenase release, MDA formation and improving myocardial contractility following ischemic injury and reperfusion [174]. In addition, ischemia also reduces cardiac mitochondrial function as represented by a decrease in oxidative phosphorylation in the rat heart, and this is further exacerbated following reperfusion of the ischemic heart [175]. Interestingly, iron is not the only metal implicated in post-ischemic injury. Data also suggest that copper is mobilised and plays an important role in the generation of ROS following ischemia [176].

Iron also appears to play a role in the progression and stability of the atherosclerotic plaque that contributes directly to IHD. Iron was first localized to the atherosclerotic plaque in patients suffering with IHD [177] and in rabbits fed a diet high in cholesterol [178]. In addition, a number of other lines of enquiry have provided further evidence for the presence of iron and iron-storage proteins associated with macrophages and foam cells in the atherosclerotic plaque [179]. Macrophages are known to be a site of iron turnover and readily take up lipids and cholesterol from the blood. It has been proposed that high iron and lipid content are toxic to the macrophage and surrounding cells, thereby expanding the atherosclerotic lesion [179]. The enhanced size and instability of the lesion contribute directly to the severity of IHD.

Iron may also have a protective role in the progression of IHD. Iron has been implicated in experimental ischemic preconditioning in the isolated rat heart in a process whereby brief (<5 min) ischemia protects the heart from a more prolonged period of ischemia [180]. Iron has been shown to induce the expression L-chain ferritin which in turn acts as a sink for reactive iron preventing iron-mediated oxidant damage [180]. The levels of myocardial ferritin immediately following ischemia in a dog experimental model were observed to be related to the degree of ischemia [181]. These findings suggest that at the cellular level, regulation of iron availability is important in the response to cardiac ischemia. Elevated serum ferritin was also observed 24 h after severe experimental brain ischemia in rats [182]. This suggests that ferritin may play a general protective role in ischemic injury by storing excess iron and reducing subsequent splanchnic oxidant stress. Patients suffering with IHD and who also exhibited a low serum iron concentration were found to be in a pro-inflammatory state. Factors such as TNFα and IL-6 were upregulated, and cardiac protective factors such as IGF-1 were downregulated when compared to IHD patients with normal serum iron [183]. These findings suggest a completely opposite role for iron to what one might expect, indicating that iron may play a cardiac protective role in patients with IHD.

5.4 Removal of Iron as a Potential Preventative Measure or Therapy for Ischemic Heart Disease

Chelation of iron using deferoxamine and dexrazoxane has been shown to improve cardiac function and energy metabolism post ischemia in rabbit and rat models of ischemia reperfusion cardiac injury [184, 185]. These data suggest that iron plays a role in the pathology of reperfusion injury, possibly by limiting the generation of oxygen free radicals [185]. The iron-chelating agent deferoxamine has also been shown to be beneficial in the recovery of sheep skeletal muscle following ischemic injury, suggesting a detrimental role of iron in the recovery process [186]. Preventing the iron from getting into the heart muscle also represents another possible therapy for ischemic heart disease and for cardiomyopathies associated with hemochromatosis. Recent studies have shown that uptake of iron by the heart muscle in patients with hemochromatosis is dependent upon L-type calcium channels [187]. L-type calcium channel blockers such as amlodipine and verapamil have been used experimentally to reduce cardiac iron overload in mice, suggesting that these agents may also be of benefit to patients with hemochromatosis [188], although whether this approach will benefit patients with IHD remains to be seen. Restricted dietary iron intake [189] and chelation of iron with deferoxamine [190] in mice and rabbits with experimentally induced atherosclerotic lesions have been shown to increase plaque stability [189] and reduce lesion size [190]. Whether iron depletion is also beneficial to atherosclerotic plaque size and stability in humans suffering with IHD remains to be determined.

5.5 *Ischemic Heart Disease and Hereditary Hemochromatosis*

Mutations in the *HFE* gene that lead to iron loading of the liver are also known to result in the deposition of excessive iron within the heart. Given that iron status may correlate with the prevalence and severity of IHD, it is not unreasonable to propose that the incidence and severity of IHD would be far greater in patients with hemochromatosis. Several studies have indicated that the two most common *HFE* mutations (C282Y and H63D) are not linked with IHD [191–193]. Experimentally, mice lacking the *Hfe* gene show increased cardiac iron loading and evidence of increased ROS generation following ischemia and reperfusion injury when compared to wild-type mice [194]. This has yet to be investigated in human studies.

5.6 *Summary*

The role of iron in IHD remains controversial. Experimental evidence in animal models of IHD and atherosclerosis would suggest that iron does have a negative impact on the progression of IHD. However, the role of iron in patients suffering with IHD remains somewhat of a mystery with more information required before a more firm conclusion is reached.

6 Concluding Remarks

While iron is an essential element required for normal cellular function, in excess it is toxic to the cell. This chapter has discussed our current knowledge of the mechanisms by which excess iron causes cellular damage leading to tissue injury and organ failure and the processes involved including hepatic fibrogenesis, the development of cirrhosis, the generation of HCC, as well as the role played by iron in IHD. There have been significant advances in our understanding of the mechanisms associated with these disease processes in hemochromatosis; however, there still remain considerable gaps in our knowledge. Some of the more vexing questions that remain include: What role does inflammation play in this non-inflammatory condition? With ferritin now appearing to play a role in inflammation associated with hepatic fibrosis, what is the source of serum ferritin and what function does it serve? What is the physiological and pathological role of the newly described ferritin receptors? In this enigmatic disease there is still much to learn about the complex interaction between resident and non-resident hepatic cells, the role of iron in tumor formation and extrahepatic disease complications and how iron influences the normal wound healing response of the liver. The precise role that iron plays in IHD is debatable and will remain so until the publication of more definitive studies. As with all pathologies described in this chapter, the role of iron remains unclear and at times controversial, with many other factors influencing the disease progression of each individual. A considerable amount of future study is still required to fully elucidate the mechanisms involved in iron-induced chronic disease.

References

1. Hampton MB, Fadeel B, Orrenius S. Redox regulation of the caspases during apoptosis. Ann N Y Acad Sci. 1998;854:328–35.
2. Videla LA, Fernandez V, Tapia G, Varela P. Oxidative stress-mediated hepatotoxicity of iron and copper: role of kupffer cells. Biometals. 2003;16:103–11.

3. Parola M, Robino G. Oxidative stress-related molecules and liver fibrosis. J Hepatol. 2001;35:297–306.
4. Pietrangelo A. Iron-induced oxidant stress in alcoholic liver fibrogenesis. Alcohol. 2003;30:121–9.
5. Wu G, Fang Y-Z, Yang S, Lupton JR, Turner ND. Glutathione metabolism and its implications for health. J Nutr. 2004;134:489–92.
6. Sies H. Oxidative stress: from basic research to clinical application. Am J Med. 1991;91:31S–8S.
7. Britton RS, Leicester KL, Bacon BR. Iron toxicity and chelation therapy. Int J Hematol. 2002;76:219–28.
8. Bacon BR, Britton RS. The pathology of hepatic iron overload: a free radical-mediated process? Hepatology. 1990;11:127–37.
9. Ramm GA, Ruddell RG. Hepatotoxicity of iron overload: mechanisms of iron-induced hepatic fibrogenesis. Semin Liver Dis. 2005;25:433–49.
10. Iancu TC, Shiloh H. Morphologic observations in iron overload: an update. Adv Exp Med Biol. 1994;356:255–65.
11. Kurz T, Terman A, Gustafsson B, Brunk UT. Lysosomes in iron metabolism, ageing and apoptosis. Histochem Cell Biol. 2008;129:389–406.
12. O'Connell MJ, Ward RJ, Baum H, Peters TJ. The role of iron in ferritin- and haemosiderin-mediated lipid peroxidation in liposomes. Biochem J. 1985;229:135–9.
13. Peters TJ, Seymour CA. Acid hydrolase activities and lysosomal integrity in liver biopsies from patients with iron overload. Clin Sci Mol Med. 1976;50:75–8.
14. Seymour CA, Peters TJ. Organelle pathology in primary and secondary haemochromatosis with special reference to lysosomal changes. Br J Haematol. 1978;40:239–53.
15. Hultcrantz R, Ahlberg J, Glaumann H. Isolation of two lysosomal populations from iron-overloaded rat liver with different iron concentration and proteolytic activity. Virchows Arch B Cell Pathol Incl Mol Pathol. 1984;47:55–65.
16. LeSage GD, Kost LJ, Barham SS, LaRusso NF. Biliary excretion of iron from hepatocyte lysosomes in the rat. A major excretory pathway in experimental iron overload. J Clin Invest. 1986;77:90–7.
17. Bacon BR, O'Neill R, Britton RS. Hepatic mitochondrial energy production in rats with chronic iron overload. Gastroenterology. 1993;105(4):1134–40.
18. Bacon BR, O'Neill R, Park CH. Iron-induced peroxidative injury to isolated rat hepatic mitochondria. J Free Radic Biol Med. 1986;2:339–47.
19. Zhao M, Antunes F, Eaton JW, Brunk UT. Lysosomal enzymes promote mitochondrial oxidant production, cytochrome c release and apoptosis. Eur J Biochem. 2003;270:3778–86.
20. Thomas C, Mackey MM, Diaz AA, Cox DP. Hydroxyl radical is produced via the Fenton reaction in submitochondrial particles under oxidative stress: implications for diseases associated with iron accumulation. Redox Rep. 2009;14:102–8.
21. Pardo Andreu GL, Inada NM, Vercesi AE, Curti C. Uncoupling and oxidative stress in liver mitochondria isolated from rats with acute iron overload. Arch Toxicol. 2009;83:47–53.
22. Halestrap AP. Calcium, mitochondria and reperfusion injury: a pore way to die. Biochem Soc Trans. 2006;34:232–7.
23. Rauen U, Petrat F, Sustmann R, de Groot H. Iron-induced mitochondrial permeability transition in cultured hepatocytes. J Hepatol. 2004;40:607–15.
24. Britton RS, O'Neill R, Bacon BR. Chronic dietary iron overload in rats results in impaired calcium sequestration by hepatic mitochondria and microsomes. Gastroenterology. 1991;101:806–11.
25. Masini A, Ceccarelli D, Trenti T, Corongiu FP, Muscatello U. Perturbation in liver mitochondrial Ca2+ homeostasis in experimental iron overload: a possible factor in cell injury. Biochim Biophys Acta. 1989;1014:133–40.
26. Garcia N, Garcia JJ, Correa F, Chavez E. The permeability transition pore as a pathway for the release of mitochondrial DNA. Life Sci. 2005;76:2873–80.
27. Walter PB, Knutson MD, Paler-Martinez A, et al. Iron deficiency and iron excess damage mitochondria and mitochondrial DNA in rats. Proc Natl Acad Sci USA. 2002;99:2264–9.
28. Pardo Andreu G, Delgado R, Velho J, et al. Mangifera indica L. Extract (vimang) inhibits Fe2+-citrate-induced lipoperoxidation in isolated rat liver mitochondria. Pharmacol Res. 2005;51:427–35.
29. Bartsch H, Nair J. Oxidative stress and lipid peroxidation-derived DNA-lesions in inflammation driven carcinogenesis. Cancer Detect Prev. 2004;28:385–91.
30. Uchida K, Szweda LI, Chae HZ, Stadtman ER. Immunochemical detection of 4-hydroxynonenal protein adducts in oxidized hepatocytes. Proc Natl Acad Sci USA. 1993;90:8742–6.
31. Tuma DJ. Role of malondialdehyde-acetaldehyde adducts in liver injury. Free Radic Biol Med. 2002;32:303–8.
32. Thiele GM, Worrall S, Tuma DJ, et al. The chemistry and biological effects of malondialdehyde-acetaldehyde adducts. Alcohol Clin Exp Res. 2001;25(5 Suppl ISBRA):218S–24S. doi:218S.
33. Kharbanda KK, Todero SL, Shubert KA, Sorrell MF, Tuma DJ. Malondialdehyde–acetaldehyde–protein adducts increase secretion of chemokines by rat hepatic stellate cells. Alcohol. 2001;25:123–8.

34. Kharbanda KK, Shubert KA, Wyatt TA, Sorrell MF, Tuma DJ. Effect of malondialdehyde–acetaldehyde–protein adducts on the protein kinase C-dependent secretion of urokinase-type plasminogen activator in hepatic stellate cells. Biochem Pharmacol. 2002;63:553–62.
35. Nair J, Carmichael PL, Fernando RC, et al. Lipid peroxidation-induced etheno-DNA adducts in the liver of patients with the genetic metal storage disorders Wilson's disease and primary hemochromatosis. Cancer Epidemiol Biomarkers Prev. 1998;7:435–40.
36. Hussain SP, Raja K, Amstad PA, et al. Increased p53 mutation load in nontumorous human liver of Wilson disease and hemochromatosis: oxyradical overload diseases. Proc Natl Acad Sci USA. 2000;97:12770–5.
37. Henle ES, Linn S. Formation, prevention, and repair of DNA damage by iron/hydrogen peroxide. J Biol Chem. 1997;272:19095–8.
38. Rosenbloom J, Castro SV, Jimenez SA. Narrative review: fibrotic diseases: cellular and molecular mechanisms and novel therapies. Ann Intern Med. 2010;152:159–66.
39. Hartley JL, Davenport M, Kelly DA. Biliary atresia. Lancet. 2009;374:1704–13.
40. Bjornsson E. The natural history of drug-induced liver injury. Semin Liver Dis. 2009;29:357–63.
41. Tsai WL, Chung RT. Viral hepatocarcinogenesis. Oncogene. 2010;29:2309–24.
42. Bataller R, Brenner DA. Liver fibrosis. J Clin Invest. 2005;115:209–18.
43. Ramm GA, Crawford DH, Powell LW, et al. Hepatic stellate cell activation in genetic haemochromatosis. Lobular distribution, effect of increasing hepatic iron and response to phlebotomy. J Hepatol. 1997;26:584–92.
44. Philippe MA, Ruddell RG, Ramm GA. Role of iron in hepatic fibrosis: one piece in the puzzle. World J Gastroenterol. 2007;13:4746–54.
45. Bridle KR, Frazer DM, Wilkins SJ, et al. Disrupted hepcidin regulation in HFE-associated haemochromatosis and the liver as a regulator of body iron homoeostasis. Lancet. 2003;361:669–73.
46. Anderson GJ, Frazer DM. Hepatic iron metabolism. Semin Liver Dis. 2005;25:420–32.
47. Bassett ML, Halliday JW, Powell LW. Value of hepatic iron measurements in early hemochromatosis and determination of the critical iron level associated with fibrosis. Hepatology. 1986;6:24–9.
48. Adams PC. Is there a threshold of hepatic iron concentration that leads to cirrhosis in C282Y hemochromatosis? Am J Gastroenterol. 2001;96:567–9.
49. Powell LW, Dixon JL, Ramm GA, et al. Screening for hemochromatosis in asymptomatic subjects with or without a family history. Arch Intern Med. 2006;166:294–301.
50. Stal P, Broome U, Scheynius A, Befrits R, Hultcrantz R. Kupffer cell iron overload induces intercellular adhesion molecule-1 expression on hepatocytes in genetic hemochromatosis. Hepatology. 1995;21:1308–16.
51. Wood MJ, Powell LW, Ramm GA. Environmental and genetic modifiers of the progression to fibrosis and cirrhosis in hemochromatosis. Blood. 2008;111:4456–62.
52. Zhao M, Laissue JA, Zimmermann A. Hepatocyte apoptosis in hepatic iron overload diseases. Histol Histopathol. 1997;12:367–74.
53. Moerman P, Pauwels P, Vandenberghe K, et al. Neonatal haemochromatosis. Histopathology. 1990;17:345–51.
54. Houglum K, Filip M, Witztum JL, Chojkier M. Malondialdehyde and 4-hydroxynonenal protein adducts in plasma and liver of rats with iron overload. J Clin Invest. 1990;86:1991–8.
55. Houglum K, Ramm GA, Crawford DH, et al. Excess iron induces hepatic oxidative stress and transforming growth factor beta1 in genetic hemochromatosis. Hepatology. 1997;26:605–10.
56. Pietrangelo A, Gualdi R, Casalgrandi G, Montosi G, Ventura E. Molecular and cellular aspects of iron-induced hepatic cirrhosis in rodents. J Clin Invest. 1995;95:1824–31.
57. Dai J, Huang C, Wu J, et al. Iron-induced interleukin-6 gene expression: possible mediation through the extracellular signal-regulated kinase and p38 mitogen-activated protein kinase pathways. Toxicology. 2004;203:199–209.
58. Hagen K, Eckes K, Melefors O, Hultcrantz R. Iron overload decreases the protective effect of tumour necrosis factor-alpha on rat hepatocytes exposed to oxidative stress. Scand J Gastroenterol. 2002;37:725–31.
59. Hagen K, Zhu C, Melefors O, Hultcrantz R. Susceptibility of cultured rat hepatocytes to oxidative stress by peroxides and iron. The extracellular matrix affects the toxicity of tert-butyl hydroperoxide. Int J Biochem Cell Biol. 1999;31:499–508.
60. Cederbaum AI. Cytochrome P450 2E1-dependent oxidant stress and upregulation of anti-oxidant defense in liver cells. J Gastroenterol Hepatol. 2006;21 Suppl 3:S22–5.
61. De Domenico I, Ward DM, Nemeth E, et al. The molecular basis of ferroportin-linked hemochromatosis. Proc Natl Acad Sci USA. 2005;102:8955–60.
62. She H, Xiong S, Lin M, et al. Iron activates NF-kappaB in kupffer cells. Am J Physiol Gastrointest Liver Physiol. 2002;283:G719–26.
63. Xiong S, She H, Sung CK, Tsukamoto H. Iron-dependent activation of NF-kappaB in kupffer cells: a priming mechanism for alcoholic liver disease. Alcohol. 2003;30:107–13.
64. Lin M, Rippe RA, Niemela O, Brittenham G, Tsukamoto H. Role of iron in NF-kappa B activation and cytokine gene expression by rat hepatic macrophages. Am J Physiol. 1997;272:G1355–1364.

65. Tsukamoto H, Rippe R, Niemela O, Lin M. Roles of oxidative stress in activation of kupffer and Ito cells in liver fibrogenesis. J Gastroenterol Hepatol. 1995;10 Suppl 1:S50–3.
66. Kobune M, Kohgo Y, Kato J, Miyazaki E, Niitsu Y. Interleukin-6 enhances hepatic transferrin uptake and ferritin expression in rats. Hepatology. 1994;19(6):1468–75.
67. Oudar O, Moreau A, Feldmann G, Scoazec JY. Expression and regulation of intercellular adhesion molecule-1 (ICAM-1) in organotypic cultures of rat liver tissue. J Hepatol. 1998;29:901–9.
68. Selzner N, Selzner M, Odermatt B, et al. ICAM-1 triggers liver regeneration through leukocyte recruitment and kupffer cell-dependent release of TNF-alpha/IL-6 in mice. Gastroenterology. 2003;124:692–700.
69. Canbay A, Feldstein AE, Higuchi H, et al. Kupffer cell engulfment of apoptotic bodies stimulates death ligand and cytokine expression. Hepatology. 2003;38:1188–98.
70. Tsukamoto H, Horne W, Kamimura S, et al. Experimental liver cirrhosis induced by alcohol and iron. J Clin Invest. 1995;96:620–30.
71. Takeyama Y, Kamimura S, Kuroiwa A, et al. Role of kupffer cell-derived reactive oxygen intermediates in alcoholic liver disease in rats in vivo. Alcohol Clin Exp Res. 1996;20(9 Suppl):335A–9A.
72. Zhang AS, Xiong S, Tsukamoto H, Enns CA. Localization of iron metabolism-related mRNAs in rat liver indicate that HFE is expressed predominantly in hepatocytes. Blood. 2004;103:1509–14.
73. Houglum K, Bedossa P, Chojkier M. TGF-beta and collagen-alpha 1 (I) gene expression are increased in hepatic acinar zone 1 of rats with iron overload. Am J Physiol. 1994;267:G908–13.
74. Solecki R, von Zglinicki T, Muller HM, Clausing P. Iron overload of spleen, liver and kidney as a consequence of hemolytic anaemia. Exp Pathol. 1983;23:227–35.
75. Bridle KR, Crawford DH, Fletcher LM, Smith JL, Powell LW, Ramm GA. Evidence for a sub-morphological inflammatory process in the liver in haemochromatosis. J Hepatol. 2003;38:426–33.
76. Deugnier YM, Loreal O, Turlin B, et al. Liver pathology in genetic hemochromatosis: a review of 135 homozygous cases and their bioclinical correlations. Gastroenterology. 1992;102:2050–9.
77. Cardoso EM, Hagen K, de Sousa M, Hultcrantz R. Hepatic damage in C282Y homozygotes relates to low numbers of CD8+ cells in the liver lobuli. Eur J Clin Invest. 2001;31:45–53.
78. Porto G, Vicente C, Teixeira MA, et al. Relative impact of HLA phenotype and CD4-CD8 ratios on the clinical expression of hemochromatosis. Hepatology. 1997;25:397–402.
79. Ruddell RG, Knight B, Tirnitz-Parker JE, et al. Lymphotoxin-beta receptor signaling regulates hepatic stellate cell function and wound healing in a murine model of chronic liver injury. Hepatology. 2009;49:227–39.
80. Smith PG, Yeoh GC. Chronic iron overload in rats induces oval cells in the liver. Am J Pathol. 1996;149:389–98.
81. Wake K, Sato T. Intralobular heterogeneity of perisinusoidal stellate cells in porcine liver. Cell Tissue Res. 1993;273:227–37.
82. Zou Z, Ekataksin W, Wake K. Zonal and regional differences identified from precision mapping of vitamin a-storing lipid droplets of the hepatic stellate cells in pig liver: a novel concept of addressing the intralobular area of heterogeneity. Hepatology. 1998;27:1098–108.
83. Friedman SL. Hepatic stellate cells: protean, multifunctional, and enigmatic cells of the liver. Physiol Rev. 2008;88:125–72.
84. Ruddell RG, Oakley F, Hussain Z, et al. A role for serotonin (5-HT) in hepatic stellate cell function and liver fibrosis. Am J Pathol. 2006;169:861–76.
85. Knittel T, Fellmer P, Muller L, Ramadori G. Bone morphogenetic protein-6 is expressed in nonparenchymal liver cells and upregulated by transforming growth factor-beta 1. Exp Cell Res. 1997;232:263–9.
86. Andriopoulos Jr B, Corradini E, Xia Y, et al. BMP6 Is a key endogenous regulator of hepcidin expression and iron metabolism. Nat Genet. 2009;41:482–7.
87. Meynard D, Kautz L, Darnaud V, et al. Lack of the bone morphogenetic protein BMP6 induces massive iron overload. Nat Genet. 2009;41:478–81.
88. Ramm GA, Li SC, Li L, et al. Chronic iron overload causes activation of rat lipocytes in vivo. Am J Physiol. 1995;268:G451–458.
89. Guido M, Rugge M, Leandro G, Fiel IM, Thung SN. Hepatic stellate cell immunodetection and cirrhotic evolution of viral hepatitis in liver allografts. Hepatology. 1997;26:310–4.
90. George DK, Ramm GA, Powell LW, et al. Evidence for altered hepatic matrix degradation in genetic haemochromatosis. Gut. 1998;42:715–20.
91. Iredale JP, Murphy G, Hembry RM, Friedman SL, Arthur MJ. Human hepatic lipocytes synthesize tissue inhibitor of metalloproteinases-1. Implications for regulation of matrix degradation in liver. J Clin Invest. 1992;90:282–7.
92. Bridle KR, Crawford DH, Ramm GA. Identification and characterization of the hepatic stellate cell transferrin receptor. Am J Pathol. 2003;162:1661–7.
93. Ramm GA, Britton RS, O'Neill R, Bacon BR. Identification and characterization of a receptor for tissue ferritin on activated rat lipocytes. J Clin Invest. 1994;94:9–15.

94. Benedetti A, Di Sario A, Casini A, et al. Inhibition of the NA(+)/H(+) exchanger reduces rat hepatic stellate cell activity and liver fibrosis: an in vitro and in vivo study. Gastroenterology. 2001;120:545–56.
95. Gardi C, Arezzini B, Fortino V, Comporti M. Effect of free iron on collagen synthesis, cell proliferation and MMP-2 expression in rat hepatic stellate cells. Biochem Pharmacol. 2002;64:1139–45.
96. Montosi G, Garuti C, Martinelli S, Pietrangelo A. Hepatic stellate cells are not subjected to oxidant stress during iron-induced fibrogenesis in rodents. Hepatology. 1998;27:1611–22.
97. Parkes JG, Liu Y, Sirna JB, Templeton DM. Changes in gene expression with iron loading and chelation in cardiac myocytes and non-myocytic fibroblasts. J Mol Cell Cardiol. 2000;32:233–46.
98. Chen TT, Li L, Chung DH, et al. TIM-2 is expressed on B cells and in liver and kidney and is a receptor for H-ferritin endocytosis. J Exp Med. 2005;202(7):955–65.
99. Li JY, Paragas N, Ned RM, et al. Scara5 is a ferritin receptor mediating non-transferrin iron delivery. Dev Cell. 2009;16:35–46.
100. Todorich B, Zhang X, Slagle-Webb B, Seaman WE, Connor JR. Tim-2 is the receptor for H-ferritin on oligodendrocytes. J Neurochem. 2008;107:1495–505.
101. Li L, Fang CJ, Ryan JC, et al. Binding and uptake of H-ferritin are mediated by human transferrin receptor-1. Proc Natl Acad Sci USA. 2010;107:3505–10.
102. Ruddell RG, Hoang-Le D, Barwood JM, et al. Ferritin functions as a proinflammatory cytokine via iron-independent protein kinase C zeta/nuclear factor kappaB-regulated signaling in rat hepatic stellate cells. Hepatology. 2009;49:887–900.
103. Kawada N, Kristensen DB, Asahina K, et al. Characterization of a stellate cell activation-associated protein (STAP) with peroxidase activity found in rat hepatic stellate cells. J Biol Chem. 2001;276:25318–23.
104. Nakatani K, Okuyama H, Shimahara Y, et al. Cytoglobin/STAP, its unique localization in splanchnic fibroblast-like cells and function in organ fibrogenesis. Lab Invest. 2004;84:91–101.
105. Xu R, Harrison PM, Chen M, et al. Cytoglobin overexpression protects against damage-induced fibrosis. Mol Ther. 2006;13:1093–100.
106. Parola M, Pinzani M, Casini A, et al. Stimulation of lipid peroxidation or 4-hydroxynonenal treatment increases procollagen alpha 1 (I) gene expression in human liver fat-storing cells. Biochem Biophys Res Commun. 1993;194:1044–50.
107. Svegliati Baroni G, D'Ambrosio L, Ferretti G, et al. Fibrogenic effect of oxidative stress on rat hepatic stellate cells. Hepatology. 1998;27:720–6.
108. Tsukamoto H. Oxidative stress, antioxidants, and alcoholic liver fibrogenesis. Alcohol. 1993;10:465–7.
109. Nieto N, Friedman SL, Cederbaum AI. Stimulation and proliferation of primary rat hepatic stellate cells by cytochrome P450 2E1-derived reactive oxygen species. Hepatology. 2002;35:62–73.
110. Parkes JG, Templeton DM. Modulation of stellate cell proliferation and gene expression by rat hepatocytes: effect of toxic iron overload. Toxicol Lett. 2003;144:225–33.
111. Olynyk JK, Khan NA, Ramm GA, et al. Aldehydic products of lipid peroxidation do not directly activate rat hepatic stellate cells. J Gastroenterol Hepatol. 2002;17:785–90.
112. Blumberg BS, Lustbader ED, Whitford PL. Changes in serum iron levels due to infection with hepatitis B virus. Proc Natl Acad Sci USA. 1981;78:3222–4.
113. Raynard B, Balian A, Fallik D, et al. Risk factors of fibrosis in alcohol-induced liver disease. Hepatology. 2002;35:635–8.
114. Powell EE, Ali A, Clouston AD, et al. Steatosis is a cofactor in liver injury in hemochromatosis. Gastroenterology. 2005;129:1937–43.
115. Parkkila S, Niemela O, Britton RS, et al. Vitamin E decreases hepatic levels of aldehyde-derived peroxidation products in rats with iron overload. Am J Physiol. 1996;270:G376–84.
116. Ramey G, Faye A, Durel B, Viollet B, Vaulont S. Iron overload in Hepc1(–/–) mice is not impairing glucose homeostasis. FEBS Lett. 2007;581:1053–7.
117. Gullo L, Corcioni E, Brancati C, et al. Morphologic and functional evaluation of the exocrine pancreas in beta-thalassemia major. Pancreas. 1993;8:176–80.
118. Lu JP, Hayashi K, Okada S, Awai M. Transferrin receptors and selective iron deposition in pancreatic B cells of iron-overloaded rats. Acta Pathol Jpn. 1991;41:647–52.
119. Kulaksiz H, Fein E, Redecker P, et al. Pancreatic beta-cells express hepcidin, an iron-uptake regulatory peptide. J Endocrinol. 2008;197:241–9.
120. Minamiyama Y, Takemura S, Kodai S, et al. Iron restriction improves type 2 diabetes mellitus in otsuka long-Evans Tokushima fatty rats. Am J Physiol Endocrinol Metab. 2010;298:E1140–9.
121. Riserus U, Sprecher D, Johnson T, et al. Activation of peroxisome proliferator-activated receptor (PPAR)delta promotes reversal of multiple metabolic abnormalities, reduces oxidative stress, and increases fatty acid oxidation in moderately obese men. Diabetes. 2008;57:332–9.
122. Lenzen S. Oxidative stress: the vulnerable beta-cell. Biochem Soc Trans. 2008;36:343–7.

123. Hucl T, Kylanpaa-Back ML, Witt H, et al. HFE genotypes in patients with chronic pancreatitis and pancreatic adenocarcinoma. Genet Med. 2007;9:479–83.
124. Ablamunits V, Baranova F, Mandrup-Poulsen T, Nerup J. In vitro inhibition of insulin release by blood mononuclear cells from insulin-dependent diabetic and healthy subjects: synergistic action of IL-1 and TNF. Cell Transplant. 1994;3:55–60.
125. el Nawawy A, Soliman AT, el Azzouni O, et al. Interleukin-1-beta, tumour necrosis factor-alpha, islet-cell antibody, and insulin secretion in children with thalassemia major on long-term blood transfusion. J Trop Pediatr. 1996;42:362–4.
126. Suvarna J, Ingle H, Deshmukh CT. Insulin resistance and beta cell function in chronically transfused patients of thalassemia major. Indian Pediatr. 2006;43:393–400.
127. Cario H, Holl RW, Debatin KM, Kohne E. Insulin sensitivity and beta-cell secretion in thalassaemia major with secondary haemochromatosis: assessment by oral glucose tolerance test. Eur J Pediatr. 2003;162:139–46.
128. El-Serag HB, Mason AC. Rising incidence of hepatocellular carcinoma in the United States. N Engl J Med. 1999;340:745–50.
129. Sangiovanni A, Del Ninno E, Fasani P, et al. Increased survival of cirrhotic patients with a hepatocellular carcinoma detected during surveillance. Gastroenterology. 2004;126:1005–14.
130. Elmberg M, Hultcrantz R, Ekbom A, et al. Cancer risk in patients with hereditary hemochromatosis and in their first-degree relatives. Gastroenterology. 2003;125:1733–41.
131. Kowdley KV. Iron, hemochromatosis, and hepatocellular carcinoma. Gastroenterology. 2004;127(5 Suppl 1):S79–86.
132. Harrison SA, Bacon BR. Relation of hemochromatosis with hepatocellular carcinoma: epidemiology, natural history, pathophysiology, screening, treatment, and prevention. Med Clin North Am. 2005;89:391–409.
133. Bradbear RA, Bain C, Siskind V, et al. Cohort study of internal malignancy in genetic hemochromatosis and other chronic nonalcoholic liver diseases. J Natl Cancer Inst. 1985;75:81–4.
134. Fargion S, Mandelli C, Piperno A, et al. Survival and prognostic factors in 212 Italian patients with genetic hemochromatosis. Hepatology. 1992;15:655–9.
135. Niederau C, Fischer R, Sonnenberg A, et al. Survival and causes of death in cirrhotic and in noncirrhotic patients with primary hemochromatosis. N Engl J Med. 1985;313:1256–62.
136. Deugnier Y, Turlin B. Iron and hepatocellular carcinoma. J Gastroenterol Hepatol. 2001;16:491–4.
137. Dumble ML, Croager EJ, Yeoh GC, Quail EA. Generation and characterization of p53 null transformed hepatic progenitor cells: oval cells give rise to hepatocellular carcinoma. Carcinogenesis. 2002;23:435–45.
138. Knight B, Tirnitz-Parker JE, Olynyk JK. C-kit inhibition by imatinib mesylate attenuates progenitor cell expansion and inhibits liver tumor formation in mice. Gastroenterology. 2008;135:969–79.
139. Shachaf CM, Kopelman AM, Arvanitis C, et al. MYC inactivation uncovers pluripotent differentiation and tumour dormancy in hepatocellular cancer. Nature. 2004;431:1112–7.
140. Borgna-Pignatti C, Vergine G, Lombardo T, et al. Hepatocellular carcinoma in the thalassaemia syndromes. Br J Haematol. 2004;124:114–7.
141. Mandishona E, MacPhail AP, Gordeuk VR, et al. Dietary iron overload as a risk factor for hepatocellular carcinoma in black Africans. Hepatology. 1998;27:1563–6.
142. Brown KE, Mathahs MM, Broadhurst KA, Weydert J. Chronic iron overload stimulates hepatocyte proliferation and cyclin D1 expression in rodent liver. Transl Res. 2006;148:55–62.
143. Chenoufi N, Loreal O, Drenou B, et al. Iron may induce both DNA synthesis and repair in rat hepatocytes stimulated by EGF/pyruvate. J Hepatol. 1997;26:650–8.
144. Hann HW, Stahlhut MW, Hann CL. Effect of iron and desferoxamine on cell growth and in vitro ferritin synthesis in human hepatoma cell lines. Hepatology. 1990;11:566–9.
145. Marrogi AJ, Khan MA, van Gijssel HE, et al. Oxidative stress and p53 mutations in the carcinogenesis of iron overload-associated hepatocellular carcinoma. J Natl Cancer Inst. 2001;93:1652–5.
146. Vautier G, Bomford AB, Portmann BC, et al. p53 Mutations in British patients with hepatocellular carcinoma: clustering in genetic hemochromatosis. Gastroenterology. 1999;117:154–60.
147. Lescoat G, Chantrel-Groussard K, Pasdeloup N, et al. Antiproliferative and apoptotic effects in rat and human hepatoma cell cultures of the orally active iron chelator ICL670 compared to CP20: a possible relationship with polyamine metabolism. Cell Prolif. 2007;40:755–67.
148. Bai X, Wu L, Liang T, et al. Overexpression of myocyte enhancer factor 2 and histone hyperacetylation in hepatocellular carcinoma. J Cancer Res Clin Oncol. 2008;134:83–91.
149. Jung JO, Gwak GY, Lim YS, Kim CY, Lee HS. Role of hepatic stellate cells in the angiogenesis of hepatoma. Korean J Gastroenterol. 2003;42:142–8.
150. Zindy PJ, L'Helgoualc'h A, Bonnier D, et al. Upregulation of the tumor suppressor gene menin in hepatocellular carcinomas and its significance in fibrogenesis. Hepatology. 2006;44:1296–307.
151. Ramm GA, Britton RS, O'Neill R, Kohn HD, Bacon BR. Rat liver ferritin selectively inhibits expression of alpha-smooth muscle actin in cultured rat lipocytes. Am J Physiol. 1996;270:G370–5.

152. Ooi LP, Crawford DH, Gotley DC, et al. Evidence that "myofibroblast-like" cells are the cellular source of capsular collagen in hepatocellular carcinoma. J Hepatol. 1997;26:798–807.
153. Bridle KR, Crawford DH, Powell LW, Ramm GA. Role of myofibroblasts in tumour encapsulation of hepatocellular carcinoma in haemochromatosis. Liver. 2001;21:96–104.
154. Budhu A, Wang XW. The role of cytokines in hepatocellular carcinoma. J Leukoc Biol. 2006;80:1197–213.
155. Porto G, De Sousa M. Iron overload and immunity. World J Gastroenterol. 2007;13:4707–15.
156. Pang YL, Zhang HG, Peng JR, et al. The immunosuppressive tumor microenvironment in hepatocellular carcinoma. Cancer Immunol Immunother. 2009;58(6):887–86.
157. Cai L, Zhang Z, Zhou L, et al. Functional impairment in circulating and intrahepatic NK cells and relative mechanism in hepatocellular carcinoma patients. Clin Immunol. 2008;129:428–37.
158. Fabio G, Zarantonello M, Mocellin C, et al. Peripheral lymphocytes and intracellular cytokines in C282Y homozygous hemochromatosis patients. J Hepatol. 2002;37:753–61.
159. Djeha A, Brock JH. Effect of transferrin, lactoferrin and chelated iron on human T-lymphocytes. Br J Haematol. 1992;80:235–41.
160. Good MF, Powell LW, Halliday JW. Iron status and cellular immune competence. Blood Rev. 1988;2:43–9.
161. Green R, Esparza I, Schreiber R. Iron inhibits the nonspecific tumoricidal activity of macrophages. A possible contributory mechanism for neoplasia in hemochromatosis. Ann N Y Acad Sci. 1988;526:301–9.
162. El-Serag HB, Marrero JA, Rudolph L, Reddy KR. Diagnosis and treatment of hepatocellular carcinoma. Gastroenterology. 2008;134:1752–63.
163. Sullivan JL. Iron and the sex difference in heart disease risk. Lancet. 1981;1:1293–4.
164. Salonen JT, Nyyssonen K, Korpela H, et al. High stored iron levels are associated with excess risk of myocardial infarction in eastern Finnish men. Circulation. 1992;86:803–11.
165. Galan P, Noisette N, Estaquio C, et al. Serum ferritin, cardiovascular risk factors and ischaemic heart diseases: a prospective analysis in the SU.VI.MAX (SUpplementation en VItamines et mineraux AntioXydants) cohort. Public Health Nutr. 2006;9:70–4.
166. Sempos CT, Looker AC, Gillum RF. Iron and heart disease: the epidemiologic data. Nutr Rev. 1996;54:73–84.
167. Sullivan JL. The iron paradigm of ischemic heart disease. Am Heart J. 1989;117:1177–88.
168. Meyers DG. The iron hypothesis – does iron cause atherosclerosis? Clin Cardiol. 1996;19:925–9.
169. Ma J, Stampfer MJ. Body iron stores and coronary heart disease. Clin Chem. 2002;48:601–3.
170. Walker AR, Walker BF, Labadarios D. High stored iron and the risk of ischemic heart disease. Circulation. 1993;88:807–8.
171. Higginson J, Gerritsen T, Walker AR. Siderosis in the bantu of southern Africa. Am J Pathol. 1953;29:779–815.
172. Seedat YK, Mayet FG, Khan S, Somers SR, Joubert G. Risk factors for coronary heart disease in the Indians of Durban. S Afr Med J. 1990;78:447–54.
173. Tanguy S, de Leiris J, Besse S, Boucher F. Ageing exacerbates the cardiotoxicity of hydrogen peroxide through the Fenton reaction in rats. Mech Ageing Dev. 2003;124:229–35.
174. Liu XK, Prasad MR, Engelman RM, Jones RM, Das DK. Role of iron on membrane phospholipid breakdown in ischemic-reperfused rat heart. Am J Physiol. 1990;259:H1101–1107.
175. van Jaarsveld H, Potgieter GM, Kuyl JM, Barnard HC, Barnard SP. The effect of desferal on rat heart mitochondrial function, iron content, and xanthine dehydrogenase/oxidase conversion during ischemia–reperfusion. Clin Biochem. 1990;23:509–13.
176. Bar-Or D, McDonald MC, Thiemermann C. Reduction of infarct size in a rat model of regional myocardial ischemia and reperfusion by the synthetic peptide DAHK. Crit Care Med. 2006;34:1955–9.
177. Smith C, Mitchinson MJ, Aruoma OI, Halliwell B. Stimulation of lipid peroxidation and hydroxyl-radical generation by the contents of human atherosclerotic lesions. Biochem J. 1992;286:901–5.
178. Thong PS, Selley M, Watt F. Elemental changes in atherosclerotic lesions using nuclear microscopy. Cell Mol Biol. 1996;42:103–10.
179. Sullivan JL. Macrophage iron, hepcidin, and atherosclerotic plaque stability. Exp Biol Med (Maywood). 2007;232:1014–20.
180. Chevion M, Leibowitz S, Aye NN, et al. Heart protection by ischemic preconditioning: a novel pathway initiated by iron and mediated by ferritin. J Mol Cell Cardiol. 2008;45:839–45.
181. Loncar R, Flesche CW, Deussen A. Myocardial ferritin content is closely related to the degree of ischaemia. Acta Physiol Scand. 2004;180:21–8.
182. Millerot E, Prigent-Tessier AS, Bertrand NM, et al. Serum ferritin in stroke: a marker of increased body iron stores or stroke severity? J Cereb Blood Flow Metab. 2005;25:1386–93.
183. Lee SD, Huang CY, Shu WT, et al. Pro-inflammatory states and IGF-I level in ischemic heart disease with low or high serum iron. Clin Chim Acta. 2006;370:50–6.
184. Ambrosio G, Zweier JL, Jacobus WE, Weisfeldt ML, Flaherty JT. Improvement of postischemic myocardial function and metabolism induced by administration of deferoxamine at the time of reflow: the role of iron in the pathogenesis of reperfusion injury. Circulation. 1987;76:906–15.

185. Ramu E, Korach A, Houminer E, et al. Dexrazoxane prevents myocardial ischemia/reperfusion-induced oxidative stress in the rat heart. Cardiovasc Drugs Ther. 2006;20:343–8.
186. Chekanov VS, Nikolaychik V, Maternowski MA, et al. Deferoxamine enhances neovascularization and recovery of ischemic skeletal muscle in an experimental sheep model. Ann Thorac Surg. 2003;75:184–9.
187. Oudit GY, Trivieri MG, Khaper N, Liu PP, Backx PH. Role of L-type Ca2+ channels in iron transport and iron-overload cardiomyopathy. J Mol Med. 2006;84:349–64.
188. Oudit GY, Sun H, Trivieri MG, et al. L-type Ca2+ channels provide a major pathway for iron entry into cardiomyocytes in iron-overload cardiomyopathy. Nat Med. 2003;9:1187–94.
189. Lee HT, Chiu LL, Lee TS, Tsai HL, Chau LY. Dietary iron restriction increases plaque stability in apolipoprotein-e-deficient mice. J Biomed Sci. 2003;10:510–7.
190. Minqin R, Rajendran R, Pan N, et al. The iron chelator desferrioxamine inhibits atherosclerotic lesion development and decreases lesion iron concentrations in the cholesterol-fed rabbit. Free Radic Biol Med. 2005;38:1206–11.
191. Campbell S, George DK, Robb SD, et al. The prevalence of haemochromatosis gene mutations in the west of Scotland and their relation to ischaemic heart disease. Heart. 2003;89:1023–6.
192. Pankow JS, Boerwinkle E, Adams PC, et al. HFE C282Y homozygotes have reduced low-density lipoprotein cholesterol: the atherosclerosis risk in communities (ARIC) study. Transl Res. 2008;152:3–10.
193. Waalen J, Felitti V, Gelbart T, Ho NJ, Beutler E. Prevalence of coronary heart disease associated with HFE mutations in adults attending a health appraisal center. Am J Med. 2002;113:472–9.
194. Turoczi T, Jun L, Cordis G, et al. HFE mutation and dietary iron content interact to increase ischemia/reperfusion injury of the heart in mice. Circ Res. 2003;92:1240–6.

Chapter 19
HFE-Associated Hereditary Hemochromatosis

Richard Skoien and Lawrie W. Powell

Keywords Arthropathy • C282Y • Cirrhosis • Diabetes • Hemochromatosis • HFE • Iron loading • Liver • Serum ferritin • Transferrin saturation

1 Introduction and Historical Perspective

The clinical phenotype of hemochromatosis – cirrhosis, diabetes, and pigmentation of the skin – has been recognized since the late nineteenth century [1]. Over the next 100 years, the molecular basis of inappropriate uptake and deposition of excessive quantities of iron in tissues became clearer. This began with the recognition of an autosomal recessive disorder linked to the short arm of chromosome 6 [2–4]. In 1996, discovery of a point mutation of the *HFE* gene [5] became an important portal to a better understanding of the genetic basis and expression of hereditary hemochromatosis.

It is now known that the C282Y mutation in HFE, in which a single base change sees tyrosine substituted for cysteine at position 282, accounts for up to 90% of cases of hemochromatosis ("classic hemochromatosis") in populations of northern European origin [6]. A second mutation, leading to the H63D substitution in the HFE protein, is quite common in a number of populations, but is usually not associated with iron loading, nor is a third, but much rarer, mutation, S65C [7]. The genes affected in a range of other genetically linked disorders (most notably juvenile hemochromatosis, TFR2-related hemochromatosis, and ferroportin-related iron overload) that behave variably like classic hereditary hemochromatosis have also been identified [8–12] and are considered in detail in Chap. 20.

HFE-related hereditary hemochromatosis is characterized by inappropriately high iron absorption and progressive body iron overload. Clinical manifestations are linked to the deposition of this iron in tissues. While the liver is most commonly affected [13], other effects include cardiac disease, diabetes mellitus, hypogonadism, arthropathy, and skin pigmentation [14–16]. Typically, a long asymptomatic phase precedes onset of symptoms in midlife related to end-organ dysfunction.

R. Skoien, M.D.
Department of Gastroenterology and Hepatology, Centre for Liver Disease Research, Princess Alexandra Hospital, The University of Queensland, Woolloongabba, QLD, Australia
e-mail: r.skoien@uq.edu.au

L.W. Powell, A.C., M.D., Ph.D. (✉)
Department of Gastroenterology and Hepatology and the Centre for the Advancement of Clinical Research, Royal Brisbane and Women's Hospital, Brisbane, QLD, Australia
e-mail: lawrie.powell@qimr.edu.au

G.J. Anderson and G. McLaren (eds.), *Iron Physiology and Pathophysiology in Humans*, Nutrition and Health, DOI 10.1007/978-1-60327-485-2_19,

Since the discovery of specific genetic mutations and the understanding of modes of inheritance, there has been significant interest in the role of screening and early identification of at-risk individuals.

There is good evidence that early identification and effective therapy, through regular venesection, can prevent disease [17, 18]. Untreated iron overload related to hemochromatosis is associated with an increased risk of hepatocellular carcinoma [19] which is mostly, but not always, related to hepatic cirrhosis [20]. Recently, there has also been interest in the presence of *HFE* gene mutations in association with other conditions [21, 22]. Hereditary or primary hemochromatosis should be distinguished from diseases which lead to a secondary iron overload state (e.g., thalassemia major, hemolytic or sideroblastic anemia, dietary or parenteral iron overload) which may also respond to iron-reduction therapy.

2 Mutation Analysis and Prevalence

The most common form of hereditary hemochromatosis is associated with mutation of the *HFE* gene located on chromosome 6. Two mutations of this gene that contribute to iron overload – C282Y and H63D – have been described.

The prevalence of the C282Y allele among Caucasian populations is 2–5% [23]. The genetic mutation probably originated more than 2,000 years ago [24] and spread through north-western Europe via Celtic or Viking migration [25–28]. This extraordinary prevalence means homozygosity for the C282Y mutation appears in 1 in 200 of those of northern European descent [27].

Inheritance of HFE-related hemochromatosis is autosomal recessive, but penetrance is variable [29]. On cross-sectional studies, normal ferritin levels have been reported in 20% of men and 40% of women homozygous for the C282Y mutation [30–33]. In a large Australian longitudinal study over 12 years of people with northern European ancestry, the proportion of male C282Y homozygotes with documented iron-overload-related disease was only 28.4% [34]. The proportion of female homozygotes with disease was only 1.2%, although 30% of all homozygotes in that study had previously undergone phlebotomy.

A second *HFE* gene mutation sees a substitution of aspartic acid for histidine at position 63 (H63D). It is more common than the C282Y mutation (15–20% allele frequency in the general population [35, 36]), and its contribution to iron overload is controversial. H63D homozygosity is rare among patients with hemochromatosis, suggesting that the mutation is not pathological. Supporting this argument is evidence that frequency of the mutation among controls and patients is similar [37]. The literature suggests that the H63D mutation has only a mild effect on iron homeostasis [38–40] and probably is a disease-related mutation with low clinical penetrance [41]. The specific contribution of the H63D mutation to iron overload without other risk factors is difficult to assess from human population studies [23].

A third mutation, S65C, has also been isolated, but there is no convincing evidence that it is linked with hereditary hemochromatosis [42]. It has been reported to interfere with H63D mutation analysis because of its close proximity, giving a false H63D homozygous result in a S65C/H63D compound heterozygote [43].

3 Symptoms and Presentation

Symptoms of classic hereditary hemochromatosis usually begin with the onset of nonspecific complaints (e.g., fatigue, joint pain). The progression from these symptoms to those related to end-organ dysfunction is inconsistent. Variable presentation in subjects with the same genotype is evidenced by the fact that in 25–30% of C282Y homozygotes, the disease never progresses beyond the biochemical phase of elevated transferrin saturation [2, 32]. A rising serum ferritin is indicative of progressive accumulation of iron in parenchymal tissues. Generally, in affected individuals, there is a gradual, stepwise trend towards organ damage which follows the relentless uptake and deposition of iron into tissues.

All patients who are homozygous for C282Y are genetically predisposed to this chain of events, but the process is influenced by many factors, and currently, it is impossible to predict phenotypic expression or its severity [34]. Examining data from a large longitudinal Australian population study [44], Allen et al. found that for C282Y homozygotes of northern European extraction, only 21 of 74 men (28.4%) and 1 of 84 women (1.2%) satisfied criteria for documented iron overload-related disease [34]. Recent studies have estimated that disease develops in 25–60% of C282Y homozygotes [45, 46].

Other studies have also described very low phenotypic penetrance of the C282Y mutation. Less than 1% of affected individuals suffered disease attributable to hereditary hemochromatosis in a cross-sectional US population study of subjects aged 20–80 years [32]. Exclusion of one quarter of homozygotes previously diagnosed with hereditary hemochromatosis may account for this finding. A Scandinavian study found no evidence of liver disease associated with hereditary hemochromatosis [47], although these results were potentially influenced by selective mortality bias. Best estimates are that a significant proportion of C282Y homozygotes will develop iron overload-related disease, although the true penetrance is lower than previously believed.

Of those who develop end-organ damage, liver involvement is common to both adult-onset (*HFE*- and *TFR2*-related disease) and juvenile hemochromatosis [2]. Cardiomyopathy and heart failure, arrhythmias, diabetes, and hypogonadotrophic hypogonadism are more prevalent in adult forms of the disease [48, 49] but may be seen also in juvenile forms where endocrine or cardiac manifestations may be the presenting complaint. Skin and joint involvement are also common in adults. This notwithstanding, early detection of abnormally high ferritin and transferrin saturation levels means that some patients are completely asymptomatic at diagnosis. In fact, the classic triad of bronzed skin, cirrhosis, and diabetes described over 100 years ago is now rare in adults diagnosed with hereditary hemochromatosis. Fatigue, malaise, and arthralgias are now the most common symptoms at presentation and are often associated with hepatomegaly and abnormal aminotransferase levels [2]. Fatigue is present in up to 60% of subjects with hemochromatosis [50] and is more common in C282Y homozygotes than controls [51], although it is nonspecific and its utility in the diagnosis of hemochromatosis has been questioned [32].

Liver fibrosis and cirrhosis due to iron overload are a significant cause of morbidity and mortality. The prevalence of cirrhosis has been reported in studies of C282Y homozygotes identified by population screening [52], health assessments [18], and family studies [53]. In these respective studies, the prevalence of cirrhosis was variable (18%, 4.2%, and 5.6% in men and 5%, 0.3%, and 1.9% in women, respectively) perhaps owing to population variation. In a population of C282Y homozygotes of northern European descent, Allen et al. reported the prevalence of fibrosis to be 13.5% and cirrhosis to be 2.7% [34]. Clinical examination reveals hepatomegaly in the vast majority (95%) of symptomatic patients [13].

Hepatocellular carcinoma (HCC) develops predominantly in male cirrhotic patients and increases in incidence with age [13, 14, 54, 55]. Different populations also seem to experience different degrees of HCC penetrance, suggesting ethnic or environmental factors also play a role [56]. *HFE* mutations do not appear to impart an increased risk of development of other malignancies [57].

Cardiac manifestations are only seen in 3–10% of symptomatic patients [14], although sequelae of iron deposition in the myocardium and conducting bundles can develop rapidly and become fatal. Of patients with overt symptoms, 35% have electrocardiographic (ECG) abnormalities, 15–30% develop congestive cardiac failure, and 20–30% suffer dysrhythmias [13].

Diabetes is an important endocrine complication of hereditary hemochromatosis. It is seen in 65% of symptomatic homozygotes [58], although the incidence of diabetes in asymptomatic patients is similar to that of controls [33, 34]. Other endocrine consequences include disruption of the hypothalamic–pituitary axis. Serum levels of testosterone are generally lower in symptomatic males, and 35–40% suffer from impotence [14, 59]. Women also exhibit lower levels of circulating luteinizing hormone and follicle-stimulating hormone, and amenorrhea affects 15% [6]. Hypothyroidism has also been described but is not as common [59].

Arthropathy is common, affecting 20–70% of symptomatic patients [14, 32, 34]. Typically, the metacarpophalangeal joints of the hands are affected. Radiological imaging shows the characteristic hook osteophytes and changes seen in pseudogout. Hips and knees are also affected and, to a lesser degree, shoulders and ankles.

4 Pathophysiology

The exact role of HFE in iron metabolism is unknown. Studies have demonstrated an association between HFE and the transferrin receptor, an interaction lost when HFE is mutated, suggesting that HFE may play a role in regulating iron entry into cells [61, 62]. However, it is its role as regulator of hepcidin that is best understood (see Chap. 9). Variable penetrance of *HFE* gene mutations has hampered the investigation of factors that modify phenotypic expression. Animal studies suggest that the C282Y mutation alone does not completely disrupt HFE function, suggesting the importance of interactions with other proteins and additional insults in the phenotypic expression of HFE mutations [63].

In the last decade, elucidation of the role of hepcidin in iron metabolism has led to a better understanding of *HFE* gene expression. As an important regulator of iron metabolism, hepcidin acts to reduce the intestinal absorption of iron and inhibits the release of iron from reticuloendothelial cells [64–66]. It has been demonstrated that C282Y homozygotes with rare hepcidin (*HAMP*) mutations are overrepresented in patients with severely elevated iron stores [67]. Heterozygous mutation of hemojuvelin (*HJV*) is also associated with more severe iron indices compared with sex- and age-matched C282Y homozygous controls.

For patients who are heterozygous for C282Y, the *HAMP* mutation appears to confer a more aggressive phenotype [67]. Indeed, the severity of iron overload may relate to the severity of the *HAMP* mutation itself and represent a "second hit" in subjects with existing C282Y homozygosity [22]. Similarly, high indices of iron status are also seen for compound heterozygotes (C282Y/H63D) with mutations of either hepcidin or hemojuvelin [68]. It is likely more genes which affect the HFE phenotype are yet to be found.

In hemochromatosis, it is believed that liver parenchymal injury results from oxidative stress resulting from iron overload and the toxic effects of redox-active iron [2]. Iron is a key molecule in the activation of hepatic stellate cells and extracellular matrix gene expression [69] leading to fibrosis. Degradation of the extracellular matrix by metalloproteinases also seems to be inhibited in hemochromatosis [70]. This topic is considered in detail in Chap. 18. There is interest, therefore, in antioxidant enzymes (e.g., GSTP1) which protect the cell from reactive oxygen species produced in response to iron overload [71, 72]. It is believed that many genetic polymorphisms for these enzymes probably exist to explain different phenotypic expression of HFE mutations. Further studies into the interaction and expression of antioxidant enzymes in iron overload are continuing.

Alcohol excess increases iron accumulation in hepatocytes and Kupffer cells [73]. This occurs via a number of mechanisms, and it seems likely, although unproven, that alcohol excess increases the penetrance of the C282Y genotype [50, 73]. Clinically, alcohol abuse certainly increases the risk of cirrhosis in C282Y homozygotes, but the molecular basis for this remains unknown. The combination of hereditary hemochromatosis and heavy alcohol use increases the risk of cirrhosis, up to tenfold, at lower total body iron levels [74–76]. There is emerging evidence that *HFE* heterozygosity itself aggravates hepatic iron loading in other diseases, such as alcoholic liver disease [77–79] and Hepatitis C [80, 81].

The pathophysiology of hemochromatosis-related diabetes mellitus is more complex than simple iron deposition causing direct damage to pancreatic islet cells. A predisposition to diabetes appears to be important as it is more likely to develop in patients with a positive family history and rarely resolves with treatment for hemochromatosis [15]. It is characterized by insulin resistance, evidenced by high circulating insulin levels, and is diagnosed in up to 65% of symptomatic patients [58].

5 Laboratory Testing and Diagnosis

The presence of symptoms and signs of iron overload should trigger an appropriate work-up for possible hereditary hemochromatosis. Unfortunately, in outside specialist centers, there is often a poor understanding of the issues surrounding diagnosis and management of hemochromatosis. In a large-scale survey of American physicians, it was discovered that a significant proportion of physicians were unaware of the population at risk for developing hemochromatosis, the pathogenesis of iron overload-associated complications, and the potential benefits of screening appropriate populations [82].

Before the discovery of the *HFE* gene mutation, hereditary hemochromatosis was diagnosed primarily by liver biopsy. Since 1996, diagnosis is based upon consistent clinical symptoms and/or signs attributable to iron overload, accompanied by a high transferrin saturation and serum ferritin level, in subjects found to be homozygous for the C282Y mutation after gene testing. Biopsy is now reserved for gaining prognostic information about the extent of liver injury, particularly the presence or absence of cirrhosis.

In cases of established hemochromatosis, an appropriate diagnostic work-up should be pursued to evaluate the degree of iron overload and the extent of other visceral and metabolic consequences of the disease [83]. Although the liver is most commonly implicated in the expression of hemochromatosis, there is considerable variation in liver enzyme abnormalities. Quantifying parenchymal iron can either be done via biopsy or other noninvasive imaging techniques.

Transferrin saturation is the best initial screening test as saturation in excess of 45% detects virtually all affected C282Y homozygotes [84]. While there is some debate surrounding the appropriate cutoff, anywhere between 45% and 70% in the literature [85], it is clear that a borderline test requires further investigation. It is acknowledged that although transferrin saturation and genotype are correlated, this association may vary by age, sex, and ethnic group [39].

Ferritin is a very sensitive test for iron overload but is nonspecific. As an acute phase reactant, levels are raised in a range of inflammatory illnesses and are also often abnormal in chronic liver disease of varying etiologies. Where possible, the ferritin level should be rechecked after the inflammatory condition has subsided or acute hepatocellular damage (e.g., alcoholic liver disease) has resolved. The serum ferritin level has, however, become an important predictor of the presence of disease related to hereditary hemochromatosis. C282Y homozygotes with a serum ferritin in excess of 1,000 μg/L are at greater risk of symptoms and disease than subjects with a lower ferritin level [34, 86]. Those with levels below this, and patients under the age of 35 years, are very unlikely to have cirrhosis [83, 87]. Arthropathy has been previously shown not to be associated with ferritin levels [53].

Measurement of these biochemical levels is generally simple and inexpensive, making them ideal screening tests, and primary carers are encouraged to maintain a high index of suspicion for hemochromatosis [88]. This is especially the case where patients have otherwise unexplained conditions or symptoms that are attributable to iron overload. Generally, it is reasonable to test for *HFE* gene status if either the transferrin saturation or serum ferritin level is high. Further diagnostic and prognostic tests should be initiated if hemochromatosis is confirmed.

For homozygous patients with a normal ferritin level and no evidence of liver disease, biochemical surveillance is appropriate with annual serum ferritin and transferrin measurements. The same surveillance principle applies for compound heterozygotes, who are at much lower risk of iron overload [89], albeit less frequently (e.g., every 3 years). About a quarter of C282Y heterozygotes will have abnormal transferrin and/or ferritin concentrations, although the latter is often due to chronic or inflammatory disease. Clinically significant iron accumulation is rare in C282Y simple heterozygosity [21].

H63D homozygosity also carries a rare risk of iron overload, and such patients should be treated like C282Y heterozygotes. Compound heterozygotes (i.e., C282Y/H63D genotype) are at higher risk of iron overload and behave phenotypically like C282Y homozygotes with considerably increased serum transferrin saturation and ferritin levels [90]. However significant iron overload is uncommon in such subjects. Obviously, H63D homozygosity and C282Y heterozygosity have implications for offspring who may be at risk of hemochromatosis depending upon their other inherited genotypes.

First-degree relatives of affected individuals should be tested for hereditary hemochromatosis [85, 91]. Symptoms, apart from lethargy, are generally far less prevalent in relatives compared to probands. Nevertheless, identification of at-risk relatives has implications for surveillance and treatment, particularly when one considers the proportion of asymptomatic patients with significant end-organ damage. There is a reasonable argument for genetic testing of the spouse of a C282Y homozygote rather than all offspring [43]. This approach could reduce the burden on genetic laboratory resources and allow offspring to be followed with less expensive biochemical surveillance.

6 Role of Liver Biopsy and Measurement of Hepatic Iron

Prior to the discovery of *HFE* gene mutations and the development of reliable genetic testing, liver biopsy played a major role in the diagnosis of hemochromatosis. Special iron stains, such as the Perls' Prussian blue test, were employed to confirm the diagnosis. Quantitative assessment of hepatic iron content (HIC; in μmol/g of liver, dry weight) is possible using biochemical testing of biopsy specimens. The calculation of the hepatic iron index (HIC divided by age) gives an objective measure with an index above 1.9 and typical iron deposition on histology being strongly suggestive of hereditary hemochromatosis, although this cutoff is not absolute [83, 92]. In cases of secondary iron overload, iron is preferentially taken up by Kupffer cells, whereas in hereditary hemochromatosis, there is virtually no iron seen in Kupffer cells and a predominantly periportal distribution of iron is typically seen.

Due to the development of other methods of estimating iron loading, biopsy has now become primarily a test of prognostic value and assessment of the severity of fibrosis is a major indication for biopsy. However, studies have identified patient and biochemical parameters that have a strong negative predictive value for fibrosis, thereby obviating the need for an invasive procedure that carries risks of sampling error [93] and a complication rate of approximately 0.5% in some series [94, 95]. Fibrosis is very uncommon where the serum ferritin is <1,000 μg/L, seen in only 1–3% of such patients [86].

In studies of patients homozygous for the C282Y mutation, no increase in hepatic fibrosis was seen in patients under 40 years of age, without hepatomegaly or abnormal liver enzymes and serum ferritin levels <1,000 μg/L [59, 87, 96]. Accordingly, it has been generally accepted that liver biopsy is only indicated in patients over 40 years, with hepatomegaly and abnormal liver enzymes, or serum ferritin levels in excess of 1,000 μg/L, or a combination of these factors [86]. Liver biopsy also serves to investigate other causes of liver disease where the diagnosis is equivocal.

Hepatic iron content can be noninvasively assessed using imaging modalities such as MRI. Using a highly T2-weighted protocol, MRI demonstrates a strong inverse relationship between T2 and iron content. In a study of over 100 patients, a strong correlation (0.98) has been shown between MRI-based and biopsy estimates of liver iron, with a prediction error comparable to the intrinsic variability of liver biopsy [97]. In another series of 112 patients, positive and negative predictive values of 100% for hemochromatosis were established for estimated hepatic iron concentrations of greater than 85 μmol/g and less than 40 μmol/g, respectively [98]. A number of studies have validated the technology [99], but the development of a quantification algorithm is complex, meaning that MRI is not universally available for this purpose [100]. MRI also appears to be sensitive and accurate in detecting cardiac iron deposition [61, 101].

7 Natural History and Disease Progression

Untreated classic hemochromatosis generally results in gradual accumulation of body iron, as evidenced by a progressive rise in serum transferrin and ferritin levels. Using data collected from surveys and standardized clinical evaluations over a 17-year period, Australian investigators found that the median transferrin saturation rose from 42% to 76% in a Caucasian cohort later found to be homozygous for C282Y [46]. Clinical features were present in only 50% of the group at diagnosis, but these symptoms and signs were not specific for hemochromatosis. Serum ferritin levels either increased or remained relatively stable in eight of ten homozygotes, but a persistent level in excess of 500 μg/L was associated with advanced fibrosis or cirrhosis. The authors concluded, therefore, that a single transferrin saturation level in patients under the age of 40 years may not adequately predict a benign course.

Parenchymal iron storage usually must exceed 10 g before organ damage ensues due to hemochromatosis. This process of insidious accumulation means that the disease does not usually become clinically apparent until middle age. In fact, it is unusual to see severe liver disease under the age of 35 years [83].

Using data from a large longitudinal study of an Australian population over 12 years, Allen et al. found that the rate of death from any cause was not increased in C282Y homozygotes compared with wild-type controls [34]. This finding is consistent with some previous reports but inconsistent with earlier work showing an increased risk of death compared to the normal population [13], although cirrhosis was probably overrepresented in that cohort. Hepatocellular carcinoma (HCC) accounts for about 30% of all deaths in hereditary hemochromatosis, and other complications of cirrhosis account for an additional 20% [13, 14].

8 Treatment

8.1 Venesection

Early work established a survival benefit for patients with hemochromatosis who undergo phlebotomy [13, 102], and venesection has now become the standard treatment [103]. Instituted before the onset of end-organ damage, phlebotomy can avoid all known complications of hemochromatosis [104]. Hepatocellular carcinoma remains a rare complication in noncirrhotic patients [20, 55].

Although venesection is effective, the effects on symptoms and signs of disease are variable [83]. Typically, skin pigmentation, abnormal serum transaminase levels, and abdominal pain are responsive to treatment with approximately 70% of patients showing improvement. Fatigue abates in 55% of patients, and 30–40% can expect some improvement in noncirrhotic fibrosis, arthralgia, impaired glucose tolerance, and cardiac manifestations. The effect of treatment on impotence is poor, with only a small proportion of patients (19%) experiencing improvement in symptoms [83].

Unfortunately, some symptoms may worsen during phlebotomy. Arthralgias worsen in 20% of patients undergoing therapy, and some patients acquire arthralgias, fatigue, or impotence (14% for each) during treatment [83].

Hepatic fibrosis can be reversed with phlebotomy [13, 105], with a recent study documenting a reduction of at least 2 METAVIR units in 47% of treated patients [17]. Cirrhosis is irreversible despite venesection, as are symptoms related to established arthritis. Once diabetes mellitus has become insulin-dependent, it is not amenable to therapy for iron overload [83]. Interestingly, the severity of portal hypertension in cirrhosis is affected by the removal of iron [106], with a reduction in variceal grade and bleeding risk.

The objective of "induction" venesection is to deplete the body of excess iron, and a regime of regular phlebotomy can be designed based upon calculations of total body iron. Each 500 mL of whole blood removed contains approximately 250 mg of iron. Patient progress can be followed using serum parameters of ferritin and MCV [103, 107], with the target being a serum ferritin level of less than 50 μg/L. Iron deficiency is indicated by a serum ferritin <25 μg/L and mandates suspension of phlebotomy. Iron-deficiency anemia should be avoided. Serum transferrin saturation levels usually remain elevated until iron stores are depleted.

Maintenance phlebotomy is performed, usually every 3 months, to keep pace with reacquisition of iron through normal dietary intake. Although animal models have shown that an iron-deficient diet reduces acute liver cell injury and attenuates chronic fibrosis [69], strict dietary iron restriction is unnecessary. Iron-rich foods, such as red meat and liver, should be avoided or significantly curtailed, however, as should iron supplements and vitamin C [83]. A small study has suggested that low-dose proton pump inhibitor therapy inhibits dietary iron absorption and may be a useful adjunctive therapy [108]. Young women, who are menstruating regularly, may not require venesection or may require less aggressive therapy. Blood from hereditary hemochromatosis patients appears to be safe for blood banks to use [109, 110], although few have allowed patients as donors to date.

8.2 *Iron Chelation*

Iron chelation by parenteral deferoxamine therapy has no advantages over phlebotomy, but it is indicated in certain circumstances. Patients with early-age onset of hemochromatosis may rapidly develop cardiac complications, particularly cardiomyopathy and arrhythmias. These conditions, often associated with *FPN1*, *TFR2*, *HJV*, or *HAMP* mutations, may require a combination of aggressive phlebotomy and iron chelation therapy. Erythrocytapheresis has been shown, in small case series, to reduce iron measures in patients with severe hemochromatosis, intolerance of phlebotomy, or coinheritance of β-thalassemia [111, 112]. Erythropoietin may augment these benefits [113, 114].

From experience in treatment for hemoglobinopathies and myelodysplastic syndromes, patients usually report lower quality of life measures with iron chelation therapy [115]. Therefore, simple, effective, nontoxic oral iron-reducing therapy has been a goal for many years. After much development and clinical trials, deferiprone (Ferriprox; LI) was licensed in Europe and elsewhere in 1999 for the treatment of secondary iron overload [116]. Side effects, however, have precluded its widespread acceptance.

More recently, the approval of deferasirox (Exjade®, ICL670) in the USA, Europe, and many other countries for the treatment of secondary iron overload, particularly due to thalassemia and sickle cell anemia, has marked a significant advance in the treatment of such disorders [117]. Deferasirox has shown good efficacy and safety in iron-overloaded subjects with a long half-life of 8–16 hours providing sustained 24-h chelation coverage [118]. However, its role in the treatment of primary iron overload and, in particular, HFE-associated hemochromatosis has not yet been established, and clinical trials are continuing. If these prove effective, it could provide a safe, effective, and convenient alternative to venesection therapy.

8.3 *Liver Transplantation*

Studies have shown that liver transplantation for hemochromatosis is associated with poorer survival than for other causes of end-stage disease [119, 120]. Late diagnosis, often at the time of transplantation, and the concurrence of hepatocellular carcinoma have been implicated as possible explanations. It has also been suggested that gross hepatic iron deposition is associated with high infection rates after transplantation. For these reasons, hemochromatosis patients should undergo intensive de-ironing by phlebotomy and possible desferrioxamine, if possible, before transplantation.

It has been speculated that differences in survival may be due to unknown functions of the *HFE* gene [121] and hepcidin [122] in the context of infection and immunological response. A multicenter US study of 260 patients with end-stage liver disease and iron overload found significantly lower 1- and 5-year survival rates (64% and 34%, respectively) for patients with hereditary hemochromatosis compared with unaffected patients [121]. A retrospective study of 153 consecutive transplant patients found a strong association between stainable iron in the explanted liver and fungal infection on multivariate analysis [123]. Although human data are scarce, it has been postulated that iron could play an important role in inhibiting phagocyte and T and B cell function.

Iron overload itself is associated with a higher risk of early mortality compared with the overall population undergoing liver transplantation. It has, however, been suggested that iron overload is associated with poorer outcome as it is a surrogate marker for advanced disease of any etiology [124].

The metabolic abnormality of hemochromatosis may be successfully reversed with liver transplantation [125–127]. Transplant patients who receive livers from donors with a normal HFE genotype do not reaccumulate iron. Normal biochemical markers post transplant also suggest that the liver itself is responsible for the basic defect in HFE-related hemochromatosis. Transplantation offers a unique model for the study of HFE expression and the pathophysiology of hemochromatosis, and further studies are awaited.

9 Early Identification and Population Screening

There has been considerable interest in markers of early, often asymptomatic, disease and the identification and treatment of potentially at-risk individuals. Diagnosis of hemochromatosis before the onset of symptoms occurs in up to 30% of patients [14], and advanced cirrhosis is detected in approximately 5% of asymptomatic sufferers [13, 128, 129]. Venesection has been shown to reverse hepatic fibrosis [18], and this underlines the importance of identifying asymptomatic homozygotes with advanced disease.

A consensus on population genetic screening has not yet been established [18, 83, 130]. Hemochromatosis, with its typically long asymptomatic phase and the capacity for serious morbidity and mortality, meets most WHO criteria for population-based screening [92]. As treatment is simple, cheap, and effective, the financial benefits of screening are obvious, although it has been suggested that any large-scale screening must be accompanied by an appropriate investigation of possible underlying liver disease [131]. Advances in the laboratory have improved throughput and turnaround times for genetic testing, making large volume screening technically feasible [42].

Due to the prevalence of *HFE* gene mutations in the general population, the clinical and public health implications of early detection strategies based upon genotype are substantial. The prevalence of HFE mutations, and C282Y in particular, is different among populations of different ethnicities [27]. Genetic screening has been variable in its utility and cost-effectiveness due to these differences [132]. Although the prevalence of the H63D mutation is higher, this mutation alone does not establish a diagnosis of hemochromatosis, and therefore, phenotypic screening has gained more support.

Early identification of asymptomatic homozygotes must be balanced against those individuals, especially heterozygotes, who may not develop disease related to iron overload. Significant anxiety related to genetic screening is variably reported in the literature [133, 134]. The recently completed Hemochromatosis and Iron Overload Screening (HEIRS) study found that genotype and phenotype were strong predictors of adverse effects on psychological well-being and health. Ethnicity and language also had an impact upon participants' responses [135]. An approach which takes these wider issues of genetic testing [136], including employment and insurance discrimination, into account is obviously necessary if population screening for HFE-related hemochromatosis is to become accepted.

Some authors have shown population phenotype screening, using transferrin saturation and ferritin levels, to be as or more cost-effective than already accepted screening strategies (e.g., for colorectal or breast cancer) [137]. The fact that intermediate biochemical levels carry uncertain significance has contributed to the controversy of population screening. The timing of screening is also problematic [60] with studies revealing that a single normal transferrin saturation at a median age of 31 years misses 60% of untreated hereditary hemochromatosis subjects [46], all of whom subsequently developed iron overload. Currently, there is no evidence that widespread population screening is appropriate [83, 138].

References

1. von Recklinghausen F. Taggeblet de. Versainumlung Deutsch Naturforsch Arzt Heidelberg 1889;62:324–25
2. Pietrangelo A. Hereditary hemochromatosis – a new look at an old disease. N Engl J Med. 2004;350:2383–97.
3. Simon M, Pawlotsky Y, Bourel M, Fauchet R, Genetet B. Letter: Idiopathic hemochromatosis associated with HL-A 3 tissular antigen. Nouv Presse Med. 1975;4:1432.
4. Simon M, Le Mignon L, Fauchet R, et al. A study of 609 HLA haplotypes marking for the hemochromatosis gene: (1) mapping of the gene near the HLA-A locus and characters required to define a heterozygous population and (2) hypothesis concerning the underlying cause of hemochromatosis-HLA association. Am J Hum Genet. 1987;41:89–105.
5. Feder JN, Gnirke A, Thomas W, et al. A novel MHC class I-like gene is mutated in patients with hereditary haemochromatosis. Nat Genet. 1996;13:399–408.
6. Adams PC, Barton JC. Haemochromatosis. Lancet. 2007;370:1855–60.
7. Swinkels DW, Janssen MC, Bergmans J, Marx JJ. Hereditary hemochromatosis: genetic complexity and new diagnostic approaches. Clin Chem. 2006;52:950–68.
8. Cazzola M, Cerani P, Rovati A, Iannone A, Claudiani G, Bergamaschi G. Juvenile genetic hemochromatosis is clinically and genetically distinct from the classical HLA-related disorder. Blood. 1998;92:2979–81.
9. Girelli D, Bozzini C, Roetto A, et al. Clinical and pathologic findings in hemochromatosis type 3 due to a novel mutation in transferrin receptor 2 gene. Gastroenterology. 2002;122:1295–302.
10. Sham RL, Phatak PD, West C, Lee P, Andrews C, Beutler E. Autosomal dominant hereditary hemochromatosis associated with a novel ferroportin mutation and unique clinical features. Blood Cells Mol Dis. 2005;34:157–61.
11. Cazzola M. Genetic disorders of iron overload and the novel "ferroportin disease". Haematologica. 2003;88:721–4.
12. Chua AC, Graham RM, Trinder D, Olynyk JK. The regulation of cellular iron metabolism. Crit Rev Clin Lab Sci. 2007;44:413–59.
13. Niederau C, Fischer R, Purschel A, Stremmel W, Haussinger D, Strohmeyer G. Long-term survival in patients with hereditary hemochromatosis. Gastroenterology. 1996;110:1107–19.
14. Adams PC, Deugnier Y, Moirand R, Brissot P. The relationship between iron overload, clinical symptoms, and age in 410 patients with genetic hemochromatosis. Hepatology. 1997;25:162–6.

15. Stocks AE, Powell LW. Pituitary function in idiopathic haemochromatosis and cirrhosis of the liver. Lancet. 1972;2:298–300.
16. Bacon BR. Hemochromatosis: diagnosis and management. Gastroenterology. 2001;120:718–25.
17. Falize L, Guillygomarc'h A, Perrin M, et al. Reversibility of hepatic fibrosis in treated genetic hemochromatosis: a study of 36 cases. Hepatology. 2006;44:472–7.
18. Powell LW, Dixon JL, Ramm GA, et al. Screening for hemochromatosis in asymptomatic subjects with or without a family history. Arch Intern Med. 2006;166:294–301.
19. Bradbear RA, Bain C, Siskind V, et al. Cohort study of internal malignancy in genetic hemochromatosis and other chronic nonalcoholic liver diseases. J Natl Cancer Inst. 1985;75:81–4.
20. Deugnier YM, Guyader D, Crantock L, et al. Primary liver cancer in genetic hemochromatosis: a clinical, pathological, and pathogenetic study of 54 cases. Gastroenterology. 1993;104:228–34.
21. Worwood M. Inherited iron loading: genetic testing in diagnosis and management. Blood Rev. 2005;19:69–88.
22. Merryweather-Clarke AT, Cadet E, Bomford A, et al. Digenic inheritance of mutations in HAMP and HFE results in different types of haemochromatosis. Hum Mol Genet. 2003;12:2241–7.
23. Tomatsu S, Orii KO, Fleming RE, et al. Contribution of the H63D mutation in HFE to murine hereditary hemochromatosis. Proc Natl Acad Sci USA. 2003;100:15788–93.
24. Ajioka RS, Kushner JP. Clinical consequences of iron overload in hemochromatosis homozygotes. Blood. 2003;101:3351–3.
25. Simon M. Genetics of hemochromatosis. N Engl J Med. 1979;301:1291–2.
26. Simon M, Alexandre JL, Fauchet R, Genetet B, Bourel M. The genetics of hemochromatosis. Prog Med Genet. 1980;4:135–68.
27. Merryweather-Clarke AT, Pointon JJ, Shearman JD, Robson KJ. Global prevalence of putative haemochromatosis mutations. J Med Genet. 1997;34:275–8.
28. Moirand R, Jouanolle AM, Brissot P, Le Gall JY, David V, Deugnier Y. Phenotypic expression of HFE mutations: a French study of 1110 unrelated iron-overloaded patients and relatives. Gastroenterology. 1999;116:372–7.
29. Bacon BR, Britton RS. Clinical penetrance of hereditary hemochromatosis. N Engl J Med. 2008;358:291–2.
30. Olynyk JK, Cullen DJ, Aquilia S, Rossi E, Summerville L, Powell LW. A population-based study of the clinical expression of the hemochromatosis gene. N Engl J Med. 1999;341:718–24.
31. Asberg A, Hveem K, Thorstensen K, et al. Screening for hemochromatosis: high prevalence and low morbidity in an unselected population of 65,238 persons. Scand J Gastroenterol. 2001;36:1108–15.
32. Beutler E, Felitti VJ, Koziol JA, Ho Ngoc J, Gelbart T. Penetrance of 845G – A (C282Y) *HFE* hereditary haemochromatosis mutation in the USA. Lancet. 2002;359:211–8.
33. Adams PC, Reboussin DM, Barton JC, et al. Hemochromatosis and iron-overload screening in a racially diverse population. N Engl J Med. 2005;352:1769–78.
34. Allen KJ, Gurrin LC, Constantine CC, et al. Iron-overload-related disease in HFE hereditary hemochromatosis. N Engl J Med. 2008;358:221–30.
35. Burt MJ, George PM, Upton JD, et al. The significance of haemochromatosis gene mutations in the general population: implications for screening. Gut. 1998;43:830–6.
36. Steinberg KK, Cogswell ME, Chang JC, et al. Prevalence of C282Y and H63D mutations in the hemochromatosis (HFE) gene in the United States. JAMA. 2001;285:2216–22.
37. Carella M, D'Ambrosio L, Totaro A, et al. Mutation analysis of the HLA-H gene in Italian hemochromatosis patients. Am J Hum Genet. 1997;60:828–32.
38. Gochee PA, Powell LW, Cullen DJ, Du Sart D, Rossi E, Olynyk JK. A population-based study of the biochemical and clinical expression of the H63D hemochromatosis mutation. Gastroenterology. 2002;122:646–51.
39. Cogswell ME, Gallagher ML, Steinberg KK, et al. HFE genotype and transferrin saturation in the United States. Genet Med. 2003;5:304–10.
40. Njajou OT, Houwing-Duistermaat JJ, Osborne RH, et al. A population-based study of the effect of the HFE C282Y and H63D mutations on iron metabolism. Eur J Hum Genet. 2003;11:225–31.
41. Beutler E. The significance of the 187G (H63D) mutation in hemochromatosis. Am J Hum Genet. 1997;61:762–4.
42. Tafe LJ, Belloni DR, Tsongalis GJ. Detection of the C282Y and H63D polymorphisms associated with hereditary hemochromatosis using the ABI 7500 fast real time PCR platform. Diagn Mol Pathol. 2007;16:112–5.
43. King C, Barton DE. Best practice guidelines for the molecular genetic diagnosis of Type 1 (HFE-related) hereditary haemochromatosis. BMC Med Genet. 2006;7:81.
44. Giles GG, English DR. The Melbourne Collaborative Cohort Study. IARC Sci Publ. 2002;156:69–70.
45. Whitlock EP, Garlitz BA, Harris EL, Beil TL, Smith PR. Screening for hereditary hemochromatosis: a systematic review for the U.S. Preventive Services Task Force. Ann Intern Med. 2006;145:209–23.
46. Olynyk JK, Hagan SE, Cullen DJ, Beilby J, Whittall DE. Evolution of untreated hereditary hemochromatosis in the Busselton population: a 17-year study. Mayo Clin Proc. 2004;79:309–13.

47. Andersen RV, Tybjaerg-Hansen A, Appleyard M, Birgens H, Nordestgaard BG. Hemochromatosis mutations in the general population: iron overload progression rate. Blood. 2004;103:2914–9.
48. Lamon JM, Marynick SP, Roseblatt R, Donnelly S. Idiopathic hemochromatosis in a young female. A case study and review of the syndrome in young people. Gastroenterology. 1979;76:178–83.
49. Cazzola M, Ascari E, Barosi G, et al. Juvenile idiopathic haemochromatosis: a life-threatening disorder presenting as hypogonadotropic hypogonadism. Hum Genet. 1983;65:149–54.
50. Waalen J, Nordestgaard BG, Beutler E. The penetrance of hereditary hemochromatosis. Best Pract Res Clin Haematol. 2005;18:203–20.
51. Allen KJ, Delatycki MB, Nisselle AE, et al. Use of community genetic screening to prevent HFE-associated hereditary haemochromatosis. Lancet. 2005;366:314–6.
52. Asberg A, Hveem K, Kannelonning K, Irgens WO. Penetrance of the C28Y/C282Y genotype of the HFE gene. Scand J Gastroenterol. 2007;42:1073–7.
53. Bulaj ZJ, Ajioka RS, Phillips JD, et al. Disease-related conditions in relatives of patients with hemochromatosis. N Engl J Med. 2000;343:1529–35.
54. Beaton MD, Adams PC. Prognostic factors and survival in patients with hereditary hemochromatosis and cirrhosis. Can J Gastroenterol. 2006;20:257–60.
55. Hiatt T, Trotter JF, Kam I. Hepatocellular carcinoma in a noncirrhotic patient with hereditary hemochromatosis. Am J Med Sci. 2007;334:228–30.
56. Willis G, Bardsley V, Fellows IW, Lonsdale R, Wimperis JZ, Jennings BA. Hepatocellular carcinoma and the penetrance of HFE C282Y mutations: a cross sectional study. BMC Gastroenterol. 2005;5:17.
57. Barton JC, Bertoli LF, Acton RT. HFE C282Y and H63D in adults with malignancies in a community medical oncology practice. BMC Cancer. 2004;4:6.
58. O'Neil J, Powell L. Clinical aspects of hemochromatosis. Semin Liver Dis. 2005;25:381–91.
59. Bacon BR, Olynyk JK, Brunt EM, Britton RS, Wolff RK. HFE genotype in patients with hemochromatosis and other liver diseases. Ann Intern Med. 1999;130:953–62.
60. Bacon BR. Diagnosis and management of hemochromatosis. Gastroenterology. 1997;113:995–9.
61. Anderson GJ. Ironing out disease: inherited disorders of iron homeostasis. IUBMB Life. 2001;51:11–7.
62. Siah CW, Ombiga J, Adams LA, Trinder D, Olynyk JK. Normal iron metabolism and the pathophysiology of iron overload disorders. Clin Biochem Rev. 2006;27:5–16.
63. Lawless MW, Mankan AK, White M, O'Dwyer MJ, Norris S. Expression of hereditary hemochromatosis C282Y HFE protein in HEK293 cells activates specific endoplasmic reticulum stress responses. BMC Cell Biol. 2007;8:30.
64. Fleming RE, Sly WS. Hepcidin: a putative iron-regulatory hormone relevant to hereditary hemochromatosis and the anemia of chronic disease. Proc Natl Acad Sci USA. 2001;98:8160–2.
65. Nicolas G, Viatte L, Lou DQ, et al. Constitutive hepcidin expression prevents iron overload in a mouse model of hemochromatosis. Nat Genet. 2003;34:97–101.
66. Fink S, Schilsky ML. Inherited metabolic disease of the liver. Curr Opin Gastroenterol. 2007;23:237–43.
67. Jacolot S, Le Gac G, Scotet V, Quere I, Mura C, Ferec C. HAMP as a modifier gene that increases the phenotypic expression of the HFE pC282Y homozygous genotype. Blood. 2004;103:2835–40.
68. Biasiotto G, Roetto A, Daraio F, et al. Identification of new mutations of hepcidin and hemojuvelin in patients with HFE C282Y allele. Blood Cells Mol Dis. 2004;33:338–43.
69. Otogawa K, Ogawa T, Shiga R, et al. Attenuation of acute and chronic liver injury in rats by iron-deficient diet. Am J Physiol Regul Integr Comp Physiol. 2008;294:R311–20.
70. George DK, Ramm GA, Powell LW, et al. Evidence for altered hepatic matrix degradation in genetic haemochromatosis. Gut. 1998;42:715–20.
71. Hayes JD, McLellan LI. Glutathione and glutathione-dependent enzymes represent a co-ordinately regulated defence against oxidative stress. Free Radic Res. 1999;31:273–300.
72. Stickel F, Osterreicher CH, Datz C, et al. Prediction of progression to cirrhosis by a glutathione S-transferase P1 polymorphism in subjects with hereditary hemochromatosis. Arch Intern Med. 2005;165:1835–40.
73. Reuben A. Alcohol and the liver. Curr Opin Gastroenterol. 2006;22:263–71.
74. Fletcher LM, Dixon JL, Purdie DM, Powell LW, Crawford DH. Excess alcohol greatly increases the prevalence of cirrhosis in hereditary hemochromatosis. Gastroenterology. 2002;122:281–9.
75. Fletcher LM, Bridle KR, Crawford DH. Effect of alcohol on iron storage diseases of the liver. Best Pract Res Clin Gastroenterol. 2003;17:663–77.
76. Powell LW. The role of alcoholism in hepatic iron storage disease. Ann N Y Acad Sci. 1975;252:124–34.
77. Alla V, Bonkovsky HL. Iron in nonhemochromatotic liver disorders. Semin Liver Dis. 2005;25:461–72.
78. Thursz M, Mantafounis D, Yallo R. Severe alcoholic liver disease is associated with the haemochromatosis gene mutant. Gastroenterology. 1997;112:A1401.
79. Frenzer A, Rudzki Z, Norton ID, Butler WJ, Roberts-Thomson IC. Heterozygosity of the haemochromatosis mutation, C282Y, does not influence susceptibility to alcoholic cirrhosis. Scand J Gastroenterol. 1998;33:1324.

80. Pacal L, Husa P, Znojil V, Kankova K. HFE C282Y gene variant is a risk factor for the progression to decompensated liver disease in chronic viral hepatitis C subjects in the Czech population. Hepatol Res. 2007;37:740–7.
81. Nahon P, Sutton A, Rufat P, et al. Liver iron, HFE gene mutations, and hepatocellular carcinoma occurrence in patients with cirrhosis. Gastroenterology. 2008;134:102–10.
82. Acton RT, Barton JC, Casebeer L, Talley L. Survey of physician knowledge about hemochromatosis. Genet Med. 2002;4:136–41.
83. Adams P, Brissot P, Powell LW. EASL International Consensus Conference on Haemochromatosis. J Hepatol. 2000;33:485–504.
84. McLaren CE, McLachlan GJ, Halliday JW, et al. Distribution of transferrin saturation in an Australian population: relevance to the early diagnosis of hemochromatosis. Gastroenterology. 1998;114:543–9.
85. Edwards CQ, Kushner JP. Screening for hemochromatosis. N Engl J Med. 1993;328:1616–20.
86. Guyader D, Jacquelinet C, Moirand R, et al. Noninvasive prediction of fibrosis in C282Y homozygous hemochromatosis. Gastroenterology. 1998;115:929–36.
87. Morrison ED, Brandhagen DJ, Phatak PD, et al. Serum ferritin level predicts advanced hepatic fibrosis among U.S. patients with phenotypic hemochromatosis. Ann Intern Med. 2003;138:627–33.
88. Hover AR, McDonnell SM, Burke W. Changing the clinical management of hereditary hemochromatosis: translating screening and early case detection strategies into clinical practice. Arch Intern Med. 2004;164:957–61.
89. Jackson HA, Carter K, Darke C, et al. HFE mutations, iron deficiency and overload in 10,500 blood donors. Br J Haematol. 2001;114:474–84.
90. Beutler E, Felitti V, Gelbart T, Ho N. The effect of HFE genotypes on measurements of iron overload in patients attending a health appraisal clinic. Ann Intern Med. 2000;133:329–37.
91. Tavill AS. Diagnosis and management of hemochromatosis AASLD practice guidelines. Hepatology. 2001;33:1321–8.
92. Powell LW. Hereditary hemochromatosis and iron overload diseases. J Gastroenterol Hepatol. 2002;17 Suppl 1:191–5.
93. Emond MJ, Bronner MP, Carlson TH, Lin M, Labbe RF, Kowdley KV. Quantitative study of the variability of hepatic iron concentrations. Clin Chem. 1999;45:340–6.
94. Angelucci E, Baronciani D, Lucarelli G, et al. Needle liver biopsy in thalassaemia: analyses of diagnostic accuracy and safety in 1184 consecutive biopsies. Br J Haematol. 1995;89:757–61.
95. Janes CH, Lindor KD. Outcome of patients hospitalized for complications after outpatient liver biopsy. Ann Intern Med. 1993;118:96–8.
96. Whittington CA, Kowdley KV. Review article: haemochromatosis. Aliment Pharmacol Ther. 2002;16:1963–75.
97. St Pierre TG, Clark PR, Chua-anusorn W, et al. Noninvasive measurement and imaging of liver iron concentrations using proton magnetic resonance. Blood. 2005;105:855–61.
98. Alustiza JM, Artetxe J, Castiella A, et al. MR quantification of hepatic iron concentration. Radiology. 2004;230:479–84.
99. Wood JC, Enriquez C, Ghugre N, et al. MRI R2 and R2* mapping accurately estimates hepatic iron concentration in transfusion-dependent thalassemia and sickle cell disease patients. Blood. 2005;106:1460–5.
100. Alustiza JM, Castiella A, De Juan MD, Emparanza JI, Artetxe J, Uranga M. Iron overload in the liver diagnostic and quantification. Eur J Radiol. 2007;61:499–506.
101. Cheong B, Huber S, Muthupillai R, Flamm SD. Evaluation of myocardial iron overload by T2* cardiovascular magnetic resonance imaging. Tex Heart Inst J. 2005;32:448–9.
102. Bomford A, Williams R. Long term results of venesection therapy in idiopathic haemochromatosis. Q J Med. 1976;45:611–23.
103. Barton JC, McDonnell SM, Adams PC, et al. Management of hemochromatosis. Hemochromatosis Management Working Group. Ann Intern Med. 1998;129:932–9.
104. Barton JC. Optimal management strategies for chronic iron overload. Drugs. 2007;67:685–700.
105. Powell LW, Kerr JF. Reversal of "cirrhosis" in idiopathic haemochromatosis following long-term intensive venesection therapy. Australas Ann Med. 1970;19:54–7.
106. Fracanzani AL, Fargion S, Romano R, et al. Portal hypertension and iron depletion in patients with genetic hemochromatosis. Hepatology. 1995;22:1127–31.
107. Bolan CD, Conry-Cantilena C, Mason G, Rouault TA, Leitman SF. MCV as a guide to phlebotomy therapy for hemochromatosis. Transfusion. 2001;41:819–27.
108. Hutchinson C, Geissler CA, Powell JJ, Bomford A. Proton pump inhibitors suppress absorption of dietary non-haem iron in hereditary haemochromatosis. Gut. 2007;56:1291–5.
109. Casella G, Biella A, Signorini S, Tramacere P, Baldini V. Hereditary hemochromatosis without organ damage: a rescue resource for blood supply? Eur J Gastroenterol Hepatol. 2004;16:1419–20.
110. Sanchez AM, Schreiber GB, Bethel J, et al. Prevalence, donation practices, and risk assessment of blood donors with hemochromatosis. JAMA. 2001;286:1475–81.

111. Conte D, Mandelli C, Cesana M, Ferrini R, Marconi M, Bianchi A. Effectiveness of erythrocytapheresis in idiopathic hemochromatosis. Report of 14 cases. Int J Artif Organs. 1989;12:59–62.
112. Cesana M, Mandelli C, Tiribelli C, Bianchi PA, Conte D. Concomitant primary hemochromatosis and beta-thalassemia trait: iron depletion by erythrocytapheresis and desferrioxamine. Am J Gastroenterol. 1989;84:150–2.
113. Kohan A, Niborski R, Daruich J, et al. Erythrocytapheresis with recombinant human erythropoietin in hereditary hemochromatosis therapy: a new alternative. Vox Sang. 2000;79:40–5.
114. Mariani R, Pelucchi S, Perseghin P, Corengia C, Piperno A. Erythrocytapheresis plus erythropoietin: an alternative therapy for selected patients with hemochromatosis and severe organ damage. Haematologica. 2005;90:717–8.
115. Abetz L, Baladi JF, Jones P, Rofail D. The impact of iron overload and its treatment on quality of life: results from a literature review. Health Qual Life Outcomes. 2006;4:73.
116. Kontoghiorghes GJ, Bartlett AN, Hoffbrand AV, et al. Long-term trial with the oral iron chelator 1,2-dimethyl-3-hydroxypyrid-4-one (L1). I. Iron chelation and metabolic studies. Br J Haematol. 1990;76:295–300.
117. Vichinsky E, Onyekwere O, Porter J, et al. A randomised comparison of deferasirox versus deferoxamine for the treatment of transfusional iron overload in sickle cell disease. Br J Haematol. 2007;136:501–8.
118. Yang LP, Keam SJ, Keating GM. Deferasirox: a review of its use in the management of transfusional chronic iron overload. Drugs. 2007;67:2211–30.
119. Kowdley KV, Hassanein T, Kaur S, et al. Primary liver cancer and survival in patients undergoing liver transplantation for hemochromatosis. Liver Transpl Surg. 1995;1:237–41.
120. Kilpe VE, Krakauer H, Wren RE. An analysis of liver transplant experience from 37 transplant centers as reported to Medicare. Transplantation. 1993;56(3):554–61.
121. Kowdley KV, Brandhagen DJ, Gish RG, et al. Survival after liver transplantation in patients with hepatic iron overload: the national hemochromatosis transplant registry. Gastroenterology. 2005;129:494–503.
122. Ashrafian H. Hepcidin: the missing link between hemochromatosis and infections. Infect Immun. 2003;71:6693–700.
123. Alexander J, Limaye AP, Ko CW, Bronner MP, Kowdley KV. Association of hepatic iron overload with invasive fungal infection in liver transplant recipients. Liver Transpl. 2006;12:1799–804.
124. Stuart KA, Fletcher LM, Clouston AD, et al. Increased hepatic iron and cirrhosis: no evidence for an adverse effect on patient outcome following liver transplantation. Hepatology. 2000;32:1200–7.
125. Crawford DH, Fletcher LM, Hubscher SG, et al. Patient and graft survival after liver transplantation for hereditary hemochromatosis: implications for pathogenesis. Hepatology. 2004;39:1655–62.
126. Kowdley KV. Liver transplantation: an "in vivo" model for the pathophysiology of hemochromatosis? Hepatology. 2004;39:1495–8.
127. Powell LW. Does transplantation of the liver cure genetic hemochromatosis? J Hepatol. 1992;16:259–61.
128. Powell LW, Dixon JL, Ramm GA, et al. The penetrance of HFE-associated hemochromatosis as assessed by clinical evaluation and liver biopsy in subjects identified by health checks, family screening or population screening. Hepatology. 2004;40:74A.
129. Adams PC, Chakrabarti S. Genotypic/phenotypic correlations in genetic hemochromatosis: evolution of diagnostic criteria. Gastroenterology. 1998;114:319–23.
130. Motulsky AG, Beutler E. Population screening in hereditary hemochromatosis. Annu Rev Public Health. 2000;21:65–79.
131. Bacon BR. Screening for hemochromatosis. Arch Intern Med. 2006;166:269–70.
132. Simsek H, Sumer H, Yilmaz E, et al. Frequency of HFE mutations among Turkish blood donors according to transferrin saturation: genotype screening for hereditary hemochromatosis among voluntary blood donors in Turkey. J Clin Gastroenterol. 2004;38:671–5.
133. Anderson RT, Wenzel L, Walker AP, et al. Impact of hemochromatosis screening in patients with indeterminate results: the hemochromatosis and iron overload screening study. Genet Med. 2006;8:681–7.
134. Delatycki MB, Allen KJ, Nisselle AE, et al. Use of community genetic screening to prevent HFE-associated hereditary haemochromatosis. Lancet. 2005;366:314–6.
135. Wenzel LB, Anderson R, Tucker DC, et al. Health-related quality of life in a racially diverse population screened for hemochromatosis: results from the Hemochromatosis and Iron Overload Screening (HEIRS) study. Genet Med. 2007;9:705–12.
136. Barlow-Stewart K, Burnett L. Ethical considerations in the use of DNA for the diagnosis of diseases. Clin Biochem Rev. 2006;27:53–61.
137. Dubois S, Kowdley KV. The importance of screening for hemochromatosis. Arch Intern Med. 2003;163:2424–6.
138. McDonnell SM, Parrish RG. Hereditary hemochromatosis and its elusive natural history. Arch Intern Med. 2003;163:2421–3.

Chapter 20
Non-HFE Hemochromatosis

Daniel F. Wallace and V. Nathan Subramaniam

Keywords African iron overload • Ferritin • Ferroportin • Hemochromatosis • Hemojuvelin • Hepcidin • Iron overload • Juvenile hemochromatosis • Transferrin receptor 2

1 Non-HFE Hemochromatosis

With the identification of the *HFE* gene in 1996, the majority of cases of hereditary hemochromatosis (HH) or type 1 HH were found to be associated with homozygosity for a mutation leading to a cysteine to tyrosine substitution (C282Y) in the HFE protein [1]. Hemochromatosis due to mutations in the *HFE* gene is the subject of Chap. 19 and is discussed in more detail there. Hemochromatosis that is not associated with mutations in HFE is termed non-HFE hemochromatosis. This is a collective term used to describe a number of other iron overload syndromes that are caused by mutations in different genes involved in regulating iron homeostasis. These iron overload syndromes vary in their phenotypic features, age of onset, and mode of inheritance. The features of each type and the role of the affected genes and proteins in iron metabolism are the subjects of this chapter and are summarized in Table 20.1.

2 Recessively Inherited Hemochromatosis

There are three other known forms of recessively inherited hemochromatosis in addition to HFE-associated hemochromatosis. Two of these have an early onset and are referred to as juvenile hemochromatosis (JH). The third is caused by mutations in the gene encoding transferrin receptor 2 (TFR2). Together with HFE, all the affected genes are involved in the regulation of the iron-regulatory hormone hepcidin. All have similar patterns of iron loading, albeit with differing severities and age at onset.

D.F. Wallace, Ph.D. • V.N. Subramaniam, Ph.D. (✉)
Membrane Transport Laboratory, Queensland Institute of Medical Research, Brisbane, QLD, Australia
e-mail: Nathan.Subramaniam@qimr.edu.au

G.J. Anderson and G. McLaren (eds.), *Iron Physiology and Pathophysiology in Humans*, Nutrition and Health, DOI 10.1007/978-1-60327-485-2_20,

Table 20.1 Summary of the clinical, biochemical, and pathological features of the different forms of non-HFE hemochromatosis

Type of HH	Gene	Inheritance	Clinical features	Laboratory findings	Liver pathology	Functional consequences of mutations
1	*HFE*	Autosomal recessive	May include fatigue, lethargy, arthropathy, skin pigmentation, liver fibrosis, diabetes mellitus, endocrine dysfunction, cardiomyopathy, hypogonadotropic hypogonadism	↑ Serum ferritin ↑ Transferrin saturation	Hepatocyte iron loading, fibrosis, cirrhosis	Impaired hepcidin regulation by iron, leading to increased intestinal iron absorption and release of iron from reticuloendothelial cells
2A	*Hemojuvelin (HJV), HFE2*	Autosomal recessive	As for HFE Earlier onset. (<30 years) Cardiomyopathy and hypogonadism more prevalent	↑ Serum ferritin ↑ Transferrin saturation	Hepatocyte iron loading, fibrosis, cirrhosis	Loss of hepcidin regulation, leading to increased intestinal iron absorption and release of iron from reticuloendothelial cells
2B	*Hepcidin (HAMP)*	Autosomal recessive	As for HFE Earlier onset (<30 years). Cardiomyopathy and hypogonadism more prevalent	↑ Serum ferritin, ↑ Transferrin saturation	Hepatocyte iron loading, fibrosis, cirrhosis	No hepcidin, leading to maximal iron absorption and release of iron from reticuloendothelial cells
3	*Transferrin Receptor 2 (TFR2)*	Autosomal recessive	As for HFE May have a slightly earlier onset	↑ Serum ferritin, ↑ Transferrin saturation	Hepatocyte iron loading, fibrosis, cirrhosis	Impaired hepcidin regulation by iron, leading to increased intestinal iron absorption and release of iron from reticuloendothelial cells
4	*Ferroportin (Fpn), SLC40A1, IREG1, MTP1*	Autosomal dominant	Typical presentation: as for HFE, except generally milder. May have mild anemia and lower tolerance to venesection	↑ Serum ferritin Normal transferrin saturation	Predominant Kupffer cell iron loading, fibrosis	Reduced ferroportin iron transport ability, leading to accumulation of iron in reticuloendothelial cells
			Atypical: as for HFE	↑ Serum ferritin ↑ Transferrin saturation	Predominant hepatocyte iron loading, fibrosis, cirrhosis	Loss of ferroportin regulation by hepcidin, leading to increased intestinal iron absorption and release of iron from reticuloendothelial cells
H-ferritin-related iron overload	H-ferritin (FTH1) 5'UTR	Autosomal dominant	Only one reported family – no clinical features reported	↑ Serum ferritin Normal transferrin saturation	Hepatocyte and Kupffer cell iron loading	Increased binding of mutant IRE to IRPs, causing downregulation of H-ferritin synthesis and corresponding upregulation of L-ferritin
African iron overload	Gene unknown	Possible genetic and dietary components	As for HFE, including liver fibrosis and diabetes mellitus	↑ Serum ferritin ↑ Transferrin saturation	Hepatocyte and Kupffer cell iron loading	Unknown

2.1 *Juvenile Hemochromatosis (Type 2 HH)*

Hemochromatosis in young people has been recognized as a distinct disorder from the adult form since before the *HFE* gene was identified [2]. Unlike the adult form or type 1 HH, JH affects both sexes equally and usually presents before the age of 30 years. The pattern of iron loading in the liver is similar to the adult form, with iron accumulation preferentially in parenchymal cells. The serum iron parameters, transferrin saturation, and serum ferritin are raised, with similar values to the adult form, but at a younger age [3]. The most prominent clinical findings in JH patients are hypogonadotropic hypogonadism and cardiomyopathy; both of these are significantly more frequent in JH than in adult-onset forms of the disease [4]. Liver involvement, including cirrhosis, is often present but is clinically less significant [3]. Other clinical features of JH are similar to HFE-HH and can include fatigue, lethargy, diabetes mellitus, skin pigmentation, and arthropathy [3, 4]. Unless early treatment to reduce iron stores is commenced, the condition can often be fatal – death normally resulting from heart failure [3]. Venesection is usually the safest and most effective treatment to reduce iron stores in hemochromatosis; however, in the face of congestive heart failure, this therapy is not recommended and iron chelators are often used. Cardiac transplantation has been used successfully in patients with end-stage iron overload – related cardiomyopathy, with combined liver transplantation in a few cases [5]. In recent years, the molecular basis of juvenile or type 2 hemochromatosis has been determined. JH can be classified into two subtypes. Type 2A is caused by mutations in *hemojuvelin* (*HJV*), also known as *HFE2* or *RGMc*, whereas type 2B is caused by mutations in the liver-expressed antimicrobial and iron-regulatory peptide *hepcidin* (*HAMP*), also known as *LEAP-1*.

2.1.1 Hemojuvelin-Associated Hemochromatosis (Type 2A HH)

After the identification of *HFE*, it was soon confirmed that JH was a distinct genetic disorder and unrelated to the adult *HFE*-related form of the disease [6]. This study utilized microsatellite markers on chromosome 6 in five Italian JH families and did not detect any linkage between these markers and the disease. Subsequently, the gene was mapped using a genome-wide linkage study in nine JH families, mostly of Italian origin, to a region on the long arm of chromosome 1 [7]. Papanikolaou et al. performed fine-mapping of the 1q21 region in 12 unrelated JH families (ten from Greece, the remaining two from France and Canada) and narrowed down the linkage interval to ~1.7 Mb. This region contained 21 annotated genes; however, no obvious candidates were apparent. Sequencing of the positional candidate genes resulted in the identification of mutations in a novel gene, termed *hemojuvelin* or *HFE2* [8]. Homozygosity or compound heterozygosity for *HJV* mutations were identified in all affected members of the 12 families studied. Six mutations were identified, with one, G320V, being present in nine of the 12 families. Lanzara et al. studied a large series of 34 patients from 29 families and identified 17 mutations. Over 40 HJV mutations have been reported to date and are illustrated in Fig. 20.1 [8–22]. The mutations are distributed throughout the length of the HJV protein. A large number of these result in frameshifts or premature termination codons and are likely to have profound effects on the structure and function of the HJV protein. The G320V mutation is significantly more prevalent and has been reported in many populations worldwide [23].

Hemojuvelin (HJV) has homology to the repulsive guidance molecule (RGM) family of proteins. Two members of this family, RGMa and RGMb (DRAGON), are expressed in the central nervous system and play important roles in neural development [24, 25]. HJV (sometimes called RGMc) is expressed predominantly in skeletal muscle, heart, and liver [8]. In keeping with other RGMs, HJV contains a carboxy-terminal glycophosphatidylinositol (GPI) anchor and can be present in a cell-associated or soluble form [26]. Urinary hepcidin levels in patients with HJV-associated JH are low relative to controls, suggesting that HJV may be involved in hepcidin regulation [8]. Knockout of HJV in mice confirmed its importance in maintaining iron homeostasis and in the regulation of

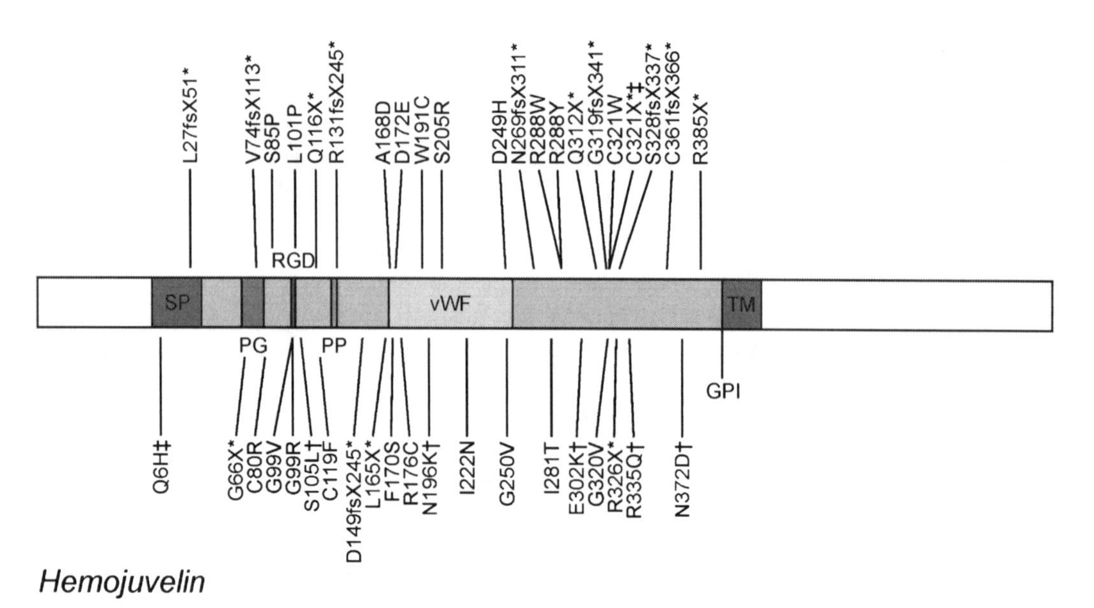

Fig. 20.1 Structure of *hemojuvelin (HJV)* mRNA and the encoded protein, showing positions of known mutations, structural domains and motifs. *SP* signal peptide, *PG* poly-glycine sequence, *RGD* RGD motif, *PP* poly-proline sequence, *vWF* partial von Willebrand type D domain, *GPI* glycophosphatidylinositol attachment point, *TM* transmembrane domain. Mutations causing juvenile hemochromatosis are depicted, including missense mutations and truncation or frameshift mutations (*). Mutations that have only been detected in the heterozygous state and may be modifiers of the HFE-hemochromatosis phenotype are indicated (†). The relevance of the Q6H mutation in causing JH is unclear as it occurred on the same allele as the C321X truncation mutation (‡) [18]

hepcidin [27, 28]. Subsequently, it has been shown that HJV is a bone morphogenetic protein (BMP) co-receptor that regulates hepcidin expression in the liver through a BMP-dependent signaling pathway [29]. BMPs are part of the transforming growth factor (TGF)-β superfamily of signaling molecules and signal to the nucleus through SMADs. Liver-specific disruption of the common mediator SMAD, Smad4, in the mouse leads to reduced hepcidin expression and iron overload [30], emphasizing the importance of the HJV-BMP-SMAD pathway in iron metabolism. HJV has also been shown to bind to neogenin, a receptor important in many cellular signaling processes [31]. Some JH mutations have been shown to disrupt the binding of HJV to either neogenin or BMP-2 [32]. Over 40 mutations in HJV have been reported to date [8–22]. How they all affect the function of HJV is not known; however, it is likely that they disrupt signaling pathways, resulting in the downregulation of hepatic hepcidin expression.

2.1.2 Hepcidin-Associated Hemochromatosis (Type 2B HH)

Although the majority of cases of JH are due to mutations in HJV, linkage to the chromosome 1q21 region was absent in two families with the typical JH phenotype. Typing of microsatellite markers on chromosome 19, in one consanguineous family, revealed homozygosity for a region around the *hepcidin* (*HAMP*) gene [33]. Sequencing of the gene revealed a single base pair deletion (93delG), causing a frameshift and potentially abnormally elongated protein [33]. A nonsense mutation (R56X) was identified in the homozygous state in the second family [33]. Mutations in hepcidin are much rarer than those in HJV, and to date, only nine have been reported (Fig. 20.2) [21, 33–41]. Two of these affect the conserved cysteine residues important in the disulfide-bonded structure of mature

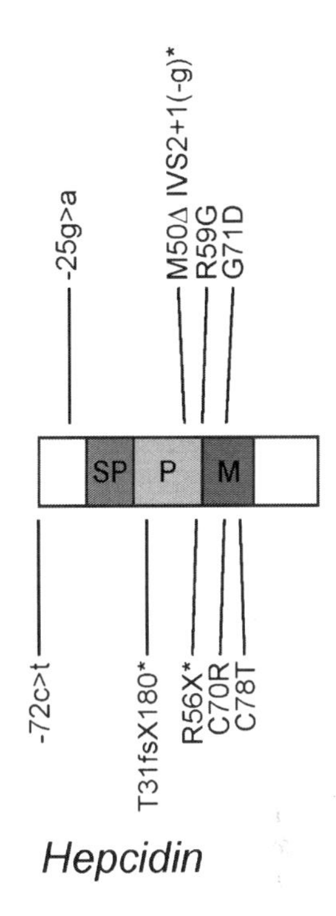

Fig. 20.2 Structure of *hepcidin (HAMP)* mRNA and the encoded protein, showing positions of known mutations and domains. *SP* signal peptide, *P* pro-region, *M* mature 25 amino acid peptide. Mutations causing juvenile hemochromatosis are depicted, including missense or single nucleotide substitution mutations and truncation or frameshift mutations (*)

hepcidin [37–39]. Some of the other mutations have been detected only in the heterozygous state and may contribute to iron loading in individuals with *HFE* mutations [34, 35]. Two studies suggested that mutations in HJV may also contribute to the severity of iron loading in patients with HFE-associated hemochromatosis [21, 22].

Hepcidin was originally identified as a liver-expressed antimicrobial peptide, also referred to as LEAP-1 [42, 43]. It is encoded as an 84 amino acid prepropeptide, possessing a signal peptide, a pro-region, and a 25 amino acid highly disulfide-bonded mature peptide. A link between hepcidin and iron metabolism was established when it was shown that iron-loaded mice had increased levels of hepatic hepcidin mRNA [44]. Transgenic mouse models have confirmed the importance of hepcidin in maintaining body iron homeostasis [45–47]. Hepcidin is expressed in hepatocytes in response to many stimuli, including iron overload and inflammation [48]. After cleavage by the prohormone convertase furin, mature hepcidin is secreted into the circulation, where it has its effect as a negative regulator of iron release from cells. Hepcidin acts by binding to the iron exporter ferroportin on the surface of cells, causing its internalization and degradation, thereby reducing iron efflux from cells [49]. The primary sites of hepcidin action include the macrophages, where iron is recycled from the breakdown of red blood cells; the duodenal mucosa, where iron is absorbed from the diet; and the liver, where iron is released from stores [50].

2.2 *TFR2-Associated Hemochromatosis (Type 3 HH)*

TFR2-associated hemochromatosis or type 3 HH was the first non-HFE form of hemochromatosis to be characterized at the molecular level [51]. Linkage analysis was used to map the locus in two Sicilian families, two members of which were originally classified as having juvenile hemochromatosis [51]. All affected members had homozygosity for markers in a region less than 1 cM in size on

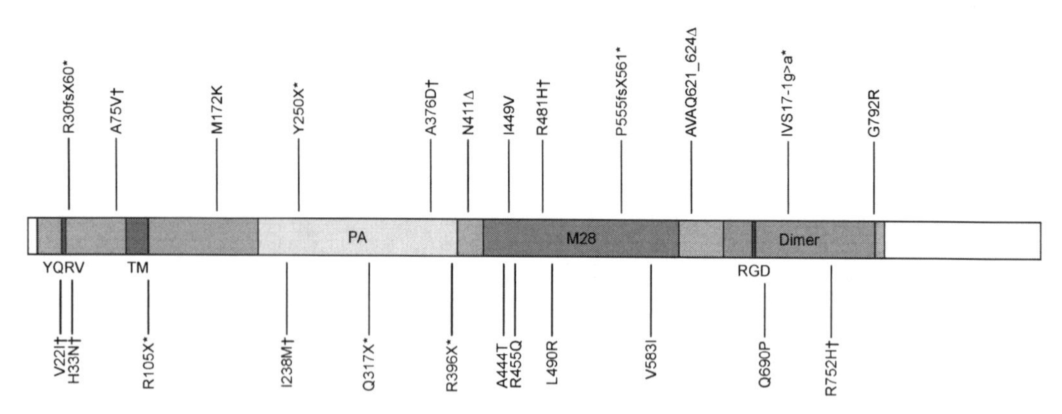

Fig. 20.3 Structure of *transferrin receptor 2 (TFR2)* mRNA and the encoded protein, showing positions of known mutations and structural domains and motifs. *YQRV* endocytosis motif, *TM* transmembrane domain, *PA* protease-associated domain, *M28* M28 peptidase domain, *Dimer* dimerization domain, *RGD* RGD motif. Mutations causing type 3 hemochromatosis are depicted, including missense mutations and truncation or frameshift mutations (*). Mutations that have only been detected in the heterozygous state and may be simple polymorphisms are indicated (†)

chromosome 7. The *TFR2* gene was located in the middle of this region, and sequence analysis revealed homozygosity for a nonsense mutation, Y250X. Several mutations in *TFR2* have now been reported in patients with non-HFE hemochromatosis from around the world. They are distributed across the entire length of the gene and are illustrated in Fig. 20.3 [36, 52–66]. TFR2-associated hemochromatosis was originally described as an adult-onset form of disease, but several reports have described patients with earlier onset and more severe disease than HFE-HH [54, 55, 63, 65]. The number of reported cases of TFR2-HH is small in comparison to HFE-HH, and hence, a direct comparison of their phenotypes is difficult. A single study compared the phenotypic features of HFE-HH, TFR2-HH, and JH. This study showed similar phenotypic features between HFE and TFR2-HH, although ascertainment bias and the small number of TFR2-HH patients studied may have affected the analysis [4]. One study reported juvenile onset hemochromatosis in two siblings who had homozygosity for a Q317X mutation in TFR2 and compound heterozygosity for the HFE mutations C282Y and H63D. Both had hypogonadotropic hypogonadism and cardiomyopathy, features typical of JH. This combination of mutations is very rare, but its occurrence can give us important insights into the functional relationship between HFE and TFR2. The JH-like phenotype in these two siblings suggests that the combination of mutations in both HFE and TFR2 are additive and result in more severe disease, akin to that caused by hemojuvelin or hepcidin.

TFR2 was originally identified as a homologue of the transferrin receptor (TFR1 or TFRC) [67]. TFR1 is an essential molecule required for the uptake of transferrin-bound iron into cells. TFR1 is ubiquitously expressed. In the erythroid bone marrow, it plays an important role in the uptake of transferrin-bound iron for the production of hemoglobin. The translation of TFR1 is controlled by cellular iron content, where the binding of iron-regulatory proteins (IRPs) to the iron-responsive element (IRE) stem-loops in the 3′-UTR of its mRNA regulates the stability of the transcript. TFR2 differs from TFR1 in its expression pattern, being expressed almost exclusively in the liver [68]. TFR2 transcripts contain no IREs and expression is not regulated by the IRE/IRP system in the same way as TFR1 [69]. TFR1 is important for development, and knockout of Tfr1 in mice results in embryonic lethality due to severe anemia. In contrast, targeted mutagenesis or knockout of Tfr2 in mice results in iron overload with phenotypic features similar to type 3 hemochromatosis in humans [70, 71]. These studies indicate that the roles of TFR1 and TFR2 in iron metabolism are quite separate. The function of TFR2, in common with other hemochromatosis genes, is thought to be in the regulation of hepatic hepcidin expression. Patients with type 3 hemochromatosis have low urinary hepcidin levels [72], and mouse models have low hepatic hepcidin expression in relation to iron stores [71, 73–75].

TFR2 is expressed on the surface of hepatocytes and may act as a sensor, monitoring the amount of circulating diferric transferrin or the iron-saturation of circulating transferrin. Treatment of hepatocyte cell lines with diferric transferrin results in stabilization of the TFR2 protein [76, 77]. Upregulation of Tfr2 protein has also been observed in animal models of dietary iron overload and HH due to knockout of Hfe [77]. Further experiments suggested that diferric transferrin increases the proportion of TFR2 targeted to the recycling endosomes and reduces the proportion targeted to the late endosomes and lysosomes for degradation [78]. A mutation, G679A, that abrogates transferrin binding to TFR2 prevents diferric transferrin-induced stabilization of TFR2, confirming that binding of TFR2 to its ligand is important for stabilization [78]. It has also been shown that the cytoplasmic domain of TFR2 is necessary for stabilization to take place [79]. Some of the mutations that cause TFR2-HH lead to loss of cell surface expression and retention of the mutant proteins in the endoplasmic reticulum [80]. The loss of cell surface expression most likely renders mutant TFR2 incapable of functioning as a sensor of diferric transferrin and unable to initiate signaling pathways resulting in the induction of hepcidin transcription.

The signaling pathway through which TFR2 regulates hepcidin has yet to be fully determined. One study has suggested that TFR2 is present in caveolin-rich lipid raft microdomains in the erythroleukemic cell line K562 and showed that activation of TFR2 by diferric transferrin can initiate signaling through p44/42-MAPK (ERK1/2) and p38-MAPK [81]. Whether these signal transduction pathways are responsible for the regulation of hepcidin by TFR2 in hepatocytes remains to be determined. The similar phenotypes of HFE-HH and TFR2-HH and the well-characterized interaction between HFE and TFR1 [82] have led to the suggestion that HFE and TFR2 may also interact in a signaling complex. Initial studies utilizing soluble forms of the proteins failed to detect any interaction between HFE and TFR2, suggesting that HFE functions by interacting with TFR1 only [83]. However, a more recent study identified an interaction between HFE and TFR2 in cells overexpressing both proteins. Another study showed that the HFE-TFR2 and HFE-TFR1 interactions are distinct, involving different protein domains and that HFE and transferrin do not compete for binding sites on TFR2 [84]. Further studies will be required to determine the functional relationship between HFE and TFR2 and the signaling pathways through which they regulate hepcidin.

3 Autosomal Dominant Hemochromatosis

There are two currently known genes involved in autosomal dominantly inherited hemochromatosis. These are the genes encoding the multiple transmembrane domain iron transporter ferroportin (*SLC40A1*) and the heavy subunit of the iron storage protein ferritin (*FTH1*). These autosomal dominant iron overload conditions differ in several aspects from the recessive forms of hemochromatosis that are caused primarily by defects in hepcidin itself or pathways regulating hepcidin expression.

3.1 Ferroportin Disease (Type 4 HH)

An autosomal dominant form of hemochromatosis was first described in a Melanesian pedigree from the Solomon Islands. Of the 81 tested members of the pedigree, 31 were found to have iron overload [85]. The iron overload syndrome was characterized by elevated transferrin saturation and serum ferritin, together with iron loading of hepatocytes and Kupffer cells, and fibrosis or cirrhosis

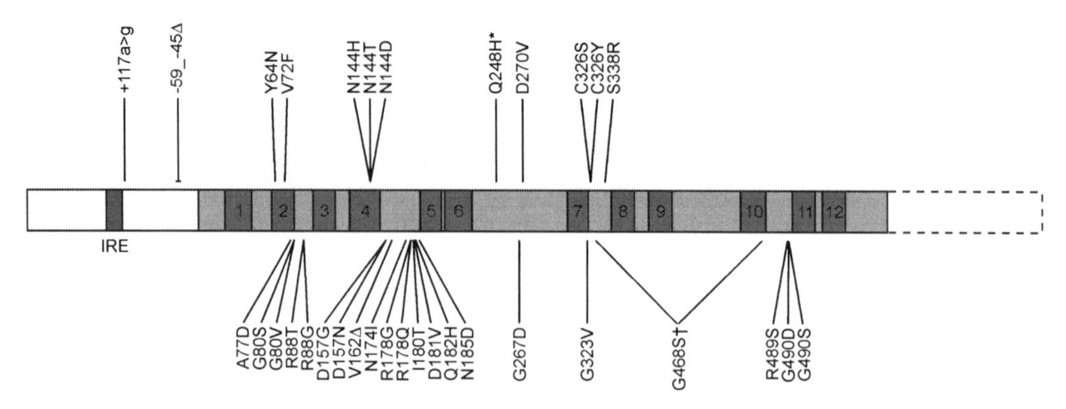

Fig. 20.4 Structure of *ferroportin (SLC40A1)* mRNA and the encoded protein, showing positions of known mutations and structural domains and motifs. *IRE* iron responsive element. Transmembrane domains are numbered and depicted in *blue*. The transmembrane organization shown is that proposed by Liu et al. with both termini of the protein oriented toward the cytoplasm [158]. Mutations causing autosomal dominant iron overload are depicted. Mutations listed below the diagram cause the typical phenotype of predominant reticuloendothelial iron loading most likely resulting from loss or reduction in iron transport ability of the protein. Mutations listed above the diagram cause the atypical phenotype of predominant hepatocyte iron loading, most likely resulting from hepcidin insensitivity of the protein. The role of the Q248H (*) variant is less clear. It is most likely a polymorphism prevalent in the African and African American populations, but has been associated with iron overload in some studies. The G468S mutation (†) results in aberrant splicing, causing truncation of ferroportin after glycine 330 and the addition of 4 irrelevant amino acids before termination

present in many of those tested [85]. This study was done before the identification of HFE; however, the iron overload syndrome was found to be unlinked to the *HFE* locus on chromosome 6 by HLA typing of affected and unaffected individuals. Whether this was the first description of ferroportin disease is unclear, as testing for *ferroportin* mutations has not been done in this pedigree. Another large pedigree with autosomal dominant hemochromatosis was described in Italy [86]. Fifteen of 53 members of the pedigree had raised serum iron indices and most had biopsy proven hepatic iron loading. The gene responsible was later found to encode the iron exporter ferroportin [87].

Mutations in ferroportin as the cause of an autosomal dominant form of hemochromatosis were established in 2001. Two groups independently identified *ferroportin* mutations in two large families with autosomal dominant non-HFE hemochromatosis [87, 88]. Genome-wide linkage analysis was performed in the two pedigrees from the Netherlands and Italy, and linkage to a region on chromosome 2 containing the *ferroportin* (*SLC40A1*, *IREG-1*, *MTP-1*, *SLC11A3*) gene was uncovered [87, 88]. Two missense mutations, A77D [87] and N144H [88], were reported associated with iron overload in the two families. To date, over 25 mutations have been reported in ferroportin (Fig. 20.4) in association with autosomal dominant iron overload [87–118]. Most have been detected only in single families, but there are some that occur in several distinct populations. The most common is the deletion of one of three valine residues (V162del), which has been reported in ferroportin disease patients from Australia [90], the UK [91, 116], Italy [92], Greece [93, 115], Austria [95], and Sri Lanka [94]. It is believed that this mutation may have occurred in multiple populations due to slippage mispairing in a repeat sequence. Another mutation that has been reported in more than one region is A77D, with cases being reported from Italy [87], Australia [89], and the UK [116]. Another mutation, N144T, was detected in a ferroportin disease patient from the Solomon Islands [96]. It is likely that this mutation may be the cause of the autosomal dominant iron overload syndrome described by Eason et al. in the Solomon Islands [85]; however, no relationship between the two families has been established [96].

With the analysis of more and more families with ferroportin disease, it has become apparent that the phenotypic features of ferroportin disease can be variable. Some cases present with features typical of classical HFE hemochromatosis, whereas others have a nonclassical phenotype. The majority of patients present with the nonclassical phenotype which is characterized by an early rise in serum ferritin, with transferrin saturation being normal or even low in the early stages of disease. Iron accumulation early in the disease almost exclusively occurs in the reticuloendothelial (RE) system. As the disease progresses, iron is deposited in the hepatocytes and this is normally accompanied by a rise in the transferrin saturation. Anemia can often be a problem in the early stages of the disease when serum iron levels are low and patients may not tolerate venesection therapy. Later in the disease, when serum iron levels are higher and the hepatocytes are iron loaded, venesection therapy is usually tolerated well. The classical HFE-like phenotype is usually characterized by an early rise in serum iron and transferrin saturation and iron deposition predominantly in the hepatocytes, with RE involvement later in the disease. Venesection therapy in these cases is usually tolerated well, with no associated anemia. Clinical features of ferroportin disease that have been reported include most of the conditions associated with other forms of hemochromatosis such as fatigue, arthritis, diabetes mellitus, impotence, arrhythmia, and hepatic fibrosis [86, 119]. Only two reported cases had fully established cirrhosis, and both of these were associated with the hepatocyte-iron phenotype [100, 109]. One report detected hepatocellular carcinoma in the absence of cirrhosis in a ferroportin disease patient. This was in an individual who carried the A77D mutation, with the RE-iron phenotype, and who had discontinued venesection treatment. Occult HBV infection may have contributed as a cofactor in this case [120].

It has been proposed that the nature of the mutation present may account for the variable phenotype. This has been backed up by cell-based studies on the functional consequences of ferroportin mutations. Some mutations affect the ability of ferroportin to transport iron, leading to a reduction in iron efflux; these include A77D, V162del, G490D, and G323V [121, 122]. These mutations are associated with the nonclassical RE-iron phenotype. Other mutant proteins retain the ability to transport iron; these include N144H, N144D, Y64N, and C326Y. However, further study has shown that these mutants are insensitive or partially insensitive to hepcidin-mediated downregulation [122, 123]. These mutations are associated with the hepatocyte-iron phenotype of ferroportin disease. Not all mutations fit neatly into this model. The Q182H and G80S mutations are associated with the RE-iron phenotype [99, 103], yet cell-based studies have shown that both mutants can effectively transport iron and internalize in response to hepcidin, although at a reduced rate [122, 124]. Further evidence for the existence of two ferroportin disease phenotypes has been supplied by MRI scanning of patients. Untreated patients carrying the A77D, V162del, and G80S mutations had iron accumulation in the liver, spleen, and spine, whereas patients carrying the N144H mutation had iron accumulation in the liver, but not in the spleen or spine [125]. This is consistent with the first group of mutations being associated with iron retention in the macrophages of the liver, spleen, and bone marrow, and N144H being associated with hepatocyte iron and relative sparing of macrophages.

It appears that the two subtypes of ferroportin disease result from either loss of function, as with the RE-iron phenotype, or gain of function, as with the hepatocyte-iron phenotype. With gain of function mutations, the ability of hepcidin to bind to ferroportin and initiate its internalization and degradation is impaired. These mutations could either directly affect the binding of hepcidin to ferroportin, as has been demonstrated for C326Y [126], or affect the mechanism responsible for internalization, as has been proposed for N144H and Q182H [127]. The net result would be a ferroportin molecule present at the cell surface and transporting iron, even in the face of iron overload and high levels of hepcidin, i.e., permanently switched on. This is a similar situation to the other forms of recessively inherited hemochromatosis that result from inappropriately low hepcidin levels and accounts for the similarity in phenotype. The loss of function mutations lead to a ferroportin molecule with an inability to transport iron. Whether the iron loading of RE cells results from haploinsufficiency for ferroportin or a dominant negative effect of mutant ferroportin on the wild-type protein

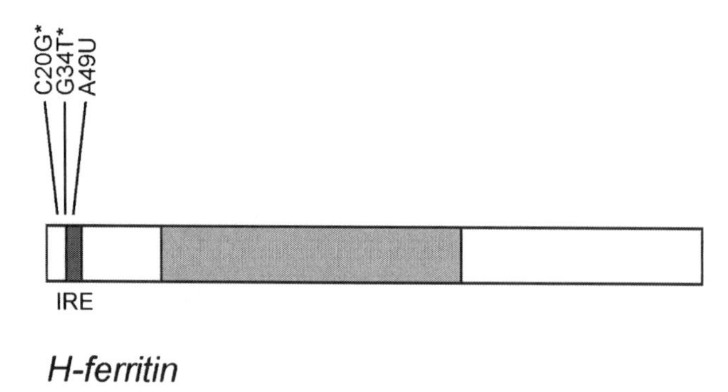

Fig. 20.5 Structure of *ferritin heavy chain (FTH1)* mRNA and the encoded protein, showing positions of known mutations and structural domains and motifs. *IRE* iron responsive element. Only one mutation causing iron overload (A49U) has been identified, affecting the function of the iron responsive element. Two mutations (*) were detected in individuals with mildly elevated ferritin, but their role in regulating ferritin and iron levels is unclear

has been debated. The dominant negative model would require functional ferroportin to exist as a dimer or multimer. Several studies have addressed this question and come up with different conclusions. Three studies have concluded that ferroportin exists as a monomer [128–130]; others have shown evidence for multimers [122, 131] and a dominant negative effect of mutant proteins on wild-type protein [132]. Many of the studies on the consequences on ferroportin mutations and the existence of multimers have had conflicting results. This may be due to the in vitro nature of the experiments, as all studies have utilized proteins overexpressed in various cell lines. Good evidence for the multimeric nature of ferroportin and the dominant negative effect of ferroportin mutations came with the characterization of a mouse model of ferroportin disease, the flatiron (*ffe*) mouse. Mice heterozygous for a H32R mutation in ferroportin (*ffe*/+) develop Kupffer cell iron loading, high serum ferritin, and low transferrin saturation, a phenotype similar to the RE-iron phenotype of ferroportin disease [133]. In contrast, mice that are heterozygous for a ferroportin-null allele have no iron loading phenotype [134]; this argues against the haploinsufficiency model. Ferroportin expression in macrophages isolated from *ffe*/+ mice was mainly intracellular, whereas wild-type macrophages had cell surface expression, a situation favoring a dominant negative effect for ferroportin mutants [133].

3.2 H-Ferritin-Associated Iron Overload

Another form of autosomal dominant iron overload is caused by a mutation in the IRE of *H-ferritin* mRNA. To date, only one family has been described with this type of iron overload [135]. The mutation, A49U, was detected in four members of a Japanese family with an autosomal dominant iron overload syndrome. The proband had a high serum ferritin level and mildly elevated transferrin saturation. Liver biopsy showed hepatocyte and Kupffer cell iron loading, and an explanted spleen showed iron loading of macrophages [135]. This pattern of iron loading is similar to that seen in the RE-iron phenotype of ferroportin disease. Functional analysis of the mutated *H-ferritin* IRE and analysis of patient liver samples suggested that the A49U mutation results in enhanced binding of IRPs to the IRE, a resultant reduction in H-ferritin translation and a concomitant increase in L-ferritin levels [135]. Another study detected two mutations in the 5'UTR of H-ferritin in a series of patients with increased iron indices. The two mutations, C20G and G34T, were detected in two individuals with only mildly elevated serum ferritin. The C20G mutation is outside the IRE sequence while G34T is located in the stem of the IRE structure (Fig. 20.5). The analysis of ferritin levels in the red blood cells of the individuals carrying the mutations revealed that neither mutation significantly affected ferritin expression or the ratio of H- to L-ferritin.

Mutations in the regulatory sequences of *H-ferritin* remain a rare cause of iron overload. In contrast, many more mutations in the IRE and regulatory sequences of *L-ferritin* have been detected. These give rise to hereditary hyperferritinemia cataract syndrome (HHCS), a condition characterized by elevated serum ferritin and bilateral cataracts, but no iron overload. The phenotypic differences between H-ferritin-associated iron overload and HHCS highlight the different roles the two ferritin subunits play in iron homeostasis.

4 African Iron Overload

Iron overload in sub-Saharan Africans has been recognized for many years [136]. Between 1925 and 1928, Strachan performed a necropsy study of 876 individuals from across southern and central Africa who had died in Johannesburg. In Strachan's MD thesis entitled "Haemosiderosis and Haemochromatosis in South African Natives with a Comment on the Etiology of Haemochromatosis," he concluded that hemochromatosis was not uncommon among native South Africans [137]. This iron overload syndrome has been referred to as African iron overload (AIO), Bantu siderosis, or dietary iron overload. The prevalence of AIO in some populations is very high and has been estimated to be up to 20% in some studies [138]. In subjects with AIO, iron is deposited in hepatocytes and Kupffer cells in the liver, as well as the spleen. The degree of iron loading is comparable to that seen in HFE-HH. Clinical consequences of the excess iron can include liver fibrosis, cirrhosis, and diabetes mellitus. Other conditions that are thought to be associated with AIO are osteoporosis, ascorbic acid deficiency (scurvy), esophageal cancer, hepatocellular carcinoma, and tuberculosis [139–141]. Originally, the iron loading was attributed to a purely dietary source. The custom of drinking a traditional beer brewed in non-galvanized steel drums or iron pots was thought to lead to dietary iron excess and consequent iron loading [142]. The iron content of the traditional beer is in the range of 50 mg/kg iron, in comparison to commercial beer which contains only 0.2 mg/kg [143]. In addition, a substantial proportion of the iron present in traditional beer is in the reduced ferrous state, making it more bioavailable and readily absorbed from the diet [138]. However, the link between iron overload and beer consumption is not perfect. Some beer drinkers do not develop iron loading and other non-beer drinkers do. Studies in pedigrees with iron overload have suggested there is a genetic component to the disease and an unidentified gene may confer susceptibility to iron loading. It was postulated that subjects homozygous for the genetic susceptibility gene could develop iron loading with normal iron intake, whereas heterozygotes could develop iron loading only when dietary iron intake was high [144]. With the availability of commercial beer, the consumption of traditionally brewed beer in southern Africa has declined considerably and is restricted mostly to rural populations. Some studies have found a higher prevalence of AIO in rural areas of southern Africa and a decline in incidence in urban areas, suggesting that traditional beer consumption is contributing to iron loading [145]. However, other studies have still found a high incidence in urban areas [146]. A study of tissue iron concentrations among victims of accidental or traumatic death in an urban hospital in Zimbabwe found high levels of iron loading, suggesting that the iron overload syndrome was present in a population where dietary iron intake was low, favoring the presence of a genetic susceptibility gene [146]. The putative African iron overload gene was shown to be unlinked to *HFE*, the gene responsible for iron overload in the majority of Europeans [147].

In the 1990s, it became apparent that iron overload could also occur in Americans of African descent. Two studies reported cases of primary iron overload in African Americans with phenotypic features similar to AIO [148, 149]. Analysis of HFE mutations in African-American hemochromatosis patients indicated that the genetic basis of iron overload in these individuals was different to most Caucasian cases and unrelated to the C282Y mutation [150]. Barton et al. sequenced several iron metabolism genes in 23 African-American patients with iron overload and concluded that iron overload in African Americans was not the result of mutations in a single gene [104].

Similarities in phenotype between AIO and ferroportin disease, namely macrophage iron loading in the liver and other organs, have led to the analysis of ferroportin mutations as the cause of iron overload in Africans and African Americans. The Q248H ferroportin variant has a high prevalence among Africans and African Americans, and several studies have evaluated this variant as a cause of iron overload in these populations. Gordeuk et al. identified Q248H in four of 19 African or African-American iron overload patients, a similar frequency to that observed in African community controls [105]. Analysis of first degree relatives and community controls led to the conclusion that Q248H may be associated with mild anemia and a tendency to iron loading. Another study looked at the Q248H variant in 19 families with AIO but failed to show an association with the condition [107]. However, this study did show an association between Q248H and an increase in serum ferritin levels when other factors influencing iron status were corrected for. They also found a strong association between Q248H carriers and reduced mean cell volume (MCV), suggesting that the variant may interfere with iron supply [107]. The role of Q248H was also assessed in African Americans enrolled in the Hemochromatosis and Iron Overload Screening Study (HEIRS). The variant was prevalent among both cases with elevated serum ferritin and controls and was associated with higher serum ferritin in males but not females [151]. These studies suggest that, although the Q248H variant of ferroportin can be associated with increased iron stores, it probably only accounts for a minority of African and African-American iron overload cases. Therefore, it is likely that other, as yet unidentified, genetic causes for iron overload exist in these populations.

5 Other Causes of Hereditary Iron Overload

Other hereditary disorders that result in iron overload include aceruloplasminemia [152] and atransferrinemia [153]. These are both rare genetic disorders resulting from a lack of circulating ceruloplasmin (Cp) or transferrin (Tf), respectively, and will not be discussed here. The cause of iron overload in some patients cannot be explained by either mutations in the *HFE* gene or the non-*HFE*-HH genes discussed in this chapter. For some, there may be other acquired conditions or environmental factors influencing iron homeostasis and resulting in iron overload. For others, there is clear evidence of familial iron overload, with more than one affected member in the same family [154]. This would suggest that other genes implicated in iron homeostasis are responsible for these non-*HFE*-related forms of HH, but these have yet to be identified. Mouse studies have revealed some novel candidate genes that may be responsible for some of the uncharacterized non-*HFE* iron overload syndromes in humans. For example, knockout of components involved in hepcidin regulation in the liver lead to iron overload. *Bmp6* knockout mice develop massive iron loading similar to that seen in JH [155, 156]. BMP6 is known to interact with HJV and is involved in hepcidin regulation through the BMP/SMAD signaling pathway [155–157]. It is possible that mutations in other genes involved in hepcidin regulation and iron homeostasis will be implicated in new forms of hereditary iron overload.

References

1. Feder JN, Gnirke A, Thomas W, et al. A novel MHC class I-like gene is mutated in patients with hereditary haemochromatosis. Nat Genet. 1996;13:399–408.
2. Lamon JM, Marynick SP, Roseblatt R, Donnelly S. Idiopathic hemochromatosis in a young female. A case study and review of the syndrome in young people. Gastroenterology. 1979;76:178–83.

3. Camaschella C. Juvenile haemochromatosis. Baillieres Clin Gastroenterol. 1998;12:227–35.
4. De Gobbi M, Roetto A, Piperno A, et al. Natural history of juvenile haemochromatosis. Br J Haematol. 2002;117:973–9.
5. Caines AE, Kpodonu J, Massad MG, et al. Cardiac transplantation in patients with iron overload cardiomyopathy. J Heart Lung Transplant. 2005;24:486–8.
6. Camaschella C, Roetto A, Cicilano M, et al. Juvenile and adult hemochromatosis are distinct genetic disorders. Eur J Hum Genet. 1997;5:371–5.
7. Roetto A, Totaro A, Cazzola M, et al. Juvenile hemochromatosis locus maps to chromosome 1q. Am J Hum Genet. 1999;64:1388–93.
8. Papanikolaou G, Samuels ME, Ludwig EH, et al. Mutations in HFE2 cause iron overload in chromosome 1q-linked juvenile hemochromatosis. Nat Genet. 2004;36:77–82.
9. Lanzara C, Roetto A, Daraio F, et al. Spectrum of hemojuvelin gene mutations in 1q-linked juvenile hemochromatosis. Blood. 2004;103:4317–21.
10. Lee P, Promrat K, Mallette C, Flynn M, Beutler E. A juvenile hemochromatosis patient homozygous for a novel deletion of cDNA nucleotide 81 of hemojuvelin. Acta Haematol. 2006;115:123–7.
11. Janosi A, Andrikovics H, Vas K, et al. Homozygosity for a novel nonsense mutation (G66X) of the HJV gene causes severe juvenile hemochromatosis with fatal cardiomyopathy. Blood. 2005;105:432.
12. Lee PL, Beutler E, Rao SV, Barton JC. Genetic abnormalities and juvenile hemochromatosis: mutations of the HJV gene encoding hemojuvelin. Blood. 2004;103:4669–71.
13. Wallace DF, Dixon JL, Ramm GA, Anderson GJ, Powell LW, Subramaniam N. Hemojuvelin (HJV)-associated hemochromatosis: analysis of HJV and HFE mutations and iron overload in three families. Haematologica. 2005;90:254–5.
14. Daraio F, Ryan E, Gleeson F, Roetto A, Crowe J, Camaschella C. Juvenile hemochromatosis due to G320V/Q116X compound heterozygosity of hemojuvelin in an Irish patient. Blood Cells Mol Dis. 2005;35:174–6.
15. Gehrke SG, Pietrangelo A, Kascak M, et al. HJV gene mutations in European patients with juvenile hemochromatosis. Clin Genet. 2005;67:425–8.
16. Aguilar-Martinez P, Lok CY, Cunat S, Cadet E, Robson K, Rochette J. Juvenile hemochromatosis caused by a novel combination of hemojuvelin G320V/R176C mutations in a 5-year old girl. Haematologica. 2007;92:421–2.
17. Koyama C, Hayashi H, Wakusawa S, et al. Three patients with middle-age-onset hemochromatosis caused by novel mutations in the hemojuvelin gene. J Hepatol. 2005;43:740–2.
18. Huang FW, Rubio-Aliaga I, Kushner JP, Andrews NC, Fleming MD. Identification of a novel mutation (C321X) in HJV. Blood. 2004;104:2176–7.
19. Filali M, Le Jeunne C, Durand E, et al. Juvenile hemochromatosis HJV-related revealed by cardiogenic shock. Blood Cells Mol Dis. 2004;33:120–4.
20. Lee PL, Barton JC, Brandhagen D, Beutler E. Hemojuvelin (HJV) mutations in persons of European, African-American and Asian ancestry with adult onset haemochromatosis. Br J Haematol. 2004;127:224–9.
21. Biasiotto G, Roetto A, Daraio F, et al. Identification of new mutations of hepcidin and hemojuvelin in patients with HFE C282Y allele. Blood Cells Mol Dis. 2004;33:338–43.
22. Le Gac G, Scotet V, Ka C, et al. The recently identified type 2A juvenile haemochromatosis gene (HJV), a second candidate modifier of the C282Y homozygous phenotype. Hum Mol Genet. 2004;13:1913–8.
23. Wallace DF, Subramaniam VN. Non-HFE haemochromatosis. World J Gastroenterol. 2007;13:4690–8.
24. Niederkofler V, Salie R, Sigrist M, Arber S. Repulsive guidance molecule (RGM) gene function is required for neural tube closure but not retinal topography in the mouse visual system. J Neurosci. 2004;24:808–18.
25. Samad TA, Srinivasan A, Karchewski LA, et al. DRAGON: a member of the repulsive guidance molecule-related family of neuronal- and muscle-expressed membrane proteins is regulated by DRG11 and has neuronal adhesive properties. J Neurosci. 2004;24:2027–36.
26. Lin L, Goldberg YP, Ganz T. Competitive regulation of hepcidin mRNA by soluble and cell-associated hemojuvelin. Blood. 2005;106:2884–9.
27. Huang FW, Pinkus JL, Pinkus GS, Fleming MD, Andrews NC. A mouse model of juvenile hemochromatosis. J Clin Invest. 2005;115:2187–91.
28. Niederkofler V, Salie R, Arber S. Hemojuvelin is essential for dietary iron sensing, and its mutation leads to severe iron overload. J Clin Invest. 2005;115:2180–6.
29. Babitt JL, Huang FW, Wrighting DM, et al. Bone morphogenetic protein signaling by hemojuvelin regulates hepcidin expression. Nat Genet. 2006;38:531–9.
30. Wang RH, Li C, Xu X, et al. A role of SMAD4 in iron metabolism through the positive regulation of hepcidin expression. Cell Metab. 2005;2:399–409.
31. Zhang AS, West Jr AP, Wyman AE, Bjorkman PJ, Enns CA. Interaction of hemojuvelin with neogenin results in iron accumulation in human embryonic kidney 293 cells. J Biol Chem. 2005;280:33885–94.
32. Kuns-Hashimoto R, Kuninger D, Nili M, Rotwein P. Selective binding of RGMc/hemojuvelin, a key protein in systemic iron metabolism, to BMP-2 and neogenin. Am J Physiol Cell Physiol. 2008;294:C994–1003.

33. Roetto A, Papanikolaou G, Politou M, et al. Mutant antimicrobial peptide hepcidin is associated with severe juvenile hemochromatosis. Nat Genet. 2003;33:21–2.
34. Jacolot S, Le Gac G, Scotet V, Quere I, Mura C, Ferec C. HAMP as a modifier gene that increases the phenotypic expression of the HFE pC282Y homozygous genotype. Blood. 2004;103:2835–40.
35. Merryweather-Clarke AT, Cadet E, Bomford A, et al. Digenic inheritance of mutations in HAMP and HFE results in different types of haemochromatosis. Hum Mol Genet. 2003;12:2241–7.
36. Biasiotto G, Belloli S, Ruggeri G, et al. Identification of new mutations of the HFE, hepcidin, and transferrin receptor 2 genes by denaturing HPLC analysis of individuals with biochemical indications of iron overload. Clin Chem. 2003;49:1981–8.
37. Delatycki MB, Allen KJ, Gow P, et al. A homozygous HAMP mutation in a multiply consanguineous family with pseudo-dominant juvenile hemochromatosis. Clin Genet. 2004;65:378–83.
38. Majore S, Binni F, Pennese A, De Santis A, Crisi A, Grammatico P. HAMP gene mutation c.208T>C (p.C70R) identified in an Italian patient with severe hereditary hemochromatosis. Hum Mutat. 2004;23:400.
39. Roetto A, Daraio F, Porporato P, et al. Screening hepcidin for mutations in juvenile hemochromatosis: identification of a new mutation (C70R). Blood. 2004;103:2407–9.
40. Matthes T, Aguilar-Martinez P, Pizzi-Bosman L, et al. Severe hemochromatosis in a Portuguese family associated with a new mutation in the 5′-UTR of the HAMP gene. Blood. 2004;104:2181–3.
41. Porto G, Roetto A, Daraio F, et al. A Portuguese patient homozygous for the −25G>A mutation of the HAMP promoter shows evidence of steady-state transcription but fails to up-regulate hepcidin levels by iron. Blood. 2005;106:2922–3.
42. Krause A, Neitz S, Magert HJ, et al. LEAP-1, a novel highly disulfide-bonded human peptide, exhibits antimicrobial activity. FEBS Lett. 2000;480:147–50.
43. Park CH, Valore EV, Waring AJ, Ganz T. Hepcidin, a urinary antimicrobial peptide synthesized in the liver. J Biol Chem. 2001;276:7806–10.
44. Pigeon C, Ilyin G, Courselaud B, et al. A new mouse liver-specific gene, encoding a protein homologous to human antimicrobial peptide hepcidin, is overexpressed during iron overload. J Biol Chem. 2001;276:7811–9.
45. Nicolas G, Bennoun M, Devaux I, et al. Lack of hepcidin gene expression and severe tissue iron overload in upstream stimulatory factor 2 (USF2) knockout mice. Proc Natl Acad Sci USA. 2001;98:8780–5.
46. Nicolas G, Bennoun M, Porteu A, et al. Severe iron deficiency anemia in transgenic mice expressing liver hepcidin. Proc Natl Acad Sci USA. 2002;99:4596–601.
47. Lesbordes-Brion JC, Viatte L, Bennoun M, et al. Targeted disruption of the hepcidin 1 gene results in severe hemochromatosis. Blood. 2006;108:1402–5.
48. Nicolas G, Chauvet C, Viatte L, et al. The gene encoding the iron regulatory peptide hepcidin is regulated by anemia, hypoxia, and inflammation. J Clin Invest. 2002;110:1037–44.
49. Nemeth E, Tuttle MS, Powelson J, et al. Hepcidin regulates cellular iron efflux by binding to ferroportin and inducing its internalization. Science. 2004;306:2090–3.
50. Rivera S, Nemeth E, Gabayan V, Lopez MA, Farshidi D, Ganz T. Synthetic hepcidin causes rapid dose-dependent hypoferremia and is concentrated in ferroportin-containing organs. Blood. 2005;106:2196–9.
51. Camaschella C, Roetto A, Cali A, et al. The gene TFR2 is mutated in a new type of haemochromatosis mapping to 7q22. Nat Genet. 2000;25:14–5.
52. Roetto A, Totaro A, Piperno A, et al. New mutations inactivating transferrin receptor 2 in hemochromatosis type 3. Blood. 2001;97:2555–60.
53. Mattman A, Huntsman D, Lockitch G, et al. Transferrin receptor 2 (TfR2) and HFE mutational analysis in non-C282Y iron overload: identification of a novel TfR2 mutation. Blood. 2002;100:1075–7.
54. Piperno A, Roetto A, Mariani R, et al. Homozygosity for transferrin receptor-2 Y250X mutation induces early iron overload. Haematologica. 2004;89:359–60.
55. Majore S, Milano F, Binni F, et al. Homozygous p.M172K mutation of the TFR2 gene in an Italian family with type 3 hereditary hemochromatosis and early onset iron overload. Haematologica. 2006;91(8 Suppl):ECR33.
56. Riva A, Mariani R, Bovo G, et al. Type 3 hemochromatosis and beta-thalassemia trait. Eur J Haematol. 2004;72:370–4.
57. Girelli D, Bozzini C, Roetto A, et al. Clinical and pathologic findings in hemochromatosis type 3 due to a novel mutation in transferrin receptor 2 gene. Gastroenterology. 2002;122:1295–302.
58. Hattori A, Wakusawa S, Hayashi H, et al. AVAQ 594–597 deletion of the TfR2 gene in a Japanese family with hemochromatosis. Hepatol Res. 2003;26:154–6.
59. Barton JC, Lee PL, West C, Bottomley SS. Iron overload and prolonged ingestion of iron supplements: clinical features and mutation analysis of hemochromatosis-associated genes in four cases. Am J Hematol. 2006;81:760–7.
60. Barton JC, Lee PL. Disparate phenotypic expression of ALAS2 R452H (nt 1407G A) in two brothers, one with severe sideroblastic anemia and iron overload, hepatic cirrhosis, and hepatocellular carcinoma. Blood Cells Mol Dis. 2006;36:342–6.

61. Lee PL, Barton JC. Hemochromatosis and severe iron overload associated with compound heterozygosity for TFR2 R455Q and two novel mutations TFR2 R396X and G792R. Acta Haematol. 2006;115:102–5.
62. Koyama C, Wakusawa S, Hayashi H, et al. Two novel mutations, L490R and V561X, of the transferrin receptor 2 gene in Japanese patients with hemochromatosis. Haematologica. 2005;90:302–7.
63. Le Gac G, Mons F, Jacolot S, Scotet V, Ferec C, Frebourg T. Early onset hereditary hemochromatosis resulting from a novel TFR2 gene nonsense mutation (R105X) in two siblings of north French descent. Br J Haematol. 2004;125:674–8.
64. Pietrangelo A, Caleffi A, Henrion J, et al. Juvenile hemochromatosis associated with pathogenic mutations of adult hemochromatosis genes. Gastroenterology. 2005;128:470–9.
65. Biasiotto G, Camaschella C, Forni GL, Polotti A, Zecchina G, Arosio P. New TFR2 mutations in young Italian patients with hemochromatosis. Haematologica. 2008;93:309–10.
66. Hsiao PJ, Tsai KB, Shin SJ, et al. A novel mutation of transferrin receptor 2 in a Taiwanese woman with type 3 hemochromatosis. J Hepatol. 2007;47:303–6.
67. Kawabata H, Yang R, Hirama T, et al. Molecular cloning of transferrin receptor 2. A new member of the transferrin receptor-like family. J Biol Chem. 1999;274:20826–32.
68. Kawabata H, Germain RS, Ikezoe T, et al. Regulation of expression of murine transferrin receptor 2. Blood. 2001;98:1949–54.
69. Fleming RE, Migas MC, Holden CC, et al. Transferrin receptor 2: continued expression in mouse liver in the face of iron overload and in hereditary hemochromatosis. Proc Natl Acad Sci USA. 2000;97:2214–9.
70. Fleming RE, Ahmann JR, Migas MC, et al. Targeted mutagenesis of the murine transferrin receptor-2 gene produces hemochromatosis. Proc Natl Acad Sci USA. 2002;99:10653–8.
71. Wallace DF, Summerville L, Lusby PE, Subramaniam VN. First phenotypic description of transferrin receptor 2 knockout mouse, and the role of hepcidin. Gut. 2005;54:980–6.
72. Nemeth E, Roetto A, Garozzo G, Ganz T, Camaschella C. Hepcidin is decreased in TFR2 hemochromatosis. Blood. 2005;105:1803–6.
73. Kawabata H, Fleming RE, Gui D, et al. Expression of hepcidin is down-regulated in TfR2 mutant mice manifesting a phenotype of hereditary hemochromatosis. Blood. 2005;105:376–81.
74. Wallace DF, Summerville L, Subramaniam VN. Targeted disruption of the hepatic transferrin receptor 2 gene in mice leads to iron overload. Gastroenterology. 2007;132:301–10.
75. Drake SF, Morgan EH, Herbison CE, et al. Iron absorption and hepatic iron uptake are increased in a transferrin receptor 2 (Y245X) mutant mouse model of hemochromatosis type 3. Am J Physiol Gastrointest Liver Physiol. 2007;292:G323–8.
76. Johnson MB, Enns CA. Diferric transferrin regulates transferrin receptor 2 protein stability. Blood. 2004;104:4287–93.
77. Robb A, Wessling-Resnick M. Regulation of transferrin receptor 2 protein levels by transferrin. Blood. 2004;104:4294–9.
78. Johnson MB, Chen J, Murchison N, Green FA, Enns CA. Transferrin receptor 2: evidence for ligand-induced stabilization and redirection to a recycling pathway. Mol Biol Cell. 2007;18:743–54.
79. Chen J, Enns CA. The cytoplasmic domain of transferrin receptor 2 dictates its stability and response to holo-transferrin in Hep3B cells. J Biol Chem. 2007;282:6201–9.
80. Wallace DF, Summerville L, Crampton EM, Subramaniam VN. Defective trafficking and localization of mutated transferrin receptor 2: implications for type 3 hereditary hemochromatosis. Am J Physiol Cell Physiol. 2008;294:C383–90.
81. Calzolari A, Raggi C, Deaglio S, et al. TfR2 localizes in lipid raft domains and is released in exosomes to activate signal transduction along the MAPK pathway. J Cell Sci. 2006;119:4486–98.
82. Parkkila S, Waheed A, Britton RS, et al. Association of the transferrin receptor in human placenta with HFE, the protein defective in hereditary hemochromatosis. Proc Natl Acad Sci USA. 1997;94:13198–202.
83. West Jr AP, Bennett MJ, Sellers VM, Andrews NC, Enns CA, Bjorkman PJ. Comparison of the interactions of transferrin receptor and transferrin receptor 2 with transferrin and the hereditary hemochromatosis protein HFE. J Biol Chem. 2000;275:38135–8.
84. Chen J, Chloupkova M, Gao J, Chapman-Arvedson TL, Enns CA. HFE modulates transferrin receptor 2 levels in hepatoma cells via interactions that differ from transferrin receptor 1-HFE interactions. J Biol Chem. 2007;282:36862–70.
85. Eason RJ, Adams PC, Aston CE, Searle J. Familial iron overload with possible autosomal dominant inheritance. Aust N Z J Med. 1990;20:226–30.
86. Pietrangelo A, Montosi G, Totaro A, et al. Hereditary hemochromatosis in adults without pathogenic mutations in the hemochromatosis gene. N Engl J Med. 1999;341:725–32.
87. Montosi G, Donovan A, Totaro A, et al. Autosomal-dominant hemochromatosis is associated with a mutation in the ferroportin (SLC11A3) gene. J Clin Invest. 2001;108:619–23.
88. Njajou OT, Vaessen N, Joosse M, et al. A mutation in SLC11A3 is associated with autosomal dominant hemochromatosis. Nat Genet. 2001;28:213–4.

89. Subramaniam VN, Wallace DF, Dixon JL, Fletcher LM, Crawford DH. Ferroportin disease due to the A77D mutation in Australia. Gut. 2005;54:1048–9.
90. Wallace DF, Pedersen P, Dixon JL, et al. Novel mutation in ferroportin1 is associated with autosomal dominant hemochromatosis. Blood. 2002;100:692–4.
91. Devalia V, Carter K, Walker AP, et al. Autosomal dominant reticuloendothelial iron overload associated with a 3-base pair deletion in the ferroportin 1 gene (SLC11A3). Blood. 2002;100:695–7.
92. Roetto A, Merryweather-Clarke AT, Daraio F, et al. A valine deletion of ferroportin 1: a common mutation in hemochromatosis type 4. Blood. 2002;100:733–4.
93. Cazzola M, Cremonesi L, Papaioannou M, et al. Genetic hyperferritinaemia and reticuloendothelial iron overload associated with a three base pair deletion in the coding region of the ferroportin gene (SLC11A3). Br J Haematol. 2002;119:539–46.
94. Wallace DF, Browett P, Wong P, Kua H, Ameratunga R, Subramaniam VN. Identification of ferroportin disease in the Indian subcontinent. Gut. 2005;54:567–8.
95. Zoller H, McFarlane I, Theurl I, et al. Primary iron overload with inappropriate hepcidin expression in V162del ferroportin disease. Hepatology. 2005;42:466–72.
96. Arden KE, Wallace DF, Dixon JL, et al. A novel mutation in ferroportin1 is associated with haemochromatosis in a Solomon Islands patient. Gut. 2003;52:1215–7.
97. Jouanolle AM, Douabin-Gicquel V, Halimi C, et al. Novel mutation in ferroportin 1 gene is associated with autosomal dominant iron overload. J Hepatol. 2003;39:286–9.
98. Rivard SR, Lanzara C, Grimard D, et al. Autosomal dominant reticuloendothelial iron overload (HFE type 4) due to a new missense mutation in the FERROPORTIN 1 gene (SLC11A3) in a large French-Canadian family. Haematologica. 2003;88:824–6.
99. Hetet G, Devaux I, Soufir N, Grandchamp B, Beaumont C. Molecular analyses of patients with hyperferritinemia and normal serum iron values reveal both L ferritin IRE and 3 new ferroportin (slc11A3) mutations. Blood. 2003;102:1904–10.
100. Wallace DF, Clark RM, Harley HA, Subramaniam VN. Autosomal dominant iron overload due to a novel mutation of ferroportin1 associated with parenchymal iron loading and cirrhosis. J Hepatol. 2004;40:710–3.
101. Robson KJ, Merryweather-Clarke AT, Cadet E, et al. Recent advances in understanding haemochromatosis: a transition state. J Med Genet. 2004;41:721–30.
102. Zaahl MG, Merryweather-Clarke AT, Kotze MJ, van der Merwe S, Warnich L, Robson KJ. Analysis of genes implicated in iron regulation in individuals presenting with primary iron overload. Hum Genet. 2004;115:409–17.
103. Corradini E, Montosi G, Ferrara F, et al. Lack of enterocyte iron accumulation in the ferroportin disease. Blood Cells Mol Dis. 2005;35:315–8.
104. Barton JC, Acton RT, Rivers CA, et al. Genotypic and phenotypic heterogeneity of African Americans with primary iron overload. Blood Cells Mol Dis. 2003;31:310–9.
105. Gordeuk VR, Caleffi A, Corradini E, et al. Iron overload in Africans and African-Americans and a common mutation in the SCL40A1 (ferroportin 1) gene. Blood Cells Mol Dis. 2003;31:299–304.
106. Beutler E, Barton JC, Felitti VJ, et al. Ferroportin 1 (SCL40A1) variant associated with iron overload in African-Americans. Blood Cells Mol Dis. 2003;31:305–9.
107. McNamara L, Gordeuk VR, MacPhail AP. Ferroportin (Q248H) mutations in African families with dietary iron overload. J Gastroenterol Hepatol. 2005;20:1855–8.
108. Kasvosve I, Gomo ZA, Nathoo KJ, et al. Effect of ferroportin Q248H polymorphism on iron status in African children. Am J Clin Nutr. 2005;82:1102–6.
109. Sham RL, Phatak PD, West C, Lee P, Andrews C, Beutler E. Autosomal dominant hereditary hemochromatosis associated with a novel ferroportin mutation and unique clinical features. Blood Cells Mol Dis. 2005;34:157–61.
110. Liu W, Shimomura S, Imanishi H, et al. Hemochromatosis with mutation of the ferroportin 1 (IREG1) gene. Intern Med. 2005;44:285–9.
111. Cremonesi L, Forni GL, Soriani N, et al. Genetic and clinical heterogeneity of ferroportin disease. Br J Haematol. 2005;131:663–70.
112. Koyama C, Wakusawa S, Hayashi H, et al. A Japanese family with ferroportin disease caused by a novel mutation of SLC40A1 gene: hyperferritinemia associated with a relatively low transferrin saturation of iron. Intern Med. 2005;44:990–3.
113. Bach V, Remacha A, Altes A, Barcelo MJ, Molina MA, Baiget M. Autosomal dominant hereditary hemochromatosis associated with two novel Ferroportin 1 mutations in Spain. Blood Cells Mol Dis. 2006;36:41–5.
114. Morris TJ, Litvinova MM, Ralston D, Mattman A, Holmes D, Lockitch G. A novel ferroportin mutation in a Canadian family with autosomal dominant hemochromatosis. Blood Cells Mol Dis. 2005;35:309–14.
115. Speletas M, Kioumi A, Loules G, et al. Analysis of SLC40A1 gene at the mRNA level reveals rapidly the causative mutations in patients with hereditary hemochromatosis type IV. Blood Cells Mol Dis. 2007;40:353–9.
116. Lim FL, Dooley JS, Roques AW, Grellier L, Dhillon AP, Walker AP. Hepatic iron concentration, fibrosis and response to venesection associated with the A77D and V162del "loss of function" mutations in ferroportin disease. Blood Cells Mol Dis. 2007;40:328–33.

117. Cunat S, Giansily-Blaizot M, Bismuth M, et al. Global sequencing approach for characterizing the molecular background of hereditary iron disorders. Clin Chem. 2007;53:2060–9.
118. Lee PL, Gelbart T, West C, Barton JC. SLC40A1 c.1402G→a results in aberrant splicing, ferroportin truncation after glycine 330, and an autosomal dominant hemochromatosis phenotype. Acta Haematol. 2007;118:237–41.
119. Njajou OT, de Jong G, Berghuis B, et al. Dominant hemochromatosis due to N144H mutation of SLC11A3: clinical and biological characteristics. Blood Cells Mol Dis. 2002;29:439–43.
120. Corradini E, Ferrara F, Pollicino T, et al. Disease progression and liver cancer in the ferroportin disease. Gut. 2007;56:1030–2.
121. Schimanski LM, Drakesmith H, Merryweather-Clarke AT, et al. In vitro functional analysis of human ferroportin (FPN) and hemochromatosis-associated FPN mutations. Blood. 2005;105:4096–102.
122. De Domenico I, Ward DM, Nemeth E, et al. The molecular basis of ferroportin-linked hemochromatosis. Proc Natl Acad Sci USA. 2005;102:8955–60.
123. Drakesmith H, Schimanski LM, Ormerod E, et al. Resistance to hepcidin is conferred by hemochromatosis-associated mutations of ferroportin. Blood. 2005;106:1092–7.
124. De Domenico I, McVey Ward D, Nemeth E, et al. Molecular and clinical correlates in iron overload associated with mutations in ferroportin. Haematologica. 2006;91:1092–5.
125. Pietrangelo A, Corradini E, Ferrara F, et al. Magnetic resonance imaging to identify classic and nonclassic forms of ferroportin disease. Blood Cells Mol Dis. 2006;37:192–6.
126. De Domenico I, Nemeth E, Nelson JM, et al. The hepcidin-binding site on ferroportin is evolutionarily conserved. Cell Metab. 2008;8:146–56.
127. De Domenico I, Ward DM, Langelier C, et al. The molecular mechanism of hepcidin-mediated ferroportin down-regulation. Mol Biol Cell. 2007;18:2569–78.
128. Pignatti E, Mascheroni L, Sabelli M, Barelli S, Biffo S, Pietrangelo A. Ferroportin is a monomer in vivo in mice. Blood Cells Mol Dis. 2006;36:26–32.
129. Schimanski LM, Drakesmith H, Talbott C, et al. Ferroportin: lack of evidence for multimers. Blood Cells Mol Dis. 2007;40:360–9.
130. Goncalves AS, Muzeau F, Blaybel R, et al. Wild-type and mutant ferroportins do not form oligomers in transfected cells. Biochem J. 2006;396:265–75.
131. De Domenico I, Ward DM, Musci G, Kaplan J. Evidence for the multimeric structure of ferroportin. Blood. 2007;109:2205–9.
132. McGregor JA, Shayeghi M, Vulpe CD, et al. Impaired iron transport activity of ferroportin 1 in hereditary iron overload. J Membr Biol. 2005;206:3–7.
133. Zohn IE, De Domenico I, Pollock A, et al. The flatiron mutation in mouse ferroportin acts as a dominant negative to cause ferroportin disease. Blood. 2007;109:4174–80.
134. Donovan A, Lima CA, Pinkus JL, et al. The iron exporter ferroportin/Slc40a1 is essential for iron homeostasis. Cell Metab. 2005;1:191–200.
135. Kato J, Fujikawa K, Kanda M, et al. A mutation, in the iron-responsive element of H ferritin mRNA, causing autosomal dominant iron overload. Am J Hum Genet. 2001;69:191–7.
136. Walker AR, Arvidsson UB. Iron intake and haemochromatosis in the Bantu. Nature. 1950;166:438–9.
137. Strachan AS. Haemosiderosis and haemochromatosis in South African natives with a comment on the etiology of haemochromatosis. Glasgow, UK: University of Glasgow; 1929.
138. Gordeuk VR, Boyd RD, Brittenham GM. Dietary iron overload persists in rural sub-Saharan Africa. Lancet. 1986;1:1310–3.
139. Seftel HC, Malkin C, Schmaman A, et al. Osteoporosis, scurvy, and siderosis in Johannesburg bantu. Br Med J. 1966;1:642–6.
140. Isaacson C, Bothwell TH, MacPhail AP, Simon M. The iron status of urban black subjects with carcinoma of the oesophagus. S Afr Med J. 1985;67:591–3.
141. Gordeuk VR, McLaren CE, MacPhail AP, Deichsel G, Bothwell TH. Associations of iron overload in Africa with hepatocellular carcinoma and tuberculosis: Strachan's 1929 thesis revisited. Blood. 1996;87:3470–6.
142. Bothwell TH, Seftel H, Jacobs P, Torrance JD, Baumslag N. Iron overload in bantu subjects; studies on the availability of iron in bantu beer. Am J Clin Nutr. 1964;14:47–51.
143. Matsha T, Brink L, van Rensburg S, Hon D, Lombard C, Erasmus R. Traditional home-brewed beer consumption and iron status in patients with esophageal cancer and healthy control subjects from Transkei, South Africa. Nutr Cancer. 2006;56:67–73.
144. Gordeuk V, Mukiibi J, Hasstedt SJ, et al. Iron overload in Africa. Interaction between a gene and dietary iron content. N Engl J Med. 1992;326:95–100.
145. MacPhail AP, Simon MO, Torrance JD, Charlton RW, Bothwell TH, Isaacson C. Changing patterns of dietary iron overload in black South Africans. Am J Clin Nutr. 1979;32:1272–8.
146. Gangaidzo IT, Moyo VM, Saungweme T, et al. Iron overload in urban Africans in the 1990s. Gut. 1999;45:278–83.
147. McNamara L, MacPhail AP, Gordeuk VR, Hasstedt SJ, Rouault T. Is there a link between African iron overload and the described mutations of the hereditary haemochromatosis gene? Br J Haematol. 1998;102:1176–8.

148. Barton JC, Edwards CQ, Bertoli LF, Shroyer TW, Hudson SL. Iron overload in African Americans. Am J Med. 1995;99:616–23.
149. Wurapa RK, Gordeuk VR, Brittenham GM, Khiyami A, Schechter GP, Edwards CQ. Primary iron overload in African Americans. Am J Med. 1996;101:9–18.
150. Monaghan KG, Rybicki BA, Shurafa M, Feldman GL. Mutation analysis of the HFE gene associated with hereditary hemochromatosis in African Americans. Am J Hematol. 1998;58:213–7.
151. Rivers CA, Barton JC, Gordeuk VR, et al. Association of ferroportin Q248H polymorphism with elevated levels of serum ferritin in African Americans in the hemochromatosis and iron overload screening (HEIRS) study. Blood Cells Mol Dis. 2007;38:247–52.
152. Harris ZL, Takahashi Y, Miyajima H, Serizawa M, MacGillivray RT, Gitlin JD. Aceruloplasminemia: molecular characterization of this disorder of iron metabolism. Proc Natl Acad Sci USA. 1995;92:2539–43.
153. Beutler E, Gelbart T, Lee P, Trevino R, Fernandez MA, Fairbanks VF. Molecular characterization of a case of atransferrinemia. Blood. 2000;96:4071–4.
154. Pelucchi S, Mariani R, Salvioni A, et al. Novel mutations of the ferroportin gene (SLC40A1): analysis of 56 consecutive patients with unexplained iron overload. Clin Genet. 2008;73:171–8.
155. Meynard D, Kautz L, Darnaud V, Canonne-Hergaux F, Coppin H, Roth MP. Lack of the bone morphogenetic protein BMP6 induces massive iron overload. Nat Genet. 2009;41:478–81.
156. Andriopoulos Jr B, Corradini E, Xia Y, et al. BMP6 is a key endogenous regulator of hepcidin expression and iron metabolism. Nat Genet. 2009;41:482–7.
157. Babitt JL, Huang FW, Xia Y, Sidis Y, Andrews NC, Lin HY. Modulation of bone morphogenetic protein signaling in vivo regulates systemic iron balance. J Clin Invest. 2007;117:1933–9.
158. Liu XB, Yang F, Haile DJ. Functional consequences of ferroportin 1 mutations. Blood Cells Mol Dis. 2005;35:33–46.

Chapter 21
Miscellaneous Iron-Related Disorders

Carole Beaumont

Keywords Cataract • Ceruloplasmin • Ferritin • Genetic diseases • Iron • Transferrin

1 The Hereditary Hyperferritinemia-Cataract Syndrome

The hereditary hyperferritinemia-cataract syndrome (HHCS, MIM #600886) is an autosomal dominant disease due to heterozygous mutations in exon 1 of the L-ferritin (*FTL*) gene present on chromosome 19q13.3–13.4. These mutations affect the iron-responsive element (IRE) of the L-ferritin mRNA and impair its interaction with the iron regulatory proteins (IRPs). It is a very mild disease with early onset cataract as the only known clinical symptom. Biologically, it is characterized by hyperferritinemia in the absence of iron overload. Serum iron and transferrin saturation are normal, and there is no evidence for tissue iron accumulation.

1.1 IRE Mutations and Deletions

HHCS was simultaneously discovered in France and in Italy in 1995. In the first two families, there was a perfect cosegregation of cataract and hyperferritinemia and these two symptoms were transmitted in the autosomal dominant mode [1, 2]. Point mutations were identified in the iron-responsive element of the L-ferritin gene. These mutations affected two different nucleotides of the IRE loop and consisted of an A40→G [3] and a G41→C [4] change in the heterozygous state (numbering from cDNA sequence in GenBank NM_000146). These and other mutations in the loop and stem of the IRE have subsequently been reported (summarized in Table 21.1 and on Fig. 21.1a), as well as partial deletion of the IRE structure (Fig. 21.1b). These mutations have been described in several European countries (France, Italy, Spain, and UK) as well as in Canada, USA, Australia and India (one large family). At least 85 families or isolated individuals with IRE mutations have been reported, and probably many more have been diagnosed. Altogether, 27 different point mutations affecting the IRE structure have been described [5], as well as four different partial deletions (Fig. 21.1b). All three possible replacements have been found at G32 and C39.

C. Beaumont, Ph.D. (✉)
INSERM U773, Centre de Recherche Biomédicale Bichat-Beaujon (CRB3),
Université Paris Diderot, Paris, France
e-mail: carole.beaumont@inserm.fr

G.J. Anderson and G. McLaren (eds.), *Iron Physiology and Pathophysiology in Humans*, Nutrition and Health, DOI 10.1007/978-1-60327-485-2_21,

Table 21.1 Summary of the point mutations identified in the L-ferritin IRE

Mutations	Country	Number of families or individuals	Ferritin range (μg/L)	Reference
C18+U22G	Italy	1	1,650	[105]
C29G	Italy	1	520–734	[106]
G32U	France	7	1,200–3,000	[12, 20]
	UK	2	1,150–1,600	[107, 108]
	Italy	1	700–1,400	[29]
	Canada	1		[109]
	Australia	1	1,550 (de novo mutation)	[13]
G32A	India	1 large family		[110]
	Netherlands	1		[111]
	Italy	2	350–1,100	[105, 112]
	France	2	1,400–1,500	[12]
G32C	UK	3	1,700–1,900	[107, 113]
	Netherlands	1		[114]
	Italy	2	1,200–1,400	[29, 115]
	France	1	1,200 (de novo mutation)	[12]
	Australia	1	2,400–2,900	[31]
C33U	Spain	4	940–1,700	[116–119]
	Italy	1	1,400	[29]
	UK	1	740	[107]
	France	3	1,400–1,500	[12]
	USA	1	1,300–1,400	[33]
C33A	France	1	1,000	[12]
U34C	France	1	1,000	[12]
C36A	UK	1	1,000	[120]
	France	1	1,600	[12]
C36G	Italy	1		[121]
A37U	Spain	1	600–1300	[122]
A37G	Italy	1		[121]
C39U	Italy	2	1,000–2,500	[29, 112]
	Italy	1	1,140 (de novo mutation)	[11]
	UK	1	1,400	[120]
	Belgium	1	820–1,100	[123]
	France	3	800–2,800	[12]
C39A	Australia	1	1400–1,800	[13]
C39G	Greece	3	900–1,500	[124]
	France	1		[125]
A40G	Spain	2	700–2,300	[126, 127]
	Italy	3	800–2,000	[29, 112]
	France	5	1,000–5,000	[12, 128]
	UK	2	1,420	[107, 129]
	Belgium	2	1,600–3,400	[123]
	Australia	1	3,200	[13]
	USA	1	1,100	[130]
G41C	Italy	2	950–2,200	[2, 29]
G43A	USA	1		[131]
G47A	France	1	2,140	[12]
G51C	Italy	1	600	[132]
	USA	1	1,200	[30]

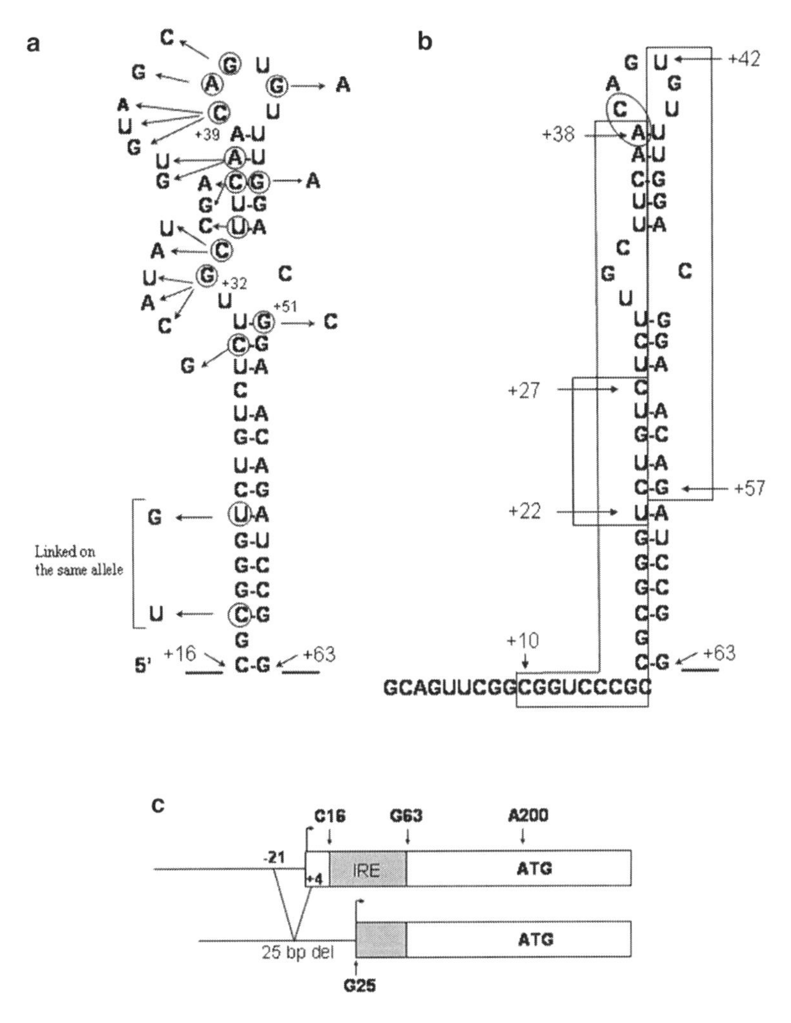

Fig. 21.1 Nucleotide sequence of the iron responsive element of the L-ferritin mRNA and position of the mutations and deletions reported in the literature. (**a**) Point mutations described on the *FTL* IRE (base changes indicated by *arrows*). (**b**) Partial deletions of the *FTL* IRE (*boxed* or *circled*); references for these differences IRE mutations/deletions can be found in Tables 21.1 and 21.2. (**c**) Schematic representation of the 25 base pair deletion encompassing the transcription start site described in [10]

In the loop, only C39, A40, and G41 have been found to be mutated, with the exception of one individual who carried a G43 mutation. This mutation abolishes a G–C base pairing with C39 which is thought to be important for RNA binding affinity [6, 7]. Interestingly, the CAGUG loop is completely conserved among all members of the IRE family [8]. Synthetic IREs with mutations at either one of these nucleotides have reduced binding affinity for the IRPs [6, 9]. However, no mutation has been reported at U42 of the loop.

The bulge in the middle of the stem also appears to be mutated frequently, with multiple mutations found at either G32 or C33. Nucleotides of the stem, between the loop and the bulge, have also been mutated (Fig. 21.1a and Table 21.1), and two mutations linked on the same allele have been found on the more distal part of the IRE structure. In addition, four deletions have been described (Fig. 21.1b and Table 21.2). One deletion removed the first half of the IRE (del C10–A38) and another the second half (del U42–G57). It is possible that the inverted repeats made by the two halves of the IRE stem might favor intrachromosomal rearrangements and subsequent deletions.

Table 21.2 Summary of the deletions identified in or upstream of the *FTL* exon 1

Deletion	Country	Number of families or individuals	Ferritin range (μg/L)	Reference
Del C10-A38	Italy	1	1,200–1,800	[133]
Del U22-C27	Italy	1	1,200–1,400	[134]
Del U42-G57	France	1	1,220	[12]
Del A38C39	Canada	1	1,845 (de novo mutation ?)	[12]
Del (−21)G3	Australia	1	880	[10]

Two internal deletions have been reported removing either six bases from U22 to C27 or deleting A38 and C39. Finally, a different 25-base pair deletion has been recently described from −21 to G3 [10], removing the proximal promoter and the transcription start site (Fig. 21.1c). Transcription was shown to start at G25 (numbering from the normal cDNA sequence), thereby removing the first part of the IRE structure. The large number of different mutations which have been identified in unrelated individuals, taken together with the observation made by some of us [11–13] that some of these mutations are de novo mutations [11, 12], suggests that the IRE structure of the L-ferritin gene is a hot spot for mutations.

1.2 HHCS, a "Translational Pathology"

Ferritin synthesis is regulated by iron at the translational level, through IRE–IRPs interactions. When iron fluxes into cells are limited, IRPs retain their native conformation and present a high RNA binding affinity for the IRE structure present in the 5′ non coding region of ferritin mRNA. IRPs binding to the ferritin IRE prevent the recruitment of the small ribosomal subunit to the ferritin mRNA and repress ferritin synthesis [14]. This mechanism had been foreshadowed by Hamish Munro in 1976 [15] and was extensively confirmed at the molecular levels several years later (for a review, see [16] and Chap. 3). Interestingly, the molecular defect in this negative translational control turned out to be the first example of a translational pathology [17].

HHCS is a dominant disease, and since half of the L-ferritin mRNA molecules bear a mutated IRE and are not subject to the normal IRP-mediated translational block, the production of L-ferritin subunits is disproportionately high (Fig. 21.2). Excess L-ferritin production has been confirmed in several tissues [3, 18], including lens and lymphoblastoid cell lines established from patients with IRE mutations.

Some in vitro studies have shown that the mutated IREs sequence have reduced binding affinity to the IRPs [19, 20]. Thermodynamic analyses have revealed that some mutations impair the stability or the secondary structures of the IRE whereas others affect the IRE–IRP interactions [19]. Identification of these natural IRE mutations and evidence that they lead to uncontrolled production of tissue ferritin have confirmed the results of prior in vitro studies that had highlighted the structural requirements of the IRE for binding to the IRPs [7, 21, 22].

1.3 Clinical Symptoms and Treatment

Hyperferritinemia and cataract are the hallmarks of HHCS. This is a very mild disease, and cataract is the only clinical symptom described so far. The hyperferritinemia reflects the increased ferritin synthesis and is clearly not indicative of iron overload. There seems to be full penetrance of the hyperferritinemia, and the age of onset and the severity of the cataract are highly variable. Lens opacification may even be absent.

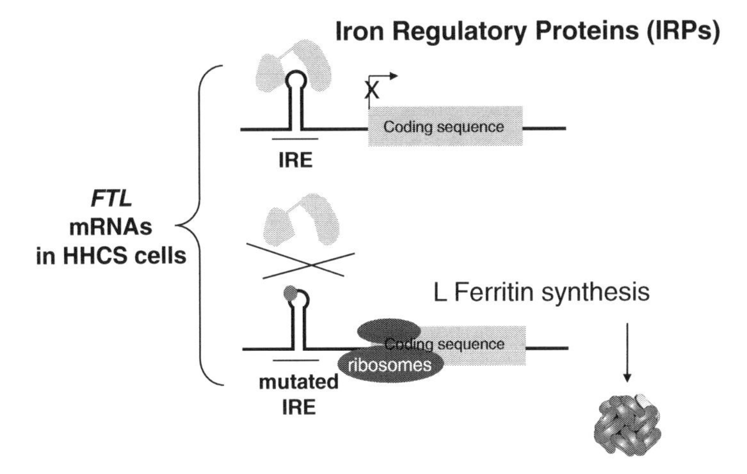

Fig. 21.2 Schematic representation of the IRE–IRP interactions on the *FTL* mRNA in cells of patients with HHCS. Two classes of *FTL* mRNAs are present in cells of patients with HHCS, due to the presence of a heterozygous mutation in the IRE sequence. When iron entry into cells is limited, wild-type *FTL* mRNA translation is repressed due to the high-affinity binding of apo-IRPs on the normal IRE sequence, whereas the mRNAs with a mutated IRE sequence do not bind the IRPs and are normally translated. This mechanism leads to the uncontrolled production of excess L-ferritin subunits which assemble into iron poor L-rich polymers

1.3.1 Hyperferritinemia

Serum ferritin consists mostly of L ferritin subunits that are N-linked glycosylated in the Golgi apparatus and are often called G subunits [23, 24]. The L-ferritin subunit has a consensus glycosylation site (NYST), the Tyr being the aminoacid at position 8 of the polypeptide chain. However, L-ferritin lacks a typical amino-terminal, hydrophobic signal sequence, and the mechanism by which it enters the secretory pathway is not known. It has been shown in rat hepatocytes that cytosolic L-ferritin is targeted to the secretory pathway during translation despite the absence of a conventional signal sequence [25]. Serum ferritin levels usually reflect an increase in tissue ferritin expression. Since ferritin synthesis is upregulated in response to increase iron stores, serum ferritin is a good indicator of tissue iron overload [26]. However, there are a number of clinical situations where increased serum ferritin levels do not necessarily reflect iron overload such as inflammation, cancer, Still's disease, and of course, HHCS [27].

In HHCS patients with IRE mutations, the presence of increased serum ferritin levels, usually above 500 μg/L, is a constant finding, although important fluctuations can be observed with time for the same individual or between several individuals within a family. For instance, one affected member of a family with an interstitial 29-base pair deletion of the IRE (del 10–38) had a progressive reduction in ferritin levels, from 2,800 μg/L at birth to 1,400 μg/L at about 1 year of age [28]. Furthermore, ferritin values ranged between 760 and 2,800 μg/L among the different members of the family. This hyperferritinemia is directly linked to the deregulated L-ferritin synthesis in tissues, and it does not reflect iron overload. Serum iron and the transferrin saturation are always normal [29]. Prior to the discovery of this syndrome, some patients underwent liver biopsy but no excess iron was detected [1]. Furthermore, several patients were mistakenly diagnosed with hereditary hemochromatosis and had repeated phlebotomies. The onset of anemia was rapid in these patients because of the lack of excess tissue iron, and, interestingly, serum ferritin values did not decrease with phlebotomy, a distinctive trait of HHCS. From the multiple family studies published in the literature, it appears that the penetrance of the IRE mutations is complete with respect to the hyperferritinemia, although this may not be the case for cataract.

1.3.2 Cataracts

L-ferritin overexpression seems to be extremely well tolerated in most tissues, except in the lens where it leads to a clinically relevant abnormality. Initially, cataract in HHCS was thought to be "congenital," as the probands from the first families reported severe visual symptoms since birth. Later, with the increasing number of observations, it became clear that the age of onset and the severity of cataract formation are quite variable and cataract is not always present at birth. For instance, a child with the 29-base pair deletion in the IRE had no lens opacities at birth nor at 1 year examination [28], despite high serum ferritin levels (1,448–1,920 μg/L). Lens opacities can be serious enough to require surgical correction in the second or third decades, or mild enough to have no detectable effect on visual acuity.

By slit-lamp examination, the cataract has a very typical pattern (Fig. 21.3), with punctuate, white breadcrumbs-like lens opacities [30], also referred to as scattered central and peripheral optic flecks [31]. In all cases, these opacities are present in the cortex and nucleus. The size and the number of these dot-like opacities increase with age and extend from the center to the periphery (Fig. 21.3 [29, 31, 32]). A large Indian family with a G32A mutation in the IRE has been reported with a very unusual presentation of bilateral sutural cataract. Y sutures in the lens were severely affected, but there were no opacities in the lens cortex or nucleus. No explanation has been found for this unusual pattern.

The ultimate mechanism leading to cataract formation in HHCS is only partially understood. It may be due either to the progressive accumulation of L-ferritin by itself or to the interaction with other(s), as yet unknown, environmental factors. Analysis of specimens from cataract surgery in an HHCS patient and age-matched controls showed that the lens from the patient contained about tenfold more L-ferritin than controls [18]. This overexpressed ferritin has been shown to form insoluble, light-diffracting, crystalline deposits with a typical polygonal appearance [33]. Several features of the lens could contribute to the formation of these ferritin crystals, including a very high protein concentration, little protein turnover and a dehydrated environment [33]. It is interesting to note that transgenic mice which overexpress L-ferritin and have a tenfold increase in the lens L-ferritin content, do not develop cataract but present with very similar ferritin crystals in the lens (C. Beaumont and D. Brooks, unpublished).

1.3.3 Diagnosis and Treatment

It is important to be aware of this disease and to consider it in the differential diagnosis of genetic hemochromatosis [27]. Hyperferritinemia, normal serum iron and normal transferrin saturation are the hallmarks of this disease. In most cases, an early onset cataract is also present, although it is not present at birth and the absence of cataract does not rule out HHCS. Similarly, the absence of family history does not preclude HHCS. Serum ferritin was not frequently measured in the past, and hyperferritinemia may have remained undetected in such families. Furthermore, de novo mutations have been observed [12]. MRI examination of the liver and HFE genotyping can rule out hereditary hemochromatosis, but the simplest way to diagnose HHCS is to perform genetic analyses. Direct sequencing of a DNA sample must encompass a larger region than initially thought because of possible upstream deletions [10]. Rapid, accurate, and reliable screening techniques such as DG-DGGE or DHPLC have also been used successfully to diagnose HHCS [34–36].

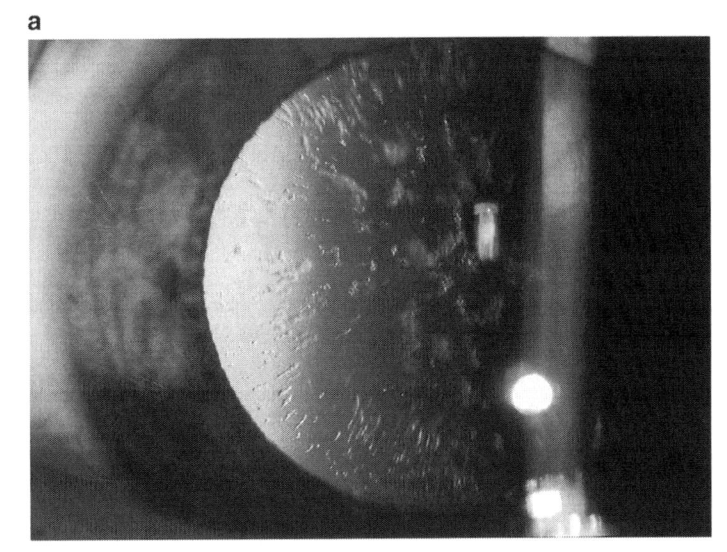

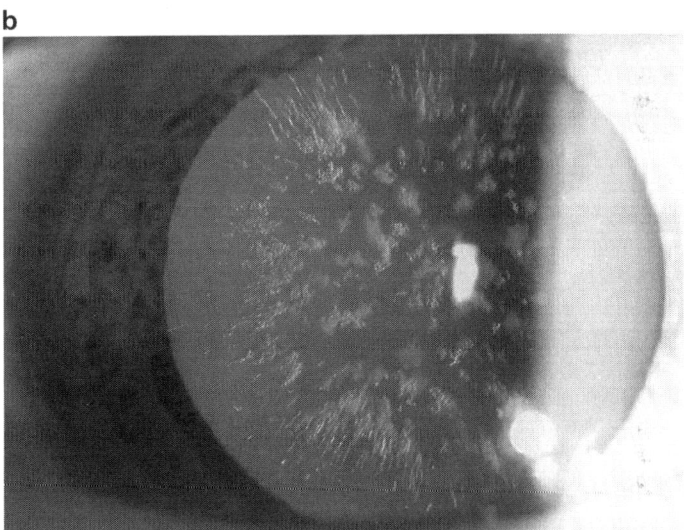

Fig. 21.3 Retroilluminated slit-lamp photograph the eye of a 19-year-old boy (**a**) and of his 46-year-old father (**b**). The picture shows the punctate white "breadcrumb" nuclear and cortical lens opacities, more pronounced in the father's lens and with additional mild nuclear sclerosis (Source: Reproduced from Chang-Godinich et al. [30]. Copyright Elsevier with permission)

There is no treatment for HHCS. An ophthalmological follow-up is recommended with cataract surgery if necessary. Treatment by venesection is to be avoided since iron deficiency anemia rapidly develops due to the lack of iron overload. Persistence of elevated serum ferritin levels during phlebotomy is a good indication of HHCS and must lead to the interruption of the treatment.

1.4 Genotype/Phenotype Correlations

There is no evidence of genotype–phenotype relationships. When the first mutations were identified, a thermodynamic analysis of the IREs suggested that differences in the effects of these mutations on the RNA–protein interaction could explain the phenotypic variability of the disease [19]. This study showed that some HHCS mutations lead to changes in the stability and secondary structure of the IRE, whereas others appear to disrupt IRP–IRE recognition with minimal effect on IRE stability.

However, now that the list of mutations has greatly increased as well as the number of individuals carrying the same mutation, it appears that there is no clear correlation between a given mutation and the severity of the disease, neither in terms of severity of the cataract nor in terms of the elevation in serum ferritin levels (Tables 21.1 and 21.2). Even the deletion of one half of the IRE structure which would be predicted to entirely suppress the IRP-mediated negative control of L-ferritin synthesis does not lead to relatively higher ferritin levels. In fact, higher ferritin levels, ranging from 3,000 to 5,000 μg/L, have been reported in patients with the A40G mutation in the IRE loop.

1.5 Other Causes of Isolated Hyperferritinemia

Hyperferritinemia with normal serum iron and normal transferrin saturation are frequently encountered in clinical practice. Once IRE mutations have been ruled out, many of these cases will remain unexplained. However, two new causes of isolated hyperferritinemia have been described recently, namely, ferroportin disease (see Chap. 20) and mutations in the L-ferritin coding sequence.

1.5.1 Ferroportin Disease

Heterozygous mutations in the ferroportin (*FPN*) gene result in an autosomal dominant disorder called "ferroportin disease" or type 4 hemochromatosis. Several different point mutations leading to an amino-acid replacement and one-codon deletion have been described so far [37]. Based on functional studies, it is now considered that these mutations belong to two categories, leading to two different diseases [38]. Some mutations will impair the hepcidin-binding site present on the extracellular part of the ferroportin molecule. In the absence of the hepcidin-mediated negative control of iron export by ferroportin, increased intestinal iron absorption and increased iron export from macrophages will lead to elevated transferrin saturation and iron loading of hepatocytes. This phenotype mimics what is found in patients with HFE mutation and defective hepcidin synthesis. It is usually a rather severe phenotype with iron overload of parenchymal cells and tissue damage. By contrast, mutations that affect the iron export function of the ferroportin protein result in milder patterns of iron loading with normal to low transferrin saturation, moderately elevated serum ferritin levels and a restricted pattern of iron overload limited to macrophages [37]. Interestingly, macrophage iron loading is generally not accompanied by fibrosis, in contrast to the most frequent form of hemochromatosis due to HFE mutations, where the iron deposits are mostly found in hepatocytes. Several studies have reported that patients with this type of ferroportin mutations do not tolerate phlebotomies and rapidly develop anemia since they fail to mobilize macrophage iron stores to support erythropoiesis, a situation reminiscent of patients with aceruloplasminemia. Patients with mutations that alter the iron export function of ferroportin will present with hyperferritinemia and normal serum iron and transferrin saturation and can be mistaken for HHCS patients [12, 39]. The absence of cataract is not informative since the age of onset of cataract is extremely variable in HHCS patients. It is only the evidence of excessive liver iron stores as determined by MRI analysis that can orientate toward a diagnosis of type 4 hemochromatosis [40] and suggest ferroportin gene sequencing.

1.5.2 L-Ferritin Mutations

Another cause of isolated hyperferritinemia was isolated recently, consisting in c.89C>T base change in the *FTL* exon 1 leading to a Thr30Ile amino acid change in the L-ferritin subunit [41]. A perfect cosegregation was observed between the mutated allele and the hyperferritinemia in the ten families that were studied. However, in this study, this mutation accounted for only 20% of the cases with isolated hyperferritinemia and the cause of the remaining hyperferritinemia remains to be determined. In these subjects with the p.Thr30Ile L-ferritin mutation, no reproducible symptoms besides increased serum ferritin could be identified.

An interesting feature in these subjects with hyperferritinemia and the Thr30Ile variant is the very high percentage of glycosylated ferritin [41]. Serum ferritin is thought to result from the secretion of a small fraction of cellular ferritin through the classical secretory pathway. In the absence of a canonical signal sequence, the A helix of the L-ferritin subunit may play a role in addressing a fraction of the molecules to the endoplasmic reticulum during translation of the mRNA. Interestingly, the substitution of the polar threonine at position 30 of L ferritin by a hydrophobic isoleucine increases the hydrophobicity of this helix.

1.6 Conclusions

We reported in 2003 a series of 52 patients with unexplained hyperferritinemia and no indication of iron overload on the basis of the serum iron indices [12]. Of these, we found 24 individuals with IRE mutations and three patients with heterozygous ferroportin mutation. Later on, we found a different type of *FTL* mutation in another 20% of these cases [41], but nowadays, we still have about half of the hyperferritinemia referred to us for molecular diagnosis of HHCS which remain unexplained. The mechanism of ferritin secretion is still poorly understood, and only its more detailed characterization will shed some light on these unexplained hyperferritinemia cases.

2 Aceruloplasminemia

Hereditary aceruloplasminemia (MIM #604290) is a rare autosomal recessive disorder of iron homeostasis caused by mutations in the ceruloplasmin (*CP*) gene. Affected individuals may present in adulthood with evidence of hepatic iron overload, diabetes, peripheral retinal degeneration, dystonia, dementia, or dysarthria. Laboratory studies demonstrate microcytic anemia, elevated serum ferritin, and a complete absence of serum CP ferroxidase activity.

2.1 Ceruloplasmin

CP is a blue, copper-binding, α2-glycoprotein that contains more than 95% of the copper present in the blood plasma. It is primarily synthesized in hepatocytes and astrocytes [42]. CP synthesized in hepatocytes is secreted into the plasma as holo-CP with six atoms of copper incorporated during biosynthesis. Copper is transported into the Golgi network by the copper-transporting ATPases ATP7B in many cell types [43]. It is subsequently incorporated into apo-CP resulting in the formation of holo-CP prior to its extracellular secretion. CP is also expressed in the central nervous system where it is mostly found on the surface of astrocytes in a glycosylphosphatidylinositol (GPI)-anchored form, resulting from alternative RNA splicing [44]. GPI-linked CP has also been described in bone marrow macrophages.

CP is encoded by a gene present on human chromosome 3q [23–25] with a length greater than 45 kb and comprising 19 exons. The encoded polypeptide has 1,046 amino acids and a molecular weight of 132 kDa. CP is involved in several pathways including copper transport (copper multi-oxidase), iron metabolism (as a ferroxidase), and oxidant defense, whereby it prevents lipid peroxidation. It belongs to the family of multi-copper oxidases which oxidize iron(II) to iron(III) without releasing radical oxygen species. It plays a major role in the mobilization of iron from parenchymal tissues by oxidizing iron and allowing its binding by apotransferrin. In mammals, hephaestin is a CP paralog, with 50% identity to Cp. It is expressed mainly in duodenal enterocytes and is as a membrane-bound enzyme which plays a role in the basolateral transport of iron from enterocytes [45]. A large deletion in hephaestin in *sla* (sex-linked anemia) mice results in reduced iron efflux from duodenal enterocytes and the development of a moderate microcytic anemia [46]. Iron export from cells requires the coordinated actions of a multi-copper ferroxidase and of ferroportin (FPN), the only known iron exporter in mammalian cells. De Domenico et al. have recently shown that cell surface localization of FPN requires the presence of secreted or GPI-linked CP, or of hephaestin. In the absence of one of these multi-copper oxidases, iron which remains bound to FPN as Fe(II) induces a conformational change that triggers ubiquitination, internalization, and degradation of FPN [47]. Loss of cell surface FPN induces iron retention. It has also been shown that in astrocytes, GPI-linked Cp is physically associated with FPN [48] and astrocytes in $Cp^{-/-}$ mice have no detectable FPN on their cell surface [47].

2.2 *Aceruloplasminemia*

Ceruloplasmin levels are decreased in Wilson's disease, in which copper cannot be incorporated into ceruloplasmin in the liver because of defects in the copper-transporting ATPase ATP7B [43]. The apoprotein devoid of copper does not have a ferroxidase activity and is rapidly degraded in the plasma [49]. However, the term aceruloplasminemia is used to designate a hereditary disease due to specific mutations in the *CP* gene. Differential diagnosis between the two diseases can easily be made on the basis of normal hepatic copper content and heavy iron overload in aceruloplasminemia. Furthermore, symptoms of aceruloplasminemia are usually not seen in Wilson's disease because the 5% residual plasma CP is sufficient to sustain plasma iron turnover [50].

2.2.1 Clinical Presentation

In 1987, Miyajima et al. [51] first described a 52-year-old woman suffering from retinal degeneration, diabetes mellitus, and neurodegeneration. Her symptoms were associated with an absence of circulating serum ceruloplasmin, elevated serum ferritin, a mild anemia, low serum iron, and profound hepatic iron overload. A mutation was identified in her *CP* gene [52]. After this first description, aceruloplasminemia has been reported mainly in Japanese patients and in some rare Caucasian whites (Table 21.1).

Patients are typically affected after the fourth to fifth decade with predominantly neurologic symptoms, and the outcome is fatal in the absence of treatment. Symptoms include subcortical dementia, dystonia, dysarthria, and movement disorders, resulting from progressive neurodegeneration of the basal ganglia [53]. In addition, ophthalmologic examination reveals iron deposition and photoreceptor loss in the peripheral regions of the retina [54]. Laboratory findings reveal low serum iron concentration, absence or near absence of CP in serum, low total serum copper concentration, and high ferritin levels. Mild anemia is frequently present [55].

2.2.2 Pathophysiology

Tissue iron overload probably results from both increased intestinal iron absorption and defective mobilization of tissue iron stores. CP is required for the oxidation of Fe(II) into Fe(III) following its export from macrophages by the iron exporter FPN and prior to its binding to apotransferrin. Recycling of heme iron by macrophages following phagocytosis and degradation of senescent erythrocytes is the major source of iron for developing erythroblasts in the bone marrow [56]. In the absence of functional CP, tissue iron efflux is reduced and iron accumulates in macrophages and hepatocytes. This results in low serum iron and mild anemia with iron-restricted erythropoiesis. This situation is known to reduce hepcidin levels and to increase intestinal iron absorption. Although this has not been demonstrated in patients with aceruloplasminemia, several studies have shown that serum hepcidin levels are abnormally low in iron-loading anemias [57, 58]. Since intestinal iron absorption relies on hephaestin to oxidize iron rather than on CP [59], patients with aceruloplasminemia are likely to have increased intestinal iron absorption, resulting in parenchymal iron overload. The unique involvement of the central nervous system distinguishes aceruloplasminemia from other inherited and acquired iron storage disorders. Neurological symptoms are not found in patients with increased intestinal iron absorption due to HFE mutations nor in thalassemia patients with heavy transfusional iron overload. CP is synthesized in astrocytes and found at the cell surface as a GPI-linked form. The distribution of iron in the brain of patients with aceruloplasminemia as seen at autopsy is limited to astrocytes and nerve cells in the basal ganglia, thalamus, and cerebellum [60]. Abnormal astrocytes, enlarged in size and with multiple nuclei, are often found. Astrocytes play a major role in brain iron metabolism, and using astrocytes derived from CP-null mice, it has been shown that ferroportin is unable to efflux iron in the absence of CP [48]. The coordinated actions of GPI-CP and FPN may be required for iron efflux from neural cells. Disruption of this balance could lead to iron accumulation in the central nervous system and development of neurological symptoms, which include involuntary movements, ataxia, and dementia, reflecting the sites of iron deposition. Excess iron functions as a potent catalyst of biologic oxidation. Several studies have shown that an increased iron concentration is associated with increased lipid peroxidation in the brain [61] and iron-loaded astrocytes were shown to react with anti-HNE and antiubiquitin antibodies [60]. Measures of brain oxygen and glucose metabolism using positron emission tomography (PET) showed a marked decrease in glucose and oxygen consumption in the entire brain of aceruloplasminemia patients [62]. Brains examined at autopsy showed that enzyme activities in the mitochondrial respiratory chain of the basal ganglia were reduced to about 50% and 43%, respectively, for complexes I and IV. Those of the cerebral and cerebellar cortices also were decreased approximately 62% and 65% [62]. These findings suggest that iron-mediated free radicals may contribute to neuronal cell damage through increased lipid peroxidation and the impairment of mitochondrial energy metabolism in aceruloplasminemia brains.

2.2.3 Molecular Defects

After the first description, aceruloplasminemia has been reported mainly in Japanese patients and more rarely in Caucasians (Table 21.3). In Japan, the incidence was estimated to be approximately one per 2,000,000 in the case of nonconsanguineous marriages [63]. More than 25 aceruloplasminemia causing mutations have been identified (Table 21.3). Some of the mutations have been found in several families throughout the world, but most of them have been detected in a single patient. Different types of mutations have been reported, including small internal deletions or insertions and splicing defects, as well as nonsense or missense mutations. Except for the missense mutations, all the other mutations lead to a frameshift and the formation of a premature stop codon. The truncated protein is retained and degraded in the endoplasmic reticulum (ER), resulting in almost complete

Table 21.3 Mutations in the human ceruloplasmin gene in aceruloplasminemia

Mutation	Exon	Predicted effects	Reference
Insertion or deletion			
607insA	3	Frameshift	[135]
1257–1258delTT	7	Truncated protein (Tyr401X)	[70]
1285 ins TACAC	7	Frameshift	[52]
1916delG–1918delG	11	Truncated protein	[69]
2389delG	13	Frameshift	[136]
2602delG	15		[137]
2917insA	17	Truncated protein	[138]
Nonsense			
Tyr694X	12	Truncated protein	[69]
Trp858X	15	Truncated protein	[139–141]
Arg882X	16	Truncated protein	[142]
Missense			
Ile28Ph	1	Reduced Cp levels	[71]
Asp58His	2		[143]
Gln146Glu	2	Reduced Cp level	[138]
Pro177Arg	3		[144]
Phe198Ser	3		[74]
Try283Ser	5		[145]
Ala331Asp	6		[55]
Gly606Glu	11		[146]
Gly631Arg	11	ER retention	[144, 147]
Gln692Lys	12		[143]
G969S	16	Half-normal Cp level	[67]
His978Gln	17	No ferroxidase activity	[142]
Splice site			
607+1G>A	3	Exon 3 skipping, splicing defect	[148]
1209-2A>G	Int6	Splicing defect, 8 bp del in mRNA, truncated protein	[149]
3019-1G>A	18	Truncated protein	[150]

absence of ceruloplasmin in the plasma. The effects of nonsense mutations including Tyr694X, Trp858X, and Arg882X were studied by transfection in CHO cultured cells [64]. The truncated Tyr694X and Trp858X proteins were found to have a rate of synthesis identical to that of wild-type CP but to be retained in the ER, inducing proteins of the ER stress pathway and eventually resulting in cell death. The Arg882X mutant was secreted normally but is likely to be unstable.

The missense mutations can affect either folding of the molecule or incorporation of the copper atoms. CP contains six integral copper ions, three of which forming a trinuclear cluster and the other three being arranged in three type I mononuclear sites. Each of the mononuclear copper ions is liganded to two histidines and a cysteine, while only histidines are required for binding of the copper ions in the trinuclear center [65]. Site-directed mutagenesis at each of the six copper-binding sites and transfection into CHO cells have shown that the synthesis and secretion of the mutant proteins is identical to that of the wild-type CP, but each mutation results in complete abrogation of copper incorporation [66]. Similarly, transfection studies of some of the natural mutants such as Gly631Arg or Gly969Ser have shown that the kinetics of the synthesis and secretion of the mutant proteins is normal, but the proteins fail to incorporate copper [60, 67]. Gly631 and Gly969 are close to His637 and His975 respectively, which are parts of type I copper-binding sites. Interestingly, the patient with the Gly969Ser mutation had apo-CP in the plasma but no detectable ferroxidase activity, whereas the patient with the Gly631Ser mutation had no detectable plasma CP. Apo-CP lacking copper ions is thought to be unstable in the plasma [49], and the reason for the unexpected stability of the Gly969Ser mutant protein is unknown. The Pro177Arg mutant was found to be retained in the ER. The mutation resides in a highly conserved 5-base pair motif, G(FLI)(LI)GP, repeated six times in the CP molecule. This motif might be critical for proper folding and subsequent trafficking of CP [60].

2.2.4 Genotype–Phenotype Relationships

Despite the presence of multiple mutations, little variation is observed in the phenotypic expression of the disease. The triad of retinal degeneration, diabetes mellitus, and neurological symptoms is almost always present in homozygous patients. Liver iron overload usually remains asymptomatic, and in contrast with other forms of hemochromatosis [68], patients with aceruloplasminemia do not develop signs of hepatic dysfunction. Although liver biopsy typically reveals marked iron accumulation within both hepatocytes and reticuloendothelial cells [67, 69], fibrosis is generally absent even in the advanced stages of the disease. While diabetes is sometimes the earliest symptom, neurological signs such as dementia, ataxia, and difficulty in walking are the major symptoms that will allow the correct diagnosis.

Some phenotypic variability can be observed within a family. For instance, Fasano et al. [70] described two siblings with the same homozygous deletion of two nucleotides causing a premature stop codon (Tyr401X). An early diagnosis of iron overload was made in the female sibling who was subsequently treated with deferoxamine. At the age of 54, her neurologic symptoms were limited to mild akinetic signs and a history of seizures. Moreover, her fasting blood glucose level never exceeded 120 mg/dL. The male sibling, who had not received any specific treatment, developed severe diabetes at the age of 32 and at 48 manifested a progressively disabling neurologic disease. Several factors can contribute to the heterogeneity in clinical symptoms such as variability in free radicals production caused by iron deposition or environmental factors such as aging.

In most cases, heterozygous individuals in the families retain half-normal CP levels and do not develop clinical signs of the disease. However, some heterozygous individuals have been reported with mild neurological symptoms, despite half-normal levels of serum CP and copper [71, 72].

Finally, five novel heterozygous CP mutations have been identified in a study cohort of 176 patients with Parkinson's disease where increased iron levels had been detected in the substantia nigra by transcranial ultrasound [73]. This observation underlies a possible role of mutations, or polymorphisms, of CP in increasing substantia nigra iron levels and in contributing to the pathogenesis of Parkinson's disease.

2.2.5 Therapeutics

Several therapeutic strategies have been tested to limit the development of hepatic and brain iron overload, with variable success. Mirayima et al. [72] observed limited progression of the neurological symptoms, reduced plasma lipid peroxidation, and a decrease of liver iron concentration in their patient following a ten-month therapy with the iron chelator deferoxamine (DFO). Loreal et al. [69] reported a one-year therapy with parenteral DFO combined with vitamin C (5 days a week) in a 62-year-old woman. This also achieved reduced liver iron burden from 250 μmol/g liver to 75 μmol/g, but the low R2* signal in brain MRI imaging was not modified, suggesting that the DFO therapy was not efficient in removing brain iron. Furthermore, there was a concomitant aggravation of the anemia leading to the cessation of the therapy. Similarly, Mariani et al. [74] found that DFO treatment was successful in removing excess iron stores from the liver, but the brain MRI signal did not change. There again aggravation of the anemia led to interruption of the chelation therapy. These authors also tried a six-month therapy with deferiprone, but the therapy was ineffective in removing iron. This is intriguing since recently deferiprone has been used successfully to reduce brain iron accumulation and neurological symptoms in Friedreich's ataxia [75]. In this disease, decreased iron–sulfur cluster and heme formation leads to mitochondrial iron accumulation and ensuing oxidative damage that primarily affects sensory neurons, the myocardium, and endocrine glands. A six-month treatment with 20–30 mg/kg/d deferiprone of nine adolescent patients with no overt cardiomyopathy reduced R2* from 18.3 s(−1) to 15.7 s(−1) ($P<.002$), specifically in dentate nuclei and proportionally to the initial R2* ($r=0.90$). Chelator treatment caused no apparent hematologic or neurologic side effects while reducing neuropathy and ataxic gait in the youngest patients [75]. Similarly, phlebotomy, which has been largely used to reduce the iron load in hemochromatotic patients, demonstrated no benefit in aceruloplasminaemia [76]. The failure of these different therapies in removing iron in aceruloplasminemia probably reflects the fact that tissue iron cannot be readily mobilized because of the defective ceruloplasmin. Kuhn et al. [77] reported the beneficial effect of oral zinc sulfate in an 18-year-old girl with a heterozygous *CP* mutation and extrapyramidal and cerebellar-mediated movement disorder, taking advantage of its antioxidant properties as well as its established effects on reducing iron absorption. Yonekawa et al. [78] obtained some success in reducing neurological symptoms following repetitive intravenous administration of commercially available fresh-frozen human plasma containing ceruloplasmin.

2.3 Animal Models

To elucidate the role of CP in iron homeostasis, in 1999, Harris and colleagues [79] created an animal model of aceruloplasminemia by disrupting the murine *Cp* gene. At 1 year of age $Cp^{-/-}$ animals displayed a three- to sixfold increase in the iron content in liver and spleen. Histological analysis of affected tissues in these mice showed abundant iron stores within reticuloendothelial cells and hepatocytes. Ferrokinetics studies in $Cp^{+/+}$ and $Cp^{-/-}$ mice revealed a striking impairment in the movement of iron out of reticuloendothelial cells and hepatocytes. However, when the same targeted *Cp* deletion was backcrossed from Swiss genetic background to a C57BL/6 background, the knockout mice displayed normal spleen iron stores, whereas liver iron stores remained elevated [80]. In addition, a spontaneous Arg435X nonsense mutation in exon 7 of the *Cp* gene in C3H/DiSnA mice was identified as a modifier of liver iron but not of spleen iron in a genetic screen of modifier genes of iron metabolism [81]. Therefore, the role of Cp in the mobilization of macrophage iron stores is not fully understood and other factors may contribute to modulating macrophage iron export.

These Cp-deficient mice have also been useful in elucidating the role of Cp in brain and retinal iron homeostasis. In $Cp^{-/-}$ mice, iron accumulation occurs mainly in astrocytes by 24 months and is accompanied by a significant loss of these cells. In contrast, Purkinje neurons and the large neurons in the deep nuclei of $Cp^{-/-}$ mice do not accumulate iron but express high levels of the iron importer divalent metal-ion transporter 1, suggesting that these cells may be iron deprived [48]. This is also accompanied by a significant reduction in the number of Purkinje neurons. These data suggest that astrocytes play a central role in the acquisition of iron from the circulation and that two different mechanisms underlie the loss of astrocytes and neurons in $Cp^{-/-}$ mice.

Patients with aceruloplasminemia develop retinal degeneration. However, this symptom is absent in $Cp^{-/-}$ mice and is only observed in double-knockout mice with inactivation of both *Cp* and *hephaestin* genes. In normal mice, Cp and hephaestin localize to Müller glia and retinal pigment epithelium, a blood-brain barrier. Mice deficient in both Cp and hephaestin show a striking age-dependent increase in retinal pigment epithelium and retinal iron, as well as retinal pigment epithelium hypertrophy, hyperplasia and death, photoreceptor degeneration, and subretinal neovascularization [82].

3 Atransferrinemia

Atransferrinemia/hypotransferrinemia (MIM #209300) is a rare genetic disorder characterized by microcytic anemia and iron overload. It was first described in 1961 [83], and since then, 13 patients have been reported. The molecular defect in the transferrin (*TF*) gene has been identified in only four of these patients; however, all these patients have in common low to undetectable levels of plasma transferrin. Human plasma TF is a 79-kDa glycoprotein produced by the liver (see also Chap. 7). Other cell types such as retinal cells [84] and oligodendrocytes [85] can synthesize TF, although they probably do not contribute to plasma TF. The human *TF* gene is located on Chr 3q22.1. The N and C termini of the molecule each contains an iron-binding site, and iron binding requires the presence of carbonate ion [86]. The anemia of patients with atransferrinemia highlights the importance of the transferrin-mediated iron delivery pathway for erythropoiesis.

3.1 Pathophysiology

Developing erythroblasts in the bone marrow rely only on the transferrin-mediated pathway for iron delivery. Low or undetectable levels of TF induce defective hemoglobin synthesis and microcytic hypochromic anemia. However, some iron is present in the plasma in a non-transferrin-bound form and is taken up by nonhematopoietic tissues, especially heart and liver. Development of tissue iron overload is exacerbated by increased intestinal iron absorption. Atransferrinemia belongs to the group of iron-loading anemias, as well as thalassemia intermedia or sideroblastic anemia. Similarly to what has been described in these diseases [87], hepcidin production is decreased in patients with atransferrinemia [88], despite the presence of iron overload. In one patient, urinary hepcidin levels were shown to rise from undetectable levels to normal values following plasma infusion, with a concomitant rise in serum iron and decrease in transferrin saturation [88].

3.2 Clinical Presentation

Microcytic hypochromic anemia and liver siderosis are the two main symptoms of this disease. Severity of the anemia is variable as well as the age of diagnosis, ranging from 2 months to 20 years of age. Since very few patients have been characterized at the molecular level, it is almost impossible to study phenotype–genotype correlation, but the residual level of plasma transferrin is probably an important feature in controlling severity of the disease. Hayashi et al. proposed that TF value below 0.2 g/L (normal 2–3.5 g/L) results in severe anemia and growth retardation, whereas patients with values above this threshold are apparently healthy [89]. The main clinical features of the disease are pallor and fatigue. Some patients have mild hepatomegaly, and liver siderosis has been documented only in several cases but is likely to be the rule, with heavy iron deposits in both Kupffer cells and hepatocytes. Two patients died at the age of seven from heart failure. In both of them, the autopsy showed marked hemosiderosis and fibrosis of liver, pancreas, thyroid, myocardium and kidney. On the reverse, several reports mention absence of bone marrow iron stores. One patient was reported to have hypothyroidism [90]. Both growth retardation and impaired mental development have been described, resolving upon therapy [89]. An increased number of infections appear to occur in patients with atransferrinemia. One patient had recurrent infections and another one died of pneumonia [91].

3.3 Molecular Defects

Only four cases have been elucidated at the molecular level. The first mutation was identified by Beutler and colleagues in a 20-year-old American woman [90]. She was found to be compound heterozygote. The first mutation was a ten-base pair deletion (cDNA 562–571del) immediately followed by a nine-base pair duplication (cDNA 572–580) in exon 5, leading to a frame shift and premature termination. The second mutation was a missense mutation in exon 12 causing an Ala477Pro amino acid change. The second patient was of Japanese origin and was a compound heterozygote with a mutated *TF* allele of paternal origin causing a Glu375Cys amino acid change and a null allele of maternal origin [92]. Sequencing of the exons and exon–intron boundaries on the null allele did not reveal any mutation, suggesting a defect in the transcription or stability of the mRNA. The third case was a Slovakian girl, diagnosed of severe hypochromic, microcytic anemia at the age of 2 months. Atransferrinemia was diagnosed and serum TF concentrations were half normal in parents, a brother, and a grandfather. She was found to be homozygous for an Asp77Asn mutation in exon 3 that probably abrogated synthesis or secretion of the molecule [93]. Consanguinity was suspected on the basis of homozygosity for the mutation and several other polymorphic sites, although not formally proven. The fourth case was a Turkish patient with severe microcytic anemia diagnosed at 4 months of age. He was homozygous for a Cys137Tyr mutation in exon 4 [94].

3.4 Therapy

The first patients that were identified were initially treated by blood transfusions. However, this induced worsening of the patient's condition and was rapidly replaced by plasma infusion, and later on by infusion of apo-TF. Monthly infusions of 500 mL of plasma provided sufficient TF to permit normal hemoglobin formation in one patient, and the infusion was preceded by a 480-mL phlebotomy to reduce the iron overload [90]. The patient, who was heavily iron overloaded at first with a liver iron concentration of 37,465 μg/g dry weight, underwent this monthly treatment for 10 years before reaching iron depletion. Monthly plasma infusion with iron chelation or phlebotomy can be sufficient to allow a good erythropoiesis and to prevent iron overload [95]. Another patient received monthly plasma infusion without phlebotomy, and serum ferritin levels declined from 1,264 to 135 μg/L. However, the patient displayed no radiological evidence of iron overload before the onset of therapy [94]. Apo-TF infusion induces a rapid rise in hemoglobin concentration within 1 week, and the effect is maintained during 4–5 months [89, 90].

3.5 *TF* Gene Polymorphisms

Multiple polymorphisms have been found in the *TF* gene and geographical *TF* allele variations have been reported in various populations. Two frequent variants named C1 and C2 have been studied into more details and found to be risk factors for Alzheimer's disease.

C2 variant is a Pro570Ser mutation arising in the native C1 allele. Frequency of C2 is 15–20% in European population, and a higher allele frequency of *TF* C2 has been proposed as a predisposing factor to Alzheimer's disease [96, 97]. However, the conformation of the two iron-binding sites is conserved between the two variants, as well as their iron-binding capacity. Another TF variant with a Gly277Ser mutation has been found associated with reduced total iron-binding capacities and a predisposition to iron deficiency in menstruating women [98]. However, another study conducted on pregnant women failed to find an increased G277S frequency in iron-deficient women [99].

3.6 Anti-TF Antibodies

Autoimmune atransferrinemia has been reported in one patient with monoclonal immunoglobulin with anti-transferrin activity. Serum iron and iron-binding capacity were extremely high (800 μg/dL, normal 270–370). There was a drastically reduced plasma iron clearance ($T_{1/2}$ of 540 min, normal 70–110), associated with iron deficiency anemia and iron overload [100]. Interestingly, two similar cases of very high serum iron and extremely high transferrin concentrations (5.4–6.5 g/L, normal 2–3.5 g/L) due to immunoglobulin with anti-TF activity were also reported, but no anemia or microcytosis were observed [101]. Plasma iron clearance was only moderately reduced (206 min) and no iron overload was observed. Differences in the affinity of the monoclonal antibodies against TF might account for these phenotypic differences.

3.7 Mouse Model

Hypotransferrinemic mice (*hpx/hpx*) carry a spontaneous mutation in the TF gene. The mutation disrupts a splice donor site at the end of exon 16 of the TF gene, resulting in the usage of a cryptic splice donor site 27-base pair upstream of the normal splice junction [102]. It has been inferred that an aberrant protein with a 9-amino-acid internal deletion circulates in plasma, albeit at a very low level, about 1% the normal amount of immunoreactive TF. New born *hpx/hpx* mice are viable but severely anemic, and they can survive for up to 2 weeks after birth without blood transfusions or TF infusions. However, they will only reach adulthood when receiving weekly injections of whole mouse serum or apo-TF. Interestingly, when the therapy is interrupted past weaning, the mice will survive and continue to grow, although they remain pale as compared to their control littermates [102]. Surviving adults will develop severe hypochromic anemia and heavy iron overload of liver, heart, and kidney. Abnormal iron accumulation also develops in adrenal medulla and the exocrine pancreas. Interestingly, spleen macrophages are free of iron deposits, a situation reminiscent of bone marrow macrophages in human patients with atransferrinemia. Iron kinetics studies with 59Fe showed that tissue distribution and clearance kinetics of iron is greatly different between *hpx* mice and control mice made iron deficient by repeated blood samplings [103]. Whereas both mouse models absorb the same amount of iron, the non-transferrin-bound iron in the *hpx* mice is rapidly cleared from the plasma and deposited into parenchymal tissues. It has also been shown that despite the heavy liver iron overload, hepcidin expression is completely suppressed in *hpx* mice [104], probably accounting for the increased intestinal absorption.

References

1. Bonneau D, Winter-Fuseau I, Loiseau MN, et al. Bilateral cataract and high serum ferritin: a new dominant genetic disorder? J Med Genet. 1995;32:778–9.
2. Girelli D, Olivieri O, De Franceschi L, Corrocher R, Bergamaschi G, Cazzola M. A linkage between hereditary hyperferritinaemia not related to iron overload and autosomal dominant congenital cataract. Br J Haematol. 1995;90:931–4.
3. Beaumont C, Leneuve P, Devaux I, et al. Mutation in the iron responsive element of the L ferritin mRNA in a family with dominant hyperferritinaemia and cataract. Nat Genet. 1995;11:444–6.
4. Girelli D, Corrocher R, Bisceglia L, et al. Molecular basis for the recently described hereditary hyperferritinemia-cataract syndrome: a mutation in the iron-responsive element of ferritin L-subunit gene (the "Verona mutation"). Blood. 1995;86:4050–3.
5. Millonig G, Muckenthaler MU, Mueller S. Hyperferritinaemia-cataract syndrome: worldwide mutations and phenotype of an increasingly diagnosed genetic disorder. Hum Genomics. 2010;4:250–62.

6. Henderson BR, Menotti E, Bonnard C, Kuhn LC. Optimal sequence and structure of iron-responsive elements. Selection of RNA stem–loops with high affinity for iron regulatory factor. J Biol Chem. 1994;269:17481–9.
7. Sierzputowska-Gracz H, McKenzie RA, Theil EC. The importance of a single G in the hairpin loop of the iron responsive element (IRE) in ferritin mRNA for structure: an NMR spectroscopy study. Nucleic Acids Res. 1995;23:146–53.
8. Theil EC. Iron regulatory elements (IREs): a family of mRNA non-coding sequences. Biochem J. 1994;304:1–11.
9. Ke Y, Wu J, Leibold EA, Walden WE, Theil EC. Loops and bulge/loops in iron-responsive element isoforms influence iron regulatory protein binding. Fine-tuning of mRNA regulation? J Biol Chem. 1998;273:23637–40.
10. Burdon KP, Sharma S, Chen CS, Dimasi DP, Mackey DA, Craig JE. A novel deletion in the FTL gene causes hereditary hyperferritinemia cataract syndrome (HHCS) by alteration of the transcription start site. Hum Mutat. 2007;28:742.
11. Arosio C, Fossati L, Vigano M, Trombini P, Cazzaniga G, Piperno A. Hereditary hyperferritinemia cataract syndrome: a de novo mutation in the iron responsive element of the L-ferritin gene. Haematologica. 1999;84:560–1.
12. Hetet G, Devaux I, Soufir N, Grandchamp B, Beaumont C. Molecular analyses of patients with hyperferritinemia and normal serum iron values reveal both L ferritin IRE and 3 new ferroportin (slc11A3) mutations. Blood. 2003;102:1904–10.
13. McLeod JL, Craig J, Gumley S, Roberts S, Kirkland MA. Mutation spectrum in Australian pedigrees with hereditary hyperferritinaemia-cataract syndrome reveals novel and de novo mutations. Br J Haematol. 2002;118:1179–82.
14. Paraskeva E, Gray NK, Schlager B, Wehr K, Hentze MW. Ribosomal pausing and scanning arrest as mechanisms of translational regulation from cap-distal iron-responsive elements. Mol Cell Biol. 1999;19:807–16.
15. Zahringer J, Baliga BS, Munro HN. Novel mechanism for translational control in regulation of ferritin synthesis by iron. Proc Natl Acad Sci USA. 1976;73:857–61.
16. Hentze MW, Kuhn LC. Molecular control of vertebrate iron metabolism: mRNA-based regulatory circuits operated by iron, nitric oxide, and oxidative stress. Proc Natl Acad Sci USA. 1996;93:8175–82.
17. Cazzola M, Skoda RC. Translational pathophysiology: a novel molecular mechanism of human disease. Blood. 2000;95:3280–8.
18. Levi S, Girelli D, Perrone F, et al. Analysis of ferritins in lymphoblastoid cell lines and in the lens of subjects with hereditary hyperferritinemia-cataract syndrome. Blood. 1998;91:4180–7.
19. Allerson CR, Cazzola M, Rouault TA. Clinical severity and thermodynamic effects of iron-responsive element mutations in hereditary hyperferritinemia-cataract syndrome. J Biol Chem. 1999;274:26439–47.
20. Martin ME, Fargion S, Brissot P, Pellat B, Beaumont C. A point mutation in the bulge of the iron-responsive element of the L ferritin gene in two families with the hereditary hyperferritinemia-cataract syndrome. Blood. 1998;91:319–23.
21. Jaffrey SR, Haile DJ, Klausner RD, Harford JB. The interaction between the iron-responsive element binding protein and its cognate RNA is highly dependent upon both RNA sequence and structure. Nucleic Acids Res. 1993;21:4627–31.
22. Leibold EA, Laudano A, Yu Y. Structural requirements of iron-responsive elements for binding of the protein involved in both transferrin receptor and ferritin mRNA post-transcriptional regulation. Nucleic Acids Res. 1990;18:1819–24.
23. Worwood M, Cragg SJ, Wagstaff M, Jacobs A. Binding of human serum ferritin to concanavalin A. Clin Sci (Lond). 1979;56:83–7.
24. Worwood M, Dawkins S, Wagstaff M, Jacobs A. The purification and properties of ferritin from human serum. Biochem J. 1976;157:97–103.
25. Ghosh S, Hevi S, Chuck SL. Regulated secretion of glycosylated human ferritin from hepatocytes. Blood. 2004;103:2369–76.
26. Worwood M. Serum ferritin. Clin Sci (Lond). 1986;70:215–20.
27. Aguilar-Martinez P, Schved JF, Brissot P. The evaluation of hyperferritinemia: an updated strategy based on advances in detecting genetic abnormalities. Am J Gastroenterol. 2005;100:1185–94.
28. Girelli D, Corrocher R, Bisceglia L, et al. Hereditary hyperferritinemia-cataract syndrome caused by a 29-base pair deletion in the iron responsive element of ferritin L-subunit gene. Blood. 1997;90:2084–8.
29. Girelli D, Bozzini C, Zecchina G, et al. Clinical, biochemical and molecular findings in a series of families with hereditary hyperferritinaemia-cataract syndrome. Br J Haematol. 2001;115:334–40.
30. Chang-Godinich A, Ades S, Schenkein D, Brooks D, Stambolian D, Raizman MB. Lens changes in hereditary hyperferritinemia-cataract syndrome. Am J Ophthalmol. 2001;132:786–8.
31. Craig JE, Clark JB, McLeod JL, et al. Hereditary hyperferritinemia-cataract syndrome: prevalence, lens morphology, spectrum of mutations, and clinical presentations. Arch Ophthalmol. 2003;121:1753–61.
32. Feys J, Nodarian M, Aygalenq P, Cattan D, Bouccara AS, Beaumont C. Hereditary hyperferritinemia syndrome and cataract. J Fr Ophtalmol. 2001;24:847–50.
33. Brooks DG, Manova-Todorova K, Farmer J, et al. Ferritin crystal cataracts in hereditary hyperferritinemia cataract syndrome. Invest Ophthalmol Vis Sci. 2002;43:1121–6.

34. Cremonesi L, Fumagalli A, Soriani N, et al. Double-gradient denaturing gradient gel electrophoresis assay for identification of L-ferritin iron-responsive element mutations responsible for hereditary hyperferritinemia-cataract syndrome: identification of the new mutation C14G. Clin Chem. 2001;47:491–7.
35. Cremonesi L, Paroni R, Foglieni B, et al. Scanning mutations of the 5 UTR regulatory sequence of L-ferritin by denaturing high-performance liquid chromatography: identification of new mutations. Br J Haematol. 2003;121:173–9.
36. Giansily M, Beaumont C, Desveaux C, Hetet G, Schved JF, Aguilar-Martinez P. Denaturing gradient gel electrophoresis screening for mutations in the hereditary hyperferritinaemia cataract syndrome. Br J Haematol. 2001;112:51–4.
37. Pietrangelo A. The ferroportin disease. Blood Cells Mol Dis. 2004;32:131–8.
38. De Domenico I, Ward DM, Musci G, Kaplan J. Iron overload due to mutations in ferroportin. Haematologica. 2006;91:92–5.
39. Cazzola M. Role of ferritin and ferroportin genes in unexplained hyperferritinaemia. Best Pract Res Clin Haematol. 2005;18:251–63.
40. Pietrangelo A, Corradini E, Ferrara F, et al. Magnetic resonance imaging to identify classic and nonclassic forms of ferroportin disease. Blood Cells Mol Dis. 2006;37:192–6.
41. Kannengiesser C, Jouanolle AM, Hetet G, et al. A new missense mutation in the L ferritin coding sequence associated with elevated levels of glycosylated ferritin in serum and absence of iron overload. Haematologica. 2009;94:335–9.
42. Hellman NE, Gitlin JD. Ceruloplasmin metabolism and function. Annu Rev Nutr. 2002;22:439–58.
43. de Bie P, Muller P, Wijmenga C, Klomp LW. Molecular pathogenesis of Wilson and Menkes disease: correlation of mutations with molecular defects and disease phenotypes. J Med Genet. 2007;44:673–88.
44. Patel BN, Dunn RJ, David S. Alternative RNA splicing generates a glycosylphosphatidylinositol-anchored form of ceruloplasmin in mammalian brain. J Biol Chem. 2000;275:4305–10.
45. Anderson GJ, Frazer DM, McKie AT, Vulpe CD. The ceruloplasmin homolog hephaestin and the control of intestinal iron absorption. Blood Cells Mol Dis. 2002;29:367–75.
46. Vulpe CD, Kuo YM, Murphy TL, et al. Hephaestin, a ceruloplasmin homologue implicated in intestinal iron transport, is defective in the sla mouse. Nat Genet. 1999;21:195–9.
47. De Domenico I, Ward DM, di Patti MC, et al. Ferroxidase activity is required for the stability of cell surface ferroportin in cells expressing GPI-ceruloplasmin. EMBO J. 2007;26:2823–31.
48. Jeong SY, David S. Age-related changes in iron homeostasis and cell death in the cerebellum of ceruloplasmin-deficient mice. J Neurosci. 2006;26:9810–9.
49. Gitlin JD, Schroeder JJ, Lee-Ambrose LM, Cousins RJ. Mechanisms of caeruloplasmin biosynthesis in normal and copper-deficient rats. Biochem J. 1992;282:835–9.
50. Roeser HP, Lee GR, Nacht S, Cartwright GE. The role of ceruloplasmin in iron metabolism. J Clin Invest. 1970;49:2408–17.
51. Miyajima H, Nishimura Y, Mizoguchi K, Sakamoto M, Shimizu T, Honda N. Familial apoceruloplasmin deficiency associated with blepharospasm and retinal degeneration. Neurology. 1987;37:761–7.
52. Harris ZL, Takahashi Y, Miyajima H, Serizawa M, MacGillivray RT, Gitlin JD. Aceruloplasminemia: molecular characterization of this disorder of iron metabolism. Proc Natl Acad Sci USA. 1995;92:2539–43.
53. McNeill A, Pandolfo M, Kuhn J, Shang H, Miyajima H. The neurological presentation of ceruloplasmin gene mutations. Eur Neurol. 2008;60:200–5.
54. He X, Hahn P, Iacovelli J, et al. Iron homeostasis and toxicity in retinal degeneration. Prog Retin Eye Res. 2007;26:649–73.
55. Perez-Aguilar F, Burguera JA, Benlloch S, Berenguer M, Rayon JM. Aceruloplasminemia in an asymptomatic patient with a new mutation. Diagnosis and family genetic analysis. J Hepatol. 2005;42:947–9.
56. Beaumont C, Canonne-Hergaux F. Erythrophagocytosis and recycling of heme iron in normal and pathological conditions; regulation by hepcidin. Transfus Clin Biol. 2005;12:123–30.
57. Origa R, Galanello R, Ganz T, et al. Liver iron concentrations and urinary hepcidin in beta-thalassemia. Haematologica. 2007;92:583–8.
58. Papanikolaou G, Tzilianos M, Christakis JI, et al. Hepcidin in iron overload disorders. Blood. 2005;105:4103–5.
59. Anderson GJ, Frazer DM. Recent advances in intestinal iron transport. Curr Gastroenterol Rep. 2005;7: 365–72.
60. Kono S, Miyajima H. Molecular and pathological basis of aceruloplasminemia. Biol Res. 2006;39:15–23.
61. Miyajima H, Takahashi Y, Serizawa M, Kaneko E, Gitlin JD. Increased plasma lipid peroxidation in patients with aceruloplasminemia. Free Radic Biol Med. 1996;20:757–60.
62. Miyajima H, Takahashi Y, Kono S, et al. Glucose and oxygen hypometabolism in aceruloplasminemia brains. Intern Med. 2002;41:186–90.
63. Miyajima H, Takahashi Y, Kono S. Aceruloplasminemia, an inherited disorder of iron metabolism. Biometals. 2003;16:205–13.

64. Kono S, Suzuki H, Oda T, et al. Cys-881 is essential for the trafficking and secretion of truncated mutant ceruloplasmin in aceruloplasminemia. J Hepatol. 2007;47:844–50.
65. Bento I, Peixoto C, Zaitsev VN, Lindley PF. Ceruloplasmin revisited: structural and functional roles of various metal cation-binding sites. Acta Crystallogr D Biol Crystallogr. 2007;63:240–8.
66. Hellman NE, Kono S, Mancini GM, Hoogeboom AJ, De Jong GJ, Gitlin JD. Mechanisms of copper incorporation into human ceruloplasmin. J Biol Chem. 2002;277:46632–8.
67. Kono S, Suzuki H, Takahashi K, et al. Hepatic iron overload associated with a decreased serum ceruloplasmin level in a novel clinical type of aceruloplasminemia. Gastroenterology. 2006;131:240–5.
68. Deugnier Y, Turlin B. Pathology of hepatic iron overload. World J Gastroenterol. 2007;13:4755–60.
69. Loreal O, Turlin B, Pigeon C, et al. Aceruloplasminemia: new clinical, pathophysiological and therapeutic insights. J Hepatol. 2002;36:851–6.
70. Fasano A, Colosimo C, Miyajima H, Tonali PA, Re TJ, Bentivoglio AR. Aceruloplasminemia: a novel mutation in a family with marked phenotypic variability. Mov Disord. 2008;23:751–5.
71. Daimon M, Susa S, Ohizumi T, et al. A novel mutation of the ceruloplasmin gene in a patient with heteroallelic ceruloplasmin gene mutation (HypoCPGM). Tohoku J Exp Med. 2000;191:119–25.
72. Miyajima H, Takahashi Y, Kamata T, Shimizu H, Sakai N, Gitlin JD. Use of desferrioxamine in the treatment of aceruloplasminemia. Ann Neurol. 1997;41:404–7.
73. Hochstrasser H, Bauer P, Walter U, et al. Ceruloplasmin gene variations and substantia nigra hyperechogenicity in Parkinson disease. Neurology. 2004;63:1912–7.
74. Mariani R, Arosio C, Pelucchi S, et al. Iron chelation therapy in aceruloplasminaemia: study of a patient with a novel missense mutation. Gut. 2004;53:756–8.
75. Boddaert N, Le Quan Sang KH, Rotig A, et al. Selective iron chelation in Friedreich ataxia: biologic and clinical implications. Blood. 2007;110:401–8.
76. Xu X, Pin S, Gathinji M, Fuchs R, Harris ZL. Aceruloplasminemia: an inherited neurodegenerative disease with impairment of iron homeostasis. Ann N Y Acad Sci. 2004;1012:299–305.
77. Kuhn J, Bewermeyer H, Miyajima H, Takahashi Y, Kuhn KF, Hoogenraad TU. Treatment of symptomatic heterozygous aceruloplasminemia with oral zinc sulphate. Brain Dev. 2007;29:450–3.
78. Yonekawa M, Okabe T, Asamoto Y, Ohta M. A case of hereditary ceruloplasmin deficiency with iron deposition in the brain associated with chorea, dementia, diabetes mellitus and retinal pigmentation: administration of fresh-frozen human plasma. Eur Neurol. 1999;42:157–62.
79. Harris ZL, Durley AP, Man TK, Gitlin JD. Targeted gene disruption reveals an essential role for ceruloplasmin in cellular iron efflux. Proc Natl Acad Sci USA. 1999;96:10812–7.
80. Cherukuri S, Potla R, Sarkar J, Nurko S, Harris ZL, Fox PL. Unexpected role of ceruloplasmin in intestinal iron absorption. Cell Metab. 2005;2:309–19.
81. Gouya L, Muzeau F, Robreau AM, et al. Genetic study of variation in normal mouse iron homeostasis reveals ceruloplasmin as an HFE-hemochromatosis modifier gene. Gastroenterology. 2007;132:679–86.
82. Hahn P, Qian Y, Dentchev T, et al. Disruption of ceruloplasmin and hephaestin in mice causes retinal iron overload and retinal degeneration with features of age-related macular degeneration. Proc Natl Acad Sci USA. 2004;101:13850–5.
83. Heilmeyer L, Keller W, Vivell O, et al. Congenital atransferrinemia in a 7-year-old girl. Dtsch Med Wochenschr. 1961;86:1745–51.
84. Yefimova MG, Jeanny JC, Guillonneau X, et al. Iron, ferritin, transferrin, and transferrin receptor in the adult rat retina. Invest Ophthalmol Vis Sci. 2000;41:2343–51.
85. Bloch B, Popovici T, Levin MJ, Tuil D, Kahn A. Transferrin gene expression visualized in oligodendrocytes of the rat brain by using in situ hybridization and immunohistochemistry. Proc Natl Acad Sci USA. 1985;82:6706–10.
86. Ponka P, Schulman HM. Acquisition of iron from transferrin regulates reticulocyte heme synthesis. J Biol Chem. 1985;260:14717–21.
87. Kearney SL, Nemeth E, Neufeld EJ, et al. Urinary hepcidin in congenital chronic anemias. Pediatr Blood Cancer. 2007;48:57–63.
88. Trombini P, Coliva T, Nemeth E, et al. Effects of plasma transfusion on hepcidin production in human congenital hypotransferrinemia. Haematologica. 2007;92:1407–10.
89. Hayashi A, Wada Y, Suzuki T, Shimizu A. Studies on familial hypotransferrinemia: unique clinical course and molecular pathology. Am J Hum Genet. 1993;53:201–13.
90. Beutler E, Gelbart T, Lee P, Trevino R, Fernandez MA, Fairbanks VF. Molecular characterization of a case of atransferrinemia. Blood. 2000;96:4071–4.
91. Heilmeyer L, Keller W, Vivell O, Betke K, Woehler F, Keiderling W. Congenital atransferrinemia. Schweiz Med Wochenschr. 1961;91:1203.
92. Asada-Senju M, Maeda T, Sakata T, Hayashi A, Suzuki T. Molecular analysis of the transferrin gene in a patient with hereditary hypotransferrinemia. J Hum Genet. 2002;47:355–9.

93. Knisely AS, Gelbart T, Beutler E. Molecular characterization of a third case of human atransferrinemia. Blood. 2004;104:2607.
94. Aslan D, Crain K, Beutler E. A new case of human atransferrinemia with a previously undescribed mutation in the transferrin gene. Acta Haematol. 2007;118:244–7.
95. Goldwurm S, Casati C, Venturi N, et al. Biochemical and genetic defects underlying human congenital hypotransferrinemia. Hematol J. 2000;1:390–8.
96. Van Rensburg SJ, Carstens ME, Potocnik FC, van der Spuy G, van der Walt BJ, Taljaard JJ. Transferrin C2 and Alzheimer's disease: another piece of the puzzle found? Med Hypotheses. 1995;44:268–72.
97. Zambenedetti P, De Bellis G, Biunno I, Musicco M, Zatta P. Transferrin C2 variant does confer a risk for Alzheimer's disease in caucasians. J Alzheimers Dis. 2003;5:423–7.
98. Lee PL, Halloran C, Trevino R, Felitti V, Beutler E. Human transferrin G277S mutation: a risk factor for iron deficiency anaemia. Br J Haematol. 2001;115:329–33.
99. Delanghe J, Verstraelen H, Pynaert I, et al. Human transferrin G277S mutation and iron deficiency in pregnancy. Br J Haematol. 2006;132:249–50.
100. Westerhausen M, Meuret G. Transferrin-immune complex disease. Acta Haematol. 1977;57:96–101.
101. Alyanakian MA, Taes Y, Bensaid M, et al. Monoclonal immunoglobulin with antitransferrin activity: a rare cause of hypersideremia with increased transferrin saturation. Blood. 2007;109:359–61.
102. Trenor III CC, Campagna DR, Sellers VM, Andrews NC, Fleming MD. The molecular defect in hypotransferrinemic mice. Blood. 2000;96:1113–8.
103. Craven CM, Alexander J, Eldridge M, Kushner JP, Bernstein S, Kaplan J. Tissue distribution and clearance kinetics of non-transferrin-bound iron in the hypotransferrinemic mouse: a rodent model for hemochromatosis. Proc Natl Acad Sci USA. 1987;84:3457–61.
104. Weinstein DA, Roy CN, Fleming MD, Loda MF, Wolfsdorf JI, Andrews NC. Inappropriate expression of hepcidin is associated with iron refractory anemia: implications for the anemia of chronic disease. Blood. 2002;100:3776–81.
105. Cazzola M, Bergamaschi G, Tonon L, et al. Hereditary hyperferritinemia-cataract syndrome: relationship between phenotypes and specific mutations in the iron-responsive element of ferritin light-chain mRNA. Blood. 1997;90:814–21.
106. Bosio S, Campanella A, Gramaglia E, et al. C29G in the iron-responsive element of L-ferritin: a new mutation associated with hyperferritinemia-cataract. Blood Cells Mol Dis. 2004;33:31–4.
107. Lachlan KL, Temple IK, Mumford AD. Clinical features and molecular analysis of seven British kindreds with hereditary hyperferritinaemia cataract syndrome. Eur J Hum Genet. 2004;12:790–6.
108. Sanders SJ, Suri M, Ross I. Hereditary hyperferritinaemia-cataract syndrome and differential diagnosis of hereditary haemochromatosis. Postgrad Med J. 2003;79:600–1.
109. Wong K, Barbin Y, Chakrabarti S, Adams P. A point mutation in the iron-responsive element of the L-ferritin in a family with hereditary hyperferritinemia cataract syndrome. Can J Gastroenterol. 2005;19:253–5.
110. Vanita V, Hejtmancik JF, Hennies HC, et al. Sutural cataract associated with a mutation in the ferritin light chain gene (FTL) in a family of Indian origin. Mol Vis. 2006;12:93–9.
111. van der Klooster JM. Hereditary hyperferritinaemia-cataract syndrome. Ned Tijdschr Geneeskd. 2003;147:1923–8.
112. Cicilano M, Zecchina G, Roetto A, et al. Recurrent mutations in the iron regulatory element of L-ferritin in hereditary hyperferritinemia-cataract syndrome. Haematologica. 1999;84:489–92.
113. Ismail AR, Lachlan KL, Mumford AD, Temple IK, Hodgkins PR. Hereditary hyperferritinemia cataract syndrome: ocular, genetic, and biochemical findings. Eur J Ophthalmol. 2006;16:153–60.
114. Simsek S, Nanayakkara PW, Keek JM, Faber LM, Bruin KF, Pals G. Two Dutch families with hereditary hyperferritinaemia-cataract syndrome and heterozygosity for an HFE-related haemochromatosis gene mutation. Neth J Med. 2003;61:291–5.
115. Campagnoli MF, Pimazzoni R, Bosio S, et al. Onset of cataract in early infancy associated with a 32G C transition in the iron responsive element of L-ferritin. Eur J Pediatr. 2002;161:499–502.
116. Garcia-Erce JA, Salvador Osuna C. Genetics of iron overloads and hereditary hyperferritinemia cataract syndrome. An Med Interna. 2003;20:213–4.
117. Ladero JM, Balas A, Garcia-Sanchez F, Vicario JL, Diaz-Rubio M. Hereditary hyperferritinemia-cataract syndrome. Study of a new family in Spain. Rev Esp Enferm Dig. 2004;96:507–11.
118. Balas A, Aviles MJ, Garcia-Sanchez F, Vicario JL. Description of a new mutation in the L-ferrin iron-responsive element associated with hereditary hyperferritinemia-cataract syndrome in a Spanish family. Blood. 1999;93:4020–1.
119. Cervera Bravo A, Sebastian Planas M, Alarabe Alarabe A, Diez Saenz A, Aviles Egea MJ, Balas Perez A. Isolated hyperferritinemia in a healthy male infant: hereditary hyperferritinemia-cataract syndrome. An Esp Pediatr. 2000;52:267–70.
120. Mumford AD, Vulliamy T, Lindsay J, Watson A. Hereditary hyperferritinemia-cataract syndrome: two novel mutations in the L-ferritin iron-responsive element. Blood. 1998;91:367–8.

121. Cremonesi L, Foglieni B, Fermo I, et al. Identification of two novel mutations in the 5′-untranslated region of H-ferritin using denaturing high performance liquid chromatography scanning. Haematologica. 2003;88: 1110–6.
122. Garcia-Erce JA, Salvador-Osuna C, Cortes T, Perez-Lungmus G. Congenital cataract syndrome and hyperferritinemia. Med Clin (Barc). 1999;112:398.
123. Ferrante M, Geubel AP, Fevery J, Marogy G, Horsmans Y, Nevens F. Hereditary hyperferritinaemia-cataract syndrome: a challenging diagnosis for the hepatogastroenterologist. Eur J Gastroenterol Hepatol. 2005;17:1247–53.
124. Papanikolaou G, Chandrinou H, Bouzas E, et al. Hereditary hyperferritinemia cataract syndrome in three unrelated families of western Greek origin caused by the C39>G mutation of L-ferritin IRE. Blood Cells Mol Dis. 2006;36:33–40.
125. Garderet L, Hermelin B, Gorin NC, Rosmorduc O. Hereditary hyperferritinemia-cataract syndrome: a novel mutation in the iron-responsive element of the L-ferritin gene in a French family. Am J Med. 2004;117:138–9.
126. Del Castillo Rueda A, Fernandez Ruano ML. Hereditary hyperferritinemia cataracts syndrome in a Spanish family caused by the A40G mutation (Paris) in the L-ferritin (FTL) gene associated with the mutation H63D in the HFE gene. Med Clin (Barc). 2007;129:414–7.
127. Perez de Nanclares G, Castano L, Martul P, et al. Molecular analysis of hereditary hyperferritinemia-cataract syndrome in a large Basque family. J Pediatr Endocrinol Metab. 2001;14:295–300.
128. Aguilar-Martinez P, Biron C, Masmejean C, Jeanjean P, Schved JF. A novel mutation in the iron responsive element of ferritin L-subunit gene as a cause for hereditary hyperferritinemia-cataract syndrome. Blood. 1996;88:1895.
129. Hughes M, Vosylius P. Dual diagnoses of hereditary hyperferritinaemia-cataract syndrome and hereditary haemochromatosis. Clin Lab Haematol. 2006;28:357–9.
130. Barton JC, Beutler E, Gelbart T. Coinheritance of alleles associated with hemochromatosis and hereditary hyperferritinemia-cataract syndrome. Blood. 1998;92:4480.
131. Phillips JD, Warby CA, Kushner JP. Identification of a novel mutation in the L-ferritin IRE leading to hereditary hyperferritinemia-cataract syndrome. Am J Med Genet A. 2005;134A:77–9.
132. Camaschella C, Zecchina G, Lockitch G, et al. A new mutation (G51C) in the iron-responsive element (IRE) of L-ferritin associated with hyperferritinaemia-cataract syndrome decreases the binding affinity of the mutated IRE for iron-regulatory proteins. Br J Haematol. 2000;108:480–2.
133. Girelli D, Piccoli P, Corrocher R. "Hyperferritinemia-cataract syndrome." Description of a new hereditary disease, from anamnesis to molecular diagnosis. Minerva Med. 1997;88:405–10.
134. Cazzola M, Foglieni B, Bergamaschi G, Levi S, Lazzarino M, Arosio P. A novel deletion of the L-ferritin iron-responsive element responsible for severe hereditary hyperferritinaemia-cataract syndrome. Br J Haematol. 2002;116:667–70.
135. Okamoto N, Wada S, Oga T, et al. Hereditary ceruloplasmin deficiency with hemosiderosis. Hum Genet. 1996;97:755–8.
136. Harris ZL, Klomp LW, Gitlin JD. Aceruloplasminemia: an inherited neurodegenerative disease with impairment of iron homeostasis. Am J Clin Nutr. 1998;67:972S–7.
137. Nagata M, Takiyama Y, Shimazaki H, Nakano I, Miyajima H. A case of aceruloplasminemia presenting as cerebellar ataxia with homozygous mutation nt2602 delG. No To Shinkei. 2004;56:885–9.
138. Bosio S, De Gobbi M, Roetto A, et al. Anemia and iron overload due to compound heterozygosity for novel ceruloplasmin mutations. Blood. 2002;100:2246–8.
139. Daimon M, Kato T, Kawanami T, et al. A nonsense mutation of the ceruloplasmin gene in hereditary ceruloplasmin deficiency with diabetes mellitus. Biochem Biophys Res Commun. 1995;217:89–95.
140. Takahashi Y, Miyajima H, Shirabe S, Nagataki S, Suenaga A, Gitlin JD. Characterization of a nonsense mutation in the ceruloplasmin gene resulting in diabetes and neurodegenerative disease. Hum Mol Genet. 1996;5:81–4.
141. Miyajima H, Kono S, Takahashi Y, Sugimoto M, Sakamoto M, Sakai N. Cerebellar ataxia associated with heteroallelic ceruloplasmin gene mutation. Neurology. 2001;57:2205–10.
142. Takeuchi Y, Yoshikawa M, Tsujino T, et al. A case of aceruloplasminaemia: abnormal serum ceruloplasmin protein without ferroxidase activity. J Neurol Neurosurg Psychiatry. 2002;72:543–5.
143. Hofmann WP, Welsch C, Takahashi Y, et al. Identification and in silico characterization of a novel compound heterozygosity associated with hereditary aceruloplasminemia. Scand J Gastroenterol. 2007;42:1088–94.
144. Hellman NE, Kono S, Miyajima H, Gitlin JD. Biochemical analysis of a missense mutation in aceruloplasminemia. J Biol Chem. 2002;277:1375–80.
145. Shang HF, Jiang XF, Burgunder JM, Chen Q, Zhou D. Novel mutation in the ceruloplasmin gene causing a cognitive and movement disorder with diabetes mellitus. Mov Disord. 2006;21:2217–20.
146. Yomono H, Kurisaki H, Murayama S, Hebisawa A, Miyajima H, Takahashi Y. An autopsy case of multiple system atrophy with a heteroallelic ceruloplasmin gene mutation. Rinsho Shinkeigaku. 2003;43:398–402.

147. Di Raimondo D, Pinto A, Tuttolomondo A, Fernandez P, Camaschella C, Licata G. Aceruloplasminemia: a case report. Intern Emerg Med. 2008;3:395–9.
148. Hatanaka Y, Okano T, Oda K, Yamamoto K, Yoshida K. Aceruloplasminemia with juvenile-onset diabetes mellitus caused by exon skipping in the ceruloplasmin gene. Intern Med. 2003;42:599–604.
149. Yazaki M, Yoshida K, Nakamura A, et al. A novel splicing mutation in the ceruloplasmin gene responsible for hereditary ceruloplasmin deficiency with hemosiderosis. J Neurol Sci. 1998;156:30–4.
150. Yoshida K, Furihata K, Takeda S, et al. A mutation in the ceruloplasmin gene is associated with systemic hemosiderosis in humans. Nat Genet. 1995;9:267–72.

Chapter 22
Iron and Liver Disease

Darrell H.G. Crawford, Linda M. Fletcher, and Kris V. Kowdley

Keywords Alcohol • Cirrhosis • Hepatitis C virus • Hepcidin • Iron • Steatosis

1 Introduction

Altered iron metabolism, as demonstrated by the presence of increased hepatic iron stores and elevated serum ferritin concentration, is a relatively common feature of various liver diseases, including hepatitis C virus infection, nonalcoholic fatty liver disease, and alcoholic liver injury. Hepatic siderosis is also present in a significant proportion of patients with end-stage liver disease. The pathophysiological basis of excess hepatic iron in these conditions is increasingly understood and relates to changes in hepcidin synthesis, altered expression of intestinal iron transporters and increased intestinal iron absorption, as well as hepatic necroinflammation with a concomitant cellular redistribution of liver iron stores. There is evidence in many of these conditions that the presence of excess iron adversely affects the natural history of liver diseases and contributes to an acceleration of disease progression and a higher rate of adverse clinical events, as well as increased mortality before and after liver transplantation. Despite this emerging evidence, therapeutic strategies designed to normalize iron indices in these conditions are not widely practiced and remain a potential area for further investigation.

2 Iron and End-Stage Liver Disease

2.1 Prevalence

Increased hepatic iron stores are commonly observed in patients with advanced cirrhosis. Ludwig et al. [1] described positive iron staining in 145 (32.4%) of 447 cirrhotic livers from a North American population. In 38 cases (8.5%), the hepatic iron index was within the hemochromatosis range, but only five subjects appeared to have homozygous hemochromatosis. In a similar study conducted in Australian patients, Stuart et al. [2] found remarkably similar results whereby 104

D.H.G. Crawford, M.D. (✉) • L.M. Fletcher, Ph.D.
Discipline of Medicine, The University of Queensland

The Gallipoli Medical Research Foundation, Greenslopes Hospital, Brisbane, QLD, Australia
e-mail: d.crawford@uq.edu.au;

K.V. Kowdley, M.D.
Center for Liver Disease, Digestive Disease Institute, Virginia Mason Medical Center, Seattle, WA, USA
e-mail: kkowdley@u.washington.edu

G.J. Anderson and G. McLaren (eds.), *Iron Physiology and Pathophysiology in Humans*,
Nutrition and Health, DOI 10.1007/978-1-60327-485-2_22,

(36.8%) of 282 explants had positive iron staining. Grade 3 or 4 staining was present in 27 (9.5%) subjects, and only four of these subjects were homozygous for the C282Y mutation in the hemochromatosis gene (*HFE*). The prevalence of iron deposition was much greater in patients with hepatocellular-type liver diseases compared to biliary diseases in both the North American and Australian populations. Similar to altered iron indices in non-cirrhotic patients, the serum ferritin concentration was higher in patients with increased hepatic iron stores. Transferrin saturation was also increased in those with higher iron stores, reflecting reduced transferrin synthesis as well altered serum iron concentration.

2.2 Pathology

In cases of advanced cirrhosis-associated iron overload, excess iron deposition appears to be greatest in hepatocytes; however, significant amounts of stainable iron are usually also present in Kupffer cells. Iron deposition of variable intensity is seen in septal macrophages, biliary epithelium, and blood vessels. Of interest, proliferating bile ductules often have heavy iron staining which is not usually seen in anatomical bile ducts, suggesting different cellular uptake mechanisms between these two structures [1, 3]. There is often substantial variability in the intensity of iron deposition and quantitative measurements of hepatic iron concentration within the same cirrhotic liver. Iron deposition is often patchy and this is caused by an uneven distribution within the parenchyma, variable degrees of steatosis, and large bands of fibrous tissue that contain little or no iron. Accurate quantification of liver iron stores in this condition is difficult and multiple sampling from different sites is necessary [2, 4].

2.3 Pathogenesis of Increased Iron Stores in End-Stage Liver Disease

As previously stated, in most patients, the increased liver iron concentration occurs independently of the common mutation in *HFE* and the prevalence of homozygosity for the C282Y mutation in hepatic explants with increased iron stores obtained at the time of liver transplantation varies from 0% to 20% [5, 6]. The pathogenesis of increased iron deposition is multifactorial and important associations include more severe liver disease, hepatocellular rather than cholestatic disease, male gender, and spur cell anemia [2, 7]. The exact mechanism by which iron accumulates most likely involves increased intestinal iron absorption as well as a redistribution of tissue storage iron from hepatocytes to Kupffer cells and macrophages. Increased intestinal iron absorption has been reported in 30–100% of patients with cirrhosis, and recent advances in the understanding of iron absorption have enabled detailed investigation of the molecular mechanisms associated with enhanced iron uptake [8–12]. Stuart et al. studied small intestinal biopsies from patients with cirrhosis and showed a threefold increased gene expression of divalent metal transporter *1 (DMT 1)* and a 1.8-fold increased ferroportin gene expression [13]. Thus, an upregulation of intestinal iron transporters may play an important role in the pathogenesis of cirrhosis-associated iron overload. These changes may be associated with reduced levels of hepcidin as Detivaud et al. [14] found that hepcidin gene expression inversely correlated with increasing fibrosis. However, Bergmann and colleagues assessed iron-related gene expression in 22 human cirrhotic livers and found similar levels of hepcidin mRNA in both control and cirrhotic livers. Furthermore, hepcidin expression correlated with hepatic iron concentration, suggesting appropriate hepcidin regulation in cirrhosis [15]. The number of control samples utilized in this study was small and they were obtained mostly from livers of patients with malignancy, which of itself may be associated with altered hepcidin expression. Whether reduced hepcidin levels account, in part, for hemosiderosis in cirrhosis remains controversial and larger studies including assays of circulating hepcidin concentration are required to fully answer this question.

The reason why iron accumulation is less common in biliary diseases compared to hepatocellular diseases is unclear. Hepatocellular diseases remain more strongly associated with iron accumulation than biliary diseases even after adjustment for severity of liver disease. There is experimental evidence that following bile duct ligation, rodents have reduced intestinal iron absorption and the underrepresentation of biliary diseases in patients with cirrhosis-associated iron overload may partly be explained by this observation. In addition, iron stores often correlate with the severity of inflammation, suggesting that damaged hepatocytes may be a source of iron or that iron acts synergistically with a number of causes of hepatocyte injury to accelerate liver damage by enhanced production of reactive oxygen species or interaction with viral proteins.

The role that non-transferrin-bound iron (NTBI) plays in the development of cirrhosis-associated iron overload is also unclear. It has been shown that NTBI is efficiently taken up by hepatocytes. The reduced synthesis of transferrin in cirrhosis and the resultant rise in transferrin saturation can increase circulating NTBI levels, and this is consistent with increased cellular iron deposition [16].

There exists an interesting association between spur cell anemia and the presence of hepatic siderosis [16–19]. Spur cell anemia is an uncommon hemolytic anemia caused by alterations in the erythrocyte membrane lecithin–phospholipid ratio resulting in acanthocytosis. In one study, 57% of patients with hepatic iron concentration greater than 80 μmol/g dry weight had spur cell anemia and the majority of patients with spur cell anemia had alcoholic liver disease. Furthermore, it is a marker of advanced disease and is associated with a poor prognosis as death usually occurs within 6 months. It is uncertain if the underlying hemolysis is associated with increased intestinal iron absorption, although this would seem a plausible reason for the association.

2.4 Prognostic Significance of Cirrhosis-Associated Iron Overload

There is emerging evidence that the presence of hemosiderosis in the cirrhotic liver has significant prognostic implications. As stated above, hemosiderosis is strongly associated with more advanced liver disease, higher Child-Pugh scores, and higher MELD scores [2]. In one study, patients with siderosis had reduced survival time without transplantation compared to patients without siderosis (23 months vs. 85 months) and patients with Child's A cirrhosis and siderosis had a much shorter time median survival time than those without siderosis [20]. The effect of siderosis on the rate of clinical deterioration and mortality remained significant after correction for severity of liver disease [20]. Furthermore, Ganne-Carrié et al. showed in a longitudinal study of 229 consecutive subjects that increased liver iron content was predictive of higher mortality in alcoholic patients [21]. More recently, it has emerged that elevated serum ferritin concentration is highly predictive of death or adverse clinical outcomes in patients awaiting liver transplantation. In a dual-center study of patients in Australia and North America, Walker et al. showed that baseline serum ferritin greater than 200 μg/L was an independent factor predicting 180-day and 1-year mortality and this effect was independent of MELD score, age, and the presence of hepatocellular carcinoma [22]. In a validation cohort, it was shown that all subjects who died awaiting liver transplantation had a baseline serum ferritin concentration greater than 500 μg/L and serum ferritin concentration and MELD were both independent predictors of waiting list mortality. The predictive value of serum ferritin may be related to its role as a measure of liver iron stores or as a marker of hepatic necroinflammatory activity. Consistent with these observations, Brandhagen et al. [5] showed that patients with significant iron loading at the time of transplant had reduced 1 and 5 year survival compared to controls (48% vs. 77%). Reduced survival was largely attributed to fungal infections.

Collectively, these observations lend significant support to the hypothesis that patients with end-stage liver disease who accumulate excess liver iron are more likely to have an adverse clinical outcome. However, these findings have not been translated into any meaningful therapeutic intervention due, in part, to the difficulties associated with venesection of patients with advanced disease. Improved understanding of the biochemical regulators of iron metabolism is likely to provide new therapeutic tools to treat excess iron accumulation, and studies of such agents in patients with cirrhosis-associated iron overload would be of great interest.

3 Nonalcoholic Fatty Liver Disease

3.1 Background

Nonalcoholic fatty liver disease (NAFLD) is the most common liver disease in the USA and many Western countries [23, 24]. Nonalcoholic steatohepatitis (NASH) is a more serious form of this disorder that affects a subgroup of these patients and may progress to cirrhosis, end-stage liver disease, and hepatocellular carcinoma. The etiopathogenesis of NASH has been proposed to occur via a number of "hits" [25]. Initially, hepatic and/or peripheral insulin resistance along with increased circulating free fatty acids combine to lead to hepatic fat accumulation which is stored in the form of triglycerides, resulting in macrovesicular steatosis. Additional sources of oxidative stress, such as mitochondrial dysfunction [26], increased activity of prooxidant cytochromes such as cytochrome P450 2E1 [27], and other factors may overwhelm antioxidant functions within hepatocytes, leading to cytotoxicity, necroinflammation, and variable degrees of fibrosis.

3.2 Pathogenesis of NASH due to Iron Overload

Excess iron deposition within the liver has been proposed as a cause of necroinflammation and fibrosis in NAFLD. The metal catalyzes the production of reactive oxygen species (ROS) via the Fenton reaction, which may lead to lipid peroxidation and activation of Kupffer cells, resulting in production of pro-inflammatory cytokines. Iron-induced toxicity within the liver is postulated to occur via activation of an oxidative stress cascade which causes damage to membranes, resulting in mitochondrial and other organelle dysfunction, cell injury, and death [27]. In addition, ROS may cause DNA damage via production of DNA adducts such as the modified guanosine base 8-hydroxydeoxyguanosine (8-OHdG). A recent study compared 38 NASH patients with iron overload to 24 patients with NAFLD. The iron-loaded NASH patients had significantly higher levels of 8-OHdG, and this was positively associated with the histologic total iron score [28]. Furthermore, iron depletion resulted in a significant decrease in 8-OHdG levels in a subset of the patients.

There are also data pointing to a relationship between body iron stores and insulin signaling; thus, iron overload may exacerbate insulin resistance, a central feature of NAFLD and NASH. Several studies have shown that hyperinsulinemia and insulin resistance with or without overt diabetes are common in patients with iron overload [29, 30]. It has been shown that increased iron stores inhibit extraction and metabolism of insulin at the level of the hepatocyte [31]. Serum iron and transferrin may play a role in adipocyte lipolysis and interfere with glucose transport [32, 33]. In vitro studies have shown that iron may reduce the affinity of insulin binding to its receptor and may reduce gene expression [34]. In fact, the unique clinical syndrome called "*I*nsulin *R*esistance-associated *H*epatic *I*ron *O*verload" (IR-HIO; also called "Dysmetabolic Hepatic Iron Overload") describes a syndrome of hepatic iron loading associated-insulin resistance, defined as body mass index of >25, diabetes, or hyperlipidemia [35]. Many of these patients also appear to have NAFLD [36].

Several human studies have examined iron depletion as a treatment for NAFLD, diabetes, and hyperferritinemia in the absence of hemochromatosis. Iron depletion appeared to improve insulin resistance, insulin secretion, and glycemic control in patients with type 2 diabetes and hyperferritinemia [37], and in patients with insulin resistance syndrome in the absence of liver disease or diabetes [38], as well as in patients with type 2 diabetes mellitus and suspected NAFLD [39]. Iron depletion was also shown to be effective in nondiabetic patients with NASH, with or without elevated serum ferritin levels [40, 41], and in patients with biopsy-proven NAFLD accompanied by hepatic iron loading [42, 43]. In summary, iron depletion appears to improve insulin resistance and liver enzyme levels in patients with NAFLD and insulin secretion in patients with type 2 diabetes and hyperferritinemia. In addition, iron has been shown to activate hepatic stellate cells, which are central to hepatic fibrogenesis and initiate the process leading to cirrhosis [44].

Heterozygosity for the common *HFE* mutations (C282Y/wild type and H63D/wild type) has been shown to be associated with increased transferrin saturation in normal individuals but does not appear to result in significant hepatic iron overload [45]. However, several studies have suggested that carriage of heterozygous *HFE* mutations may be associated with increased hepatic iron deposition and may contribute to liver injury in NASH. In an Australian study, George and colleagues found that a surprisingly high proportion of 51 NASH patients (31.4%) were either C282Y homozygotes or C282Y/H63D compound heterozygotes compared to 12% in 2,375 population controls [46]. Furthermore, the presence of hepatic iron was an independent risk factor for advanced hepatic fibrosis in this cohort. This seminal study has been followed by a number of others examining the prevalence of *HFE* mutations in NAFLD and NASH, as well as the contribution of *HFE* mutations to hepatic iron deposition and advanced histologic features of NAFLD.

Bonkovsky and colleagues examined a cohort of patients with NASH from the Boston area and found that the prevalence of the H63D mutation was higher among the NASH patients than in a historical control population [47]. Another Australian study concluded that Caucasian patients with NASH were more likely to carry the C282Y mutation, although presence of these mutations was not associated with increased risk of advanced disease [48]. A number of additional studies [49–53] have examined the role of *HFE* mutations in NAFLD, and six of eight studies performed in countries with predominantly Caucasian populations have concluded that *HFE* mutations are more common among patients with NASH or NAFLD. By contrast, studies in populations where the common *HFE* mutations are infrequent (Brazil, China, Japan) have concluded that these mutations do not contribute to the development of NAFLD or NASH [54–57]. A subsequent meta-analysis did not find a higher overall prevalence among patients with NAFLD [58]. It is likely that ascertainment bias, lack of a similar control population, case definition, and sample size influence the discrepancies in the literature with regard to the prevalence of *HFE* mutations in patients with NAFLD and NASH.

Several studies have now also examined the relationship between *HFE* mutations and the presence of NASH or severe NASH (defined as increased histologic activity and/or advanced hepatic fibrosis) with disparate results. Five studies reported that hepatic iron stores among patients with *HFE* mutations and NASH are increased compared to those without *HFE* mutations [46, 49–52]. Two studies have found a positive relationship between *HFE* mutations and advanced hepatic fibrosis in NASH [47, 49]. In the original study, George et al. found that hepatic iron content, but not presence of the C282Y mutation, was a risk factor for advanced hepatic fibrosis [46]. However, an important confounding variable in these early studies is that insulin resistance or type 2 diabetes was also associated with advanced hepatic fibrosis [48, 49, 52, 53]. Based on the previous data that increased iron stores are associated with insulin resistance, it is possible that *HFE* mutations may contribute to the pathogenesis of NASH either directly by increasing body iron stores or indirectly through iron-related tissue injury. One study examined the relationship between hepatic iron content and subsequent liver disease complications. Younossi et al. measured the hepatic iron concentration of archived liver biopsy specimens from 65 patients with NAFLD [59]. These authors did not find a relationship between iron content and subsequent complications. However, these data should be interpreted with caution given the small sample size. We have recently published a population-based examination of the relationship between serum transferrin saturation (TS) and subsequent cirrhosis-related hospitalization or death [60]. In comparison to those with low TS (<40%) and low alcohol consumption (≤1 drink/day) who had an incidence of cirrhosis/liver cancer of 70/100,000 person-years, the incidence of cirrhosis and liver cancer was increased in persons with elevated TS (≥40%) and low alcohol consumption (154/100,000; adjusted hazard ratio, 2.2; 95% confidence interval, 1.3–3.8). Although this study did not specifically examine patients with NAFLD, these data support the concept that body iron stores may contribute to liver disease complications even in the absence of alcohol intake.

We reported that presence of the C282Y mutation was associated with advanced hepatic fibrosis in a cohort of 126 patients with NASH ascertained from several centers in the USA and Canada [49]. Data from 126 NASH subjects were collected from six North American centers. The prevalence of heterozygous C282Y and H63D *HFE* mutations was 14.3% and 21.4%, respectively. Among Caucasians, the prevalence of the C282Y mutation (both the C282Y/wild type and C282Y/H63D) was significantly higher in subjects with NASH (21.6%) compared to the expected prevalence based on previous studies in the general population (11.4% and 12%) [61, 62]. These results suggest that subjects carrying the C282Y mutation may be at increased risk for NASH.

Patients with *HFE* mutations were also more likely to have stainable hepatic iron compared with wild-type subjects (28% vs. 19%, *NS*), and C282Y heterozygotes and C282Y/H63D compound heterozygotes were more likely to have stainable iron in the liver compared with WT subjects (43%, $p=0.058$ and 80%, $p=0.009$, respectively, vs. 19% for *HFE* wild type). Caucasian patients with the C282Y mutation were more likely to have stainable hepatic iron compared to wild-type subjects (50% vs. 15%, $p=0.012$). C282Y heterozygotes were also more likely to have bridging fibrosis or cirrhosis (44% vs. 21%, $p=0.05$) compared with patients with other *HFE* genotypes. A history of diabetes mellitus was independently associated with advanced fibrosis on multivariable regression (OR, 3.90; 95% CI, 1.55–9.84; $p=0.004$). C282Y heterozygosity showed a positive association with advanced hepatic fibrosis (OR, 2.35; 95% CI, 0.82–6.75; $p=0.112$), especially among Caucasians ($n=98$) (OR, 2.97; 95% CI, 0.97–9.14; $p=0.057$) but these trends did not reach significance. A subsequent preliminary study found that reticuloendothelial system (RES) cell iron deposition was independently associated with NASH and more severe histologic features in a large cohort from the NASH Clinical Research Network [63].

A recent large study by Valenti et al. has been another addition to the literature examining the relationship between *HFE* mutations and NAFLD [64]. A total of 587 Italian patients with NAFLD and 187 control subjects were studied. Inclusion criteria included elevated serum liver enzymes and steatosis with or without hyperferritinemia. The presence of "predominantly hepatocellular" iron deposition was associated a hepatic fibrosis stage >1 (95% confidence interval, 1.2–2.3) compared to those without hepatic iron deposition. However, the presence of *HFE* mutations was not associated with an increased risk of fibrosis stage >1 or with hepatic fibrosis or advanced hepatic fibrosis. As discussed in an accompanying editorial, a number of factors such as case definition and prevalence of *HFE* mutations may explain the differences between this study and previous results. Nevertheless, these data support further investigation of the effect of even mild or moderate iron loading in the liver as a pathogenetic factor in NAFLD and NASH.

4 Iron and Alcoholic Liver Disease

4.1 Background

The role of alcohol in the development of iron overload has been the source of considerable interest over an extend period of time. Indeed, the view was held for many years that hemochromatosis was a form of alcoholic or nutritional liver injury unrelated to any underlying genetic abnormality.

An improved understanding of the mechanisms of interaction between alcohol and iron is of considerable importance because both alcoholic liver disease and genetic hemochromatosis are common diseases and alcohol and iron act synergistically to exacerbate hepatocyte injury and liver fibrogenesis. The relationship between alcohol, iron, and liver disease has constantly been re-evaluated as researchers incorporate landmark discoveries related to genetics and biochemistry of these hepatotoxins into existing paradigms. The identification of the underlying genetic abnormality responsible for most cases of hereditary hemochromatosis; the discovery of specific iron transporters in enterocytes, Kupffer cells, and hepatocytes; as well as the recognition that hepcidin is a master controller of iron metabolism have all given greater clarity to our understanding of the unique interactions that exist between alcohol and iron.

The exact prevalence of excess hepatic iron in patients with alcoholic liver disease is uncertain. Studies of explants show that 65% of livers obtained from patients with a primary diagnosis of alcoholic liver disease have positive iron staining as determined by Perls' Prussian blue analysis [1, 2]. In general, this is associated with a modest increase in hepatic iron concentration – usually less than 80 μmol/g dry weight. In mild cases of alcoholic liver disease, iron is preferentially seen in hepatocytes compared to Kupffer cells and this may relate to a direct suppressive effect of alcohol on hepcidin gene expression. In later stages of disease, stainable iron is predominantly found in Kupffer cells and macrophages with lesser intensity of staining in hepatocytes. This redistribution of iron is thought to represent release of iron from damaged hepatocytes.

The true clinical significance of this observation is unclear, but some studies have shown that increased hepatic iron content is associated with greater mortality in patients with alcoholic cirrhosis [21]. Furthermore, patients with fully expressing hereditary hemochromatosis often have consumed alcohol in excess of 60 g/day. The presence of two toxic insults may potentiate more aggressive disease, and hemochromatosis subjects who consume more than 60 g/day are approximately nine times more likely to develop cirrhosis than those who drink less than this amount [65].

4.2 *Pathogenesis*

It is clear that most affected patients do not carry mutations in genes known to be involved in iron metabolism and the accumulation of iron in the majority of patients with alcoholic liver disease occurs independently of any known genetic abnormality. The pathogenesis of iron overload in alcoholic liver injury is multifactorial and due to direct effects of alcohol on proteins involved in iron metabolism, as well as nonspecific changes in iron metabolism associated with the presence of cirrhosis [66]. Studies of liver explants show that liver iron loading occurs in alcoholic liver disease as well as a variety of other liver diseases, including chronic viral hepatitis, autoimmune hepatitis, and alpha-1-antitrypsin deficiency. As discussed earlier in this chapter, cirrhosis per se promotes increased liver iron stores, and an increased hepatic iron concentration seen in those patients with alcoholic liver disease and cirrhosis is due, in part, to this phenomenon. Of more interest have been recent studies confirming an alcohol-mediated downregulation of the expression of the iron regulatory peptide hepcidin, a response consistent with increased iron absorption [67]. In male rats pair fed an alcoholic liquid diet for 12 weeks, Bridle et al. [68] showed that hepcidin gene expression was reduced sixfold compared with pair fed control animals. In mice treated with ethanol 10–20% for 7 days, Harrison-Findik et al. [69] showed that ethanol metabolism downregulated hepcidin mRNA and protein expression and this effect was abolished by inhibiting alcohol-metabolizing enzymes by the addition of 4-methylpyrazole. The downregulation in hepcidin expression was accompanied by elevated duodenal DMT-1 and ferroportin protein expression, and all of these effects were abolished by the addition of antioxidants. This suggests that alcohol-mediated oxidative stress is an important cause of the altered iron metabolism seen in alcohol-related liver injury. Furthermore, alcohol suppressed the upregulation of hepcidin mRNA expression induced by excess iron in the carbonyl iron model of iron overload, suggesting that alcohol negates the protective effect of increased hepcidin in states of iron loading [70].

The precise molecular signaling pathways which account for the downregulation of hepcidin expression by alcohol are of considerable interest. Hepcidin expression is mediated through a range of interconnecting pathways. Pathways that positively regulate hepcidin transcription include the iron responsive HFE and TfR2 pathways, the interleukin 6/STAT3 (IL6/STAT3) pathway that responds to inflammatory stimuli, and the hemojuvelin/bone morphogenic protein/SMAD pathway that appears to be required for setting basal hepcidin levels [71–74]. Negative regulators of hepcidin include anemia and hypoxia [75]. Inhibition of CEBPα activity by alcohol is involved in the downregulation of hepcidin gene expression and treatment with alcohol abolished the iron-induced upregulation of CEBPα DNA-binding activity [70]. Thus, inhibition of C/EBPα DNA-binding activity by alcohol is almost certain to play an important role in the alcohol-induced suppression of hepcidin expression.

It has also been suggested that hepatic hypoxia may play an important pathophysiological role in alcohol-related liver iron accumulation [76, 77]. Hypoxia-inducible factors (HIFs) are central regulators of the cellular response to hypoxia. Under hypoxic conditions, HIF-1α is stabilized and translocates to the nucleus where it binds to HIF-1β. The complex functions as a transcriptional activator for several genes containing hypoxia response elements within their promoter/enhancer regions. It modulates the expression of more than 100 genes involved in angiogenesis, cell survival, and iron metabolism by upregulating their expression in hypoxic regions. Hepcidin transcription is decreased when hypoxia is present, and chronic alcohol exposure leads to hypoxia in the oxygen-poor pericentral regions of the liver [78, 79].

It is proposed that the HIF complex binds to and negatively transactivates the hepcidin promoter [80, 81]. Increased levels of HIF-1α have been demonstrated in alcohol-fed rodents in association with downregulated hepcidin gene expression, suggesting that the hypoxic pathway may play a role in the altered iron homeostasis observed in alcoholic liver injury [76].

The biochemical mechanisms of toxicity in iron overload and alcohol-induced liver injury are remarkably similar and involve the generation of reactive oxygen species leading to lipid peroxidation, stellate cell activation, and progressive hepatic fibrosis [82–86]. Studies in humans strongly support the hypothesis that the combination of alcohol and iron accelerates liver injury. However, studies of alcohol/iron co-toxicity in animal models have not consistently demonstrated evidence of significant pathological sequelae. In most studies to date, the administration of alcohol to animals has not resulted in a significant increase in hepatic iron despite the aforementioned changes in the expression of the many proteins involved in iron metabolism. It is likely that this reflects the relatively short timeframe over which these studies are conducted. For example, it is well known in humans with *HFE*-associated hemochromatosis that the hepatic iron concentration increases very slowly over time and may not rise to pathological levels until the third decade, despite the genetic abnormality being present since birth. It is likely that animals need to be fed on alcohol for a much longer period of time to demonstrate an increase in hepatic iron concentration. It also has been difficult to generate models of progressive liver injury in rodent models investigating the effects of iron/alcohol co-toxicity. Tsukamoto et al. [87] were able to induce significant liver injury by feeding rats small amounts of iron in addition to intragastric alcohol. However, it is difficult to induce significant liver injury or generate products of lipid peroxidation in the traditional Leiber de Carli model of alcohol consumption, and this has hindered studies of pathological complications related to alcohol and iron co-toxicity. Achieving a higher hepatic iron concentration in the setting of a sustained period of alcohol exposure in combination with a significant inflammatory response in an animal model is a desirable quality if the pathophysiological basis of liver injury mediated by a combination of iron and alcohol is to be fully understood.

5 Hepatitis C Virus Infection

5.1 Background

It has been known for almost two decades that chronic hepatitis C (CHC) infection may be associated with elevated serum iron values and that mild to moderately increased storage iron may be present in the liver among patients with CHC. There is growing evidence that iron deposition in the liver may contribute to oxidative stress and facilitate carcinogenesis. *HFE* mutations have also been proposed as cofactors for liver disease progression in CHC, presumably via increased iron absorption and deposition in the liver. Studies of phlebotomy therapy in CHC have consistently shown improvement in serum liver biochemical tests, surrogate markers of fibrogenesis, and possibly stabilization of fibrosis. However, there are, as yet, no conclusive data that iron depletion via phlebotomy improves sustained virologic responses to interferon and ribavirin-based therapies. There remains a paucity of data examining whether iron depletion therapy slows the progression of liver disease in patients with cirrhosis or reduces the incidence of hepatocellular carcinoma among patients with CHC.

Di Bisceglie and colleagues are credited with the initial observation that over one third of patients with CHC have elevated serum iron levels and that CHC is associated with increased stainable iron in both RES cells and hepatocytes [88]. Subsequent larger studies confirmed that RES cell iron deposition was common in CHC, especially among patients with cirrhosis, and was associated with increased histologic severity [89].

5.2 Pathogenesis

A major proposed mechanism for increased iron loading in patients with CHC is the presence of *HFE* mutations. Several cross-sectional studies have examined the relationship between carriage of *HFE* mutations, pattern and degree of hepatic iron deposition, and histologic features of severity in patients with CHC. As in NAFLD and NASH, some studies have found *HFE* mutations, in particular the C282Y mutation, to be associated with increased stainable iron and/or advanced hepatic fibrosis [90–94], while others have not [89, 95–99]. In general, the C282Y mutation rather than the H63D mutation appears more likely to have a pathogenetic role [91, 93]. The most recent data supporting a role for increased iron deposition among CHC patients with *HFE* mutations are from the HALT-C study, a long-term trial in patients with advanced fibrosis. *HFE* mutations were found to be associated with increased hepatic iron content in 363 patients, all with advanced hepatic fibrosis. This study confirmed the findings of several previous reports that C282Y or H63D heterozygosity is associated with hepatic iron loading in CHC patients [90, 91, 100–102]. We previously examined the relationship between *HFE* mutations, hepatic iron concentration, and disease severity in a cohort of almost 400 patients with CHC, approximately half of whom had end-stage liver disease [90]. The prevalence of *HFE* mutations was not increased among CHC patients with end-stage liver disease when compared to patients with compensated liver disease. Additionally, there was no difference in hepatic iron concentration between patients with and without *HFE* mutations (although hepatic iron concentration was higher in men in both groups). However, among patients with compensated liver disease, CHC patients with *HFE* mutations (especially the C282Y heterozygous mutation) had significantly higher hepatic iron concentration compared to wild-type patients [90]. Other studies have found divergent results. Two studies have reported that the heterozygous H63D mutation is associated with both increased fibrosis stage and presence of cirrhosis [92, 94]. However, the majority of studies have suggested that the C282Y heterozygous mutation is more strongly associated with advanced fibrosis than the H63D mutation. Smith et al. reported that mean fibrosis stage was significantly higher among C282Y heterozygotes compared to wild-type patients (3.6 vs. 1.5) [91]. Cirrhosis was also present more often in those with the *HFE* mutation (40%) compared to those without (8.7%). We similarly found that any *HFE* mutation (C282Y and H63D) was strongly associated with bridging fibrosis or cirrhosis in individuals with compensated liver disease (OR, 18; 95% CI, 1.7–193) [90]. The odds ratio for presence of advanced fibrosis in association with C282Y was 30 (95% CI, 1.8–484) compared to 22 (95% CI, 1.8–267) for H63D mutations [90]. More importantly, carriage of *HFE* mutations was independently associated with advanced fibrosis after adjustment for gender, age and duration of disease [90]. Gehrke et al. also found an association between C282Y mutations and advanced fibrosis (OR, 2.5; 95% CI, 1.0–6.3; $p<0.05$) [93]. Geier and colleagues described a strong association between carriage of the C282Y mutation and hepatic fibrosis (OR, 4.58; 95% CI, 1.13–18.52; $p=0.026$) [22, 94]. Erhardt et al. also found a significant association between C282Y heterozygotes and cirrhosis with an odds ratio of 5.9 (95% CI, 1.6–22.6; $p<0.009$) [92]. Although a handful of studies have concluded that the C282Y mutation is not a modifier gene in CHC [95, 96, 99], the bulk of the evidence suggests that heterozygous C282Y individuals with CHC infection are most likely to have more severe hepatocellular injury and fibrosis.

There is additional evidence that iron deposition in the liver as a consequence of *HFE* mutations may contribute to disease progression. Two studies found that the C282Y mutation was associated with hepatocellular carcinoma among CHC patients [103, 104], although two other studies did not confirm this association [105, 106]. In a previous cross-sectional study of over 5,000 patients with end-stage liver disease undergoing liver transplantation, iron overload in the liver explant was independently associated with hepatocellular carcinoma among patients with CHC [107].

Iron depletion via phlebotomy has been explored as a means to slow down the progression of liver disease. Phlebotomy treatment resulted in reduction in serum liver enzymes in previously treated and untreated patients, and iron depletion prior to treatment resulted in improved sustained virologic responses to interferon monotherapy and showed improvement in hepatic necroinflammation in previously treated nonresponder patients [108]. One long-term study of iron depletion demonstrated a significant reduction in risk of hepatocellular carcinoma compared to a control group (8.6% vs. 39%, OR 0.57) [109]. The mechanism may be linked to reduction in DNA damage as manifested by reduced 8-OHdG levels [110].

In summary, there appears to be sufficient evidence that increased hepatic iron stores may be a cofactor in the progression of chronic liver disease due to CHC. Carriage of *HFE* mutations, especially the C282Y polymorphism, is associated with increased hepatic iron content compared to wild-type patients. There are also substantial data showing that *HFE* mutations are associated with advanced hepatic fibrosis in patients with CHC, although some studies have not confirmed these findings.

Van Thiel and colleagues first reported that CHC patients who responded to interferon monotherapy had significantly lower hepatic iron concentration compared to those who did not clear HCV [111]. Subsequent studies did not find hepatic iron to be a predictor of response to interferon and ribavirin combination therapy [112]. Although iron depletion via phlebotomy does not improve response to interferon and ribavirin therapy, preliminary studies suggest that iron depletion improves hepatic necroinflammation and may reduce the incidence of hepatocellular carcinoma.

Acknowledgment KVK is supported in part by NIH grant DK-02957.

References

1. Ludwig J, Hashimoto E, Porayko MK, Moyer TP, Baldus WP. Hemosiderosis in cirrhosis: a study of 447 native livers. Gastroenterology. 1997;112:882–8.
2. Stuart KA, Fletcher LM, Clouston AD, et al. Increased hepatic iron and cirrhosis: no evidence for an adverse effect on patient outcome following liver transplantation. Hepatology. 2000;32:1200–6.

3. Searle J, Kerr JFR, Halliday JW, Powell L. Iron storage disease. In: MacSween R, Anthony PP, Scheuer PJ, Portman BC, Burt AD, editors. Pathology of the liver, vol. 1. 3rd ed. London: Churchill Livingstone; 1994. p. 219–41.
4. Deugnier Y, Turlin B, Quilleuc D, et al. A reappraisal of hepatic siderosis in patients with end stage cirrhosis: practical implication for the diagnosis of hemochromatosis. Am J Surg Pathol. 1997;21:669–75.
5. Brandhagen DJ, Alvarez W, Therneau TM, et al. Iron overload in cirrhosis-HFE genotypes and outcome after liver transplantation. Hepatology. 2000;31:456–60.
6. Parolin MB, Batts KP, Wiesner RH, et al. Liver allograft iron accumulation in patients with and without pretransplantation hepatic hemosiderosis. Liver Transpl. 2002;8:331–9.
7. Pascoe A, Kerlin P, Steadman C, et al. Spur cell anemia and hepatic iron stores in patients with alcoholic liver disease undergoing orthotopic liver transplantation. Gut. 1999;45:301–5.
8. Conrad ME, Berman A, Crosby WH. Iron kinetics in Laennec's cirrhosis. Gastroenterology. 1962;43:385–90.
9. Friedman BI, Schafer JW, Schiff L. Increased iron[59] absorption in patients with hepatic cirrhosis. J Nucl Med. 1966;7:594–602.
10. Williams R, Williams HS, Scheuer PJ, Pitcher CS, Loiseau E, Sherlock S. Iron absorption and siderosis in chronic liver disease. Q J Med. 1967;141:151–66.
11. Deller DJ. Iron[59] absorption measurement by whole body counting: studies in alcoholic cirrhosis, hemochromatosis and pancreatitis. Am J Dig Dis. 1965;10:248–58.
12. Duane P, Raja KB, Simpson RJ, Peters TJ. Intestional iron absorption in chronic alcoholics. Alcohol Alcohol. 1992;27:539–44.
13. Stuart KA, Anderson GJ, Frazer DM, et al. Increased duodenal expression of divalent metal transporter 1 and iron-regulated gene 1 in cirrhosis. Hepatology. 2004;39:492–9.
14. Detivaud L, Nemeth E, Boudjema K, et al. Hepcidin levels in humans are correlated with hepatic iron stores, hemoglobin levels and hepatic function. Blood. 2005;106:746–8.
15. Bergman OM, Mathahs MM, Broadhurst KA, et al. Altered expression of iron regulatory genes in cirrhotic human livers: clues to the cause of hemosiderosis? Lab Invest. 2008;88:1349–57.
16. Kohgo Y, Ohtake T, Ikuta K, et al. Iron accumulation in alcoholic liver diseases. Alcohol Clin Exp Res. 2005;29(11 Suppl):189S–93.
17. Stillman AE, Giordano GF. Spur cell anemia associated with extra-hepatic biliary obstruction. Am J Gastroenterol. 1983;78:589–92.
18. Hitchins R, Naughton L, Kerlin P, Cobcroft R. Spur cell anemia (acanthocytosis) complicating idiopathic hemochromatosis. Pathology. 1988;20:59–61.
19. Silber R, Amarosi E, Chowe J, Kayden HJ. Spur shaped erythrocytes in Laennec's cirrhosis. N Engl J Med. 1966;275:639–43.
20. Kayali Z, Ranguelov R, Mitros F, et al. Hemosiderosis is associated with accelarated decompensation and decreased survival in patients with cirrhosis. Liver Int. 2005;25:41–8.
21. Ganne-Carrié N, Christidis C, Chastang C, et al. Liver iron is predictive of death in alcoholic cirrhosis: a multivariate study of 229 consecutive patients with alcoholic and/or hepatitis C virus cirrhosis: a prospective follow up study. Gut. 2000;46:277–82.
22. Walker NM, Stuart KA, Nicol JA, Ryan RJ, Fletcher LM, Crawford DHG. Serum ferritin concentration predicts mortality and adverse liver-related clinical events in patients listed for liver transplantation. Hepatology. 2010;51:1683–91.
23. Lazo M, Clark JM. The epidemiology of nonalcoholic fatty liver disease: a global perspective. Semin Liver Dis. 2008;28:339–50.
24. Adams LA, Lindor KD. Nonalcoholic fatty liver disease. Ann Epidemiol. 2007;17:863–9.
25. Day CP, James OF. Steatohepatitis: a tale of two "hits"? Gastroenterology. 1998;114:842–5.
26. Sanyal AJ, Campbell-Sargent C, Mirshahi F, et al. Nonalcoholic steatohepatitis: association of insulin resistance and mitochondrial abnormalities. Gastroenterology. 2001;120:1183–92.
27. Emery MG, Fisher JM, Chien JY, et al. CYP2E1 activity before and after weight loss in morbidly obese subjects with nonalcoholic fatty liver disease. Hepatology. 2003;38:428–35.
28. Fujita N, Miyachi H, Tanaka H, et al. Iron overload is associated with hepatic oxidative damage to DNA in nonalcoholic steatohepatitis. Cancer Epidemiol Biomarkers Prev. 2009;18:424–32.
29. Fernandez-Real JM, Lopez-Bermejo A, Ricart W. Cross-talk between iron metabolism and diabetes. Diabetes. 2002;51:2348–54.
30. Barton JC, Acton RT, Leiendecker-Foster C, et al. Characteristics of participants with self-reported hemochromatosis or iron overload at HEIRS study initial screening. Am J Hematol. 2008;83:126–32.
31. Niederau C, Berger M, Stremmel W, et al. Hyperinsulinaemia in non-cirrhotic haemochromatosis: impaired hepatic insulin degradation? Diabetologia. 1984;26:441–4.
32. Rumberger JM, Peters Jr T, Burrington C, Green A. Transferrin and iron contribute to the lipolytic effect of serum in isolated adipocytes. Diabetes. 2004;53:2535–41.

33. Green A, Basile R, Rumberger JM. Transferrin and iron induce insulin resistance of glucose transport in adipocytes. Metabolism. 2006;55:1042–5.
34. Fargion S, Dongiovanni P, Guzzo A, Colombo S, Valenti L, Fracanzani AL. Iron and insulin resistance. Aliment Pharmacol Ther. 2005;22 Suppl 2:61–3.
35. Mendler MH, Turlin B, Moirand R, et al. Insulin resistance-associated hepatic iron overload. Gastroenterology. 1999;117:1155–63.
36. Moirand R, Mendler MH, Guillygomarch A, Brissot P, Deugnier Y. Non-alcoholic steatohepatitis with iron: part of insulin resistance-associated hepatic iron overload? J Hepatol. 2000;33:1024–6.
37. Fernandez-Real JM, Penarroja G, Castro A, Garcia-Bragado F, Hernandez-Aguado I, Ricart W. Blood letting in high-ferritin type 2 diabetes: effects on insulin sensitivity and beta-cell function. Diabetes. 2002;51:1000–4.
38. Guillygomarch A, Mendler MH, Moirand R, et al. Venesection therapy of insulin resistance-associated hepatic iron overload. J Hepatol. 2001;35:344–9.
39. Facchini FS, Hua NW, Stoohs RA. Effect of iron depletion in carbohydrate-intolerant patients with clinical evidence of nonalcoholic fatty liver disease. Gastroenterology. 2002;122:931–9.
40. Valenti L, Fracanzani AL, Fargion S. Effect of iron depletion in patients with nonalcoholic fatty liver disease without carbohydrate intolerance. Gastroenterology. 2003;124:866–7.
41. Valenti L, Fracanzani AL, Dongiovanni P, et al. Iron depletion by phlebotomy improves insulin resistance in patients with nonalcoholic fatty liver disease and hyperferritinemia: evidence from a case–control study. Am J Gastroenterol. 2007;102:1251–8.
42. Aigner E, Theurl I, Theurl M, et al. Pathways underlying iron accumulation in human nonalcoholic fatty liver disease. Am J Clin Nutr. 2008;87:1374–83.
43. Sumida Y, Kanemasa K, Fukumoto K, et al. Effect of iron reduction by phlebotomy in Japanese patients with nonalcoholic steatohepatitis: a pilot study. Hepatol Res. 2006;36:315–21.
44. Ramm GA, Crawford DH, Powell LW, Walker NI, Fletcher LM, Halliday JW. Hepatic stellate cell activation in genetic haemochromatosis: lobular distribution, effect of increasing hepatic iron and response to phlebotomy. J Hepatol. 1997;26:584–92.
45. Pedersen P, Milman N. Genetic screening for HFE hemochromatosis in 6,020 Danish men: penetrance of C282Y, H63D, and S65C variants. Ann Hematol. 2009;88:775–84.
46. George DK, Goldwurm S, MacDonald GA, et al. Increased hepatic iron concentration in nonalcoholic steatohepatitis is associated with increased fibrosis. Gastroenterology. 1998;114:311–8.
47. Bonkovsky HL, Jawaid Q, Tortorelli K, et al. Non-alcoholic steatohepatitis and iron: increased prevalence of mutations of the HFE gene in non-alcoholic steatohepatitis. J Hepatol. 1999;31:421–9.
48. Chitturi S, Weltman M, Farrell GC, et al. HFE mutations, hepatic iron, and fibrosis: ethnic-specific association of NASH with C282Y but not with fibrotic severity. Hepatology. 2002;36:142–9.
49. Nelson JE, Bhattacharya R, Lindor KD, et al. HFE C282Y mutations are associated with advanced hepatic fibrosis in Caucasians with nonalcoholic steatohepatitis. Hepatology. 2007;46:723–9.
50. Fargion S, Mattioli M, Fracanzani AL, et al. Hyperferritinemia, iron overload, and multiple metabolic alterations identify patients at risk for nonalcoholic steatohepatitis. Am J Gastroenterol. 2001;96:2448–55.
51. Valenti L, Dongiovanni P, Fracanzani AL, et al. Increased susceptibility to nonalcoholic fatty liver disease in heterozygotes for the mutation responsible for hereditary hemochromatosis. Dig Liver Dis. 2003;35:172–8.
52. Bugianesi E, Manzini P, D'Antico S, et al. Relative contribution of iron burden, HFE mutations, and insulin resistance to fibrosis in nonalcoholic fatty liver. Hepatology. 2004;39:179–87.
53. Loria P, Lonardo A, Carulli N. Relative contribution of iron burden, HFE mutations, and insulin resistance to fibrosis in nonalcoholic fatty liver. Hepatology. 2004;39:1748–9.
54. Deguti MM, Sipahi AM, Gayotto LC, et al. Lack of evidence for the pathogenic role of iron and HFE gene mutations in Brazilian patients with nonalcoholic steatohepatitis. Braz J Med Biol Res. 2003;36:739–45.
55. Yamauchi N, Itoh Y, Tanaka Y, et al. Clinical characteristics and prevalence of GB virus C, SEN virus, and HFE gene mutation in Japanese patients with nonalcoholic steatohepatitis. J Gastroenterol. 2004;39:654–60.
56. Dhillon BK, Das R, Garewal G, et al. Frequency of primary iron overload and HFE gene mutations (C282Y, H63D and S65C) in chronic liver disease patients in North India. World J Gastroenterol. 2007;13:2956–9.
57. Duseja A, Das R, Nanda M, Das A, Garewal G, Chawla Y. Nonalcoholic steatohepatitis in Asian Indians is neither associated with iron overload nor with HFE gene mutations. World J Gastroenterol. 2005;11:393–5.
58. Hernaez R, Yeung E, Clark JM, Kowdley KV, Brancati FL, Kao WL. HFE and nonalcoholic fatty liver disease: a systematic review and meta-analysis. Hepatology. 2009;50 Suppl 4:781A.
59. Younossi ZM, Gramlich T, Bacon BR, et al. Hepatic iron and nonalcoholic fatty liver disease. Hepatology. 1999;30:847–50.
60. Ioannou GN, Weiss NS, Kowdley KV. Relationship between transferrin-iron saturation, alcohol consumption, and the incidence of cirrhosis and liver cancer. Clin Gastroenterol Hepatol. 2007;5:624–9.
61. Beutler E, Felitti V, Gelbart T, Ho N. The effect of HFE genotypes on measurements of iron overload in patients attending a health appraisal clinic. Ann Intern Med. 2000;133:329–37.

62. Adams PC, Reboussin DM, Barton JC, et al. Hemochromatosis and iron-overload screening in a racially diverse population. N Engl J Med. 2005;352:1769–78.
63. Nelson JE, Wilson L, Brunt EM, et al. Hepatic iron deposition in reticuloendothelial cells but not hepatocytes is associated with more severe NASH: results from the NASH clinical research network. International BioIron Society Meeting 2009. Am J Hematol. 2009;84:E373–4.
64. Valenti L, Fracanzani AL, Bugianesi E, et al. HFE genotype, parenchymal iron accumulation, and liver fibrosis in patients with nonalcoholic fatty liver disease. Gastroenterology. 2010;138:905–12.
65. Fletcher LM, Dixon JL, Purdie DM, et al. Excess alcohol greatly increases the prevalence of cirrhosis in hereditary hemochromatosis. Gastroenterology. 2002;122:281–9.
66. Fletcher LM, Bridle K, Crawford DHG. Effect of alcohol on iron storage diseases of the liver. Best Pract Res Clin Gastroenterol. 2003;17:663–77.
67. Nicolas G, Bennoun M, Devaux I, et al. Lack of hepcidin gene expression and severe tissue iron overload in upstream stimulatory factor 2 (USF2) knockout mice. Proc Natl Acad Sci USA. 2001;98:8780–5.
68. Bridle KR, Cheung T, Murphy TL, et al. Hepcidin is down-regulated in alcoholic liver injury: implications for the pathogenesis of alcoholic liver disease. Alcohol Clin Exp Res. 2006;30:106–12.
69. Harrison-Findik DD, Schafer D, Klein E, et al. Alcohol metabolism-mediated oxidative stress down-regulates hepcidin transcription and leads to increased duodenal iron transporter expression. J Biol Chem. 2006;281:22974–82.
70. Harrison-Findik DD, Klein E, Crist C, Evans J, Timchenko N, Gollan J. Iron-mediated regulation of liver hepcidin expression in rats and mice is abolished by alcohol. Hepatology. 2007;46:1979–85.
71. Gao J, Chen J, Kramer M, Tsukamoto H, Zhang AS, Enns CA. Interaction of the hereditary hemochromatosis protein HFE with transferrin receptor 2 is required for transferrininduced hepcidin expression. Cell Metab. 2009;9:217–27.
72. Courselaud B, Pigeon C, Inoue Y, et al. C/EBPα regulates hepatic transcription of hepcidin, an anti-microbial peptide regulator of iron metabolism. Cross-talk between C/EBP pathway and iron metabolism. J Biol Chem. 2002;277:41163–70.
73. Heinrich PC, Behrmann I, Muller-Newen G, Schoaper F, Graeve L. Interleukin-6-type cytokine signalling though the gp 130/Jak/STAT pathway. Biochem J. 1998;334:297–314.
74. Yu PB, Hong CC, Sachidanandan C, et al. Dorsomorphin inhibits BMP signals required for embryogenesis and iron metabolism. Nat Chem Biol. 2007;4:33–41.
75. Nicolas G, Chauvet C, Viatte L, et al. The gene encoding the iron regulatory peptide hepcidin is regulated by anemia, hypoxia, and inflammation. J Clin Invest. 2002;110:1037–44.
76. Heritage ML, Murphy TL, Bridle KR, Anderson GJ, Crawford DHG, Fletcher LM. Hepcidin regulation in wild-type and Hfe knockout mice in response to alcohol consumption: evidence for an alcohol induced hypoxic response. Alcohol Clin Exp Res. 2009;33:1391–400.
77. Shah YM, Matsubara T, Ito S, Yim SH, Gonzalez FJ. Intestinal hypoxia-inducible transcription factors are essential for iron absorption following iron deficiency. Cell Metab. 2009;9:152–64.
78. Arteel GE, Iimuro Y, Yin M, Raleigh JA, Thurman RG. Chronic enteral ethanol treatment causes hypoxia in rat liver tissue in vivo. Hepatology. 1997;25:920–6.
79. Li J, French B, Wu Y, et al. Liver hypoxia and lack of recovery after reperfusion at high blood alcohol levels in the intragastric feeding model of alcohol liver disease. Exp Mol Pathol. 2004;77:184–92.
80. Peyssonnaux C, Nuzet V, Johnson RS. Role of the hypoxia inducible factors HIF in iron metabolism. Cell Cycle. 2008;7:28–32.
81. Peyssonnaux C, Zinkernagel AS, Schuepback RA, et al. Regulation of iron homeostasis by the hypoxia-inducible transcription factors (HIFs). J Clin Invest. 2007;117:1926–32.
82. Leiber CS. Alcoholic liver disease: new insights in pathogenesis lead to new treatments. J Hepatol. 2000;32:113–28.
83. Bacon BR, Britton RS. The pathology of hepatic iron overload: a free radical-mediated process? Hepatology. 1990;11:127–37.
84. Pietrangelo A. Iron, oxidative stress and liver fibrogenesis. J Hepatol. 1998;29 Suppl 1:8–13.
85. Nimela O, Parkkila S, Britton RS, Brunt E, Janney C, Bacon B. Hepatic lipid peroxidation in hereditary hemochromatosis and alcohol liver injury. J Lab Clin Med. 1999;133:451–60.
86. Britton RS, Bacon BR. Hereditary hemochromatosis and alcohol: a fibrogenic cocktail. Gastroenterology. 2002;122:563–75.
87. Tsukamoto H, Horne W, Kamimura S, et al. Experimental liver cirrhosis induced by alcohol and iron. J Clin Invest. 1995;95:620–30.
88. Di Bisceglie AM, Axiotis CA, Hoofnagle JH, Bacon BR. Measurements of iron status in patients with chronic hepatitis. Gastroenterology. 1992;102:2108–13.
89. Hezode C, Cazeneuve C, Coue O, et al. Liver iron accumulation in patients with chronic active hepatitis C: prevalence and role of hemochromatosis gene mutations and relationship with hepatic histological lesions. J Hepatol. 1999;31:979–84.

90. Tung BY, Emond MJ, Bronner MP, Raaka SD, Cotler SJ, Kowdley KV. Hepatitis C, iron status, and disease severity: relationship with HFE mutations. Gastroenterology. 2003;124:318–26.
91. Smith BC, Gorve J, Guzail MA, et al. Heterozygosity for hereditary hemochromatosis is associated with more fibrosis in chronic hepatitis C. Hepatology. 1998;27:1695–9.
92. Erhardt A, Maschner-Olberg A, Mellenthin C, et al. HFE mutations and chronic hepatitis C: H63D and C282Y heterozygosity are independent risk factors for liver fibrosis and cirrhosis. J Hepatol. 2003;38:335–42.
93. Gehrke S, Stremmel W, Mathes I, Riedel H, Bents K, Kallinowski B. Hemochromatosis and transferrin receptor gene polymorphisms in chronic hepatitis C: impact on iron status, liver injury, and HCV genotype. J Mol Med. 2003;81:780–7.
94. Geier A, Reugels M, Weiskirchen R, et al. Common heterozygous hemochromatosis gene mutations are risk factors for inflammation and fibrosis in chronic hepatitis C. Liver Int. 2004;24:285–94.
95. Thorburn D, Curry G, Spooner R, et al. The role of iron and haemochromatosis gene mutations in the progression of liver disease in chronic hepatitis C. Gut. 2002;50:248–52.
96. Lal P, Fernandes H, Koneru B, Albanese E, Hameed M. C282Y mutation and hepatic iron status in hepatitis C and cryptogenic cirrhosis. Arch Pathol Lab Med. 2000;124:1632–5.
97. Pirisi M, Scott CA, Avellini C, et al. Iron deposition and progression of disease in chronic hepatitis C. Am J Clin Pathol. 2000;113:546–54.
98. Negro F, Samii K, Rubbia-Brandt L, et al. Hemochromatosis gene mutations in chronic hepatitis C patients with and without liver siderosis. J Med Virol. 2000;60:21–7.
99. Hohler T, Leininger S, Kohler HH, Schirmacher P, Galle PR. Heterozygosity for the hemochromatosis gene in liver diseases – prevalence and effects on liver histology. Liver. 2000;20:482–6.
100. Piperno A, Vergani A, Malosio D, et al. Hepatic iron overload in patients with chronic viral hepatitis: role of HFE gene mutations. Hepatology. 1998;28:1105–9.
101. Bonkovsky HL, Troy N, McNeal K, et al. Iron and HFE or TfR1 mutations as comorbid factors for development and progression of chronic hepatitis C. J Hepatol. 2002;37:848–54.
102. Kazemi-Shirazi L, Datz C, Maier-Dobersberger T, et al. The relation of iron status and hemochromatosis gene mutations in patients with chronic hepatitis C. Gastroenterology. 1999;116:127–34.
103. Cauza E, Peck-Radosavljevic M, Ulrich-Pur H, et al. Mutations of the HFE gene in patients with hepatocellular carcinoma. Am J Gastroenterol. 2003;98:442–7.
104. Hellerbrand C, Poppl A, Hartmann A, Scholmerich J, Lock G. HFE C282Y heterozygosity in hepatocellular carcinoma: evidence for an increased prevalence. Clin Gastroenterol Hepatol. 2003;1:279–84.
105. Lauret E, Rodriguez M, Gonzalez S, et al. HFE gene mutations in alcoholic and virus-related cirrhotic patients with hepatocellular carcinoma. Am J Gastroenterol. 2002;97:1016–21.
106. Boige V, Castera L, de Roux N, et al. Lack of association between HFE gene mutations and hepatocellular carcinoma in patients with cirrhosis. Gut. 2003;52:1178–81.
107. Ko C, Siddaiah N, Berger J, et al. Prevalence of hepatic iron overload and association with hepatocellular cancer in end-stage liver disease: results from the National Hemochromatosis Transplant Registry. Liver Int. 2007;27:1394–401.
108. Di Bisceglie AM, Bonkovsky HL, Chopra S, et al. Iron reduction as an adjuvant to interferon therapy in patients with chronic hepatitis C who have previously not responded to interferon: a multicenter, prospective, randomized, controlled trial. Hepatology. 2000;32:135–8.
109. Kato J, Miyanishi K, Kobune M, et al. Long-term phlebotomy with low-iron diet therapy lowers risk of development of hepatocellular carcinoma from chronic hepatitis C. J Gastroenterol. 2007;42:830–6.
110. Kato J, Kobune M, Nakamura T, et al. Normalization of elevated hepatic 8-hydroxy-2 -deoxyguanosine levels in chronic hepatitis C patients by phlebotomy and low iron diet. Cancer Res. 2001;61:8697–702.
111. Van Thiel DH, Friedlander L, Fagiuoli S, Wright HI, Irish W, Gavaler JS. Response to interferon α therapy is influenced by the iron content of the liver. J Hepatol. 1994;20:410–5.
112. Rulyak SJ, Eng SC, Patel K, McHutchinson JG, Gordon SC, Kowdley K. Relationships between hepatic iron content and virologic response in chronic hepatitis C patients treated with interferon and ribavirin. Am J Gastroenterol. 2005;100:332–7.

Chapter 23
Neuropathology and Iron: Central Nervous System Iron Homeostasis

Sarah J. Texel, Xueying Xu, Sokhon Pin, and Z. Leah Harris

Keywords Alzheimer's disease • Friedreich's ataxia • Iron • NBIA • Neurodegeneration • Neuron • Pantothenate kinase deficiency • Parkinson's disease • Restless leg syndrome

1 Introduction

The cells of the central nervous system, and in particular neurons, are metabolically active cells with a high iron requirement. The mechanism(s) by which iron is trafficked across the blood–brain barrier has yet to be fully elucidated. A great interest in central nervous system iron homeostasis is derived from the increasing incidence of neurodegenerative disorders over the last decade. Advances in clinical imaging and the ability to differentiate iron from other metals utilizing magnetic resonance imaging (MRI) has permitted radiological confirmation of brain iron accumulation in patients presenting with neurodegenerative symptoms. The observation that brain iron content increases with aging and is associated with neuropathology has led to a heightened interest in the role of iron in these conditions. The potential for iron to not only participate in but enhance oxidative stress coupled with the concomitant increased tissue iron burden in Parkinson's disease, Alzheimer's disease, and aging has led numerous investigators to study the relationship between iron, oxidative injury, and neurodegeneration. The recent identification of many of the proteins required for systemic cellular iron metabolism within the central nervous system (CNS) and the subsequent characterization of neurodegenerative disorders attributed to mutations in these proteins have even further highlighted the critical role of iron in CNS functioning.

S.J. Texel, M.S.
Department of Neuroscience, Johns Hopkins University, Baltimore, MD, USA
e-mail: texelsj@mail.nih.gov, stexel1@jhmi.edu

X. Xu, M.D., Ph.D. • S. Pin, B.S., MBiotech.
Department of Anesthesiology and Critical Care Medicine, Johns Hopkins University, Baltimore, MD, USA
e-mail: xxu@mymail.aacc.edu; sokhonp@yahoo.com

Z.L. Harris, M.D. (✉)
Department of Pediatrics, Vanderbilt University, Nashville, TN, USA
e-mail: zena.harris@Vanderbilt.edu

G.J. Anderson and G. McLaren (eds.), *Iron Physiology and Pathophysiology in Humans*,
Nutrition and Health, DOI 10.1007/978-1-60327-485-2_23,

2 Iron and the Central Nervous System

Whereas for decades it has been clear that iron is an essential nutrient, the exact role for iron in CNS development and functioning has been less well understood. The first description of iron in a whole brain was made by Zaleski in 1886 who, after immersing brain sections in 2% potassium ferrocyanide followed by staining in 1% hydrochloric acid, revealed that gray matter contained more iron than white matter, that much of the iron was present as a ferric salt, and that the iron appeared to be independent of hemoglobin [1]. Adaptations of the original "Berlin blue" stain by Perls for identifying ferric iron and Fe^{3+} salts by Nguyen-Legros allowed for much more detailed histochemical analysis of iron in the brain [2, 3]. The original histochemical analysis identified ferric iron based on both its abundance and the oxidation artifact of Fe^{2+} that occurs as part of the tissue fixation process. Scientists were able to identify iron throughout the brain in neurons, astrocytes, oligodendroglia, axons, microglia, and myelin sheaths [4–7]. Distinguishing whether that tissue iron is in a Fe^{2+} or Fe^{3+} state has not been possible and that determination has remained difficult and somewhat elusive, although recent fluorescent probes may be helpful in this regard. Irrespective of its oxidation state, it is clearly established that neurons need iron. Iron appears to have an essential role in myelination, neuroectodermal development, and the synthesis and secretion of many neuromodulators and enzymes critical for neuronal, glial, and microglial function.

Iron facilitates myelination as an essential component in the biosynthesis of lipids and cholesterol [8]. In addition to normal myelination, iron is required for cytochrome *c* oxidase function, an iron-dependent enzyme involved in oxidative phosphorylation and a quantifiable marker of neuronal metabolic activity [9]. Iron is a prerequisite for the neurotransmitter synthesis and is required for the activity of tyrosine hydroxylase and tryptophan hydroxylase [10]. Tyrosine hydroxylase, an iron-containing monooxygenase that uses a tetrahydropterin cofactor, catalyzes the hydroxylation of tyrosine in catecholamine biosynthesis [10]. The enzyme is a homotetramer, and each monomer contains a single nonheme iron atom. The role of iron in this enzyme is not understood; however, tyrosine hydroxylase mutants lacking iron are enzymatically inactive [11]. Iron, incorporated into heme, is the backbone of the mitochondrial electron transport chain and is essential for cellular metabolism. Iron is an essential component of cytochromes a and b, iron–sulfur complexes of the respiratory chain (including aconitase), and is a cofactor for tryptophan hydroxylase, ribonucleotide reductase, and succinate dehydrogenase [12].

Although the body's need for iron has been well established, excess iron is harmful and, as such, iron homeostasis is tightly regulated. In 1896, Fenton successfully oxidized malic acid by exposing the acid to a solution containing both ferrous iron and hydrogen peroxide [13]. However, it was not until 1932 that Haber and Weiss identified the active species in Fenton chemistry to be the free OH radical generated by the iron-catalyzed dissociation of hydrogen peroxide [14]. To accommodate both the critical need for iron and the toxicity of this transition metal owing to its potential to generate reactive oxygen species, a complex system of balances has developed in the body.

Four separate "iron cycles" exist in the body: the "systemic" cycle (involving the gut, bone marrow, and liver), the "central nervous system" cycle (retina and brain), the "placenta" cycle, and the "testicular" cycle. Behind every blood barrier, distinct iron proteins are synthesized: transferrin, DMT1 (divalent metal-ion transporter 1/SLC11A2: solute carrier family 11a member 2), and ceruloplasmin [15]. Transferrin (Tf) is the primary plasma protein responsible for binding diferric iron and delivering it to cells via transferrin receptor-mediated endocytosis. Ceruloplasmin (Cp) is a ferroxidase necessary for the oxidation of Fe^{2+} to Fe^{3+} prior to its binding to Tf. DMT1 is a Fe^{2+} iron transporter present on the apical membrane of polarized epithelial cells and the endosomal membranes of most cells.

To enter the CNS, iron must cross one of two separate membranes: the blood–brain barrier (BBB) or the blood–CSF–brain (BCSF) interface. Diferric transferrin binds to the transferrin receptor 1 (TfR1)

a

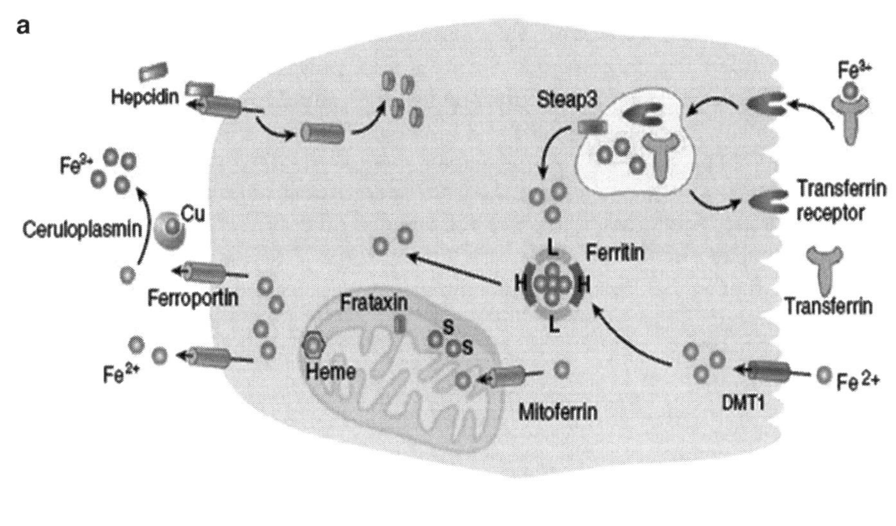

b

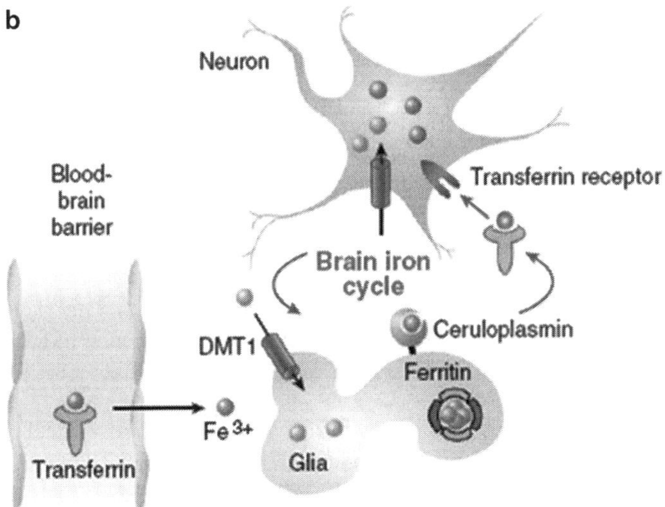

Fig. 23.1 Model for iron trafficking in both the systemic (**a**) and central nervous system (**b**) iron cycles. Iron uptake occurs via the transferrin–transferrin receptor 1-mediated pathway or a non-transferrin-mediated mechanism, possibly mediated in part by DMT1. Once inside the cell, Fe^{2+} is either stored in ferritin, utilized by the cell, or exported via ferroportin, the sole iron export protein. Ferroportin is stabilized by ceruloplasmin and is regulated by hepcidin. Ceruloplasmin oxidizes Fe^{2+} to Fe^{3+} for its subsequent binding to transferrin. The same process occurs in the brain where GPI-linked ceruloplasmin resides on the astrocytes most intimately associated with the microvasculature. Iron binds transferrin synthesized and secreted by oligodendrocytes for delivery to the neuron (Source: Reproduced with permission from [16])

on the blood–brain barrier, and iron is endocytosed into brain capillary endothelial cells. Iron in the Fe^{2+} form likely exits these cells via ferroportin that is expressed on BBB endothelial cells, neurons, oligodendrocytes, astrocytes, the choroid plexus, and ependymal cells. Following transport, iron is likely oxidized by either a perivascular astrocyte-specific ceruloplasmin or secreted ceruloplasmin or another nonspecific ferroxidase. The abundant expression of TfR1 throughout the CNS, and specifically on neurons, suggests that neurons can acquire iron through the classic transferrin/TfR1 endocytosis pathway (Fig. 23.1).

Studies on iron transport in the hypotransferrinemic mouse (hpx) have revealed that neurons acquire iron via both TfR1-mediated endocytosis and a non-transferrin-bound iron (NTBI) mechanism [17].

Homozygote (hpx/hpx) mice had an equivalent radioiron uptake relative to control and heterozygote (+/hpx) mice 24 h following the intravenous injection of radiolabeled iron. One candidate NTBI transporter is DMT1. Mice engineered to lack Dmt1 are viable, anemic, and without gross CNS defects [18]. Their phenotype suggests that DMT1 is essential for gut and bone marrow iron demands to be met but that alternative methods of iron delivery take over in the placenta, liver, and brain. The molar excess of CSF iron to transferrin in the CNS is consistent with a significant role for NTBI transport in this system, but does not prove such a role.

Whether iron enters the neuron either through the transferrin/TfR1 pathway or via Tf-independent means, the iron is ultimately either used for metabolic purposes or incorporated into ferritin for storage [19]. Unlike neurons, glial cells lack TfR1 but have abundant ferritin and are the professional iron storage cells of the CNS [20]. Still to be identified are the mechanisms by which neurons sense and communicate their own iron status. It is interesting that a unique GPI-linked melanotransferrin is found in cerebral endothelial cells [21]. Perhaps they play a role in sensing iron levels?

The basolateral membrane iron exporter ferroportin (FPN) has been characterized in the CNS, and it is expressed on BBB endothelial cells, neurons, oligodendrocytes, astrocytes, the choroid plexus, and ependymal cells [22]. FPN acts in conjunction with ceruloplasmin (Cp) to facilitate iron release. Cp is a multicopper enzyme with ferroxidase activity that oxidizes Fe^{2+} to Fe^{3+} for subsequent binding to transferrin. It is both synthesized and secreted by astrocytes and is found predominantly as a GPI-linked protein on the astrocyte cell surface [23]. It is important to note that the astrocytes expressing ceruloplasmin are those that are most intimately associated with the vasculature. The foot processes of these astrocytes extend great distances and can be localized adjacent to neurons. Cp is also found in ependymal cells, the choroid plexus, substantia nigra, Purkinje cells, and the granule cell layer of the cerebellum. Hephaestin, another multicopper oxidase and ceruloplasmin homologue, is abundantly expressed in the mouse central nervous system and is found on neurons, ependymal cells, the choroid plexus, neuronal bodies in the hippocampus, corpus callosum oligodendrocytes, glial cell bodies in the cortex, substantia nigra (pars compacta), Purkinje cells and the granule cell layer of the cerebellum. We speculate that the abundant expression of both ceruloplasmin and hephaestin within the central nervous system reflects not only their requirement for appropriate FPN localization and function [24], but also their ability to act as ferroxidases and cuprous oxidases, to act as antioxidants (through superoxide and hydrogen peroxide inactivation), and their role in NO/nitrite homeostasis.

The potential for oxidative stress in the face of free Fe^{2+} coupled with the evidence that iron accumulates with aging and neurodegeneration sets the stage for the discussion of the role of iron in neurobiology. Neurodegenerative diseases, as diverse as Alzheimer's disease, Parkinson's disease, Huntington's disease, aceruloplasminemia, and amyotrophic lateral sclerosis, share a conspicuous common feature: selective neuronal loss. The mechanism(s) of this neuronal loss and the basis for the selective vulnerability of certain neuron populations are unknown. These diseases also are noteworthy for increased brain iron accumulation. The abnormal accumulation of iron in the brain does not appear to be a result of increased dietary iron, but rather a disruption in the complex process of cellular iron regulation. Whether the iron deposition is a cause or result of the neuronal loss remains to be determined.

Much of our understanding of regional brain iron acquisition comes from studies of iron deficiency in adults and children. Moos et al. observed that neurons in rat brains express TfR1 in a biphasic pattern with peaks during embryogenesis and in adulthood [25]. During the immediate postnatal period, iron is shuttled for myelinogenesis, glial cell proliferation, and expansion of synaptic number. During this time period, neurons have no detectable TfR1 on their surface. Presumably, adequate iron storage during embryonic development sustains the neurons during this period. During iron deficiency, neurons increase their expression of TfR1 [26]; astrocytes, oligodendrocytes, and microglia in the same brains do not. This suggests that in the postnatal brain, neuronal iron supply is limited and might explain the susceptibility of neurons to a limited iron supply in those neurodegenerative disorders where iron trafficking is disrupted.

Below, we introduce the reader to neurodegenerative syndromes associated with brain iron accumulation and discuss the mechanisms of disease as it relates to disruptions of iron homeostasis. It is interesting to note that as an aging society, our interest in neurodegeneration has gained significant attention. Possible environmental confounders; therapeutic interventions, both allopathic and homeopathic; and the role of nutrition in the development of these disorders are gaining public attention. It is the characterization of the mechanisms regulating central nervous system iron metabolism that will ultimately provide answers.

3 Friedreich's Ataxia

First described by Nikolaus Friedreich in the 1860s, Friedreich's ataxia (FA) is an autosomal recessive, inherited ataxia with sensory loss most commonly associated with GAA trinucleotide repeats in the first noncoding intron of the FRDA1 gene [27]. It is the most common inherited ataxia, with an estimated prevalence of 1/50,000, most patients present in adolescence with muscle weakness, gait disturbances, sensory loss, arreflexia, dysarthria, and cardiomyopathy. The disease is progressive and fatal. A later-onset form of the disease, VLOFA (very-late-onset FA), occurs in 25% of those diagnosed with FA and represents a more slowly progressing form of the disease. Deafness, diabetes, scoliosis, dysphagia, bladder dysfunction, and optic atrophy are also associated with the disease. Within 5 years of the onset of disease, most patients with FA develop neurologic abnormalities consistent with dorsal root ganglia, posterior column, corticospinal tract, dorsal spinocerebellar tract, and cerebellar degeneration. They lose proprioception and develop spasticity and significant proximal muscle weakness, and as the disease advances, distal limb muscle weakness and wasting occurs. Cognition is usually spared. Patients become wheelchair dependent usually within 10 years of diagnosis.

FA is readily distinguished from other inherited ataxia syndromes by the following: (1) While a host of neurodegenerative ataxia diseases have been identified with trinucleotide repeats, only FA has a GAA repeat (Huntington's disease, for example, is characterized by a CAG repeat); (2) only FA is an intron expansion repeat; (3) FA is an autosomal recessive disorder whereas most others are autosomal dominant (i.e., Charcot–Marie–Tooth type 1); and (4) FA is associated with both skeletal and cardiac muscle disease and most affected individuals die from their hypertrophic cardiomyopathy. Recently, ataxia with oculomotor apraxia (AOA) type 1 was found to map to the same locus as FA (chromosome 9p13.3), and this locus is now referred to as FRDA2 [28]. It remains to be determined if this represents a unique locus or if AOA type 1 is a variant of FA.

The severity of disease in FA is determined by the level of frataxin protein. This in turn is determined by the number of GAA repeat sequences in intron 1 of the FRDA1 gene. The hyperexpansion repeats inhibit transcription [29]. If both alleles are affected by hyperexpansion repeats, severe disease occurs. Milder forms of the disease are associated with mutations in one allele and hyperexpansion repeats in the other. Individuals with 5–33 GAA repeats are phenotypically normal. Those with 34–66 GAA repeats, either interrupted by $(GAGGAA)_n$ sequences or uninterrupted, represent a "borderline" situation. Disease has been identified in some cases, but the vast majority of cases have been identified in parents of affected children. These "premutation" alleles are likely capable of expansion into full penetrance alleles based on their somatic instability. Disease-causing FA occurs with greater than 66 GAA repeats, and up to 1,700 GAA repeats have been identified. The majority of FA patients that have been genetically screened as having between 600 and 1,200 GAA repeats. To date, the most common disease-causing point mutation in a single FRDA allele with a hyperexpanded second allele is I154F. The disease severity with this single allelic point mutation is identical to disease caused when hyperexpanded repeats affect both alleles. Another single allelic mutation associated with milder disease when in combination with a hyperexpanded allele is G130V. Whereas one would predict larger expansion repeats to be associated with worse disease, individuals with

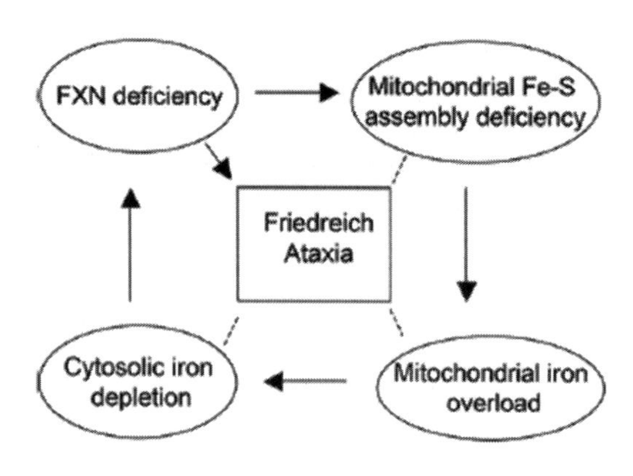

Fig. 23.2 Model for the role of iron homeostasis in the pathogenesis of Friedreich's ataxia. This model hypothesizes that increased mitochondrial iron results in depleted cytosolic iron stores which further downregulates frataxin expression by decreasing iron-responsive frataxin transcription (Source: Reproduced with permission from [33])

VLOFA have been identified that are homozygote for 800+ GAA repeats, making predictions about disease severity imperfect. A specific form of FA observed in an Acadian population has further revealed the imprecise genotype–phenotype correlation that exists in this disease. FA in Acadians is characterized by a later age of onset, later age of wheelchair use, and less incidence of cardiomyopathy. Similarly, FA with retained reflexes (FARR) and spastic paraparesis without ataxia are later-onset, clinically less severe forms of the disease.

Elegant work in *Saccharomyces cerevisiae* studying the yeast frataxin homologue, Yfh1, has provided considerable input into our current molecular and mechanistic understanding of the disease [30]. Despite considerable research, the exact sequence of events that lead to the neuropathology in FA still remains unclear. We now know that frataxin is a ubiquitously expressed protein critical for iron–sulfur cluster assembly such that a lack of frataxin manifests as a disruption of mitochondrial iron homeostasis that uniquely affects specific tissues [31]. Frataxin is a small protein that has been shown to bind several ferrous iron atoms. Frataxin is also able to bind the iron–sulfur cluster scaffold protein ISCU and the heme biosynthetic enzyme ferrochelatase [32]. Thus, it appears that frataxin likely acts as a chaperone donating ferrous iron for incorporation into nascent iron–sulfur clusters as they are assembled on ISCU. Why there is a predilection for cardiac, dorsal root ganglia, and large sensory neurons to be affected is unknown, but perhaps, it reflects the increased mitochondrial activity in the cells in these regions. It is unclear if the mitochondrial iron accumulation is a primary or secondary event. A frataxin deficiency is associated with mitochondrial dysfunction, reduced mitochondrial DNA, reduced antioxidant levels, and increased redox-mediated cellular damage. Iron appears to be trapped in a mitochondrial compartment that is not accessible to iron-dependent proteins and mitochondrial cytochromes, and aconitase has decreased activity levels [33]. Thus, two potential mechanisms for cell damage include Fenton chemistry/oxyradical injury and iron deficiency. Iron-dependent regulation of frataxin expression creates a vicious cycle: The mitochondrial iron overload induces decreased frataxin expression and leads to more severe cytosolic iron deficiency [33] (Fig. 23.2).

Current therapies for FA involve targeting the abnormal accumulation of iron in the mitochondria and the resulting mitochondrial oxyradical injury and subsequent mitochondrial respiratory defects. Free radical scavengers such as coenzyme Q10, vitamin E, idebenone (a coenzyme Q10 analogue) and MitoQ (a mitochondrial-targeted idebenone), and iron chelators have been used with some success [34–36]. Therapies directed at increasing cellular frataxin levels are also being initiated [37]. It is likely that therapies will also be proposed in the future that will increase heat-shock proteins that may be able to offer redundant chaperone function and help mitochondrial iron trafficking and homeostasis.

4 Alzheimer's Disease

Since it was first described by Alois Alzheimer over a century ago, Alzheimer's disease (AD) has become the major neurodegenerative disease worldwide [38]. AD is distinguished by a progressive loss of memory and an inclusive deterioration of mental faculties and abilities [39]. The dementia in AD has been correlated with extensive neuronal death and degeneration, thought to be caused by deposition of protein aggregates in the cells [40]. Two specific groups of protein aggregates are associated with AD and are considered hallmarks of the disease: neuritic plaques and neurofibrillary tangles (NFT) [39, 40]. It is important to keep in mind that these aggregations or lesions also occur in nondiseased aged brains, though in much lower numbers, and that the lesions in AD are more likely a result of the disease, not the underlying cause [41]. Each of the protein aggregates has a specific composition which provides clues to the homeostatic mechanisms disrupted in AD.

Neuritic plaques were first discovered in 1930 by Divry, who used a dye bound to amyloid [39]. Plaques are extracellular protein aggregates composed mainly of beta-amyloid (Aβ) peptides resulting from the cleavage of a larger protein, amyloid precursor protein (APP), by secretase enzymes [39]. The normal role for APP is not known but has been proposed to be a neurotrophin, vesicle trafficker, or a serine protease inhibitor [40]. Two sizes of the Aβ peptide can result depending on the type of secretase that cleaves APP. One is 40 amino acids in length, and the other is 42 amino acids long [40]. The Aβ-42 has been shown to be more hydrophobic and thus more amenable to aggregation [42]. There has been a great deal of research that focuses on mutations in the APP gene that would cause increased production of Aβ or would confer an increased self-aggregation of the Aβ peptide [39, 40]. These mutations, and those in other proteins that affect Aβ processing, have been implicated in the familial form of AD (FAD) and show direct genetic inheritance patterns. FAD, however, only accounts for 5–10% of all incidences of AD, and thus, Aβ production and processing is not a complete answer for AD pathophysiology [43].

Unlike plaques, NFTs are intracellular aggregates composed of hyperphosphorylated tau [39]. Tau is a microtubule-associated protein that functions in the reinforcement of the cytoskeleton, and its ability to bind microtubules is modulated by phosphorylation and dephosphorylation [40]. The hyperphosphorylation of tau interferes with microtubule binding [44]. These hyperphosphorylated taus instead have a tendency to aggregate into paired helices. Tau aggregates may contribute to cell death by loss of microtubule stabilization or by physically blocking axonal transport [45]. Tau aggregations are found in a variety of other neurodegenerative diseases and, like plaques, cannot be held solely responsible for the pathophysiology of AD [45].

One commonality of all neurodegenerative diseases is oxidative stress and the production of reactive oxygen species (ROS) [46]. The involvement of iron in Fenton chemistry is a large contributor of oxidative stress and there is speculation that iron plays a large role in the pathophysiology of AD [46]. It is well known that brain iron levels increase with age, and since a major risk factor for AD is old age, it has led researchers to consider that modifications in iron levels and distribution may be a contributing factor to AD [47]. Increased iron levels have been shown to be present in areas such as the hippocampus and cerebral cortex, areas that are known to be affected in AD [48]. Upon closer examination of post-mortem brain tissue, iron can be found in association with senile plaques [49] and NFTs [47]. Specific histidine and tyrosine residues at the N terminus of Aβ have been shown to be able to bind iron [47], and the binding of iron to Aβ has been shown to lead to the production of ROS [50] and promote AB aggregation. Replacing the histidine residues of Aβ, thereby abolishing the iron binding motif, has been shown to reduce aggregation [51]. Iron may also play a role in APP translation as it has been shown that the mRNA for APP contains an iron-responsive element in its 5′ untranslated region [52]. It is easy for one to imagine how increased levels of APP protein caused by high iron levels may add to AD pathophysiology.

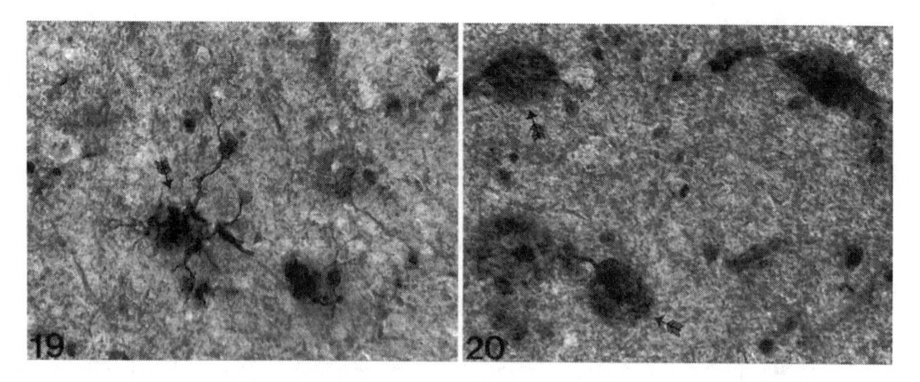

Fig. 23.3 A Perls' stain is used to show intense iron deposits (*left*) in cells and processes involved in the senile plaque and also the diffuse iron staining (*right*) associated with the plaques (Source: Reproduced with permission from [61])

Studies have also demonstrated that tau can bind iron. Increased iron can be found in NFTs and has been associated with increased levels of oxidative stress [53]. Increased levels of oxidative stress can be found in neurons that lack NTFs, indicating that oxidative stress might set the stage for NFT formation. Other than direct interaction with tau, iron has been shown to affect kinase activity, which could play a role in disruption of tau phosphorylation [54]. Increased iron levels are likely present in diseased brain areas because plaque accumulation can lead to microglia activation. Microglia have been shown to react to superoxide by the release of iron from ferritin stores [55]. In addition, the lysosomal degradation of malfunctioning mitochondria, which is prevalent in AD, can cause the release of iron into already ailing neurons [47, 56]. Iron accumulation then leads to cellular dysfunction which can further increase iron load and result in more cell damage.

Advances in technology have made it possible not only to get a more precise mapping of iron levels in brain tissue but also to be able to distinguish between specific iron compounds [57]. A surprising discovery using these advanced techniques has been the amount of a ferromagnetic iron oxide, called biogenic magnetite, in areas of iron accumulation [46]. Biogenic magnetite, although not considered a common iron compound, has been found to be present in brain tissue [58]. The level of biogenic magnetite is elevated in AD brains [59] and was the main form of iron in brain areas with prominent iron accumulation. Levels of biogenic magnetite are of great consequence because this form of iron can produce free ferrous iron that is able to participate in ROS generation through Fenton reactions [60]. Thus, not only the amount and location but also the form of excess iron may be important factors in the pathophysiology of AD (Fig. 23.3).

Although it has been over 100 years since AD was first described, there are few drugs approved by the FDA for its treatment [39]. Most of these drugs are cholinesterase inhibitors, which act to reduce the breakdown of acetylcholine, a common neurotransmitter [39]. The drugs are effective in slowing AD progression, but not preventing it, because AChR stimulation increases the release of soluble APP from cells, thus reducing the production of Aβ. As more of the molecular mechanisms of AD have been discovered, more experimental treatment options have been studied. Among these experimental treatment options is the use of iron chelators [46]. Clinical trials with common iron chelators such as desferrioxamine (DFO), ethylenediaminetetraacetic acid (EDTA), and clioquinol have demonstrated their ability to decrease cognitive decline and Aβ levels [62, 63]. The toxicity of clioquinol and hydrophobicity of DFO, preventing it from crossing the BBB, have led to the search for better chelators that were not only safe but could also easily access the brain. One group has synthesized a range of novel chelators that are derivatives of the iron chelator VK-28 and are conjugated to the neuroprotective moiety of the drugs rasagiline and selegiline commonly used to treat Parkinson's disease [62]. These drugs, which can cross the BBB and are nontoxic, have shown the ability *in vitro* to regulate Aβ production and be neuroprotective against Aβ toxicity. Other naturally occurring iron chelators, such as plant polyphenol flavonoids, are also being investigated for their potential use in AD treatment [62, 63]. The advantages of these substances, in addition to their non-toxic nature and ability to cross the BBB, are that they are naturally occurring and function as anti-oxidant, anti-inflammatory, and neuroprotective agents [63]. One such substance is EGCG, which is a component found in green tea. Preliminary *in vitro* and in vivo animal studies have shown that EGCG has the ability to prevent neurodegeneration, reduce APP translation, and increase secretion of soluble APP which causes a decrease in Aβ levels [63]. These experiments lend hope for better treatment options in the future not just for AD but for all neurodegenerative diseases where oxidative stress and transition metals may play a role in pathophysiology.

As with most neurodegenerative diseases, the pathophysiology of AD is complex. While recent evidence convincingly shows that iron accumulation plays a role in AD progression, there is most likely a variety of components that act together to cause AD. Also, it should not be forgotten that other transition metals may also have a hand in generating oxidative stress and neurodegeneration. Thus any successful treatment for such an intricate disease is likely to include a multi-approach treatment.

5 Parkinson's Disease

In 1817, James Parkinson, a British physician, encountered a novel motor disease, which caused a resting tremor and a loss of muscle strength [38]. Today, this disease, aptly named Parkinson's disease (PD), is one of the most common neurodegenerative diseases, second only to Alzheimer's disease [64] in prevalence. PD is characterized by the selective loss and depletion of pigmented dopaminergic neurons in the substantia nigra pars compacta (SNpc) in the basal ganglia, a brain area intricately involved in motor control. A hallmark of PD is cytoplasmic protein aggregates called Lewy bodies (LBs) [65]. These LBs are made up of lipids and proteins, with α-synuclein protein aggregates being a major component [66, 67]. A variety of gene loci, Park1–13, Park1 being α-synuclein, have been found mutated in familial forms of PD [66]. Many of the functions for these loci are still unknown, and even though much time has been spent investigating the genetic causes of PD, most PD cases are sporadic, with $< 10\%$ of cases having a genetic component [66]. PD has also been linked to environmental factors such as prolonged iron exposure [68] and mitochondrial "neurotoxins" such as 1-methyl-4-phenyl-1,2,3,6-tetrahydropyridine (MPTP) [67].

A challenge in studying PD has been trying to find a good animal model. Most of the current animal models used are MPTP toxin-treated animals or transgenic mice containing a mutation in one of the crucial associated loci [68]. As in most neurodegenerative diseases, oxidative stress and production of reactive oxygen species (ROS) are believed to play a role in the pathophysiology of PD [66]. The role of iron in the generation of both oxidative stress and production of ROS has led to much research on the role iron dysregulation may play in PD.

It is generally accepted that the substantia nigra (SN) is a critical area of the brain that is affected in PD. Along with the basal ganglia, the SN has the highest iron concentration/dry tissue weight of the brain and in many cases is greater than that of the liver [69, 70]. Such high concentrations of iron in the SN are explained by the requirement for iron as a necessary cofactor for the rate-limiting enzyme in the production of dopamine – tyrosine hydroxylase [71]. Dopaminergic neurons of the midbrain are the main source of dopamine (DA) in the mammalian central nervous system. Although dopaminergic neurons correspond to less than 1% of the total number of brain neurons and their numbers are few, they play an important role in regulating several aspects of basic brain function including voluntary movement and a broad array of behavioral processes such as motor behavior, motivation, working memory, mood, addiction, and stress. The effect of iron deficiency on dopamine

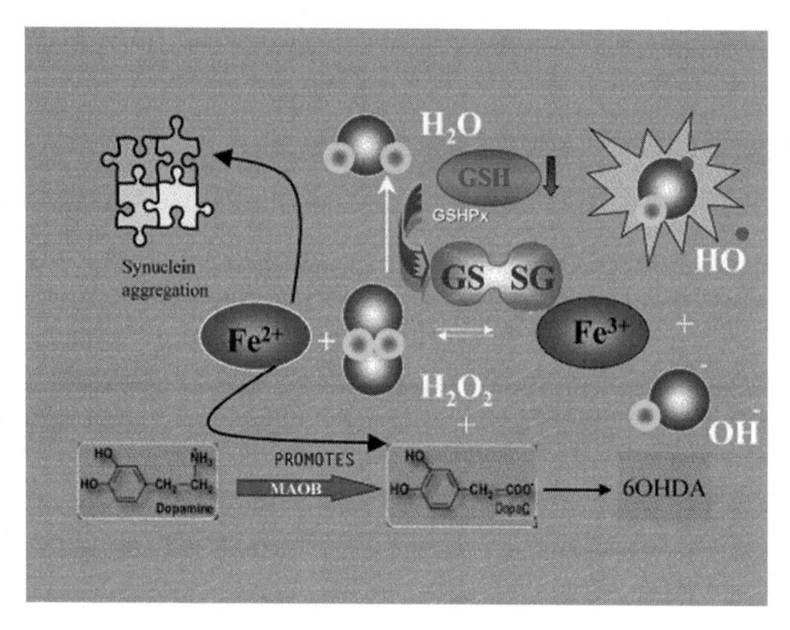

Fig. 23.4 Model of the role of iron in Parkinson's disease. Iron appears to be a catalyst for α-synuclein aggregation in addition to participating in oxyradical formation. Iron-induced oxidative stress further potentiates Lewy body formation and likely increases the tendency for Lewy-body aggregation (Source: Reproduced with permission from [78])

production in the SN has been well documented. It has been demonstrated that iron deficiency results in a reduction in D1 and D2 dopamine receptor density. If this deficiency occurs early in CNS development, it can lead to dramatic learning disabilities associated with lack of dopamine production [70].

While a certain concentration of iron is important in the SN, SN iron levels of PD patients can be up to 35% higher than in nondiseased brain [72]. A closer examination of iron levels in dopaminergic neurons of PD patients revealed excess iron confined to dopaminergic neurovesicles. This neurovesicular iron storage can be reduced by inhibiting dopamine synthesis, suggesting that dopamine is a player in iron regulation that might be disrupted in PD [73]. Additional experiments lend fuel to the argument that iron plays a role in the pathophysiology of PD. It has been shown that iron accumulates in melanized dopamine neurons and interneurons, and it is generally accepted that ROS production by this excess iron is a cause for the degeneration and death of these neurons [9, 74]. However, whether iron accumulation is a primary cause of the disease or just a secondary effect of a larger pathogenic mechanism remains to be elucidated.

One of the most convincing groups of experiments that point to iron being a primary cause of PD describes the interactions of iron and α-synuclein. *In vitro* studies have shown that Fe^{3+} can cause wild-type α-synuclein to aggregate and form short, thick fibrils which differ from the type of fibrils induced by Cu^{2+}, another transition metal implicated in PD pathophysiology, suggesting a fibril morphology specific to iron [75]. Thermodynamic experiments have also demonstrated that binding kinetics of α-synuclein suggest one binding site for iron [76]. Further, it has recently been predicted, by use of computer-generated folding of α-synuclein mRNA, that the 5′ region of the gene contains an iron-responsive element, meaning that α-synuclein may be under posttranscriptional control by iron levels [77]. While these experiments are not definitive proof, they are highly suggestive that increased iron levels can cause the aggregation of α-synuclein present in Lewy bodies of PD patients (Fig. 23.4).

Dopaminergic neurons are believed to be particularly prone to oxidative stress due to their high rate of oxygen metabolism, low levels of antioxidants, and high iron content. Unique to dopamine is the ability to generate toxic ROS spontaneously in the presence of Fe^{2+} or via a monoamine oxidase (MAO)-catalyzed reaction which generates hydrogen peroxide, oxygen radicals, semiquinones, and quinones [79, 80]. Conceivably, conditions that increase brain iron concentrations, while antioxidant capabilities are limited and/or maximally consumed, could result in selective dopaminergic neuronal loss. The bigger question with most neurodegenerative diseases is not how iron is causing the generation of ROS but what is causing the iron buildup. One of the causes of excess iron might be due to a failure in iron storage. Changes in the main iron storage protein, ferritin, have been studied in PD patients, and it has been found that there is a decrease in L-ferritin subunits in the SN [81]. These results indicate that changes in the composition of the ferritin shell in PD may lead to increased efflux of iron [81]. Studies have also shown that iron levels in the SN go beyond the binding capacity of the ferritin present, and this may be due to sustained IRP1 binding activity to the ferritin mRNA which prevents the upregulation of ferritin in the face of accumulating iron levels [82, 83]. Also, it has been shown that the expression of the H-ferritin subunit decreases with normal aging, and this may compound an already faulty iron storage system that occurs in PD patients [84].

In the SN, there are specific neurons that contain neuromelanin (NM), a pigment in the melanin family that can bind and store iron, which may be the main iron storage for these cells [84, 85]. Release of iron from NM has been shown to fuel mitochondrial oxidative stress causing dysfunction of mitochondria and proteasomes [86]. Study of the involvement of neuromelanin in the pathogenesis of Parkinson's disease suggests that iron released from neuromelanin increases oxidative stress in mitochondria. Subsequent mitochondrial dysfunction ensues resulting in dopaminergic neuronal death. Neuromelanin is associated with increased oxidative stress, but synthetic melanin is not. Further, superoxide dismutase and desferrioxamine completely suppress the presumed iron-mediated oxidative stress. In fact, close examination of NM pigment levels in PD patients have shown simpler, less dense iron aggregate cores compared to controls, suggesting less iron in the NM–iron aggregates consistent with increased pathological iron release in PD [87]. Another possible source of excess iron might come from NM and ferritin pools that are released by dying neurons. These in turn might recruit activated microglia that could further add to iron levels [84, 88].

Other iron-related proteins have also been reported to be modulated in PD models. Rats treated with 6-hydroxydopamine (6-OHDA), an SN-specific lesion model in which the animal becomes PD-like after 6 weeks, show reduced protein and mRNA expression of the iron exporter ferroportin and the ferroxidase hephaestin after only 1 day of treatment [89]. This model suggests another explanation for increased iron levels (i.e., impaired iron release) and its link to the development of PD [89]. Other researchers treating C6 cells with 6-OHDA demonstrated an upregulation of the IRE + form of DMT1, an important iron transporter, suggesting increased iron uptake in this system [90]. Mutations in the ferritin H subunit, ceruloplasmin, IRP2, and HFE have also been found in single PD patients, strengthening the link between iron dysregulation and PD pathophysiology [91].

A cure for PD has yet to be discovered, and current treatment aims to reduce symptoms and delay progression of the disease. Current PD treatment involves agents that either enhance dopamine transmission or mimic the agonist effects of dopamine [67]. It is common, however, for these drugs to lose their therapeutic effects after prolonged treatment, and thus, much time has been invested in finding better ways to treat PD [67]. One of main targets of experimental therapy is reducing oxidative damage by ROS. Certain compounds, such as melatonin and vitamins A, C, and E, are thought to have nonspecific antioxidant and radical scavenging properties that would protect neurons [67]. Selenium, a trace metal, is thought to enhance the antioxidant properties of glutathione peroxidase, which in turn reduces the levels of hydrogen peroxide that can form ROS when interacting with iron [67]. A disruption in complex I in the mitochondria of PD patients suggested that supplementation of coenzyme Q10, a mitochondrial cofactor and antioxidant, might be neuroprotective. Indeed, *in vitro* experiments on primary dopaminergic neurons showed that administration of coenzyme Q10 was able to reduce cell death [92]. As in AD, many novel iron chelators that are able to cross the blood–brain barrier have been shown to be able to reduce iron levels and neuronal death [93, 94]. This neuroprotective effects might also result from the chelators' ability to decrease the inhibition of proteasomes and microglia activation [94]. Although these experimental treatments have shown promise, they are still a long way from being used clinically to treat PD, and research into new treatments for PD will continue.

As with many neurodegenerative diseases, treatment of PD is challenging. In many cases, this is due to the fact that by the time it has been diagnosed, the disease has progressed quite far, and there is a lot of degeneration that cannot be reversed. Thus advancements in early diagnosis of such diseases may have a large impact on treatment. Iron is an attractive biomarker, whose changes in metabolism and storage can often be found before hallmark disease symptoms. Further research in understanding the link between iron dysregulation and PD may lead to better and more efficient treatment options.

6 Parkinson's Disease, Alzheimer's Disease, and Hereditary Hemochromatosis

The term hereditary hemochromatosis (HH) is applied to a family of iron-loading disorders resulting from mutations in proteins which regulate body iron intake. By far the most common of these disorders is that associated with mutations in the *HFE* gene (Chap. 19), and hereafter, the abbreviation HH will be used to represent that disease. Two mutations in the *HFE* gene have been associated with HH, but the one leading to the C282Y substitution is responsible for almost all cases of iron loading. Homozygosity for C282Y is around 1:200 in people of northern European descent, but the penetrance of disease that manifests with overt clinical pathology associated with iron overload is significantly less. Are HH individuals at increased risk of CNS disease due to their systemic iron loading? Is the incidence of neurodegeneration increased in a population with systemic iron overload – symptomatic or not? Alternatively – does CNS iron overload occur in patients with systemic iron overload, or does systemic iron overload increase "oxidative risk" and herald an increase in neurodegeneration? The HFE gene product colocalizes with β-2 microglobulin, and the β-2 microglobulin null mouse is a model of HFE iron overload. A study by Moos et al. [95] concluded that high circulating levels of iron did not result in an increase in brain iron accumulation in these mice. Histological examination of the brains of β-2 microglobulin null mice and controls, including basal ganglia and substantia nigra, were indistinguishable. Nonetheless, studies with AD and PD patients have been less conclusive. The studies on mice have the good fortune of evaluating a specific phenotype on an identical genotype living under tight environmental control. Human studies are inconclusive, in large part due to factors difficult to control: variability in disease presentation, environmental influences, sample size, and the unrecognized significance of additional genetic polymorphisms.

The association between HFE gene mutations, Parkinson's disease, and Alzheimer's disease was evaluated in a Portuguese cohort that included 130 individuals with AD, 132 PD patients, 55 patients with mild cognitive impairment (MCI), and 115 age-matched normal controls [96]. All those enrolled in the study were screened for the HFE mutations C282Y and H63D (a common HFE mutation but one that is rarely associated with iron loading). While no difference in genotype or allelic frequencies were identified between AD and MCI patients, the C282Y heterozygote state was significantly overrepresented among PD patients relative to the controls and other clinical groups (13.6% vs. 5%). The C282Y carrier state did not affect onset of disease, duration of symptoms, or survival. The results of this study were in contrast to previous publications suggesting no link between PD and HFE. The French Parkinson's Disease Genetic Study Group screened 216 patients with PD and 193 matched controls to analyze potential polymorphisms and/or mutations in five iron-related genes (transferrin, TfR1, HFE, frataxin, and lactoferrin) [97]. No differences for any allele frequencies were identified, except for transferrin [97]. Two separate studies examining a potential link between PD and HFE have also failed to identify a connection [98, 99]. In a study by Berg et al. [99], no variations in HFE mutation frequency were identified in patients with diagnosed PD who also had hyperechogenicity of their substantia nigra consistent with increased iron accumulation. In a study by Aamodt et al. [98], 400 Norwegian patients with PD were screened, and no significant differences in gene frequencies were identified. Despite an initial suggestion for increased frequency of PD in individuals with C282Y mutations [100], subsequent studies have questioned these findings.

The data supporting a link between AD and HFE appear more convincing than those presented for PD and HFE. Despite no differences in HFE and AD frequencies in the Portuguese study described above, the OPTIMA study identified four patient "risk sets" based on biochemical and genetic testing that were designated either a higher risk or lower risk for AD [101–103]. In the low-risk groups (infrequent disease risk and less early onset AD before 65 years of age), HFE genetic variation played no role. High-risk sets (higher incidence of disease, younger age of presentation) were significant for biochemical serum abnormalities (low folate, low B12, elevated total homocysteine) and overrepresentation of specific genetic allelic risks: APOE4 (apolipoprotein E E4 allele), AR1 (androgen receptor 1), and Tf-C2 (transferrin C2 allele). HFE mutation status played no role in elevating risk, although compound heterozygosity for the C282Y and H63D mutations approached significance [101–103]. However, in a separate study, synergy between Tf-C2 and HFE C282Y was identified and compound heterozygosity for HFE C282Y and H63D increased the risk for AD five times over each single variation [101–103]. In short, there is no clear-cut association between AD, PD, and HFE, however, it is clear that specific allelic variations increase the risk for neuronal oxidative stress.

7 Restless Leg Syndrome

Restless leg syndrome (RLS) became a familiar disease only recently, especially in cases of insomnia, but it was first described in the late 1600s by Thomas Willis, a British physician [104]. Willis described symptoms that were "so great a restlessness … that the diseased are no more able to sleep than if they were in a place of the greatest torture" [104]. Since Willis' first publication on RLS, much research and clinical characterization of the disease has occurred. The International RLS Study Group has identified the core criteria for diagnosis of RLS [105, 106]: "(1) an urge to move, usually due to uncomfortable sensations that occur primarily in the legs, (2) motor restlessness, expressed as activity that relieves the urge to move, (3) worsening of symptoms by relaxation, and (4) variability over the course of the day–night cycle, with symptoms worse in the evening and early in the night" [106]. This is a disease that affects approximately 10% of the population, with the exception of Asian populations where the incidence of RLS seems to be much lower [105, 106]. Due to its high incidence and the impact that RLS has on sleep quality, there is a major effort to identify the mechanism responsible for the disorder and to develop potential therapeutic interventions for RLS symptoms.

RLS can be categorized as either primary or secondary. The primary or idiopathic form was first described by Ekbom in 1945 who demonstrated a strong familial component in RLS [107]. A study looking at 238 RLS patients and their first degree relatives identified strong evidence that RLS is inherited in an autosomal dominant fashion [108] and three distinct loci have been linked to RLS in three separate families, RLS-1, RLS-2, and RLS-3 [108–111]. Secondary or sporadic RLS is known to be associated with conditions leading to iron deficiency. This has been shown to be the case during pregnancy, renal failure, and anemia, where RLS symptoms can be reversed by correcting the iron deficit. Symptomatic presentation of RLS does not differ between primary or secondary forms, and this has led many to believe that iron metabolism dysregulation may be a common thread in all cases of RLS [108–111].

Continuing research has highlighted many reasons why the dysregulation of iron metabolism is an attractive candidate for the etiology of RLS. The control of the spinal flexor reflex, whose activity is believed to be exaggerated in RLS, is modulated by dopamine [112] and iron plays a large role in dopamine synthesis. Iron is a necessary cofactor for the rate-limiting enzyme in catecholamine production – tyrosine hydroxylase [113]. Animal models have revealed that iron deficiency can lead to a decreased D1 and D2 dopamine receptor concentration and to a decrease in the dopamine transporter density in striatal areas [114–116]. Another factor implicating iron homeostasis is that plasma iron concentrations fluctuate with a circadian rhythm, where iron levels at night drop down to half of daytime values [117]. Studies have correlated the time point of lowest serum iron with the time point of the most intense RLS symptoms [116, 117]. Due to the role of iron in dopamine synthesis, it is not surprising that tyrosine hydroxylase, the dopamine transporter, and dopamine D1 and D2 receptors also follow a circadian rhythm with lower levels in brain tissue at night [117].

Early attempts to characterize iron deficiency in RLS relied on serum ferritin levels, and many studies were able to show an inverse correlation between the severity of RLS symptoms and serum ferritin levels [118–120]. The reliability of this correlation has been challenged as other experiments have shown no reduction in serum ferritin in patients with RLS. Because much of the emphasis for RLS symptoms has examined dopamine metabolism and production in the brain, many researchers thought to look at cerebral spinal fluid (CSF) ferritin levels. While serum ferritin levels reflect body iron storage, CSF ferritin levels likely represent a more accurate method to evaluate central nervous system iron storage and metabolism. Patients with RLS have decreased CSF ferritin and increased CSF transferrin levels compared to controls, while the serum levels of ferritin and transferrin did not differ [121–123]. Recent experiments have further analyzed CSF ferritin and have shown that the levels of both the H and L subunits are decreased in RLS, although only in early and not late-onset disease [124]. A reduced iron content in the substantia nigra (SN) of patients with RLS has also been demonstrated [125, 126].

While these studies strengthen the argument for the role of iron in RLS, they do not point to a mechanism. Electrophysiological measurements of motor and sensory nerve conduction groups in the periphery, spinal cord, and brainstem of iron deficient anemia patients are similar to controls, suggesting that, despite the anemia and presumably an anemia-associated decrease in brain iron in RLS patients, any dysfunction in nerve conduction is unlikely to be related to iron levels [127]. Neuromelanin cells isolated from the SN of RLS patients showed decreased ferritin, DMT1, TfR1, and ferroportin protein [128]. In addition, these experiments also showed reduced IRP1, but not IRP2, activity and protein levels in RLS patients. Further linking RLS and iron deficiency, Wang et al. showed a decrease in Thy-1 in the SN of RLS patients [129]. Thy-1 is a cell adhesion molecule that has shown to play a role in regulating secretory and neurotransmitter vesicle release and stabilizing synapses [130–132]. Thy-1 is important developmentally where it plays a role in the formation of axonal projections from the SN to the striatum [130–132]. Rats on a low-iron diet have decreased Thy-1 levels in the brain. Similarly, decreased iron levels in the SN of RLS patients correlate with decreased Thy-1 in the same area and suggest a mechanism for how low brain iron levels could disrupt dopamine transmission [130–132]. Other experiments have suggested a mechanism involving the iron regulatory peptide hepcidin. In RLS patients, there are decreased levels of prohepcidin in CSF but increased levels in neuromelanin cells, SN, and the putamen [133] (Fig. 23.5). However, this result is difficult to interpret as levels of prohepcidin do not reflect accurately levels of the bioactive mature peptide.

There are a variety of treatments prescribed for RLS. The most common are levodopa and other dopamine agonists [135]. These medications act by interacting with dopamine receptors and mimicking increased dopamine signaling. Anticonvulsants have been administered to treat RLS based on

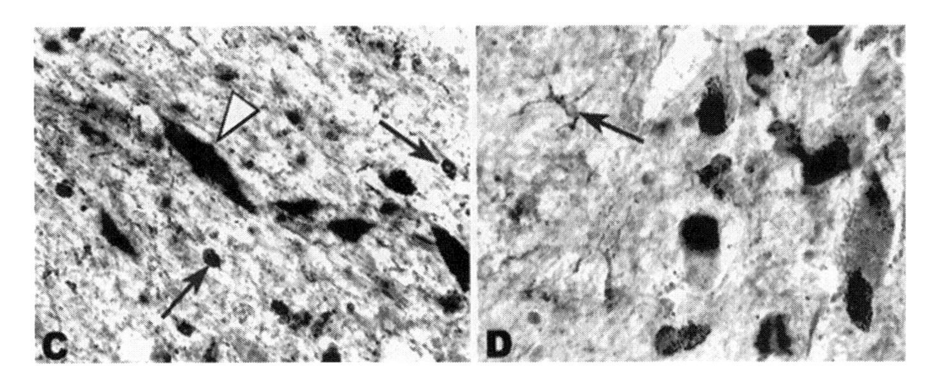

Fig. 23.5 Perls' stain in control brain (*left*) demonstrates neuromelanin-containing cells in dark brown (indicated by *white arrow head*) and oligodendrocytes containing iron (stained blue, indicated by *black arrows*). Perls' stain in the RLS brain (*right*) shows no staining for neuromelanin and a blue iron-positive cell (indicated by the *black arrow*) unlike the positive oligodendrocytes seen in the control brain (Source: Reproduced with permission from [134])

experimental data suggesting that GABA modulates dopamine and serotonin release [136]. Opioids were the first treatment for RLS suggested by Willis, but the mechanism of action is not understood. Benzodiazepines have also been used to treat RLS, but, like opioids, they have given mixed results in clinical trials. Due to the large involvement serum iron levels seem to play in RLS, supplemental iron administration has been studied as an alternative to pharmaceutical treatment of RLS. Patients with serum ferritin levels less than 50 μg/L are encouraged to take iron supplements [137–140]. However, studies on the use of iron supplementation to treat RLS have been contradictory. Some studies have shown no benefit of iron, especially in those patients that do not show a significant iron deficit. On the other hand, other experiment data have reported considerable improvement of RLS symptoms after iron supplementation [138–140]. Despite the variety of treatment options for RLS, there is little treatment consensus, and none of the options explored so far have proven to be 100% effective.

8 Pantothenate Kinase Deficiency (PANK2)

"Neurodegeneration with brain iron accumulation (NBIA)" was proposed by Susan Hayflick in the mid-1990s as an umbrella term to describe a group of progressive extrapyramidal disorders with radiographic evidence of iron accumulation in the brain, usually in the basal ganglia. The Hayflick lab recently characterized the gene defect in Hallervorden–Spatz syndrome (HSS). For decades, the name HSS had been used to represent a group of clinical disorders that were defined by neurodegeneration with radiographically confirmed iron accumulation in the central nervous system. However, with the identification of the "classical" HSS gene, it was clear that many of the disorders were genetically different, and this prompted the broader classification of NBIA to be developed. No longer called Hallervorden–Spatz, pantothenate kinase–associated neurodegeneration (PKAN) accounts for the majority of NBIA cases and is caused by an autosomal recessive inborn error of coenzyme A metabolism associated with mutations in the PANK2 gene (pantothenate kinase 2) [141]. PKAN is characterized by dystonia and pigmentary retinopathy in children or speech and neuropsychiatric disorders coupled with dystonia in adults. In addition, a specific pattern on brain MRI, called the eye-of-the-tiger sign, is virtually pathognomonic for the disease (Fig. 23.6) [141]. Identification of this major NBIA gene has led to more accurate clinical delineation of the diseases that comprise this group. For the purposes of this chapter, the only other NBIA disorder included

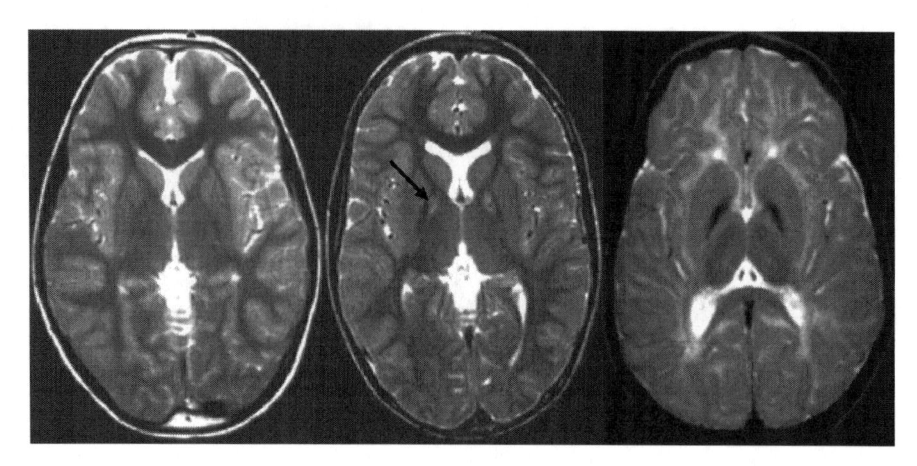

Fig. 23.6 T2-weighted brain magnetic resonance imaging (*MRI*) of a normal brain (*left*), the classic "eye-of-the-tiger" sign characteristic of PKAN (*center, arrow*), and the MRI of a typical non-PKAN form of NBIA with the hypointense signal in the globus pallidus (*right*) (Source: Reproduced with permission from [142])

will be non-PKAN NBIA associated with mutations in PLA2G6 (PLAN or PLA2G6-associated neurodegeneration). It is now known that a significant number of patients suffering from infantile neuroaxonal dystrophy (INAD) and Karak syndrome are a result of PLAN [143]. The neuroferritinopathy syndrome and aceruloplasminemia are frequently included under the NBIA heading, but are discussed elsewhere.

Classic PKAN is characterized by onset of disease symptoms before age 6, gait abnormalities, dystonia, dysarthria, rigidity, spasticity, and hyperreflexia secondary to corticospinal tract involvement. Progression is rapid and uniformly fatal. T2-weighted brain magnetic resonance imaging (MRI) reveals bilateral anteromedial hyperdensity surrounded by regions of hypointensity in the medial globus pallidus, the "eye-of-the-tiger" sign (Fig. 23.6). Optic atrophy or pigmentary retinopathy and an autosomal recessive pattern of inheritance are highly associated [142]. Like other ataxia syndromes associated with brain iron accumulation, clinical disease presentation for patients with atypical PKAN is variable, with a later age of onset, slower progression of deterioration, and less severe motor involvement. Dysarthria predominates, and psychiatric abnormalities are more common.

Pantothenate kinases are essential for coenzyme A biosynthesis and subsequent CoA utilization in multiple critical energy pathways, including fatty acid synthesis and metabolism, energy metabolism, glutathione metabolism, and neurotransmitter synthesis. Unlike the other pantothenate kinases, the PANK2 protein is targeted to the mitochondria. The current hypothesis of PKAN pathogenesis is based on both tissue-specific coenzyme A deficiency and the accumulation of cysteine-containing secondary metabolites [144]. Establishing a link between a PANK2- and CoA-deficient state, high cysteine-containing secondary metabolite accumulation and disrupted iron homeostasis are somewhat more complicated. The Hayflick group proposes cysteine-rich metabolites, N-pantothenoylcysteine and N-pantetheine, that chelate and bind the iron. However, further data are needed in order to decipher a mechanism and develop a model for the neurodegeneration [144].

Infantile neuroaxonal dystrophy (INAD) is a neuroaxonal dystrophy that presents in infancy with motor regression and profound hypotonia. Affected infants have axonal degeneration with distended axons, often identified as "spheroid bodies" histologically in both the central and peripheral nervous system [145]. INAD patients develop progressive motor and sensory deficits. Some affected individuals also have been noted to have elevated brain iron concentrations in the globus pallidus. Genome-wide linkage studies and subsequent candidate gene sequencing identified mutations in PLA2G6. Karak syndrome, originally named for brothers in Karak, Jordan, presents in early childhood

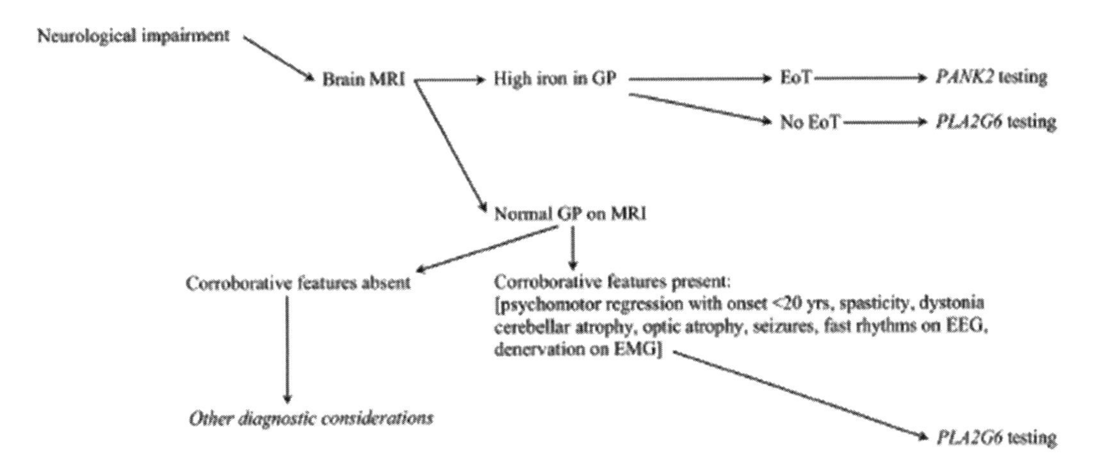

Fig. 23.7 Diagnostic scheme for NBIA. Other diagnostic considerations would include measuring serum ceruloplasmin and ferritin (Source: Reproduced with permission from [142])

with cerebellar ataxia that progresses to HSS/PKAN, including a classic "eye-of-the-tiger" MRI, but lacks PANK2 mutations. Based on the similarity to patients with INAD that have globus pallidus iron accumulation on T2-weighted MRI, individuals with Karak syndrome were also screened and found to have PLAN (PLA2G6-associated neurodegeneration) [145]. That there are INAD and Karak-like cases that do not have PLAN emphasizes that a wide spectrum of diseases is classified under NBIA banner (Fig. 23.7).

PLA2G6 is a calcium-independent phospholipase A2 that catalyzes glycerophospholipid hydrolysis, usually generating arachidonic acid and lysophospholipid [143, 145]. In this capacity, the phospholipase A2 enzymes maintain a delicate balance in the levels of phosphatidycholine expressed in cell membranes and thereby regulate and maintain cellular membrane integrity. This balance is maintained through their action opposing cytidylylphosphocholine transferase [145]. Mutations in PLA2G6 therefore lead to an increased expression of membrane phosphatidylcholine and resultant structural abnormalities in the cell membrane [143]. The mechanism by which a mutation in PLA2G6 results in NBIA remains unknown. Many authors have hypothesized that both PANK2 and PLA2G6 are critical for membrane integrity and cellular energy metabolism, but a common theme remains elusive.

9 Conclusion

That iron plays a role in neurodegeneration is indisputable. The striking similarity in presentation for many of the NBIA disorders, Alzheimer's disease, and Parkinson's disease further suggests a common final pathway for neuronal cell death despite different primary insults. The selective vulnerability of specific cell types and regions of the central nervous system has yet to be elucidated. Noninvasive imaging technology beyond MRI (e.g., magnetic resonance spectroscopy and magnetic resonance relaxometry) is poised to assist in further delineating and quantifying concentrations of metals and other chemicals, biochemical alterations, and regional differences within small brain regions. Only with mechanistic insight will successful and targeted therapeutic interventions be available. The diseases highlighted here represent those whose link to iron has been extensively studied, but it is important to mention that in recent years, the involvement of iron in other neurological diseases such as autism, attention deficit disorder/attention deficit and hyperactivity disorder (ADD/ADHD), and amyotrophic lateral sclerosis (ALS) has gained some attention. While many complex neurodegenerative diseases result from a convergence of multiple insults, the growing research and interest on a final pathway catalyzed by a disruption in iron homeostasis is significant. The role of iron and nutrition in aging and disease, antioxidant defense, and redox chemistry will become pivotal to our understanding of iron-mediated neurodegeneration.

References

1. Koeppen AH. The history of iron in the brain. J Neurol Sci. 1995;134(Suppl):1–9.
2. Jimenez Brundelet P. The combined perls-hematoxylin-eosin stain. Stain Technol. 1973;48:173–5.
3. Nguyen-Legros J, Bizot J, Bolesse M, Pulicani JP. "Diaminobenzidine black" as a new histochemical demonstration of exogenous iron. Histochemistry. 1980;66:239–44.
4. Ke Y, Qian ZM. Brain iron metabolism: neurobiology and neurochemistry. Prog Neurobiol. 2007;83:149–73.
5. Dringen R, Bishop GM, Koeppe M, Dang TN, Robinson SR. The pivotal role of astrocytes in the metabolism of iron in the brain. Neurochem Res. 2007;32:1884–90.
6. Shoham S, Youdim MB. Iron involvement in neural damage and microgliosis in models of neurodegenerative diseases. Cell Mol Biol. 2000;46:743–60.
7. Gelman BB. Iron in CNS disease. J Neuropathol Exp Neurol. 1995;54:477–86.
8. Connor JR, Menzies SL. Relationship of iron to oligodendrocytes and myelination. Glia. 1996;17:83–93.
9. Whitnall M, Richardson DR. Iron: a new target for pharmacological intervention in neurodegenerative diseases. Semin Pediatr Neurol. 2006;13:186–97.
10. Lange SJ, Que Jr L. Oxygen activating nonheme iron enzymes. Curr Opin Chem Biol. 1998;2:159–72.
11. Fitzpatrick PF. Tetrahydropterin-dependent amino acid hydroxylases. Annu Rev Biochem. 1999;68:355–81.
12. Fitzpatrick PF. The aromatic amino acid hydroxylases. Adv Enzymol Relat Areas Mol Biol. 2000;74:235–94.
13. Merli C, Petrucci E, Da Pozzo A, Pernetti M. Fenton-type treatment: state of the art. Ann Chim. 2003;93:761–70.
14. Koppenol WH. The Haber-Weiss cycle – 70 years later. Redox Rep. 2001;6:229–34.
15. Vassiliev V, Harris ZL, Zatta P. Ceruloplasmin in neurodegenerative diseases. Brain Res Brain Res Rev. 2005;49:633–40.
16. Madsen E, Gitlin JD. Copper and iron disorders of the brain. Annu Rev Neurosci. 2007;30:317–37.
17. Craven CM, Alexander J, Eldridge M, Kushner JP, Bernstein S, Kaplan J. Tissue distribution and clearance kinetics of non-transferrin-bound iron in the hypotransferrinemic mouse: a rodent model for hemochromatosis. Proc Natl Acad Sci USA. 1987;84:3457–61.
18. Gunshin H, Fujiwara Y, Custodio AO, Direnzo C, Robine S, Andrews NC. Slc11a2 is required for intestinal iron absorption and erythropoiesis but dispensable in placenta and liver. J Clin Invest. 2005;115:1258–66.
19. Morgan EH, Moos T. Mechanism and developmental changes in iron transport across the blood–brain barrier. Dev Neurosci. 2002;24:106–13.
20. Moos T. Brain iron homeostasis. Dan Med Bull. 2002;49:279–301.
21. Karkan D, Pfeifer C, Vitalis TZ, et al. A unique carrier for delivery of therapeutic compounds beyond the blood–brain barrier. PLoS One. 2008;3:e2469.
22. Moos T, Rosengren Nielsen T. Ferroportin in the postnatal rat brain: implications for axonal transport and neuronal export of iron. Semin Pediatr Neurol. 2006;13:149–57.
23. Jeong SY, David S. Glycosylphosphatidylinositol-anchored ceruloplasmin is required for iron efflux from cells in the central nervous system. Biol Chem. 2003;278:27144–8.
24. De Domenico I, Ward DM, di Patti MC, et al. Ferroxidase activity is required for the stability of cell surface ferroportin in cells expressing GPI-ceruloplasmin. EMBO J. 2007;26:2823–31.
25. Moos T, Oates PS, Morgan EH. Expression of transferrin mRNA in rat oligodendrocytes is iron-independent and changes with increasing age. Nutr Neurosci. 2001;4:15–23.
26. Moos T, Rosengren Nielsen T, Skjørringe T, Morgan EH. Iron trafficking inside the brain. J Neurochem. 2007;103:1730–40.
27. Pandolfo M. Iron and Friedreich ataxia. J Neural Transm Suppl. 2006;70:143–6.
28. Christodoulou K, Deymeer F, Serdaroğlu P, et al. Mapping of the second Friedreich's ataxia (FRDA2) locus to chromosome 9p23–p11: evidence for further locus heterogeneity. Neurogenetics. 2001;3:127–32.
29. Pandolfo M. Friedreich ataxia: detection of GAA repeat expansions and frataxin point mutations. Methods Mol Med. 2006;126:197–216.
30. Knight SA, Kim R, Pain D, Dancis A. The yeast connection to Friedreich ataxia. Am J Hum Genet. 1999;64:365–71.

31. Rouault TA, Tong WH. Iron-sulfur cluster biogenesis and human disease. Trends Genet. 2008;24:398–407.
32. Wilson RB. Iron dysregulation in Friedreich ataxia. Semin Pediatr Neurol. 2006;13:166–75.
33. Li K, Besse EK, Ha D, Kovtunovych G, Rouault TA. Iron-dependent regulation of frataxin expression: implications for treatment of Friedreich ataxia. Hum Mol Genet. 2008;17:2265–73.
34. Babady NE, Carelle N, Wells RD, et al. Advancements in the pathophysiology of Friedreich's Ataxia and new prospects for treatments. Mol Genet Metab. 2007;92:23–35.
35. Cooper JM, Schapira AH. Friedreich's ataxia: coenzyme Q10 and vitamin E therapy. Mitochondrion. 2007;7(Suppl. 1):S127–35.
36. Lodi R, Tonon C, Calabrese V, Schapira AH. Friedreich's ataxia: from disease mechanisms to therapeutic interventions. Antioxid Redox Signal. 2006;8:438–43.
37. Calabrese V, Cornelius C, Mancuso C, et al. Cellular stress response: a novel target for chemoprevention and nutritional neuroprotection in aging, neurodegenerative disorders and longevity. Neurochem Res. 2008;33:2444–71.
38. Cote L, Crutcher MD. The basal ganglia. In: Kandel ER, Schwartz JH, Jessell TM, editors. Principles of neural science. 3rd ed. Norwalk: Appleton and Lange; 1998. p. 647.
39. Suh YH, Checler F. Amyloid precursor protein, presenilins, and alpha-synuclein: molecular pathogenesis and pharmacological applications in Alzheimer's disease. Pharmacol Rev. 2002;54:469–525.
40. Maccioni RB, Munoz JP, Barbeito L. The molecular bases of Alzheimer's disease and other neurodegenerative disorders. Arch Med Res. 2001;32:367–81.
41. Castellani RJ, Lee HG, Zhu X, Nunomura A, Perry G, Smith MA. Neuropathology of Alzheimer disease: pathognomonic but not pathogenic. Acta Neuropathol. 2006;111:503–9.
42. Jarrett JT, Berger EP, Lansbury Jr PT. The carboxy terminus of the beta amyloid protein is critical for the seeding of amyloid formation: implications for the pathogenesis of Alzheimer's disease. Biochemistry. 1993;32:4693–7.
43. Rosenberg RN. The molecular and genetic basis of AD: the end of the beginning: the 2000 Wartenberg lecture. Neurology. 2000;54:2045–54.
44. Maccioni RB, Cambiazo V. Role of microtubule-associated proteins in the control of microtubule assembly. Physiol Rev. 1995;75:835–64.
45. Goedert M, Spillantini MG. A century of Alzheimer's disease. Science. 2006;314:777–81.
46. Castellani RJ, Moreira PI, Liu G, et al. Iron: the redox-active center of oxidative stress in Alzheimer disease. Neurochem Res. 2007;32:1640–5.
47. Adlard PA, Bush AI. Metals and Alzheimer's disease. J Alzheimers Dis. 2006;10:145–63.
48. Smith MA, Harris PL, Sayre LM, Perry G. Iron accumulation in Alzheimer disease is a source of redox-generated free radicals. Proc Natl Acad Sci USA. 1997;94:9866–8.
49. Lovell MA, Robertson JD, Teesdale WJ, Campbell JL, Markesbery WR. Copper, iron and zinc in Alzheimer's disease senile plaques. J Neurol Sci. 1998;158:47–52.
50. Dikalov SI, Vitek MP, Maples KR, Mason RP. Amyloid beta peptides do not form peptide-derived free radicals spontaneously, but can enhance metal-catalyzed oxidation of hydroxylamines to nitroxides. J Biol Chem. 1999;274:9392–9.
51. Atwood CS, Moir RD, Huang X, et al. Dramatic aggregation of Alzheimer abeta by cu(II) is induced by conditions representing physiological acidosis. J Biol Chem. 1998;273:12817–26.
52. Rogers JT, Randall JD, Cahill CM, et al. An iron-responsive element type II in the 5′-untranslated region of the Alzheimer's amyloid precursor protein transcript. J Biol Chem. 2002;277:45518–28.
53. Sayre LM, Perry G, Harris PL, Liu Y, Schubert KA, Smith MA. In situ oxidative catalysis by neurofibrillary tangles and senile plaques in Alzheimer's disease: a central role for bound transition metals. J Neurochem. 2000;74:270–9.
54. Harris FM, Brecht WJ, Xu Q, Mahley RW, Huang Y. Increased tau phosphorylation in apolipoprotein E4 transgenic mice is associated with activation of extracellular signal-regulated kinase: modulation by zinc. J Biol Chem. 2004;279:44795–801.
55. Yoshida T, Tanaka M, Sotomatsu A, Hirai S, Okamoto K. Activated microglia cause iron-dependent lipid peroxidation in the presence of ferritin. Neuroreport. 1998;9:1929–33.
56. Hirai K, Aliev G, Nunomura A, et al. Mitochondrial abnormalities in Alzheimer's disease. J Neurosci. 2001;21:3017–23.
57. Collingwood J, Dobson J. Mapping and characterization of iron compounds in Alzheimer's tissue. J Alzheimers Dis. 2006;10:215–22.
58. Kirschvink JL, Kobayashi-Kirschvink A, Woodford BJ. Magnetite biomineralization in the human brain. Proc Natl Acad Sci USA. 1992;89:7683–7.
59. Hautot D, Pankhurst QA, Khan N, Dobson J. Preliminary evaluation of nanoscale biogenic magnetite in Alzheimer's disease brain tissue. Proc Biol Sci. 2003;270(Suppl. 1):S62–4.
60. Dobson J. Magnetic iron compounds in neurological disorders. Ann N Y Acad Sci. 2004;1012:183–92.

61. Connor JR, Menzies SL, St Martin SM, Mufson EJ. A histochemical study of iron, transferrin, and ferritin in Alzheimer's diseased brains. J Neurosci Res. 1992;31:75–83.
62. Amit T, Avramovich-Tirosh Y, Youdim MB, Mandel S. Targeting multiple Alzheimer's disease etiologies with multimodal neuroprotective and neurorestorative iron chelators. FASEB J. 2008;22:1296–305.
63. Mandel S, Amit T, Bar-Am O, Youdim MB. Iron dysregulation in Alzheimer's disease: multimodal brain permeable iron chelating drugs, possessing neuroprotective–neurorescue and amyloid precursor protein-processing regulatory activities as therapeutic agents. Prog Neurobiol. 2007;82:348–60.
64. Levenson CW. Iron and Parkinson's disease: chelators to the rescue? Nutr Rev. 2003;61:311–3.
65. Burke RE, Kholodilov NG. Programmed cell death: does it play a role in Parkinson's disease? Ann Neurol. 1998;44(3 Suppl. 1):S126–33.
66. Thomas B, Beal MF. Parkinson's disease. Hum Mol Genet. 2007;16(Spec No. 2):R183–94.
67. Singh N, Pillay V, Choonara YE. Advances in the treatment of Parkinson's disease. Prog Neurobiol. 2007;81:29–44.
68. Berg D, Hochstrasser H. Iron metabolism in parkinsonian syndromes. Mov Disord. 2006;21:1299–310.
69. Hallgren B, Sourander P. The effect of age on the non-haemin iron in the human brain. J Neurochem. 1958;3:41–51.
70. Berg D. Disturbance of iron metabolism as a contributing factor to SN hyperechogenicity in Parkinson's disease: implications for idiopathic and monogenetic forms. Neurochem Res. 2007;32:1646–54.
71. Youdim MB, Green AR. Iron deficiency and neurotransmitter synthesis and function. Proc Nutr Soc. 1978;37:173–9.
72. Sofic E, Riederer P, Heinsen H, et al. Increased iron (III) and total iron content in post mortem substantia nigra of parkinsonian brain. J Neural Transm. 1988;74:199–205.
73. Ortega R, Cloetens P, Deves G, Carmona A, Bohic S. Iron storage within dopamine neurovesicles revealed by chemical nano-imaging. PLoS One. 2007;2:e925.
74. Oakley AE, Collingwood JF, Dobson J, et al. Individual dopaminergic neurons show raised iron levels in Parkinson disease. Neurology. 2007;68:1820–5.
75. Bharathi, Indi SS, Rao KS. Copper- and iron-induced differential fibril formation in alpha-synuclein: TEM study. Neurosci Lett. 2007;424:78–82.
76. Bharathi, Rao KS. Thermodynamics imprinting reveals differential binding of metals to alpha-synuclein: relevance to Parkinson's disease. Biochem Biophys Res Commun. 2007;359:115–20.
77. Friedlich AL, Tanzi RE, Rogers JT. The 5′-untranslated region of Parkinson's disease alpha-synuclein messengerRNA contains a predicted iron responsive element. Mol Psychiatry. 2007;12:222–3.
78. Kaur D, Andersen J. Does cellular iron disregulation play a causative role in Parkinson's disease? Ageing Res Rev. 2004;3:327–43.
79. Halliwell B, Gutteridge JM. Biologically relevant metal ion-dependent hydroxyl radical generation. An update. FEBS Lett. 1992;307:108–12.
80. Graham DG, Tiffany SM, Bell Jr WR, Gutknecht WF. Autoxidation versus covalent binding of quinones as the mechanism of toxicity of dopamine, 6-hydroxydopamine, and related compounds toward C1300 neuroblastoma cells in vitro. Mol Pharmacol. 1978;14:644–53.
81. Koziorowski D, Friedman A, Arosio P, Santambrogio P, Dziewulska D. ELISA reveals a difference in the structure of substantia nigra ferritin in Parkinson's disease and incidental lewy body compared to control. Parkinsonism Relat Disord. 2007;13:214–8.
82. Thompson K, Menzies S, Muckenthaler M, et al. Mouse brains deficient in H-ferritin have normal iron concentration but a protein profile of iron deficiency and increased evidence of oxidative stress. J Neurosci Res. 2003;71:46–63.
83. Faucheux BA, Martin ME, Beaumont C, et al. Lack of up-regulation of ferritin is associated with sustained iron regulatory protein-1 binding activity in the substantia nigra of patients with Parkinson's disease. J Neurochem. 2002;83:320–30.
84. Fasano M, Bergamasco B, Lopiano L. Modifications of the iron-neuromelanin system in Parkinson's disease. J Neurochem. 2006;96:909–16.
85. Zecca L, Zucca FA, Albertini A, Rizzio E, Fariello RG. A proposed dual role of neuromelanin in the pathogenesis of Parkinson's disease. Neurology. 2006;67(Suppl. 2):S8–11.
86. Shamoto-Nagai M, Maruyama W, Yi H, et al. Neuromelanin induces oxidative stress in mitochondria through release of iron: mechanism behind the inhibition of 26S proteasome. J Neural Transm. 2006;113:633–44.
87. Lopiano L, Chiesa M, Digilio G, et al. Q-band EPR investigations of neuromelanin in control and Parkinson's disease patients. Biochim Biophys Acta. 2000;1500:306–12.
88. Gerlach M, Double KL, Youdim MB, Riederer P. Potential sources of increased iron in the substantia nigra of parkinsonian patients. J Neural Transm Suppl. 2006;70:133–42.
89. Wang J, Jiang H, Xie JX. Ferroportin1 and hephaestin are involved in the nigral iron accumulation of 6-OHDA-lesioned rats. Eur J Neurosci. 2007;25:2766–72.
90. Song N, Jiang H, Wang J, Xie JX. Divalent metal transporter 1 up-regulation is involved in the 6-hydroxydopamine-induced ferrous iron influx. J Neurosci Res. 2007;85:3118–26.

91. Berg D, Hochstrasser H, Schweitzer KJ, Riess O. Disturbance of iron metabolism in Parkinson's disease – ultrasonography as a biomarker. Neurotox Res. 2006;9:1–13.
92. Kooncumchoo P, Sharma S, Porter J, Govitrapong P, Ebadi M. Coenzyme Q(10) provides neuroprotection in iron-induced apoptosis in dopaminergic neurons. J Mol Neurosci. 2006;28:125–41.
93. Jiang H, Luan Z, Wang J, Xie J. Neuroprotective effects of iron chelator desferal on dopaminergic neurons in the substantia nigra of rats with iron-overload. Neurochem Int. 2006;49:605–9.
94. Zhu W, Xie W, Pan T, et al. Prevention and restoration of lactacystin-induced nigrostriatal dopamine neuron degeneration by novel brain-permeable iron chelators. FASEB J. 2007;21:3835–44.
95. Moos T, Trinder D, Morgan EH. Cellular distribution of ferric iron, ferritin, transferrin and divalent metal transporter 1 (DMT1) in substantia nigra and basal ganglia of normal and beta2-microglobulin deficient mouse brain. Cell Mol Biol (Noisy-le-Grand). 2000;46:549–61.
96. Guerreiro RJ, Bras JM, Santana I, et al. Association of HFE common mutations with Parkinson's disease, Alzheimer's disease and mild cognitive impairment in a Portuguese cohort. BMC Neurol. 2006;6:24–32.
97. Borie C, Gasparini F, Verpillat P, et al. French Parkinson's disease genetic study group. Association study between iron-related genes polymorphisms and Parkinson's disease. J Neurol. 2002;249:801–4.
98. Aamodt AH, Stovner LJ, Thorstensen K, Lydersen S, White LR, Aasly JO. Prevalence of haemochromatosis gene mutations in Parkinson's disease. J Neurol Neurosurg Psychiatry. 2007;78:315–7.
99. Akbas N, Hochstrasser H, Deplazes J, et al. Screening for mutations of the HFE gene in Parkinson's disease patients with hyperechogenicity of the substantia nigra. Neurosci Lett. 2006;407:16–9.
100. Dekker MC, Giesbergen PC, Njajou OT, et al. Mutations in the hemochromatosis gene (HFE), Parkinson's disease and parkinsonism. Neurosci Lett. 2003;348:117–9.
101. Robson KJ, Lehmann DJ, Wimhurst VL, et al. Synergy between the C2 allele of transferrin and the C282Y allele of the haemochromatosis gene (HFE) as risk factors for developing Alzheimer's disease. J Med Genet. 2004;41:261–5.
102. Lehmann DJ, Worwood M, Ellis R, et al. Iron genes, iron load and risk of Alzheimer's disease. J Med Genet. 2006;43:e52.
103. Corder EH, Beaumont H. Susceptibility groups for Alzheimer's disease (OPTIMA cohort): integration of gene variants and biochemical factors. Mech Ageing Dev. 2007;128:76–82.
104. Willis T. De Anima Brutorum. London: Wells and Scot; 1672.
105. Ryan M, Slevin JT. Restless legs syndrome. Am J Health Syst Pharm. 2006;63:1599–612.
106. Allen R. International Restless Legs Syndrome Study Group. http://www.irlssg.org. Accessed 24.05.2008.
107. Ekbom K-A. Restless legs: a clinical study. Acta Med Scand. 1945;158(Suppl. 1):1–123.
108. Winkelmann J, Muller-Myhsok B, Wittchen HU, et al. Complex segregation analysis of restless legs syndrome provides evidence for an autosomal dominant mode of inheritance in early age at onset families. Ann Neurol. 2002;52:297–302.
109. Desautels A, Turecki G, Montplaisir J, Sequeira A, Verner A, Rouleau GA. Identification of a major susceptibility locus for restless legs syndrome on chromosome 12q. Am J Hum Genet. 2001;69:1266–70.
110. Bonati MT, Ferini-Strambi L, Aridon P, Oldani A, Zucconi M, Casari G. Autosomal dominant restless legs syndrome maps on chromosome 14q. Brain. 2003;126:1485–92.
111. Chen S, Ondo WG, Rao S, Li L, Chen Q, Wang Q. Genomewide linkage scan identifies a novel susceptibility locus for restless legs syndrome on chromosome 9p. Am J Hum Genet. 2004;74:876–85.
112. Bara-Jimenez W, Aksu M, Graham B, Sato S, Hallett M. Periodic limb movements in sleep: state-dependent excitability of the spinal flexor reflex. Neurology. 2000;54:1609–16.
113. Sachdev P. The neuropsychiatry of brain iron. J Neuropsychiatry Clin Neurosci. 1993;5:18–29.
114. Eisensehr I, Ehrenberg BL, Rogge Solti S, Noachtar S. Treatment of idiopathic restless legs syndrome (RLS) with slow-release valproic acid compared with slow-release levodopa/benserazid. J Neurol. 2004;251:579–83.
115. Erikson KM, Jones BC, Beard JL. Iron deficiency alters dopamine transporter functioning in rat striatum. J Nutr. 2000;130:2831–7.
116. Erikson KM, Jones BC, Hess EJ, Zhang Q, Beard JL. Iron deficiency decreases dopamine D1 and D2 receptors in rat brain. Pharmacol Biochem Behav. 2001;69:409–18.
117. Scales WE, Vander AJ, Brown MB, Kluger MJ. Human circadian rhythms in temperature, trace metals, and blood variables. J Appl Physiol. 1988;65:1840–6.
118. Garcia-Borreguero D, Larrosa O, de la Llave Y, Granizo JJ, Allen R. Correlation between rating scales and sleep laboratory measurements in restless legs syndrome. Sleep Med. 2004;5:561–5.
119. Earley CJ, Heckler D, Allen RP. Repeated IV doses of iron provides effective supplemental treatment of restless legs syndrome. Sleep Med. 2005;6:301–5.
120. O'Keeffe ST, Gavin K, Lavan JN. Iron status and restless legs syndrome in the elderly. Age Ageing. 1994;23:200–3.
121. Sun ER, Chen CA, Ho G, Earley CJ, Allen RP. Iron and the restless legs syndrome. Sleep. 1998;21:371–7.
122. Kryger MH, Otake K, Foerster J. Low body stores of iron and restless legs syndrome: a correctable cause of insomnia in adolescents and teenagers. Sleep Med. 2002;3:127–32.

123. O'Keeffe ST. Iron deficiency with normal ferritin levels in restless legs syndrome. Sleep Med. 2005;6:281–2.
124. Mizuno S, Mihara T, Miyaoka T, Inagaki T, Horiguchi J. CSF iron, ferritin and transferrin levels in restless legs syndrome. J Sleep Res. 2005;14:43–7.
125. Earley CJ, Allen RP, Beard JL, Connor JR. Insight into the pathophysiology of restless legs syndrome. J Neurosci Res. 2000;62:623–8.
126. Godau J, Schweitzer KJ, Liepelt I, Gerloff C, Berg D. Substantia nigra hypoechogenicity: definition and findings in restless legs syndrome. Mov Disord. 2007;22:187–92.
127. Akyol A, Kiylioglu N, Kadikoylu G, Bolaman AZ, Ozgel N. Iron deficiency anemia and restless legs syndrome: is there an electrophysiological abnormality? Clin Neurol Neurosurg. 2003;106:23–7.
128. Connor JR, Wang XS, Patton SM, et al. Decreased transferrin receptor expression by neuromelanin cells in restless legs syndrome. Neurology. 2004;62:1563–7.
129. Wang X, Wiesinger J, Beard J, et al. Thy1 expression in the brain is affected by iron and is decreased in restless legs syndrome. J Neurol Sci. 2004;220:59–66.
130. Jeng CJ, McCarroll SA, Martin TF, et al. Thy-1 is a component common to multiple populations of synaptic vesicles. J Cell Biol. 1998;140:685–98.
131. Almqvist P, Carlsson SR, Hardy JA, Winblad B. Regional and subcellular distribution of thy-1 in human brain assayed by a solid-phase radioimmunoassay. J Neurochem. 1986;46:681–5.
132. Shults CW, Kimber TA. Thy-1 immunoreactivity distinguishes patches/striosomes from matrix in the early postnatal striatum of the rat. Brain Res Dev Brain Res. 1993;75:136–40.
133. Clardy SL, Wang X, Boyer PJ, Earley CJ, Allen RP, Connor JR. Is ferroportin-hepcidin signaling altered in restless legs syndrome? J Neurol Sci. 2006;247:173–9.
134. Connor JR, et al. Neuropathological examination suggests impaired brain iron acquisition in restless legs syndrome. Neurology. 2003;61:304–9.
135. Garcia-Borreguero D, Larrosa O, de la Llave Y, Verger K, Masramon X, Hernandez G. Treatment of restless legs syndrome with gabapentin: a double-blind, cross-over study. Neurology. 2002;59:1573–9.
136. Zucconi M, Coccagna G, Petronelli R, Gerardi R, Mondini S, Cirignotta F. Nocturnal myoclonus in restless legs syndrome effect of carbamazepine treatment. Funct Neurol. 1989;4:263–71.
137. Ineck B, Mason BJ, Thompson EG. Anemias. In: DiPiro JT, Talbert RL, Yee GC, et al., editors. Pharmacotherapy: a pathophysiologic approach. 6th ed. New York: McGraw-Hill; 2005. p. 1814.
138. Silber MH. Calming restless legs. Sleep. 2004;27:839–41.
139. Davis BJ, Rajput A, Rajput ML, Aul EA, Eichhorn GR. A randomized, double-blind placebo-controlled trial of iron in restless legs syndrome. Eur Neurol. 2000;43:70–5.
140. Earley CJ, Heckler D, Allen RP. The treatment of restless legs syndrome with intravenous iron dextran. Sleep Med. 2004;5:231–5.
141. Hayflick SJ, Hartman M, Coryell J, Gitschier J, Rowley H. Brain MRI in neurodegeneration with brain iron accumulation with and without PANK2 mutations. Am J Neuroradiol. 2006;27:1230–3.
142. Hayflick SJ. Neurodegeneration with brain iron accumulation: from genes to pathogenesis. Semin Pediatr Neurol. 2006;13:182–5.
143. Morgan NV, Westaway SK, Morton JE, et al. PLA2G6, encoding a phospholipase A2, is mutated in neurodegenerative disorders with high brain iron. Nat Genet. 2006;38:752–4.
144. Gregory A, Hayflick SJ. Neurodegeneration with brain iron accumulation. Folia Neuropathol. 2005;43:286–96.
145. Kurian MA, Morgan NV, MacPherson L, et al. Phenotypic spectrum of neurodegeneration associated with mutations in the PLA2G6 gene (PLAN). Neurology. 2008;70:1623–9.

Chapter 24
Iron Metabolism in Cancer and Infection

Sergei Nekhai and Victor R. Gordeuk

Keywords Anemia of chronic disease • Cancer • Cell cycle • HIV • Infection • Malaria • Microbial growth

1 Iron and the Cell Cycle

Progression through the G1, S, G2, and M phases of the cell cycle is regulated by sets of Cdks bound to corresponding cyclins (reviewed in [1]). Transition through the G1 phase is regulated by Cdk4/cyclin D1 and by Cdk6/cyclin D3. Cdk2/cyclin E is active at the late G1 phase and is responsible for the G1/S transition. Progression through the S phase is regulated by Cdk2/cyclin A. DNA synthesis during the S phase critically relies on the enzymatic activity of ribonucleotide reductase [2]. The S/G2 transition is regulated by Cdk1/cyclin A. Cdk1/cyclin B is responsible for the G2/M transition and for the completion of mitosis.

1.1 Ribonucleotide Reductase

Ribonucleotide reductase, the rate limiting enzyme for DNA synthesis and therefore critical for the S phase of the cell cycle, is composed of two subunits [2]. The R1 subunit of ribonucleotide reductase binds substrate and the R2 subunit contains nonheme iron which is important for enzymatic activity [2]. Inhibition of the enzymatic activity of R2 by iron chelators 311 and desferrioxamine inhibited growth of a number of cancer cell lines [3]. Recent studies have suggested that iron depletion influences the control of the cell cycle and angiogenesis and may suppress metastasis [4].

1.2 Cdk2

Cdk2 is positively regulated by the binding of cyclin E (G1/S transition) or cyclin A (S-phase transition) and by Cdk7-mediated phosphorylation of Thr160 [1]. Negative regulation of Cdk2 includes its association with the p21 (CIP1/WAF1) and p27 (Kip1) inhibitory proteins and phosphorylation of

S. Nekhai, Ph.D.
Center for Sickle Cell Disease, Division of Hematology and Oncology, Department of Medicine, Howard University, Washington, DC, USA

V.R. Gordeuk, M.D. (✉)
Sickle Cell Center, Division of Hematology and Oncology, Department of Medicine, University of Illinois at Chicago, Chicago, IL, USA
e-mail: vgordeuk@uic.edu

G.J. Anderson and G. McLaren (eds.), *Iron Physiology and Pathophysiology in Humans*, Nutrition and Health, DOI 10.1007/978-1-60327-485-2_24,

Tyr15 by Weel kinase [5]. Iron chelators reduce p21 protein levels through the inhibition of translocation of p21 (CIP1/WAF1) mRNA from the nucleus to cytosol and induction of ubiquitin-independent proteosomal degradation of p21 [6]. Desferrioxamine markedly increased p27Kip1 expression but not p21 (CIP1/WAF1) and the induction of p27Kip1 was accompanied by an increased level of transforming growth factor beta1 [7]. Cdk2 activity is dramatically inhibited by iron chelators [8, 9]. The mechanism of Cdk2 inhibition could be related to the expression of the cyclin-dependent kinase inhibitors p21 or p27. Iron depletion by DpT-based iron chelators increased expression of p21 [4]. A lipid-soluble iron chelator desferri-exochelin (D-Exo) caused reversible cell cycle arrest in normal human mammary epithelial cells by inhibiting binding of cyclins A and E to Cdk2 [8]. In contrast, D-Exo increased binding of cyclin E and cyclin A to Cdk2 and also increased binding of p21 to Cdk2 in MCF-7 breast cancer cells resulting in apoptosis [8]. Iron depletion caused G1 arrest in fibroblasts that was due to elevated levels of the cyclin-dependent kinase inhibitor p27(Kip1) and inhibition of Cdk2 activity [10]. Iron depletion removing iron from prolyl hydroxylase, decreasing the activity of prolyl hydroxylase and increasing HIF-1α and HIF-2α protein levels [11]. An earlier study showed that hypoxia-induced G1 cell cycle arrest required retinoblastoma protein (Rb) and not p53 or p21, and that hypoxia facilitates transcription of p27 through an HIF-1-independent region of its proximal promoter thereby inhibiting Cdk2 activity and maintaining Rb hypophosphorylation [12]. But more recent studies showed that hypoxia-induced p27 protein expression was abrogated by RNAi-mediated knockdown of HIF-1a [13] suggesting that HIF-1a might be critical for the induction of p27. In our recent study, we found that the activity of Cdk9 (see more details in HIV section) is inhibited when cells are cultured at 3% oxygen [14], or treated with iron chelators [9]. Because Cdk9 regulates most if not all RNA polymerase II-mediated transcription [15], iron chelation is likely to have a general transcription inhibitory effect. Iron depletion also led to decreased expression of cyclins D1, D2, D3, A, and B1 and Cdk4 [4, 16]. Cdk2 but not cyclin E expression was decreased in cells treated with DFO and 311 [16]. It is possible that the decrease of Cdk2 activity observed in cells treated with iron chelators is related to the inability of Cdk2 to bind to cyclin E or cyclin A. This deregulation of Cdk2 interaction with its cyclins could be due to increased interaction of Cdk2 with p21 or p27 or changes in Cdk2 phosphorylation.

2 Iron and Cancer

Iron may be involved in cancerogenesis through promoting the formation of reactive oxygen species (ROS) and increased mutation rate of DNA. In a longitudinal survey of more than 14,000 adults in NHANESI, the mean total iron-binding capacity was significantly lower and transferrin saturation significantly higher among men who developed cancer compared to those who remained free of cancer, and the risk of cancer was elevated in women with a high transferrin saturation [17]. Further follow-up of this cohort indicated that for men and women combined, the risk of cancer occurrence in the participants with transferrin saturation >40% was 1.81 times the risk in those with transferrin saturation <30%, and corresponding relative risk for mortality from cancer was 1.73 [18]. These results are consistent with the hypothesis that higher body iron stores increase the risk of cancer.

2.1 Gastrointestinal Cancer

Epithelial cells of the gastrointestinal tract undergo active cell division and constant shedding [19]. The cells are exposed to dietary heme, an important source of body iron, and serve as a separation barrier in the intestinal lumen. Inactivation of a homeobox transcription factor, CDX2, in mice resulted in development of colonic polyps, and low level of CDX2 expression is often seen in poorly differentiated colon carcinomas in humans [20]. On the other hand, overexpression of CDX2 in transgenic mice promotes intestinal metaplasia, and CDX2 expression is found in intestinal metaplasia in stomach and esophagus [20]. Gene array analysis of gene targets of CDX2 identified the ceruloplasmin-related iron transport protein hephaestin (HEPH) [20]. Intracellular iron induces the expression of CDX2 and HEPH simultaneously, and HEPH participates in the export of iron [20]. Although about half of the cases of diagnosed colorectal cancer have no association with anemia [21], low levels of iron correlate with incidence of gastrointestinal cancer [22]. Therefore, chronically low iron levels might contribute to the deregulation of CDX2 and production of undifferentiated colon endothelial cells.

Iron overload related to the consumption of home-brewed beer in Africa has been implicated as a risk factor for esophageal cancer [23, 24], although this association has been questioned [25]. There is conflicting epidemiologic evidence whether increased iron stores are associated with the development of colorectal cancer [17, 26]. Formation of ROS, DNA repair, cell growth and glutathione (GSH) was analyzed in human colon tumor cells treated with ferric nitrilotriacetate (Fe-NTA). ROS formation was increased in cells treated with 1 mM concentration of Fe-NTA as detected with the peroxide-labile fluorescent dye, carboxy-dichlorodihydrofluorescine-diacetate [27]. Treatment with 25 μM Fe-NTA was associated with increased cell growth [27]. Analysis of the effect of 100–250 μM concentrations of Fe-NTA in primary nontransformed colon cells and in a preneoplastic colon adenoma cell line showed increased DNA damage [28], suggesting that increased iron might induce early stages of colorectal cancerogenesis. Analysis of high dietary iron on colon carcinogenesis in mouse injected intraperitoneally with the colonotropic carcinogen, azoxymethane, showed an increase in tumorgenesis with high dietary iron compared to low dietary iron [29]. No tumors were observed in mice receiving only dietary iron, suggesting that iron may promote tumor growth but be unable to initiate tumor formation [29]. Analysis of biomarkers in colon epithelium showed increased proliferation and apoptosis in response to iron but no difference in biomarkers of oxidative stress, suggesting that elevated dietary iron may promote carcinogenesis through mechanisms independent of oxidative stress [29].

2.2 *Hepatocellular Carcinoma*

Among more than 5,000 patients undergoing liver transplantation, iron overload was associated with hepatocellular carcinoma (HCC), suggesting a possible carcinogenic or cocarcinogenic role for iron in chronic liver disease [30]. HCC was reported in a patient with genetic hemochromatosis in the absence of cirrhosis suggesting that increased iron can potentially cause HCC in noncirrhotic hemochromatosis [31]. Dietary iron overload that occurs commonly in parts of sub-Saharan Africa is associated with an increased risk for HCC [32–34] likely due to chronic necroinflammatory hepatic disease [35]. Administration of aflatoxin B(1) (AFB(1)) to rats along with iron showed multiplicative effects on the rate of mutagenesis [36], suggesting a potential synergistic effect of dietary AFB(1) and dietary iron on the development of HCC. Correlation analysis of serum transferrin-iron saturation (TS) and the incidence of hospitalizations or deaths related to cirrhosis and liver cancer showed an association between elevated serum TS and increased incidence of cirrhosis or liver cancer especially with the elevated alcohol consumption [37].

Aberrant hypermethylation of CpG islands in the promoters and subsequent epigenetic silencing of the corresponding gene might be among the molecular mechanisms of HCC. Analysis of methylation of frequently methylated RASSF1A, cyclin D2, p16(INK4a), GSTpi1, SOCS-1, and APC genes in patients with HFE-mediated hemochromatosis showed different extent of methylation of these genes and also transcriptional downregulation of RASSF1A, cyclin D2, GSTpi1, and SOCS-1 [38].

Thus severe iron overload might be directly related to epigenetic gene silencing that is characteristic of HCC and changes in DNA methylation patterns might be useful for the early detection of HCC [38]. Chronic hepatitus C viral (HCV) infection may be associated with increased liver iron stores. Transgenic mice that expressed HCV polyprotein and fed with an excess-iron diet developed HCC in 45% of cases compared to none in nontransgenic mice and transgenic mice with normal dietary iron [39]. Proteomic analysis of changes in the expression of proteins in the liver of mice fed an iron-rich diet identified 30 liver proteins including enzymes involved in the urea cycle, fatty acid oxidation, and the methylation cycle [40].

2.3 *Pancreatic Adenocarcinoma*

Analysis of HFE mutations C282Y and H63D in patients with chronic pancreatitis and pancreatic adenocarcinoma showed no significant differences in heterozygosity for either mutations in patients with alcoholic, idiopathic, or familial pancreatitis, or pancreatic adenocarcinoma in comparison with corresponding controls [41].

2.4 *Breast Cancer*

In a cohort of almost 50,000 Canadian women, no association of iron or heme iron intake with risk of breast cancer was found in women consuming alcohol or in women who had ever used hormone replacement therapy [42]. However, polymorphism analysis of enzymes that are involved in removal of iron-mediated reactive oxygen species showed an increased risk of breast cancer in women with high iron intake who carried genotypes that potentially result in higher levels of iron-generated oxidative stress [43].

2.5 *Other Forms of Cancer*

Transferrin receptor 2 (Tfr2) expression is restricted to the liver and intestines in normal tissue whereas it is expressed in cells derived from ovarian cancer, colon cancer, and glioblastoma [44]. In leukemic and melanoma cell lines, Tfr2 expression is inversely correlated to the expression of Tfr1 [44]. Increased iron downregulates total Tfr2 levels in some cell types whereas in the other cell types iron downregulates membrane-bound Tfr2 but not the total amount of Tfr2 [44]. Iron depletion increased Tfr2 expression suggesting that decreased iron in cancer cells may be the cause of increased Tfr2 expression, although the direct effect of Tfr2 on the cancer cells remains to be determined.

Invasiveness and metastasic aggressiveness of head and neck squamous cell carcinoma (HNSCC) has been linked to overexpression of matrix metalloproteinase-9 (MMP-9). Treatment of neck squamous carcinoma cell lines, OM-2 and HN-22, with ferric ammonium sulfate increased both RNA and protein expression of MMP-9 [45]. The induction of MMP-9 was mediated by activated protein-1 (AP-1) transcription factor that was activated by signaling through extracellular signal-regulated kinase (ERK1/2) and Akt [45]. Thus, iron might influence the development of head and neck squamous cell carcinoma.

2.6 Iron as a Target for Cancer Therapy

Patients with widespread neuroblastoma (NB) frequently have elevated serum ferritin levels, and anti-NB effects of the iron chelator DFO have been reported. The effect of DFO on human bone marrow NB cells from two untreated children with Evans Stage IV disease was examined. DFO caused dose- and time-dependent cytotoxicity of NB cells, with maximal killing at exposure to 50 μm DFO for 72 h. Cytotoxicity was prevented by cotreatment with stoichiometric amounts of iron salts and reversible by removal of DFO or addition of iron salts within 48 h of treatment. Additionally, DFO inhibited clonal growth of human bone marrow NB cells in methylcellulose in a time- and dose-dependent manner. These effects were also prevented by cotreatment with iron salts. Thus, DFO seems to have antitumor effects on human NB cells which appear to be related to iron deprivation [46].

Lymphoblastoma CEM-T cell growth is inhibited by 311 (2-hydroxy-1-naphthylaldehyde benzoyl hydrazone) and deferoxamine (DFO) [3]. Tyrosyl radical signal of the R2 subunit of ribonucleotide reductase was analyzed by electron spin resonance and shown to be reduced in CEM cells treated with iron chelators suggesting that ribonucleotide reductase is a target of iron chelators [3]. Overexpression of the R2 subunit in CEM decreased the sensitivity to 311 but not to DFO suggesting the R2 might be a primary target for 311 [3].

The oral tridentate iron chelator, deferasirox (ICL670), is approved for use in the United States [47]. ICL670 demonstrated potent antiproliferative effects for rat and human hepatoma cells and was found to be four-times more efficient than the bidentate iron chelator CP20 (deferiprone) [48]. ICL670 decreased DNA synthesis and significantly reduced the number of cells in G2-M phase [48]. Interestingly, while ICL670 inhibited polyamine biosynthesis, CP20 increased polyamine biosynthesis, suggesting distinct mechanisms of action of ICL670 and CP20 [48].

A group of novel di-2-pyridylketone thiosemicarbazone (DpT)-based iron chelators and especially Dp44mT were shown to exhibit marked antiproliferative efficacy in vitro and antitumor activity in vivo [49]. Dp44mT upregulated the metastasis suppressor Ndrg1 in the tumor but not in the liver [50]. Animals treated with Dp44mT showed little alteration in hematological and biochemical indices at the chelator doses of 0.4–0.75 mg/kg per day that were required to induce antitumor activity [50]. Treatment of control mice with Triapine, an iron chelator that has entered phase II clinical trials [51], resulted in hematological toxicity at the doses that were required to achieve antitumor activity [50]. This observation correlates with evidence of anemia and methemoglobinemia in patients treated with Triapine [51]. Of note, the higher doses of Dp44mT (0.75 mg/kg per day) resulted in cardiac fibrosis likely due to Fe accumulation in the heart [50]. Combined treatment with Dp44mT and DFO allowed avoidance of fibrosis [50]. At a lower dose of 0.4 mg/kg per day over 7 weeks Dp44mT was well tolerated, indicating its potential for in vivo use.

3 Iron and Microbial Growth

Iron is essential for bacterial growth and these microorganisms produce siderophores to acquire iron from the environment. Iron is a cofactor for several enzymes in both microbes and in their eukaryotic hosts. The stringent regulation of iron uptake, which is necessary to prevent toxicity, is a challenge for pathogens that reside within the endocytic pathway of mammalian cells. Endosomes and lysosomes tend to be gradually depleted of iron by host transporters. For example, Nramp1 (Slc11a1) is a proton efflux pump that translocates Fe^{2+} and Mn^{2+} ions from macrophage lysosomes/phagolysosomes into the cytosol. Mutations in Nramp1 cause susceptibility to infection with the bacteria *Salmonella* and *Mycobacteria* and the protozoan *Leishmania*, suggesting that a pool of intraphagosomal iron is necessary for the intracellular growth of these pathogens. *Salmonella* and *Mycobacteria* express iron transporter systems that effectively compete with host transporters for iron. *Leishmania amazonensis* expresses LIT1, a ZIP family membrane Fe(2+) transporter, that is required for intracellular growth and virulence [52]. There is a vast literature on the role of iron in microbial infections. Only a small sampling is provided in this chapter.

3.1 Yersinia Pestis

Yersinia pestis is the etiologic agent of plague. Without appropriate treatment, the pathogen rapidly causes septicemia, the terminal and fatal phase of the disease. In order to identify bacterial genes that are essential during septicemic plague in humans, transcriptome analysis was performed on the fully virulent *Y. pestis* CO92 strain grown in either decomplemented human plasma or Luria-Bertani medium. *Y. pestis* genes involved in 12 iron-acquisition systems and one iron-storage system (bfr, bfd) were specifically induced in human plasma. Of these, the ybt and tonB genes (encoding the yersiniabactin siderophore virulence factor and the siderophore transporter, respectively) were induced at 37° C, i.e., under conditions mimicking the mammalian environment [53].

3.2 Helicobacter Pylori

Helicobacter pylori is a prevalent, worldwide, chronic infection that is linked to the development of peptic ulcer disease, gastric malignancy, and dyspeptic symptoms. There is evidence to support a relationship of *H. pylori* with iron deficiency anemia, but this association remains controversial [54]. Treatment of *H. pylori* may enhance the efficacy of oral iron therapy in iron deficiency anemia patients with *H. pylori*-positive chronic gastritis.

3.3 Bordetella

Whooping cough is a reemerging infectious disease of the respiratory tract. Iron has been found to induce substantial phenotypic changes in this pathogen. Using an in vitro model for bacterial attachment it was shown that the attachment capacity of *Bordetella pertussis* to epithelial respiratory cells is enhanced under iron stress conditions. Attachment is mediated by iron-induced surface-exposed proteins with sialic acid-binding capacity. Some of these iron-induced surface-associated proteins are immunogenic and may represent attractive vaccine candidates [55]. Colonization by *Bordetella bronchiseptica* results in a variety of inflammatory respiratory infections in animals and humans. For successful colonization, *B. bronchiseptica* must acquire iron from the infected host. Utilization of host heme iron in hemoglobin and myoglobin by *B. bronchiseptica* requires expression of BhuR, an outer membrane protein. BhuR appears to be a hemin receptor [56].

3.4 Tuberculosis

Tuberculosis (TB) caused by the pathogen *Mycobacterium tuberculosis* infects one-third of the world population. Despite 50 years of available drug treatments, TB continues to increase at a significant rate. The failure to control TB stems in part from the expense of delivering treatment to infected individuals and from complex treatment regimens [57]. A number of studies indicate that increased iron status enhances tuberculosis infection [33, 58–62]. Siderophore molecules used for iron acquisition are potential new therapeutic targets because pathogen survival and virulence is directly related to iron availability. A key host defense mechanism is the production of siderocalins that sequester iron-laden siderophores and *M. tuberculosis* replicates poorly in the absence of these siderophores. "Dominant negative" mycobactin siderophore analogues inhibit bacterial growth. Several groups have developed agents that directly inhibit enzymes involved in siderophore synthesis. Another approach is to target the iron dependent regulator protein (IdeR) that represses siderophore synthesis genes and virulence factors when sustainable iron levels have been achieved. Loss of the repression leads to iron excess and oxidative damage. In contrast, greater IdeR repression at low iron levels attenuates *M. tuberculosis* virulence in mice. Small peptides that either enhance IdeR repression or inhibit IdeR dimerization demonstrate that IdeR activity can be rationally modulated [63].

3.5 Hepatitis C

Increased iron deposition in liver is more common in patients with chronic hepatitis C as compared to hepatitis B virus infected patients or uninfected controls [64]. Moreover, nonresponse to treatment with ribavirin and interferon was correlated with increased liver iron [64]. Analysis of hepcidin mRNA expression in liver samples showed significantly lower hepcidin expression in HCV(+) patients than in HBV(+) patients, suggesting that deregulation of hepcidin may contribute to iron overload in patients with chronic hepatitis C [65]. Iron chelation therapy with deferiprone (L1) (DFP) in thalassemic patients of which about 50% were positive for HCV showed significant decrease in serum ferritin after 6 and 12 months of treatment [66].

3.6 HIV

3.6.1 HIV-1-Associated Anemia

Infection with HIV-1 subtype C led to a twofold increase in the prevalence of anemia to about 50% [67]. The hypoxic response is an important component of the body's reaction to impaired tissue perfusion, chronic pulmonary complications and the low hemoglobin concentrations of sickle cell disease (SCD) and other types of anemia. HIV-1 latency might result from decreased activities of cellular factors that are required for HIV-1 replication in T cells that grow under physiological conditions. Physiological oxygen levels (3–6% O_2) are significantly lower than the atmospheric 21% O_2 and this difference might have a profound effect on the activity of cellular proteins. For example, iron regulatory protein (IRP) –2 is a predominant regulator of mammalian iron metabolism at 3–6% O_2, whereas at 21% O_2 IRP-2 is degraded and iron metabolism is regulated by IRP-1 [68]. Primary T cells cultured at 3–6% O_2 maintain the intracellular redox environment as opposed to the T cells cultured at 21% O_2 in which the intracellular redox state is significantly altered [69]. Hypoxic stimulation results in increased levels of HIF1. HIF-1 is a global mediator of the mammalian transcriptional response to hypoxia. HIF-1 is a heterodimer composed of alpha and beta subunits [70]. HIF-1α is hydroxylated on Pro-402 and Pro-564 residues by prolyl hydroxylases and hydroxylated HIF-1α is targeted for degradation by von Hippel-Lindau tumor suppressor protein (VHL), a component of an E3 ubiquitin ligase complex [71, 72]. HIF-1 is part of a widespread O_2-sensing mechanism providing transcriptional regulation of the genes for α_{1B}-adrenergic receptor, adrenomedullin, angiopoietin

1 and 2, endothelin 1, erythropoietin, heme oxygenase-1, NOS 1 (nNOS), NOS 2 (iNOS), NOS 3 (eNOS), plasminogen activator inhibitor 1 (PAI-1), transforming growth factor β1, vascular endothelial growth factor (VEGF), VEGF receptor FLT-1, several glycolytic enzymes, and many others [73]. Sickle cell disease (SCD) is characterized by upregulation of the hypoxic response due to the marked anemia and to the vasoocclusive episodes. Interestingly, it has been suggested that progression of HIV-1 infection occurs more slowly in SCD patients [74]. Among HIV-1-infected SCD patients there were about 40% long-term nonprogressors as compared to only 5% of nonprogressors in a racially matched control group [74]. It is possible that comparing the hypoxic response in SCD disease and in normal subjects could be useful in elucidating the mechanisms of HIV-1 replication at hypoxia.

3.6.2 Cellular Iron Activates NF-κB

Influx of low molecular weight iron activates IκB kinase (IKK) in hepatic macrophages [75–77]. The IKK activation by iron involves beta-activated kinase-1 (TAK1), NF-kB-inducing kinase, phosphatidylinositol 3-kinase (PI3K), and mitogen-activated protein kinase –1 (MEK1). Filipin III, a caveolae inhibitor, abrogated iron-induced TAK1 and IKK activation. These studies indicated that TAK1, PI3K, and p21ras physically interact in caveolae to initiate signal transduction and activate IKK by iron [75].

3.6.3 Iron and HIV

The multifunctional Nef protein of HIV-1 is important for progression to AIDS. One action of Nef is to downregulate surface MHC I molecules, helping infected cells to evade immunity. Nef also downregulates the macrophage-expressed HFE, which regulates iron homeostasis and is mutated in the iron-overloading disorder hemochromatosis. In model cell lines, Nef reroutes HFE to a perinuclear structure that overlaps the trans-Golgi network, causing a 90% reduction of surface HFE. This activity requires a Src-kinase-binding proline-rich domain of Nef and a conserved tyrosine-based motif in the cytoplasmic tail of HFE. HIV-1 infection of ex vivo macrophages similarly downregulates naturally expressed surface HFE in a Nef-dependent manner. The effect of Nef expression on cellular iron was explored. Iron and ferritin accumulation were increased in HIV-1-infected ex vivo macrophages expressing wild-type HFE, but this effect was lost with Nef-deleted HIV-1 or when infecting macrophages from hemochromatosis patients expressing mutated HFE. The iron accumulation in HIV-1-infected HFE-expressing macrophages was paralleled by an increase in cellular HIV-1-gag expression. Thus, HIV-1 may regulate cellular iron metabolism through Nef and HFE, possibly benefiting viral growth [78].

3.6.4 Cellular Iron Influences HIV-1

Increased iron stores correlated with faster HIV-1 progression in HIV-1- positive thalassemia major patients, in HIV-positive patients who were administered oral iron, and in HIV-positive subjects with haptoglobin 2-2 polymorphism associated with higher iron stores [79]. Moreover, a retrospective study of bone marrow macrophage iron in HIV-positive patients suggested that survival is shorter with higher iron stores [79]. In cultured T cells, excess of iron stimulated HIV-1 viral replication, whereas iron chelation with desferrioxamine (DFO) lowered viral replication as measured by decreased p24 levels and reverse transcriptase (RT) activity [80]. Treatment of monocyte-derived macrophages and peripheral blood lymphocytes (PBL) with DFO or deferiprone (CP20) reduced expression of p24 and also cellular proliferation [81]. The orally active bidentate chelators CP502 and CP511 decreased HIV-1 replication and cellular proliferation in a manner similar to DFO and CP20 [82]. Thus, reduction of HIV-1 replication by DFO or by hydroxypyridinone bidentate chelators may be due to the inhibition of cellular proliferation rather than by a direct antiviral action. Iron chelation has been shown to inhibit NF-κB activation [83, 84] and the subsequent replication of HIV-1, as measured by p24 antigen production and RT measurements in peripheral blood mononuclear cells [83].

3.6.5 Cellular Iron and Hypoxia Influence HIV-1 Transcription

Expression of the HIV-1 provirus requires host cell transcription factors as well as the viral Tat protein [85]. HIV-1 promoter contains two NF-κB binding sites that regulate basal HIV-1 transcription [86]. In latently infected T cells, proinflammatory cytokines (such as TNFα) induce NF-κB and activate HIV-1 promoter. One explanation for HIV-1 latency is lack of transcriptional factors required for the efficient HIV-1 transcription, such as NF-κB and HIV-1 Tat [87]. NF-κB promotes efficient initiation of HIV-1 transcription in a model of postintegration HIV-1 latency [88]. In the absence of Tat, however, sustained phosphorylation of RNAPII CTD and efficient transcription elongation was impaired by the action of an okadaic acid-sensitive phosphatase [88]. Activation of HIV-1 transcription occurs with the remodeling of a single nucleosome, nuc-1 located immediately downstream of the HIV transcription start site through posttranslational acetylation of histones [89]. Transactivation responsive (TAR) RNA element (nucleotides +1 to +82) is important for induction of HIV-1 transcription by Tat. Tat interacts with the bulge of transactivation response (TAR) RNA, a hairpin-loop structure at the 5′-end of all nascent viral transcripts [90–92]. Tat transcriptional activity is regulated by Tat-associated kinase, Cdk9/cyclin T1 [93–96] and also by Tat-associated histone acetyl transferases [97–99]. In human primary monocytes, cyclin T1 protein expression is low but can be induced by treatment of macrophages with lipopolysaccharide (LPS) through posttranscriptional mechanisms [100]. In late-differentiated macrophages cyclin T1 undergoes proteasome-mediated proteolysis, but HIV-1 infection later in differentiation results in the reinduction of cyclin T1 [101]. Cellular activity of Cdk9/cyclinT1 is negatively regulated by 7SK RNA [102, 103]. Inhibition of Cdk9/cyclinT1 activity by 7SK RNA is mediated by the binding of the inhibitory HEXIM1 protein [104, 105]. HEXIM1 binds to cyclin T1 and prevents binding of HIV-1 Tat to the N-terminus of cyclin T1 [105]. HIV-1 transcription is inducible by Tat only at G1 phase, while at G2 phase it is Tat-independent [106, 107]. Tat associates with a protein complex containing Cdk2 [108]. Cdk2/cyclin E binds the CTD of RNAP II, associates with transcriptional elongation complexes, and phosphorylates Tat in vitro [109]. The significance of these findings was verified with the use of the pharmacological Cdk2 inhibitor, CYC202, that inhibited Cdk2/cyclin E kinase activity and HIV-1 replication in T cells, monocytes, and PBMCs [110]. Inhibition of Cdk2 expression by siRNA resulted in loss of Tat-induced transcription from the HIV-1 promoter and suppression of viral replication [111]. Tat is phosphorylated by Cdk2 on Ser16 and Ser46 in cultured cells, and mutations of these residues prevented HIV-1 transcription [112]. HIV-1 transcription was inhibited by ICL670 and 311 in CEM-T cells, 293T, and HeLa cells [9]. The chelators decreased cellular activity of CDK2 and reduced HIV-1 Tat phosphorylation by CDK2 [9]. The chelators also significantly reduced association of CDK9 with cyclin T1 and reduced phosphorylation of Ser-2 residues of RNA polymerase II C-terminal domain [9], suggesting that the mechanism of inhibition includes deregulation of CDK2 and CDK9. HIV-1 transcription was inhibited in the cells cultured at 3% O_2 compared to 21% O_2 [14]. At 3% O_2, the activity of CDK9/cyclin T1 was inhibited and Sp1 activity was reduced, whereas the activity of other host cell factors including CDK2 and NF-κB was not affected [14].

3.7 *Malaria Infection*

3.7.1 Iron Pathways of the Malaria Parasite

Many metabolic pathways of the erythrocytic malaria parasite are dependent on iron, including enzymes involved in DNA synthesis [113–115], de novo synthesis of heme [116], and normal mitochondrial function and electron transport [117, 118]. *Plasmodium falciparum* iron regulatory-like protein (PfIRPa) has homology to both mammalian iron regulatory proteins and aconitases and is capable of binding RNA iron response elements. Differential digitonin permeabilization of isolated trophozoites with subsequent Western blot analysis suggested that the localization of PfIRPa is predominantly in the membranous compartments of the parasite, such as the mitochondrion. Immunofluorescence analysis showed that PfIRPa colocalizes with heat shock protein 60, a mitochondrial marker, and is also present in the parasitic cytosol/food vacuole. Under conditions favoring the formation of an iron-sulfur cluster, recombinant PfIRPa (rPfIRPa) had aconitase activity, with an overall catalytic efficiency similar in magnitude to human cytosolic IRP1/aconitase and human mitochondrial aconitase. PfIRPa immunoprecipitated from parasite lysates also had aconitase activity [119].

3.7.2 Acquisition of Iron by the Intraerythrocytic Parasite

How the intraerythrocytic phase parasite acquires iron has not yet been determined, and several possible sources have been postulated. The intraerythrocytic parasite lying within a parasitophorous vacuole obtains nutrients by ingesting host cell cytoplasm including hemoglobin by taking up molecules from the outer medium as well [120]. Host hemoglobin is degraded in the food vacuole of the parasite, and heme liberated in this process is polymerized to form hemozoin [121]. Iron bound to host transferrin in the plasma does not appear to be taken up directly by parasitized red cell [122, 123]. Iron derived from host hemoglobin undergoing proteolysis in the food vacuole of the parasite is a theoretical source of iron [124]. However, heme released through proteolysis is efficiently polymerized to form hemozoin, and it is not clear that heme is broken down to release iron for the parasite's needs. The possibility that host erythrocyte ferritin serves as a source of iron for the parasite has not been investigated in detail [125]. In one study, parasitized erythrocytes that were incubated with ferritin in the medium internalized the ferritin and ferritin appeared in the parasitophorous vacuole [126]; however, the growth of malaria was inhibited rather than promoted.

3.7.3 Reticulocyte and Erythrocyte Labile Iron and the Growth of Plasmodia

While not all studies are in agreement [127], several investigations have suggested that intraerythrocytic parasites utilize erythrocyte labile iron for their growth [122, 128]. In support of this possible source, gel filtration and ultrafiltration studies on hemolysates of rat red cells parasitized with *Plasmodium berghei* revealed a labile pool of iron that is chelatable by preincubation of the intact cells with the iron chelator, desferrioxamine [122]. Further evidence in support of this hypothesis was obtained by monitoring the concentration of labile iron in parasitized and nonparasitized erythrocytes with the fluorescent iron-sensing probe, calcein. Labile iron pools were lower in parasitized than nonparasitized erythrocytes, suggesting that labile iron of the host red cell may be either utilized or stored during plasmodial growth [128]. On the other hand, two studies found that when iron-chelating agents are introduced into the cytoplasm of erythrocytes but not into the parasite compartment within the parasitophorous vacuole, no plasmodial growth inhibition occurs [127, 129].

A plasmodial ortholog of DMT-1 is expressed on the parasite plasma membrane, and could conceivably be the means of transporting host labile iron into the parasite cytosol [125]. The mean (SD) labile iron concentration of erythrocytes in control individuals has been reported to be 1.3 μM (0.7) [130]. The merozoites of *Plasmodium vivax* invade only reticulocytes [131] and certain strains of *P. falciparum* invade reticulocytes and young erythrocytes preferentially to older erythrocytes [132]. Reticulocytes have a threefold higher labile iron pool than mature erythrocytes [133]. Whether the higher labile iron level of reticulocytes contributes to their enhanced ability to sustain infection by malaria parasites is not known.

3.7.4 NTBI as a Source of Plasmodial Iron

Virtually all iron present in the plasma is bound to transferrin under normal circumstances, but in conditions of iron overload an iron fraction that is not bound to transferrin may be present. Such non-transferrin-bound iron (NTBI) has been described in thalassemia major and intermedia [134, 135], hereditary hemochromatosis [136, 137], sickle cell anemia with transfusional iron overload [138], African iron overload [139], and other conditions. NTBI in the plasma would be expected to be toxic [134], has been implicated in the formation of potentially toxic oxygen derivatives and in the acceleration of lipid peroxidation [140], and is associated with abnormal liver function tests in African iron overload [139]. The precise nature of serum NTBI is not known, but some of this fraction may be present in the form of ferric citrate [137]. The liver and other organs such as the heart rapidly take up NTBI, and this uptake is many times faster than that of physiologic transferrin-bound iron [141–143]. Uptake by the liver may be mediated by divalent metal transporter 1 (DMT1) [144].

3.7.5 NTBI and the Hepatic Phase of Plasmodial Growth

Treating BALB/c mice with ferric ammonium citrate reportedly promotes the hepatic development of *Plasmodium yoelii* in vivo and in vitro due to increased penetration of the parasite into hepatocytes [145]. Conversely, several iron chelators inhibit the growth of *P. yoelii* in murine hepatocyte cultures [146, 147] and of *P. falciparum* in human hepatocyte cultures [147] by inhibiting liver schizogony [147]. These results are consistent with the need of a labile iron fraction for the hepatic phase of malaria. It seems reasonable that increased levels of NTBI in the plasma associated with iron therapy or iron supplementation may enhance the growth of the hepatic phase of human malaria, but experimental evidence for this is lacking.

3.7.6 NTBI and the Erythrocytic Phase of Plasmodial Growth

One study indicated that transferrin-independent uptake of ^{55}Fe-NTA and ^{55}Fe-citrate occurred in both plasmodium-infected and uninfected erythrocytes in culture in a time-, temperature-, and concentration-dependent manner. Some of the iron taken up in this manner was associated with the parasites obtained after mechanical lysis of the erythocytes, indicating that this iron is delivered to the intracellular organism [148].

3.7.7 Elevated Transferrin Saturations Correlate with Deep Coma in Children with Cerebral Malaria: Possible Association with NTBI

Some degree of intravascular hemolysis is common in acute malaria [149] and, although not measured in the setting of malaria, circulating NTBI is increased in other hematologic conditions characterized by intravascular hemolysis [150]. Furthermore, NTBI levels correlate strongly with transferrin saturation in a variety of conditions [139, 150, 151]. Endothelial adhesion proteins such as ICAM-1, the expression of which may be induced by NTBI [152, 153], have been implicated in the pathogenesis of cerebral malaria [154]. To determine if the elevated transferrin saturations found in some patients with severe malaria are associated with an adverse outcome in cerebral malaria, we retrospectively measured baseline saturations in stored serum samples from 81 Zambian children with strictly defined cerebral malaria [155]. The children had been treated with quinine, sulfadoxine-pyrimethamine, and intravenous infusions of either placebo (n=39) or the iron chelator, desferrioxamine B (n=42). More than one-third of children in both the placebo- and iron chelator–treated groups had transferrin saturations exceeding 43%, which is three standard deviations above the expected mean for age. Among children receiving quinine and placebo, those with elevated transferrin saturations had a delayed estimated median time to recover full consciousness (68.2 h) compared with those with saturations 43% (25.4 h; *P*=.006). The addition of iron chelation to quinine therapy in children with high saturations appeared to hasten recovery (*P*=0.046). These findings are consistent with the possibility that increased transferrin saturations, possibly reflecting the presence of NTBI in some cases, may be associated with delayed recovery from coma during standard therapy for cerebral malaria. These findings also suggest that addition of an iron chelator, which would bind any NTBI, can hasten recovery from coma.

3.7.8 Antimalarial Activity of Iron Chelators

Several classes of iron-chelating compounds suppress the growth of *P. falciparum* in erythrocytes in vitro, including naturally occurring siderophores produced by microorganisms to acquire iron from the environment. The antimalarial iron chelators can be placed into two major mechanisms of action: (1) the withholding of iron from plasmodial metabolic pathways by iron III chelators such as desferrioxamine [156] and, (2) the formation of complexes with iron that are toxic to the parasite by iron II chelators such as bipyridyl [157]. Specific agents that have antimalarial activity include desferrioxamine, a naturally occurring trihydroxamic acid derived from cultures of *Streptomyces pilosus* that is widely available for clinical use as an iron chelator [127, 156], and deferiprone, a neutral bidentate ligand with a high specificity for ferric iron, that is in less widespread use [158]. A number of iron chelators, including desferrioxamine, also inhibit the hepatic phase of plasmodial growth [128, 147]. The antimalarial activity of desferrioxamine has been confirmed in animal models of malaria [122].

3.7.9 Iron Chelation Therapy for Human Malaria

At least eight clinical studies of the use of iron chelators in the treatment of malaria in humans have been published. These include two studies of desferrioxamine as a single agent in adults with asymptomatic *P. falciparum* parasitemia [159, 160], one study of deferiprone as a single agent in adults with asymptomatic parasitemia [161], a study of desferrioxamine as a single agent in adults with uncomplicated clinical malaria [162], a study of desferrioxamine in addition to chloroquine for symptomatic malaria [163], a study of desferrioxamine in addition to artesunate in symptomatic malaria [164], and two studies of desferrioxamine in combination with standard quinine therapy for cerebral malaria in Zambian children [165, 166]. Desferrioxamine as a single agent has discernible antimalarial activity in humans as a single agent, but it does not effect a radical cure [159, 160, 162]. In contrast, deferiprone at an acceptable dose as a single agent did not have a clinical effect [161].

3.7.10 Desferrioxamine as Adjunctive Therapy for Cerebral Malaria

While the pathophysiology of cerebral malaria is incompletely understood, obstruction of the cerebral microvasculature by *P. falciparum*-infected erythrocytes leading to ischemia, microhemorrhage, and free radical formation probably contributes to the development of this condition. Desferrioxamine inhibits peroxidant damage to the central nervous system [167], and therefore it is conceivable that this agent might protect the central nervous system in the setting of cerebral malaria. In a prospective, randomized, double-blind trial of desferrioxamine or placebo added to standard quinine treatment but no loading dose of quinine in 83 children with cerebral malaria, the addition of desferrioxamine to conventional therapy shortened the time to clearance of parasitemia and the time to recovery of full consciousness in children with deep coma, each by about twofold [166]. In a follow-up study, 352 children followed the same study design except that a loading dose of quinine was given [165]. Overall mortality and parasite clearance were not different between the two treatment arms. The lack of a positive effect of desferrioxamine on parasite clearance in this study, in contrast to the earlier work [166], might be attributable to the impact of a loading dose of quinine used in the present study but not in the previous one. Our data indicate that a loading dose of quinine has a substantial benefit in the treatment of cerebral malaria [168], and a relatively delayed beneficial effect of desferrioxamine in cerebral malaria may have been masked by the loading dose of quinine.

References

1. Morgan DO. Cyclin-dependent kinases: engines, clocks, and microprocessors. Annu Rev Cell Dev Biol. 1997;13:261–291.
2. Tsimberidou AM, Alvarado Y, Giles FJ. Evolving role of ribonucleoside reductase inhibitors in hematologic malignancies. Expert Rev Anticancer Ther. 2002;2:437–448.
3. Green DA, Antholine WE, Wong SJ, Richardson DR, Chitambar CR. Inhibition of malignant cell growth by 311, a novel iron chelator of the pyridoxal isonicotinoyl hydrazone class: effect on the R2 subunit of ribonucleotide reductase. Clin Cancer Res. 2001;7:3574–3579.
4. Richardson DR. Molecular mechanisms of iron uptake by cells and the use of iron chelators for the treatment of cancer. Curr Med Chem. 2005;12:2711–2729.
5. Coulonval K, Bockstaele L, Paternot S, Roger PP. Phosphorylations of cyclin-dependent kinase 2 revisited using two-dimensional gel electrophoresis. J Biol Chem. 2003;278:52052–52060.
6. Fu D, Richardson DR. Iron chelation and regulation of the cell-cycle: two mechanisms of post-transcriptional regulation of the universal cyclin-dependent kinase inhibitor p21CIP1/WAF1 by iron depletion. Blood. 2007; 110:752–761.
7. Yoon G, Kim HJ, Yoon YS, Cho H, Lim IK, Lee JH. Iron chelation-induced senescence-like growth arrest in hepatocyte cell lines: association of transforming growth factor beta1 (TGF-beta1)-mediated p27Kip1 expression. Biochem J. 2002;366:613–621.
8. Pahl PM, Reese SM, Horwitz LD. A lipid-soluble iron chelator alters cell cycle regulatory protein binding in breast cancer cells compared to normal breast cells. J Exp Ther Oncol. 2007;6:193–200.
9. Debebe Z, Ammosova T, Jerebtsova M, et al. Iron chelators ICL670 and 311 inhibit HIV-1 transcription. Virology. 2007;367:324–33.
10. Wang G, Miskimins R, Miskimins WK. Regulation of p27(Kip1) by intracellular iron levels. Biometals. 2004;17:15–24.
11. Semenza GL. Hypoxia-inducible factor 1 (HIF-1) pathway. Sci STKE 2007;2007:cm8.
12. Gardner LB, Li Q, Park MS, Flanagan WM, Semenza GL, Dang CV. Hypoxia inhibits G1/S transition through regulation of p27 expression. J Biol Chem. 2001;276:7919–7926.
13. Horree N, Gort EH, van der Groep P, Heintz AP, Vooijs M, van Diest PJ. Hypoxia-inducible factor 1 alpha is essential for hypoxic p27 induction in endometrioid endometrial carcinoma. J Pathol. 2008;214:38–45.
14. Charles S, Ammosova T, Cardenas J, et al. Regulation of HIV-1 transcription at 3% versus 21% oxygen concentration. J Cell Physiol. 2009;221:469–479.
15. Pumfery A, de la Fuente C, Berro R, Nekhai S, Kashanchi F, Chao SH. Potential use of pharmacological cyclin-dependent kinase inhibitors as anti-HIV therapeutics. Curr Pharm Des. 2006;12:1949–1961.

16. Gao J, Richardson DR. The potential of iron chelators of the pyridoxal isonicotinoyl hydrazone class as effective antiproliferative agents, IV: the mechanisms involved in inhibiting cell-cycle progression. Blood. 2001;98:842–850.
17. Stevens RG, Jones DY, Micozzi MS, Taylor PR. Body iron stores and the risk of cancer. N Engl J Med. 1988;319:1047–1052.
18. Stevens RG, Graubard BI, Micozzi MS, Neriishi K, Blumberg BS. Moderate elevation of body iron level and increased risk of cancer occurrence and death. Int J Cancer. 1994;56:364–369.
19. Oates PS, West AR. Heme in intestinal epithelial cell turnover, differentiation, detoxification, inflammation, carcinogenesis, absorption and motility. World J Gastroenterol. 2006;12:4281–4295.
20. Hinoi T, Gesina G, Akyol A, et al. CDX2-regulated expression of iron transport protein hephaestin in intestinal and colonic epithelium. Gastroenterology. 2005;128:946–961.
21. Masson S, Chinn DJ, Tabaqchali MA, Waddup G, Dwarakanath AD. Is anaemia relevant in the referral and diagnosis of colorectal cancer? Colorectal Dis. 2007;9:736–739.
22. Killip S, Bennett JM, Chambers MD. Iron deficiency anemia. Am Fam Physician. 2007;75:671–678.
23. Isaacson C, Bothwell TH, MacPhail AP, Simon M. The iron status of urban black subjects with carcinoma of the oesophagus. S Afr Med J. 1985;67:591–593.
24. MacPhail AP, Simon MO, Torrance JD, Charlton RW, Bothwell TH, Isaacson C. Changing patterns of dietary iron overload in black South Africans. Am J Clin Nutr. 1979;32:1272–1278.
25. Matsha T, Brink L, van Rensburg S, Hon D, Lombard C, Erasmus R. Traditional home-brewed beer consumption and iron status in patients with esophageal cancer and healthy control subjects from Transkei, South Africa. Nutr Cancer. 2006;56:67–73.
26. Kabat GC, Miller AB, Jain M, Rohan TE. A cohort study of dietary iron and heme iron intake and risk of colorectal cancer in women. Br J Cancer. 2007;97:118–122.
27. Knobel Y, Glei M, Osswald K, Pool-Zobel BL. Ferric iron increases ROS formation, modulates cell growth and enhances genotoxic damage by 4-hydroxynonenal in human colon tumor cells. Toxicol In Vitro. 2006;20:793–800.
28. Knobel Y, Weise A, Glei M, Sendt W, Claussen U, Pool-Zobel BL. Ferric iron is genotoxic in non-transformed and preneoplastic human colon cells. Food Chem Toxicol. 2007;45:804–811.
29. Ilsley JN, Belinsky GS, Guda K, et al. Dietary iron promotes azoxymethane-induced colon tumors in mice. Nutr Cancer. 2004;49:162–169.
30. Ko C, Siddaiah N, Berger J, et al. Prevalence of hepatic iron overload and association with hepatocellular cancer in end-stage liver disease: results from the national hemochromatosis transplant registry. Liver Int. 2007;27:1394–1401.
31. Hiatt T, Trotter JF, Kam I. Hepatocellular carcinoma in a noncirrhotic patient with hereditary hemochromatosis. Am J Med Sci. 2007;334:228–230.
32. Moyo VM, Makunike R, Gangaidzo IT, et al. African iron overload and hepatocellular carcinoma (HA-7-0-080). Eur J Haematol. 1998;60:28–34.
33. Gordeuk VR, McLaren CE, MacPhail AP, Deichsel G, Bothwell TH. Associations of iron overload in Africa with hepatocellular carcinoma and tuberculosis: Strachan's 1929 thesis revisited. Blood. 1996;87:3470–3476.
34. Mandishona E, MacPhail AP, Gordeuk VR, et al. Dietary iron overload as a risk factor for hepatocellular carcinoma in Black Africans. Hepatology. 1998;27:1563–1566.
35. Kew MC, Asare GA. Dietary iron overload in the African and hepatocellular carcinoma. Liver Int. 2007;27:735–741.
36. Asare GA, Bronz M, Naidoo V, Kew MC. Interactions between aflatoxin B1 and dietary iron overload in hepatic mutagenesis. Toxicology. 2007;234:157–166.
37. Ioannou GN, Weiss NS, Kowdley KV. Relationship between transferrin-iron saturation, alcohol consumption, and the incidence of cirrhosis and liver cancer. Clin Gastroenterol Hepatol. 2007;5:624–629.
38. Lehmann U, Wingen LU, Brakensiek K, et al. Epigenetic defects of hepatocellular carcinoma are already found in non-neoplastic liver cells from patients with hereditary haemochromatosis. Hum Mol Genet. 2007;16:1335–1342.
39. Furutani T, Hino K, Okuda M, et al. Hepatic iron overload induces hepatocellular carcinoma in transgenic mice expressing the hepatitis C virus polyprotein. Gastroenterology. 2006;130:2087–2098.
40. Petrak J, Myslivcova D, Man P, et al. Proteomic analysis of hepatic iron overload in mice suggests dysregulation of urea cycle, impairment of fatty acid oxidation, and changes in the methylation cycle. Am J Physiol Gastrointest Liver Physiol. 2007;292:G1490–G1498.
41. Hucl T, Kylanpaa-Back ML, Witt H, et al. HFE genotypes in patients with chronic pancreatitis and pancreatic adenocarcinoma. Genet Med. 2007;9:479–483.
42. Kabat GC, Miller AB, Jain M, Rohan TE. Dietary iron and heme iron intake and risk of breast cancer: a prospective cohort study. Cancer Epidemiol Biomarkers Prev. 2007;16:1306–1308.
43. Hong CC, Ambrosone CB, Ahn J, et al. Genetic variability in iron-related oxidative stress pathways (Nrf2, NQ01, NOS3, and HO-1), iron intake, and risk of postmenopausal breast cancer. Cancer Epidemiol Biomarkers Prev. 2007;16:1784–1794.

44. Calzolari A, Oliviero I, Deaglio S, et al. Transferrin receptor 2 is frequently expressed in human cancer cell lines. Blood Cells Mol Dis. 2007;39:82–91.
45. Kaomongkolgit R, Cheepsunthorn P, Pavasant P, Sanchavanakit N. Iron increases MMP-9 expression through activation of AP-1 via ERK/Akt pathway in human head and neck squamous carcinoma cells. Oral Oncol. 2008;44:587–594.
46. Becton DL, Bryles P. Deferoxamine inhibition of human neuroblastoma viability and proliferation. Cancer Res. 1988;48:7189–7192.
47. Porter JB. Deferasirox: an effective once-daily orally active iron chelator. Drugs Today (Barc). 2006;42:623–637.
48. Lescoat G, Chantrel-Groussard K, Pasdeloup N, Nick H, Brissot P, Gaboriau F. Antiproliferative and apoptotic effects in rat and human hepatoma cell cultures of the orally active iron chelator ICL670 compared to CP20: a possible relationship with polyamine metabolism. Cell Prolif. 2007;40:755–767.
49. Kalinowski DS, Richardson DR. Future of toxicology–iron chelators and differing modes of action and toxicity: the changing face of iron chelation therapy. Chem Res Toxicol. 2007;20:715–720.
50. Whitnall M, Howard J, Ponka P, Richardson DR. A class of iron chelators with a wide spectrum of potent antitumor activity that overcomes resistance to chemotherapeutics. Proc Natl Acad Sci USA. 2006;103:14901–14906.
51. Kalinowski DS, Richardson DR. The evolution of iron chelators for the treatment of iron overload disease and cancer. Pharmacol Rev. 2005;57:547–583.
52. Huynh C, Andrews NW. Iron acquisition within host cells and the pathogenicity of Leishmania. Cell Microbiol. 2008;10:293–300.
53. Chauvaux S, Rosso ML, Frangeul L, et al. Transcriptome analysis of Yersinia pestis in human plasma: an approach for discovering bacterial genes involved in septicaemic plague. Microbiology. 2007;153:3112–3124.
54. Chey WD, Wong BC. American college of gastroenterology guideline on the management of helicobacter pylori infection. Am J Gastroenterol. 2007;102:1808–1825.
55. Vidakovics ML, Lamberti Y, Serra D, Berbers GA, van der Pol WL, Rodriguez ME. Iron stress increases Bordetella pertussis mucin-binding capacity and attachment to respiratory epithelial cells. FEMS Immunol Med Microbiol. 2007;51:414–421.
56. Mocny JC, Olson JS, Connell TD. Passively released heme from hemoglobin and myoglobin is a potential source of nutrient iron for Bordetella bronchiseptica. Infect Immun. 2007;75:4857–4866.
57. Murillo AC, Li HY, Alber T, et al. High throughput crystallography of TB drug targets. Infect Disord Drug Targets. 2007;7:127–139.
58. Gordeuk VR, Moyo VM, Nouraie M, et al. Circulating cytokines in pulmonary tuberculosis according to HIV status and dietary iron content. Int J Tuberc Lung Dis. 2009;13:1267–1273.
59. Lounis N, Truffot-Pernot C, Grosset J, Gordeuk VR, Boelaert JR. Iron and Mycobacterium tuberculosis infection. J Clin Virol. 2001;20:123–126.
60. Boelaert JR, Vandecasteele SJ, Appelberg R, Gordeuk VR. The effect of the host's iron status on tuberculosis. J Infect Dis. 2007;195:1745–1753.
61. Kasvosve I, Gomo ZA, Mvundura E, et al. Haptoglobin polymorphism and mortality in patients with tuberculosis. Int J Tuberc Lung Dis. 2000;4:771–775.
62. Gangaidzo IT, Moyo VM, Mvundura E, et al. Association of pulmonary tuberculosis with increased dietary iron. J Infect Dis. 2001;184:936–939.
63. Monfeli RR, Beeson C. Targeting iron acquisition by Mycobacterium tuberculosis. Infect Disord Drug Targets. 2007;7:213–220.
64. Fujita N, Sugimoto R, Urawa N, et al. Hepatic iron accumulation is associated with disease progression and resistance to interferon/ribavirin combination therapy in chronic hepatitis C. J Gastroenterol Hepatol. 2007;22:1886–1893.
65. Fujita N, Sugimoto R, Takeo M, et al. Hepcidin expression in the liver: relatively low level in patients with chronic hepatitis C. Mol Med. 2007;13:97–104.
66. Taher A, Chamoun FM, Koussa S, et al. Efficacy and side effects of deferiprone (L1) in thalassemia patients not compliant with desferrioxamine. Acta Haematol. 1999;101:173–177.
67. Mlisana K, Auld SC, Grobler A, et al. Anaemia in acute HIV-1 subtype C infection. PLoS One. 2008;3:e1626.
68. Meyron-Holtz EG, Ghosh MC, Rouault TA. Mammalian tissue oxygen levels modulate iron-regulatory protein activities in vivo. Science. 2004;306:2087–2090.
69. Atkuri KR, Herzenberg LA, Niemi AK, Cowan T. Importance of culturing primary lymphocytes at physiological oxygen levels. Proc Natl Acad Sci USA. 2007;104:4547–4552.
70. Lee JW, Bae SH, Jeong JW, Kim SH, Kim KW. Hypoxia-inducible factor (HIF-1)alpha: its protein stability and biological functions. Exp Mol Med. 2004;36:1–12.
71. Maxwell PH, Wiesener MS, Chang GW, et al. The tumour suppressor protein VHL targets hypoxia-inducible factors for oxygen-dependent proteolysis. Nature. 1999;399:271–275.

72. Salceda S, Caro J. Hypoxia-inducible factor 1alpha (HIF-1alpha) protein is rapidly degraded by the ubiquitin-proteasome system under normoxic conditions. Its stabilization by hypoxia depends on redox-induced changes. J Biol Chem. 1997;272:22642–22647.
73. Manalo DJ, Rowan A, Lavoie T, et al. Transcriptional regulation of vascular endothelial cell responses to hypoxia by HIF-1. Blood. 2005;105:659–669.
74. Bagasra O, Steiner RM, Ballas SK, et al. Viral burden and disease progression in HIV-1-infected patients with sickle cell anemia. Am J Hematol. 1998;59:199–207.
75. Chen L, Xiong S, She H, Lin SW, Wang J, Tsukamoto H. Iron causes interactions of TAK1, p21ras, and phosphatidylinositol 3-kinase in caveolae to activate IkappaB kinase in hepatic macrophages. J Biol Chem. 2007;282:5582–5588.
76. Xiong S, She H, Takeuchi H, et al. Signaling role of intracellular iron in NF-kappaB activation. J Biol Chem. 2003;278:17646–17654.
77. Xiong S, She H, Tsukamoto H. Signaling role of iron in NF-kappa B activation in hepatic macrophages. Comp Hepatol. 2004;3(Suppl 1):S36.
78. Drakesmith H, Chen N, Ledermann H, Screaton G, Townsend A, Xu XN. HIV-1 Nef down-regulates the hemochromatosis protein HFE, manipulating cellular iron homeostasis. Proc Natl Acad Sci USA. 2005;102:11017–11022.
79. Gordeuk VR, Delanghe JR, Langlois MR, Boelaert JR. Iron status and the outcome of HIV infection: an overview. J Clin Virol. 2001;20:111–115.
80. Traore HN, Meyer D. The effect of iron overload on in vitro HIV-1 infection. J Clin Virol. 2004;31(Suppl 1):S92–S98.
81. Georgiou NA, van der Bruggen T, Oudshoorn M, Nottet HS, Marx JJ, van Asbeck BS. Inhibition of human immunodeficiency virus type 1 replication in human mononuclear blood cells by the iron chelators deferoxamine, deferiprone, and bleomycin. J Infect Dis. 2000;181:484–490.
82. Georgiou NA, van der Bruggen T, Oudshoorn M, Hider RC, Marx JJ, van Asbeck BS. Human immunodeficiency virus type 1 replication inhibition by the bidentate iron chelators CP502 and CP511 is caused by proliferation inhibition and the onset of apoptosis. Eur J Clin Invest. 2002;32(Suppl 1):91–96.
83. Sappey C, Boelaert JR, Legrand-Poels S, Forceille C, Favier A, Piette J. Iron chelation decreases NF-kappa B and HIV type 1 activation due to oxidative stress. AIDS Res Hum Retroviruses. 1995;11:1049–1061.
84. Li L, Frei B. Iron chelation inhibits NF-{kappa}B-mediated adhesion molecule expression by inhibiting p22phox protein expression and NADPH oxidase activity. Arterioscler Thromb Vasc Biol. 2006;26:2638–2643.
85. Nekhai S, Jeang K-T. Transcriptional and post-transcriptional regulation of HIV-1 gene expression: role of cellular factors for Tat and Rev. Future Microbiol. 2006;1:417–426.
86. Pereira LA, Bentley K, Peeters A, Churchill MJ, Deacon NJ. A compilation of cellular transcription factor interactions with the HIV-1 LTR promoter. Nucleic Acids Res. 2000;28:663–668.
87. Lassen K, Han Y, Zhou Y, Siliciano J, Siliciano RF. The multifactorial nature of HIV-1 latency. Trends Mol Med. 2004;10:525–531.
88. Williams SA, Kwon H, Chen LF, Greene WC. Sustained induction of NF-kappa B is required for efficient expression of latent human immunodeficiency virus type 1. J Virol. 2007;81:6043–6056.
89. Van Lint C, Quivy V, Demonte D, et al. Molecular mechanisms involved in HIV-1 transcriptional latency and reactivation: implications for the development of therapeutic strategies. Bull Mem Acad R Med Belg. 2004;159:176–189.
90. Dingwall C, Ernberg I, Gait MJ, et al. Human immunodeficiency virus 1 tat protein binds trans-activation-responsive region (TAR) RNA in vitro. Proc Natl Acad Sci USA. 1989;86:6925–6929.
91. Feng S, Holland EC. HIV-1 tat trans-activation requires the loop sequence within tar. Nature. 1988;334:165–167.
92. Berkhout B, Jeang KT. Trans activation of human immunodeficiency virus type 1 is sequence specific for both the single-stranded bulge and loop of the trans-acting-responsive hairpin: a quantitative analysis. J Virol. 1989;63:5501–5504.
93. Herrmann CH, Rice AP. Lentivirus Tat proteins specifically associate with a cellular protein kinase, TAK, that hyperphosphorylates the carboxyl-terminal domain of the large subunit of RNA polymerase II: candidate for a Tat cofactor. J Virol. 1995;69:1612–1620.
94. Yang X, Gold MO, Tang DN, et al. TAK, an HIV Tat-associated kinase, is a member of the cyclin-dependent family of protein kinases and is induced by activation of peripheral blood lymphocytes and differentiation of promonocytic cell lines. Proc Natl Acad Sci USA. 1997;94:12331–12336.
95. Zhu Y, Pe'ery T, Peng J, et al. Transcription elongation factor P-TEFb is required for HIV-1 tat transactivation in vitro. Genes Dev. 1997;11:2622–2632.
96. Garber ME, Wei P, Jones KA. HIV-1 Tat interacts with cyclin T1 to direct the P-TEFb CTD kinase complex to TAR RNA. Cold Spring Harb Symp Quant Biol. 1998;63:371–380.

97. Kiernan RE, Vanhulle C, Schiltz L, et al. HIV-1 tat transcriptional activity is regulated by acetylation. EMBO J. 1999;18:6106–6118.
98. Ott M, Schnolzer M, Garnica J, et al. Acetylation of the HIV-1 Tat protein by p300 is important for its transcriptional activity. Curr Biol. 1999;9:1489–1492.
99. Deng L, de la Fuente C, Fu P, et al. Acetylation of HIV-1 Tat by CBP/P300 increases transcription of integrated HIV-1 genome and enhances binding to core histones. Virology. 2000;277:278–295.
100. Liou LY, Herrmann CH, Rice AP. HIV-1 infection and regulation of Tat function in macrophages. Int J Biochem Cell Biol. 2004;36:1767–1775.
101. Liou LY, Herrmann CH, Rice AP. Human immunodeficiency virus type 1 infection induces cyclin T1 expression in macrophages. J Virol. 2004;78:8114–8119.
102. Nguyen VT, Kiss T, Michels AA, Bensaude O. 7SK small nuclear RNA binds to and inhibits the activity of CDK9/cyclin T complexes. Nature. 2001;414:322–325.
103. Yang Z, Zhu Q, Luo K, Zhou Q. The 7SK small nuclear RNA inhibits the CDK9/cyclin T1 kinase to control transcription. Nature. 2001;414:317–322.
104. Yik JH, Chen R, Nishimura R, Jennings JL, Link AJ, Zhou Q. Inhibition of P-TEFb (CDK9/Cyclin T) kinase and RNA polymerase II transcription by the coordinated actions of HEXIM1 and 7SK snRNA. Mol Cell. 2003;12:971–982.
105. Michels AA, Nguyen VT, Fraldi A, et al. MAQ1 and 7SK RNA interact with CDK9/cyclin T complexes in a transcription-dependent manner. Mol Cell Biol. 2003;23:4859–4869.
106. Kashanchi F, Agbottah ET, Pise-Masison CA, et al. Cell cycle-regulated transcription by the human immunodeficiency virus type 1 Tat transactivator. J Virol. 2000;74:652–660.
107. Nekhai S, Shukla RR, Fernandez A, Kumar A, Lamb NJ. Cell cycle-dependent stimulation of the HIV-1 promoter by Tat-associated CAK activator. Virology. 2000;266:246–256.
108. Nekhai S, Zhou M, Fernandez A, et al. HIV-1 Tat-associated RNA polymerase C-terminal domain kinase, CDK2, phosphorylates CDK7 and stimulates Tat-mediated transcription. Biochem J. 2002;364:649–657.
109. Deng L, Ammosova T, Pumfery A, Kashanchi F, Nekhai S. HIV-1 Tat interaction with RNA polymerase II C-terminal domain (CTD) and a dynamic association with CDK2 induce CTD phosphorylation and transcription from HIV-1 promoter. J Biol Chem. 2002;277:33922–33929.
110. Agbottah E, de La Fuente C, Nekhai S, et al. Antiviral activity of CYC202 in HIV-1-infected cells. J Biol Chem. 2005;280:3029–3042.
111. Ammosova T, Berro R, Kashanchi F, Nekhai S. RNA interference directed to CDK2 inhibits HIV-1 transcription. Virology. 2005;341:171–178.
112. Ammosova T, Berro R, Jerebtsova M, et al. Phosphorylation of HIV-1 Tat by CDK2 in HIV-1 transcription. Retrovirology. 2006;3:78.
113. Chakrabarti D, Schuster SM, Chakrabarti R. Cloning and characterization of subunit genes of ribonucleotide reductase, a cell-cycle-regulated enzyme, from Plasmodium falciparum. Proc Natl Acad Sci USA. 1993;90:12020–12024.
114. Rubin H, Salem JS, Li LS, et al. Cloning, sequence determination, and regulation of the ribonucleotide reductase subunits from Plasmodium falciparum: a target for antimalarial therapy. Proc Natl Acad Sci USA. 1993;90:9280–9284.
115. Krungkrai J, Cerami A, Henderson GB. Purification and characterization of dihydroorotate dehydrogenase from the rodent malaria parasite Plasmodium berghei. Biochemistry. 1991;30:1934–1939.
116. Bonday ZQ, Taketani S, Gupta PD, Padmanaban G. Heme biosynthesis by the malarial parasite. Import of delta-aminolevulinate dehydrase from the host red cell. J Biol Chem. 1997;272:21839–21846.
117. Krungkrai J, Krungkrai SR, Suraveratum N, Prapunwattana P. Mitochondrial ubiquinol-cytochrome c reductase and cytochrome c oxidase: chemotherapeutic targets in malarial parasites. Biochem Mol Biol Int. 1997;42:1007–1014.
118. Petmitr S, Krungkrai J. Mitochondrial cytochrome b gene in two developmental stages of human malarial parasite plasmodium falciparum. Southeast Asian J Trop Med Public Health. 1995;26:600–605.
119. Hodges M, Yikilmaz E, Patterson G, et al. An iron regulatory-like protein expressed in Plasmodium falciparum displays aconitase activity. Mol Biochem Parasitol. 2005;143:29–38.
120. Pouvelle B, Spiegel R, Hsiao L, et al. Direct access to serum macromolecules by intraerythrocytic malaria parasites. Nature. 1991;353:73–75.
121. Slater AF, Cerami A. Inhibition by chloroquine of a novel haem polymerase enzyme activity in malaria trophozoites. Nature. 1992;355:167–169.
122. Hershko C, Peto TE. Deferoxamine inhibition of malaria is independent of host iron status. J Exp Med. 1988;168:375–387.
123. Peto TE, Thompson JL. A reappraisal of the effects of iron and desferrioxamine on the growth of plasmodium falciparum 'in vitro': the unimportance of serum iron. Br J Haematol. 1986;63:273–280.
124. Gabay T, Ginsburg H. Hemoglobin denaturation and iron release in acidified red blood cell lysate–a possible source of iron for intraerythrocytic malaria parasites. Exp Parasitol. 1993;77:261–272.

125. Scholl PF, Tripathi AK, Sullivan DJ. Bioavailable iron and heme metabolism in Plasmodium falciparum. Curr Top Microbiol Immunol. 2005;295:293–324.
126. Burns ER, Pollack S. *P. falciparum* infected erythrocytes are capable of endocytosis. In Vitro Cell Dev Biol. 1988;24:481–486.
127. Loyevsky M, Lytton SD, Mester B, Libman J, Shanzer A, Cabantchik ZI. The antimalarial action of desferal involves a direct access route to erythrocytic (Plasmodium falciparum) parasites. J Clin Invest. 1993;91:218–224.
128. Loyevsky M, John C, Dickens B, Hu V, Miller JH, Gordeuk VR. Chelation of iron within the erythrocytic Plasmodium falciparum parasite by iron chelators. Mol Biochem Parasitol. 1999;101:43–59.
129. Scott MD, Ranz A, Kuypers FA, Lubin BH, Meshnick SR. Parasite uptake of desferroxamine: a prerequisite for antimalarial activity. Br J Haematol. 1990;75:598–602.
130. Darbari D, Loyevsky M, Gordeuk V, et al. Fluorescence measurements of the labile iron pool of sickle erythrocytes. Blood. 2003;102:357–364.
131. Galinski MR, Medina CC, Ingravallo P, Barnwell JW. A reticulocyte-binding protein complex of Plasmodium vivax merozoites. Cell. 1992;69:1213–1226.
132. Pasvol G, Weatherall DJ, Wilson RJ. The increased susceptibility of young red cells to invasion by the malarial parasite Plasmodium falciparum. Br J Haematol. 1980;45:285–295.
133. Prus E, Fibach E. The labile iron pool in human erythroid cells. Br J Haematol. 2008;142:301–307.
134. Hershko C, Graham G, Bates GW, Rachmilewitz EA. Non-specific serum iron in thalassaemia: an abnormal serum iron fraction of potential toxicity. Br J Haematol. 1978;40:255–263.
135. Anuwatanakulchai M, Pootrakul P, Thuvasethakul P, Wasi P. Non-transferrin plasma iron in beta-thalassaemia/Hb E and haemoglobin H diseases. Scand J Haematol. 1984;32:153–158.
136. Batey RG, Lai Chung Fong P, Shamir S, Sherlock S. A non-transferrin-bound serum iron in idiopathic hemochromatosis. Dig Dis Sci. 1980;25:340–346.
137. Grootveld M, Bell JD, Halliwell B, Aruoma OI, Bomford A, Sadler PJ. Non-transferrin-bound iron in plasma or serum from patients with idiopathic hemochromatosis. Characterization by high performance liquid chromatography and nuclear magnetic resonance spectroscopy. J Biol Chem. 1989;264:4417–4422.
138. Wang WC, Ahmed N, Hanna M. Non-transferrin-bound iron in long-term transfusion in children with congenital anemias. J Pediatr. 1986;108:552–557.
139. McNamara L, MacPhail AP, Mandishona E, et al. Non-transferrin-bound iron and hepatic dysfunction in African dietary iron overload. J Gastroenterol Hepatol. 1999;14:126–132.
140. Gutteridge JM, Rowley DA, Griffiths E, Halliwell B. Low-molecular-weight iron complexes and oxygen radical reactions in idiopathic haemochromatosis. Clin Sci (Lond). 1985;68:463–467.
141. Baker E, Baker SM, Morgan EH. Characterisation of non-transferrin-bound iron (ferric citrate) uptake by rat hepatocytes in culture. Biochim Biophys Acta. 1998;1380:21–30.
142. Brissot P, Wright TL, Ma WL, Weisiger RA. Efficient clearance of non-transferrin-bound iron by rat liver. Implications for hepatic iron loading in iron overload states. J Clin Invest. 1985;76:1463–1470.
143. Link G, Pinson A, Hershko C. Heart cells in culture: a model of myocardial iron overload and chelation. J Lab Clin Med. 1985;106:147–153.
144. Shindo M, Torimoto Y, Saito H, et al. Functional role of DMT1 in transferrin-independent iron uptake by human hepatocyte and hepatocellular carcinoma cell, HLF. Hepatol Res. 2006;35:152–162.
145. Goma J, Renia L, Miltgen F, Mazier D. Iron overload increases hepatic development of Plasmodium yoelii in mice. Parasitology. 1996;112:165–168.
146. Loyevsky M, Sacci Jr JB, Boehme P, Weglicki W, John C, Gordeuk VR. Plasmodium falciparum and Plasmodium yoelii: effect of the iron chelation prodrug dexrazoxane on in vitro cultures. Exp Parasitol. 1999;91:105–114.
147. Stahel E, Mazier D, Guillouzo A, et al. Iron chelators: in vitro inhibitory effect on the liver stage of rodent and human malaria. Am J Trop Med Hyg. 1988;39:236–240.
148. Sanchez-Lopez R, Haldar K. A transferrin-independent iron uptake activity in Plasmodium falciparum-infected and uninfected erythrocytes. Mol Biochem Parasitol. 1992;55:9–20.
149. Ekvall H, Arese P, Turrini F, et al. Acute haemolysis in childhood falciparum malaria. Trans R Soc Trop Med Hyg. 2001;95:611–617.
150. von Bonsdorff L, Lindeberg E, Sahlstedt L, Lehto J, Parkkinen J. Bleomycin-detectable iron assay for non-transferrin-bound iron in hematologic malignancies. Clin Chem. 2002;48:307–314.
151. Walter PB, Macklin EA, Porter J, et al. Inflammation and oxidant-stress in beta-thalassemia patients treated with iron chelators deferasirox (ICL670) or deferoxamine: an ancillary study of the Novartis CICL670A0107 trial. Haematologica. 2008;93:817–825.
152. Kartikasari AE, Georgiou NA, Visseren FL, van Kats-Renaud H, van Asbeck BS, Marx JJ. Endothelial activation and induction of monocyte adhesion by nontransferrin-bound iron present in human sera. FASEB J. 2006;20:353–355.

153. Kartikasari AE, Georgiou NA, Visseren FL, van Kats-Renaud H, van Asbeck BS, Marx JJ. Intracellular labile iron modulates adhesion of human monocytes to human endothelial cells. Arterioscler Thromb Vasc Biol. 2004;24:2257–2262.
154. Tripathi AK, Sullivan DJ, Stins MF. Plasmodium falciparum-infected erythrocytes increase intercellular adhesion molecule 1 expression on brain endothelium through NF-kappaB. Infect Immun. 2006;74:3262–3270.
155. Gordeuk VR, Thuma PE, McLaren CE, et al. Transferrin saturation and recovery from coma in cerebral malaria. Blood. 1995;85:3297–3301.
156. Raventos-Suarez C, Pollack S, Nagel RL. Plasmodium falciparum: inhibition of in vitro growth by desferrioxamine. Am J Trop Med Hyg. 1982;31:919–922.
157. Scheibel LW, Adler A. Antimalarial activity of selected aromatic chelators. Mol Pharmacol. 1980;18:320–325.
158. Heppner DG, Hallaway PE, Kontoghiorghes GJ, Eaton JW. Antimalarial properties of orally active iron chelators. Blood. 1988;72:358–361.
159. Gordeuk VR, Thuma PE, Brittenham GM, et al. Iron chelation as a chemotherapeutic strategy for falciparum malaria. Am J Trop Med Hyg. 1993;48:193–197.
160. Gordeuk VR, Thuma PE, Brittenham GM, et al. Iron chelation with desferrioxamine B in adults with asymptomatic Plasmodium falciparum parasitemia. Blood. 1992;79:308–312.
161. Thuma PE, Olivieri NF, Mabeza GF, et al. Assessment of the effect of the oral iron chelator deferiprone on asymptomatic Plasmodium falciparum parasitemia in humans. Am J Trop Med Hyg. 1998;58:358–364.
162. Bunnag D, Poltera AA, Viravan C, Looareesuwan S, Harinasuta KT, Schindlery C. Plasmodicidal effect of desferrioxamine B in human vivax or falciparum malaria from Thailand. Acta Trop. 1992;52:59–67.
163. Traore O, Carnevale P, Kaptue-Noche L, et al. Preliminary report on the use of desferrioxamine in the treatment of Plasmodium falciparum malaria. Am J Hematol. 1991;37:206–208.
164. Looareesuwan S, Wilairatana P, Vannaphan S, et al. Co-administration of desferrioxamine B with artesunate in malaria: an assessment of safety and tolerance. Ann Trop Med Parasitol. 1996;90:551–554.
165. Thuma PE, Mabeza GF, Biemba G, et al. Effect of iron chelation therapy on mortality in Zambian children with cerebral malaria. Trans R Soc Trop Med Hyg. 1998;92:214–218.
166. Gordeuk V, Thuma P, Brittenham G, et al. Effect of iron chelation therapy on recovery from deep coma in children with cerebral malaria. N Engl J Med. 1992;327:1473–1477.
167. Sadrzadeh SM, Anderson DK, Panter SS, Hallaway PE, Eaton JW. Hemoglobin potentiates central nervous system damage. J Clin Invest. 1987;79:662–664.
168. van der Torn M, Thuma PE, Mabeza GF, et al. Loading dose of quinine in African children with cerebral malaria. Trans R Soc Trop Med Hyg. 1998;92:325–331.

Section V
Clinical Diagnosis and Therapy

Chapter 25
Estimation of Body Iron Stores

Mark Worwood

Keywords Hemoglobin • Quantitative phlebotomy • Red cell indices • Serum ferritin • Serum iron • Soluble transferrin receptor • TIBC • Tissue iron concentration • Transferrin saturation

1 Introduction

1.1 Body Iron and Iron Stores

In quantitative terms, hemoglobin is the most important pool of iron in the body comprising up to 80% of the 3–4 g total body iron in young women and about 60% in men. Much of the remaining iron (0–2 g) is found in ferritin and hemosiderin in the liver, spleen, and bone marrow, and this is referred to as "storage iron." This may be used to regenerate hemoglobin after blood loss whether physiological, pathological, or as a result of trauma.

1.2 Investigating Human Iron Metabolism

In practice, most investigations can be reduced to two questions: Is the person anemic? Is the absence of stored iron the cause of the anemia? To answer the first question, the blood hemoglobin concentration is usually measured. To answer the second question, a variety of tests can be applied. Often, additional questions must be asked. For example, although adequate amounts of storage iron appear to be present, is it available for hemoglobin synthesis? Is there an excess of storage iron?

1.3 Iron Status

Normal iron status implies a level of hemoglobin synthesis which is not limited by the supply of iron and the presence of a small reserve of "storage iron" to cope with normal physiological functions [1]. The ability to survive the acute loss of blood (iron) which may result from injury is also an

M. Worwood, M.D. (✉)
Emeritus Professor, Cardiff University, Cardiff, Wales, UK
e-mail: mworwood@aol.com

G.J. Anderson and G. McLaren (eds.), *Iron Physiology and Pathophysiology in Humans*, Nutrition and Health, DOI 10.1007/978-1-60327-485-2_25,

Table 25.1 Disorders of iron metabolism

Iron deficiency	Caused by low intake	Usually due to a diet of low bioavailability in combination with increased physiological requirements
	Due to increased physological requirements	Rapid growth in early childhood and in adolescence
	Due to blood loss	Physiological (e.g., menstruation)
		Pathological (e.g., gastrointestinal bleeding)
	Due to malabsorption of iron	Reduced gastric acid secretion (e.g., after partial gastrectomy)
		Reduced duodenal absorptive area (e.g., in celiac disease)
	"Functional" iron deficiency	Storage iron is present but cannot be supplied rapidly enough for heme synthesis, e.g., during erythropoietin treatment in chronic renal failure
Redistribution of iron	Macrophage iron accumulation	Inflammatory, infectious or malignant diseases ("anemia of chronic disease")
Iron overload	Increased iron absorption	Hereditary hemochromatosis (commonly homozygosity for HFE C282Y, but sometimes involving other genes)
		Ineffective erythropoiesis (e.g., severe thalassemia syndromes, sideroblastic anemias)
		Sub-Saharan iron overload ("Bantu siderosis") – an unknown genetic susceptibility in combination with increased dietary iron
		Other rare inherited disorders (e.g., congenital atransferrinemia)
		Due to inappropriate iron therapy (rare)
	Multiple blood transfusions in refractory anemias	e.g., thalassemia major, sickle-cell anemia, and aplastic and myelodysplastic anemias

advantage. The limits of normality are difficult to define and some argue that physiological normality is the presence of only a minimal amount of storage iron [2], but the extremes of iron-deficiency anemia and iron overload are well understood.

Apart from too little or too much iron in the body, there is also the possibility of a maldistribution. An example is anemia associated with inflammation or infection where there is both a partial failure of erythropoiesis and of iron release from phagocytic cells in liver, spleen and bone marrow which leads to iron accumulation in these cells. Occasionally, further investigations into iron loss, iron absorption, and flow rates within the body are also required.

1.4 Disorders of Iron Metabolism

Clinical aspects of iron metabolism are reviewed in several other chapters in this volume and are summarized in Table 25.1.

2 Methods for Assessing Iron Status

There are two ways of identifying threshold values for iron deficiency or iron overload for many of the analytes discussed here. The first is to identify subjects with iron deficiency or iron overload and to establish the range of values found for each group. This approach has rarely been applied, although ferritin in iron deficiency provides one example. The second approach is to measure concentrations

Table 25.2 Hemoglobin cutoff values [4]

Age or gender group	Hemoglobin (g/L)
Children 6 months to 59 months	110
Children 5–11 years	115
Children 12–14 years	120
Nonpregnant women (above 15 years of age)	120
Pregnant women	110
Men (above 15 years of age)	130

Hemoglobin concentrations are influenced by smoking and altitude (>1,000 m) (see [4]). There are also genetic influences. In the USA, individuals of African extraction with adequate iron stores have Hb values 5–10 g/L lower than those of European origin

in otherwise healthy subjects in a particular population living under the same environmental conditions, and to define iron deficiency or iron overload as values below or above two standard deviations of the distribution median for the analyte. This has been used for many of the analytes being considered here.

2.1 Hemoglobin

The measurement of hemoglobin concentration depends on the conversion of hemoglobin to cyanmethemoglobin and determination of the absorbance at 540 nm. An international standard is available for calibration (WHO International Standard Hemiglobincyanide, NIBSC code 98/708 http://www.nibsc.ac.uk), and the measurement is included in the analysis provided by electronic blood cell counters. Portable hemoglobin readers are available but should be evaluated against a standardized method [3].

Anemia has been defined as a hemoglobin concentration below two standard deviations of the distribution mean for hemoglobin in an otherwise healthy population of the same gender and age. Cutoff values for age and gender groups are shown in Table 25.2. The WHO criteria of anemia are in widespread use, despite evidence of significant racial differences in normal hemoglobin values (Table 25.2). Hemoglobin has been widely used to assess iron deficiency (low iron stores). However, the sensitivity of these measurements is poor because anemia associated with nutritional iron deficiency is usually mild, resulting in extensive overlap between healthy and iron-deficient subjects. In developing countries, poverty, malnutrition, and infection are associated with a high prevalence of the anemia of chronic disease, which often exceeds that caused by iron-deficiency anemia [5, 6].

2.2 Red Cell Indices

Modern automated cell counters provide a rapid and sophisticated way of detecting the changes in red cells which accompany a reduced supply of iron to the bone marrow: low mean cell volume (MCV) and mean cell hemoglobin (MCH), an increased percentage of hypochromic red cells, and an increased red cell distribution width (RDW). In principle, the reticulocyte hemoglobin content (CHr) provides an early indication of functional iron deficiency [7]. At present, the clinical utility of percentage hypochromic cells and CHr is limited as these measures are only available on the ADVIA analyzers (Bayer Diagnostics). However, the corresponding indices provided by the Sysmex XE 2100 series analyzers, RBC-Y and RET-Y, show good correlations with HYPO and CHr respectively [8–10]. Further tests are usually necessary to identify iron deficiency (absence of storage iron) in anemia associated with acute or chronic disease (see later).

2.3 *Tissue Iron Stores*

2.3.1 Quantitative Phlebotomy

A direct way of measuring iron stores is by quantitative phlebotomy (removing up to 500 mL blood/week until anemia develops). If blood is removed at a rate of 450 mL/week (c 220 mg Fe/week), most of the iron used to regenerate hemoglobin is obtained from the stores (ferritin and hemosiderin) rather than by absorption [11] and the total amount removed is the amount of iron available for hemoglobin synthesis at the start of phlebotomy. Quantitative phlebotomy has been applied to validate the concept that serum ferritin concentrations in normal subjects reflect the level of available storage iron [12]. Phlebotomy is used to deplete iron stores in patients with genetic hemochromatosis and, if the amount of blood removed is measured accurately, provides a reliable measure of the initial iron load [13].

2.3.2 Tissue Iron Concentrations

The liver and bone marrow are quantitatively important, and relatively accessible storage sites and the amount of iron present can be estimated either visually, using the Prussian-Blue reaction on tissue sections, or chemically. With the exception of genetic hemochromatosis, there is generally a good relationship between iron concentrations in liver and bone marrow [14]. Methods for chemical and histological assessment of tissue iron concentration have been described in detail [11]. Today, liver iron concentration is usually determined on dried needle biopsy samples using atomic absorption spectrometry (see for example [15]). Mean liver nonheme iron concentrations lie between 5 and 20 μmol/g dry weight (80 and 300 μg/g wet weight [16]). Chemical determination of liver iron concentration is most widely applied for the demonstration of iron overload and allows the important distinction to be made between the relatively minor elevations of liver nonheme iron often found in patients with liver disease and iron overload associated with inherited hemochromatosis. The hepatic iron index is the liver iron concentration in μmol/g dry weight divided by the age in years. A value >1.9 indicates iron overload [17]. Note, however, that there is considerable variability when concentrations are compared from several sites in the same liver [15].

Estimation of iron concentration in bone marrow is, by contrast, usually by staining [18] and is usually applied to the detection of iron deficiency. In particular, assessing marrow iron in macrophages distinguishes between "true" iron deficiency and other chronic disorders where iron is present within reticuloendothelial cells. Although often referred to as the "gold standard," the semiquantitative estimation of storage iron in the bone marrow is technically demanding [19, 20] and is subject to considerable interobserver variation [21]. Stuart-Smith et al. [22] compared the uses of trephine bone marrow specimens with aspirates and concluded that "aspirate smears reflect bone marrow iron stores more reliably than formic acid decalcified trephine biopsy sections." They suggested that the preparation of Perls' stained sections should be confined to cases in which aspirate samples are inadequate for iron assessment and no obvious hemosiderin is present in an H&E stained section.

Noninvasive methods including MRI are increasingly important in detection of overload in the liver, heart and spleen.

2.3.3 Serum Ferritin

Early studies of circulating ferritin were concerned with the role of ferritin as a vasodepressor as determined with a bioassay. This research into the biological activity of ferritin contributed to understanding of the function and metabolism of ferritin [23], but there has been little interest in the topic since.

Circulating ferritin iron concentrations were first reported by Reissmann and Dietrich [24] who measured precipitated iron after incubation of serum with a rabbit antibody to human liver ferritin. Ferritin was only found in serum from patients with acute liver disease. Reissmann and Dietrich found no evidence of any relationship between the concentration of ferritin and blood pressure, pulse rate, or urinary output and concluded that ferritinemia was a symptom of hepatocellular necrosis. There was little interest in circulating ferritin until the advent of the immunoradiometric assay (below), although other methods for detecting circulating ferritin were described. Circulating ferritin has also been called α_2-H-antigen and β-fetoprotein (for review of these early studies see [25]).

Immunoassays for Serum Ferritin

The development of a sensitive immunoradiometric assay (IRMA) allowed the detection of ferritin protein in normal serum and plasma [26]. Early assays, both RIA (labeled ferritin) and IRMA (labeled antibody), have been described in detail [27]. Later, these assays were supplanted by enzyme-linked immunoassays (ELISA) with colorimetric and fluorescent substrates or by antibodies with chemiluminescent labels. Serum ferritin is included in the latest batch and random-access automated analyzers for immunoassay.

The use of a reference ferritin preparation to calibrate the assay is recommended, and most commercial systems have been calibrated against the international standard. The current reference material is the third WHO standard (reagent 94/578, http://www.nibsc.ac.uk/).

Ferritin Concentrations and Iron Stores

Our knowledge of tissue iron concentrations in normal subjects is largely derived from measurements of nonheme iron concentrations in the liver from accident victims. Serum ferritin concentrations reflect liver iron concentrations [28] with relatively high values at birth, low values throughout childhood, and an increase after adolescence. Good correlations have been found between serum ferritin concentrations and storage iron mobilized by phlebotomy [12], stainable iron in the bone marrow [29], and the concentration of both nonheme iron and ferritin in the bone marrow [30].

Serum ferritin concentrations are normally within the range 15–300 μg/L, are lower in children than adults, and from puberty to middle age mean concentrations are higher in men than in women. Mean concentrations and ranges throughout life are given in Fig. 25.1a. The mother's iron status appears to have relatively little influence on cord serum concentrations, mean values for which are in the range 100–200 μg/L. A study using stable isotopes of iron showed that transfer of dietary iron to the fetus was regulated in response to maternal iron status and suggests that the iron needs of the fetus take priority over maternal requirements [33]. In a sample of Australian office workers, blood donation and alcohol intake influenced serum ferritin concentrations along with diet in women [34]. A significant association with alcohol consumption in both men and women has been confirmed in the Health Survey for England [35], and ferritin levels also increased with increasing body mass index. In older men and women, mean concentrations are similar. In elderly, unselected patients, high levels of ferritin are often associated with disease [36]. High concentrations of serum ferritin are found in iron overload but infection, inflammation and tissue damage also raise ferritin concentrations (see below).

Serum Ferritin and Iron Deficiency

A threshold of 15 μg/L, below which iron stores are absent, was derived by measuring serum ferritin concentrations in patients with iron-deficiency anemia – defined as microcytic anemia, with either an absence of stainable iron in the bone marrow or a subsequent response to therapeutic iron [25].

Hallberg et al. [37] measured serum ferritin concentrations in healthy women with no stainable iron in the bone marrow and also suggested a threshold of 15 μg/L. Milman et al. [29] found that a serum ferritin concentration of 20 μg/L showed the highest diagnostic efficiency for identifying "reduced" (not absent) iron stores. Table 25.3 shows cutoff values for ferritin derived from population data.

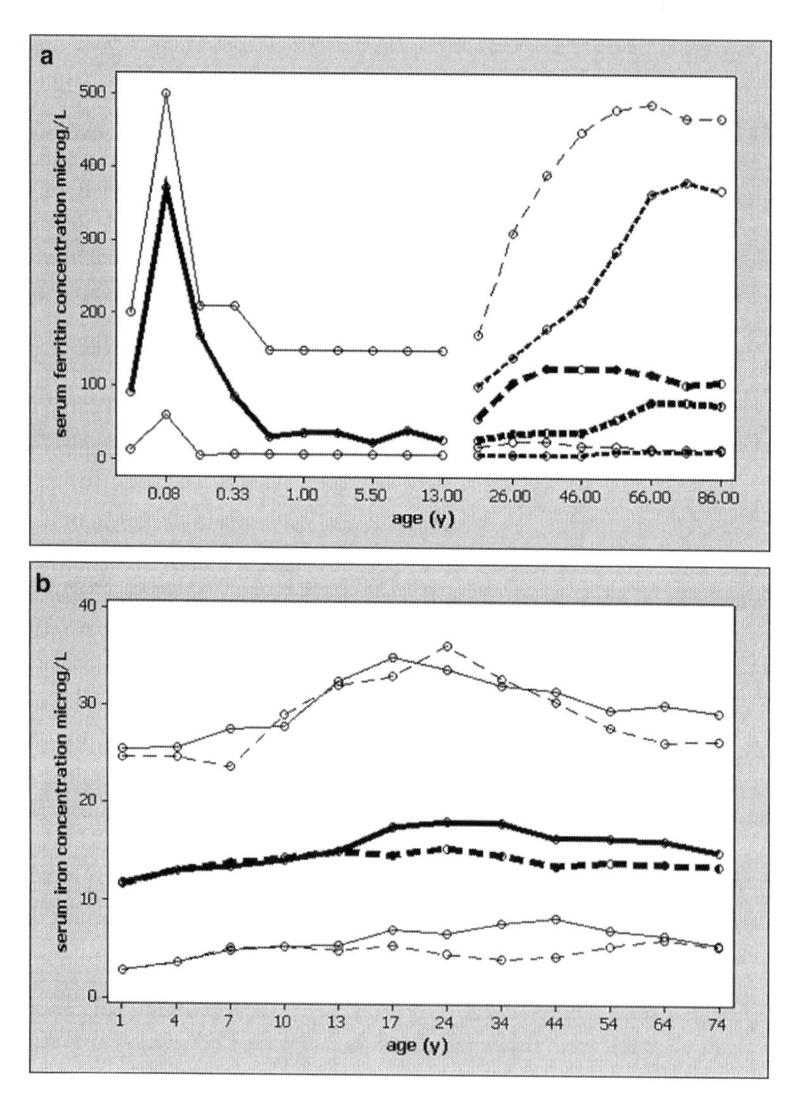

Fig. 25.1 Median concentrations of (**a**) serum ferritin, (**b**) serum iron, (**c**) TIBC, (**d**) transferrin saturation, and (**e**) sTfR, and variation with age. Also shown are 2.5 and 97.5 percentiles. (**a**) Serum ferritin concentrations are similar in infants and children for males and females and values are taken from the table in Worwood [28]. The *left-hand side* of the figure refers to children. Median values are shown by the *thick* with the 2.5 and 97.5 percentiles by the *thin lines*. Adult concentrations are shown on the *right-hand side* and are from Custer et al. [31]. These refer to US subjects with normal values for all analytes apart from serum ferritin. The *thick dotted lines* are for men and women with the *thinner lines* showing 2.5 and 97.5 percentiles. The highest values are always for men. (**b–d**) Values for serum iron, TIBC, and transferrin saturation are taken from NHANES III (http://www.cdc.gov/nchs/data/series/sr_11/sr11_247.pdf) and refer to all race/ethnic groups. The *solid lines* refer to men, and the *dotted lines* refer to women. The data for sTfR are taken from Choi et al. [32]. The *lines* refer to both men and women

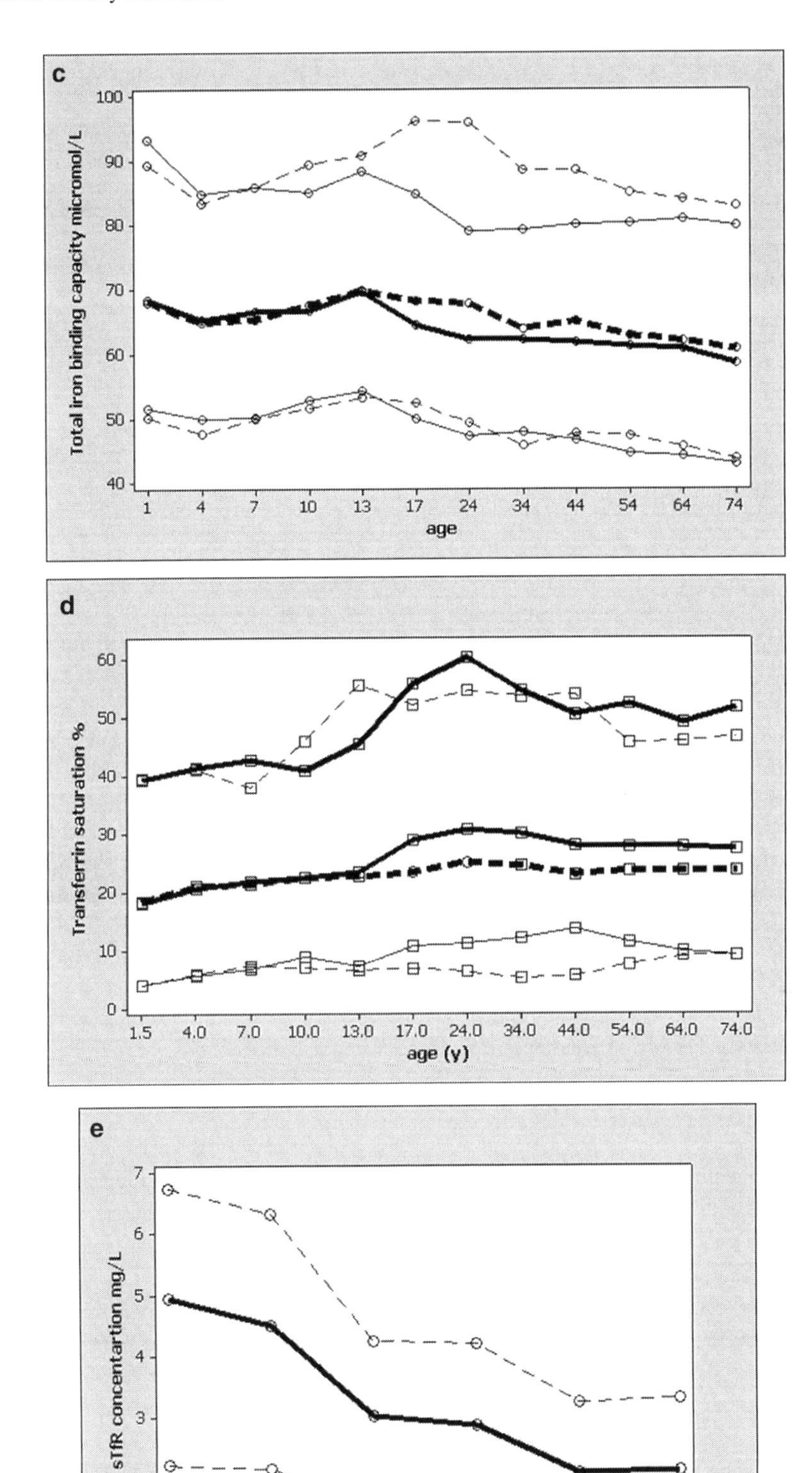

Fig. 25.1 (continued)

Table 25.3 Recommended thresholds for detecting iron deficiency (absence of storage iron) in adults

NHANES III 1988–1994 [38]		WHO 2001 [4]	
Age years	Serum ferritin μg/L	Age years	Serum ferritin μg/L
1–2	<10		
3–5	<10	<5	<12
6–11	<12	>5	<15
12–15	<12		
>16	<12		

Biochemistry and Physiology of Plasma Ferritin

Immunologically, plasma ferritin resembles liver or spleen ferritin and is recognized by antibodies raised against these ferritins. Purified serum ferritin from patients with iron overload had a relatively low iron content (0.02–0.07 μg Fe/μg) [39, 40] and a mean of 0.06 μg Fe/μg protein by immunoprecipitation from serum [41]. In the liver and spleen of iron-overloaded patients, the iron content of ferritin is >0.2 μg Fe/μg protein [42]. However, several authors have claimed that serum ferritin has a much higher iron content. Tenkate et al. [43] purified ferritin by immunoprecipitation and measured the iron content by atomic absorption spectrophotometry. They found a mean iron saturation of ferritin of 24% (0.13 μg Fe/μg protein) in normal serum and suggested that the extensive purification used in earlier studies would lead to loss of iron. Herbert et al. [44] claimed that measurement of serum ferritin iron by a similar procedure provided an accurate assessment of the whole range of human body iron status, unconfounded by inflammation. Later, Nielsen et al. [45] determined the iron content of serum ferritin from patients with iron overload and tissue damage using the method of Tenkate et al. [43]. The iron saturation found was about 5%, and the assay of ferritin iron was of little value in the diagnosis of iron overload. Yamanshi et al. [46] found concentrations from 0.02 to 0.04 μg Fe/μg ferritin protein in serum samples with ferritin concentrations greater than 2,000 μg/L.

It should be remembered that in 1956, Reissmann and Dietrich only detected ferritin iron in the circulation after liver necrosis [24]. In terms of methodology, specific antibodies and effective washing of the immunoprecipitate are essential if ferritin iron is to be accurately measured.

Glycosylation

On isoelectric focusing, both native and purified serum ferritin contain a wide range of isoferritins covering the pI range found in human tissues [39, 47]; yet on anion exchange chromatography, serum ferritin is apparently a relatively basic isoferritin [39]. The reason for this is glycosylation. In normal serum, about 60% of ferritin binds to concanavalin A [48], whereas tissue ferritins do not bind. Incubation with neuraminidase converts the acidic ferritins of serum to the more basic isoferritins, but the pI of acidic heart ferritin is unaffected [49]. A carbohydrate containing G subunit in addition to the H and L subunits has also been identified in purified preparations of serum ferritin [40, 50].

Origin of Serum Ferritin and Clearance from the Circulation

These findings suggest that some ferritin may enter the circulation by secretion rather than release from damaged cells. In a hepatocyte cell line there was direct evidence of regulated secretion of glycosylated ferritin [51]. In vivo, much of the secreted ferritin may originate from phagocytic cells degrading hemoglobin. When there is tissue damage, direct release of cytosolic ferritin through damaged cell membranes becomes important. In patients with ferritinemia resulting from necrosis of the liver, the plasma ferritin shows reduced binding to concanavalin A. Findings in patients with thalassemia intermedia and in the early stages of hemochromatosis confirm the importance of phagocytic cells as the origin of circulating ferritin (see below).

Another explanation for the differences between plasma and tissue ferritins may be differential clearance from the circulation. [^{131}I]-labeled plasma ferritin was removed only slowly [$T½<24$ h] from the plasma after intravenous injection into normal subjects [52], but [^{131}I]-labeled spleen ferritin was cleared very rapidly [$T½$ approx 9 min] [53]. Such rapid clearance may be due to interaction with ferritin receptors on hepatocytes [54] which appear to have a higher affinity for liver ferritin than serum ferritin, at least in the rat. Rapid clearance may also be initiated by interaction with ferritin-binding proteins in the plasma [55–57]. Of the isoferritins released into the plasma, the ones which normally accumulate are L_{24} molecules and glycosylated molecules which are rich in L subunits and again contain little iron. The L_{24} molecules take up iron slowly in vitro and have been termed "natural apoferritin" [58]. The glycosylated protein may have little opportunity to acquire iron during secretion. These molecules may accumulate because clearance by receptors or interaction with binding proteins requires at least some H subunits.

Serum Ferritin Concentrations Exceeding 10,000 μg/L

The factors controlling plasma ferritin concentrations are: synthesis, release from cells, and the rate of clearance from the plasma. There are no instances yet known where very high ferritin concentrations are due to abnormalities in ferritin clearance, although this has been suggested in the case of Still's disease [59], but abnormalities in both synthesis and release occur.

In iron overload, serum ferritin concentrations are unlikely to exceed 4,000 μg/L in the absence of concomitant liver damage [27], but in liver necrosis, there may be ferritin concentrations in excess of 50,000 μg/L [60]. The stimulation of synthesis by a combination of iron and cytokines can lead to ferritin concentrations >20,000 μg/L in adult onset Still's disease [61]. In the reactive hemophagocytic syndrome, there is inappropriate activation of monocytes leading to hemophagocytosis and cytokine release. Ferritin concentrations of up to 400,000 μg/L have been reported in children [62, 63] and adults [64]. Patients with AIDS may also have the reactive hemophagocytosis syndrome, and high concentrations may also occur in AIDS patients with disseminated histoplasmosis [65]. It is likely that the percentage of glycosylated ferritin will always be low where total concentrations exceed 10,000 μg/L as in iron overload synthesis reaches a maximum of 4,000 μg/L [27]. These very high ferritin concentrations therefore reflect release of cytosolic ferritin from damaged cells. However, in adult Still's disease, the percentage of glycosylated ferritin was low even when the disease was in remission, and it has been suggested that percentage glycosylated ferritin may be a useful diagnostic tool in this condition [59].

High Serum Ferritin Concentrations and Congenital Cataract

An interesting cause of elevated ferritin concentration in the absence of iron overload is that associated with inherited cataract formation. It has now been demonstrated that mutations in the "stem loop" structure of the ferritin L subunit may lead to synthesis of the "L" subunit of ferritin that is no longer regulated by iron concentration (Chap. 21). This causes elevated serum ferritin concentrations (c 1,000 μg/L) in the absence of iron overload.

2.4 Serum Iron/Total Iron-Binding Capacity and Percentage Saturation

Iron exchange in the body is mediated by transferrin (Chap. 7), and transferrin iron has been measured for many years for diagnosis of iron deficiency and overload. The International Committee for Standardization in Hematology (Expert Panel on Iron) has recommended a reference method for serum iron [66], and a similar method was recommended by the NCCLS (USA) [67]. The simultaneous precipitation of serum proteins and the release of iron from transferrin in the presence of a reducing agent are followed by centrifugation to remove denatured protein and detection of the ferrous iron in the supernatant with a chromogen. The method minimizes nonspecific absorbance caused by interference with serum proteins and interference from heme iron or copper. Methods in which iron is released from transferrin without precipitating serum proteins have obvious advantages in terms of automation [68]. Procedures for measuring serum iron are available for most clinical chemistry autoanalyzers.

Measurement of the serum iron concentration alone provides little useful clinical information because of the considerable variation from hour to hour and day to day in normal individuals (see below). Transferrin iron is only 0.1% of the total body iron, and the transferrin iron pool turns over 10–20 times each day. Changes in supply and demand due to infection, inflammation, or surgery therefore cause rapid changes in serum iron concentration. Normal ranges for serum iron concentration are given in Fig. 25.1b and change little with age in adult life. Low concentrations are found in iron-deficiency anemia and high concentrations in iron overload. However, many hospital patients have a low serum iron concentration which is a response to inflammation, infection, or surgery, and does not necessarily indicate an absence of storage iron. High concentrations are found in liver disease, hypoplastic conditions, ineffective erythropoiesis, and iron overload [69, 70].

More information may be obtained by measuring both the serum iron concentration and the total iron-binding capacity (TIBC), from which the percentage of transferrin saturation with iron may be calculated. The TIBC is a measurement of transferrin concentration and may be estimated by saturating the transferrin iron-binding capacity with excess iron and removing the excess with solid magnesium carbonate, charcoal, or an ion exchange resin. This is followed by determination of the iron content of the saturated serum. The unsaturated iron-binding capacity (UIBC) may be determined by methods which detect iron remaining and able to bind to chromogen, after adding an excess of iron to the serum [68]. Protocols for clinical chemistry analyzers often include a method for UIBC. An alternative approach is to measure transferrin directly by immunological assay. Bandi et al. [71] reported great variability among a number of immunochemical assays for transferrin. However, others have found a good correlation between the chemical and immunological TIBC [72, 73], although the latter found that when TIBC was calculated as the sFe+UIBC, values were lower than the direct TIBC. Transferrin concentrations (g/L) may be converted to TIBC (μmol/L) by multiplying by 25.

Normal ranges for both TIBC and transferrin saturation are given in Fig. 25.1c, d. A raised TIBC is characteristic of a deficiency of storage iron, and values are low in patients with iron overload. In principle, measurement of TIBC or transferrin concentration should be a sensitive and reliable method for detecting both iron deficiency [74] and iron overload as transferrin synthesis is tightly controlled by iron levels through the IRP/IRE system (Chap. 3) and levels are not subject to the rapid changes seen for serum iron concentration. However, reliable reference ranges for the several ways of measuring TIBC are not available. Furthermore, there is a relatively small amplitude of variation in transferrin concentration over the extremes of iron deficiency and iron overload (c 1–3 g/dL) compared with that for serum iron (c 1–40 μmol/L) and serum ferritin (c 5–1,000 μg/L).

The most widely used indicator of transport iron is the transferrin saturation, and a saturation of 16% or less is usually considered to indicate an inadequate iron supply for erythropoiesis [75]. Measurements based on serum iron have largely been replaced by the assay of serum ferritin for detecting iron deficiency, but in diagnosing idiopathic hemochromatosis, it is essential to measure both the serum iron concentration and the TIBC or transferrin concentration (see below).

2.5 Transferrin Index

Beilby et al. [76] have recommended that the transferrin saturation is replaced by the "transferrin index." This is the serum iron concentration (μmol/L) divided by the transferrin concentration (determined immunologically and expressed as μmol/L). They claimed that the transferrin index had better precision than the transferrin saturation and showed greater specificity for detecting iron overload than the transferrin saturation. However, the transferrin index has attracted little use.

2.6 Non-Transferrin Bound Iron

The measurement of TIBC or transferrin may sometimes lead to an apparent saturation of greater than 100% if there is non-transferrin-bound iron (NTBI) present in the serum. Such non-transferrin iron may be tissue ferritin if there is significant liver damage which releases ferritin into the blood and some of the ferritin iron may be assayed in the determination of serum iron [66]. Other low-molecular-weight forms of iron may also be present in iron-overloaded patients.

Non-transferrin-bound iron (NTBI) is nonheme iron which is not bound to transferrin in plasma. It is present when the transferrin iron-binding capacity is saturated, but may also be detected at lower transferrin saturations. Its nature is still unclear, but the term is not usually taken to refer to the small amounts of iron in ferritin in the plasma. It is potentially toxic, leading to free radical generation. The term "labile plasma iron" (LPI) has been used by Cabantchik [77] to refer to the toxic component of NTBI.

The presence of TBI was first suggested by Hershko [78] and later confirmed by the same group [79]. Initially, work was carried out on serum from patients with thalassemia major [80]. NTBI was later detected in patients with hemochromatosis who may also have saturated transferrin in serum [81, 82]. Somewhat surprisingly, NTBI has been detected in patients with only partially saturated transferrin [81, 83, 84].

A number of assays have been used to measure NTBI. The first assay used EDTA as an iron (III) scavenging molecule [79], but later, it was clear that nitrilotriacetic acid was a more effective chelator in that it removed less iron from transferrin [85]. A third method employs bathophenanthroline [86]. Another problem with the use of chelators is that they will also deliver iron to apotransferrin or transferrin with one iron-binding site occupied. The chelated NTBI must be separated from serum proteins and can then be detected by a range of methods, including colorimetry and HPLC. In order to overcome the problem of donation of iron to transferrin, cobalt(III) has been used to block vacant iron-binding sites [87].

The bleomycin method [88] depends on the reduction of Fe(III) to Fe(II) which is then chelated by bleomycin. This complex generates hydroxyl radicals which damage DNA added as a substrate. Damaged DNA is detected by its reaction with thiobarbituric acid and the pink color detected. The reduction of Fe(III) to Fe(II) by ascorbic acid is a critical step, and hemolysis must be avoided. The technique has been modified for a 96-well microtiter plate format, although this method gives low values [89].

The third general method was introduced by Cabantchik and involves the quenching of fluorescence due to an iron chelator by NTBI iron. In the first assay, NTBI is bound by desferrioxamine coating the wells of a 96-well plate [90]. Bound iron is detected by adding the metal sensor calcein. It is added as the Fe–calcein complex which is nonfluorescent. During a 2-h incubation, the remaining bound desferrioxamine removes iron from the calcein complex and the fluorescence increases. Fluorescence is inversely proportional to the amount of NTBI in the serum. In a later procedure, NTBI is released by oxalate and binding to transferrin prevented by the addition of Gallium (III). NTBI is detected by the reduction of fluorescence of fluorescein-labeled apotransferrin [91].

These methods probably measure different things as was demonstrated in a recent "round robin" study of NTBI [92]. NTBI has been detected in patients with iron overload (with or without saturated transferrin), in subjects heterozygous for hemochromatosis, and also in patients with heart disease [93], diabetes [94, 95] and renal failure [96]. In the study of Lee et al., the level of NTBI showed a strong correlation with severity of diabetes. Despite considerable interest, measurements of NTBI are not in routine diagnostic use.

2.7 *Erythrocyte Protoporphyrin (EP)*

This assay has been performed for many years as a screening test for lead poisoning. More recently, there has been considerable interest in its use in evaluating the iron supply to the bone marrow. The "free" protoporphyrin concentration of red blood cells increases in iron deficiency and is usually present as the zinc complex. A widely used technique directly measures the fluorescence of zinc protoporphyrin (ZPP), usually in μmol/mol heme, in an instrument called a hematofluorometer [97]. The small sample size (about 20 μL of venous or skin-puncture blood), simplicity, rapidity, and reproducibility within a laboratory are advantages. Furthermore, the test has an interesting retrospective application. Because it takes some weeks for a significant proportion of the circulating red blood cells to be replaced with new cells, it is possible to make a diagnosis of iron-deficiency anemia some time after iron therapy has commenced. Chronic diseases that reduce the serum iron concentration, but do not reduce iron stores, also increase protoporphyrin levels [98].

Evaluation of EP and ZPP levels is complicated by the use of several units of measurement: μg EP/dL whole blood, μg EP/dL red cells, μg EP/g Hb, and μmol EP/mol Hb.

To convert between the various units used to express protoporphyrin levels, the following calculations apply:

μg EP/dL red cell = (μg EP/dL whole blood)/hematocrit
From μg EP/dL red cell to μg EP/g Hb multiply by 0.037
From μg EP/dL red cell to μmol EP/mol heme multiply by 0.87

These factors are based on an assumed normal mean cell hemoglobin concentration, although this may be measured in individual samples and an appropriate factor calculated.

In adults, EP levels remain relatively constant with increasing age – median value approximately 42 μg/dL red blood cells in males and 47 μg/dL red blood cells in females (NHANES III http://www.cdc.gov/nchs/data/series/sr_11/sr11_247.pdf). The threshold for iron-deficient erythropoiesis is approximately 80 μg/dL red blood cells. For ZPP the normal range in adults is <80 μmol/mol heme, but concentrations are lower if washed red cells are assayed. Mean values in normal women are slightly higher than in men. The measurement of erythrocyte protoporphyrin levels as an indicator of iron deficiency has particular advantages in pediatric hematology and in large-scale surveys in which the small sample size and simplicity of the test are important. Reference ranges derived from large populations of healthy adults are not available, but pediatric reference ranges have been determined in 6,478 subjects (0–17 years) by Soldin et al. [99]. Mean ZPP values declined with age, and a diurnal variation was noted with ZPP concentrations being higher between 18.00 and midnight.

However, in the general clinical laboratory, ZPP provides less information about iron storage levels in anemic patients than the serum ferritin assay [100].

2.8 *Red Cell Ferritin*

Erythrocyte ferritin is but a tiny residue of that present in nucleated red cells in the bone marrow. Normal erythroblasts contain ferritin which is immunologically more similar to heart than liver ferritin (i.e., ferritin rich in H subunits), and mean concentrations are about 10 fg ferritin protein/cell [101]. Concentrations decline in late erythroblasts, decline further in reticulocytes, and only about 10 ag/cell (10^{-18} g/cell) remains in the erythrocyte (measured with antibodies to L ferritin) again with somewhat higher levels detected with antibodies to H-type ferritin [102]. Red cell ferritin concentrations have been measured in many disorders of iron metabolism, usually with antibodies to L ferritin. Red cell ferritin levels reflect the iron supply to the erythroid marrow and tend to vary inversely with red cell protoporphyrin levels [102]. Thus in patients with rheumatoid arthritis and anemia, low values of red cell ferritin are found in those with microcytosis and low serum iron concentrations regardless of the serum ferritin levels. Red cell ferritin levels do not therefore necessarily indicate levels of storage iron. High levels of red cell ferritin are also found in thalassemia, megaloblastic anemia, and myelodysplastic syndromes presumably indicating a disturbance of erythroid iron metabolism in these conditions.

Despite possible diagnostic advantages such as differentiation between hereditary hemochromatosis and alcoholic liver disease [103], the assay of red cell ferritin has seen little routine application. This is because it is necessary to have fresh blood in order to prepare red cells free of white cells (which have much higher ferritin levels).

2.9 *Serum Soluble Transferrin Receptor (sTfR)*

In 1986, Kohgo et al. [104] reported that transferrin receptors were detectable in plasma by immunoassay. Since then, there has been much investigation of the physiological and diagnostic significance of circulating serum transferrin receptors [105]. The protein is derived by proteolysis at the cell membrane and circulates bound to transferrin. Plasma concentrations reflect the number of cellular receptors and, for patients with adequate iron stores, the number of nucleated red cells in the bone marrow. As the number of cellular transferrin receptors per cell increases in iron deficiency, concentrations also rise when erythropoiesis becomes iron limited.

2.9.1 Erythropoiesis

The function of the TfR in delivering iron to the immature red cell immediately suggested an application in the clinical laboratory for the assay of circulating sTfR. The use of the assay to monitor changes in the rate of erythropoiesis has been explored by several authors [106–108]. When iron supply is not limiting, the assay can provide a replacement for ferrokinetic investigations which required the injection of radioactive iron [109]. In reviewing the applications of serum transferrin receptor assays, Beguin [110] concluded that soluble TfR represents a valuable quantitative assay of marrow erythropoietic activity as well as a marker of tissue iron deficiency

2.9.2 Iron Deficiency

When normal subjects are subjected to quantitative phlebotomy, sFn concentrations fall steadily as iron stores are depleted, but there is little change in sTfR concentration. As iron stores become exhausted (sFn <15 μg/L), the iron supply to the erythroid marrow becomes limited. Erythroblasts respond with increased surface TfR numbers, and sTfR levels rise and continue rising as hemoglobin concentrations fall [111]. In this study, the increased rate of erythropoeisis during phlebotomy had little effect on sTfR levels as long as iron stores were adequate; so most of the increase in sTfR level was ascribed to iron deficiency rather than increased erythropoiesis. Only 250 mL of blood was removed per week instead of the 450 mL/week usually removed during treatment of hemochromatosis; higher rates may cause an immediate increase in sTfR levels during phlebotomy. In infants (8–15 months) sTfR concentration increased as the severity of iron deficiency increased [112].

The ratio of sTfR/sFn gives a linear relationship with storage iron that is of potentially great value in assessing iron stores in epidemiological studies. This ratio is defined as the logarithm of the concentrations in micrograms per liter of serum transferrin receptor/serum ferritin [113]. Note that several other sTfR/ferritin ratios are in use for diagnosing iron deficiency: transferrin receptor (mg/L)/$\log_{10}$ ferritin (μg/L) [114] and a transferrin/ferritin molar ratio [115].

2.9.3 Reference Ranges

sTfR concentrations are high in neonates and decline until adult concentrations are reached at about 18 years (Fig. 25.1e). Concentrations are similar in normal men and women [116] unlike serum ferritin concentrations, which are lower in women before the menopause (Fig. 25.1a). sTfR concentrations with different assay systems cannot be directly compared as reference ranges differ (see below).

2.9.4 Assays for the Serum Transferrin Receptor

Three enzyme immunoassay kits for the determination of serum transferrin receptor concentrations have been evaluated for the Medical Devices Agency [117]. All have been used in the investigation of iron deficiency – Ramco [118], R&D [116, 119], and Orion [120]. All have been approved for diagnostic purposes in the USA by the FDA.

The different reference ranges in the three commercial assays reflect the differences in preparations of transferrin receptor used to raise antibodies and as a standard in the various assays. There was some assay drift but acceptable intra-assay coefficient of variation (CV%) values. The determined sensitivity was adequate for clinical purposes for the three assay systems. There are differences in both units and absolute amounts for serum transferrin receptor concentrations. For four kits evaluated [117, 121, 122], there were four different units (nmol/L, μg/mL, mg/L, kU/L) and four different normal ranges (despite the equivalence of μg/mL and mg/L). At the present time, sTfR is not included in the national external quality control schemes for the UK. Automated assays are now available on platforms for immunoassay used in clinical chemistry laboratories. Pfeiffer et al. [123] found that STfR concentrations determined with an immunoturbidimetric assay (Roche Hitachi) showed acceptable correlation with two ELISA assays. Nevertheless, values obtained were lower and the Roche Hitachi assay showed superior performance in predicting iron deficiency.

A WHO reference reagent for the serum transferrin receptor has now been established, and an international collaborative study showed that using this reagent as a standard markedly improved agreement between methods. Currently available commercial assays are listed in this report [124].

2.10 Serum and Urine Hepcidin Concentrations

Hepcidin plays a major role in iron metabolism, particularly in the regulation of iron absorption and the release of iron from macrophages (see Chap. 9). Not only is synthesis controlled by iron status but also by infection and inflammation. Reliable assays for serum hepcidin are now being developed. However, the role of hepcidin in the differential diagnosis of both iron deficiency and iron overload is not yet clear, although a number of useful diagnostic applications are being investigated [125]. An international round robin of urinary and plasma hepcidin assays demonstrated that absolute concentrations vary widely. However, analytical variation was generally low and similar for the six methods included in the study [126].

3 Methodological and Biological Variability of Assays

These assays vary greatly in methodological and biological stability (see survey in [68]). Hemoglobin concentrations are stable and a simple and well-standardized method ensures relatively low day-to-day variation in individuals (2–4%). Automated cell counters analyze at least 10,000 cells, and this reduces errors. Immunoassays have higher methodological variation. For ferritin, the coefficient of variation (CV) is about 5%, and this coupled with some physiological variation gives an overall coefficient of variation for serum ferritin for an individual over a period of weeks of the order of 15%. There is, however, little evidence of any significant diurnal variation in serum ferritin concentration [127]. Cooper and Zlotkin [128] found lower variability for serum transferrin receptor than for ferritin. The serum iron determination is an example of extremes with low methodological variation coupled with extreme physiological variability giving an overall "within subject" CV of approximately 30% when venous samples are taken at the same time of day. A diurnal rhythm has been reported with higher values in the morning than in late afternoon when the concentration may fall to 50% of the morning value [69]. The circadian fluctuation may be due largely to variation in the release of iron from the reticuloendothelial system to the plasma. Higher variability for Hb and ferritin was reported by Borel et al. [129] and may be due to their use of capillary blood and plasma. Pootrakul et al. [130] found that the mean plasma ferritin concentration was slightly higher in capillary specimens than in venous specimens and that within and between samples, variations were approximately three times greater. Variability was less in capillary serum but still greater than venous serum. In contrast, Cooper and Zlotkin [128] found lower variability for ferritin and transferrin receptor in both capillary serum and plasma compared with venous serum and plasma.

These results would suggest that for population studies [38, 128, 131, 132] or in the assessment of patients [129], either a multiparameter analysis is required or the assay of several samples. However, in special circumstances, single samples may provide adequate information for prospective epidemiologic studies. Zeleniuch-Jacquotte et al. [115] found that serum ferritin, sTfR, and prohepcidin levels were stable during a 2-year period in postmenopausal women.

4 The Predictive Value of Indicators of Iron Stores

The major diagnostic application of the various measures of iron status is in the differential diagnosis of hypochromic anemia. The large amount of iron present as hemoglobin means that the degree of any anemia must always be considered in assessing iron status. An overall reduction in body iron accompanies reduced amounts of hemoglobin in iron-deficiency anemia. In other anemias, including the anemia of chronic disease and the megaloblastic anemias, iron is redistributed from the red cells

Table 25.4 Methods for assessment of body iron stores and confounding factors

Measurement	Reference range (adults)	Diagnostic use	Confounding factors
Tissue (liver) biopsy iron (chemical assay)	3–33 μg/g dry weight	Confirmation of iron overload	Potential for sampling error on needle biopsy when <0.5 mg or liver is nodular
Bone marrow (Perls' stain)	Grade	Graded as absent, present or increased. Most commonly used to differentiate ACD from IDA	Adequate sample required Considerable observer variation
Quantitative phlebotomy	<2 g Fe	Treatment of genetic hemochromatosis	
Urine chelatable Fe (after IM injection of desferrioxamine)	<2 mg/24 h	Rarely used but may provide confirmation of iron overload	
Imaging			
MRI		Becoming available both for hepatic and cardiac iron deposition	Machines widely available but special analysis and software required
SQUID[a]		Quantitation of liver iron overload	Not generally available
Serum ferritin (sFn)	15–300 μ/L	Correlated with body iron stores from deficiency to overload	Increased: as acute phase protein and by release of tissue ferritin after organ damage (particularly liver disease) Decreased: vitamin C deficiency
Serum iron (sFe)	10–30 μmol/L	Low values in iron deficiency, high values in iron overload. TS is more sensitive and specific	Labile; use of fasting, morning sample reduces normal daily variation Reduced in acute and chronic disease
Total iron-binding capacity (TIBC)	47–70 μmol/L	High values characteristic of tissue iron deficiency. Low values in iron overload. May also be calculated from transferrin concentration (Tf g/L × 25)	Rarely used on its own
Transferrin saturation (TS) [sFe/TIBC × 100]	16–50%	Low values in iron deficiency, high values in iron overload. Raised TS is an early indicator of iron accumulation in genetic hemochromatosis	See sFe (above)
Serum transferrin receptor (sTfR)	2.8–8.5 mg/L[b]	Increased sTfR indicates impaired iron supply to the bone marrow. Useful for identifying early iron deficiency. In ACD, sTfR only increases in presence of tissue iron deficiency	sTfR concentration related to extent of erythroid activity as well as iron supply to cells
Red cell zinc protoporphyrin (ZPP)	<80 μmol/mol Hb	Increased ZPP indicates impaired iron supply to the bone marrow	May be affected by other causes of impaired iron incorporation into heme (sideroblastic anemias, lead poisoning)
Red cell ferritin ("L" type)	3–40 ag/cell	Reduced red cell ferritin indicates impaired iron supply to the bone marrow	As above – also requires removal of white cells before assay

[a] See text

[b] Units and reference ranges are specific to method (see text)

to macrophage iron stores, with a corresponding increase in marrow stainable iron and serum ferritin. No single measurement of iron status is ideal for all clinical circumstances since all are affected by confounding factors (Table 25.4).

The anemia of chronic disorders combines normal or increased iron stores (reflected by an increased serum ferritin) and a reduced tissue iron supply (low serum iron and low to normal TIBC with a low transferrin saturation). Although serum ferritin is an acute phase reactant, values below 50 μg/L are usually associated with absent iron stores in rheumatoid arthritis, renal disease, and inflammatory bowel disease. Serum transferrin receptor levels may also provide valuable diagnostic information on iron deficiency in chronic disease.

Despite years of investigations, there is little reliable comparative information. The main reason for this is the difficulty of distinguishing between the presence and absence of storage iron. Most investigators have used the grade of storage iron in the bone marrow as a "gold standard." This is an invasive procedure and so limits drastically the number of patients investigated. It is often difficult to justify bone marrow aspiration to determine a patient's iron status and even more difficult in the case of normal volunteers. Furthermore, bone marrow aspiration followed by staining for iron is not a reproducible procedure. Observer error [21] inadequate specimens and lack of correlation with response to iron therapy [133] have been described. An alternative is to demonstrate a response in hemoglobin concentration to oral iron therapy and this has been the method of choice in pediatric practice.

4.1 *Iron-Deficiency Anemia in Adults*

This is anemia due to a decline in the iron content of the body caused by blood loss or inadequate iron intake. Menstrual blood loss is the most common cause of IDA in premenopausal women, but blood loss from the GI tract or malabsorption are common causes in men and postmenopausal women. Colonic cancer, gastric cancer, and celiac disease may present with IDA, and it is essential to exclude these conditions as the cause of IDA in men and postmenopausal women [134].

Almost all the analytes show a high sensitivity and specificity for distinguishing between subjects with iron-deficiency anemia and those with iron stores and normal hemoglobin levels in the absence of any other disease process. Guyatt et al. [135] conducted a systematic review of the diagnostic value of the various laboratory tests for the diagnosis of iron deficiency and concluded that serum ferritin was the most powerful test for simple iron deficiency and also for iron deficiency in hospital patients. However, the serum transferrin receptor was not included.

4.2 *Iron Deficiency in Infancy and Childhood*

In infants, diagnostic thresholds for iron-deficiency and iron deficiency anemia are not universally agreed. There are rapid changes in iron status in the first year of life as fetal hemoglobin is replaced by Hb A. The serum ferritin concentration is a less useful guide to iron deficiency than in adults partly because of the rapid decline in concentration in the first 6 months and the low concentrations generally found in children over 6 months of age. In a study of healthy breast-fed infants from Honduras and Sweden, Domellof et al. [136] evaluated the Hb response to oral iron supplementation. At 4–6 months, the initial Hb concentration did not predict a response to iron therapy. At 6 months, Hb, MCV, and ZPP predicted the response but sFn and sTfr did not. Suggested cutoffs for iron deficiency (two standard deviations for iron replete infants) are given in Table 25.5.

Margolis et al. [137] found that the best predictor of response was the initial Hb concentration, although sensitivity was only 66% and specificity 60%. sFn, TS and erythrocyte protoporphyrin had even lower efficiencies, and a combination of the various measures made little improvement.

Table 25.5 Suggested cutoff values for iron deficiency at 4, 6, and 9 months based on iron-replete, breast-fed infants [137]

	4 months	6 months	9 months
Hb (g/L)	<105	<105	<100
MCV (fL)	<73	<71	<71
ZPP (µmol/mol heme)	>75	>75	>90
Ferritin (µg/L)	<20	<9	<5
TfR (mg/L)[a]	>11	>11	>11

[a] Ramco assay (cannot be compared directly with other assays but should relate to the assay of Flowers et al. [138]). For infants (8–15 months) the upper reference value (95% CI) for sTfR is 13.5 mg/L [112]

Hershko et al. [139] studied children in villages from the Golan Heights (Israel) and concluded that erythrocyte protoporphyrin was a more reliable index of iron deficiency than serum ferritin and serum iron. They suggested that a significant incidence of chronic disease affected both ferritin and iron values. ZPP provides a useful indicator of iron-deficient erythropoiesis, although high values may indicate lead poisoning rather than iron deficiency. The small sample volume for ZPP determination is also an advantage in pediatric practice.

A recent report confirms the effect of low-level infection on measures of iron status. Abraham et al. [140] studied 101 healthy 11-month-old infants. On the morning of blood sampling, slight clinical signs of airway infection were observed for 42 infants. Extensive blood analyses were done, including high-sensitivity CRP. CRP measured by the routine methods gave values of <6 mg/L for all infants, but with the high-sensitivity assay, values were higher for many infants with symptoms of airway infection. Serum iron concentration was depressed in these children and correlated significantly with CRP level. When a further blood sample was taken, serum ferritin concentration was higher for the sample with the higher CRP level, serum iron was reduced, but sTfR and transferrin levels were unaffected.

Lopez et al. [141] studied sTfR, sTfR/ferritin ratio (µg/µg), and sTfR-$\log_{10}$ ferritin (called the TfR-F index by Punnonen et al. [114]) in 368 children aged 1–10 years. These included 206 healthy children, 60 with iron-deficiency anemia and 102 with anemia and infectious disease including 58 meeting the criteria for iron-deficiency anemia (microcytic anemia with two of three indicators of iron deficiency – ferritin, EP and TS). The iron deficient children responded to oral iron. Children with thalassemia trait were excluded. Ferritin, sTfR, and sTfR log ferritin index were reliable ways to identify children with infection who were also iron deficient but the sTfR/ferritin ratio showed very low sensitivity.

4.3 Pregnancy

In early pregnancy, serum ferritin concentrations usually provide a reliable indication of iron deficiency. Hemodilution in the second and third trimesters of pregnancy reduces the concentrations of all measures of iron status and means that the threshold values for iron deficiency established in nonpregnant women are not appropriate. In principle, determination of values as ratios (ZPP umol/mol heme, transferrin saturation and sTfR/ferritin) should be more reliable, but there is little evidence for this. Although it has been claimed that sTfR measurements provide a sensitive indicator of iron deficiency in pregnancy [142], questions remain about decreased erythropoiesis in early pregnancy as this may mask iron deficiency at this time [118, 143]. Increases in sTfR in later pregnancy relate to increased erythropoiesis as well as iron depletion [144]. In healthy, nonanemic women supplemented with iron [144], serum iron, TS, and sFn fell from the first to the third trimester and increased after delivery; TIBC increased during pregnancy and fell after delivery. sTfR concentrations showed a substantial increase (approx. twofold) during pregnancy, and this probably reflects increased erythropoiesis [144]. In contrast, Carriaga et al. [142] had reported that the mean sTfR concentration of pregnant women in the third trimester did not differ from that in nonpregnant women and that sTfR concentration was not influenced by pregnancy per se. Choi et al. [144] suggest that different assays and different ages in the control groups may explain this discrepancy. Measurement of sTfR did not enhance the sensitivity and specificity for the detection of iron-deficiency anemia in pregnant women from Malawi where anemia and chronic disease are very prevalent [145]. Milman et al. [146] have reported geometric means and reference intervals for many analytes for over 400 pregnant women from Denmark. These were relatively prosperous women who were healthy and had normal pregnancies and normal deliveries in any previous pregnancy. They all received oral iron at several dose levels. In addition to the full blood count, serum ferritin and sTfR levels were reported. Ferritin levels declined between 18 and 32 weeks and had increased at 8 week after delivery. sTfR levels increased from 18 to 32 weeks and remained high.

The Institute of Medicine (USA) has recommended that iron deficiency in the first and second trimester be identified by Hb < 11.0 g/dL and ferritin < 20 μg/L [147]. Women with decreased iron stores only should receive lower doses of oral iron than those who are also anemic. In the third trimester, all women should receive supplemental iron. Other guidelines recommend supplementation for all women throughout pregnancy [148, 149].

4.4 *β-Thalassemia Trait*

A common cause of microcytic anemia is β-thalassemia trait. Measurement of serum ferritin and hemoglobin A_2 usually allows a distinction between iron-deficiency anemia and β-thalassemia trait. A number of red cell "discrimination indices" have been devised to avoid the extra expense of ferritin and HbA_2, but, along with measurements of red cell indices including RDW, these have not proved to be sufficiently reliable to replace measurement of ferritin and hemoglobin A_2 [150, 151]. RDW does not discriminate.

4.5 *Detection of Iron Deficiency in Acute or Chronic Disease*

In clinical practice, there are two different questions (a) Is there a lack of RES storage iron in a patient with inflammation, infection, malignancy, or renal failure? (b) Is here "functional iron deficiency" – an inadequate iron supply to the bone marrow despite the presence of storage iron in reticuloendothelial cells? This is often encountered in patients on dialysis for chronic renal failure receiving erythropoietin to correct renal anemia. In this setting, the iron demands of the erythropoietin-driven marrow outstrip the ability of the RES to release storage iron.

4.5.1 Lack of Storage Iron

A number of studies where stainable iron in the bone marrow has been examined and the sensitivity and specificity of various assays compared are summarized in Table 25.6. Despite some inconsistencies, some general points may be made from this analysis and studies referred to earlier:

1. Conventional red cell parameters – Hb, MCV, MCH, and reticulocyte count – do not distinguish between the presence and absence of bone marrow iron in patients with chronic disease.
2. The serum iron concentration is usually low in chronic disease, and although the TIBC (or transferrin concentration) is higher for patients with no storage iron, neither this measurement nor the transferrin saturation derived from the serum iron and TIBC provides useful discrimination.

Table 25.6 Sensitivity/specificity for the diagnosis of iron deficiency in the presence of chronic disease in adults (iron stores determined by staining for iron in bone marrow).

	Study (ref)											
Test	[152]	[153]	[7]	[154]	[114]	[155]	[156]	[157]	[158]	[159]	[119]	[160]
MCV	–	–	0.32/0.93	L	0.86[a]	–	–	0.42/0.83	–	–	–	–
MCH	–	–	–	–	–	0.71/0.71[a]	–	–	–	–	–	–
% Hypo	–	–	–	–	–	0.77/0.90	–	–	–	–	–	–
CHr	–	–	0.74/0.73	–	–	–	–	–	–	–	–	–
Serum iron	–	–	–	L	0.68	L	–	–	NS	–	–	–
TIBC	–	–	–	L	0.84[b]	L	–	–	–	–	–	<0.65[a]
% Saturation	–	–	0.65/0.70	L	0.79[c]	L	–	0.38–0.89	–	–	–	<0.65[a,c]
Serum ferritin	0.79/0.97	0.870[a]	0.52/0.93	90/75	0.89	0.86/0.90	1.00/0.81	0.25/0.99	0.94/0.95	0.60/0.90	0.92/0.98	0.83[a] (0.75/0.75)
Red cell ferritin	–	–	–	L	–	–	–	–	–	0.82/0.83	–	0.68[a]
ZPP	0.74/0.94		–	–	–	L	–	–	–	–	–	–
STfR	0.63/0.81	0.704	–	–	0.98	L	1.00/0.84	0.71/0.74	0.61/0.68	–	0.92/0.84	0.69[a]
sTfR/log ferritin	0.74/0.97	0.865	–	–	1.00	–	1.00/0.97	0.67/0.93	–	–	–	–

Note: Optimum diagnostic thresholds selected vary

L lower sensitivity/specificity than serum ferritin, individually or in combination. The combination of ferritin and ESR or CRP did not improve efficiency

[a] Area under receiver operating characteristics (ROC) curve

[b] Transferrin concentration (equivalent to TIBC, see text)

[c] Transferrin Index (equivalent to % saturation, see text)

3. In chronic disease, serum ferritin concentrations reflect storage iron levels, but concentrations are higher than in normal subjects. It is necessary to set a threshold of 30–60 μg/L in order to distinguish between the presence and absence of storage iron. Even with this limit, sensitivity is low.
4. Combinations of serum ferritin, ESR, or CRP either in a discriminant analysis [161] or logistic regression [154] provide only marginal improvement in the ability to detect a lack of storage iron.
5. The serum transferrin receptor level also discriminates between the presence and absence of storage iron, although there is disagreement as to whether or not the assay is superior to serum ferritin. Several studies show that the sTfR/$\log_{10}$ sFn ratio provides superior discrimination to either test on its own. The use of Log sFn decreases the influence of serum ferritin (and thus the acute phase response) on the overall ratio. Although the sTfR/sFn ratio is an excellent measure of iron stores in healthy subjects, its use may not be appropriate for clinical applications. When the assay of sTfR is generally available on high-throughput immunoanalyzers, the sTfR/log sFn ratio may provide a useful discriminator for identifying the coexistence of iron deficiency in chronic disease. However, this will also require standardization of units and ranges for the various sTfR assays if the use of the ratio is to gain wide acceptance (see above).
6. Measurements of percentage hypochromic erythrocytes or reticulocyte hemoglobin content also provide reasonable sensitivity and specificity, but few comparative studies have been reported.

4.5.2 Functional Iron Deficiency

Here, the diagnostic question is to identify those patients with a functional iron deficiency who will require parenteral iron therapy to respond to erythropoietin with an acceptable rise in Hb concentration. The percentage hypochromic erythrocytes is a good predictor of response [133, 162]. Fishbane et al. [163] concluded that "CHr is a markedly more stable analyte than serum ferritin or transferrin saturation, and iron management based on CHr results in similar hematocrit and epoetin dosing while significantly reducing IV iron exposure." They did not include percentage hypochromic cells in their analysis. Fernandez-Rodriguez [160] assessed the sensitivity and specificity of sFn, TIBC, TS index, RBC Fn, and sTfR in 63 patients with anemia and chronic renal failure undergoing dialysis with anemia. They were not being treated with erythropoietin. Storage iron was assessed by bone marrow iron staining. For serum ferritin a cutoff value of 121 μg/L gave a sensitivity and specificity of 75%. Efficiency was lower for sTfR and RBC ferritin. MCV, TS index, and TIBC showed the lowest values for sensitivity and specificity [160]. For anemic patients with myeloma and lymphoma, the percentage hypochromic red cells proved to be more reliable than transferrin saturation, serum ferritin, and sTfR in recognizing iron-deficient erythropoiesis before erythropoietin treatment and in predicting response to treatment [164].

4.5.3 Treatment of Iron-Deficiency Anemia

Oral iron therapy at conventional doses (ferrous sulfate 200 mg three three times daily provides 195 mg elemental iron per day) has little immediate effect on serum ferritin levels which rise slowly as the hemoglobin concentration increases. However, with twice the dose (120 ng Fe three times daily), there was a rapid rise of serum ferritin over a few days, although ferritin levels remain within the normal range. This probably does not represent an immediate increase in storage iron [165]. Intravenous iron causes a rapid rise to concentrations that may be above the normal range and ferritin concentrations then gradually drop back to the normal range [166].

4.6 Genetic Hemochromatosis

Iron overload in hemochromatosis starts with enhanced iron absorption, leading to an increase in plasma iron concentration and transferrin saturation and increasing iron concentration in liver parenchymal cells. As serum ferritin concentrations reflect iron concentration in macrophages [167], and macrophages accumulate little iron initially, the serum ferritin concentration might be expected to remain normal during the early stages of iron accumulation. Transferrin saturation is therefore the most efficient test for detecting initial iron accumulation in genetic hemochromatosis [168]. An alternative is the unsaturated iron-binding capacity. This is a test that is readily automated and provides a similar efficiency to the transferrin saturation [169–172]. In hospital patients, the transferrin saturation may be depressed by chronic or acute infection or inflammation leading to false-negative results [173]. In the absence of inflammation, infection, or liver disease, serum ferritin usually provides a reasonable indication of the degree of iron loading.

A TS >50% will identify over 80% of healthy men homozygous for C282Y, but only a minority of women [170, 172], although in the HEIRS study, more than half of female homozygotes had TS >45% [174]. Thresholds for diagnosis have varied – in the case of TS from 45% to 62% – in the various guidelines on the diagnosis and management of hemochromatosis that have been published.

Normal concentrations of sTfR have been reported for patients with genetic hemochromatosis (although some had been venesected) and also in African iron overload [107, 175]. In contrast, lower mean values of sTfR were found in subjects with a raised transferrin saturation [176, 177]. However, there was considerable overlap with the normal range of sTfR concentration and measurement of sTfR in iron overload is unlikely to be of diagnostic value.

4.7 Secondary Iron Overload

The major diagnostic aims are the determination of the degree of iron overload and monitoring the success of chelation therapy in removing iron. Reliable methods are quantitation of liver iron concentration on biopsy samples (an invasive procedure) and the newly developed MRI and magnetic susceptibility measurements. In patients with homozygous β-thalassemia, serum ferritin shows a correlation with both liver iron concentration [178] and amount of blood transfused [27], although this does not apply in patients deficient in ascorbic acid [179]. However, in general clinical practice, serum ferritin has limited value in predicting liver iron concentrations in both thalassemia major [180] and patients with sickle-cell disease on chronic transfusions [181]. In patients with thalassemia intermedia who do not require transfusion, serum ferritin concentrations tend to underestimate the liver iron concentration, and this may lead to delay in instituting effective iron chelation therapy [182].

In practice, serum ferritin concentrations provide a combined index of storage iron levels and liver damage and give useful information for monitoring progress. The aim of chelation is to reduce both tissue iron levels and tissue damage. Reduction of serum ferritin to 1,000 μg/L is a realistic aim.

5 Assessing the Iron Status of Populations and Any Response to Iron Supplementation

At a meeting held in Geneva in 2004, a WHO and CDC expert consultation evaluated the best methods for assessing the iron status of populations and of the response to an intervention such as food fortification with iron [6]. The meeting recommended that blood hemoglobin and serum ferritin are the most useful indicators of the impact of programs to control iron deficiency. The main problem with the use of ferritin lies in the fact that it is affected by inflammation due to infection and chronic

Table 25.7 The interpretation of low serum ferritin and high transferrin receptor concentrations during population surveys [6]

Percentage of serum ferritin values below threshold[a]	Percentage of transferrin receptor values above threshold[b]	Interpretation
<20% (low) <30% for pregnant women	<10% (low)	Iron deficiency is not prevalent
<20% (low)	≥10% (high)	Iron deficiency is prevalent; inflammation is prevalent
≥20% (high)	≥10% (high)	Iron deficiency is prevalent
≥20% (high) ≥30% for pregnant women	<10% (low)	Mild iron deficiency may be prevalent

[a] World Health Organization [4]
[b] Use thresholds recommended by manufacturer of assay until an international reference standard is available

disease, so it is less useful to assess the prevalence of iron deficiency than to estimate a change brought about by a program. Because of this, the consultation recommended that to assess iron deficiency, the transferrin receptor, in addition to hemoglobin and ferritin, should be measured (Table 25.7). The value of this approach has not been confirmed. Despite many attempts, methods of correcting serum ferritin concentrations for the effect of inflammation or infection have not been successful. C-reactive protein (CRP) is commonly used as an indicator of inflammation, but CRP has a rapid response to an acute inflammatory stimulus compared to ferritin [183]. Beard et al. [184] found that in areas with a low prevalence of inflammation, neither CRP nor α_1-acid glycoprotein predicted high ferritin concentrations accurately. They concluded that where the prevalence of inflammation is <10%, this has little influence on the distribution of ferritin. In order to allow for the affect of infection, the WHO has recommended a cutoff of 30 μg/L for the identification of iron deficiency in children with infection/inflammation [4]. No corresponding adult threshold was suggested.

The value of the serum transferrin receptor ratio Log (sTfR in μg/L/ferritin μg/L) to assess body iron in population surveys has been demonstrated in several studies [113]. The group was unable to recommend general application of this until standardization of the assay had been achieved.

6 Conclusions

The investigation of iron metabolism begins with the measurement of blood hemoglobin concentration and red cell indices. Anemia, with hypochromic red cells, is a result of a reduced iron supply to the bone marrow. If this is a result of a reduction in total body iron in an otherwise healthy subject (iron-deficiency anemia), there will be a low serum ferritin concentration (<15 μg/L).

If total body iron is not reduced, the hypochromic anemia may be due to a disturbance in hemoglobin synthesis (thalassemia or sideroblastic anemia) or, more commonly, may result from acute or chronic disease. In this case, the serum ferritin concentration will be normal or elevated.

Ferritin synthesis is also increased by the cytokines released during infection and inflammation, and serum ferritin concentrations up to 60 μg/L may be found in subjects with acute or chronic disease and an absence of storage iron. In subjects with ferritin concentrations of around 60–100 μg/L (and a raised level of CRP or a raised ESR), it should be remembered that iron stores may not be adequate for hemoglobin regeneration once the inflammation subsides.

In general hematological practice, assay of serum iron and transferrin saturation, ZPP, and sTfR are less sensitive and specific than the assay of serum ferritin. The use of discriminant analysis, algorithms, or logistic regression of ferritin with CRP concentration or ESR does not enhance the accuracy of diagnosis significantly.

In the detection of early iron accumulation in hemochromatosis, measurement of transferrin saturation is the test of choice. In hospital patients, transferrin saturation may be depressed and the test should be repeated once the patient has recovered from surgery, infection, or inflammation. Serum ferritin provides a useful indication of the level of storage iron in genetic hemochromatosis and a useful way of monitoring iron stores during chelation therapy for iron removal after multiple blood transfusions.

References

1. British Nutrition Foundation. Report of the task force. Iron – nutritional and physiological significance. London: Chapman and Hall; 1995.
2. Sullivan JL. The iron hypothesis: claim vs. hypothesis. Vasc Med. 2000;5:127–8.
3. Bain BJ, Lewis SM, Bates I. Basic haematological techniques. In: Lewis SM, Bain BJ, Bates I, editors. Dacie and Lewis practical haematology. Philadelphia: Churchill Livingstone; 2006. p. 25–57.
4. World Health Organization. Iron deficiency anemia. Assessment, prevention, and control. A guide for programme managers; 2001.
5. Assessing the iron status of populations. Report of a joint World Health Organization/Centers for Disease Control and Prevention technical consultation on the assessment of iron status at the population level Geneva, Switzerland; 2004.
6. World Health Organization. WHO/CDC expert consultation agrees on best indicators to assess iron deficiency, a major cause of anaemia; 2004.
7. Mast AE, Blinder MA, Lu Q, Flax S, Dietzen DJ. Clinical utility of the reticulocyte hemoglobin content in the diagnosis of iron deficiency. Blood. 2002;99:1489–91.
8. David O, Grillo A, Ceoloni B, et al. Analysis of red cell parameters on the Sysmex XE 2100 and ADVIA 120 in iron deficiency and in uraemic chronic disease. Scand J Clin Lab Invest. 2006;66:113–20.
9. Thomas L, Franck S, Messinger M, Linssen J, Thome M, Thomas C. Reticulocyte hemoglobin measurement – comparison of two methods in the diagnosis of iron-restricted erythropoiesis. Clin Chem Lab Med. 2005;43:1193–202.
10. Brugnara C, Schiller B, Moran J. Reticulocyte hemoglobin equivalent (Ret He) and assessment of iron-deficient states. Clin Lab Haematol. 2006;28:303–8.
11. Torrance JD, Bothwell TH. Tissue iron stores. In: Cook JD, editor. Iron. New York: Churchill Livingstone; 1980. p. 90–115.
12. Walters GO, Miller FM, Worwood M. Serum ferritin concentration and iron stores in normal subjects. J Clin Pathol. 1973;26:770–2.
13. Dooley J, Worwood M. Guidelines on diagnosis and therapy: genetic haemochromatosis. British Committee for Standards in Haematology. http://www.bshguidelines.com/documents/haemochromatosis_200.pdf.
14. Gale E, Torrance J, Bothwell T. The quantitative estimation of total iron stores in human bone marrow. J Clin Invest. 1963;42:1076–82.
15. Villeneuve JP, Bilodeau M, Lepage R, Cote J, Lefebvre M. Variability in hepatic iron concentration measurement from needle-biopsy specimens. J Hepatol. 1996;25:172–7.
16. Charlton RW, Hawkins DM, Mavor WO, Bothwell TH. Hepatic iron storage concentrations in different population groups. Am J Clin Nutr. 1970;23:358–71.
17. Bassett ML, Halliday JW, Powell LW. Value of hepatic iron measurements in early hemochromatosis and determination of the critical iron level associated with fibrosis. Hepatology. 1986;6:24–9.
18. Swirsky D, Bain BJ. Erythrocyte and leucocyte cytochemistry. In: Lewis SM, Bain BJ, Bates I, editors. Dacie and Lewis practical haematology. Philadelphia: Churchill Livingstone/Elsevier; 2006. p. 311–33.
19. Barron BA, Hoyer JD, Tefferi A. A bone marrow report of absent stainable iron is not diagnostic of iron deficiency. Ann Hematol. 2001;80:166–9.
20. Hughes DA, Stuart-Smith SE, Bain BJ. How should stainable iron in bone marrow films be assessed? J Clin Pathol. 2004;57:1038–40.
21. Bentley DP, Williams P. Serum ferritin concentration as an index of storage iron in rheumatoid arthritis. J Clin Pathol. 1974;27:786–8.
22. Stuart-Smith SE, Hughes DA, Bain BJ. Are routine iron stains on bone marrow trephine biopsy specimens necessary? J Clin Pathol. 2005;58:269–72.
23. Shorr E. Intermediary metabolism and biological activities of ferritin. Harvey Lect. 1956;50:112–53.
24. Reissmann KR, Dietrich MR. On the presence of ferritin in the peripheral blood of patients with hepatocellular disease. J Clin Invest. 1956;35:588–95.
25. Worwood M. Serum ferritin. CRC Crit Rev Clin Lab Sci. 1979;10:171–204.
26. Addison GM, Beamish MR, Hales CN, Hodgkins M, Jacobs A, Llewellin P. An immunoradiometric assay for ferritin in the serum of normal subjects and patients with iron deficiency and iron overload. J Clin Pathol. 1972;25:326–9.

27. Worwood M, Cragg SJ, Jacobs A, McLaren C, Ricketts C, Economidou J. Binding of serum ferritin to concanavalin A: patients with homozygous beta thalassaemia and transfusional iron overload. Br J Haematol. 1980;46:409–16.
28. Worwood M. Ferritin in human-tissues and serum. Clin Haematol. 1982;11:275–307.
29. Milman N, Strandberg N, Visfelt J. Serum ferritin in healthy Danes: relation to marrow haemosiderin iron stores. Dan Med Bull. 1983;30:115–20.
30. Oertel J, Bombik BM, Stephan M, Gerhartz H. Ferritin in bone marrow and serum in iron deficiency and iron overload. Blut. 1978;37:113–17.
31. Custer EM, Finch CA, Sobel RE, Zettner A. Population norms for serum ferritin. J Lab Clin Med. 1995;126:88–94.
32. Choi JW, Pai SH, Im MW, Kim SK. Change in transferrin receptor concentrations with age. Clin Chem. 1999;45:1562–3.
33. O'Brien KO, Zavaleta N, Abrams SA, Caulfield LE. Maternal iron status influences iron transfer to the fetus during the third trimester of pregnancy. Am J Clin Nutr. 2003;77:924–30.
34. Leggett BA, Brown NN, Bryant SJ, Duplock L, Powell LW, Halliday JW. Factors affecting the concentrations of ferritin in serum in a healthy Australian population. Clin Chem. 1990;36:1350–5.
35. White A, Nicolas G, Foster K. Health survey for England 1991. Her Majesty's Stationary Office; 1993.
36. Touitou Y, Proust J, Carayon A, et al. Plasma ferritin in old age. Influence of biological and pathological factors in a large elderly population. Clin Chim Acta. 1985;149:37–45.
37. Hallberg L, Bengtsson C, Lapidus L, Lindstedt G, Lundberg P-A, Hulten L. Screening for iron deficiency: an analysis based on bone-marrow examinations and serum ferritin determinations on a population sample of women. Br J Haematol. 1993;85:787–98.
38. Looker AC, Dallman PR, Carroll MD, Gunter EW, Johnson CL. Prevalence of iron deficiency in the United States. JAMA. 1997;277:973–6.
39. Worwood M, Dawkins S, Wagstaff M, Jacobs A. The purification and properties of ferritin from human serum. Biochem J. 1976;157:97–103.
40. Cragg SJ, Wagstaff M, Worwood M. Detection of a glycosylated subunit in human serum ferritin. Biochem J. 1981;199:565–71.
41. Pootrakul P, Josephson B, Huebers HA, Finch CA. Quantitation of ferritin iron in plasma, an explanation for non-transferrin iron. Blood. 1988;71:1120–3.
42. Wagstaff M, Worwood M, Jacobs A. Properties of human tissue isoferritins. Biochem J. 1978;173:969–77.
43. Tenkate J, Wolthuis A, Westerhuis B, Vandeursen C. The iron content of serum ferritin: physiological importance and diagnostic value. Eur J Clin Chem Clin Biochem. 1997;35:53–6.
44. Herbert V, Jayatilleke E, Shaw S, Rosman AS, Giardina P. Serum ferritin iron, a new test, measures human body iron stores unconfounded by inflammation. Stem Cells. 1997;15:291–6.
45. Nielsen P, Gunther U, Durken M, Fischer R, Dullmann J. Serum ferritin iron in iron overload and liver damage: correlation to body iron stores and diagnostic relevance. J Lab Clin Med. 2000;135:413–18.
46. Yamanishi H, Iyama S, Fushimi R, Amino N. Interference of ferritin in measurement of serum iron concentrations: comparison by five methods. Clin Chem. 1996;42:331–2.
47. McKeering LV, Halliday JW, Caffin JA, Mack U, Powell LW. Immunological detection of isoferritins in normal human serum and tissue. Clin Chim Acta. 1976;67:189–97.
48. Worwood M, Cragg SJ, Wagstaff M, Jacobs A. Binding of human serum ferritin to concanavalin A. Clin Sci. 1979;56:83–7.
49. Cragg SJ, Wagstaff M, Worwood M. Sialic acid and the microheterogeneity of human serum ferritin. Clin Sci. 1980;58:259–62.
50. Santambrogio P, Cozzi A, Levi S, Arosio P. Human serum ferritin G-peptide is recognized by anti-L ferritin subunit antibodies and concanavalin-A. Br J Haematol. 1987;65:235–7.
51. Ghosh S, Hevi S, Chuck SL. Regulated secretion of glycosylated human ferritin from hepatocytes. Blood. 2004;103:2369–76.
52. Worwood M, Cragg SJ, Williams AM, Wagstaff M, Jacobs A. The clearance of 131I-human plasma ferritin in man. Blood. 1982;60:827–33.
53. Cragg SJ, Covell AM, Burch A, Owen GM, Jacobs A, Worwood M. Turnover of 131I-human spleen ferritin in plasma. Br J Haematol. 1983;55:83–92.
54. Adams PC, Powell LW, Halliday JW. Isolation of a human hepatic ferritin receptor. Hepatology. 1988;8:719–21.
55. Covell AM, Jacobs A, Worwood M. Interaction of ferritin with serum – implications for ferritin turnover. Clin Chim Acta. 1984;139:75–84.
56. Bellotti V, Arosio P, Cazzola M, et al. Characteristics of a ferritin-binding protein present in human-serum. Br J Haematol. 1987;65:489–93.
57. Santambrogio P, Massover WH. Rabbit serum alpha-2-macroglobulin binds to liver ferritin – association causes a heterogeneity of ferritin molecules. Br J Haematol. 1989;71:281–90.

58. Arosio P, Yokota M, Drysdale JW. Characterization of serum ferritin in iron overload: possible identity to natural apoferritin. Br J Haematol. 1977;36:199–207.
59. Vignes S, Le Moel G, Fautrel B, Wechsler B, Godeau P, Piette JC. Percentage of glycosylated serum ferritin remains low throughout the course of adult onset Still's disease. Ann Rheum Dis. 2000;59:347–50.
60. Prieto J, Barry M, Sherlock S. Serum ferritin in patients with iron overload and with acute and chronic liver diseases. Gastroenterology. 1975;68:525–33.
61. Ota T, Higashi S, Suzuki H, Eto S. Increased serum ferritin levels in adult Still's disease [letter]. Lancet. 1987;1:562–3.
62. Esumi N, Ikushima S, Todo S, Imashuku S. Hyperferritinemia in malignant histiocytosis, virus-associated hemophagocytic syndrome and familial erythrophagocytic lymphohistiocytosis. A survey of pediatric cases. Acta Paediatr Scand. 1989;78:268–70.
63. Esumi N, Ikushima S, Hibi S, Todo S, Imashuku S. High serum ferritin level as a marker of malignant histiocytosis and virus-associated hemophagocytic syndrome. Cancer. 1988;61:2071–6.
64. Koduri PR, Shah PC, Goyal V. Elevated serum ferritin levels: associated diseases and clinical significance. Am J Med. 1996;101:121–2.
65. Kirn DH, Fredericks D, Mccutchan JA, Stites D, Shuman M. Marked elevation of the serum ferritin is highly specific for disseminated histoplasmosis in AIDS. AIDS. 1995;9:1204–5.
66. Iron Panel of the International Committee for Standardization in Haematology. Revised recommendations for the measurement of serum iron in human blood. Br J Haematol. 1990;75:615–16.
67. National Committee for Clinical Laboratory Standards. Determination of serum iron and total iron-binding capacity: proposed standard. Document H17-P 1990;10: Villanova, PA.
68. Worwood M. Iron deficiency anaemia and iron overload. In: Lewis SM, Bain BJ, Bates I, editors. Dacie and Lewis practical haematology. 10th ed. Philadelphia: Church Livingstone Elsevier; 2006. p. 131–60.
69. Bothwell TH, Charlton RW, Cook JD, Finch CA. Iron metabolism in man. Oxford: Blackwell Scientific Publications; 1979.
70. Brink B, Disler P, Lynch S, Jacobs P, Charlton R, Bothwell T. Patterns of iron storage in dietary iron overload and idiopathic hemochromatosis. J Lab Clin Med. 1976;88:725–31.
71. Bandi ZL, Schoen I, Bee DE. Immunochemical methods for measurement of transferrin in serum – effects of analytical errors and inappropriate reference intervals on diagnostic utility. Clin Chem. 1985;31:1601–5.
72. Huebers HA, Eng MJ, Josephson BM, et al. Plasma iron and transferrin iron-binding-capacity evaluated by colorimetric and immunoprecipitation methods. Clin Chem. 1987;33:273–7.
73. Yamanishi H, Iyama S, Yamaguchi Y, Kanakura Y, Iwatani Y. Total iron-binding capacity calculated from serum transferrin concentration or serum iron concentration and unsaturated iron-binding capacity. Clin Chem. 2003;49:175–8.
74. Hawkins RC. Total iron binding capacity or transferrin concentration alone outperforms iron and saturation indices in predicting iron deficiency. Clin Chim Acta. 2007;380:203–7.
75. Bainton DF, Finch CA. The diagnosis of iron deficiency anemia. Am J Med. 1964;37:62–70.
76. Beilby J, Olynyk J, Ching S, et al. Transferrin index: an alternative method for calculating the iron saturation of transferrin. Clin Chem. 1992;38:2078–81.
77. Cabantchik ZI, Breuer W, Zanninelli G, Cianciulli R. LPI-labile plasma iron in iron overload. Best Pract Res Clin Haematol. 2005;18:277–87.
78. Hershko C. Study of chelating agent diethylenetriaminepentaacetic acid using selective radioiron probes of reticuloendothelial and parenchymal iron stores. J Lab Clin Med. 1975;85:913–21.
79. Hershko C, Graham G, Bates GW, Rachmilewitz EA. Nonspecific serum iron in thalassemia – abnormal serum iron fraction of potential toxicity. Br J Haematol. 1978;40:255–63.
80. Graham G, Bates GW, Rachmilewitz EA, Hershko C. Nonspecific serum iron in thalassemia – quantitation and chemical-reactivity. Am J Hematol. 1979;6:207–17.
81. Gutteridge JM, Rowley DA, Griffiths E, Halliwell B. Low-molecular-weight iron complexes and oxygen radical reactions in idiopathic haemochromatosis. Clin Sci. 1985;68:463–7.
82. Batey RG, Lai CF, Shamir S, Sherlock S. Non-transferrin bound serum iron in idiopathic haemochromatosis. Dig Dis Sci. 1980;25:340–6.
83. Aruoma OI, Bomford A, Polson RJ, Halliwell B. Nontransferrin-bound iron in plasma from hemochromatosis patients: effect of phlebotomy therapy. Blood. 1988;72:1416–19.
84. De Valk B, Addicks MA, Gosriwatana I, Lu S, Hider RC, Marx JJM. Non-transferrin-bound iron is present in serum of hereditary haemochromatosis heterozygotes. Eur J Clin Invest. 2000;30:248–51.
85. Singh S, Hider RC, Porter JB. A direct method for quantification of non-transferrin-bound iron. Anal Biochem. 1990;186:320–3.
86. Nilsson UA, Bassen M, Savman K, Kjellmer I. A simple and rapid method for the determination of "free" iron in biological fluids. Free Radic Res. 2002;36:677–84.

87. Gosriwatana I, Loreal O, Lu S, Brissot P, Porter J, Hider RC. Quantification of non-transferrin-bound iron in the presence of unsaturated transferrin. Anal Biochem. 1999;273:212–20.
88. Evans PJ, Halliwell B. Measurement of iron and copper in biological systems – bleomycin and copper-phenanthroline assays. Methods Enzymol. 1994;233:82–92.
89. Sahlstedt L, Ebeling F, von Bonsdorff L, Parkkinen J, Ruutu T. Non-transferrin-bound iron during allogeneic stem cell transplantation. Br J Haematol. 2001;113:836–8.
90. Breuer W, Ronson A, Slotki IN, Abramov A, Hershko C, Cabantchik ZI. The assessment of serum nontransferrin-bound iron in chelation therapy and iron supplementation. Blood. 2000;95:2975–82.
91. Breuer W, Cabantchik ZI. A fluorescence-based one-step assay for serum non transferrin-bound iron. Anal Biochem. 2001;299:194–202.
92. Jacobs EMG, Hendriks JCM, van Tits BLJH, et al. Results of an international round robin for the quantification of serum non-transferrin-bound iron: need for defining standardization and a clinically relevant isoform. Anal Biochem. 2005;341:241–50.
93. van der A DL, Marx JJM, Grobbee DE, et al. Non-transferrin-bound iron and risk of coronary heart disease in postmenopausal women. Circulation. 2006;113:1942–9.
94. Lee DH, Liu DY, Jacobs DR, et al. Common presence of non-transferrin-bound iron among patients with type 2 diabetes. Diabetes Care. 2006;29:1090–5.
95. Van Campenhout A, Van Campenhout C, Lagrou AR, Moorkens G, De Block C, Keenoy B. Iron-binding antioxidant capacity is impaired in diabetes mellitus. Free Radic Biol Med. 2006;40:1749–55.
96. Prakash M, Upadhya S, Prabhu R. Serum non-transferrin bound iron in hemodialysis patients not receiving intravenous iron. Clin Chim Acta. 2005;360:194–8.
97. Labbe RF, Vreman HJ, Stevenson DK. Zinc protoporphyrin: a metabolite with a mission. Clin Chem. 1999;45:2060–72.
98. Hastka J, Lasserre JJ, Schwarzbeck A, Strauch M, Heier HE. Zinc protoporphyrin in anemia of chronic disorders. Blood. 1993;81:1200–4.
99. Soldin OP, Miller M, Soldin SJ. Pediatric reference ranges for zinc protoporphyrin. Clin Biochem. 2003;36:21–5.
100. Zanella A, Gridelli L, Berzuini A, et al. Sensitivity and predictive value of serum ferritin and free erythrocyte protoporphyrin for iron-deficiency. J Lab Clin Med. 1989;113:73–8.
101. Hodgetts J, Hoy TG, Jacobs A. Iron uptake and ferritin synthesis in human erythroblasts. Clin Sci. 1986;70:53–7.
102. Cazzola M, Dezza L, Bergamaschi G, et al. Biologic and clinical significance of red cell ferritin. Blood. 1983;62:1078–87.
103. Cazzola M, Ascari E. Red cell ferritin as a diagnostic tool. Br J Haematol. 1986;62:209–13.
104. Kohgo Y, Nishisato T, Kondo H, Tsushima N, Niitsu Y, Urushshizaki I. Circulating transferrin receptor in human serum. Br J Haematol. 1986;64:277–81.
105. Cook JD, Skikne BS, Baynes RD. Serum transferrin receptor. Annu Rev Med. 1993;44:63–74.
106. Kohgo Y, Niitsu Y, Kondo H, et al. Serum transferrin receptor as a new index of erythropoiesis. Blood. 1987;70:1955–8.
107. Huebers HA, Beguin Y, Pootrakul P, Einspahr D, Finch CA. Intact transferrin receptors in human plasma and their relation to erythropoiesis. Blood. 1990;75:102–7.
108. Beguin Y, Clemons GK, Pootrakul P, Fillet G. Quantitative assessment of erythropoiesis and functional classification of anemia based on measurements of serum transferrin receptor and erythropoietin. Blood. 1993;81:1067–76.
109. Cavill I, Ricketts C. Human iron kinetics. In: Jacobs A, Worwood M, editors. Iron in biochemistry and medicine II. London: Academic Press; 1980. p. 573–604.
110. Beguin Y. Soluble transferrin receptor for the evaluation of erythropoiesis and iron status. Clin Chim Acta. 2003;329:9–22.
111. Skikne BS, Flowers C, Cook JD. Serum transferrin receptor: a quantitative measure of tissue iron deficiency. Blood. 1990;75:1870–6.
112. Olivares M, Walter T, Cook JD, Hertrampf E, Pizarro F. Usefulness of serum transferrin receptor and serum ferritin in diagnosis of iron deficiency in infancy. Am J Clin Nutr. 2000;72:1191–5.
113. Cook JD, Flowers CH, Skikne BS. The quantitative assessment of body iron. Blood. 2003;101:3359–64.
114. Punnonen K, Irjala K, Rajamaki A. Serum transferrin receptor and its ratio to serum ferritin in the diagnosis of iron deficiency. Blood. 1997;89:1052–7.
115. Zeleniuch-Jacquotte A, Zhang Q, Dai JS, et al. Reliability of serum assays of iron status in postmenopausal women. Ann Epidemiol. 2007;17:354–8.
116. Allen J, Backstrom KR, Cooper JA, et al. Measurement of soluble transferrin receptor in serum of healthy adults. Clin Chem. 1998;44:35–9.

117. Worwood M, Ellis RD, Bain BJ. Three serum transferrin receptor ELISAs. MDA/2000/09. Norwich UK, Her Majesty's Stationary Office; 2000.
118. Akesson A, Bjellerup P, Berglund M, Bremme K, Vahter M. Serum transferrin receptor: a specific marker of iron deficiency in pregnancy. Am J Clin Nutr. 1998;68:1241–6.
119. Mast AE, Blinder MA, Gronowski AM, Chumley C, Scott MG. Clinical utility of the soluble transferrin receptor and comparison with serum ferritin in several populations. Clin Chem. 1998;44:45–51.
120. Suominen P, Punnonen K, Rajamaki A, Irjala K. Evaluation of new immunoenzymometric assay for measuring soluble transferrin receptor to detect iron deficiency in anemic patients. Clin Chem. 1997;43:1641–6.
121. Akesson A, Bjellerup P, Vahter M. Evaluation of kits for measurement of the soluble transferrin receptor. Scand J Clin Lab Invest. 1999;59:77–81.
122. Kuiperkramer EPA, Huisman CMS, Vanraan J, Vaneijk HG. Analytical and clinical implications of soluble transferrin receptors in serum. Eur J Clin Chem Clin Biochem. 1996;34:645–9.
123. Pfeiffer CM, Cook JD, Mei ZG, Cogswell ME, Looker AC, Lacher DA. Evaluation of an automated soluble transferrin receptor (sTfR) assay on the Roche Hitachi analyzer and its comparison to two ELISA assays. Clin Chim Acta. 2007;382:112–16.
124. Thorpe SJ, Heath A, Sharp G, Cook J, Ellis R, Worwood M. A WHO reference reagent for the Serum Transferrin Receptor (sTfR): international collaborative study to evaluate a recombinant soluble transferrin receptor preparation. Clin Chem Lab Med. 2010;48:815–20.
125. Bergamaschi G, Villani L. Serum hepcidin: a novel diagnostic tool in disorders of iron metabolism. Haematologica. 2009;94:1631–3.
126. Kroot JJC, Hendriks JCM, Laarakkers CMM, et al. (Pre)analytical imprecision, between-subject variability, and daily variations in serum and urine hepcidin: implications for clinical studies. Anal Biochem. 2009;389:124–9.
127. Dawkins S, Cavill I, Ricketts C, Worwood M. Variability of serum ferritin concentration in normal subjects. Clin Lab Haematol. 1979;1:41–6.
128. Cooper MJ, Zlotkin SH. Day-to-day variation of transferrin receptor and ferritin in healthy men and women. Am J Clin Nutr. 1996;64:738–42.
129. Borel MJ, Smith SM, Derr J, Beard JL. Day-to-day variation in iron-status indices in healthy men and women. Am J Clin Nutr. 1991;54:729–35.
130. Pootrakul P, Skikne BS, Cook JD. The use of capillary blood for measurements of circulating ferritin. Am J Clin Nutr. 1983;37:307–10.
131. Dallman PR. Diagnosis of anemia and iron-deficiency – analytic and biological variations of laboratory tests. Am J Clin Nutr. 1984;39:937–41.
132. Wiggers P, Dalhoj J, Hyltoft Petersen P, Blaabjerg O, Horder M. Screening for haemochromatosis: influence of analytical imprecision, diagnostic limit and prevalence on test validity. Scand J Clin Lab Invest. 1991;51:143–8.
133. Tessitore N, Solero GP, Lippi G, et al. The role of iron status markers in predicting response to intravenous iron in haemodialysis patients on maintenance erythropoietin. Nephrol Dial Transplant. 2001;16:1416–23.
134. Goddard AF, McIntyre AS, Scott BB. Guidelines for the management of iron deficiency anaemia. Gut. 2000;46:A1–5.
135. Guyatt G, Oxman AD, Ali M, Willan A, Mcilroy W, Patterson C. Laboratory diagnosis of iron-deficiency anemia – an overview. J Gen Intern Med. 1992;7:145–53.
136. Domellof M, Dewey KG, Lonnerdal B, Cohen RJ, Hernell O. The diagnostic criteria for iron deficiency in infants should be reevaluated. J Nutr. 2002;132:3680–6.
137. Margolis HS, Huntley Hardison H, Bender TR, Dallman PR. Iron deficiency in children: the relationship between pretreatment laboratory tests and subsequent hemoglobin response to iron therapy. Am J Clin Nutr. 1981;34:2158–68.
138. Flowers CH, Skikne BS, Covell AM, Cook JD. The clinical measurement of serum transferrin receptor. J Lab Clin Med. 1989;114:368–77.
139. Hershko C, Baror D, Gaziel Y, et al. Diagnosis of iron-deficiency anemia in a rural-population of children – relative usefulness of serum ferritin, red-cell protoporphyrin, red-cell indexes, and transferrin saturation determinations. Am J Clin Nutr. 1981;34:1600–10.
140. Abraham K, Muller C, Gruters A, Wahn U, Schweigert FJ. Minimal inflammation, acute phase response and avoidance of misclassification of vitamin A and iron status in infants – importance of a high-sensitivity C-reactive protein (CRP) assay. Int J Vitam Nutr Res. 2003;73:423–30.
141. Lopez MAV, Molinos FL, Carmona ML, et al. Serum transferrin receptor in children: usefulness for determinating the nature of anemia in infection. J Pediatr Hematol Oncol. 2006;28:809–15.
142. Carriaga MT, Skikne BS, Finley B, Cutler B, Cook JD. Serum transferrin receptor for the detection of iron deficiency in pregnancy. Am J Clin Nutr. 1991;54:1077–81.
143. Akesson A, Bjellerup P, Berglund M, Bremme K, Vahter M. Soluble transferrin receptor: longitudinal assessment from pregnancy to postlactation. Obstet Gynecol. 2002;99:260–6.

144. Choi JW, Im MW, Pai SH. Serum transferrin receptor concentrations during normal pregnancy. Clin Chem. 2000;46:725–7.
145. Vandenbroek NR, Letsky EA, White SA, Shenkin A. Iron status in pregnant women: which measurements are valid? Br J Haematol. 1998;103:817–24.
146. Milman N, Bergholt T, Byg KE, Eriksen L, Hvas AM. Reference intervals for haematological variables during normal pregnancy and postpartum in 434 healthy Danish women. Eur J Haematol. 2007;79:39–46.
147. Institute of Medicine. Iron deficiency anemia: recommended guidelines for the prevention, detection and management among U.S. children and women of childbearing age. Washington, DC: National Academy Press; 1993.
148. Centers for Disease Control and Prevention. Recommendations to prevent and control iron deficiency in the United States. MMWR Recomm Rep. 1998;47:1–29.
149. American Academy of Pediatrics. Guidelines for perinatal care. Elk Grove Village: The Academy; 1997.
150. Ntaios G, Chatzinikolaou A, Saouli Z, et al. Discrimination indices as screening tests for beta-thalassemic trait. Ann Hematol. 2007;86:487–91.
151. Ferrara M, Capozzi L, Russo R, Bertocco F, Ferrara D. Reliability of red blood cell indices and formulas to discriminate between beta thalassemia trait and iron deficiency in children. Hematology. 2010;15:112–15.
152. van Tellingen A, Kuenen JC, de Kieviet W, van Tinteren H, Kooi MLK, Vasmel WLE. Iron deficiency anaemia in hospitalised patients: value of various laboratory parameters – differentiation between IDA and ACD. Neth J Med. 2001;59:270–9.
153. Lee EJ, Oh EJ, Park YJ, Lee HK, Kim BK. Soluble transferrin receptor (sTfR), ferritin, and sTfR/log ferritin index in anemic patients with nonhematologic malignancy and chronic inflammation. Clin Chem. 2002;48:1118–21.
154. Kotru M, Rusia U, Sikka M, Chaturvedi S, Jain AK. Evaluation of serum ferritin in screening for iron deficiency in tuberculosis. Ann Hematol. 2004;83:95–100.
155. Kurer SB, Seifert B, Michel B, Ruegg R, Fehr J. Prediction of iron-deficiency in chronic inflammatory rheumatic disease anemia. Br J Haematol. 1995;91:820–6.
156. Bultink IEM, Lems WF, de Stadt RJV, et al. Ferritin and serum transferrin receptor predict iron deficiency in anemic patients with rheumatoid arthritis. Arthritis Rheum. 2001;44:979–81.
157. Means RT, Allen J, Sears DA, Schuster SJ. Serum soluble transferrin receptor and the prediction of marrow aspirate iron results in a heterogeneous group of patients. Clin Lab Haematol. 1999;21:161–7.
158. Joosten E, Van Loon R, Billen J, Blanckaert N, Fabri R, Pelemans W. Serum transferrin receptor in the evaluation of the iron status in elderly hospitalized patients with anemia. Am J Hematol. 2002;69:1–6.
159. Balaban EP, Sheehan RG, Demian RA, Frenkel EP. Evaluation of bone marrow iron stores in anemia associated with chronic disease: a comparative study of serum and red cell ferritin. Am J Hematol. 1993;42:177–81.
160. Fernandez-Rodriguez AM, Guindeo-Casasus MC, Molero-Labarta T, et al. Diagnosis of iron deficiency in chronic renal failure. Am J Kidney Dis. 1999;34:508–13.
161. Ahluwalia N, Lammikeefe CJ, Bendel RB, Morse EE, Beard JL, Haley NR. Iron-deficiency and anemia of chronic disease in elderly women – a discriminant-analysis approach for differentiation. Am J Clin Nutr. 1995;61:590–6.
162. Macdougall IC, Cavill I, Hulme B, et al. Detection of functional iron-deficiency during erythropoietin treatment – a new approach. BMJ. 1992;304:225–6.
163. Fishbane S, Galgano C, Langley RC, Canfield W, Maesaka JK. Reticulocyte hemoglobin content in the evaluation of iron status of hemodialysis patients. Kidney Int. 1997;52:217–22.
164. Katodritou E, Terpos E, Zervas K, et al. Hypochromic erythrocytes (%): a reliable marker for recognizing iron-restricted erythropoiesis and predicting response to erythropoietin in anemic patients with myeloma and lymphoma. Ann Hematol. 2007;86:369–76.
165. Wheby MS. Effect of iron therapy on serum ferritin levels in iron-deficiency anemia. Blood. 1980;56:138–40.
166. Blunden RW, Lloyd JV, Rudzki Z, Kimber RJ. Changes in serum ferritin levels after intravenous iron. Ann Clin Biochem. 1981;18:215–17.
167. Worwood M. Ferritin. Blood Rev. 1990;4:259–69.
168. Edwards CQ, Griffen LM, Bulaj ZJ, Ajioka RS, Kushner JP. The iron phenotype of hemochromatosis heterozygotes. In: Barton JC, Edwards CQ, editors. Hemochromatosis: genetics, pathophysiology, diagnosis and treatment. Cambridge: Cambridge University Press; 2000. p. 411–18.
169. Adams PC, Kertesz AE, Mclaren CE, Bamford A, Chakrabarti S. Population screening for haemochromatosis: a comparison of unbound iron binding capacity, transferrin saturation and C282Y genotyping in 5211 voluntary blood donors. Hepatology. 2000;31:1160–4.
170. Jackson HA, Carter K, Darke C, et al. HFE mutations, iron deficiency and overload in 10 500 blood donors. Br J Haematol. 2001;114:474–84.
171. Murtagh LJ, Whiley M, Wilson S, Tran H, Bassett ML. Unsaturated iron binding capacity and transferrin saturation are equally reliable in detection of HFE hemochromatosis. Am J Gastroenterol. 2002;97:2093–9.
172. Adams PC, Reboussin DM, Press RD, et al. Biological variability of transferrin saturation and unsaturated iron-binding capacity. Am J Med. 2007;120:999.e1–7.

173. Distante S. Phenotypic expression of the HFE gene mutauion (C282Y) among the hospitalised population. Gut. 2000;47:575–9.
174. Adams PC, Reboussin DM, Barton JC, et al. Hemochromatosis and iron-overload screening in a racially diverse population. N Engl J Med. 2005;352:1769–78.
175. Baynes RD, Cook JD, Bothwell TH, Friedman BM, Meyer TE. Serum transferrin receptor in hereditary hemochromatosis and African siderosis. Am J Hematol. 1994;45:288–92.
176. Khumalo H, Gomo ZAR, Moyo VM, et al. Serum transferrin receptors are decreased in the presence of iron overload. Clin Chem. 1998;44:40–4.
177. Looker AC, Loyevsky M, Gordeuk VR. Increased serum transferrin saturation is associated with lower serum transferrin receptor concentration. Clin Chem. 1999;45:2191–9.
178. Letsky EA, Miller F, Worwood M, Flynn DM. Serum ferritin in children with thalassemia regularly transfused. J Clin Pathol. 1974;27:652–5.
179. Chapman RWG, Hussain MAM, Gorman A, et al. Effect of ascorbic-acid deficiency on serum ferritin concentration in patients with beta-thalassemia major and iron overload. J Clin Pathol. 1982;35:487–91.
180. Angelucci E, Baronciani D, Lucarelli G, et al. Needle liver-biopsy in thalassemia – analyses of diagnostic-accuracy and safety in 1184 consecutive biopsies. Br J Haematol. 1995;89:757–61.
181. Karam LB, Disco D, Jackson SM, et al. Liver biopsy results in patients with sickle cell disease on chronic transfusions: poor correlation with ferritin levels. Pediatr Blood Cancer. 2008;50:62–5.
182. Pakbaz Z, Fischer R, Fung E, Nielsen P, Harmatz P, Vichinsky E. Serum ferritin underestimates liver iron concentration in transfusion independent thalassemia patients as compared to regularly transfused thalassemia and sickle cell patients. Pediatr Blood Cancer. 2007;49:329–32.
183. Feelders RA, Vreugdenhil G, Eggermont AMM, Kuiper-Kramer PA, van Eijk HG, Swaak AJG. Regulation of iron metabolism in the acute-phase response: interferon gamma and tumour necrosis factor alpha induce hypoferraemia, ferritin production and a decrease in circulating transferrin receptors in cancer patients. Eur J Clin Invest. 1998;28:520–7.
184. Beard JL, Murray-Kolb LE, Rosales FJ, Solomons NW, Angelilli ML. Interpretation of serum ferritin concentrations as indicators of total-body iron stores in survey populations: the role of biomarkers for the acute phase response. Am J Clin Nutr. 2006;84:1498–505.

Chapter 26
Genetic Testing for Disorders of Iron Homeostasis

James C. Barton, Pauline L. Lee, and Corwin Q. Edwards

Keywords Anemia • Ferroportin • Hemochromatosis • Hemojuvelin • Hepcidin • Iron overload • Iron-refractory iron-deficiency anemia • Matripase-2 • Sideroblastic anemia

1 Introduction

Iron homeostasis in health is maintained by the controlled absorption of iron from the small intestine that equals daily iron losses and meets iron requirements for erythropoiesis. The susceptibility to develop iron overload is increased in persons in whom absorption of dietary iron is increased. Deleterious mutations in genes that encode proteins that control or mediate iron absorption, transport, or storage cause diverse primary iron overload syndromes, e.g., *HFE* hemochromatosis. Similarly, heritable and acquired forms of anemia characterized by ineffective erythropoiesis and increased production of growth/differentiation factor 15 enhance iron absorption by the small intestine in the absence of other mutations or chronic erythrocyte transfusion, e.g., X-linked sideroblastic anemia. Mutations in genes that encode transferrin or matripase-2 may lead to iron-deficient erythropoiesis that is refractory to iron therapy. In this chapter, principal methods to detect and evaluate mutations associated with heritable disorders of iron homeostasis are reviewed, and deleterious mutations of genomic DNA associated with these disorders are tabulated.

2 Sample Collection and Preparation

All mutation analysis methods require the acquisition and preparation of suitable samples of genomic DNA. The clinical evaluation of subjects with iron overload disorders is typically performed by extracting DNA from a readily available source such as blood leukocytes ("buffy coat"). Blood samples are anticoagulated in EDTA and transported to the laboratory, preferably on wet ice or at

J.C. Barton, M.D. (✉)
Southern Iron Disorders Center,
Department of Medicine, University of Alabama at Birmingham,
Birmingham, AL, USA
e-mail: ironmd@dnamail.com

P.L. Lee, Ph.D.
Department of Molecular and Experimental Medicine, The Scripps Research Institute, La Jolla, CA, USA

C.Q. Edwards, M.D.
Departments of Medicine, Intermountain Medical Center and University of Utah, Salt Lake City, USA

G.J. Anderson and G. McLaren (eds.), *Iron Physiology and Pathophysiology in Humans*,
Nutrition and Health, DOI 10.1007/978-1-60327-485-2_26,

room temperature (within one day after venipuncture). Many laboratories use commercially available DNA extraction kits; other laboratories employ their own DNA isolation protocols. DNA of the best quantity and quality is obtained soon after blood collection; blood can be stored at 4°C, if necessary. DNA can be extracted from as little as 200 µL of whole blood or from leukocyte pellets from using commercially available DNA extraction kits. In general, non-column-based methods process larger amounts of blood and yield more DNA than column-based methods. In some cases, sufficient DNA suitable for analysis can be obtained from saliva, buccal swabs, or other sources. DNA is quantified by measuring the absorbance at 260 nm, using the conversion of one A_{260} O.D. unit of double-stranded DNA=50 µg/mL. Regardless of the method of collection or subsequent analysis, it is usually necessary to amplify the quantity of available DNA using the polymerase chain reaction (PCR) and suitable oligonucleotide primers. Mutation analysis of clinical specimens also requires selection of a gene(s) of interest, based on the clinical and iron phenotype of the subject and his/her first-degree family members, and the availability of suitable DNA oligonucleotide probes.

3 Methods of Mutation Analysis

3.1 Allele-Specific Oligonucleotide Hybridization (ASOH)

This is an economical, efficient method for genotyping a large number of subjects or to examine population frequencies of known mutations or polymorphisms. ASOH requires the least amount of specialized equipment (water bath, oven that can maintain 42°C, X-ray film developer). ASOH technique involves amplification of the DNA region containing the reported polymorphism, and spotting the amplified product without purification on a nitrocellulose membrane. After denaturation and neutralization of the amplified DNA on the membrane, the membrane is hybridized with either ^{32}P-labeled wild-type or mutant 18-bp probes spanning the polymorphism. After hybridizing the membrane, the unbound probe is washed to remove the mismatched but not the matched probe. The hybridized probe is then visualized by radioautography or phosphorimaging. An alternative to using ^{32}P-labeled probes is the use of biotin-labeled probes. Basic ASOH has been used to detect mutations of *HFE* [1], *TFR2* [2], and *SLC40A1* [3, 4].

3.2 Fluorescent Techniques

Mutation and SNP analyses can be performed using TaqMan® (ABI, Foster City, CA) methods. These are useful for large-scale population studies that examine gene frequencies and can be used instead of ASOH. TaqMan® technology requires a LightCycler® and specially designed amplification primers and probes. The costs of consumables, reagents, and equipment needed for TaqMan® methods are significantly higher than for ASOH. The TaqMan® method is useful for genes like *HFE* in which mutations such as C282Y occur at high frequency [5].

3.3 Reverse Hybridization Strip-Based Assay

This proprietary technique can detect 14 known *HFE* (V53M, V59M, H63D, H63H, S65C, Q127H, E168Q, E168X, W169X, C282Y, Q283P) and *TFR2* (E60X, M172K, Y250X) mutations (ViennaLab Labordiagnostika GmbH, Austria). A multiplex PCR amplification is performed with biotinylated primers to amplify *HFE* exons 2–4 and *TFR2* exons 2, 4, and 6. The amplified product is then hybridized to the test strip with an array of allele-specific probes, and mutations are detected with a colorimetric enzyme assay [6].

3.4 Restriction Fragment Length Polymorphism (RFLP)

RFLP analysis is suitable for laboratories that do not have ready access to automatic sequencing, and only if analysis of specific mutations is needed, i.e., family members of affected individuals with previously identified common *HFE* mutations or other hemochromatosis-associated alleles, regardless of gene. With this technique, restriction enzymes either digest or do not digest the amplified product containing the mutant allele(s). Amplification of DNA is performed under standard conditions, restriction digestion is performed as recommended by the manufacturers, and separation and staining of the DNA products by size are performed using polyacrylamide/TBE gels with molecular weight markers with a separation range of 75 bp–1 kb. RFLP has been used for the genetic analysis of common *HFE* mutations [7] and to detect previously identified *HJV* mutations [8].

3.5 Direct Sequencing

This method is applicable to all genes of interest. The iron phenotype of the proband and pattern of inheritance in the kinship under study usually permit a prudent selection of genes for direct sequencing. DNA amplifications are performed in a reaction mix containing template DNA, primers, Taq polymerase, PCR buffer, and bovine serum albumin. PCR buffers supplied with various Taq DNA polymerases can also be used. Different buffers and conditions may result in vastly different yields of amplified DNA product. In our experience, the presence of ammonium sulfate and the absence of DMSO are optimal.

Amplification conditions are described in detail elsewhere for each gene [9]. After DNA amplification, DNA products are electrophoresed on a polyacrylamide/TBE gel with molecular weight markers in the range of 75 bp–1 kb to ensure that the DNA products are of the expected size. The remainder of amplified product is purified using QIAquick PCR columns (Qiagen, Inc., Valencia, CA) or a similar cleanup product. Direct sequencing is then performed on an automatic DNA sequencer utilizing the same and/or internal primers. For the sake of brevity, we define only internal primers when needed to obtain complete coverage of the region.

3.6 Denaturing High-Performance Liquid Chromatography (dHPLC)

These methods are ideal for scanning genes for novel mutations and for analyzing many samples at relatively low cost. dHPLC can also be used for genotyping specific mutations or polymorphisms. The major limitation to dHPLC analyses is that few laboratories are equipped with this specialized, expensive equipment. dHPLC identifies only the presence of a heteroduplex that arises from mismatched alleles. Accordingly, dHPLC requires mixing samples with control homozygous wild-type DNA in order to identify homozygous and hemizygous mutations. Once the presence of a heteroduplex is identified, it may be necessary to sequence the amplified DNA to identify the mutation. Amplification of DNA for dHPLC analyses must be performed with a high-fidelity Taq polymerase, and buffers that lack carrier protein (i.e., bovine serum albumin) and organic solvents (i.e., DMSO).

After DNA amplification, samples must be denatured and cooled slowly in order to generate heteroduplex complexes. The dHPLC method described here was established using the Transgenomic WAVE dHPLC system with a DNASep™ C_{18} reverse phase-column [9]. Other dHPLC protocols have been used for large-scale mutation detection in numerous exons of hemochromatosis-associated genes [10].

4 Selection of Genes for Analysis

Clinical features of patients with iron overload and the pattern of inheritance of iron overload phenotypes within kinships under study should be evaluated to determine the most direct and economical means of mutation analysis. Transferrin saturation is usually elevated in patients with *HFE, HJV, TFR2, HAMP*, or "gain-of-function" *SLC40A1* hemochromatosis. Hyperferritinemia without elevated transferrin saturation values is typical of patients with "loss-of-function" *SLC40A1* alleles or mutations in the iron-responsive element of *FTL*. Severe iron overload in children, adolescents, or young adults is typically caused by *HJV, TFR2*, or *HAMP* hemochromatosis, whereas severe iron overload in *HFE* hemochromatosis usually occurs in adults of middle age or older. Anemia is sometimes present in persons with iron overload associated with "loss-of-function" ferroportin hemochromatosis, and in most persons with atransferrinemia, *DMT1* mutations, *GLXR* mutations, X-linked sideroblastic anemia, congenital dyserythropoietic anemias, and pyruvate kinase deficiency. In geographic regions where thalassemia is common, persons with iron overload may co-inherit thalassemia alleles and mutations that directly affect iron absorption. Neurologic abnormalities are typical of persons with iron overload due to aceruloplasminemia or neuroferritinopathy.

HFE, HJV, TFR2, and *HAMP* hemochromatosis are transmitted as autosomal recessive disorders; heterozygotes usually have little or no evidence of iron overload. *HFE* C282Y homozygosity occurs predominantly in Caucasians of European ancestry. Pseudodominant patterns of inheritance sometimes occur in white *HFE* hemochromatosis kinships due to the high prevalence of *HFE* C282Y or H63D in the general background populations, or in *HJV, TFR2*, and *HAMP* hemochromatosis due to consanguinity or founder effects in relatively isolated geographic areas. Dominant patterns of inheritance occur in *SLC40A1* (ferroportin) hemochromatosis, and perturbations in iron and iron protein metabolism caused by deleterious mutations in genes that encode ferritin light chain (*FTL*, hereditary hyperferritinemia-cataract syndrome, neuroferritinopathy) and ferritin heavy chain (*FTH1*, Japanese autosomal dominant iron overload). Patterns of inheritance in families with X-linked sideroblastic anemia and *ALAS2* mutations may be typical of other X-linked disorders or exhibit pseudodominance due to disease expression in females with skewed X-inactivation. In unusual cases, it may be desirable to sequence all iron-related genes for which analyses are feasible, especially if initial analyses reveal that the most likely genes do not have a mutation(s) that would explain the clinical phenotype.

5 Pathogenicity of Mutations

Several criteria should be used to establish the pathogenicity of a previously undescribed mutation as a causative agent of or contributor to chronically increased iron absorption and consequent iron overload. Firstly, the mutation(s) should segregate with iron overload phenotypes in kinships, and the pattern of inheritance of iron phenotypes should be consistent with that previously described for mutations in the corresponding gene(s). Secondly, the mutation should significantly alter a highly conserved amino acid in the encoded protein. Determinations of amino acid conservation can be made by comparing orthologous sequences in man with those readily available in other mammals, lower vertebrates such as *Xenopus* or zebrafish, or with invertebrates such as *Caenorhabditis elegans*.

Thirdly, most highly conserved amino acids lie in intracellular or extracellular domains known to be crucial for normal function of corresponding proteins. In many cases, deleterious mutations encode a protein that has less functional capacity than the wild-type homologue (although "gain-of-function" mutations also occur). Accordingly, point mutations may result in qualitative changes of amino acid charge or sulfhydryl linkages in the encoded protein resulting in conformational changes in the protein structure. Deletions, insertions, or premature stop-codon triplets may cause frameshifts that affect protein stability or cellular localization. Mutations in iron-responsive elements or promoter regions alter expression levels of qualitatively normal protein. Synonymous mutations do not result in qualitative or quantitative changes in protein expression, although some synonymous mutations may be linked to mutations that produce a clinically detectable phenotype.

Fourthly, most deleterious mutations have been detected only in single kinships and are rare in the corresponding general population. Therefore, the allele frequency of newly discovered mutations should be determined in a sample of 50 or more population control subjects and compared to that in persons with iron overload phenotypes unexplained by previously reported mutations. Fifthly, some missense mutations occur as polymorphisms (e.g., *HFE* C282Y in European Caucasians, *SLC40A1* Q248H in Native Africans and African Americans) but have very low penetrance. Therefore, it is necessary to compare iron phenotypes in large cohorts of persons with and without these mutations from appropriate population samples to ascertain their effects on iron phenotypes. Finally, in vitro expression of the mutated gene and its wild-type counterpart permit functional assessments of the encoded mutant protein. Functional studies can be performed in vivo by creating mouse, zebrafish, or other animal models in which the mutation is simulated.

Mutations in some genes that are almost certainly pathogenic have been discovered in screening venues, often in persons whose iron phenotype is normal. Accordingly, it should not be asserted that the mutations are deleterious until they are discovered to segregate with iron overload in families or until they are demonstrated to alter protein function in laboratory expression models. It is widely acknowledged that other genes and mutations that affect iron overload phenotypes await discovery.

6 Inheritance of Mutations in Two or More Iron-Related Genes

This circumstance has been reported most frequently in persons with both a deleterious mutation(s) in a non-*HFE* iron-related gene, and heterozygosity or homozygosity for a *HFE* polymorphism such as C282Y or H63D. Most individuals have been described in the context of case and family reports or small case series. Some persuasive cases have been labeled as "digenic" hemochromatosis involving *HFE* C282Y homozygosity or heterozygosity and a *HAMP* mutation [11]. *ALAS2* P520L appears to enhance iron phenotype in C282Y homozygotes and in patients with other iron overload disorders [12]. In an exceptional man heterozygous for a *SLC40A1* mutation and hemizygous for a *ALAS2* mutation, iron overload due to the respective mutations may have been additive [13]. Nonetheless, analyses of population data or laboratory models that provide rigorous proof that mutations in the two genes account for additive or multiplicative effects on iron absorption in the same individual are usually lacking. Overall, it seems unlikely that heterozygosity for *HFE* C282Y or H63D has sufficient penetrance to induce or alter phenotypes reasonably attributable to mutations in non-*HFE* genes.

7 Modifier Mutations in *HFE* C282Y Homozygotes

HFE C282Y is the most common mutation that has a significant effect on iron absorption and metabolism, yet its penetrance in C282Y homozygotes to cause an iron overload phenotype is relatively low. Putative "modifier" genes have been reported in various case and family studies of C282Y homozygotes, but the strength of the conclusions have necessarily been limited by the small numbers of subjects available for analysis. Other studies have sought to identify mutations in iron-related genes that could explain iron phenotype heterogeneity in adults with C282Y homozygosity in a broader scope: cohorts of C282Y homozygotes diagnosed in medical care or ascertained in screening programs. Few mutations in non-*HFE* genes that represent plausible explanations of phenotype heterogeneity have been demonstrated in the latter studies. The results of analyses of tumor necrosis factor-alpha and mitochondrial DNA alleles as possible "modifiers" of C282Y homozygosity phenotypes are inconsistent. Genome-wide association scans and quantitative trait loci heritability analyses nonetheless provide substantial evidence that genetic regions (other than those generally recognized) have significant influences on iron phenotypes. It is also likely that diverse acquired disorders, dietary factors, and environmental conditions also act as "modifiers" of C282Y homozygosity, although the relationship of most of these to the expression of *HFE* hemochromatosis is poorly understood.

8 Ethical, Legal, and Social Issues

Some clinicians rely on DNA analyses to assess the risk of single-mutation disorders such as familial breast and colon cancer, hemochromatosis, and Huntington disease. In *HFE* hemochromatosis, the capability to prevent disease due to iron overload is great, but the risk that subjects with a "positive" genetic test will develop severe iron overload is relatively low. Many patients and their physicians are concerned about the possibility that employment and insurance discrimination will occur as a consequence of DNA testing. Informal reports of insurance denial and increased premium rates are common among individuals with *HFE* hemochromatosis without end organ damage; further investigation reveals that only some of these incidents are related to hemochromatosis [14]. The overall proportion of hemochromatosis patients with active insurance, their quality of life, and their psychological well-being were similar to those of siblings without hemochromatosis [14].

The most contentious circumstance occurs when genetic testing detects a genotype that is associated with hemochromatosis. Such information is sometimes used by both health and life insurance carriers to exclude individuals from coverage or to increase their insurance premiums based on the theoretical increased risk of medical care needs or disease-related complications. Thus, legislation to protect individuals against "labeling" and genetic discrimination has been advocated [15]. The need for such legislation is predicated on the perceived discrimination associated with early diagnosis. During counseling, adult patients should be informed that discrimination with respect to obtaining health, life, and disability income insurance, and employment is possible [16]. In the USA, some states require written informed consent before any type of genetic testing can be performed. In the USA, the Genetic Information Nondiscrimination Act ("GINA") of 2009 expands protections for Americans from being treated unfairly by insurers or employers due to differences in their DNA.

Identification of a hemochromatosis-associated genotype permits monitoring of iron stores and institution of therapy to reduce body iron before organ dysfunction occurs. Genetic testing in the course of work-up for suspected hemochromatosis can be a useful adjunct to confirm the diagnosis, often abrogating the need for invasive testing such as liver biopsy. Although at least one negative emotional impact was seen in individuals undergoing *HFE* mutation analysis during screening in the HEIRS Study, there was no significant overall physical or mental harm [17, 18].

It is generally recommended that minors not be tested for adult-onset heritable disorders. In *HFE* hemochromatosis, disease manifestations rarely occur before the age of 30 years in subjects identified in medical care or in population screening [19, 20], and the rate of penetrance of severe iron overload is low in adults of middle age. Testing minors for iron-related mutations, particularly those of *HFE*, is not justified unless phenotyping reveals substantive abnormalities that need further understanding or management. If early age-of-onset hemochromatosis were detected in a child or his/her sibling(s), especially that possibly related to *HJV*, *TFR2*, *HAMP*, or *SLC40A1* mutations, testing should be performed and interpreted by qualified persons. In other cases, testing can usually be postponed until the individual is an adult and can make his/her informed decision. In routine care delivery, the concerns of testing of cord blood samples or neonates to detect subjects with at-risk hemochromatosis and iron overload genotypes are similar to those for testing minors.

9 Deleterious Mutations in Iron-Related Genes

This section comprises a compilation of data on pathogenic and some non-pathogenic mutations in genes associated with iron overload disorders. Mutations that cause X-linked sideroblastic anemia are also included.

9.1 HFE Hemochromatosis

The *HFE* gene (OMIM +235200, chromosome 6p21.3) comprises six exons. Human HFE protein predicted from the cDNA sequence is composed of 343 amino acids and has a molecular weight of ~48 kDa; multiple splice variants have been described. HFE is a human leukocyte antigen (HLA)-like protein that associates with β_2-microglobulin, modulates transferrin binding to transferrin receptor, and positively modulates hepatic expression of hepcidin through interaction with transferrin receptor-2. (Table 26.1). *HFE* hemochromatosis is an autosomal recessive disorder with low penetrance. Many non-synonymous mutations of the *HFE* gene have been reported. *HFE* C282Y is the most common known mutation that significantly affects iron metabolism. Two other common *HFE* mutations (H63D, S65C) are sometimes associated with iron overload, usually mild. The *HFE* C282Y and H63D mutations most often occur in trans (different chromosomes), but there are few reports in which they were detected in *cis* (on a single chromosome) [42, 43]. An *Alu*-mediated deletion of *HFE* may be relatively common in Sardinia [40, 41]. Most other deleterious *HFE* mutations are rare, occur only in specific families, and are not detected by routine allele-specific mutation analyses available through most reference laboratories. It is likely that additional pathogenic *HFE* mutations will be found in the future, but they will almost certainly be uncommon.

9.2 Hemojuvelin (HJV) Hemochromatosis

The term "juvenile hemochromatosis" (JH) (OMIM #602390) is used to describe rare forms of hereditary hemochromatosis characterized by severe iron overload, heart failure, and hypogonadotrophic hypogonadism in children, adolescents, or adults less than 30 years of age. JH is associated with an autosomal recessive pattern of inheritance in most kinships. Most persons with JH have two mutations of the hemojuvelin gene (*HJV*) on chromosome 1q (OMIM *608374). Hemojuvelin is homologous to the repulsive guidance molecule (RGM) family of proteins, and is highly expressed in heart, liver, and skeletal muscle. The major hemojuvelin isoform is predicted to encode a 426-amino acid membrane-localized protein characterized by a RGD motif and a von Willebrand type D domain; this glycosylphosphatidylinositol-linked membrane protein (GPI-hemojuvelin) is an essential upstream regulator of hepcidin. Hemojuvelin cleavage is essential for its membrane localization, and the loss of hemojuvelin membrane localization is central to the pathogenesis of JH. *HJV* may regulate hepcidin synthesis through signaling pathways that involve bone morphogenetic proteins and their subsequent effects on receptor SMADs and co-SMAD4 [44]. All *HJV* mutations discovered

Table 26.1 Mutations of the hemochromatosis gene (*HFE*)[a]

Exon	cDNA alteration	Protein alteration	Phenotype[b]	References
2	88C→T	L30L	0	[21]
2	128G→A+187C→G	G43D+H63D	1	[22]
2	138T→G	L46W	1	[23]
2	157G→A	V53M	0	[24]
2	175G→A	V59M	0	[24]
2	187C→G	H63D	1	[25]
2	189T→C	H63H	0	[24]
2	193A→T	S65C	1	[26]
2	196 C→T	R66C	2	[21]
2	211C→T	R74X	2	[27]
2	277G→C	G93R	1	[28]
2	277del	G93fs	2	[29]
2	314T→C	I105T	1	[28]
	IVS2(+4)T→C	–	0	[30]
3	381A→C	Q127H	0	[24]
3	385G→A	D129N	0	[23]
3	414T→G	Y138X	2	[23]
3	471del	A158fs	2	[31]
3	478del	P160fs	2	[32]
3	502G→C	E168Q	1	[6]
3	502G→T	E168X	2	[33]
3	506G→A	W169X	2	[33]
	IVS3(+1)G→T	(Null allele)	2	[34]
	IVS3(+21)T→C	–	0	[21]
4	636G→C	V212V	0	[35]
4	671G→A	R224G	2	[21]
4	689A→T	Y230F	2	[23]
4	696C→T	P232P	0	[21]
4	814G→T	V272L	0	[36]
4	829G→A	E277K	0	[35]
4	845G→A	C282Y	2	[25]
4	845G→C	C282S	2	[37]
4	848A→C	Q283P	2	[38]
4	867C→G	L289L	0	[21]
	IVS4(+37)A→G	–	0	[24]
	IVS4(+109)A→G	–	0	–
	IVS4(+115)T→C	–	0	[24]
5	989G→T	R330M	2	[24]
	IVS5(+1)G→A	–	0	[39]

[a]Deletion of *HFE* (Chr6 g.(26 175 442)_g.(26 208 186)del) in subject of Sardinian ancestry was associated with a phenotype that is similar to that of *HFE* C282Y homozygotes [40, 41]
[b]Phenotype: 0=none known, 1=probably weak effect on iron homeostasis, 2=probably strong effect on iron homeostasis

in patients with iron overload phenotypes and two *HJV* mutations encode ineffective forms of mutant hemojuvelin ("loss-of-function" mutations). Juvenile hemochromatosis associated with mutations in hemojuvelin is inherited in an autosomal recessive manner and is highly penetrant.

The most common pathogenic *HJV* mutation is G320V; this allele accounted for two-thirds of *HJV* mutations in French, Greek, and Italian JH patients and their families, and has been reported in many other populations [8, 45–48]. Many other *HJV* mutations have been detected only in single families (Table 26.2). Many persons with JH phenotypes occur in consanguineous marriages, or

Table 26.2 *HJV* mutations associated with juvenile hemochromatosis phenotypes[a]

Exon	cDNA alteration	Protein alteration	Race/ethnicity, other comments	References
2	18G→C	Q6H[b]		[49]
2	81Gdel	L27fsX51	English/Irish	[50]
3	160A→T	R54X	African American	[51]
3	196G→T	G66X		[52]
3	205insGGA	insG70		[53]
3	220del G	V74fsX113	European	[54]
3	238T→C	C80R	European	[53]
3	253T→C	S85P	European	[54]
3	295G→A	G99R	European	[54]
3	296G→T	G99V	European	[48]
3	302T→C	L101P	European	[53, 54]
3	314C→T	S105L		[55]
3	346C→T	Q116X		[56]
3	356G→T	C119F	European	[57]
3	391–403del	R131fsX245		[54]
3	445del G	D149fsX245		[54]
3	503C→A	A168D		[54]
3	509T→C	F170S		[54]
3	516C→G	D172E		[54]
3	526C→T	R176C	European	[58]
3	573G→T	W191C		[54]
3	588T→G	N196K		[59]
3	615C→G	S205R		[54]
4	665T→A	I222N		[48, 60]
4	700-703AAGdel	K234del	European	[9]
4	745G→C	D249H	Asian	[61]
4	749G→T	G250V		[54]
4	806–807ins A	N269fsX311		[54]
4	842T→C	I281T	European	[48]
4	862C→T	R288W		[54, 62]
4	904G→A	E302K		[55]
4	934C→T	Q312X	Asian	[61]
4	954–955ins G	G319fsX341		[54]
4	959G→T	G320V	European	[48, 54]
4	963C→G	C321W	European	[53]
4	963C→A	C321X[b]	Asian	[49]
4	976C→T	R326X		[48]
4	980–983 delTCTC	S328fsX337	Slovakian	[57]
4	1004G→A	R335Q		[55]
4	1080delC	C361fsX366	European	[48]
4	1114A→G	N372D		[55]
4	1153C→T	R385X	European	[54]

[a]Data adapted in part from Beutler and Beutler 2002 [63] and Wallace and Subramaniam [64]
[b]*HJV* Q6H and C321X were detected on the same chromosome

reside in isolated communities or populations in which the prospect of marriages among distant relatives is relatively great. JH has been described in identical twins [46]. Most JH cases have been described in whites from European populations [23, 45–48], but few patients in different kinships appear to be closely related by geography or ethnicity. *HJV* mutations and JH phenotypes have also been described in families of sub-Saharan African descent [51, 53], in Japanese kinships [61], and in other Asian populations [65].

9.3 Transferrin Receptor-2 (TFR2) Hemochromatosis

TFR2 hemochromatosis (OMIM #604250) is a rare autosomal recessive disorder characterized by elevated serum iron measures, parenchymal iron deposition, and complications of iron overload. In individual cases, the *TFR2* hemochromatosis phenotype may resemble that of *HFE* hemochromatosis or *HJV* hemochromatosis. The TFR2-alpha transcript contains 18 exons, including a cytosolic domain, a transmembrane domain, a protease-associated domain, and a transferrin receptor-like dimerization region. Pathogenic mutations that occur in each of these regions have been described (Table 26.3). The beta transcript lacks exons 1 through 3 and has an additional 142 bases at the

Table 26.3 Pathogenic mutations of the transferrin receptor-2 gene *TFR2*[a,b]

Exon/intron	cDNA alteration	Protein alteration	Race/ethnicity, other comments	References
2	64G→A	V22I	Italian subject with "altered iron status"; may be polymorphism	[21]
2	88-89insC	E60X[c]	Italian, including one with beta-thalassemia trait	[66, 67]
3	313C→T	R105X	North French	[68]
4	515T→A	M172K	Italian	[66, 69]
6	750C→G	Y250X	Several Sicilian, Italian families	[70, 71]
7	(Not reported)	Q317X	Italian	[72]
7	1186C→T	R396X	Scotch-Irish American; in *cis* with G792R	[73]
9	1231–3 del	del411H	Italian	[74]
10	1330G→A	A444T	Italian	[74]
10	1364G→A	R455Q	Asian; Scotch-Irish American; may be polymorphism	[73, 75]
11	1403G→A	R468H	Taiwanese	[76, 86]
11	1469T→G	L490R	Japanese	[77]
14	1665delC	V561X (P555fsX561; S556AfsX6)	Japanese	[77]
16	del1861-1872	delAVAQ594-597[d]	Italian; Japanese	[78, 79]
17	2069A→C	Q690P	Portuguese	[80]
IVS17+5636G→A	IVS17+5636G→A	–	Italian	[74]
18	2374G→A	G792R	Scotch-Irish American, in *cis* with R396X; French, not in *cis* with another mutation	[73, 81]

[a] All mutations were reported to cause or were associated with iron overload phenotypes as homozygosity or compound heterozygosity with other deleterious *TFR2* alleles

[b] Some *TFR2* mutations are unproven to cause iron overload. These include H33N (exon 2; Italian) [74]; A75V (exon 2; Italian) [21]; IVS3+49C→A (Italian; polymorphism) [74]; D189N (exon 4; Native American/white with hemochromatosis and *HAMP* promoter mutation –443C→T) [82]; I238M (exon 5; white, Chinese, Japanese subjects with, without iron overload; polymorphism in Asian population at a frequency of 0.0192; not associated with increased transferrin saturation or ferritin levels in heterozygotes or an I238M homozygote) [2, 23, 77, 83]; F280L (exon 6; Portuguese) [23]; IVS–9T→A (Portuguese) [23]; I449V (exon 10; heterozygosity in white American without iron overload) [84]; R455G (exon 10; heterozygosity in American with *HFE* C282Y homozygosity) [75]; D590D (exon 16; polymorphism in white American population at a frequency of 0.037; not associated with increased transferrin saturation or ferritin levels in heterozygotes); A617A (exon 16; white Americans; polymorphism in Asians (allele frequency 0.33); not associated with increased transferrin saturation or ferritin levels in heterozygotes; in Italians, allele frequencies were 0.11 in controls and 0.14 in hemochromatosis patients) [2, 85]; R678P (exon 17; French) [81]; and M705HfsX87 (exon 18; French) [81]

[c] There are reports of two corresponding mutations: c.ins88C (p.R30PfsX31) [66]; and c.313C→T (p.R105X) [68] The former was subsequently reported by Wallace and Subramaniam as R30fsX60 [64]

[d] Identified by Beutler as A621–Q624 [63], and by Camaschella as 1902–1213del (AVAQ621–624del) [86]

5-prime end of exon 4. Experiments in mice demonstrated that transferrin receptor-2 continues to mediate uptake of transferrin-bound iron by the liver after the classical transferrin receptor is down-regulated by iron overload [87]. Although TFR2 binds to holo-transferrin, it does so at much lower affinity than transferrin receptor-1. HFE binds to TFR2 in a region that does not overlap with the holo-transferrrin binding site. A complex of TFR2 and HFE promotes expression of hepcidin.

In 2000, Camaschella and colleagues described persons with hemochromatosis phenotypes in two unrelated Sicilian families who had mutations in *TFR2* [70]. The typical pattern of genetic transmission is autosomal recessive with moderate or complete penetrance. Many pathogenic mutations have been detected only in single kinships. Some mutations have been detected in consanguineous kinships. Some deleterious mutations, especially *TFR2* Y250X and R455Q, have appeared in individuals or kindreds who were not closely related (Table 26.3), suggesting that these mutations may have arisen more than once or may occur at low frequency in some populations. In one man, *TFR2* R396X and G792R probably occurred on the same haplotype [73].

TFR2 hemochromatosis has been reported in subjects of European and Asian ancestry (Table 26.3). *TFR2* Y250X was not identified in large samples of persons of various race/ethnicity (including African Americans), with or without iron overload and related conditions [2, 88, 89]. *TFR2* AVAQ594-597del was not detected in 100 healthy Italian controls [78]. Other population testing programs have detected few pathologic or other *TFR2* alleles [21, 90, 91]. Sequencing *TFR2* in persons who reported having or were proven to have hemochromatosis or iron overload confirms that pathologic *TFR2* mutations are rare [2, 75, 82]. *TFR2* I238M is a polymorphism detected in an Asian population sample at a frequency of ~0.0192. The prevalence of *TFR2* I238M in Asian subjects with and without iron overload phenotypes is similar, and simple heterozygosity for I238M was not associated with an increase in transferrin saturation or ferritin levels in control subjects [2]. To date, other *TFR2* mutations have not been associated with a hemochromatosis or iron overload phenotype (Table 26.4).

Table 26.4 *TFR2* mutations not proven to cause iron overload

Exon or intervening sequence	Amino acid substitution	Race/ethnicity, other comments	References
2	H33N	Italian; not expected to be pathologic	[74]
2	A75V	Italian	[21]
IVS3+49C→A	–	Italian; polymorphism	[74]
4	D189N	Native American/white reported having hemochromatosis; also had *HAMP* promoter mutation –443C→T	[82]
5	I238Ma	White, Chinese, Japanese subjects with, without iron overload; polymorphism	[2, 23, 77, 83]
6	F280L	Portuguese	[23]
IVS–9T→A	–	Portuguese	[23]
10	I449V	heterozygosity in white American without iron overload	[92]
10	R455G	Heterozygosity in American with *HFE* C282Y homozygosity	[75]
15	V583I	Heterozygosity in white American without iron overload	[84]
16	D590D[b]	White American	[2]

[a] Polymorphism in Asian population at a frequency of 0.0192; not associated with increased transferrin saturation or ferritin levels in heterozygotes or an I238M homozygote [2]

[b] Polymorphism in white American population at a frequency of 0.037; not associated with increased transferrin saturation or ferritin levels in heterozygotes [2]

[c] Polymorphism in Asian population (allele frequency 0.33); not associated with increased transferrin saturation or ferritin levels in heterozygotes [2]. In Italian subjects, allele frequencies were 0.11 in controls and 0.14 in hemochromatosis patients [83]

9.4 Hepcidin (HAMP) Hemochromatosis

Hepcidin, an antimicrobial peptide produced by hepatocytes, is a central negative regulator of iron absorption that is encoded by the *HAMP* gene on chromosome 19q13. The precursor of hepcidin comprises 84 amino acids, from which three active peptides of 25, 22, and 20 amino acids, respectively, are produced by protease cleavage [93, 94]. The 25- and 20-amino acid peptides represent the major forms [93]. Eight highly conserved cysteine residues form four disulfide bonds, the critical basis for a rigid structure of the final peptide [95]. The *HAMP* promoter contains consensus sequences for the transcription factor CCAAT/enhancer binding protein-α (CEBP/α) that confers liver tissue specificity [96]. The *HAMP* promoter also responds to interleukin-6 (IL-6), and has two bone morphogenetic protein-responsive elements (BMP-RE) that bind a receptor SMADs1/5/8 and co-SMAD4 protein complex [9, 97–99]. Hepcidin expression is decreased in *HFE*, *TFR2*, and "gain-of-function" *SLC40A1* hemochromatosis and increased in "loss-of-function" *SLC40A1* hemochromatosis in the absence of *HAMP* mutations [100–105].

HAMP hemochromatosis occurs in at least two defined patterns of inheritance. The first pattern is an autosomal recessive disorder (OMIM #602390) that often resembles *HJV* hemochromatosis. These deleterious *HAMP* mutations are rare and have been reported in consanguineous kinships [65, 106–109] (Table 26.5). *HAMP* –25G→A has been reported in apparently unrelated Portuguese kinships [108, 111]. In a consanguineous Australian kinship, both a father and his daughter were *HAMP* C78T homozygotes, resulting in a pseudodominant pattern of inheritance [107].

The second pattern of inheritance is "digenic" hemochromatosis associated with co-inheritance of a pathogenic *HAMP* mutation and *HFE* C282Y. Such configurations were first reported in *HFE* C282Y homozygotes who were tested for *HAMP* alleles [11]. In a cohort of 392 French *HFE* homozygotes with hemochromatosis phenotypes, Jacolot and colleagues found that five were also heterozygous for a *HAMP* mutation (R59G, G71D, or R56X)[112]. Biasiotto et al. tested 136 C282Y homozygous, 43 heterozygous, 42 C282Y/H63D compound heterozygous, and 62 control Italian subjects for *HAMP* mutations using denaturing high-performance liquid chromatography (dHPLC). Abnormally high indices of iron status were found in a C282Y/H63D heterozygote who also had *HAMP* –72C→T; the iron phenotype of another C282Y/H63D compound heterozygote who also had *HAMP* G71D was normal [21]. In the HEIRS Study, dHPLC analysis of 191 C282Y homozygotes identified in screening was performed; two were heterozygous for *HAMP* mutations. One had the *HAMP* promoter mutation –72C→T and the other had *HAMP* R59G; both study participants had high transferrin saturation and serum ferritin values [110]. In the same study, *HAMP* –153C→T was not detected in any of 191 *HFE* C282Y homozygotes [10]. *HAMP* mutations that would account for iron overload were not detected in a group of white, Asian, and African-American subjects with and without iron overload [116].

HAMP G71D was detected in the general English population at an allele frequency of 0.3% [11]. In the HEIRS Study, the allele frequencies of *HAMP* R59G in white controls and *HAMP* G71D in Hispanic controls were 0.7% and 0.6%, respectively. *HAMP* –153C→T was not detected in 100 French subjects with normal serum iron and hemoglobin measures [98]. In the HEIRS Study, *HAMP* –153C→T occurred in a single Hispanic participant, but was not detected in large cohorts of white, African American, or Asian study participants [110]. Taken together, these observations indicate *HAMP* mutations are uncommon in general populations and account for little of the iron phenotype heterogeneity in persons with or without *HFE* C282Y [10].

9.5 Ferroportin (SLC40A1) Hemochromatosis

Mutations in the *SLC40A1* gene that encodes ferroportin (OMIM *604653) cause an uncommon, heterogeneous group of iron overload disorders characterized by an autosomal dominant pattern of inheritance (OMIM #606069). *SLC40A1* mutations cause two major iron overload phenotype patterns,

Table 26.5 Pathogenic mutations of the hepcidin gene (*HAMP*)

Promoter/exon	cDNA alteration	Protein alteration	Genotypes with high iron phenotypes	Region/Ethnicity	References
–	c.–153C→T[a]	–	Digenic with C282Y	French, US Hispanic	[98, 110]
–	–72C→T	–	Digenic with C282Y[b]	Italian, US whites	[10, 59]
–	–25G→A (+14G→A, 5' UTR)[c]	–	Homozygosity	Portuguese	[108, 111]
1	93delG	G32fs (T31fsX180)[d]	Homozygosity	Italian/Greek	[106]
2	148-IVS2(+1) delATGG[e]	M50fs	Digenic with C282Y	English	[11]
2	126–127delAG	R42Sfs[f]	Homozygosity	Pakistani	[65]
3	166C→T[g]	R56X	Homozygosity; digenic with C282Y	Italian/Greek	[106, 112]
3	175C→G	R59G	Digenic with C282Y	French, US white	[10, 112]
3	208T→C	C70R[h]	Homozygosity; digenic with C282Y	Italian	[109, 113]
3	212G→A	G71D	Digenic with C282Y	English, Italian, US Hispanic	[10, 11, 59]
3	233G→A	C78T[f, h]	Homozygosity	Australian	[107]

[a] In vitro, *HAMP* –153C→T decreased transcriptional activity of the promoter, altered its IL-6 responsiveness, and prevented binding of SMAD1/5/8/4 protein complex to the bone morphogenetic protein-responsive element (BMP-RE) of *HAMP* [98]

[b] Two Italian subjects with this mutation also had beta-thalassemia trait, hepatitis C, and iron overload [114]

[c] This mutation creates a new initiation codon at position +14 of the 5 UTR, which induces a shift of the reading frame and the generation of an abnormal protein. In one patient, this protein was probably unstable or otherwise degraded, as it was not found on bidirectional protein gel electrophoresis [108, 115]. In another patient, there was detectable hepcidin, suggesting that the start of translation was maintained at the original ATG with some normal protein production [111]

[d] This deletion resulted in a frameshift and, if mutated RNA achieved translation, generated an abnormal elongated prohepcidin peptide of 179 amino acids, in contrast to the normal hepcidin propeptide of 84 amino acids [106]

[e] This four-nucleotide ATGG deletion (last codon of exon 2 (M50)) and first base of the splice donor site of intron 2 (IVS+1(-G)) causes a 4-bp frameshift. The mutation was predicted to result in retention of the splice consensus site but alteration of the reading frame, extending it beyond the end of the normal transcript [11]

[f] Homozygosity for *HAMP* R42Sfs or C78T abrogates production of normally functional hepcidin [107]

[g] This mutation affects a propeptide cleavage site

[h] This mutation affects a highly conserved cysteine residues that form disulfide bonds crucial for normal structure and function of mature hepcidin

each depending on the particular mutation and its effect on the function of the transcribed ferroportin protein (Table 26.6). The pattern of inheritance of ferroportin hemochromatosis is due to a dominant negative effect of the mutant ferroportin that prevents the normal function of wild-type (normal) ferroportin and is not due to haploinsufficiency [117]. Most reported ferroportin mutations are restricted to single families, and are relatively uncommon (Table 26.7). Although the geographic extent of the various reported mutations is worldwide, only a few specific mutations have been identified in diverse populations. The most prevalent of these is V162del; this mutation has been reported in kinships from Australia, UK, Italy, Greece, Sri Lanka, and Austria [102, 133–137]. It has been proposed that this mutation has occurred independently, several times, due to slippage mispairing in a repeat sequence [64]. The A77D mutation has been described in iron overload patients from Italy, Australia, and India [121–123]. The common Q248H allele occurs as a polymorphism in persons who reside in diverse areas of sub-Saharan Africa and in African Americans (Table 26.6), but increased risk of iron overload in Q248H heterozygotes, if any, is minimal [3, 4, 147, 149, 150].

Table 26.6 Characteristics of two major hemochromatosis phenotypes due to altered ferroportin protein activity

Characteristic	"Loss of function"	"Gain of function"
Representative mutations	A77D, V162del, G490D	Y64N, C326Y, N144D, N144H
Mechanism of action of abnormal ferroportin	Abnormal ferroportin trafficking	Hepcidin resistance
Location of altered portion of ferroportin[a]	Mostly intracellular	Mostly extracellular
Hepcidin levels	Elevated	Normal but disproportionately low for degree of iron loading
Iron absorption	Secondarily increased	Increased due resistance of ferroportin to hepcidin binding
Transferrin saturation	Normal or mildly subnormal	Elevated
Serum ferritin level	Normal to very elevated	Elevated
Iron-limited erythropoiesis	In some cases	No
Predominant sites of iron retention or deposition	Macrophages	Hepatocytes, other parenchymal cells

[a]The mutation *SLC40A1* A77D affects a transmembrane portion of the ferroportin molecule, and is associated with a "mixed" phenotype. Other *SLC40A1* mutations reported to be associated with "mixed" or both iron phenotypes ("gain of function" and "loss of function") include R88T, N144H, N174I, R178G, N185D, R489S, G490S, and G490D

9.6 Hereditary Hyperferritinemia-Cataract Syndrome (HHCS) due to IRE Mutations of Ferritin Light Chain Gene (FTL)

HHCS is an autosomal dominant disorder characterized by increased serum L-ferritin levels and bilateral cataracts, in the absence of iron overload (OMIM #600886). Binding of iron-responsive proteins (IRPs) to iron-responsive elements (IREs) normally represses translation of their corresponding *cis* genes. Heterogeneous mutations in the IRE of L-ferritin reduce the binding affinity to IRPs and thereby diminish the negative control of L-ferritin synthesis. This leads to the constitutive up-regulation of ferritin L-chain synthesis characteristic of HHCS [151].

More than 35 *FTL* mutations have been identified in HHCS kinships (Table 26.8). Most persons reported to have HHCS have western European ancestry. Most mutations are restricted to single kindreds and are not present in members of the general population, although some mutations have been detected in multiple geographic areas or in persons of diverse race/ethnicity (Table 26.8). There are no reports of HHCS or *FTL* mutation analysis in most other race/ethnicity groups, and thus it cannot be assumed that HHCS is a disorder that occurs predominantly in European whites. Most reported *FTL* mutations associated with HHCS are single nucleotide substitutions. Point mutations or deletions in the CAGUGU RNA sequence of the apical loop greatly decrease binding of the mutant IRE with IRPs. The deletion del22-27 is predicted to introduce a novel loop in the upper stem of the IRE structure very close to the lateral bulge that would markedly reduce binding to IRPs [158]. Clusters of mutations affect nucleotides 22, 32–33, and 36–42 [156].

The estimated prevalence of HHCS in southeast Australia is approximately 1/200,000 [161]. This estimate is probably conservative, because serum ferritin is not routinely measured by ophthalmologists investigating cataracts (including congenital cataracts) [161]. Some *FTL* IRE mutations result in mild hyperferritinemia and clinically insignificant cataract [186]. HHCS was not detected in 135 Swiss persons whose cataracts required excision and lens implants on or before age 51 years [187]. Three of 52 DNA samples from French patients referred for molecular diagnosis of HHCS revealed ferroportin mutations [132]. The results of three studies of highly selected subjects also suggest that L-ferritin IRE mutations typical of HHCS are collectively rare [155, 188]. Testing "at-risk" subjects is probably much more productive than general population screening.

Table 26.7 Geographic distribution and race/ethnicity of persons with ferroportin gene (*SLC40A1*) mutations[a]

Promoter/exon	cDNA alteration	Protein alteration	Location or race/ethnicity	References
	−59–45del	–	French	[58]
	−188A→G	–	Japanese	[118]
3	190T→C	Y64N	Japanese	[119]
3	214G→T	V72F	Italian	[120]
3	230C→A	A77D	Italian; Indian; Australia	[121–123]
3	238G→A	G80S	Italian	[124, 125]
3	239G→T	G80V	Italian	[126]
3	262A→G	R88G	French	[58]
3	263G→C	R88T	Spanish	[127]
5	430A→C	N144H	Dutch	[128]
5	430A→G	N144D	Australian	[129]
5	431A→C	N144T	Solomon Islander	[130]
5	"758A→T"	I152F	Italian	[131]
5	"744A→G"	D157G	French	[132]
5	469G→A	D157N	Italian	[120]
5	484–486delGTT	V162del	Australia, UK, Italy, Greece, Sri Lanka, Austria	[102, 133–137]
6	521A→T	N174I	Italian	[124, 125]
6	532C→A	R178G	Greek	[138]
6	539T→C	I180T	Spanish	[127]
6	"846A→T"	D181V	Italian	[126]
6	546G→T	Q182H	French	[132]
6	533G→A	R178Q	French	[58]
6	553A→G	N185D	Scandinavian	[139]
6	698T→C	L233P	Italian	[131]
7	"1104G→A"	G267D	Chinese	[126]
7	809A→T	D270V	Black South African	[140]
7	968G→T	G323V	French	[132]
7	977G→C	C326S	USA	[141]
7	977G→A	C326Y	Thailand	[65, 142]
7	1014T→G	S338R	New Zealand	[64]
7	1402G→A	G468S[b]	Scottish-Irish (USA)[a]	[143]
8	1466G→A	R489K	English	[144]
8	1467A→C	R489S	Japanese	[119]
8	1468G→A	G490S[c]	French	
8	1469G→A	G490D[c]	Caucasian-Asian	[145]
8	1502A→G	Y501C	Italian	[146]

[a] *SLC40A1* Q248H (c.744G→T) occurs as a polymorphism in Native Africans and in African Americans; persons with this allele may have slightly higher serum ferritin levels than those without Q248H [3, 4, 147]. *SLC40A1* G339D (c.1016G→A), L384M (c.1148T→A), and L384B (c.1149T→G) are also common in African Americans, but have no defined association with abnormal iron measures [4]. *SLC40A1* L384M (c.1149T→A) and L384V (c.1149T→G) were detected in Italian blood donors at frequencies of 10% and 5%, respectively [148]. Pathogenicities of *SLC40A1* F405S (c.1214T→C) (ENSEMBL database), M432V (c.1294A→G), P443L (c.1328C→T), and R561G (c.1681A→G)(NCBI SNP database) are unreported

[b] This allele, a splice site mutation, caused premature truncation of ferroportin transcription at amino acid 330 and, thus, is the functional equivalent of G330X [143]

[c] Identical cDNA alterations were reported for these different protein alterations

Table 26.8 *FTL* IRE mutations associated with hereditary hyperferritinemia-cataract syndrome[a]

Mutation	Race/ethnicity[b]	References
c.-220_-196del25[c]	Australian	[152]
10C→G	Italian	[153]
10_38del29	Italian	[154]
14G→C	Italian	[155]
16C→U	Italian	[153]
18C→T	Italian	[156]
[18C→T]+[22T→G]	Italian	[157]
22T→G	Italian	[157]
22_27del6	Italian	[158]
29C→G	Italian	[159]
32G→A	Italian, French, Indian	[132, 157, 160]
32G→C	French, Australian	[132, 161–163]
32G→T	French, Canadian, Italian	[132, 164, 165]
32G→U	Australian	[161]
33C→A	French	[132]
33C→T	American, French, Spanish	[132, 166–168]
33C→U	Spanish	[169]
34T→C	French	[132]
36C→A	English, French	[132, 170]
36C→G	Italian	[153]
37A→C	Italian	[156]
37A→G	Italian	[153]
37A→T	Spanish	[168]
38_39delAC	French	[132]
39C→A	Australian	[161]
39C→G	French, Greek	[171, 172]
39C→T	Italian, French	[132, 173]
39C→U	English, Italian	[170, 174]
40A→G	French, Basque, American, Australian, Spanish	[132, 161, 175–179]
[40A→C]+[41G→C]	Italian	[155]
41G→C	Italian	[180]
42_57del16	French	[132, 181]
43G→A	American	[182]
47G→A	French	[132]
51G→C	American, Italian	[183, 184]
56A→T	French	[156]
56del1	Italian	[153]
90C→U	Italian	[153]

[a] Names of mutations are those previously reported in the literature. Numbering is from the first transcripted nucleotide

[b] Mutations are informally denoted by names of cities in which they were first identified and characterized include 10_38del29, Verona-2; [18C→T]+[22T→G], Pavia-2; 32G→A, Pavia-1; 32G→U, Paris-2; 36C→A, London-2; 37A→T, Zaragoza; 39C→U, London-1; 40A→G, Paris-1; and 41G→C, Verona-1

[c] This mutation consists of a 25-bp deletion encompassing the transcription start site designated c.-220_-196del25, where nucleotide +1 is the A of the ATG translation initiation start site (Genbank accession NM_000146.3) [152]. An Italian subject with a mutation in the ATG start codon of L-ferritin had no hematological or neurological symptoms [185]

Table 26.9 Pathogenic *FTL* mutations in neuroferritinopathy

cDNA alteration[a]	Race/ethnicity	References
458dupA	French	[198]
460insA	English/Cumbrian, French	[189, 190, 199]
469_484dup16nt	Japanese	[196]
474G→A	Portuguese/Gypsy	[194]
498insTC	French	[200]
641_642dup4nt	Japanese	[201]
646insC	French-Canadian/Dutch	[195]

[a]Each mutation occurs in exon 4 of *FTL*

9.7 Neuroferritinopathies

Neuroferritinopathy (OMIM #606159), also known as adult-onset basal ganglia disease, is an adult-onset, progressive movement disorder caused by mutations in the coding region of the ferritin light chain gene (*FTL*, chromosome 19q13.3–q13.4). Persons with neuroferritinopathy have abnormal ferritin light chain polypeptide, decreased serum ferritin concentrations, and accumulation of iron in the basal ganglia. Curtis and colleagues first described this syndrome in an English kinship in 2001. They also coined the commonly used term "neuroferritinopathy" [189]. Subsequent identification and study of other subjects have revealed further data on the genotypes, phenotypes, and epidemiology associated with neuroferritinopathy.

All reported pathogenic *FTL* mutations associated with neuroferritinopathy are rare [189–197] (Table 26.9). *FTL* 460InsA was the first mutation reported and has been described in the greatest number of cases. Most of these cases occurred in a geographic cluster in Cumbria that was traced to a common ancestor [189–191]. *FTL* 460InsA has also been identified in other English [200] and French [190] patients. All reported pathogenic *FTL* mutations associated with neuroferritinopathy involve exon 4. Most mutations are insertions in exon 4 that result in frameshifts. These mutations alter the reading frame, lengthen the C-terminus of ferritin light chain polypeptide, and disrupt protein folding and stability. As a consequence, ferritin dodecahedron structure is altered, causing accumulation of ferritin and iron [200], primarily in central neurons. L-ferritin probably has no effect on systemic iron metabolism and neuroferritinopathy is probably not a consequence of haploinsufficiency of L-ferritin, but likely results from gain-of-function mutations in the *FTL* gene [185, 200].

9.8 Another FTL Coding Region Mutation Syndrome

Persons heterozygous for the coding region mutation *FTL* T30II have elevated serum levels of glycosylated ferritin, report no specific symptoms, and lack iron overload, ocular cataracts, and neurologic abnormality [202]. It has been postulated that *FTL* T30II increases the efficacy of L-ferritin secretion by increasing the hydrophobicity of the N-terminal "A" alpha helix [202].

9.9 Iron Overload due to IRE Mutations of Ferritin Heavy Chain Gene (FTH1)

Ferritin H- and L-chains form a shell of 24 subunits that stores iron. Each type of chain has a distinct role in iron storage [203]. The H-chain is encoded by the *FTH1* gene (chromosome 11q12-q13) and the L-chain by the *FTL* gene (19q13.13-13.4) [204, 205]. Ferritin H-subunits generate ferroxidase activity essential for incorporation of iron into the protein shell, whereas L-subunits facilitate iron core formation [203]. A common cytosolic protein, iron regulatory protein (IRP), binds to the iron-responsive element (IRE) of the 5' untranslated regions (UTRs) of the H- and L-subunit RNAs, and thus controls the synthesis of both proteins [206–210].

In 2001, Kato and colleagues described a unique Japanese family in which a mutation in the H-ferritin IRE caused hyperferritinemia and autosomal dominant iron overload (OMIM + 134770) [211]. The mutation was a single A→U conversion at position 49 (A49U) in the second residue of the five-base IRE loop sequence (CAGUG) of the H-ferritin subunit. This mutation was not detected in the genomic DNA of 42 unrelated control subjects [211]. In vitro studies revealed that the mutated IRE had a higher binding affinity to IRP than did the wild-type probe [212]. The novel A49U mutation accounts for hereditary iron overload, presumably related to impairment of the ferroxidase activity generated by the H-ferritin subunit. It is probable that other families will eventually be identified who have autosomal dominant iron overload caused by the same or other IRE mutations of H-ferritin.

9.10 Hereditary Aceruloplasminemia

Hereditary aceruloplasminemia (OMIM #604290) is a rare autosomal recessive disorder due to mutations of *Cp*, the gene that encodes the copper-binding protein ceruloplasmin (Cp). The *Cp* gene is located on the long arm of chromosome 3 (3q23–q24) and comprises 20 exons. Cp is a plasma metalloprotein, an alpha-2 glycoprotein polypeptide of 1,046 amino acids. A member of the multicopper oxidase enzyme family, Cp, the principal copper transport protein in plasma, is synthesized in hepatocytes and functions as a ferroxidase. In Cp deficiency, ferrous iron is not oxidized, so iron is not transported from storage cells into plasma. This causes iron accumulation within storage cells. Aceruloplasminemia is associated with the accumulation of excessive storage iron in most tissues, including the occurrence of heavy iron deposits in the retina, liver, pancreas, and basal ganglia. The first report of hereditary aceruloplasminemia was published in 1987 in Japan [213].

The frequency of homozygosity for deleterious *Cp* mutations in non-consanguineous marriages in Japan was estimated to be one per 2,000,000 population [214]. Aceruloplasminemia has been reported in several countries including Japan, China, Ireland, Belgium, France, Italy, and the USA [215]. More Japanese patients have been reported than any other nationality. Altogether, about 60 patients with hereditary aceruloplasminemia have been described [215].

About 40 *Cp* mutations have been reported in 60 patients in 46 families with aceruloplasminemia worldwide [215, 216]. Many of the reported *Cp* mutations occur in single kinships [214]. In Japan, 4,990 healthy adults were screened using serum Cp measurements. Subsequent *Cp* sequencing in subjects with subnormal serum Cp detected three mutations (5-bp insertion in exon 7, one heterozygote; one-bp deletion in exon 14, two heterozygotes; nonsense mutation in exon 15, one homozygote and two heterozygotes). The estimated frequency of these mutations was 70 per 100,000 [217]. The mutations in aceruloplasminemia kindreds include nonsense, missense, base-pair insertions, base-pair deletions, and splice site, frameshift, and truncation stop-codon mutations involving different *Cp* exons and introns [215]. In a tabulation of 21 *Cp* mutations, abnormal variants were detected in eleven exons and one intron [215].

Cp mutations in patients with aceruloplasminemia are diverse. Consequently, the only feasible way to substantiate a genetic diagnosis in newly diagnosed individuals is to sequence the *Cp* gene. This is neither commercially available nor practical for routine patient care. In contrast, most persons with *HFE* hemochromatosis with iron overload in many countries have the C282Y missense mutation, and thus a single, inexpensive mutation analysis will identify a high proportion of patients. Many different *Cp* mutations cause a similar neurologic phenotype, and siblings with the same genotype may have a different neurologic phenotype [215].

9.11 ALAS2 Sideroblastic Anemia

X-linked sideroblastic anemias (XLSA) are characterized by impaired mitochondrial iron metabolism, "ringed" sideroblasts and increased erythropoiesis. In some cases, these disorders cause parenchymal iron overload similar to that of hemochromatosis [218]. Mutations in the *ALAS2* gene that encodes erythroid-specific 5-aminolevulinate synthase (ALA synthase) account for the most common group of these disorders (OMIM #300751). *ALAS2* missense mutations result in single amino acid changes in ALA synthase, the first enzyme of the heme biosynthesis pathway that catalyzes the pyridoxal 5'-phosphate-dependent condensation of glycine and succinyl-CoA to yield 5-aminolevulinic acid (Table 26.10). The same *ALAS2* promoter region mutation was detected in two unrelated kinships, and premature stop-codon and *de novo* frameshift mutations, respectively, were identified in two other families (Table 26.10). Approximately two-thirds of probands are hemizygous men [227]. In apparently rare cases, hemizygous males do not have a XLSA phenotype [249]. The remaining third of patients comprise heterozygous women who have variable degrees of unbalanced inactivation of chromosome X [227, 240]. In some kinships, men and women are affected, and pedigree analysis may suggest autosomal dominant transmission [227]. In other kinships, only heterozygous women are affected, hinting that the mutation is fatal *in utero* or in early life to male hemizygotes [250–253]. In kindreds with X-linked anemia without identifiable *ALAS2* mutations, another chromosome X locus is implicated [254, 255].

ALAS2 mutations are uncommon, and most XLSA kinships are not consanguineous. Most mutations occur in single kinships. A possible exception is *ALAS2* P520L, an allele detected in several iron overload kinships, some with anemia and others without [12]. P520L alone has no anemia- or iron-associated phenotype, but it acts by an unknown mechanism to modify the severity of other heritable iron overload disorders [12]. In one family, *ALAS2* P520L occurred on the same haplotype as *ALAS2* R560H [12]. Mutations in the triplet codon for the arginine^{452} residue of ALA synthase and a promoter mutation appear to have arisen independently in unrelated kindreds (Table 26.10). Many reported kinships have been Caucasian, although this disorder has also been described in Japanese [232, 236, 241], Chinese [247], and African Americans [219, 256, 257]. *ALAS2* mutation analysis or gene sequencing is not available commercially, although some research laboratories will perform this testing. Routine clinical laboratory methods and pedigree analysis are sufficient for diagnosis and management in most kinships.

9.12 ABCB7 Sideroblastic Anemia

Hereditary sideroblastic anemia with ataxia (XLSA/A) is characterized by hypochromic, microcytic anemia; non-progressive cerebellar ataxia manifest in infancy or early childhood; and lack of systemic iron overload. This rare disorder is due to mutations in the gene *ABCB7* on chromosome X that encodes ATP-binding cassette, subfamily B, member 7. The family of ABC transporters consists of a large group of adenosine triphosphate-dependent transmembrane proteins that specifically transport a wide variety of substrates across cell and organelle membranes [258–260]. *ABCB7* is an ortholog of the yeast *ATM1* gene, the product of which localizes to the mitochondrial inner membrane and is involved in iron homeostasis. ABCB7 functions as a mitochondrial iron–sulfur (Fe/S) cluster transporter. *ABCB7* positively regulates the expression of extramitochondrial thioredoxin and the intramitochondrial iron–sulfur-containing protein, ferrochelatase, in erythroid precursors, and thus influences normal heme synthesis [261, 262]. The precise mechanism by which *ABCB7* mutations impair neurologic development or lead to neurologic injury is unknown.

There are three Caucasian families with documented pathogenic *ABCB7* mutations; there was no consanguinity in these kindreds [255, 263, 264]. The kinships show typical disease manifestations

Table 26.10 *ALAS2* mutations associated with X-linked sideroblastic anemia[a]

Exon	cDNA alteration	Protein alteration	Anemia	Pyridoxine responsiveness	References
(promoter)	–206C→G[b]		Mild	None/Partial	[219, 220]
5	CD506–507(–C)[c]	del169Cfs	Severe	None	[221]
5	514G→A	M154I	?	?	[222]
5	527G→T	D159Y	Severe	Partial	[223]
5	527G→A	D159N	?	Partial?	[224]
5	533A→G	T161A	?	?	[225]
5	547C→A	F165L	Severe	Partial	[226]
5	560C→A	R170S	Severe	Partial	[227]
5	560C→T	R170C	?	Partial	[228]
5	561G→A	R170H	Mild	None	[229]
5	561G→T	R170L	Severe	Partial	[230]
5	566G→A	A172T	Severe	Complete	[231]
5	621A→T	D190V	Moderate	None	[232]
5	647T→C	Y199H	Moderate	Partial	[233]
5	662C→T	R204term	Severe	None	[234, 235]
5	663G→A	R204Q	Severe	Partial	[236]
6	731C→T	R227C	Moderate	None	[234]
6	802T→C	S251P	Severe	?	[237]
6	839G→A	D263N	Severe	Probable	[227]
7	880C→G	C276W	Severe	None	[234]
7	918T→C	I289T	Severe	Responsive	[238]
7	923G→A	G291S	Severe	Complete	[239]
7	947A→C	K299Q	Severe	Complete	[231]
8	1103G→A	G351R	Moderate	Complete	[227]
8	1215C→G	T388S	Severe	Complete	[239]
9	1236G→A	C395Y	Severe	Complete	[240]
9	1245G→A	G398D	Severe	None	[234]
9	1283C→T	R411C	Severe	Partial	[233, 241, 242]
9	1284G→A	R411H	Moderate	Partial	[234]
9	1299G→A	G416D	Moderate	Partial	[243]
9	1331A→G	M426V	Severe	Complete	[232]
9	1358C→T	R436W	Severe	None	[234, 244]
9	1395G→A	R448Q	Mild-moderate	None/Partial	[228, 233, 243]
9	1406C→A	R452S	Moderate	Partial	[243]
9	1407C→T	R452C	Mild	Partial	[228, 233, 243]
9	1407C→A	R452H	Mild-severe	None/Partial	[227, 228, 245, 246]
9	1479T→A	I476N	Severe	Complete	[247]
10	1574A→T	T508S	Moderate	?	[227]
10	1601C→T	R517C	Severe	None	[234]
10		P520L[d]	Anemia absent	Anemia absent	[12]
10	1622C→G	H524D	Severe	Partial	[248]
11	1731G→A	R560H	Severe	Partial	[12]
11	1754A→G	S568G	Moderate to severe	Partial	[236]

[a] Adapted in part from Bottomley [227]

[b] This promoter mutation was associated with sideroblastic anemia and iron overload in Welsh and African American kinships. In the former, ALAS2 mRNA levels in the proband's erythroid precursors were reduced 87%. The mutation occurred in or near three different putative transcription factor binding sites of unknown importance; the region affected by the mutation may be a receptor for an erythroid regulatory element

[c] Predicted to cause premature truncation 60 amino acids distal

[d] P520L alone has no phenotype but modifies the severity of other heritable iron overload disorders. In one family, P520L occurred on the same haplotype as *ALAS2* R560H [12]

in males hemizygous for *ABCB7* mutations, no abnormalities in their siblings without *ABCB7* mutations, and mild erythrocyte abnormalities in their heterozygous mothers. No heterozygous women with neurologic manifestations due to skewed X-inactivation have been reported, but differences in lyonization could account for anemia phenotype disparities in hemizygous women in two kinships [220, 265]. Each novel *ABCB7* missense mutation occurred in exon 10 and each changed a highly conserved amino acid. The resulting protein alterations are I400M [255], V411L [263], and E433K [264]. Each mutation affected a relatively short span of 34 consecutive amino acids in a region of the protein involved in binding and transport of substrate. These respective *ABCB7* mutations were not detected in population control subjects [255, 263, 264].

9.13 GLRX Sideroblastic Anemia

Normal erythropoiesis depends on iron-reactive protein (IRP) function and production of iron–sulfur (Fe/S) clusters. Located on chromosome 5q14 [266], *GLRX5* encodes glutaredoxin, a glutathione (GSH)-dependent hydrogen donor for ribonucleotide reductase that also catalyzes glutathione-disulfide oxidoreduction reactions in the presence of NADPH and glutathione reductase [267]. In 2007, Camaschella and colleagues described a man in his 60s who had sideroblastic anemia, severe iron overload, cirrhosis, diabetes mellitus, and hyperpigmentation. He had an explanatory, pathogenic mutation in the *GLRX5* gene. This patient's kinship was consanguineous. This suggested that he had an autosomal recessive disorder. Sequencing of his *GLRX5* gene using genomic DNA revealed that he was homozygous for an A→G transition at position 294 in the third nucleotide of the last codon of *GLRX5* exon 1. The CAA→CAG substitution does not change the encoded glutamine at position 98. The change affects the penultimate nucleotide of exon 1, and therefore, it was predicted that the mutation would interfere with correct RNA splicing [268]. Amplification products of *GLRX5* cDNA from the patient's blood mononuclear cells were much lower than in controls. Analysis of *GLRX* expression by quantitative RT-PCR showed significantly decreased levels in the proband than in healthy subjects. Compatible with a splicing defect, unspliced fragments encompassing the exon–intron junctions were amplified from the patient's cDNA [268]. Based on the biochemical and clinical phenotype, it was hypothesized that IRP2, less degraded by low levels of heme, contributed to the repression of erythroblast ferritin and ALA synthase and thereby increased mitochondrial iron deposition. It was also hypothesized that iron chelation could redistribute iron to erythroblast cytosol, decrease IRP2 excess, and improve heme synthesis and anemia [268].

9.14 Thiamine-Responsive Megaloblastic Anemia Syndrome (TRMA)

This disorder, also known as Rogers syndrome [269], is an early-onset, autosomal recessive disorder defined by megaloblastic anemia, diabetes mellitus, and sensorineural deafness. Examination of the bone marrow reveals megaloblastic anemia with erythroblasts, many of which contain iron-filled mitochondria (ringed sideroblasts). TRMA is due to mutations in the gene *SLC19A2* (chromosome 1q23.3) that encodes thiamine transporter protein 1. Diverse *SLC19A2* mutations have been identified in patients with TRMA [270, 271]. Clinical phenotypes are also heterogeneous. Patients represent diverse race/ethnicity groups.

Table 26.11 Transferrin (*TF*) genotypes in hereditary atransferrinemia[a]

Genotype	Clinical presentation	Country	References
Compound heterozygosity for A477P (exon 12; c.1429G→C) and 188fsX215 (exon 5; c.562_571del 572_580dup)[b,c]	20-year-old woman with anemia, heavy menstrual bleeding	USA	[283]
Compound heterozygosity for E394K (exon 9; c.1180G→A) and inferred maternal null allele[d]	7-year-old boy with pallor	Japan	[284–286]
Homozygosity for D77N (exon 3; c.229G→A)[c]	2-month-old girl with severe anemia	Slovakia	[287–289]
Homozygosity for C137Y (exon 4; c.410A→G)[c]	4-month-old girl with severe anemia	Turkey	[290]

[a] Mutations are indicated as cDNA nucleotide substitutions (or other alterations). We used the recommended nomenclature [291, 292] in which the A of the upstream ATG is counted as nucleotide number 1 and the initiator methionine is amino acid number 1 [289], as suggested by Beutler and colleagues [283, 289]

[b] *TF* A477P involves a highly conserved site. *TF* 188fsX215 resulted in a stop codon 27 amino acids downstream [283]

[c] Reported or previously unreported non-deleterious *TF* polymorphisms, especially single nucleotide polymorphisms, were also discovered in these patients [283, 290]

[d] No mutation was found in either the coding region or the exon–intron boundaries, suggesting an abnormality in the transcription or stability of mRNA of maternal allele origin

9.15 Erythropoietic Protoporphyria

Mild hypochromic, microcytic anemia is common in persons with erythropoietic protoporphyria, a heterogeneous disorder due to mutations in the *FECH* gene (chromosome 18q21.3) that encodes ferrochelatase. Bone marrow examination in a few patients revealed ringed sideroblasts [272, 273].

9.16 Mitochondrial Myopathy and Sideroblastic Anemia (MLASA)

This is a rare autosomal recessive oxidative phosphorylation disorder specific to skeletal muscle and bone marrow that is due to mutations in the gene *PSU1* (chromosome 12q24.33) that encodes pseudouridine synthase-1 [274–281]. Mitochondrial DNA is normal [279]. Several MLASA kinships have been consanguineous; the disorder has been reported in several race/ethnicity groups.

9.17 Hereditary Atransferrinemia

Hereditary atransferrinemia (OMIM #209300) is a rare disorder characterized by severe quantitative or functional deficiency of transferrin. As a consequence, there is reduced delivery of iron to erythroid cells in the marrow, reduced hemoglobin synthesis, increased iron absorption, and severe iron overload of parenchymal organs. In 1961, Heilmeyer and colleagues described atransferrinemia in a girl who had severe hypochromic anemia at age 3 months and severe, progressive generalized iron overload [282]. Other patients with similar abnormalities have been reported subsequently, and explanatory mutations in the gene that encodes transferrin (*TF;* chromosome 3q21) have been demonstrated in four cases (Table 26.11). Phenotypic heterogeneity in patients with hereditary atransferrinemia is due in part to *TF* genotype (Table 26.11). Cases of acquired or secondary atransferrinemia or hypotransferrinemia have also been described in patients with diverse underlying conditions.

Patients diagnosed on phenotypic grounds have been described from Germany [282], Slovakia [287–289], Japan [284–286], Mexico [293, 294], France [295], Samoa [296], Italy [297], USA [283], and Turkey [290]. Two siblings have been described in each of the kinships from Japan and Mexico. In all kinships, it is assumed that atransferrinemia was transmitted as an autosomal recessive disorder. This assumption has been substantiated in four kinships in which deleterious *TF* mutations have been demonstrated. Consanguinity has been reported or inferred in some kinships [282, 289, 290]. This is consistent with demonstration of homozygosity for a deleterious *TF* allele in two respective probands [289, 290]. There is no known relationship between the various kinships in which hereditary atransferrinemia has been reported, and this agrees with the different deleterious *TF* mutations detected across the kinships (Table 26.11).

Deleterious *TF* alleles are typically not detected in population samples [283, 289, 290]. In a Portuguese kinship, however, a transferrin null allele was discovered in a case of disputed paternity [298]. The mother and putative father were heterozygous for transferrin null alleles, and their transferrin levels were 40–41% of normal [298]. Null transferrin alleles have also been described in German and Finnish kinships [299–301].Polymorphisms of *TF* are common [302], and some patients with hereditary atransferrinemia have had known or previously unreported *TF* polymorphisms, in addition to deleterious *TF* alleles [283, 289]. Five *TF* polymorphisms were not associated with any significant changes in iron metabolism, nor did they appear to influence the expression of hemochromatosis [302].

9.18 Divalent Metal Transporter-1 (DMT1) Iron Overload

DMT1 is a member of the "natural-resistance-associated macrophage protein" (*Nramp*) family. DMT1 is upregulated by dietary iron deficiency, is expressed strongly on the microvillus membranes of duodenal enterocytes at the villus tips, and is a key mediator of iron absorption [303, 304]. DMT1 also mediates iron transfer from endosomes into the cytosol of developing erythroid cells. The *SLC11A2* gene that encodes DMT1 is located on chromosome 12q13 (OMIM *604653) [305]. In 2004 and 2005, Priwitzerova and colleagues described a Czech female in a consanguineous kinship who had severe hypochromic, microcytic anemia; erythroid hyperplasia; abnormal erythroid maturation; elevated serum iron concentration; normal to slightly increased serum ferritin level; and markedly increased serum transferrin receptor levels at age 3 months [306, 307]. In 2005, Mims and colleagues reported that this woman was homozygous for a mutation in *SLC11A2* [308]. Similar phenotypes in two siblings were reported by Shahidi and colleagues in 1964 [309].

The anemia–iron overload syndrome associated with inheritance of two abnormal *SLC11A2* alleles is transmitted as an autosomal recessive trait. Consanguinity was reported in one of the three families and was associated with homozygosity for a missense mutation of *SLC11A2* [306]. Each of the three kinships had European ancestry (Czech, Italian, and French, respectively), although this may reflect an increased awareness of hemochromatosis and other iron overload disorders due to the predominance of *HFE* mutations in European peoples. Five pathogenic mutations have been described in three probands with the clinical syndrome. The Czech patient was homozygous for *SLC11A2* E399D. The ultimate nucleotide of exon 12 of *SLC11A2* encodes a highly conserved glutamic acid residue that was changed to an aspartic acid residue due to the E399D missense mutation. The predominant effect of this mutation was preferential skipping of exon 12 during processing of pre-messenger RNA (mRNA) [307]. The E399D substitution has no effect on protein expression and function in vitro [307], and was stable and had normal targeting and trafficking to the membrane [310]. This suggests that the mutated protein has a modest amount of activity in vivo [310].

In the Italian patient, a 3-bp deletion in *SLC11A2* intron 4 (c.310-3_5del CTT) resulted in a splicing abnormality. The second abnormal allele in this patient was the missense mutation R416C [311]. In vitro studies indicate that R416C is a "loss of function" mutation [312]. The French proband was a compound heterozygote, a GTG deletion in exon 5 leading to the V114 in-frame deletion in transmembrane domain 2, and the missense mutation G212V in exon 8 [313]. Variability of function of mutant DMT1 proteins largely accounts for the phenotypic heterogeneity that has been observed among the few reported patients with DMT1 anemia–iron overload syndrome.

SLC11A2 mutations have been investigated as possible "modifiers" of iron overload phenotypes in persons with hemochromatosis associated with *HFE* C282Y homozygosity. In one study, *SLC11A2* mutations were sought using sequencing in C282Y homozygotes with clinical disease, in C282Y homozygotes with normal or low serum ferritin levels and no iron overload disease, in persons without common *HFE* mutations who had high ferritin and transferrin saturation levels, and in normal control subjects without common *HFE* mutations [314]. No *SLC11A2* mutations were found that explained differences in iron phenotypes in these subjects [314]. In another study, the presence of four specific mutations/polymorphisms within the *SLC11A2* gene (1245T/C, 1303C/A, IVS4+44C/A, IVS15Ex16-16C/G) was evaluated in C282Y homozygotes and in control subjects without common *HFE* mutations using standard PCR techniques [315]. There were no significant differences in the allele frequencies of the IVS4+44C/A, 1303C/A, 1254T/C, and IVS15Ex16-16C/G polymorphisms in the patient cohort and in the control cohort. The commonest haplotypes identified were CCTC: IVS4C+44C, 1303C, 1254T, IVS15ex16-16C; ACCC: IVS4C+44A, 1303C, 1254C, IVS15ex16-16C; and ACTG: IVS4C+44A, 1303C, 1254T, IVS15ex16-16G. Similarly, there were no significant differences in the frequencies of these three haplotypes in the patient cohorts (regardless of the degree of hepatic iron deposition) and in the control cohort. Accordingly, it appears that common *SLC11A2* polymorphisms do not influence hemochromatosis phenotypes in persons with *HFE* C282Y homozygosity. In French-Canadian subjects with restless leg syndrome (RLS), a disorder characterized by abnormal brain iron metabolism, sequencing of *SLC11A2* from selected patients did not detect pathogenic mutation(s) [316]. Further studies did not find any association between ten single nucleotide polymorphisms (SNPs), spanning the entire *SLC11A2* gene region, and the presence or absence of RLS. Two *SLC11A2* intronic SNPs were positively associated with RLS in patients with a history of anemia [316].

9.19 Iron-Refractory Iron-Deficiency Anemia (IRIDA)

The term IRIDA (OMIM #206200) is used to describe rare heritable forms of iron deficiency characterized by hypochromic, microcytic anemia; reticulocytopenia; iron-deficient erythropoiesis; low serum iron and transferrin saturation levels despite demonstrable marrow, spleen, or hepatic iron stores; partial block of intestinal absorption of inorganic iron; subnormal responses to intravenously administered iron; and inappropriately normal or elevated serum hepcidin levels (urine and serum protein; liver mRNA) [317]. IRIDA is associated with an autosomal recessive pattern of inheritance in most kinships. Most persons with IRIDA have two mutations of the *TMPRSS6* gene (OMIM *609682; transmembrane protein, serine 6) on chromosome 22q12-q13 that encodes matripase-2 [318]. Northern blot analysis of multiple human tissues revealed expression of a 3.5-kb *TMPRSS6* transcript exclusively in fetal and adult liver. Immunofluorescence and Western blot analysis of COS-7 cells transfected with *TMPRSS6* showed that matripase-2 localizes to the cell membrane. Matriptase-2 possesses all the typical motifs of the family of transmembrane serine proteases, including a transmembrane domain, a LDL receptor class A (LDLRA) domain, a scavenger receptor cysteine-rich (SRCR) domain, and a serine protease domain [318]. Normal matriptase-2 represses hepcidin by cleaving hemojuvelin, a regulator of hepcidin, on plasma membrane. Mutational inactivation of matriptase-2 causes iron-deficiency anemia in mice and humans [319]. Deleterious mutations of

Table 26.12 Pathogenic mutations of the *TMPRSS6* gene[a,b,c]

Exon/intron	cDNA alteration	Protein alteration	Affected domain	Region/ethnicity	References
3	467C→A+468C→T	A118D		Spanish	[321]
	497delT	Frameshift (L166X+36) and premature termination		Dutch	[322]
IVS6+1G→C		S288fs	CUB1	Sardinia	[323]
8	911→T	S304L	CUB1	Swiss	[324]
9	1065→A	Y355X	CUB2	African American	[325]
10	1179→G	Y393X	CUB2	English	[326]
11	1324→A	G442R	CUB2	Northern European	[325]
12	1383delA	E461fs	LDLRA-1	African American	[325]
12	1336→T	R446W	LDLRA-1		[322]
12-13	1435–1524del (deletion of 1054 nucleotides including intron 12)	D478–K508 del	LDLRA-1/-2	Swiss	[324]
13	1561G→A	D521N	LDLRA-2	French; Northern European	[317, 320]
13	1564G→A	E522K	LDLRA-3	French	[320]
IVS13+1G→A		E527fs	Protease	Northern European	[322, 325]
15	1795C→T	R599X	Protease	English	[326]
15	1813delG	A605fs	Protease	Northern European	[325]
15	1868G→C	S623T	Protease (mutation in last nucleotide of exon 15 (Aggt→ACgt) causes a splicing defect)	Italian	[324]
IVS15-1C→G		D622fs	Protease		[325]
16	1906_1907insGC	K636fs	Protease	Turkish	[325]
16		L674F	Protease		[322]
16	2172_2173insCCCC	P686fs	Protease	Spanish	[321]
IVS16+1G→C		G713fs	Protease	Nigerian	[325]
IVS17-1G→C	2278-2402del	760Gfs Splice site mutation	Protease	Indian	[327]
18	2320C→T	R774C	Protease	African American	[325]

[a]CUB=C1r/C1s, urchin embryonic growth factor, and bone morphogenetic protein 1; LDLRA=low-density lipoprotein receptor class A

[b]Beutler et al. detected the uncommon non-synonymous polymorphisms G228D, R446W, and V795I (allele frequencies 0.0074, 0.023, and 0.0074, respectively), of which R446W appeared to be overrepresented in persons with anemia [322]

[c]*TMPRSS6* V736A (2207T→C) is associated with lower serum iron levels, lower hemoglobin levels, smaller erythrocytes, and more variability in erythrocyte size than *TMPRSS6* V736 [328, 329].

TMPRSS6 result in abnormal matripase-2 that typically interacts with hemojuvelin but has reduced or absent protease activity. Thus, hemojuvelin cleavage and export are diminished [320].

All *TMPRSS6* mutations discovered in patients with IRIDA phenotypes and two *TMPRSS6* mutations encode ineffective forms of mutant matripase-2 ("loss-of-function" mutations) and thus cause dysregulation of hepcidin (Table 26.12). Some reported patients with IRIDA phenotypes are compound heterozygotes for novel *TMPRSS6* mutations; heterozygosity for a single deleterious *TMPRSS6* mutation was detected in two IRIDA probands [325]. Homozygosity for a *TMPRSS6* mutation has been detected in four kinships; some were consanguineous [323, 325, 326].

Genome-wide association studies in Europeans and Indian Asians demonstrate that common *TMPRSS6* variants influence serum iron levels, hemoglobin levels, and erythrocyte size [328–331]. The SNP most strongly associated with lower serum iron concentration is rs4820268 (*TMPRSS6* exon 13) [328, 329]; rs4820268 results in a nonsynonymous (V736A) change in the serine protease domain of *TMPRSS6* and a blood hemoglobin concentration 0.13 g/dL (95% CI 0.09–0.17 g/dL) lower per copy of mutant allele than in persons without this allele. This allele was also associated with lower hemoglobin levels, smaller erythrocytes, and more variability in erythrocyte (higher red blood cell distribution width) [329].

References

1. Beutler E, Gelbart T. Large-scale screening for *HFE* mutations: methodology and cost. Genet Test. 2000;4:131–42.
2. Lee PL, Halloran C, West C, Beutler E. Mutation analysis of the transferrin receptor-2 gene in patients with iron overload. Blood Cells Mol Dis. 2001;27:285–9.
3. Barton JC, Acton RT, Rivers CA, et al. Genotypic and phenotypic heterogeneity of African Americans with primary iron overload. Blood Cells Mol Dis. 2003;31:310–9.
4. Beutler E, Barton JC, Felitti VJ, et al. Ferroportin 1 (*SCL40A1*) variant associated with iron overload in African-Americans. Blood Cells Mol Dis. 2003;31:305–9.
5. Bernard PS, Ajioka RS, Kushner JP, Wittwer CT. Homogeneous multiplex genotyping of hemochromatosis mutations with fluorescent hybridization probes. Am J Pathol. 1998;153:1055–61.
6. Oberkanins C, Moritz A, de Villiers JN, Kotze MJ, Kury F. A reverse-hybridization assay for the rapid and simultaneous detection of nine *HFE* gene mutations. Genet Test. 2000;4:121–4.
7. Aslam S, Standen GR. Rapid diagnosis of asymptomatic hereditary haemochromatosis by detection of the Cys282Tyr mutation in the *HLA-H* gene. Postgrad Med J. 1997;73:573–4.
8. Barton JC, Rivers CA, Niyongere S, Bohannon SB, Acton RT. Allele frequencies of hemojuvelin gene (*HJV*) I222N and G320V missense mutations in white and African American subjects from the general Alabama population. BMC Med Genet. 2004;5:29.
9. Lee PL, Beutler E. Regulation of hepcidin and iron-overload disease. Annu Rev Pathol. 2009;4:489–515.
10. Barton JC, LaFreniere S, Leiendecker-Foster C, et al. *HFE*, *SLC40A1*, *HAMP*, *HJV*, *TFR2*, and *FTL* mutations detected by denaturing high-performance liquid chromatography after iron phenotyping and *HFE* C282Y and H63D genotyping in 785 HEIRS study participants. Am J Hematol. 2009;84:710–4.
11. Merryweather-Clarke AT, Cadet E, Bomford A, et al. Digenic inheritance of mutations in *HAMP* and *HFE* results in different types of haemochromatosis. Hum Mol Genet. 2003;12:2241–7.
12. Lee PL, Barton JC, Rao SV, Acton RT, Adler BK, Beutler E. Three kinships with *ALAS2* P520L (c. 1559C→T) mutation, two in association with severe iron overload, and one with sideroblastic anemia and severe iron overload. Blood Cells Mol Dis. 2006;36:292–7.
13. Sussman NL, Lee PL, Dries AM, Schwartz MR, Barton JC. Multi-organ iron overload in an African-American man with *ALAS2* R452S and *SLC40A1* R561G. Acta Haematol. 2008;120:168–73.
14. Shaheen NJ, Lawrence LB, Bacon BR, et al. Insurance, employment, and psychosocial consequences of a diagnosis of hereditary hemochromatosis in subjects without end organ damage. Am J Gastroenterol. 2003;98:1175–80.
15. Hudson KL. Prohibiting genetic discrimination. N Engl J Med. 2007;356:2021–3.
16. Acton RT, Harman L. Genetic counseling for hemochromatosis. In: Barton JC, Edwards CQ, editors. Hemochromatosis: genetics, pathophysiology, diagnosis and treatment. Cambridge University Press, Cambridge. 2000;574–582.
17. Hall MA, Barton JC, Adams PC, et al. Genetic screening for iron overload: no evidence of discrimination at 1 year. J Fam Pract. 2007;56:829–34.
18. Power TE, Adams PC, Barton JC, et al. Psychosocial impact of genetic testing for hemochromatosis in the HEIRS Study: a comparison of participants recruited in Canada and in the United States. Genet Test. 2007;11:55–64.
19. Barton JC, Felitti VJ, Lee P, Beutler E. Characteristics of *HFE* C282Y homozygotes younger than age 30 years. Acta Haematol. 2004;112:219–21.
20. Barton JC, Acton RT, Leiendecker-Foster C, et al. *HFE* C282Y homozygotes aged 25–29 years at HEIRS Study initial screening. Genet Test. 2007;11:269–75.
21. Biasiotto G, Belloli S, Ruggeri G, et al. Identification of new mutations of the *HFE*, hepcidin, and transferrin receptor 2 genes by denaturing HPLC analysis of individuals with biochemical indications of iron overload. Clin Chem. 2003;49:1981–8.
22. Dupradeau FY, Pissard S, Coulhon MP, et al. An unusual case of hemochromatosis due to a new compound heterozygosity in *HFE* (p.[Gly43Asp;His63Asp] + [Cys282Tyr]): structural implications with respect to binding with transferrin receptor 1. Hum Mutat. 2008;29:206.

23. Mendes AI, Ferro A, Martins R, et al. Non-classical hereditary hemochromatosis in Portugal: novel mutations identified in iron metabolism-related genes. Ann Hematol. 2009;88:229–34.
24. de Villiers JN, Hillermann R, Loubser L, Kotze MJ. Spectrum of mutations in the *HFE* gene implicated in haemochromatosis and porphyria. Hum Mol Genet. 1999;8:1517–22.
25. Feder JN, Gnirke A, Thomas W, et al. A novel MHC class I-like gene is mutated in patients with hereditary haemochromatosis. Nat Genet. 1996;13:399–408.
26. Henz S, Reichen J, Liechti-Gallati S. *HLA-H* gene mutations and haemochromatosis: the likely association of H63D with mild phenotype and the detection of S65C, a novel variant in exon 2. J Hepatol. 1997;26:57A.
27. Beutler E, Griffin MJ, Gelbart T, West C. A previously undescribed nonsense mutation of the *HFE* gene. Clin Genet. 2002;61:40–2.
28. Barton JC, Sawada-Hirai R, Rothenberg BE, Acton RT. Two novel missense mutations of the *HFE* gene (I105T and G93R) and identification of the S65C mutation in Alabama hemochromatosis probands. Blood Cells Mol Dis. 1999;25:147–55.
29. Barton JC, West C, Lee PL, Beutler E. A previously undescribed frameshift deletion mutation of *HFE* (c.del277; G93fs) associated with hemochromatosis and iron overload in a C282Y heterozygote. Clin Genet. 2004;66:214–6.
30. Beutler E, West C. New diallelic markers in the HLA region of chromosome 6. Blood Cells Mol Dis. 1997;23:219–29.
31. Cukjati M, Koren S, Curin SV, Vidan-Jeras B, Rupreht R. A novel homozygous frameshift deletion c.471del of *HFE* associated with hemochromatosis. Clin Genet. 2007;71:350–3.
32. Pointon JJ, Lok CY, Shearman JD, et al. A novel *HFE* mutation (c.del478) results in nonsense-mediated decay of the mutant transcript in a hemochromatosis patient. Blood Cells Mol Dis. 2009;43:194–8.
33. Piperno A, Arosio C, Fossati L, et al. Two novel nonsense mutations of *HFE* gene in five unrelated italian patients with hemochromatosis. Gastroenterology. 2000;119:441–5.
34. Wallace DF, Dooley JS, Walker AP. A novel mutation of *HFE* explains the classical phenotype of genetic hemochromatosis in a C282Y heterozygote. Gastroenterology. 1999;116:1409–12.
35. Bradbury R, Fagan E, Payne SJ. Two novel polymorphisms (E277K and V212V) in the haemochromatosis gene *HFE*. Hum Mutat. 2000;15:120.
36. The UK Haemochromatosis Consortium. A simple genetic test identifies 90% of UK patients with haemochromatosis. Gut. 1997;41:841–4.
37. Rosmorduc O, Poupon R, Nion I, et al. Differential *HFE* allele expression in hemochromatosis heterozygotes. Gastroenterology. 2000;119:1075–86.
38. Le Gac G, Dupradeau FY, Mura C, et al. Phenotypic expression of the C282Y/Q283P compound heterozygosity in *HFE* and molecular modeling of the Q283P mutation effect. Blood Cells Mol Dis. 2003;30:231–7.
39. Steiner M, Ocran K, Genschel J, et al. A homozygous *HFE* gene splice site mutation (IVS5+1G/A) in a hereditary hemochromatosis patient of Vietnamese origin. Gastroenterology. 2002;122:789–95.
40. Le Gac G, Gourlaouen I, Ronsin C, et al. Homozygous deletion of *HFE* produces a phenotype similar to the *HFE* p.C282Y/p.C282Y genotype. Blood. 2008;112:5238–40.
41. Pelucchi S, Mariani R, Bertola F, Arosio C, Piperno A. Homozygous deletion of *HFE*: the Sardinian hemochromatosis? Blood. 2009;113:3886.
42. Best LG, Harris PE, Spriggs EL. Hemochromatosis mutations C282Y and H63D in 'cis' phase. Clin Genet. 2001;60:68–72.
43. Lucotte G, Champenois T, Semonin O. A rare case of a patient heterozygous for the hemochromatosis mutation C282Y and homozygous for H63D. Blood Cells Mol Dis. 2001;27:892–3.
44. Truksa J, Peng H, Lee P, Beutler E. Bone morphogenetic proteins 2, 4, and 9 stimulate murine hepcidin 1 expression independently of Hfe, transferrin receptor 2 (Tfr2), and IL-6. Proc Natl Acad Sci USA. 2006;103:10289–93.
45. Roetto A, Totaro A, Cazzola M, et al. Juvenile hemochromatosis locus maps to chromosome 1q. Am J Hum Genet. 1999;64:1388–93.
46. Kaltwasser JP. Juvenile hemochromatosis. In: Barton JC, Edwards CQ, editors. Hemochromatosis: genetics, pathophysiology, diagnosis and treatment. Cambridge: Cambridge University Press; 2000. p. 318–25.
47. Barton JC, Rao SV, Pereira NM, et al. Juvenile hemochromatosis in the southeastern United States: a report of seven cases in two kinships. Blood Cells Mol Dis. 2002;29:104–15.
48. Papanikolaou G, Samuels ME, Ludwig EH, et al. Mutations in *HFE2* cause iron overload in chromosome 1q-linked juvenile hemochromatosis. Nat Genet. 2004;36:77–82.
49. Huang FW, Rubio-Aliaga I, Kushner JP, Andrews NC, Fleming MD. Identification of a novel mutation (C321X) in *HJV*. Blood. 2004;104:2176–7.
50. Lee P, Promrat K, Mallette C, Flynn M, Beutler E. A juvenile hemochromatosis patient homozygous for a novel deletion of cDNA nucleotide 81 of hemojuvelin. Acta Haematol. 2006;115:123–7.
51. Murugan RC, Lee PL, Kalavar MR, Barton JC. Early age-of-onset iron overload and homozygosity for the novel hemojuvelin mutation *HJV* R54X (exon 3; c.160→T) in an African American male of West Indies descent. Clin Genet. 2008;74:88–92.

52. Janosi A, Andrikovics H, Vas K, et al. Homozygosity for a novel nonsense mutation (G66X) of the *HJV* gene causes severe juvenile hemochromatosis with fatal cardiomyopathy. Blood. 2005;105:432.
53. Lee PL, Barton JC, Brandhagen D, Beutler E. Hemojuvelin (*HJV*) mutations in persons of European, African-American and Asian ancestry with adult onset haemochromatosis. Br J Haematol. 2004;127:224–9.
54. Lanzara C, Roetto A, Daraio F, et al. Spectrum of hemojuvelin gene mutations in 1q-linked juvenile hemochromatosis. Blood. 2004;103:4317–21.
55. Le Gac G, Scotet V, Ka C, et al. The recently identified type 2A juvenile haemochromatosis gene (*HJV*), a second candidate modifier of the C282Y homozygous phenotype. Hum Mol Genet. 2004;13:1913–8.
56. Daraio F, Ryan E, Gleeson F, Roetto A, Crowe J, Camaschella C. Juvenile hemochromatosis due to G320V/Q116X compound heterozygosity of hemojuvelin in an Irish patient. Blood Cells Mol Dis. 2005;35:174–6.
57. Gehrke SG, Pietrangelo A, Kascak M, et al. *HJV* gene mutations in European patients with juvenile hemochromatosis. Clin Genet. 2005;67:425–8.
58. Aguilar-Martinez P, Lok CY, Cunat S, Cadet E, Robson K, Rochette J. Juvenile hemochromatosis caused by a novel combination of hemojuvelin G320V/R176C mutations in a 5-year old girl. Haematologica. 2007;92:421–2.
59. Biasiotto G, Roetto A, Daraio F, et al. Identification of new mutations of hepcidin and hemojuvelin in patients with *HFE* C282Y allele. Blood Cells Mol Dis. 2004;33:338–43.
60. Lee PL, Beutler E, Rao SV, Barton JC. Genetic abnormalities and juvenile hemochromatosis: mutations of the *HJV* gene encoding hemojuvelin. Blood. 2004;103:4669–71.
61. Koyama C, Hayashi H, Wakusawa S, et al. Three patients with middle-age-onset hemochromatosis caused by novel mutations in the hemojuvelin gene. J Hepatol. 2005;43:740–2.
62. Filali M, Le Jeunne C, Durand E, et al. Juvenile hemochromatosis *HJV*-related revealed by cardiogenic shock. Blood Cells Mol Dis. 2004;33:120–4.
63. Beutler L, Beutler E. Hematologically important mutations: iron storage diseases. Blood Cells Mol Dis. 2004;33:40–4.
64. Wallace DF, Subramaniam VN. Non-*HFE* haemochromatosis. World J Gastroenterol. 2007;13:4690–8.
65. Lok CY, Merryweather-Clarke AT, Viprakasit V, et al. Iron overload in the Asian community. Blood. 2009;114:20–5.
66. Roetto A, Totaro A, Piperno A, et al. New mutations inactivating transferrin receptor 2 in hemochromatosis type 3. Blood. 2001;97:2555–60.
67. Riva A, Mariani R, Bovo G, et al. Type 3 hemochromatosis and beta-thalassemia trait. Eur J Haematol. 2004;72:370–4.
68. Le Gac G, Mons F, Jacolot S, Scotet V, Ferec C, Frebourg T. Early onset hereditary hemochromatosis resulting from a novel *TFR2* gene nonsense mutation (R105X) in two siblings of north French descent. Br J Haematol. 2004;125:674–8.
69. Majore S, Milano F, Binni F, et al. Homozygous p.M172K mutation of the *TFR2* gene in an Italian family with type 3 hereditary hemochromatosis and early onset iron overload. Haematologica. 2006;91:ECR33.
70. Camaschella C, Roetto A, Cali A, et al. The gene *TFR2* is mutated in a new type of haemochromatosis mapping to 7q22. Nat Genet. 2000;25:14–5.
71. Piperno A, Roetto A, Mariani R, et al. Homozygosity for transferrin receptor-2 Y250X mutation induces early iron overload. Haematologica. 2004;89:359–60.
72. Pietrangelo A, Caleffi A, Henrion J, et al. Juvenile hemochromatosis associated with pathogenic mutations of adult hemochromatosis genes. Gastroenterology. 2005;128:470–9.
73. Lee PL, Barton JC. Hemochromatosis and severe iron overload associated with compound heterozygosity for *TFR2* R455Q and two novel mutations *TFR2* R396X and G792R. Acta Haematol. 2006;115:102–5.
74. Biasiotto G, Camaschella C, Forni GL, Polotti A, Zecchina G, Arosio P. New *TFR2* mutations in young Italian patients with hemochromatosis. Haematologica. 2008;93:309–10.
75. Hofmann WK, Tong XJ, Ajioka RS, Kushner JP, Koeffler HP. Mutation analysis of transferrin-receptor 2 in patients with atypical hemochromatosis. Blood. 2002;100:1099–100.
76. Hsiao PJ, Tsai KB, Shin SJ, et al. A novel mutation of transferrin receptor 2 in a Taiwanese woman with type 3 hemochromatosis. J Hepatol. 2007;47:303–6.
77. Koyama C, Wakusawa S, Hayashi H, et al. Two novel mutations, L490R and V561X, of the transferrin receptor 2 gene in Japanese patients with hemochromatosis. Haematologica. 2005;90:302–7.
78. Girelli D, Bozzini C, Roetto A, et al. Clinical and pathologic findings in hemochromatosis type 3 due to a novel mutation in transferrin receptor 2 gene. Gastroenterology. 2002;122:1295–302.
79. Hattori A, Wakusawa S, Hayashi H, et al. AVAQ 594–597 deletion of the *TfR2* gene in a Japanese family with hemochromatosis. Hepatol Res. 2003;26:154–6.
80. Mattman A, Huntsman D, Lockitch G, et al. Transferrin receptor 2 (*TfR2*) and *HFE* mutational analysis in non-C282Y iron overload: identification of a novel *TfR2* mutation. Blood. 2002;100:1075–7.
81. Jouanolle AM, Mosser A, David V, et al. Early onset iron overload in two patients presenting with new mutations in *TFR2*. The Second Congress of the International BioIron Society 2007;72.

82. Barton JC, Acton RT, Leiendecker-Foster C, et al. Characteristics of participants with self-reported hemochromatosis or iron overload at HEIRS study initial screening. Am J Hematol. 2008;83:126–32.
83. Chan V, Wong MS, Ooi C, et al. Can defects in transferrin receptor 2 and hereditary hemochromatosis genes account for iron overload in HbH disease? Blood Cells Mol Dis. 2003;30:107–11.
84. Barton JC, Lee PL, West C, Bottomley SS. Iron overload and prolonged ingestion of iron supplements: clinical features and mutation analysis of hemochromatosis-associated genes in four cases. Am J Hematol. 2006;81:760–7.
85. Meregalli M, Pellagatti A, Bissolotti E, Fracanzani AL, Fargion S, Sampietro M. Molecular analysis of the *TFR2* gene: report of a novel polymorphism (1878C→T). Hum Mutat. 2000;16:532.
86. Camaschella C, Roetto A. *TFR2*-Related hereditary hemochromatosis [Type 3 hereditary hemochromatosis]. In: Pagon RA, Bird TO, Dolan CR, et al., editors. Gene reviews. Seattle: University of Washington; 2006.
87. Fleming RE, Migas MC, Holden CC, et al. Transferrin receptor 2: continued expression in mouse liver in the face of iron overload and in hereditary hemochromatosis. Proc Natl Acad Sci USA. 2000;97:2214–9.
88. Barton EH, West PA, Rivers CA, Barton JC, Acton RT. Transferrin receptor-2 (*TFR2*) mutation Y250X in Alabama Caucasian and African American subjects with and without primary iron overload. Blood Cells Mol Dis. 2001;27:279–84.
89. Dereure O, Esculier C, Aguilar-Martinez P, Dessis D, Guillot B, Guilhou JJ. No evidence of Y250X transferrin receptor type 2 mutation in patients with porphyria cutanea tarda. A study of 38 cases. Dermatology. 2002; 204:158–9.
90. De Gobbi M, Daraio F, Oberkanins C, et al. Analysis of *HFE* and *TFR2* mutations in selected blood donors with biochemical parameters of iron overload. Haematologica. 2003;88:396–401.
91. Mariani R, Salvioni A, Corengia C, et al. Prevalence of HFE mutations in upper Northern Italy: study of 1132 unrelated blood donors. Dig Liver Dis. 2003;35:479–81.
92. Barton JC, Lee PL. Disparate phenotypic expression of *ALAS2* R452H (nt 1407G→A) in two brothers, one with severe sideroblastic anemia and iron overload, hepatic cirrhosis, and hepatocellular carcinoma. Blood Cells Mol Dis. 2006;36:342–6.
93. Park CH, Valore EV, Waring AJ, Ganz T. Hepcidin, a urinary antimicrobial peptide synthesized in the liver. J Biol Chem. 2001;276:7806–10.
94. Krause A, Neitz S, Magert HJ, et al. LEAP-1, a novel highly disulfide-bonded human peptide, exhibits antimicrobial activity. FEBS Lett. 2000;480:147–50.
95. Hunter HN, Fulton DB, Ganz T, Vogel HJ. The solution structure of human hepcidin, a peptide hormone with antimicrobial activity that is involved in iron uptake and hereditary hemochromatosis. J Biol Chem. 2002;277:37597–603.
96. Courselaud B, Pigeon C, Inoue Y, et al. C/EBPalpha regulates hepatic transcription of hepcidin, an antimicrobial peptide and regulator of iron metabolism. Cross-talk between C/EBP pathway and iron metabolism. J Biol Chem. 2002;277:41163–70.
97. Truksa J, Peng H, Lee P, Beutler E. Different regulatory elements are required for response of hepcidin to interleukin-6 and bone morphogenetic proteins 4 and 9. Br J Haematol. 2007;139:138–47.
98. Island ML, Jouanolle AM, Mosser A, et al. A new mutation in the hepcidin promoter impairs its BMP response and contributes to a severe phenotype in *HFE* related hemochromatosis. Haematologica. 2009;94:720–4.
99. Truksa J, Lee P, Beutler E. Two BMP responsive elements, STAT, and bZIP/HNF4/COUP motifs of the hepcidin promoter are critical for BMP, SMAD1, and HJV responsiveness. Blood. 2009;113:688–95.
100. Gehrke SG, Kulaksiz H, Herrmann T, et al. Expression of hepcidin in hereditary hemochromatosis: evidence for a regulation in response to the serum transferrin saturation and to non-transferrin-bound iron. Blood. 2003;102:371–6.
101. Nemeth E, Roetto A, Garozzo G, Ganz T, Camaschella C. Hepcidin is decreased in *TFR2* hemochromatosis. Blood. 2005;105:1803–6.
102. Zoller H, McFarlane I, Theurl I, et al. Primary iron overload with inappropriate hepcidin expression in V162del ferroportin disease. Hepatology. 2005;42:466–72.
103. Ganz T, Nemeth E. Regulation of iron acquisition and iron distribution in mammals. Biochim Biophys Acta. 2006;1763:690–9.
104. Origa R, Galanello R, Ganz T, et al. Liver iron concentrations and urinary hepcidin in beta-thalassemia. Haematologica. 2007;92:583–8.
105. Piperno A, Girelli D, Nemeth E, et al. Blunted hepcidin response to oral iron challenge in *HFE*-related hemochromatosis. Blood. 2007;110:4096–100.
106. Roetto A, Papanikolaou G, Politou M, et al. Mutant antimicrobial peptide hepcidin is associated with severe juvenile hemochromatosis. Nat Genet. 2003;33:21–2.
107. Delatycki MB, Allen KJ, Gow P, et al. A homozygous *HAMP* mutation in a multiply consanguineous family with pseudo-dominant juvenile hemochromatosis. Clin Genet. 2004;65:378–83.
108. Matthes T, Aguilar-Martinez P, Pizzi-Bosman L, et al. Severe hemochromatosis in a Portuguese family associated with a new mutation in the 5′-UTR of the *HAMP* gene. Blood. 2004;104:2181–3.

109. Roetto A, Daraio F, Porporato P, et al. Screening hepcidin for mutations in juvenile hemochromatosis: identification of a new mutation (C70R). Blood. 2004;103:2407–9.
110. Barton JC, Leiendecker-Foster C, Li H, et al. *HAMP* promoter mutation nc.-153C→T in 785 HEIRS Study participants. Haematologica. 2009;94:1465.
111. Porto G, Roetto A, Daraio F, et al. A Portuguese patient homozygous for the −25G→A mutation of the *HAMP* promoter shows evidence of steady-state transcription but fails to up-regulate hepcidin levels by iron. Blood. 2005;106:2922–3.
112. Jacolot S, Le Gac G, Scotet V, Quere I, Mura C, Ferec C. *HAMP* as a modifier gene that increases the phenotypic expression of the *HFE* pC282Y homozygous genotype. Blood. 2004;103:2835–40.
113. Majore S, Binni F, Pennese A, De Santis A, Crisi A, Grammatico P. *HAMP* gene mutation c.208T→C (p.C70R) identified in an Italian patient with severe hereditary hemochromatosis. Hum Mutat. 2004;23:400.
114. Valenti L, Pulixi EA, Arosio P, et al. Relative contribution of iron genes, dysmetabolism and hepatitis C virus (HCV) in the pathogenesis of altered iron regulation in HCV chronic hepatitis. Haematologica. 2007;92:1037–42.
115. Rideau A, Mangeat B, Matthes T, Trono D, Beris P. Molecular mechanism of hepcidin deficiency in a patient with juvenile hemochromatosis. Haematologica. 2007;92:127–8.
116. Lee PL, Gelbart T, West C, Halloran C, Felitti V, Beutler E. A study of genes that may modulate the expression of hereditary hemochromatosis: transferrin receptor-1, ferroportin, ceruloplasmin, ferritin light and heavy chains, iron regulatory proteins (IRP)-1 and −2, and hepcidin. Blood Cells Mol Dis. 2001;27:783–802.
117. De Domenico I, Ward DM, Musci G, Kaplan J. Iron overload due to mutations in ferroportin. Haematologica. 2006;91:92–5.
118. Liu W, Shimomura S, Imanishi H, et al. Hemochromatosis with mutation of the ferroportin 1 (*IREG1*) gene. Intern Med. 2005;44:285–9.
119. Koyama C, Wakusawa S, Hayashi H, et al. A Japanese family with ferroportin disease caused by a novel mutation of *SLC40A1* gene: hyperferritinemia associated with a relatively low transferrin saturation of iron. Intern Med. 2005;44:990–3.
120. Pelucchi S, Mariani R, Salvioni A, et al. Novel mutations of the ferroportin gene (*SLC40A1*): analysis of 56 consecutive patients with unexplained iron overload. Clin Genet. 2008;73:171–8.
121. Montosi G, Donovan A, Totaro A, et al. Autosomal-dominant hemochromatosis is associated with a mutation in the ferroportin (*SLC11A3*) gene. J Clin Invest. 2001;108:619–23.
122. Subramaniam VN, Wallace DF, Dixon JL, Fletcher LM, Crawford DH. Ferroportin disease due to the A77D mutation in Australia. Gut. 2005;54:1048–9.
123. Agarwal S, Sankar VH, Tewari D, Pradhan M. Ferroportin (*SLC40A1*) gene in thalassemic patients of Indian descent. Clin Genet. 2006;70:86–7.
124. Corradini E, Montosi G, Ferrara F, et al. Lack of enterocyte iron accumulation in the ferroportin disease. Blood Cells Mol Dis. 2005;35:315–8.
125. De Domenico I, McVey WD, Nemeth E, et al. Molecular and clinical correlates in iron overload associated with mutations in ferroportin. Haematologica. 2006;91:1092–5.
126. Cremonesi L, Forni GL, Soriani N, et al. Genetic and clinical heterogeneity of ferroportin disease. Br J Haematol. 2005;131:663–70.
127. Bach V, Remacha A, Altes A, Barcelo MJ, Molina MA, Baiget M. Autosomal dominant hereditary hemochromatosis associated with two novel Ferroportin 1 mutations in Spain. Blood Cells Mol Dis. 2006;36:41–5.
128. Njajou OT, Vaessen N, Joosse M, et al. A mutation in *SLC11A3* is associated with autosomal dominant hemochromatosis. Nat Genet. 2001;28:213–4.
129. Wallace DF, Clark RM, Harley HA, Subramaniam VN. Autosomal dominant iron overload due to a novel mutation of ferroportin1 associated with parenchymal iron loading and cirrhosis. J Hepatol. 2004;40:710–3.
130. Arden KE, Wallace DF, Dixon JL, et al. A novel mutation in ferroportin1 is associated with haemochromatosis in a Solomon Islands patient. Gut. 2003;52:1215–7.
131. Girelli D, De Domenico I, Bozzini C, et al. Clinical, pathological, and molecular correlates in ferroportin disease: a study of two novel mutations. J Hepatol. 2008;49:664–71.
132. Hetet G, Devaux I, Soufir N, Grandchamp B, Beaumont C. Molecular analyses of patients with hyperferritinemia and normal serum iron values reveal both L ferritin IRE and 3 new ferroportin (*slc11A3*) mutations. Blood. 2003;102:1904–10.
133. Cazzola M, Cremonesi L, Papaioannou M, et al. Genetic hyperferritinaemia and reticuloendothelial iron overload associated with a three base pair deletion in the coding region of the ferroportin gene (*SLC11A3*). Br J Haematol. 2002;119:539–46.
134. Devalia V, Carter K, Walker AP, et al. Autosomal dominant reticuloendothelial iron overload associated with a 3-base pair deletion in the ferroportin 1 gene (*SLC11A3*). Blood. 2002;100:695–7.
135. Roetto A, Merryweather-Clarke AT, Daraio F, et al. A valine deletion of ferroportin 1: a common mutation in hemochromastosis type 4. Blood. 2002;100:733–4.

136. Wallace DF, Pedersen P, Dixon JL, et al. Novel mutation in ferroportin1 is associated with autosomal dominant hemochromatosis. Blood. 2002;100:692–4.
137. Wallace DF, Browett P, Wong P, Kua H, Ameratunga R, Subramaniam VN. Identification of ferroportin disease in the Indian subcontinent. Gut. 2005;54:567–8.
138. Speletas M, Kioumi A, Loules G, et al. Analysis of *SLC40A1* gene at the mRNA level reveals rapidly the causative mutations in patients with hereditary hemochromatosis type IV. Blood Cells Mol Dis. 2008;40:353–9.
139. Morris TJ, Litvinova MM, Ralston D, Mattman A, Holmes D, Lockitch G. A novel ferroportin mutation in a Canadian family with autosomal dominant hemochromatosis. Blood Cells Mol Dis. 2005;35:309–14.
140. Zaahl MG, Merryweather-Clarke AT, Kotze MJ, van der Merwe S, Warnich L, Robson KJ. Analysis of genes implicated in iron regulation in individuals presenting with primary iron overload. Hum Genet. 2004;115:409–17.
141. Sham RL, Phatak PD, West C, Lee P, Andrews C, Beutler E. Autosomal dominant hereditary hemochromatosis associated with a novel ferroportin mutation and unique clinical features. Blood Cells Mol Dis. 2005;34:157–61.
142. Robson KJ, Merryweather-Clarke AT, Cadet E, et al. Recent advances in understanding haemochromatosis: a transition state. J Med Genet. 2004;41:721–30.
143. Lee PL, Gelbart T, West C, Barton JC. SLC40A1 c.1402G a results in aberrant splicing, ferroportin truncation after glycine 330, and an autosomal dominant hemochromatosis phenotype. Acta Haematol. 2007;118:237–41.
144. Griffiths W, Mayr R, McFarlane I, et al. Clinical presentation and molecular pathophysiology of autosomal dominant hemochromatosis caused by a ferroportin mutation. Hepatology. 2010;51:788–95.
145. Jouanolle AM, Douabin-Gicquel V, Halimi C, et al. Novel mutation in ferroportin 1 gene is associated with autosomal dominant iron overload. J Hepatol. 2003;39:286–9.
146. Letocart E, Le Gac G, Majore S, et al. A novel missense mutation in SLC40A1 results in resistance to hepcidin and confirms the existence of two ferroportin-associated iron overload diseases. Br J Haematol. 2009;147:379–85.
147. Gordeuk VR, Caleffi A, Corradini E, et al. Iron overload in Africans and African-Americans and a common mutation in the *SCL40A1* (ferroportin 1) gene. Blood Cells Mol Dis. 2003;31:299–304.
148. Duca L, Delbini P, Nava I, Vaja V, Fiorelli G, Cappellini MD. Mutation analysis of hepcidin and ferroportin genes in Italian prospective blood donors with iron overload. Am J Hematol. 2009;84:592–3.
149. Barton JC, Acton RT, Lee PL, West C. *SLC40A1* Q248H allele frequencies and Q248H-associated risk of non-*HFE* iron overload in persons of sub-Saharan African descent. Blood Cells Mol Dis. 2007;39:206–11.
150. Rivers CA, Barton JC, Gordeuk VR, et al. Association of ferroportin Q248H polymorphism with elevated levels of serum ferritin in African Americans in the Hemochromatosis and Iron Overload Screening (HEIRS) Study. Blood Cells Mol Dis. 2007;38:247–52.
151. Roetto A, Bosio S, Gramaglia E, Barilaro MR, Zecchina G, Camaschella C. Pathogenesis of hyperferritinemia cataract syndrome. Blood Cells Mol Dis. 2002;29:532–5.
152. Burdon KP, Sharma S, Chen CS, Dimasi DP, Mackey DA, Craig JE. A novel deletion in the *FTL* gene causes hereditary hyperferritinemia cataract syndrome (HHCS) by alteration of the transcription start site. Hum Mutat. 2007;28:742.
153. Cremonesi L, Paroni R, Foglieni B, et al. Scanning mutations of the 5'UTR regulatory sequence of L-ferritin by denaturing high-performance liquid chromatography: identification of new mutations. Br J Haematol. 2003;121:173–9.
154. Girelli D, Corrocher R, Bisceglia L, et al. Hereditary hyperferritinemia-cataract syndrome caused by a 29-base pair deletion in the iron responsive element of ferritin L-subunit gene. Blood. 1997;90:2084–8.
155. Cremonesi L, Fumagalli A, Soriani N, et al. Double-gradient denaturing gradient gel electrophoresis assay for identification of L-ferritin iron-responsive element mutations responsible for hereditary hyperferritinemia-cataract syndrome: identification of the new mutation C14G. Clin Chem. 2001;47:491–7.
156. Ferrari F, Foglieni B, Arosio P, et al. Microelectronic DNA chip for hereditary hyperferritinemia cataract syndrome, a model for large-scale analysis of disorders of iron metabolism. Hum Mutat. 2006;27:201–8.
157. Cazzola M, Bergamaschi G, Tonon L, et al. Hereditary hyperferritinemia-cataract syndrome: relationship between phenotypes and specific mutations in the iron-responsive element of ferritin light-chain mRNA. Blood. 1997;90:814–21.
158. Cazzola M, Foglieni B, Bergamaschi G, Levi S, Lazzarino M, Arosio P. A novel deletion of the L-ferritin iron-responsive element responsible for severe hereditary hyperferritinaemia-cataract syndrome. Br J Haematol. 2002;116:667–70.
159. Bosio S, Campanella A, Gramaglia E, et al. C29G in the iron-responsive element of L-ferritin: a new mutation associated with hyperferritinemia-cataract. Blood Cells Mol Dis. 2004;33:31–4.
160. Vanita V, Hejtmancik JF, Hennies HC, et al. Sutural cataract associated with a mutation in the ferritin light chain gene (*FTL*) in a family of Indian origin. Mol Vis. 2006;12:93–9.
161. Craig JE, Clark JB, McLeod JL, et al. Hereditary hyperferritinemia-cataract syndrome: prevalence, lens morphology, spectrum of mutations, and clinical presentations. Arch Ophthalmol. 2003;121:1753–61.

162. Campagnoli MF, Pimazzoni R, Bosio S, et al. Onset of cataract in early infancy associated with a 32G→C transition in the iron responsive element of L-ferritin. Eur J Pediatr. 2002;161:499–502.
163. Ismail AR, Lachlan KL, Mumford AD, Temple IK, Hodgkins PR. Hereditary hyperferritinemia cataract syndrome: ocular, genetic, and biochemical findings. Eur J Ophthalmol. 2006;16:153–60.
164. Wong K, Barbin Y, Chakrabarti S, Adams P. A point mutation in the iron-responsive element of the L-ferritin in a family with hereditary hyperferritinemia cataract syndrome. Can J Gastroenterol. 2005;19:253–5.
165. Martin ME, Fargion S, Brissot P, Pellat B, Beaumont C. A point mutation in the bulge of the iron-responsive element of the L ferritin gene in two families with the hereditary hyperferritinemia-cataract syndrome. Blood. 1998;91:319–23.
166. Brooks DG, Manova-Todorova K, Farmer J, et al. Ferritin crystal cataracts in hereditary hyperferritinemia cataract syndrome. Invest Ophthalmol Vis Sci. 2002;43:1121–6.
167. Ladero JM, Balas A, Garcia-Sanchez F, Vicario JL, Diaz-Rubio M. Hereditary hyperferritinemia-cataract syndrome. Study of a new family in Spain. Rev Esp Enferm Dig. 2004;96:510–1.
168. Garcia Erce JA, Cortes T, Cremonesi L, Cazzola M, Perez-Lungmus G, Giralt M. Hyperferritinemia-cataract syndrome associated to the *HFE* gene mutation. Two new Spanish families and a new mutation (A37T: "Zaragoza"). Med Clin (Barc). 2006;127:55–8.
169. Balas A, Aviles MJ, Garcia-Sanchez F, Vicario JL. Description of a new mutation in the L-ferrin iron-responsive element associated with hereditary hyperferritinemia-cataract syndrome in a Spanish family. Blood. 1999;93:4020–1.
170. Mumford AD, Vulliamy T, Lindsay J, Watson A. Hereditary hyperferritinemia-cataract syndrome: two novel mutations in the L-ferritin iron-responsive element. Blood. 1998;91:367–8.
171. Garderet L, Hermelin B, Gorin NC, Rosmorduc O. Hereditary hyperferritinemia-cataract syndrome: a novel mutation in the iron-responsive element of the L-ferritin gene in a French family. Am J Med. 2004;117:138–9.
172. Papanikolaou G, Chandrinou H, Bouzas E, et al. Hereditary hyperferritinemia cataract syndrome in three unrelated families of western Greek origin caused by the C39→G mutation of L-ferritin IRE. Blood Cells Mol Dis. 2006;36:33–40.
173. Arosio C, Fossati L, Vigano M, Trombini P, Cazzaniga G, Piperno A. Hereditary hyperferritinemia cataract syndrome: a de novo mutation in the iron responsive element of the L-ferritin gene. Haematologica. 1999;84:560–1.
174. Cicilano M, Zecchina G, Roetto A, et al. Recurrent mutations in the iron regulatory element of L-ferritin in hereditary hyperferritinemia-cataract syndrome. Haematologica. 1999;84:489–92.
175. Beaumont C, Leneuve P, Devaux I, et al. Mutation in the iron responsive element of the L ferritin mRNA in a family with dominant hyperferritinaemia and cataract. Nat Genet. 1995;11:444–6.
176. Aguilar-Martinez P, Biron C, Masmejean C, Jeanjean P, Schved JF. A novel mutation in the iron responsive element of ferritin L-subunit gene as a cause for hereditary hyperferritinemia-cataract syndrome. Blood. 1996;88:1895.
177. Barton JC, Beutler E, Gelbart T. Coinheritance of alleles associated with hemochromatosis and hereditary hyperferritinemia-cataract syndrome. Blood. 1998;92:4480.
178. de Perez N, Castano L, Martul P, et al. Molecular analysis of hereditary hyperferritinemia-cataract syndrome in a large Basque family. J Pediatr Endocrinol Metab. 2001;14:295–300.
179. Del Castillo RA, Fernandez Ruano ML. Hereditary hyperferritinemia cataracts syndrome in a Spanish family caused by the A40G mutation (Paris) in the L-ferritin (*FTL*) gene associated with the mutation H63D in the *HFE* gene. Med Clin (Barc). 2007;129:414–7.
180. Girelli D, Corrocher R, Bisceglia L, et al. Molecular basis for the recently described hereditary hyperferritinemia-cataract syndrome: a mutation in the iron-responsive element of ferritin L-subunit gene (the "Verona mutation"). Blood. 1995;86:4050–3.
181. Feys J, Nodarian M, Aygalenq P, Cattan D, Bouccara AS, Beaumont C. Hereditary hyperferritinemia syndrome and cataract. J Fr Ophtalmol. 2001;24:847–50.
182. Phillips JD, Warby CA, Kushner JP. Identification of a novel mutation in the L-ferritin IRE leading to hereditary hyperferritinemia-cataract syndrome. Am J Med Genet A. 2005;134:77–9.
183. Chang-Godinich A, Ades S, Schenkein D, Brooks D, Stambolian D, Raizman MB. Lens changes in hereditary hyperferritinemia-cataract syndrome. Am J Ophthalmol. 2001;132:786–8.
184. Camaschella C, Zecchina G, Lockitch G, et al. A new mutation (G51C) in the iron-responsive element (IRE) of L-ferritin associated with hyperferritinaemia-cataract syndrome decreases the binding affinity of the mutated IRE for iron-regulatory proteins. Br J Haematol. 2000;108:480–2.
185. Cremonesi L, Cozzi A, Girelli D, et al. Case report: a subject with a mutation in the ATG start codon of L-ferritin has no haematological or neurological symptoms. J Med Genet. 2004;41:e81.
186. Girelli D, Bozzini C, Zecchina G, et al. Clinical, biochemical and molecular findings in a series of families with hereditary hyperferritinaemia-cataract syndrome. Br J Haematol. 2001;115:334–40.
187. Rosochova J, Kapetanios A, Pournaras C, Vadas L, Samii K, Beris P. Hereditary hyperferritinaemia cataract syndrome: does it exist in Switzerland? Schweiz Med Wochenschr. 2000;130:324–8.

188. Bozzini C, Galbiati S, Tinazzi E, Aldigeri R, De Matteis G, Girelli D. Prevalence of hereditary hyperferritinemia-cataract syndrome in blood donors and patients with cataract. Haematologica. 2003;88:219–20.
189. Curtis AR, Fey C, Morris CM, et al. Mutation in the gene encoding ferritin light polypeptide causes dominant adult-onset basal ganglia disease. Nat Genet. 2001;28:350–4.
190. Chinnery PF, Curtis AR, Fey C, et al. Neuroferritinopathy in a French family with late onset dominant dystonia. J Med Genet. 2003;40:e69.
191. Chinnery PF, Crompton DE, Birchall D, et al. Clinical features and natural history of neuroferritinopathy caused by the *FTL1* 460InsA mutation. Brain. 2007;130:110–9.
192. Costa MC, Teixeira-Castro A, Constante M, et al. Exclusion of mutations in the *PRNP*, *JPH3*, *TBP*, *ATN1*, *CREBBP*, *POU3F2* and *FTL* genes as a cause of disease in Portuguese patients with a Huntington-like phenotype. J Hum Genet. 2006;51:645–51.
193. Foglieni B, Ferrari F, Goldwurm S, et al. Analysis of ferritin genes in Parkinson disease. Clin Chem Lab Med. 2007;45:1450–6.
194. Maciel P, Cruz VT, Constante M, et al. Neuroferritinopathy: missense mutation in *FTL* causing early-onset bilateral pallidal involvement. Neurology. 2005;65:603–5.
195. Mancuso M, Davidzon G, Kurlan RM, et al. Hereditary ferritinopathy: a novel mutation, its cellular pathology, and pathogenetic insights. J Neuropathol Exp Neurol. 2005;64:280–94.
196. Ohta E, Nagasaka T, Shindo K, et al. Neuroferritinopathy in a Japanese family with a duplication in the ferritin light chain gene. Neurology. 2008;70:1493–4.
197. Wild EJ, Mudanohwo EE, Sweeney MG, et al. Huntington's disease phenocopies are clinically and genetically heterogeneous. Mov Disord. 2008;23:716–20.
198. Devos D, Tchofo P, Vuillaume I, et al. Clinical features and natural history of neuroferritinopathy caused by the 458dupA *FTL* mutation. Brain. 2009;132:e109.
199. Mir P, Edwards MJ, Curtis AR, Bhatia KP, Quinn NP. Adult-onset generalized dystonia due to a mutation in the neuroferritinopathy gene. Mov Disord. 2005;20:243–5.
200. Vidal R, Miravalle L, Gao X, et al. Expression of a mutant form of the ferritin light chain gene induces neurodegeneration and iron overload in transgenic mice. J Neurosci. 2008;28:60–7.
201. Kubota A, Hida A, Ichikawa Y, et al. A novel ferritin light chain gene mutation in a Japanese family with neuroferritinopathy: description of clinical features and implications for genotype-phenotype correlations. Mov Disord. 2008;24:441–5.
202. Kannengiesser C, Jouanolle AM, Hetet G, et al. A new missense mutation in the L ferritin coding sequence associated with elevated levels of glycosylated ferritin in serum and absence of iron overload. Haematologica. 2009;94:335–9.
203. Harrison PM, Arosio P. The ferritins: molecular properties, iron storage function and cellular regulation. Biochim Biophys Acta. 1996;1275:161–203.
204. Hentze MW, Rouault TA, Caughman SW, Dancis A, Harford JB, Klausner RD. A cis-acting element is necessary and sufficient for translational regulation of human ferritin expression in response to iron. Proc Natl Acad Sci USA. 1987;84:6730–4.
205. McGill JR, Naylor SL, Sakaguchi AY, et al. Human ferritin H and L sequences lie on ten different chromosomes. Hum Genet. 1987;76:66–72.
206. Eisenstein RS. Iron regulatory proteins and the molecular control of mammalian iron metabolism. Annu Rev Nutr. 2000;20:627–62.
207. Hentze MW, Caughman SW, Rouault TA, et al. Identification of the iron-responsive element for the translational regulation of human ferritin mRNA. Science. 1987;238:1570–3.
208. Leibold EA, Munro HN. Cytoplasmic protein binds in vitro to a highly conserved sequence in the 5 untranslated region of ferritin heavy- and light-subunit mRNAs. Proc Natl Acad Sci USA. 1988;85:2171–5.
209. Theil EC. Ferritin: structure, gene regulation, and cellular function in animals, plants, and microorganisms. Annu Rev Biochem. 1987;56:289–315.
210. Thomson AM, Rogers JT, Leedman PJ. Iron-regulatory proteins, iron-responsive elements and ferritin mRNA translation. Int J Biochem Cell Biol. 1999;31:1139–52.
211. Kato J, Fujikawa K, Kanda M, et al. A mutation, in the iron-responsive element of H ferritin mRNA, causing autosomal dominant iron overload. Am J Hum Genet. 2001;69:191–7.
212. Kawanaka M, Kinoyama S, Niiyama G, et al. A case of idiopathic hemochromatosis which occurred in three siblings with high level of serum CA 19–9. Nippon Shokakibyo Gakkai Zasshi. 1998;95:910–5.
213. Miyajima H, Nishimura Y, Mizoguchi K, Sakamoto M, Shimizu T, Honda N. Familial apoceruloplasmin deficiency associated with blepharospasm and retinal degeneration. Neurology. 1987;37:761–7.
214. Miyajima H, Kohno S, Takahashi Y, Yonekawa O, Kanno T. Estimation of the gene frequency of aceruloplasminemia in Japan. Neurology. 1999;53:617–9.
215. McNeill A, Pandolfo M, Kuhn J, Shang H, Miyajima H. The neurological presentation of ceruloplasmin gene mutations. Eur Neurol. 2008;60:200–5.

216. Hofmann WP, Welsch C, Takahashi Y, et al. Identification and in silico characterization of a novel compound heterozygosity associated with hereditary aceruloplasminemia. Scand J Gastroenterol. 2007;42:1088–94.
217. Miyajima H, Takahashi Y, Kamata T, Shimizu H, Sakai N, Gitlin JD. Use of desferrioxamine in the treatment of aceruloplasminemia. Ann Neurol. 1997;41:404–7.
218. Bottomley SS. Iron overload in sideroblastic and other non-thalassemic anemias. In: Barton JC, Edwards CQ, editors. Hemochromatosis: genetics, pathophysiology, diagnosis and treatment. Cambridge: Cambridge University Press; 2000. p. 442–52.
219. Barton JC, Lee PL, Bertoli LF, Beutler E. Iron overload in an African American woman with SS hemoglobinopathy and a promoter mutation in the X-linked erythroid-specific 5-aminolevulinate synthase (*ALAS2*) gene. Blood Cells Mol Dis. 2005;34:226–8.
220. Bekri S, May A, Cotter PD, et al. A promoter mutation in the erythroid-specific 5-aminolevulinate synthase (*ALAS2*) gene causes X-linked sideroblastic anemia. Blood. 2003;102:698–704.
221. Cortesao E, Vidan J, Pereira J, Goncalves P, Ribeiro ML, Tamagnini G. Onset of X-linked sideroblastic anemia in the fourth decade. Haematologica. 2004;89:1261–3.
222. Zhu P, Wang M, Shi Y, et al. Pathogenic gene linkage analysis and hemopoietic characteristics in a kindred with sideroblastic anemia. Zhonghua Yi Xue Yi Chuan Xue Za Zhi. 1999;16:22–5.
223. Hurford MT, Marshall-Taylor C, Vicki SL, et al. A novel mutation in exon 5 of the *ALAS2* gene results in X-linked sideroblastic anemia. Clin Chim Acta. 2002;321:49–53.
224. Furuyama K, Harigae H, Kinoshita C, et al. Late-onset X-linked sideroblastic anemia following hemodialysis. Blood. 2003;101:4623–4.
225. Zhu P, Bu D. A novel mutation of the *ALAS2* gene in a family with X-linked sideroblastic anemia. Zhonghua Xue Ye Xue Za Zhi. 2000;21:478–81.
226. Cotter PD, Rucknagel DL, Bishop DF. X-linked sideroblastic anemia: identification of the mutation in the erythroid-specific delta-aminolevulinate synthase gene (*ALAS2*) in the original family described by Cooley. Blood. 1994;84:3915–24.
227. Bottomley SS. Iron overload in sideroblastic and other non-thalassemic anemias. In: Greer JP, Foerster J, Lukens JN, Rogers GM, Paraskevas F, Glader BE, editors. Wintrobe's clinical hematology. Philadelphia: Lippincott Williams & Wilkins; 2004. p. 1011–33.
228. Furuyama K, Sassa S. Multiple mechanisms for hereditary sideroblastic anemia. Cell Mol Biol. 2002;48:5–10.
229. May A, Bishop DF. The molecular biology and pyridoxine responsiveness of X-linked sideroblastic anaemia. Haematologica. 1998;83:56–70.
230. Edgar AJ, Vidyatilake HM, Wickramasinghe SN. X-linked sideroblastic anaemia due to a mutation in the erythroid 5-aminolaevulinate synthase gene leading to an arginine170 to leucine substitution. Eur J Haematol. 1998;61:55–8.
231. Cotter PD, May A, Fitzsimons EJ, et al. Late-onset X-linked sideroblastic anemia. Missense mutations in the erythroid delta-aminolevulinate synthase (*ALAS2*) gene in two pyridoxine-responsive patients initially diagnosed with acquired refractory anemia and ringed sideroblasts. J Clin Invest. 1995;96:2090–6.
232. Furuyama K, Fujita H, Nagai T, et al. Pyridoxine refractory X-linked sideroblastic anemia caused by a point mutation in the erythroid 5-aminolevulinate synthase gene. Blood. 1997;90:822–30.
233. Cotter PD, May A, Li L, et al. Four new mutations in the erythroid-specific 5-aminolevulinate synthase (*ALAS2*) gene causing X-linked sideroblastic anemia: increased pyridoxine responsiveness after removal of iron overload by phlebotomy and coinheritance of hereditary hemochromatosis. Blood. 1999;93:1757–69.
234. Bottomley SS, Wise PD, Wasson EG, Carpenter NJ. X-linked sideroblastic anemia in ten female probands due to *ALAS2* mutations and skewed X chromosome inactivation. Am J Hum Genet. 1998;63(Suppl):A352.
235. Anderson KE, Sassa S, Bishop DF, Desnick RJ. Disorders of heme biosynthesis: X-linked sideroblastic anemia and the porphyrias. In: Scriver CR, Beaudet AL, Sly WS, et al., editors. The metabolic and molecular basis of inherited disease, 8th ed, McGraw-Hill, New York. 2001;8:2991–3062.
236. Harigae H, Furuyama K, Kimura A, et al. A novel mutation of the erythroid-specific delta-aminolaevulinate synthase gene in a patient with X-linked sideroblastic anaemia. Br J Haematol. 1999;106:175–7.
237. Rivera CE, Heath AP. Identification of a new mutation in erythroid-specific δ-aminolevulinate synthase in a patient with congential sideroblastic anemia. Blood. 1999;94(Suppl):19b.
238. Percy MJ, Cuthbert RJ, May A, McMullin MF. A novel mutation, Ile289Thr, in the *ALAS2* gene in a family with pyridoxine responsive sideroblastic anaemia. J Clin Pathol. 2006;59:1002.
239. Prades E, Chambon C, Dailey TA, Dailey HA, Briere J, Grandchamp B. A new mutation of the *ALAS2* gene in a large family with X-linked sideroblastic anemia. Hum Genet. 1995;95:424–8.
240. Cazzola M, May A, Bergamaschi G, Cerani P, Rosti V, Bishop DF. Familial-skewed X-chromosome inactivation as a predisposing factor for late-onset X-linked sideroblastic anemia in carrier females. Blood. 2000;96:4363–5.
241. Furuyama K, Uno R, Urabe A, et al. R411C mutation of the *ALAS2* gene encodes a pyridoxine-responsive enzyme with low activity. Br J Haematol. 1998;103:839–41.
242. Bishop DF, Cotter PD, May Aea. A novel mutation in exon 9 of the erythroid 5-aminolevulinate synthase gene shows phenotypic variablility lead to X-linked sideroblastic anemia in two unrelated male children but to the late-onset form of this disorder in an unrelated female. Am J Hum Genet. 1996;59(Suppl):A248.

243. Bottomley SS, May BK, Cox TC, Cotter PD, Bishop DF. Molecular defects of erythroid 5-aminolevulinate synthase in X-linked sideroblastic anemia. J Bioenerg Biomembr. 1995;27:161–8.
244. Aivado M, Gattermann N, Rong A, et al. X-linked sideroblastic anemia associated with a novel *ALAS2* mutation and unfortunate skewed X-chromosome inactivation patterns. Blood Cells Mol Dis. 2006;37:40–5.
245. Edgar AJ, Losowsky MS, Noble JS, Wickramasinghe SN. Identification of an arginine[452] to histidine substitution in the erythroid 5-aminolaevulinate synthetase gene in a large pedigree with X-linked hereditary sideroblastic anaemia. Eur J Haematol. 1997;58:1–4.
246. Koc S, Bishop DF, Li Lea. Iron overload in pyridoxine-responsive X-linked sideroblastic anemia: greater severity in a heterozygote tha in her hemizygoous brother. Blood. 1997;90(Suppl):16b.
247. Cotter PD, Baumann M, Bishop DF. Enzymatic defect in "X-linked" sideroblastic anemia: molecular evidence for erythroid delta-aminolevulinate synthase deficiency. Proc Natl Acad Sci USA. 1992;89:4028–32.
248. Edgar AJ, Wickramasinghe SN. Hereditary sideroblastic anaemia due to a mutation in exon 10 of the erythroid 5-aminolaevulinate synthase gene. Br J Haematol. 1998;100:389–92.
249. Cazzola M, May A, Bergamaschi G, Cerani P, Ferrillo S, Bishop DF. Absent phenotypic expression of X-linked sideroblastic anemia in one of 2 brothers with a novel ALAS2 mutation. Blood. 2002;100:4236–8.
250. Pasanen AV, Salmi M, Vuopio P, Tenhunen R. Heme biosynthesis in sideroblastic anemia. Int J Biochem. 1980;12:969–74.
251. Lee GR, MacDiarmid WD, Cartwright GE, Wintrobe MM. Hereditary, X-linked, sideroachrestic anemia. The isolation of two erythrocyte populations differing in Xga blood type and porphyrin content. Blood. 1968;32:59–70.
252. Weatherall DJ, Pembrey ME, Hall EG, Sanger R, Tippett P, Gavin J. Familial sideroblastic anaemia: problem of Xg and X chromosome inactivation. Lancet. 1970;2:744–8.
253. Peto TE, Pippard MJ, Weatherall DJ. Iron overload in mild sideroblastic anaemias. Lancet. 1983;1:375–8.
254. Cox TC, Kozman HM, Raskind WH, May BK, Mulley JC. Identification of a highly polymorphic marker within intron 7 of the *ALAS2* gene and suggestion of at least two loci for X-linked sideroblastic anemia. Hum Mol Genet. 1992;1:639–41.
255. Allikmets R, Raskind WH, Hutchinson A, Schueck ND, Dean M, Koeller DM. Mutation of a putative mitochondrial iron transporter gene (*ABC7*) in X-linked sideroblastic anemia and ataxia (XLSA/A). Hum Mol Genet. 1999;8:743–9.
256. Prasad AS, Tranchida L, Konno ET, et al. Hereditary sideroblastic anemia and glucose-6-phosphate dehydrogenase deficiency in a Negro family. J Clin Invest. 1968;47:1415–24.
257. Collins TS, Arcasoy MO. Iron overload due to X-linked sideroblastic anemia in an African American man. Am J Med. 2004;116:501–2.
258. Higgins CF. ABC transporters: from microorganisms to man. Annu Rev Cell Biol. 1992;8:67–113.
259. Higgins CF. The ABC of channel regulation. Cell. 1995;82:693–6.
260. Dean M, Allikmets R. Evolution of ATP-binding cassette transporter genes. Curr Opin Genet Dev. 1995;5: 779–85.
261. Kispal G, Csere P, Prohl C, Lill R. The mitochondrial proteins Atm1p and Nfs1p are essential for biogenesis of cytosolic Fe/S proteins. EMBO J. 1999;18:3981–9.
262. Taketani S, Kakimoto K, Ueta H, Masaki R, Furukawa T. Involvement of ABC7 in the biosynthesis of heme in erythroid cells: interaction of ABC7 with ferrochelatase. Blood. 2003;101:3274–80.
263. Maguire A, Hellier K, Hammans S, May A. X-linked cerebellar ataxia and sideroblastic anaemia associated with a missense mutation in the *ABC7* gene predicting V411L. Br J Haematol. 2001;115:910–7.
264. Bekri S, Kispal G, Lange H, et al. Human *ABC7* transporter: gene structure and mutation causing X-linked sideroblastic anemia with ataxia with disruption of cytosolic iron-sulfur protein maturation. Blood. 2000;96:3256–64.
265. Pagon RA, Bird TD, Detter JC, Pierce I. Hereditary sideroblastic anaemia and ataxia: an X linked recessive disorder. J Med Genet. 1985;22:267–73.
266. Padilla CA, Bajalica S, Lagercrantz J, Holmgren A. The gene for human glutaredoxin (*GLRX*) is localized to human chromosome 5q14. Genomics. 1996;32:455–7.
267. Padilla CA, Martinez-Galisteo E, Barcena JA, Spyrou G, Holmgren A. Purification from placenta, amino acid sequence, structure comparisons and cDNA cloning of human glutaredoxin. Eur J Biochem. 1995;227:27–34.
268. Camaschella C, Campanella A, De Falco L, et al. The human counterpart of zebrafish *shiraz* shows sideroblastic-like microcytic anemia and iron overload. Blood. 2007;110:1353–8.
269. Porter FS, Rogers LE, Sidbury Jr JB. Thiamine-responsive megaloblastic anemia. J Pediatr. 1969;74:494–504.
270. Raz T, Labay V, Baron D, et al. The spectrum of mutations, including four novel ones, in the thiamine-responsive megaloblastic anemia gene *SLC19A2* of eight families. Hum Mutat. 2000;16:37–42.
271. Labay V, Raz T, Baron D, et al. Mutations in *SLC19A2* cause thiamine-responsive megaloblastic anaemia associated with diabetes mellitus and deafness. Nat Genet. 1999;22:300–4.
272. Scott AJ, Ansford AJ, Webster BH, Stringer HC. Erythropoietic protoporphyria with features of a sideroblastic anaemia terminating in liver failure. Am J Med. 1973;54:251–9.

273. Rademakers LH, Koningsberger JC, Sorber CW, de la Baart F, Van Hattum J, Marx JJ. Accumulation of iron in erythroblasts of patients with erythropoietic protoporphyria. Eur J Clin Invest. 1993;23:130–8.
274. Zeharia A, Fischel-Ghodsian N, Casas K, et al. Mitochondrial myopathy, sideroblastic anemia, and lactic acidosis: an autosomal recessive syndrome in Persian Jews caused by a mutation in the PUS1 gene. J Child Neurol. 2005;20:449–52.
275. Bykhovskaya Y, Casas K, Mengesha E, Inbal A, Fischel-Ghodsian N. Missense mutation in pseudouridine synthase 1 (*PUS1*) causes mitochondrial myopathy and sideroblastic anemia (MLASA). Am J Hum Genet. 2004;74:1303–8.
276. Casas K, Bykhovskaya Y, Mengesha E, et al. Gene responsible for mitochondrial myopathy and sideroblastic anemia (MSA) maps to chromosome 12q24.33. Am J Med Genet A. 2004;127:44–9.
277. Casas KA, Fischel-Ghodsian N. Mitochondrial myopathy and sideroblastic anemia. Am J Med Genet A. 2004;125:201–4.
278. Fernandez-Vizarra E, Berardinelli A, Valente L, Tiranti V, Zeviani M. Nonsense mutation in pseudouridylate synthase 1 (PUS1) in two brothers affected by myopathy, lactic acidosis and sideroblastic anaemia (MLASA). J Med Genet. 2007;44:173–80.
279. Inbal A, Avissar N, Shaklai M, et al. Myopathy, lactic acidosis, and sideroblastic anemia: a new syndrome. Am J Med Genet. 1995;55:372–8.
280. Patton JR, Bykhovskaya Y, Mengesha E, Bertolotto C, Fischel-Ghodsian N. Mitochondrial myopathy and sideroblastic anemia (MLASA): missense mutation in the pseudouridine synthase 1 (PUS1) gene is associated with the loss of tRNA pseudouridylation. J Biol Chem. 2005;280:19823–8.
281. Rawles JM, Weller RO. Familial association of metabolic myopathy, lactic acidosis and sideroblastic anemia. Am J Med. 1974;56:891–7.
282. Heilmeyer L, Keller W, Vivell O, Betke K, Woehler F, Keiderling W. Congenital atransferrinemia. Schweiz Med Wochenschr. 1961;91:1203.
283. Beutler E, Gelbart T, Lee P, Trevino R, Fernandez MA, Fairbanks VF. Molecular characterization of a case of atransferrinemia. Blood. 2000;96:4071–4.
284. Goya N, Miyazaki S, Kodate S, Ushio B. A family of congenital atransferrinemia. Blood. 1972;40:239–45.
285. Sakata T. A case of congenital atransferrinemia. Shonika Shinryo. 1969;32:1523.
286. Asada-Senju M, Maeda T, Sakata T, Hayashi A, Suzuki T. Molecular analysis of the transferrin gene in a patient with hereditary hypotransferrinemia. J Hum Genet. 2002;47:355–9.
287. Cap J, Lehotska V, Mayerova A. Congenital atransferrinemia in a 11-month-old child. Cesk Pediatr. 1968;23:1020–5.
288. Hromec A, Payer Jr J, Killinger Z, Rybar I, Rovensky J. Congenital atransferrinemia. Dtsch Med Wochenschr. 1994;119:663–6.
289. Knisely AS, Gelbart T, Beutler E. Molecular characterization of a third case of human atransferrinemia. Blood. 2004;104:2607.
290. Aslan D, Crain K, Beutler E. A new case of human atransferrinemia with a previously undescribed mutation in the transferrin gene. Acta Haematol. 2007;118:244–7.
291. den Dunnen JT, Antonarakis SE. Mutation nomenclature extensions and suggestions to describe complex mutations: a discussion. Hum Mutat. 2000;15:7–12.
292. Antonarakis SE, Nomenclature Working Group. Recommendations for a nomenclature system for human gene mutations. Hum Mutat. 1998;11:1–3.
293. Loperena L, Dorantes S, Medrano E, et al. Hereditary atransferrinemia. Bol Med Hosp Infant Mex. 1974;31:519–35.
294. Dorantes-Mesa S, Marquez JL, Valencia-Mayoral P. Iron overload in hereditary atransferrinemia. Bol Med Hosp Infant Mex. 1986;43:99–101.
295. Walbaum R. Congenital transferrin deficiency. Lille Med. 1971;16:1122–4.
296. Hamill RL, Woods JC, Cook BA. Congenital atransferrinemia. A case report and review of the literature. Am J Clin Pathol. 1991;96:215–8.
297. Goldwurm S, Casati C, Venturi N, et al. Biochemical and genetic defects underlying human congenital hypotransferrinemia. Hematol J. 2000;1:390–8.
298. Espinheira R, Geada H, Mendonca J, Reys L. Alpha-1-antitrypsin and transferrin null alleles in the Portuguese population. Hum Hered. 1988;38:372–4.
299. Weidinger S, Cleve H, Schwarzfischer F, Postel W, Weser J, Gorg A. Transferrin subtypes and variants in Germany; further evidence for a Tf null allele. Hum Genet. 1984;66:356–60.
300. Püshel K, Krüger A, Soder R. Further evidence of a silent Tf allele. 12th International Congress Society Forensic Haemog. Vienna; 1987.
301. Lukka M, Enholm C. A silent transferrin allele in a Finnish family. Hum Hered. 1985;35:157–60.
302. Lee PL, Ho NJ, Olson R, Beutler E. The effect of transferrin polymorphisms on iron metabolism. Blood Cells Mol Dis. 1999;25:374–9.
303. Gunshin H, Mackenzie B, Berger UV, et al. Cloning and characterization of a mammalian proton-coupled metal-ion transporter. Nature. 1997;388:482–8.

304. Hubert N, Hentze MW. Previously uncharacterized isoforms of divalent metal transporter (DMT)-1: implications for regulation and cellular function. Proc Natl Acad Sci USA. 2002;99:12345–50.
305. Vidal S, Belouchi AM, Cellier M, Beatty B, Gros P. Cloning and characterization of a second human *NRAMP* gene on chromosome 12q13. Mamm Genome. 1995;6:224–30.
306. Priwitzerova M, Pospisilova D, Prchal JT, et al. Severe hypochromic microcytic anemia caused by a congenital defect of the iron transport pathway in erythroid cells. Blood. 2004;103:3991–2.
307. Priwitzerova M, Nie G, Sheftel AD, Pospisilova D, Divoky V, Ponka P. Functional consequences of the human *DMT1* (*SLC11A2*) mutation on protein expression and iron uptake. Blood. 2005;106:3985–7.
308. Mims MP, Guan Y, Pospisilova D, et al. Identification of a human mutation of *DMT1* in a patient with microcytic anemia and iron overload. Blood. 2005;105:1337–42.
309. Shahidi NT, Nathan DG, Diamond LK. Iron deficiency anemia associated with an error of iron metabolism in two siblings. J Clin Invest. 1964;43:510–21.
310. Lam-Yuk-Tseung S, Mathieu M, Gros P. Functional characterization of the E399D *DMT1/NRAMP2/SLC11A2* protein produced by an exon 12 mutation in a patient with microcytic anemia and iron overload. Blood Cells Mol Dis. 2005;35:212–6.
311. Iolascon A, D'Apolito M, Servedio V, Cimmino F, Piga A, Camaschella C. Microcytic anemia and hepatic iron overload in a child with compound heterozygous mutations in DMT1 (*SCL11A2*). Blood. 2006;107:349–54.
312. Lam-Yuk-Tseung S, Camaschella C, Iolascon A, Gros P. A novel R416C mutation in human *DMT1* (*SLC11A2*) displays pleiotropic effects on function and causes microcytic anemia and hepatic iron overload. Blood Cells Mol Dis. 2006;36:347–54.
313. Beaumont C, Delaunay J, Hetet G, Grandchamp B, de Montalembert M, Tchernia G. Two new human *DMT1* gene mutations in a patient with microcytic anemia, low ferritinemia, and liver iron overload. Blood. 2006;107:4168–70.
314. Lee P, Gelbart T, West C, Halloran C, Beutler E. Seeking candidate mutations that affect iron homeostasis. Blood Cells Mol Dis. 2002;29:471–87.
315. Kelleher T, Ryan E, Barrett S, O'Keane C, Crowe J. *DMT1* genetic variability is not responsible for phenotype variability in hereditary hemochromatosis. Blood Cells Mol Dis. 2004;33:35–9.
316. Xiong L, Dion P, Montplaisir J, et al. Molecular genetic studies of *DMT1* on 12q in French-Canadian restless legs syndrome patients and families. Am J Med Genet B Neuropsychiatr Genet. 2007;144:911–7.
317. Ramsay AJ, Hooper JD, Folgueras AR, Velasco G, Lopez-Otin C. Matriptase-2 (*TMPRSS6*): a proteolytic regulator of iron homeostasis. Haematologica. 2009;94:840–9.
318. Park TJ, Lee YJ, Kim HJ, Park HG, Park WJ. Cloning and characterization of *TMPRSS6*, a novel type 2 transmembrane serine protease. Mol Cells. 2005;19:223–7.
319. Silvestri L, Pagani A, Nai A, De Domenico I, Kaplan J, Camaschella C. The serine protease matriptase-2 (*TMPRSS6*) inhibits hepcidin activation by cleaving membrane hemojuvelin. Cell Metab. 2008;8:502–11.
320. Silvestri L, Guillem F, Pagani A, et al. Molecular mechanisms of the defective hepcidin inhibition in *TMPRSS6* mutations associated with iron-refractory iron deficiency anemia. Blood. 2009;113:5605–8.
321. Ramsay AJ, Quesada V, Sanchez M, et al. Matriptase-2 mutations in iron-refractory iron deficiency anemia patients provide new insights into protease activation mechanisms. Hum Mol Genet. 2009;18:3673–83.
322. Beutler E, Van Geet C, Te Loo DM, et al. Polymorphisms and mutations of human *TMPRSS6* in iron deficiency anemia. Blood Cells Mol Dis. 2010;44:16–21.
323. Melis MA, Cau M, Congiu R, et al. A mutation in the *TMPRSS6* gene, encoding a transmembrane serine protease that suppresses hepcidin production, in familial iron deficiency anemia refractory to oral iron. Haematologica. 2008;93:1473–9.
324. Tchou I, Diepold M, Pilotto PA, Swinkels D, Neerman-Arbez M, Beris P. Haematologic data, iron parameters and molecular findings in two new cases of iron-refractory iron deficiency anaemia. Eur J Haematol. 2009;83:595–602.
325. Finberg KE, Heeney MM, Campagna DR, et al. Mutations in *TMPRSS6* cause iron-refractory iron deficiency anemia (IRIDA). Nat Genet. 2008;40:569–71.
326. Guillem F, Lawson S, Kannengiesser C, Westerman M, Beaumont C, Grandchamp B. Two nonsense mutations in the *TMPRSS6* gene in a patient with microcytic anemia and iron deficiency. Blood. 2008;112:2089–91.
327. Edison ES, Athiyarath R, Rajasekar T, Westerman M, Srivastava A, Chandy M. A novel splice site mutation c.2278 (−1) G→C in the *TMPRSS6* gene causes deletion of the substrate binding site of the serine protease resulting in refractory iron deficiency anaemia. Br J Haematol. 2009;147:766–9.
328. Chambers JC, Zhang W, Li Y, et al. Genome-wide association study identifies variants in *TMPRSS6* associated with hemoglobin levels. Nat Genet. 2009;41:1170–2.
329. Tanaka T, Roy CN, Yao W, et al. A genome-wide association analysis of serum iron concentrations. Blood. 2010;115:94–6.
330. Ganesh SK, Zakai NA, van Rooij FJ, et al. Multiple loci influence erythrocyte phenotypes in the CHARGE Consortium. Nat Genet. 2009;41:1191–8.
331. Benyamin B, Ferreira MA, Willemsen G, et al. Common variants in *TMPRSS6* are associated with iron status and erythrocyte volume. Nat Genet. 2009;41:1173–5.

Chapter 27
The Properties of Therapeutically Useful Iron Chelators

Robert C. Hider and Yong Min Ma

Keywords Deferasirox • Deferiprone • Deferoxamine • Iron chelators • pFe^{3+} value

1 Introduction

Although iron is essential for the proper functioning of all living cells, it is toxic when present in excess. In the presence of molecular oxygen, "loosely bound" iron is able to redox cycle between the two most stable oxidation states, iron(II) and iron(III), thereby generating oxygen-derived free radicals, such as the hydroxyl radical [1]. Hydroxyl radicals are highly reactive and capable of interacting with most types of biological molecules, including sugars, lipids, proteins and nucleic acids, resulting in peroxidative tissue damage [2]. The uncontrolled production of such highly reactive species is undesirable, and thus, a number of protective strategies are adopted by cells to prevent their formation. One of the most important is the tight control of iron storage, transport and distribution. In fact, iron metabolism in man is highly conservative with the majority of iron being recycled within the body. Since man lacks a physiological mechanism for eliminating iron, iron homeostasis is largely achieved by the regulation of iron absorption. In addition, the levels of many of the proteins involved in iron transport, storage and catalysis are controlled by body iron levels.

In the normal individual, iron levels are under extremely tight control, and there is little opportunity for iron-catalyzed, free radical-generating reactions to occur. However, there are situations when the iron status can change either locally, as in ischemic tissue, or systematically, as with genetic hemochromatosis or transfusion-induced iron overload. In such circumstances, the elevated levels of iron ultimately lead to free radical-mediated tissue/organ damage and eventual death. Deferoxamine B (DFO) [**1**] (compounds are identified by a bold number in square brackets), the most widely used iron chelator in hematology over the past 30 years, has a major disadvantage of being orally inactive [3], and consequently, there is a need for an orally active iron-chelating agent.

When designing iron chelators for clinical application, the properties governing metal selectivity and ligand–metal complex stability are paramount. In theory, chelating agents can be designed for

R.C. Hider, Ph.D. (✉)
Department of Pharmacy, Institute of Pharmaceutical Science, King's College, London, UK
e-mail: robert.hider@kcl.ac.uk

Y.M. Ma, Ph.D.
Institute of Pharmaceutical Science, King's College London, London, UK
e-mail: yong_min.ma@kcl.ac.uk

G.J. Anderson and G. McLaren (eds.), *Iron Physiology and Pathophysiology in Humans*, Nutrition and Health, DOI 10.1007/978-1-60327-485-2_27,

Table 27.1 Metal affinity constants for selected ligands

Ligand	Log cumulative stability constant					
	Fe(III)	Al(III)	Ga(III)	Cu(II)	Zn(II)	Fe(II)
DFO [**1**]	30.6	25.0	27.6	14.1	11.1	7.2
2,2′-Bipyridyl [**2**]	16.3	–	7.7	16.9	13.2	17.2
1,10-Phenanthroline [**3**]	14.1	–	9.2	21.4	17.5	21.0
N,N-Dimethyl-2,3-dihydroxybenzamide (DMB) [**7**]	40.2	–	–	24.9	13.5	17.5
Acetohydroxamic acid [**8**]	28.3	21.5	–	7.9	9.6	8.5
Deferiprone [**12**]	37.4	35.8	32.6	21.7	13.5	12.1
EDTA [**13**]	25.1	16.5	21.0	18.8	16.5	14.3
DTPA [**14**]	28.0	18.6	25.5	21.6	18.4	16.5

Data sourced from Martell and Smith (1974–1989) [4]

either the iron(II) (ferrous) or the iron(III) (ferric) oxidation state. Ligands that prefer iron(II) contain "soft" donor atoms, exemplified by nitrogen-containing ligands, such as 2,2′-bipyridyl [**2**] and 1,10-phenanthroline [**3**]. Although these compounds are selective for iron(II) over iron(III), they retain an appreciable affinity for other biologically important bivalent metals, such as copper(II) and zinc(II) ions (Table 27.1). Thus, the design of a nontoxic iron(II)-selective ligand is extremely difficult and indeed may not be possible. In contrast, iron(III)-selective ligands, typically oxyanions and notably hydroxamates and catecholates, are generally more selective for tribasic metal cations over dibasic cations (Table 27.1). Most tribasic cations, for instance aluminum(III) and gallium(III), are not essential for living cells, and thus in practice, iron(III) is a suitable target for "clinical chelator" design. An additional advantage of high-affinity iron(III) chelators is that, under aerobic conditions, they will chelate iron(II) and facilitate autoxidation to iron(III) [5]. Thus, high-affinity iron(III)-selective ligands bind both iron(III) and iron(II) under most physiological conditions. Siderophores, compounds possessing a high affinity for iron(III) and produced by microorganisms for scavenging iron from the environment, utilize the above principle [6]. Typically, they are hexadentate in design and utilize catechol or hydroxamate as ligands, for instance enterobactin [**4**], deferriferrichrome [**5**] and DFO [**1**]. The stereochemistry of these molecules is such that the coordination sphere of iron(III) is completely occupied by oxygen-containing ligands, for example ferrioxamine B (Fig. 27.1). The selectivity of these molecules for iron(III) over iron(II) is enormous, leading to extremely low redox potentials, for example enterobactin –750 mV and DFO –468 mV [7].

2 Design Features of Iron(III) Chelators

In order to identify an ideal iron(III) chelator for clinical use, careful design consideration is essential, and a range of specifications must be considered, such as metal selectivity and affinity, kinetic stability of the complex, bioavailability and toxicity.

2.1 Thermodynamic Stability of Iron(III) Complexes

Ligands can be structurally classified according to the number of donor atoms that each molecule possesses. When a ligand contains two or more donor atoms, they are termed bidentate, tridentate, bis bidentate, hexadentate, or, generally, multidentate. The coordination requirements of iron(III) are

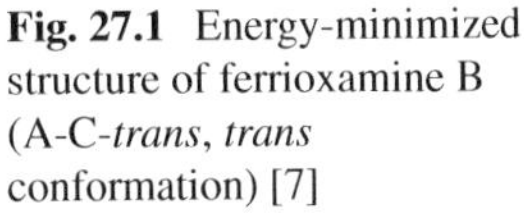

Fig. 27.1 Energy-minimized structure of ferrioxamine B (A-C-*trans*, *trans* conformation) [7]

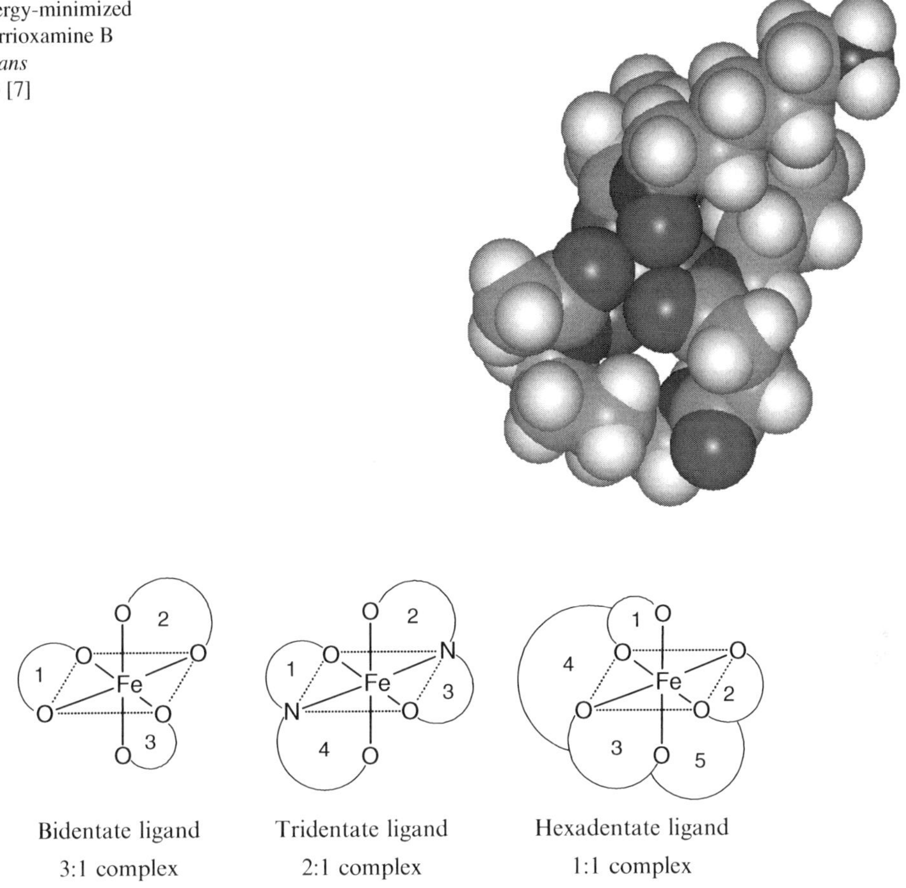

Fig. 27.2 Schematic representation of chelate ring formation in metal–ligand complexes

best satisfied by six donor atoms ligating in an octahedral fashion to the metal center. A factor of great importance relating to the stability of a metal complex is the number and size of chelate rings formed in the resultant ligand–metal complex. The most favorable chelate ring sizes consist of five or six atoms. The number of chelating rings can be enhanced by increasing the number of donor atoms attached to a single chelator; for example, a metal ion with coordination number six may form three rings with a bidentate ligand or five rings with a hexadentate ligand (Fig. 27.2). Thus, in order to maximize the thermodynamic stability of the iron(III) complex, it is necessary to incorporate all six donors into a single molecular structure, thereby creating a hexadentate ligand. This increase in stability is largely associated with the entropic changes that occur on going from free ligand and solvated free metal to the ligand–metal complex (Scheme 27.1). Significantly, the majority of natural siderophores are hexadentate ligands.

The overall stability constant trends for bidentate and hexadentate ligands are typified by the bidentate ligand *N,N*-dimethyl-2,3-dihydroxybenzamide (DMB)[**7**] and the hexadentate congener MECAM [**6**], where a differential of 3 log units in stability is observed (Table 27.2). Similarly, comparison of the stability constants of the bidentate ligand acetohydroxamic acid [**8**] with that of the linear hexadentate ligand DFO [**1**] demonstrates a difference of 2.3 log units (Table 27.2). Although MECAM binds iron(III) three orders of magnitude more tightly than its bidentate analogue DMB, other hexadentate catechols, for instance enterobactin, bind iron(III) even more tightly (log stability constant=49).

$$Fe(H_2O)_6 + 3\,L_B \underset{}{\overset{\beta_3}{\rightleftharpoons}} Fe(L_B)_3 + 6\,H_2O$$

$$Fe(H_2O)_6 + 2\,L_T \underset{}{\overset{\beta_2}{\rightleftharpoons}} Fe(L_T)_2 + 6\,H_2O$$

$$Fe(H_2O)_6 + L_H \underset{}{\overset{K_1}{\rightleftharpoons}} FeL_H + 6\,H_2O$$

L_B, bidentate; L_T, tridentate; L_H, hexadentate ligand

Scheme 27.1 The complex formation of iron(III) with bidentate, tridentate and hexadentate ligands (charges omitted for clarity)

Table 27.2 A comparison of the pFe^{3+} values and iron(III) stability constants for bidentate and hexadentate ligands

Ligand	pFe^{3+a}	Log stability constant
N,N-Dimethyl-2,3-dihydroxybenzamide (DMB) [**7**]	15	40.2
MECAM [**6**]	28	43
Acetohydroxamic acid [**7**]	13	28.3
DFO [**1**]	26	30.6

[a] $pFe^{3+} = -\log[Fe^{3+}]$ when $[Fe^{3+}]_{total} = 10^{-6}$ M and $[ligand]_{total} = 10^{-5}$ M at pH 7.4

Under biological conditions, a parameter which is generally more useful than the conventional stability constant for comparison of chelators is the pM value or, specifically for iron(III), the pFe^{3+} value [8, 9]. pFe^{3+} is defined as the negative logarithm of the concentration of the free iron(III) in solution. For clinically relevant conditions, pFe^{3+} values are typically calculated for total $[ligand] = 10^{-5}$ M and total $[iron] = 10^{-6}$ M at pH 7.4. The comparison of ligands under these conditions is useful, as the pFe^{3+} value, unlike the stability constant log K or log β_3, takes into account the effects of ligand protonation and denticity as well as differences in metal–ligand stoichiometries. The comparison of the pFe^{3+} values for hexadentate and bidentate ligands (Table 27.2) reveals that hexadentate ligands are far superior scavengers when compared with their bidentate counterparts. Indeed, when the influence of pH is monitored, the overall shift in pFe^{3+} values becomes even clearer (Fig. 27.3). The pFe^{3+} versus pH plot provides a useful method of comparing the ability of chelators to bind iron(III) at different pH values. For a ligand to dominate iron(III) chelation in aqueous media, it must produce a pFe^{3+} curve above that corresponding to the hydroxide anion. The larger the difference, the stronger the chelator and the larger the pFe^{3+} value.

The formation of a complex will also be dependent on both free metal and free ligand concentration and as such will be sensitive to concentration changes. Thus, the degree of dissociation for a *tris*-bidentate ligand–metal complex is dependent on $[ligand]^3$, while the hexadentate ligand–metal complex dissociation is only dependent on $[ligand]^1$ (Scheme 27.2). Hence, the dilution sensitivity of complex dissociation follows the order hexadentate < tridentate < bidentate. It is probably for this reason that the majority of natural siderophores are hexadentate compounds and can therefore scavenge iron(III) efficiently at low metal and low ligand concentrations [6].

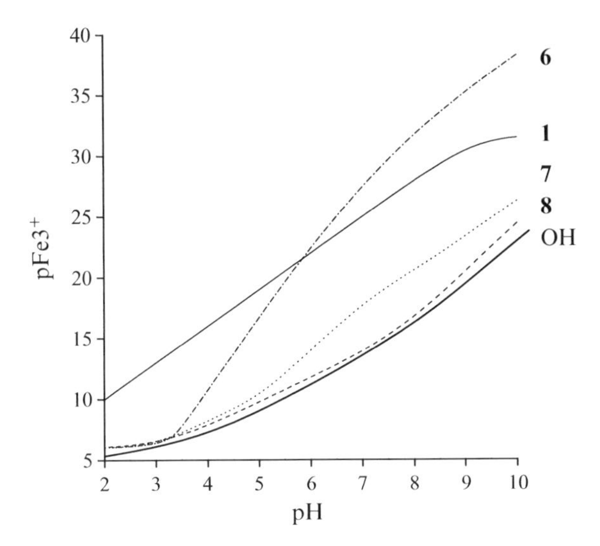

Fig. 27.3 Influence of pH on pFe^{3+} values of DFO [**1**], MECAM [**6**], *N,N*-dimethyl-2,3-dihydroxybenzamide [**7**], acetohydroxamic acid [**8**] and hydroxide anion. $[Fe^{3+}]_{total} = 10^{-6}$ M; $[Ligand]_{total} = 10^{-5}$ M

Scheme 27.2 Dissociation of bidentate, tridentate and hexadentate ligand–iron(III) complexes

$$Fe(L_B)_3 \underset{}{\overset{K'_d}{\rightleftharpoons}} Fe^{III} + 3\,L_B \qquad K'_d = \frac{[Fe^{III}][L_B]^3}{[Fe(L_B)^3]}$$

$$Fe(L_T)_2 \underset{}{\overset{K''_d}{\rightleftharpoons}} Fe^{III} + 2\,L_T \qquad K''_d = \frac{[Fe^{III}][L_T]^2}{[Fe(L_T)_2]}$$

$$FeL_H \underset{}{\overset{K'''_d}{\rightleftharpoons}} Fe^{III} + L_H \qquad K'''_d = \frac{[Fe^{III}][L_H]}{[FeL_H]}$$

L_B, bidentate; L_T, tridentate; L_H, hexadentate ligand

2.2 *Iron(III) Ligand Selection*

High-spin iron(III) is a spherically symmetrical tripositive cation of radius 0.65 Å. By virtue of the resulting high charge density, iron(III) forms most stable bonds with ligands containing weakly polarizable atoms, such as oxygen. It is for this reason that the majority of siderophores utilize dioxo ligands, such as catechol and hydroxamate. The affinity of such compounds for iron(III) reflects the pKa values of the chelating oxygen atoms: the higher the affinity for iron(III), the higher the pKa value (Table 27.3).

2.2.1 Catechols

Catechol moieties possess a high affinity for iron(III). This extremely strong interaction with tripositive metal cations results from the high electron density of both oxygen atoms. However, this high charge density is also associated with the high affinity for protons (pKa values, 12.1 and 8.4). Thus, the

Table 27.3 pKa values and affinity constants of dioxobidentate ligands for iron(III)

Ligand	Structure	pKa_1	pKa_2	$Log\beta_3$	pFe^{3+}
N,N-Dimethyl-2,3-dihydroxybenzamide (DMB) [**7**]	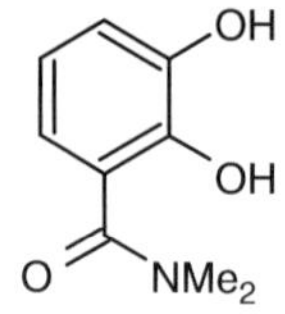	8.4	12.1	40.2	15
Acetohydroxamic acid [**8**]	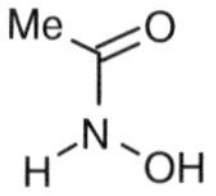	–	9.4	28.3	13
2-Methyl-3-hydroxy-pyran-4-one (maltol) [**9**]	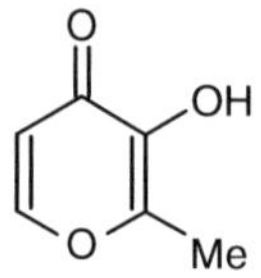	–	8.7	28.5	15
1-Hydroxypyridin-2-one [**10**]	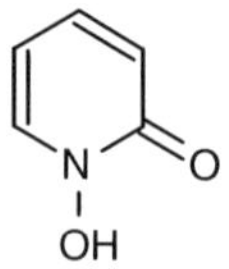	–	5.8	27	16
1-Methyl-3-hydroxy-pyridin-2-one [**11**]	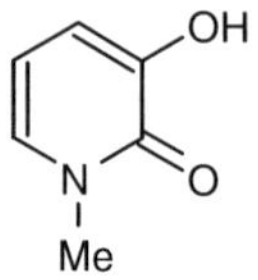	0.2	8.6	32	16
1,2-Dimethyl-3-hydroxy-pyridin-4-one (deferiprone) [**12**]	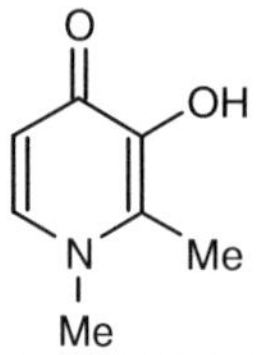	3.6	9.9	37.4	20

$pFe^{3+} = -\log[Fe^{3+}]$ when $[Fe^{3+}]_{total} = 10^{-6}$ M and $[ligand]_{total} = 10^{-5}$ M at pH 7.4

binding of cations by catechol has marked pH sensitivity [10]. The complexes forming at pH 7.0 each bear a net charge and, consequently, are unlikely to permeate membranes by simple diffusion. Therefore, these charged iron complexes will tend to be trapped in intracellular compartments. For simple bidentate catechols, the 2:1 complex is the dominant form in the pH range 5.5–7.5 (Fig. 27.4a). With such complexes, the iron atom is not completely protected from the solvent and, consequently, is able to interact with hydrogen peroxide or oxygen, possibly resulting in the generation of hydroxyl radicals. An additional problem with catechol-based ligands is their susceptibility towards oxidation [10].

2.2.2 Hydroxamates

The hydroxamate moiety possesses a lower affinity for iron than catechol. However, it has the advantage of forming neutral *tris*-complexes with iron(III) which are, in principle, able to permeate membranes by non-facilitated diffusion. The selectivity of hydroxamates, like catechols, favors tribasic cations over dibasic cations (Table 27.1). Because of the relatively low protonation constant (pKa ~9), hydrogen ion interference at physiological pH is less pronounced than for that of catechol ligands;

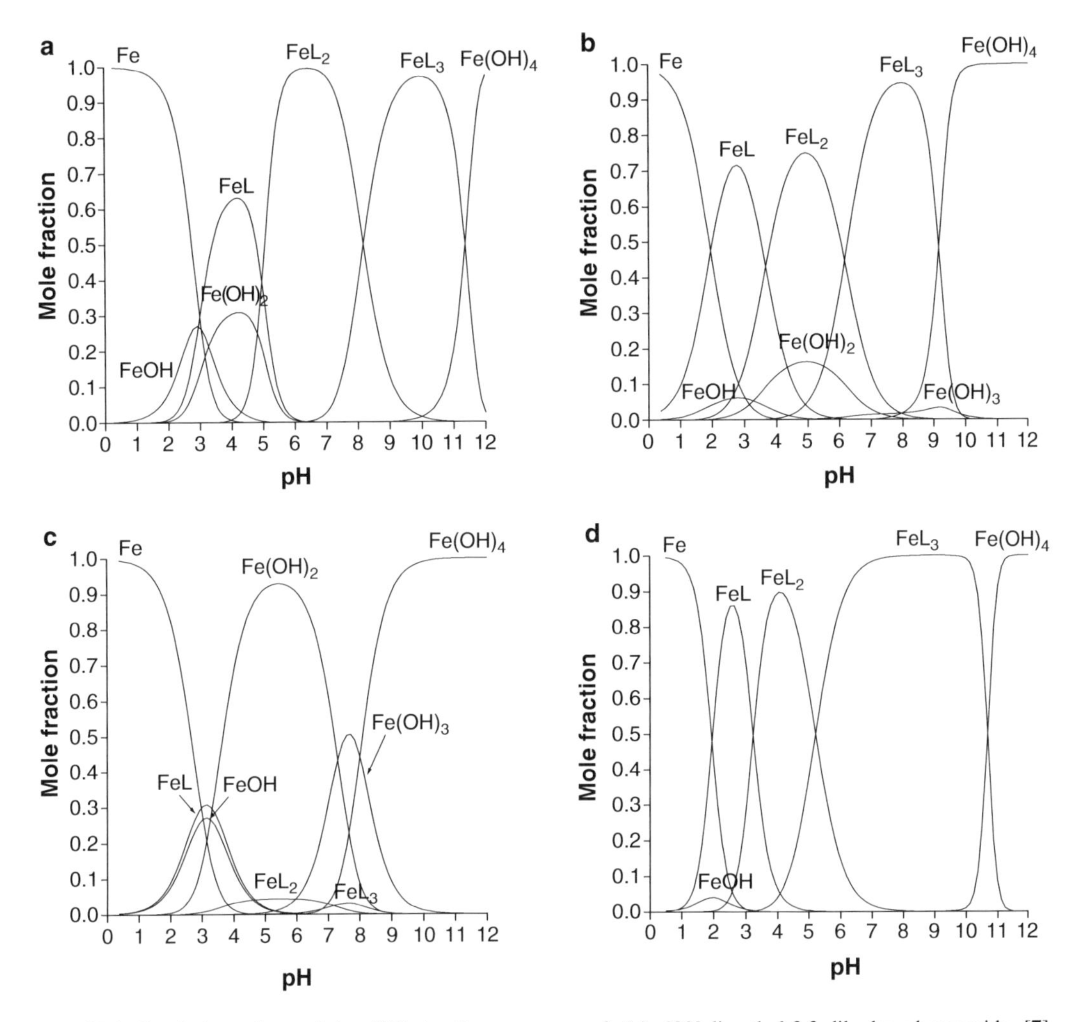

Fig. 27.4 Speciation plots of iron(III) in the presence of (**a**) *N,N*-dimethyl-2,3-dihydroxybenzamide [**7**], $[Fe^{3+}]_{total} = 1 \times 10^{-6}$ M; [Ligand] = 1×10^{-5} M; (**b**) acetohydroxamic acid [**8**], $[Fe^{3+}]_{total} = 1 \times 10^{-6}$ M; [Ligand] = 1×10^{-4} M; (**c**) acetohydroxamic acid [**8**], $[Fe^{3+}]_{total} = 1 \times 10^{-6}$ M; [Ligand] = 1×10^{-5} M; (**d**) 1,2-dimethyl-3-hydroxypyridin-4-one [**12**], $[Fe^{3+}]_{total} = 1 \times 10^{-6}$ M; [Ligand] = 1×10^{-5} M

consequently, the 3:1 complex predominates at pH 7.0 when sufficient ligand is present (Fig. 27.4b). However, the affinity of a simple bidentate hydroxamate ligand for iron is insufficient to solubilize iron(III) at pH 7.4 at clinically achievable concentrations (Fig. 27.4c); thus, only bis bidentate and hexadentate hydroxamates are likely to be effective iron(III) scavengers under such conditions. Many hydroxamates are metabolically labile and are only poorly absorbed via the oral route. Numerous approaches have been taken to address this problem; however, to date no suitable hydroxamate derivative has been identified which possesses a comparable activity to that of subcutaneous DFO.

2.2.3 Hydroxypyridinones

Hydroxypyridinones (HPOs) combine characteristics of both hydroxamate and catechol groups, forming five-membered chelate rings in which the metal is coordinated by two vicinal oxygen atoms. The hydroxypyridinones are monoprotic acids at pH 7.0 and thus form neutral *tris*-iron(III) complexes.

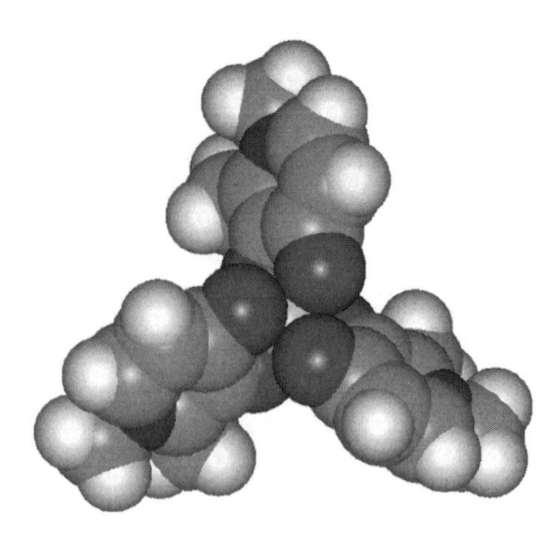

Fig. 27.5 Energy-minimized structure of the 3:1 iron(III) complex of 1,2-dimethyl-3-hydroxypyridin-4-one [**12**]

The affinity of such compounds for iron(III) reflects the pKa values of the chelating oxygen atoms: the higher the affinity for iron(III), the higher the pKa value (Table 27.3). There are three classes of metal-chelating HPO ligands, namely 1-hydroxypyridin-2-one [**10**], 3-hydroxypyridin-2-one [**11**] and 3-hydroxypyridin-4-one [**12**]. Of these, the pyridin-4-ones possess the highest affinity for iron(III) (Table 27.3) and are selective for tribasic metal cations over dibasic cations (Table 27.1). The surprisingly high pKa value of the carbonyl function of 3-hydroxypyridin-4-ones results from extensive delocalization of the lone pair associated with the ring nitrogen atom. The pyridin-4-ones form neutral 3:1 complexes with iron(III) (Fig. 27.5), which are stable over a wide range of pH values (Fig. 27.4d). Although catechol derivatives possess higher β_3 values than those of 3-hydroxypyridin-4-one, the corresponding pFe^{3+} values are lower (Table 27.3). This difference is due to the relatively high affinity of catechol for protons. Thus, of all dioxygen ligand classes, 3-hydroxypyridin-4-ones possess the greatest affinity for iron(III) in the physiological pH range [5–8], as indicated by their respective pFe^{3+} values (Table 27.3).

2.2.4 Aminocarboxylates

Aminocarboxylate ligands are excellent iron(III)-chelating agents. Several polycarboxylate ligands, such as ethylenediaminetetraacetic acid (EDTA) [**13**] and diethylenetriaminepentaacetic acid (DTPA) [**14**], have been widely investigated for their iron-chelating abilities. However, the selectivity of these molecules for iron(III) is relatively poor (Table 27.1). This lack of selectivity leads to zinc depletion in patients receiving aminocarboxylate-based ligands such as DTPA.

2.2.5 Hydroxycarboxylates

Hydroxycarboxylate ligands are strong chelating agents, which are more selective for iron(III) than the corresponding aminocarboxylates due to all the coordinating atoms being oxygen. The interaction between iron(III) and citrate [**15**] has been well characterized [11], but by virtue of its tridentate nature, a large number of complexes have been identified [12]. In contrast, hexadentate hydroxycarboxylate ligands, for instance staphloferrin [**16**] and rhizoferrin [**17**], have simple iron(III) complex chemistries dominated by the formation of 1:1 complexes [13].

3 Critical Features for Clinical Application

3.1 Lipophilicity and Molecular Weight

In order for a chelating agent to exert its pharmacological effect, a drug must be able to reach the target sites at sufficient concentration. Hence, the key property for an orally active iron chelator is its ability to be efficiently absorbed from the gastrointestinal tract and to cross biological membranes, thereby gaining access to the desired target sites such as the liver. There are three major factors which influence the ability of a compound to freely permeate a lipid membrane, namely lipophilicity, ionization state and molecular size.

In order to achieve efficient oral absorption, the chelator should possess appreciable lipid solubility which may facilitate the molecule to penetrate the gastrointestinal tract (partition coefficient greater than 0.2) [14]. However, highly lipid-soluble chelators can also penetrate most cells and critical barriers such as the blood-brain and placental barriers, thereby enhancing possible toxic side effects. Membrane permeability can also be affected by the ionic state of the compound. Uncharged molecules penetrate cell membranes more rapidly than charged molecules. It is for this reason that aminocarboxylate-containing ligands are unlikely to possess high oral activity.

Molecular size is another critical factor which influences the rate of drug absorption [15, 16]. Non-facilitated diffusion is generally considered to be dominant for drugs with molecular weights <200. The transcellular route involves diffusion into the enterocyte and thus utilizes some 95% of the surface of the small intestine. In contrast, the paracellular route only utilizes a small fraction of the total surface area, and the corresponding flux via this route is much smaller. The "cut-off" molecular weight for the paracellular route in the human small intestine is approximately 400, and this route is unlikely to be quantitatively important for molecules with molecular weights >200. There is no clear "cut-off" value for the transcellular route, but as judged by PEG permeability, penetration falls off rapidly with molecular weights >500 [17]. Thus in order to achieve greater than 70% absorption, subsequent to oral application, the chelator molecular weight probably needs to be less than 500. This molecular weight limit provides a considerable restriction on the choice of chelator and may effectively exclude hexadentate ligands from consideration; most siderophores, for instance DFO, have molecular weights in the range 500–900. Although EDTA has a molecular weight of only 292, it is too small to fully encompass the chelated iron, thereby facilitating the potential toxicity of the metal. Bidentate and tridentate ligands, by virtue of their much lower molecular weights, are predicted to possess higher absorption efficiencies. The fraction of the absorbed dose for a range of bidentate 3-hydroxypyridin-4-ones has typically been found to fall between 60% and 90%.

3.2 Chelator Disposition

The metabolic properties of chelating agents also play a critical role in determining both their efficacy and toxicity. It is important to ensure that the agent is not degraded to metabolites which lack the ability to bind iron. Such properties will inevitably require the use of higher chelator levels, thereby increasing the risk of inducing toxicity. Chelators are likely to be more resistant to metabolism if their backbones lack ester and amide links and, to a lesser extent, hydroxamate links. The catechol function is a disadvantage with respect to metabolism as there are numerous enzymes specifically designed to modify the catechol entity, for instance catechol-*O*-methyl transferase and tyrosinase.

Ideally, for maximal scavenging effect, a chelator must be present within the extracellular fluids at a reasonable concentration (10–25 μM) and for a sufficient length of time to ensure interception of iron from both the extracellular and intracellular pools. Compounds with short plasma half-lives are thus likely to be less effective due to the limited pool of chelatable iron present within the body at any one time. DFO possesses a very short plasma half-life, and it is for this reason that the molecule is administered via an infusion pump.

3.3 Toxicity

The toxicity associated with iron chelators originates from a number of factors, including inhibition of iron-containing metalloenzymes, lack of metal selectivity (which may lead to the deficiency of other physiologically important metals, such as zinc(II)), redox cycling of iron complexes between iron(II) and iron(III) (thereby generating free radicals), and the kinetic lability of the iron complex, leading to iron redistribution.

3.3.1 Metal Selectivity

An ideal iron chelator should be highly selective for iron(III) in order to minimize chelation of other biologically essential metal ions which could lead to deficiency with prolonged usage. Unfortunately, many ligands that possess a high affinity for iron(III) may also have appreciable affinities for other metals, such as zinc(II), this being especially so with carboxylate- and nitrogen-containing ligands. However, this is less of a problem with the oxygen-containing bidentate catechol, hydroxamate and hydroxypyridinone ligand families which possess a strong preference for tribasic over dibasic cations (Table 27.1).

Although, in principle, competition with copper(II) could be a problem, under most biological conditions, it is not so, as copper is extremely tightly bound to proteins and the unbound intracellular fraction is reported to be less than 10^{-20} M [18]. Copper is exchanged between proteins via specialized high-affinity chaperone molecules.

3.3.2 Complex Structure

In order to prevent free radical production, iron should be coordinated in such a manner as to avoid direct access of oxygen and hydrogen peroxide. Most hexadentate ligands, such as DFO, are kinetically inert and reduce hydroxyl radical production to a minimum by entirely masking the surface of the iron (Fig. 27.1). However, not all hexadentate ligands are of sufficient dimensions to entirely mask the surface of the bound iron, in which case the resulting complex may enhance the ability of iron to generate free radicals. This phenomenon is particularly marked at neutral or alkaline pH values when the solubility of noncomplexed iron(III) is severely limited. The classic example of this type of behavior is demonstrated by EDTA, where a seventh coordination site is occupied by a water molecule [19]. This water molecule is kinetically labile and is capable of rapidly exchanging with oxygen, hydrogen peroxide and many other ligands present in biological media.

In contrast to the kinetically stable ferrioxamine complex (Fig. 27.1), bidentate and tridentate ligands are kinetically more labile, and the iron(III) complexes tend to dissociate at low ligand concentrations (Scheme 27.3). Partial dissociation of bi- and tridentate ligand–iron complexes renders the iron(III) cation surface accessible to other ligands. The concentration dependence of 3-hydroxypyridin-4-one iron complex speciation is minimal at pH 7.4 when the ligand concentration is above 1 μM due to the relatively high affinity of the ligand for iron(III). Thus, bidentate 3-hydroxypyridin-4-ones behave more like hexadentate ligands as the 3:1 complex is the dominant species at pH 7.4 (Fig. 27.4d) and the iron atom is completely coordinated (Fig. 27.5).

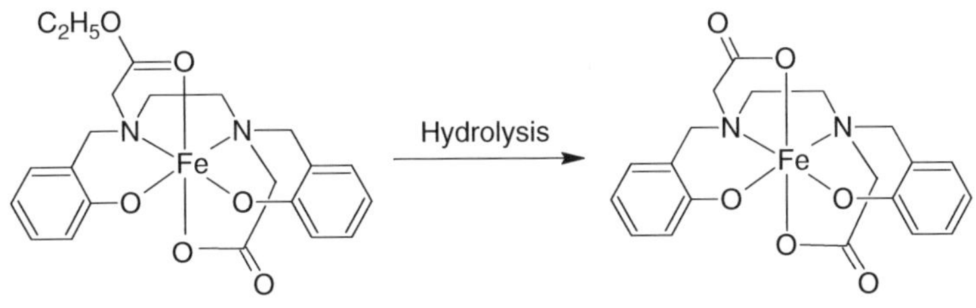

HBED monoester (**21**) : Fe(III) complex — Hydrolysis → HBED (**20**) : Fe(III) complex

Scheme 27.3 The ester hydrolysis of the iron(III) complex of the monoethyl ester derivative of HBED [**21**], leading to the formation of HBED [**20**]

3.3.3 Redox Activity

Chelators that bind both iron(II) and iron(III) are capable of redox cycling, a property that has been utilized by a wide range of enzymes and industrial catalysts. However, this is an undesirable property for iron-scavenging molecules as redox cycling can lead to the production of hydroxyl radicals. Significantly, the high selectivity of siderophores for iron(III) over iron(II) renders redox cycling under biological conditions unlikely. Chelators which utilize nitrogen tend to possess lower redox potentials, and the coordinated iron can be reduced enzymatically under biological conditions. Such complexes may redox cycle under aerobic conditions, generating oxygen radicals. Ideally, a therapeutic iron chelator will lock iron in the iron(III) state, thereby preventing redox activity.

3.3.4 Enzyme Inhibition

In general, iron chelators do not directly inhibit heme-containing enzymes due to the inaccessibility of porphyrin-bound iron to chelating agents. In contrast, many non-heme iron-containing enzymes, such as the lipoxygenase and aromatic hydroxylase families, and ribonucleotide reductase are susceptible to chelator-induced inhibition [20]. Lipoxygenases are generally inhibited by hydrophobic chelators; therefore, the introduction of hydrophilic characteristics into a chelator tends to minimise such inhibitory potential. Although this relationship holds with hydroxypyridinones, where the size of the alkyl substitution is increased in the 1-position of the pyridinone ring, in an essentially linear manner, it is less evident for compounds with large substituents in the 2-position. In fact, the variation in the inhibitory properties of the HPO chelators possessing different R_2 substituents is more dependent on the size of the substituent than the lipophilicity of the chelator. The introduction of a hydrophilic substituent at the 2-position of hydroxypyridinones markedly reduces the inhibitory properties, in general, presumably due to steric interference of the chelation process at the enzyme active site [21]. In contrast, lipophilicity is reported to be the dominant factor in controlling the ability of HPO chelators to inhibit mammalian tyrosine hydroxylase, hydrophilic chelators ($\text{LogP} \leq -1.0$) tending to be relatively weak inhibitors of this enzyme. Clearly, by careful modification of their physicochemical properties, iron chelators can be designed to exert minimal inhibitory influence on many metalloenzymes.

3.3.5 Hydrophilicity

Although bidentate and tridentate ligands possess a clear advantage over hexadentate ligands with respect to oral bioavailability, their enhanced ability to permeate membranes renders them potentially more toxic. Thus, the penetration of the blood–brain barrier (BBB) is one of the likely side effects associated with bidentate and tridentate ligands. The ability of a compound to penetrate the BBB is critically dependent on the partition coefficient as well as the molecular weight. BBB permeability is predicted to be low for most hexadentate compounds, by virtue of their higher molecular weight. With low-molecular-weight molecules (MW <300), penetration is largely dependent on the lipophilicity, and molecules with partition coefficients <0.05 tend to penetrate inefficiently. Thus, chelators with partition coefficients lower than this critical value are predicted to show poor entry into the central nervous system. Indeed, brain penetration of 3-hydroxypyridin-4-ones is strongly dependent on their lipophilicity [22], a clear correlation being observed between BBB permeability and the percentage polar surface area of the molecule. Thus, 1,ω-hydroxyalkyl hydroxypyridinones (e.g. [**18**]) penetrate the BBB much more slowly than the simple 1-alkyl derivatives (e.g. [**19**]). These results suggest that the biological distribution pattern of the HPOs can be significantly altered by simple modification of chemical structure without compromising their pharmacological function (selective iron chelation).

4 Iron(III) Chelators Currently Under Investigation for Clinical Use

4.1 Hexadentate Chelators

4.1.1 Deferoxamine

Naturally occurring siderophores provide excellent models for the development of therapeutic useful iron chelators. Indeed, deferoxamine (DFO) [**1**], a growth-promoting agent secreted by the microorganism *Streptomyces pilosus*, is presently widely used for the clinical treatment of chronic iron overload. DFO is a *tris*-hydroxamic acid derivative and chelates ferric iron in a 1:1 molar ratio. It possesses an extremely high affinity for iron(III) and a much lower affinity for other metal ions present in biological fluids, such as zinc, calcium and magnesium (Table 27.1). Although DFO is a large and a highly hydrophilic molecule ($D_{7.4}$=0.01), it gains entry into the liver via a facilitated transport system. It can therefore interact with both hepatocellular and extracellular iron, promoting urinary and biliary iron excretion [23]. Ferrioxamine, the DFO–iron complex (Fig. 27.1), is kinetically inert and possesses a relatively low lipophilicity and thus is unlikely to enter cells. This property reduces the potential of iron redistribution. However, DFO is far from being an ideal therapeutic agent due to its oral inactivity and rapid renal clearance (plasma half-life of 5–10 min) (Table 27.4). In order to achieve sufficient iron excretion, it has to be administered subcutaneously or intravenously for 8–12 h a day, 5–7 days a week. Consequently, patient compliance with this expensive and cumbersome regimen is often poor.

In an attempt to improve the oral bioavailability of this chelator, a range of DFO prodrugs obtained via esterification of the labile hydroxamate functions have been investigated [24]. However, only

Table 27.4 Comparison of deferoxamine, deferasirox and deferiprone

	Deferoxamine	Deferasirox	Deferiprone
Iron chelator ratio of stable complex at pH 7.4	1:1	1:2	1:3
$\log D_{7.4}$ of ligand	−2	1.0	−0.77
Molecular weight of free ligand/iron complex	560/613	373/798	139/470
Ionization state of iron complex at pH 7.4	1^+	3^-	0
pFe^{3+}	26	22.5	20.6
Plasma half-life	5–10 min	8–16 h	1–2 h
Typical dosage (mg/kg/day)	40	20–40	75–100

marginal improvement in oral activity was found with tetra-acyl derivatives, and none have been identified which possess comparable activity to that of subcutaneous DFO. Several strategies centered on modification of the DFO backbone have also been pursued [25]. Unfortunately, no lead compound has yet emerged for further development.

4.1.2 Aminocarboxylates

DTPA [**14**] is an aminocarboxylate hexadentate ligand and has been used in patients who develop toxic side effects with DFO. Due to its net charge at neutral pH, DTPA is largely confined to extracellular compartments in vivo and is excreted in the urine within 24 h of administration. DTPA is not orally active and, due to its relative lack of selectivity for iron(III), leads to zinc depletion. Consequently, zinc supplementation is required to prevent the toxic sequelae of such depletion.

In order to enhance the selectivity of the aminocarboxylate ligands for iron(III), several analogues which contain both carboxyl and phenolic ligands have been designed [26]. A particularly useful compound is *N,N′*-bis(2-hydroxybenzyl)-ethylenediamine-*N,N′*-diacetic acid (HBED) [**20**], which is significantly more effective than DFO when given intramuscularly to iron-overloaded rats [27]. It binds ferric iron strongly with an overall stability constant (log K_1) of 40 and a pFe^{3+} value of 31, rendering this molecule a potent ligand for chelation of iron in vivo. Unfortunately, HBED is not efficiently absorbed via the oral route in man because of the zwitterionic nature of the molecule. Consequently, a considerable effort has been placed into the design of HBED ester prodrugs. Pitt et al. demonstrated oral activity for a number of HBED diester derivatives [28]; however, the rate of hydrolysis of simple alkyl esters was found to be slow, particularly in primate, and the efficacy of the compounds, disappointing. In addition, many of the compounds were found to be neurotoxic, the esters apparently crossing the blood-brain barrier. Significantly, this series of compounds possesses a relatively small molecular weight (MW <500) as compared with the majority of hexadentate ligands. These investigations were extended to include a wider range of ester and amide derivatives [29], and a compound of particular interest was found to be the HBED monoethyl ester [**21**], which possesses good oral availability [30]. The reasons for the efficacy of this compound are probably manifold, including a disruption of intramolecular H-bonding, thereby improving water solubility; an enhancement of partition constant; the ability of the monoester to bind iron(III); and the activation of ester hydrolysis of the resulting iron(III) complex (Scheme 27.3). Unfortunately, by virtue of the presence of the two nitrogen ligands, HBED retains a relatively high affinity for zinc (Log $K_1 = 18.4$) and therefore would be predicted to induce undesirable side effects due to the coordination of endogenous zinc. The monoester [**21**] was not developed for clinical studies due to adverse toxicity of the molecule.

4.1.3 Catechols

Hexadentate tricatechols are iron(III) chelators par excellence, enterobactin [**4**] typifying the group. However, such molecules possess a relatively high molecular weight, and therefore, their oral bioavailability is poor, particularly at clinically useful doses. A further complication with such molecules is that they adopt a high net negative charge when coordinated to iron(III), which tends to minimize their rate of efflux by non-facilitated diffusion. A number of synthetic analogues have been prepared, which retain the high affinity for iron(III) typical of enterobactin and yet are more stable under biological conditions, for instance MECAM [**6**]. Unfortunately, many of these hexadentate catechols bind to the enterobactin receptor expressed by many pathogenic organisms and hence will supply iron to such bacteria, an undesirable feature for clinical use [31].

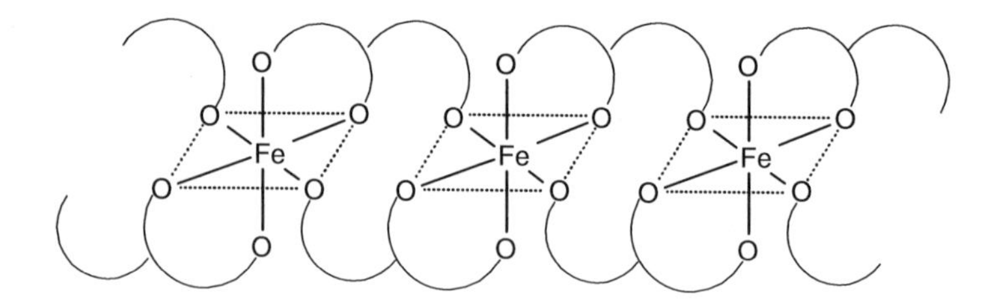

Scheme 27.4 Schematic representation of the polymerization of a tridentate iron complex

4.1.4 Hydroxypyridinones

Hexadentate siderophore analogues can be constructed by derivatizing prototype bidentate hydroxypyridinones and attaching them to suitable molecular frameworks. Although enterobactin [**4**] has an extremely high stability constant for iron(III), the effectiveness of this molecule and its analogues under acid conditions is limited by their weak acid nature and the required loss of six protons on binding iron(III). In contrast, hydroxypyridinones are stronger acids than catechols, and since they are monoprotic, hexadentate ligands formed from three such units only loose three protons on formation of a six-coordinated complex. Thus, hexadentate HPOs compete well with hexadentate catechols at neutral pH values. Another potential advantage of these molecules is that they are not recognized by siderophore receptors and are therefore less likely to donate iron to pathogenic organisms.

Several hexadentate ligands based on the 1-hydroxypyridin-2-one and the 3-hydroxypyridin-2-one moiety have been investigated, such as [**22**] [32], [**23**] [33] and [**24**] [34]. Although the pFe^{3+} values of the hexadentate ligands were significantly higher (approximately 7 and 8 log units) than those of the corresponding bidentate ligands, a clear decrease in the formation constants of up to 2 log units was observed with the hexadentate ligands when compared to the bidentate analogues, indicating the lack of ligand predisposition for metal binding. In order to provide the correct geometry for metal binding, it is important to attach the molecular scaffold to the *ortho* position to the chelating oxygens. A synthetic route which adopts this strategy has been developed for constructing hexadentate ligands from the 3-hydroxypyridin-4-one unit. This method leads to hexadentate 3-hydroxypyridin-4-ones [**25**] which possess the appropriate geometry for iron chelation and thus bind iron(III) with greater affinity than any of the previously prepared oligomeric hydroxypyridinones [35].

By virtue of their higher molecular weight, hexadentate pyridinones, like siderophores, possess low oral bioavailability.

4.2 *Tridentate Chelators*

A potential problem associated with all tridentate ligands is that, unlike bidentate and most hexadentate compounds, there is a possibility of polymeric structure formation (Scheme 27.4). Such structures are difficult to clear via the kidney and are likely to become trapped within cells. Without exception, tridentate ligands with a high affinity for iron(III) include a nitrogen atom as a ligand.

4.2.1 Desferrithiocins

Desferrithiocin (DFT) [**26**] is a siderophore isolated from *Streptomyces antibioticus*. It forms a 2:1 complex with iron(III) at neutral pH using a phenolate oxygen, a carboxylate oxygen and a nitrogen atom as ligands [36]. It possesses a high affinity for ferric iron (Log $\beta_2 = 29.6$); however, by virtue of the presence of the nitrogen and carboxylate ligands, it also binds zinc tightly. Long-term studies of DFT in normal rodents and dogs at low doses have shown toxic side effects [37]. A range of synthetic

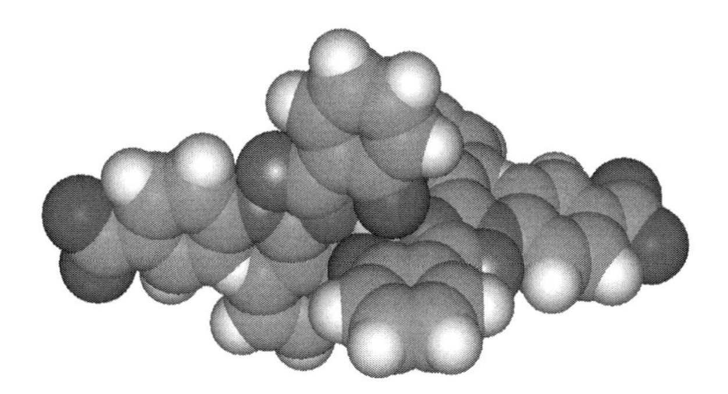

Fig. 27.6 Energy-minimized structure of the 2:1 iron(III) complex of deferasirox [**28**]

analogues of DFT have been prepared, and recently a PEG-conjugated analogue has been demonstrated to possess excellent iron-scavenging properties in both rodents and primates [38]. Compound [**27**] has been reported to be particularly effective and is currently in clinical trials.

4.2.2 Triazoles

Triazoles have been investigated as ligands by Novartis [39]. These compounds chelate iron(III) with two phenolate oxygens and one triazolyl nitrogen. The lead compound 4-(3,5-bis(2-hydroxy-phenyl)-1*H*-1,2,4-triazol-1-yl)benzoic acid (deferasirox; [**28**]) possesses a pFe^{3+} value of 22.5 and is extremely hydrophobic, with a logP value of 3.8 and a $logD_{7.4}$ value of 1.0 (Table 27.4) [40]. As a result, it can penetrate membranes easily and possesses good oral availability. It is highly effective at removing iron from iron-loaded animals and is the current lead orally active iron chelator of Novartis [41].

The high hydrophobicity of this chelator is undesirable; indeed, the logP value indicates that deferasirox is predicted to accumulate in tissue and to gain access to a wide variety of cells. However, the extremely high logP value also ensures that deferasirox binds to plasma proteins, and this property will, to some extent, limit body distribution. Deferasirox is efficiently extracted by the liver; indeed, virtually all induced iron excretion is via the bile, very little being excreted in the urine [40]. The triazole [**28**] forms a 2:1 iron complex (Fig. 27.6) which possesses a net charge of 3^- and a molecular weight over 800. Should such a complex form intracellularly, it is possible that, as with tricatechols, the iron will remain trapped within the cell. The triazoles can exist in two conformations: one, a tridentate structure; and the alternate, a bis bidentate structure with a strong tendency to form polymeric complexes (Scheme 27.5). The latter conformation favors zinc(II) binding since 50% of the coordinating ligands are nitrogen [42]. Despite these apparent drawbacks, deferasirox is currently widely investigated in clinical trials [43, 44].

4.2.3 PIH Analogues

Pyridoxal isonicotinoyl hydrazone (PIH) [**29**], together with a wide range of analogues, has been subjected to extensive evaluation as iron(III) chelators. Many have been demonstrated to be orally active in rodents. The efficiency of in vivo iron removal increases with lipophilicity of both the ligand and the iron complex, but as more lipophilic chelators are likely to be associated with enhanced toxicity, log P values close to unity are preferred. Many of the PIH analogues are uncharged at neutral pH values and therefore gain ready access to cells; indeed, salicylaldehyde isonicotinoyl hydrazone (SIH) [**30**] gains entry to a range of cell types more rapidly than most other chelators, including the smaller hydroxypyridinones [45]. The binding of iron(III) by PIH and related ligands is complicated because of the existence of a number of dissociable protons both in the free and coordinated

a

Tridentate conformation

b

bis bidentate conformation

Scheme 27.5 Two possible conformations of the triazole derivatives (**a**) the tridentate conformation and (**b**) the bis bidentate conformation. The bis bidentate structure has a strong tendency to form polymeric complexes via the two opposing bidentate sites

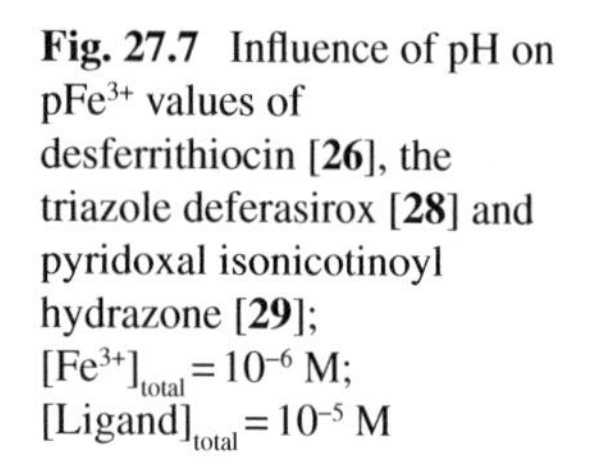

Fig. 27.7 Influence of pH on pFe^{3+} values of desferrithiocin [**26**], the triazole deferasirox [**28**] and pyridoxal isonicotinoyl hydrazone [**29**]; $[Fe^{3+}]_{total} = 10^{-6}$ M; $[Ligand]_{total} = 10^{-5}$ M

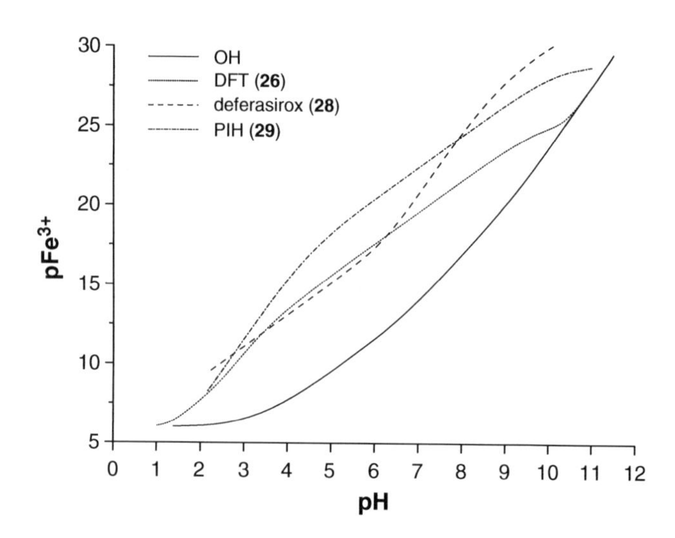

states. Nevertheless, the 2:1 complex is the favored species over the pH range of 4–8, and the affinity for iron(III) compares well with other tridentate ligands (Fig. 27.7).

PIH was selected for human balance studies because the two components of the condensed molecule, isoniazid and pyridoxal, have been safely used to treat tuberculosis. No significant toxicity was observed at a dose of 30 mg kg^{-1} day^{-1} for 6 days, but iron excretion at this dose was insufficient to produce negative iron balance. This dose is much lower than those used in animals (typically >100 mg kg^{-1}), and ideally, the study should be repeated at a higher dose. However, the two nitrogen atoms in the coordinating sphere of the complex (Fig. 27.8) enable PIH analogues to bind iron(II) with appreciable affinity and will therefore facilitate redox cycling.

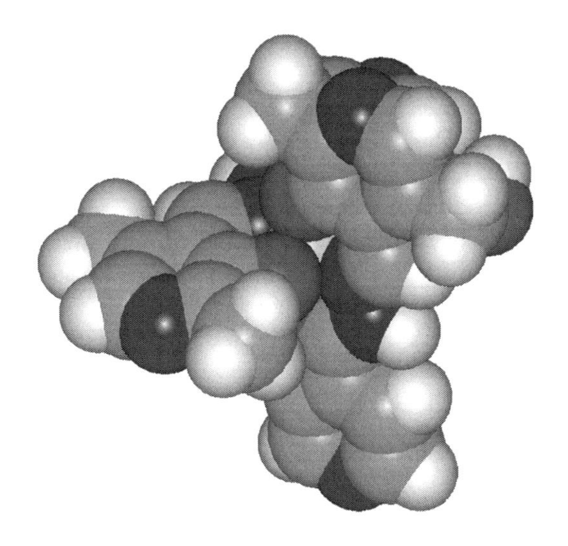

Fig. 27.8 Energy-minimised structure of the 2:1 iron(III) complex of pyridoxal isonicotinoyl hydrazone [**29**]

4.3 Bidentate Chelators

On the basis of selectivity and affinity, particularly considering the pFe^{3+} value, 3-hydroxypyridin-4-one is the optimal bidentate ligand for the chelation of iron(III) over the pH range of 6.0–9.0 (Table 27.3) [46].

4.3.1 Dialkylhydroxypyridinones

The 1,2-dimethyl derivative (deferiprone) [**12**] is currently available for clinical use (marketed by Apotex Inc., Toronto, Canada, as Ferriprox™). The dose required to keep a previously well-chelated patient in negative iron balance with Ferriprox™ is relatively high, in the region of 75 to 100 mg/kg/day [47]. One of the major reasons for the limited efficacy of deferiprone in clinical use is that it undergoes extensive phase II metabolism in the liver. The 3-hydroxyl functionality, which is crucial for scavenging iron, is a prime target for glucuronidation. Urinary recovery studies conducted on deferiprone in man have shown that >85% of the administered dose is recovered in the urine as the non-chelating 3-*O*-glucuronide conjugate [48]. By virtue of the neutral nature of the iron–deferiprone complex (Table 27.4), deferiprone is able to remove elevated levels of iron from cardiac and endocrine tissue [49]. Deferiprone is used worldwide and has been reported to be a highly effective iron chelator in many clinical situations [50, 51]. Indeed, deferiprone has recently found application in the treatment of Friedreich's ataxia [52, 53].

The 1,2-diethyl 3-hydroxypyridin-4-one (CP94, [**19**]) has also been investigated [52–56]. This chelator has been found to be more efficient at iron removal than deferiprone in several mammalian species. The presumed reason for the greater efficacy of CP94 in the rat is its unusual phase I metabolic pathway which leads to the formation of the 2-(1′-hydroxyethyl) metabolite [**31**] [48]. This metabolite does not undergo further phase II metabolism to form a glucuronide conjugate and hence retains the ability to chelate iron. Promising results obtained in rat models led to the limited clinical evaluation of CP94 in thalassemic patients. Unfortunately, the metabolism of CP94 in man does not parallel that of the rat, the main urinary metabolite of CP94 in man being the 3-*O*-glucuronide conjugate (>85%) [55]. Extensive conversion to this metabolite was found to severely limit clinical efficacy.

4.3.2 "High pFe^{3+}" Hydroxypyridinones

Chelators with high pFe^{3+} values are predicted to scavenge iron more effectively at low ligand concentrations. In order to further improve chelation efficacy and minimize drug-induced toxicity, considerable effort has been applied to the design of novel hydroxypyridinones with enhanced pFe^{3+} values [9, 57]. Novartis synthesized a range of bidentate hydroxypyridinone ligands, which possess an aromatic substituent at the 2-position. The aromatic group is reported to stabilize the resulting iron complex and hence increase the pFe^{3+} values. The lead compound [**32**] was found to be orally active [58] and highly effective at removing iron from both the iron-loaded rat and marmoset. In a parallel study, it has been demonstrated that the introduction of a 1′-hydroxyalkyl group [**31**] [9] or an amido function [**33**] [57] at the 2-position of 3-hydroxypyridin-4-ones enhances the affinity for iron(III) in the pH range 5–8. This effect results from stabilizing the ionized species due to the combined effect of intramolecular hydrogen bonding between the 2-(1′-hydroxyl) group or the 2-amido substituent with the adjacent 3-hydroxyl function and electron withdrawal from the pyridinone ring. Although such an effect reduces the overall iron(III) stability constant, it also reduces the pKa values of the chelating function. These combined changes result in an increase in the corresponding pFe^{3+} values. Interestingly, the Novartis compound [**32**] also possesses a 1′-hydroxyl group at the 2-position, and this is almost certainly responsible for the observed enhanced pFe^{3+} value.

These novel high pFe^{3+} HPOs show great promise in their ability to remove iron under in vivo conditions. [**33**] is a highly effective compound ($pFe^{3+}=22.8$), when compared with deferiprone ($pFe^{3+}=20.6$). It is highly hydrophilic ($D_{7.4}=0.17$) and yet experiences good oral absorption and liver extraction, as demonstrated by its high efficacy in animal models. Such low lipophilicity will severely limit the distribution of the chelator, which in turn could possibly minimize the potential toxicity. Furthermore, the improved efficacy could lead to the use of lower doses, which again would be predicted to be associated with lower toxicity.

5 Conclusions

During the past 30 years, many attempts have been directed towards the design of nontoxic, orally active iron chelators, but only two clinically useful compounds have emerged to date, deferiprone and deferasirox (Table 27.4). Since 2000, a number of significant advances have been made, and it is likely that other more efficacious orally active chelators will join these two compounds. The successful introduction of such compounds will impact considerably on the therapeutic outcome and quality of life for the thalassemic and sickle cell population. There is a potential for iron chelation in a wider range of clinical situations, and once an orally active chelator has been clinically proven in thalassemic patients, such compounds will almost certainly find application for the treatment of other disease states, possibly including neurodegeneration [59, 60].

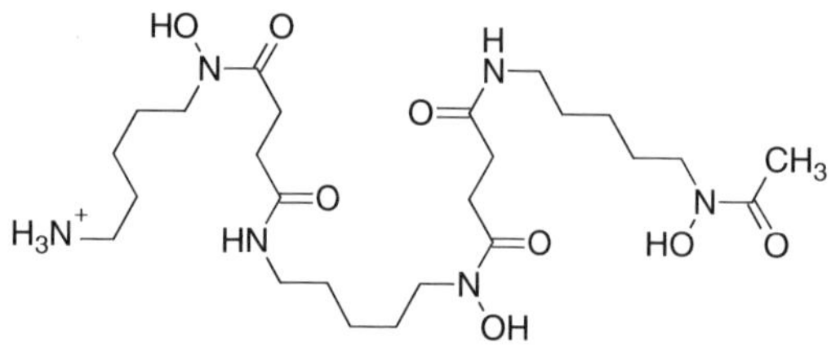

(1)

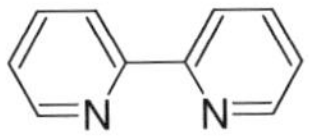

(2) 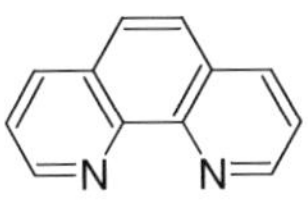 (3)

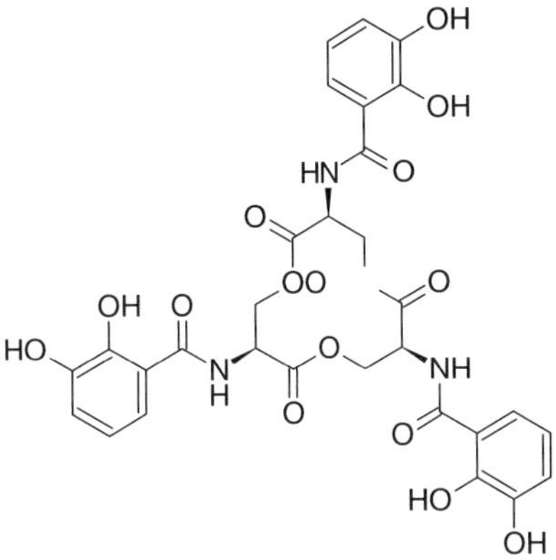

(4) 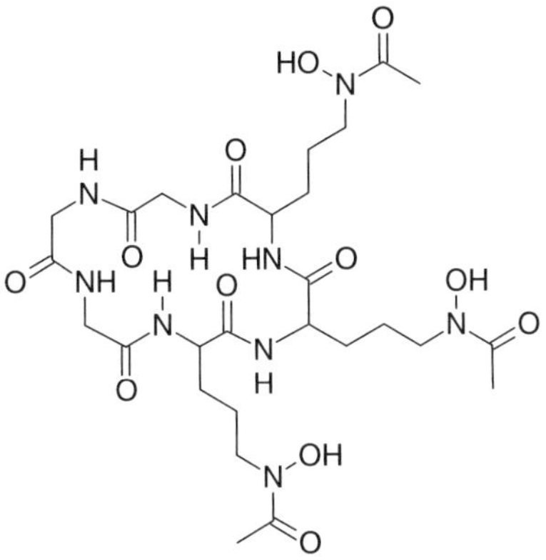 (5)

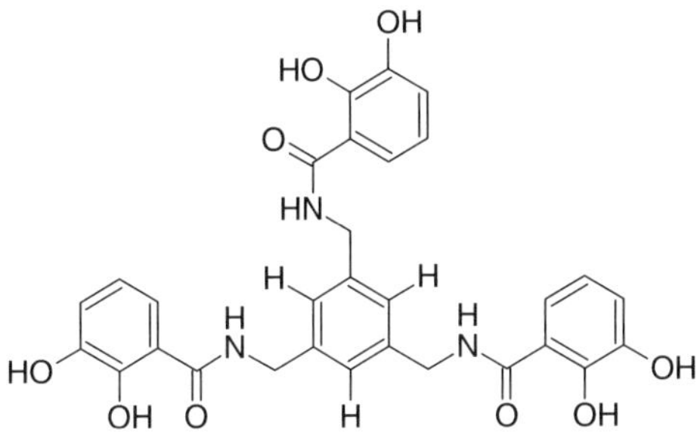

(6)

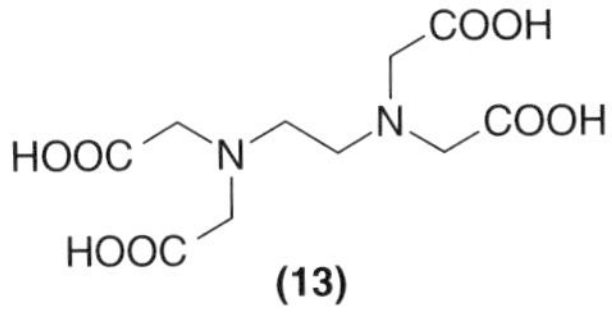

(13)

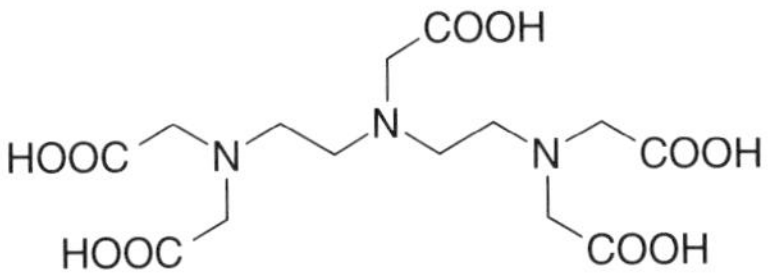

(14)

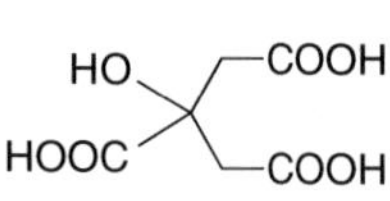

HO COOH
HOOC COOH

(15)

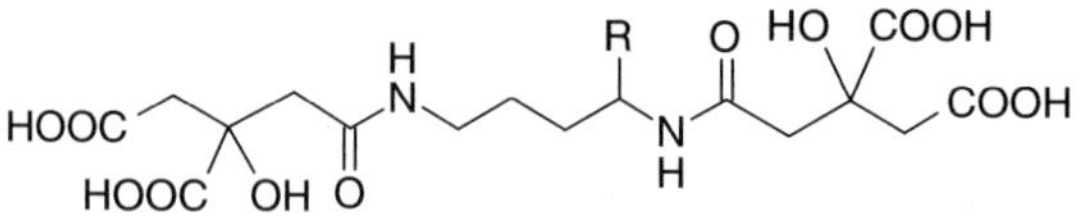

H R O HO COOH
HOOC N COOH
N
HOOC OH O H

(16) R = H

(17) R = COOH

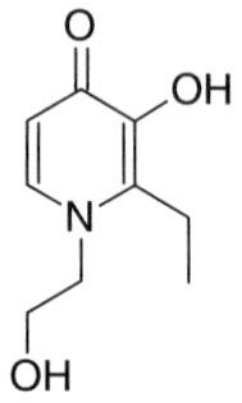

OEt
O O OH
O OH O OH
N N
N N
OH

(18) 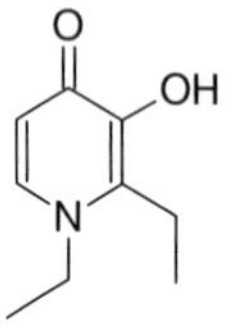 (19) 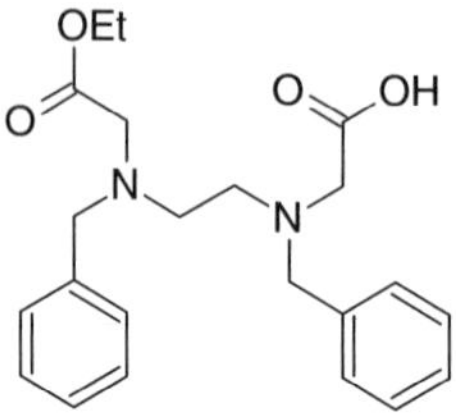 (21)

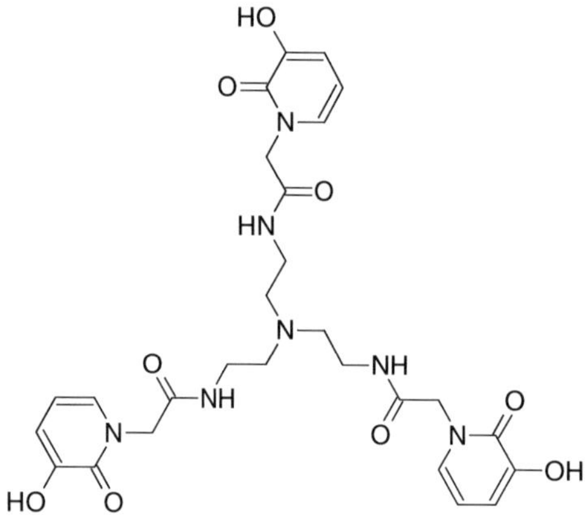

HO
O
N
O
HN
N
O NH
NH
N O N O
HO O OH

(22)

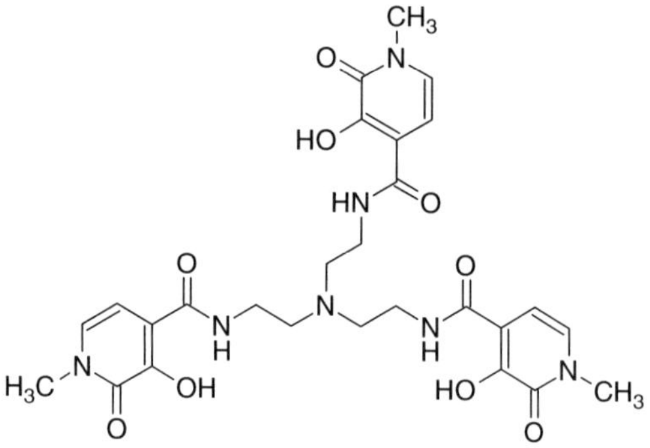

CH3
O N
HO
HN O
O O
N N N
H H
H3C N OH HO N CH3
O O

(23)

OH
N O
O
H N
H H O
HO O N N
N N
O O
OH

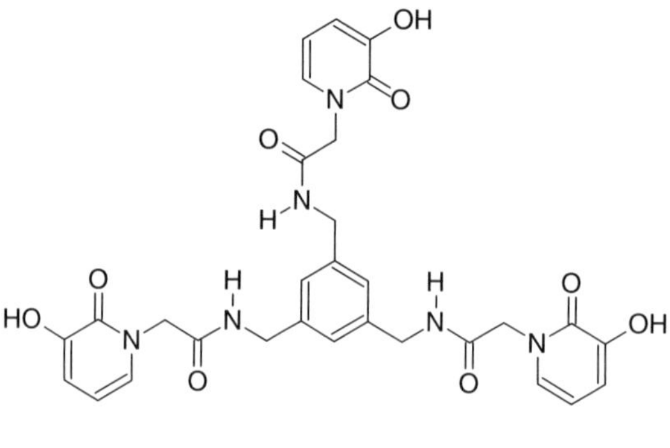

(24)

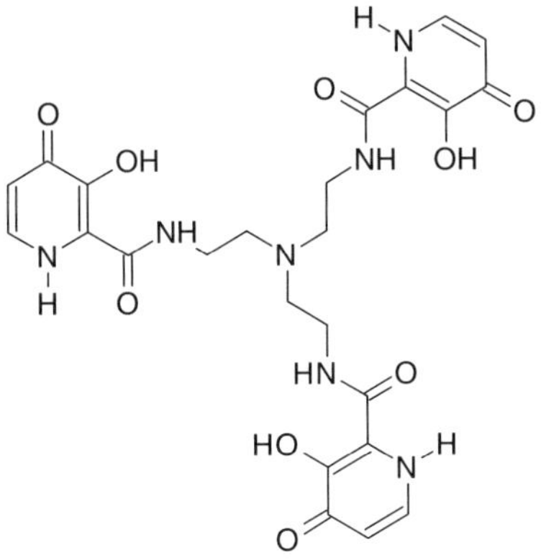

(25)

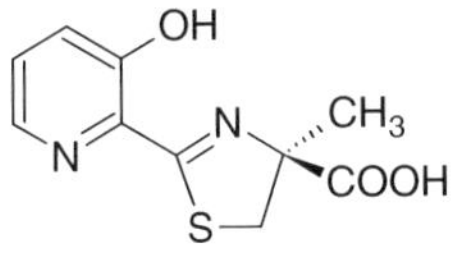

(26) 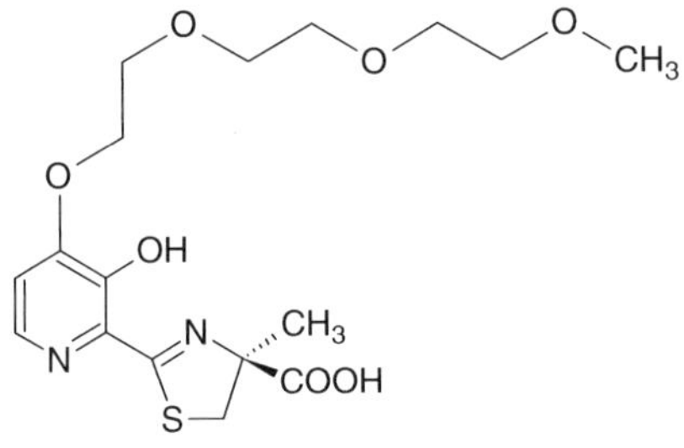 **(27)** 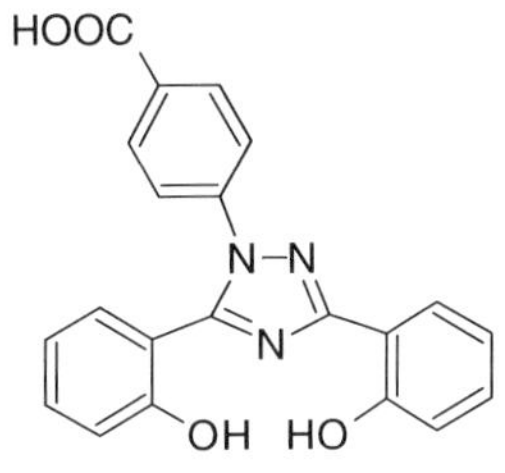 **(28)**

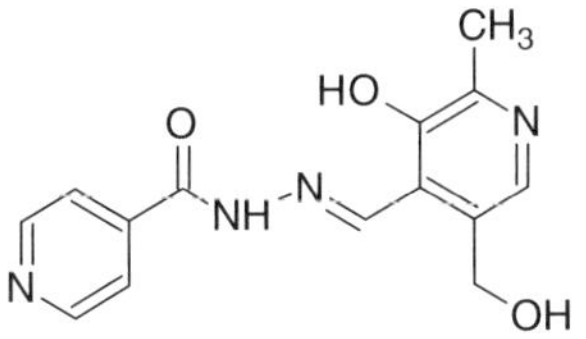

(29) 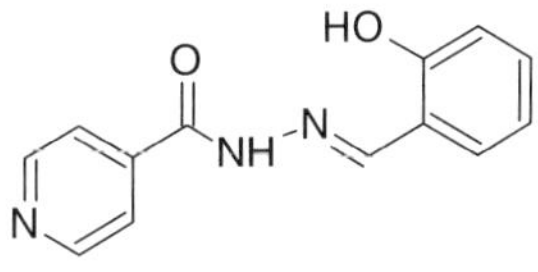 **(30)**

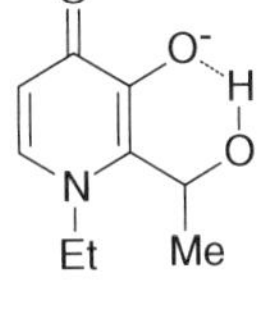

(31) 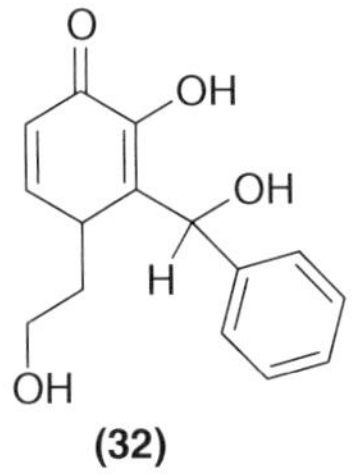 **(32)** 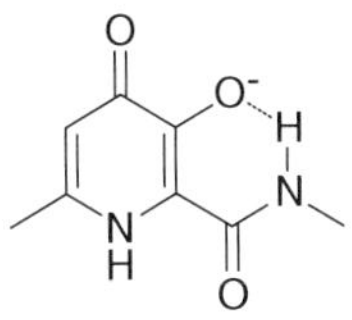 **(33)**

References

1. Halliwell B, Gutteridge JMC. Free radicals in biology and medicine. 4th ed. Oxford: Clarendon; 2007.
2. Crichton RR. Inorganic biochemistry of iron metabolism from molecular mechanisms to clinical consequences. 2nd ed. New York: Wiley; 2001.
3. Hershko C, Konijn AM, Link G. Iron chelators for thalassaemia. Br J Haematol. 1998;101:399–406.
4. Martell AE, Smith RM. Critical stability constant, vol. 1–6. London: Plenum Press; 1974–1989.
5. Harris DC, Aisen P. Facilitation of Fe(II) autoxidation by Fe(III) complexing agents. Biochim Biophys Acta. 1973;329:156–8.
6. Hider RC, Kong X. Chemistry and biology of siderophores. Nat Prod Rep. 2010;27:637–57.
7. Borgias B, Hugi AD, Raymond KN. Isomerization and solution structures of desferrioxamine B complexes of Al^{3+} and Ga^{3+}. Inorg Chem. 1989;28:3538–45.
8. Raymond KN, Muller G, Matzanke BF. Complexation of iron by siderophores: a review of their solution and structural chemistry and biological function. Top Curr Chem. 1984;58:49–102.
9. Liu ZD, Khodr HH, Liu DY, Lu SL, Hider RC. Synthesis, physicochemical characterisation and biological evaluation of 2-(1′-hydroxyalkyl)-3-hydroxypyridin-4-ones: novel iron chelators with enhanced pFe^{3+} values. J Med Chem. 1999;42:4814–23.
10. Hider RC, Mohd-Nor AR, Silver J, Morrison IEG, Rees LVC. Model compounds for microbial iron-transport compounds. Part 1. Solution chemistry and mössbauer study of iron(II) and iron(III). Complexes from phenolic and catecholic system. J Chem Soc Dalton Trans. 1981;2:609–22.
11. Gautier-Luneau I, Merle C, Phanon D, et al. New trends in the chemistry of iron(III) citrate complexes: correlations between X-ray structures and solution species probed by electrospray mass spectrometry and kinetics of iron uptake from citrate by iron chelators. Chemistry. 2005;11:2207–19.
12. Silva AMN, Kong X, Parkin MC, Cammack R, Hider RC. Iron(III) citrate speciation in aqueous solution. Dalton Trans. 2009;40:8616–25.
13. Carrano CJ, Drechsel H, Kaiser D, et al. Coordination chemistry of the carboxylate type siderophore rhizoferrin: the iron(III) complex and its metal analogs. Inorg Chem. 1996;35:6429–36.
14. Tilbrook GS, Hider RC. Iron chelators for clinical use. In: Sigel A, Sigel H, editors. Metal irons in biological systems, Iron transport and storage in microorganisms, plants and animals, vol. 35. New York: Marcel Dekker; 1998. p. 691–730.
15. Holander D, Ricketts D, Boyd CAR. Importance of probe molecular geometry in determining intestinal permeability. Can J Gastroenterol. 1988;2:35A–8.
16. Fagerholm U, Nilsson D, Knutson L, Lennernas H. Jejunal permeability in humans in vivo and rats in situ: investigation of molecular size selectivity and solvent drag. Acta Physiol Scand. 1999;165:315–24.
17. Kim M. Absorption of polyethylene glycol oligomers (330–1122 Da) is greater in the jejunum than in the ileum of rats. J Nutr. 1996;126:2172–8.
18. O'Halloran TV. Transition-metals in control of gene-expression. Science. 1993;261:715–25.
19. Lind MD, Hamor MJ, Hamor TA, Hoard JL. Stereochemistry of ethylene diaminetetroaceto complexes. Inorg Chem. 1964;3:34–43.
20. Hider RC. Potential protection from toxicity by oral iron chelators. Toxicol Lett. 1995;82–3:961–7.
21. Liu ZD, Kayyali R, Hider RC, Porter JB, Theobald AE. Design, synthesis, and evaluation of novel 2-substituted 3-hydroxypyridin-4-ones: structure-activity investigation of metalloenzyme inhibition by iron chelators. J Med Chem. 2002;45:631–9.
22. Habgood MD, Liu ZD, Dehkordi LS, Khodr HH, Abbott J, Hider RC. Investigation into the correlation between the structure of hydroxypyridinones and blood-brain barrier permeability. Biochem Pharmacol. 1999;57:1305–10.
23. Hershko C, Grady RW, Cerami A. Mechanism of iron chelation in the hypertransfused rat: definition of two alternative pathways of iron mobilisation. J Lab Clin Med. 1978;92:144–9.
24. Peter HH. Industrial aspects of iron chelators: pharmaceutical application. In: Spik G, Montreuil J, Crichton RR, Mazurier J, editors. Proteins of iron storage and transport. Amsterdam: Elsevier; 1985. p. 293–303.
25. Bergeron RJ, Wiegand J, McManis JS, Perumal PT. Synthesis and biological evaluation of hydroxamate-based iron chelators. J Med Chem. 1991;34:3182–7.
26. Martell AE, Motekaitis RJ, Clarke ET. Synthesis of N,N′-di(2-hydroxybenzyl)ethylenediamine-N,N′-diacetic (HBED) derivatives. Can J Chem. 1986;64:449–56.
27. Bergeron RJ, Wiegand J, Brittenham GM. HBED: a potential alternative to deferoxamine for iron-chelating therapy. Blood. 1998;91:1446–52.
28. Pitt CG, Bao Y, Thompson J, Wani MC, Rosenkrantz H, Metterville J. Esters and lactones of phenolic amino carboxylic acids: prodrugs for iron chelation. J Med Chem. 1986;29:1231–7.

29. Gasparini F, Leutert T, Farley DL. N,N′-bis(2-hydroxybenzyl)ethylene-diamine-N,N′-diacetic acid derivatives as chelating agents. International Patent WO 95/16663; 1995.
30. Lowther N, Tomlinson B, Fox R, Faller B, Sergejew T, Donnelly H. Caco-2 cell permeability of a new (hydroxybenzyl)ethylenediamine oral iron chelator: correlation with physicochemical properties and oral activity. J Pharm Sci. 1998;87:1041–5.
31. Guterman SK, Morris PM, Tannenberg WJK. Feasibility of enterochelin as an iron-chelating drug: studies with human serum and a mouse model system. Gen Pharm. 1978;9:123–7.
32. Streater M, Taylor PD, Hider RC, Porter JB. Novel 3-hydroxyl-2(1 H)-pyridinones. Synthesis, iron(III) chelating properties and biological activity. J Med Chem. 1990;33:1749–55.
33. Xu JD, Kullgren B, Durbin PW, Raymond KN. Specific sequestering agents for the actinides. 28: synthesis and initial evaluation of multidentate 4-carbamoyl-3-hydroxy-1-methyl-2(1 H)-pyridinone ligands for in vivo plutonium(IV) chelation. J Med Chem. 1995;38:2606–14.
34. Rai BL, Khodr H, Hider RC. Synthesis, physico-chemical and iron(III)-chelating properties of novel hexadentate 3-hydroxy-2(1H)pyridinone ligands. Tetrahedron. 1999;55:1129–42.
35. Piyamongkol S, Zhou T, Liu ZD, Khodr HH, Hider RC. Design and characterisation of novel hexadentate 3-hydroxypyridin-4-one ligands. Tetrahedron Lett. 2005;46:1333–6.
36. Hahn FN, McMurry TJ, Hugi A, Raymond KN. Coordination chemistry of microbial iron transport. 42: structural and spectroscopic characterisation of diastereometric Cr(III) and Co(III) complexes of desferrithiocin. J Am Chem Soc. 1990;112:1854–60.
37. Bergeron RJ, Wiegand J, McManis JS, Bharti N, Singh S. Desferrithiocin analogues and nephrotoxicity. J Med Chem. 2008;51:5993–6004.
38. Bergeron RJ, Wiegand J, Bharti N, Singh S, Rocca JR. Impact of the 3,6,9-trioxadecyloxy group on desazadesferrithiocin analogue iron clearance and organ distribution. J Med Chem. 2007;50:3302–13.
39. Lattmann R, Acklin P. Substituted 3,5-diphenyl-1,2,4-triazoles and their use as pharmaceutical metal chelators. International Patent WO 97/49395; 1997.
40. Nick HP, Acklin P, Faller B, et al. A new, potent, orally active iron chelator. In: Badman DG, Bergeron RJ, Brittenham GM, editors. Iron chelators: new development strategies. Florida: The Saratoga Group; 2000. p. 311–31.
41. Steinhauser S, Heinz U, Bartholoma M, Weyhermuller T, Nick H, Hegetschweiler K. Complex formation of ICL670 and related ligands with Fe(II) and Fe(III). Eur J Inorg Chem. 2004;21:4177–92.
42. Heinz U, Hegetschweiler K, Acklin P, Faller B, Lattmann R, Schnebli HP. 4-[3,5-Bis(2-hydroxyphenyl)-1,2,4-triazol-1-yl]benzoic acid: a novel efficient and selective iron(III) complexing agent. Angew Chem Int Ed. 1999;38:2568–70.
43. Porter JB. Monitoring and treatment of iron overload: state of the art and new approaches. Semin Hematol. 2005;42(2 Suppl. 1):S14–8.
44. Pennell DJ, Porter JB, Cappellini MD, et al. Efficacy of defersirox in reducing and preventing cardiac iron overload in β-thalassemia. Blood. 2010;115:2364–71.
45. Zanninelli G, Glickstein H, Breuer W, et al. Chelation and mobilization of cellular iron by different classes of chelators. Mol Pharmacol. 1997;51:842–52.
46. Liu ZD, Hider RC. Design of clinically useful iron(III)-selective chelators. Med Res Rev. 2002;22:26–64.
47. Balfour JAB, Foster RH. Deferiprone – a review of its clinical potential in iron overload in beta-thalassaemia major and other transfusion-dependent diseases. Drugs. 1999;58:553–78.
48. Singh S, Epemolu O, Dobbin PS, et al. Urinary metabolic profiles in man and rat of 1,2-dimethyl- and 1,2-diethyl substituted 3-hydroxypyridin-4-ones. Drug Metab Dispos. 1992;20:256–61.
49. Borgna-Pignatti C, Cappellini MD, De Stefano P, et al. Cardiac morbidity and mortality in deferoxamine- or deferiprone-treated patients with thalassemia major. Blood. 2006;107:3733–7.
50. Maggio A, D'Amico G, Morabito A, et al. Deferiprone versus deferoxamine in patients with thalassemia major: a randomized clinical trial. Blood Cells Mol Dis. 2002;28:196–208.
51. Neufeld EJ. Oral chelators deferasirox and deferiprone for transfusional iron overload in thalassemia major: new data, new questions. Blood. 2006;107:3436–41.
52. Boddaert N, Le Quan Sang KH, Rotig A, et al. Selective iron chelation in Friedreich ataxia: biologic and clinical implications. Blood. 2007;110:401–8.
53. Sohn YS, Breuer W, Munnich A, Cabantchik ZI. Redistribution of accumulated cell iron: a modality of chelation with therapeutic implications. Blood. 2008;111:1690–9.
54. Porter JB, Morgan J, Hoyes KP, Burke LC, Huehns ER, Hider RC. Relative oral efficacy and acute toxicity of hydroxypyridin-4-one iron chelators in mice. Blood. 1990;76:2389–96.
55. Porter JB, Abeysinghe RD, Hoyes KP, et al. Contrasting interspecies efficacy and toxicology of 1,2-diethyl-3-hydroxypyridin-4-one CP94, relates to differing metabolism of the iron chelating site. Br J Haematol. 1993;85:159–68.

56. Porter JB, Singh S, Katherine PH, Epemolu O, Abeysinghe RD, Hider RC. Lessons from preclinical and clinical studies with 1,2-diethyl-3-hydroxypyridin-4-one, CP94 and related compounds. Adv Exp Med Biol. 1994;356:361–70.
57. Piyamongkol S, Ma YM, Kong X, et al. Amido-3-hydroxypyridin-4-ones as iron(III) ligands. Chem-Eur J. 2010;16:6374–81.
58. Lowther N, Fox P, Faller B, et al. In vitro and in situ permeability of a 'second generation' hydroxypyridinone oral iron chelator: correlation with physico-chemical properties and oral activity. Pharm Res. 1999;16:434–40.
59. Gaeta A, Hider RC. The crucial role of metal ions in neurodegeneration: the basis for a promising therapeutic strategy. Br J Pharmacol. 2005;146:1041–59.
60. Molina-Holgado F, Gaeta A, Francis PT, Williams RJ, Hider RC. Neuroprotective actions of deferiprone in cultured cortical neurons and SHSY-5Y cells. J Neurochem. 2008;105:2466–76.

Chapter 28
Clinical Use of Iron Chelators

John B. Porter and Chaim Hershko

Keywords Chelation therapy • Chelator • Deferasirox • Deferiprone • Deferoxamine • Heart • Iron overload • Liver • Non-transferrin-bound iron • Toxicity

1 Causes and Rates of Iron Overloading

1.1 Normal Iron Homeostasis

Iron is one of the most common elements in nature and, as a transition metal, is essential for the functioning of proteins involved in oxidative energy production, oxygen transport, mitochondrial respiration, inactivation of harmful oxygen radicals and DNA synthesis. Because of its poor solubility, living organisms were compelled to develop efficient mechanisms for the transport and storage of iron, but there is no natural mechanism for the excretion of excess iron in humans. In recent years, elegant mechanisms have been discovered which are responsible for the translational control of proteins involved in iron transport and storage [1]. The recent discovery of hepcidin, a regulator of iron absorption and recycling produced by hepatocytes [2], allows new insights into the mechanism of iron homeostasis in health and disease (see Chap. 9). The main components of this regulatory mechanism are described in Fig. 28.1.

1.2 Increased Iron Absorption

Normal iron homeostasis fails to prevent the harmful accumulation of iron in two major disease categories (a) in inherited hemochromatosis syndromes where abnormal hepcidin regulation results in increased intestinal iron absorption (Chaps. 19 and 20) and (b) in iron-loading anemias such as

J.B. Porter, M.A., M.D., FRCP, FRCPath
Department of Hematology, University College London, London, UK
e-mail: j.porter@ucl.ac.uk

C. Hershko, M.D. (✉)
Department of Hematology, Shaare Zedek Medical Center and Hebrew University of Jerusalem, Jerusalem, Israel
e-mail: hershko@szmc.org.il

G.J. Anderson and G. McLaren (eds.), *Iron Physiology and Pathophysiology in Humans*, Nutrition and Health, DOI 10.1007/978-1-60327-485-2_28,

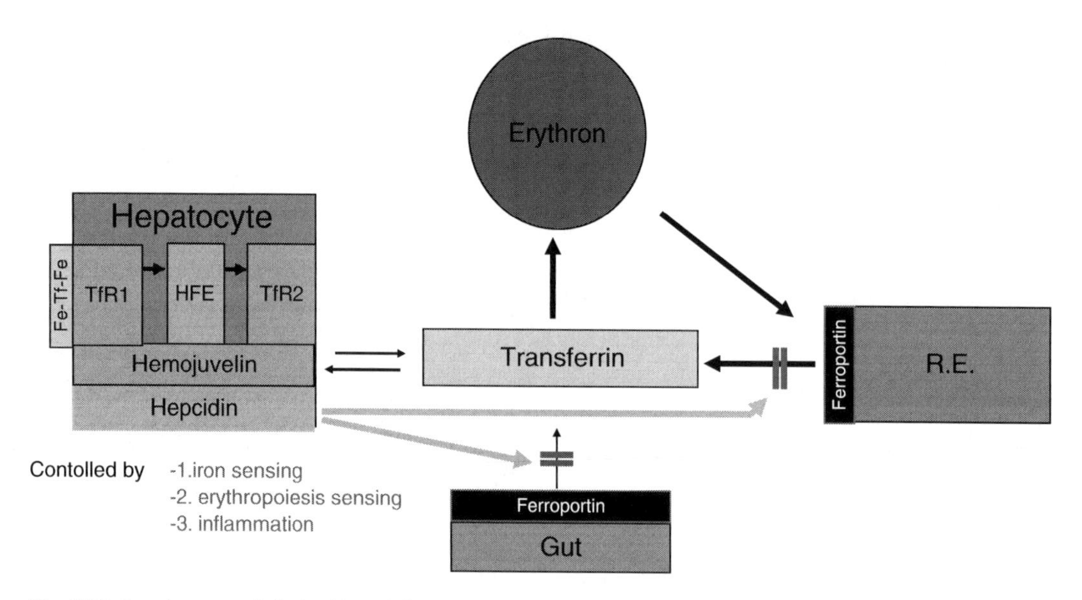

Fig. 28.1 Iron homeostasis in health and disease. The bulk of iron requirements are derived from efficient recycling of senescent erythrocytes by the macrophage system, with limited contribution of absorbed intestinal iron. Hepcidin controls these two sources of incoming iron by its association with ferroportin preventing iron influx. Hepcidin production in turn is controlled by three distinct regulatory mechanisms: iron sensing, erythropoiesis sensing and inflammation. Iron sensing involves the binding of diferric transferrin to transferrin receptor 1 (*TfR1*) initiating the translocation of HFE from TfR1 to TfR2 and its subsequent interaction with hemojuvelin [1, 2]

thalassaemia major where transfusional iron overload is aggravated by increased iron absorption, caused by increased rates of ineffective erythropoiesis [3, 4] (Chap. 16). The rate of increased iron loading is variable, depending on the underlying genetic basis, but is generally a fraction of the rate seen with transfusional iron loading. Humans cannot increase iron excretion to compensate for iron overload; so this must be removed therapeutically. The most simple and effective method for removing or preventing the accumulation of excess iron in hereditary hemochromatosis is by repeated phlebotomies (see Chap. 19). However, in inherited or acquired iron-loading anemias, phlebotomies are impractical, and alternative methods, such as the use of iron chelators to enhance urinary or fecal iron excretion, have been developed.

1.3 Iron Loading from Transfusion

Approximately 200 mg of iron is present in a pint (420 mL) of donated blood, or about 1.08 mg of iron per 1 mL of pure red blood cells (i.e. hematocrit 1.0). The amount of iron transfused can thus be calculated by multiplying the volume of blood product transfused by 1.08 and then by the hematocrit of the transfused product. Recent work has shown that there is considerable variability in the iron loading rate both within a given diagnosis and between diagnoses [5, 6]. In thalassaemia major (TM), the mean transfusional iron loading rate is 0.4 mg/kg/day [5], but this varies considerably, with 20% of patients <0.3 mg/kg/day, about 60% receiving 0.3–0.5 mg/kg/day, and a further 20% receiving >0.5 mg/kg/day. Chelation response both to deferasirox (DFS) and deferoxamine (DFO) has been shown to be dependent on the transfusion category that patients fall into. Thus the planned dose of chelation therapy can be tailored to the transfusion rate of each patient [5]. The average rate of transfusional iron loading is less in sickle-cell disease (SCD) (0.22 mg/kg/day) [7] than in TM, and this is further decreased by using an exchange transfusion procedure, although this effect varies considerably depending on the exchange procedure used. In MDS, the average rate of iron loading (0.28 mg/kg/day) is less than in TM although there is considerable overlap between these conditions [6]. Iron chelation must at least match these iron loading rates.

2 Toxicities from Iron Overload

Iron is highly reactive because this metal can easily alternate between iron(III) and iron(II) redox states under clinically relevant conditions. This results in the gain and loss of electrons which can generate harmful free radicals. These have unpaired electrons that can damage many molecules such as lipid membranes, organelles and DNA. Cell death, as well as the generation of fibrosis, can result. In health, iron is 'kept safe' by binding to molecules such as transferrin, but in iron overload, the capacity to bind iron is exceeded both within cells and in the plasma compartment. This 'free iron' will cause damage to many tissues in the body and will be fatal unless treated by iron chelation therapy.

Repeated blood transfusions lead to increasing saturation of transferrin and ultimately to the presence of iron species in the plasma that are not bound to transferrin, so-called non-transferrin-bound iron (NTBI) [8]. These species are likely to be heterogeneous, consisting of iron citrate monomers, oligomers and polymers, as well as protein-bound forms [9, 10]. Plasma NTBI (or subfractions of it) has long been known to generate lipid peroxidation [11]. An assay has been developed for this redox active subfraction, which has been termed labile plasma iron (LPI) [12]. There is evidence that some NTBI species are taken into myocardium and endocrine tissues through L-type voltage-dependent calcium channels [13] that are not present on all tissues, and this is likely to explain the pattern of tissue iron deposition in transfusional iron overload.

The consequences of transfusional iron overload are best described in TM, where transfusional iron loading begins within a few months of birth. Untreated transfusional iron overload in TM is fatal in the second decade of life, usually from cardiac failure or arrhythmia [14, 15]. Infection is the second commonest cause of death in thalassaemia patients. Iron overload also causes anterior pituitary damage with hypogonadism and poor growth. Endocrine complications, namely diabetes, hypothyroidism and hypoparathyroidism, are also important complications, the frequencies of which have been steadily receding since the introduction of DFO chelation therapy in the late 1970s. Liver disease with fibrosis and eventually cirrhosis is also a serious complication. Hepatoma from the effects of iron overload with or without the additional risks from hepatitis is increasingly seen [16], as chelated patients may now live beyond the fifth and sixth decades of life. In other conditions associated with iron overload, the complications are less well defined although there is evidence for endocrine disorders [17] and myocardial iron loading [18, 19] in multi-transfused MDS patients. Although overall survival is significantly worse in iron-overloaded MDS patients compared with untransfused MDS patients [20, 21], an independent effect of the iron loading is not certain without prospective studies. In SCD, however, increased iron loading is not seen without blood transfusion, but liver fibrosis and cirrhosis are recognized features of uncontrolled iron overload [22, 23]. There may be a possible decreased tendency to endocrine disturbances [24, 25] or to myocardial iron deposition [26–28] in the face of transfusional iron overload in SCD. However, it is not yet clear whether the apparently lower frequency of these complications in patients with otherwise similar levels of total body iron loading is a consequence of differences in the rates and duration of iron overload, or whether some fundamental differences between TM and SCD exist with respect to iron distribution to these tissues.

3 Monitoring of Iron Overload and Its Consequences

Estimation of iron load using liver iron and serum ferritin has recently been supplemented by the possibility of examining body iron distribution using MRI techniques. An understanding of how these measures indicate risk from iron overload is of key importance to tailoring chelation on an individual basis.

3.1 Liver Iron Concentration (LIC)

Normal LIC values are up to 1.8 mg/g dry wt, and levels up to 7 mg/g dry wt are seen in some non-thalassaemic populations without apparent adverse effects [29]. Body iron stores can be predicted from the LIC using the formula: total body iron stores in mg/kg = 10.6 x the LIC (in mg/g dry wt) [30]. In unchelated patients, high LIC values predict an increased risk of myocardial iron deposition [18, 19], but once chelation therapy has been initiated, this simple relationship no longer exists [31]. This is because iron is removed faster from the liver than from the heart [32] and because increments in liver iron precede those of heart iron. Despite this, high LIC values (above 15–20mg/g dry wt) have been linked to worsening prognosis [33, 34], liver fibrosis progression [35] or liver function abnormalities [19].

Liver biopsy of adequate size (<1 mg/g dry weight, 4 mg wet wt or about a 2.5-cm core length) was the method most commonly used to quantitate liver iron until recently. Complication rates are very low in expert hands, using ultrasound guidance [36]. However, many centers perform biopsies at insufficient frequency and samples are often inadequate in size and quality. Values are also unreliable in the presence of cirrhosis. A further problem in standardization has been that the relative measurements of wet and dry weights of samples vary considerably between laboratories. Non-invasive standardized methodology has therefore been desirable.

Magnetic susceptometry [37] (SQUID) has thus far been very expensive with only four working machines worldwide. Standardization between these devices has been problematic [38]. The current development of room-temperature handheld susceptometric devices would have wider applications. MRI techniques are now available [39, 40], and these rely on the general principle that tissue iron exerts a paramagnetic effect on surrounding tissues that affects the relaxation time of molecules excited by the application of a magnetic field. One such method (R2, FerriScan) is available in a standardized and validated format that approximates linearity over a clinically useful range [39]. This is registered in the EU and USA and can utilise widely available MRI equipment with little extra training of local staff [39]. Not all MRI measures give comparable LIC values however. The T2* method that was developed for heart iron measurement has also been used to estimate LIC, but as currently calibrated, gives LIC values a half of those obtained by biopsy or FerriScan [41].

3.2 Serum Ferritin

Serum ferritin, which is iron free below serum levels of 3,000 μg/L, is derived mainly from macrophages, thus reflecting the iron stores in this compartment [42]. Above this value, an increasing proportion is iron rich and is derived from hepatocytes [42]. Serum ferritin is a useful predictor of body iron stores as well as trends in iron removal with chelation therapy, but has its limitations. It has been shown that variations in body iron stores account for only about 57% of the variability in plasma ferritin [43]. Inflammation increases serum ferritin independently of the body iron, so that a sudden increase in serum ferritin should prompt a search for hepatitis, other infections or inflammatory conditions. The relationship between serum ferritin and iron stores is similar in thalassaemia major and sickle-cell disease [43] provided serum values are taken several weeks away from a vaso-occlusive sickle crisis [44]. In thalassaemia intermedia, however, serum ferritin tends to underestimate the degree of iron overloading [45]. A further problem is that many 'kits' for measuring serum ferritin are optimized for identifying iron deficiency, and care must be taken at high ferritin values to ensure that dilutions allow measurements within the linear range of the assay. Another issue that needs greater attention is that the relationship between serum ferritin and body iron stores may vary with the chelator being used [46]. Recent work suggests that deferiprone (DFP) is associated with lower serum ferritin (SF) relative to liver iron concentrations (LIC) than deferoxamine and deferasirox [47]. It is clear however that if the ferritin is maintained below 2,500 μg/L (with DFO) on a long-term basis, this is associated with a significantly lower risk of cardiac disease and death [16, 34, 48–50]. However, lower ferritin levels are desirable, and there is evidence that long-term maintenance of serum ferritin closer to 1,000 μg/L has additional benefits [16].

3.3 Monitoring of the Heart

Sequential monitoring of LVEF identifies patients at high risk of developing clinical heart failure; when LVEF fell below reference value, there was a 35-fold increased risk of clinical cardiac failure and death with a median interval to progression of 3.5 years, allowing time for intensification of chelation therapy [50]. This approach required a reproducible method for determination of LVEF (such as MUGA or now using MRI), and echocardiography was too operator dependent for this purpose. Furthermore, there was clearly a need to identify high-risk patients before a fall in LVEF developed. MRI was initially used to evaluate myocardial iron in MDS patients using a signal intensity ratio method [19]. A significant advance in understanding began when myocardial T2* was used to compare LVEF with this measure. Myocardial T2* values <20 ms, the lowest value found in healthy individuals, were in TM patients associated with an increased risk of the LVEF below reference values [31]. This publication also showed a linear correlation of liver 1/T2* with LIC by biopsy [31]. More recently, the relationship between myocardial iron concentration and myocardial T2* has been elucidated using postmortem myocardial material and T2* measurement in iron-overloaded patients [51]. The mean global myocardial iron causing severe heart failure in 10 patients was 5.98 mg/g dry weight (range, 3.2–9.5 mg/g). The relationship between risk of heart failure and mT2* has now been further elucidated in prospective studies [52]. T2* values <10 ms are associated with 160-fold increased risk of development of clinical heart failure in the next 12 months. This risk increases progressively with T2* values <10 ms, so that the proportion of patients developing heart failure in the next 12 months at mT2* of 8–10 ms, 6–8 ms and <6 ms was 18%, 31% and 52% respectively. The value of mT2* monitoring is supported by a recent report in a cohort of TM patients monitored for 10 years using mT2*, in which iron-mediated cardiomyopathy was no longer a leading cause of death and the proportion of patients with mT2* <20 ms fell from 60% to 1% over the decade [53], although other factors such as chelation options may have contributed to this improved outcome. mT2* monitoring has now been established and validated internationally [54] and is now recommended as a part of yearly monitoring of multi-transfused patients at risk of developing myocardial iron loading.

3.4 Urinary Iron Excretion

Urinary iron excretion in response to DFO was initially used as a way of quantitating iron overload [55]. The variability in daily iron excretion necessitates repeated determinations however. Furthermore the proportion of fecal excretion with DFO is highly variable, 30–100% [56]. There is effectively only fecal iron excretion with DFS, making urinary estimation unhelpful.

3.5 Plasma Non-Transferrin-Bound Iron

There are a variety of assays for NTBI that give variable reference ranges but generally correlate with each other [57]. An assay measuring a labile subfraction (the component capable of accelerating oxidation of a fluorophore, termed LPI assay) [12] is convenient for measuring iron in the presence of chelators. Progressive removal of this subfraction has been seen with DFP [58] and DFS [59]. Removal of LPI is maintained 24 h per day with DFS [11], consistent with the notion that continuous chelation minimizes exposure to NTBI species [60]. A prognostic or pathophysiological significance for any given 'cut-off' value has yet to be demonstrated in prospective studies, however. There are interesting differences in NTBI and LPI values between disease states. For example, plasma NTBI is lower in SCD than TM at matched levels of iron loading [61, 62]. Labile plasma iron (LPI) levels are also low in SCD and aplastic anemia, compared to other forms of transfusional iron overload, such as TM and MDS, despite similar serum ferritin values [63].

3.6 Other Markers of Organ Dysfunction

The earliest consequence of iron overload manifested in transfused children is hypogonadotropic hypogonadism, which although not fatal, has severe consequences for growth, sexual development, fertility and osteoporosis. Close monitoring of growth and sexual development in children is therefore vital so that chelation can be intensified before irreversible effects ensue. In older patients, monitoring for impaired glucose tolerance may identify patients at most risk of developing diabetes. Monitoring for hypothyroidism and hypoparathyroidism is also advisable, particularly in adults. Although there is evidence from retrospective analysis in patients with very low ferritin values [64] that damage to these tissues can be reversed, prevention of these complications by adequate control of body iron at all times is the optimal strategy.

4 Objectives of Chelation Therapy

Chelation therapy should aim to maintain body iron stores at safe levels at all times and at the lowest doses that are consistent with avoiding toxicity from chelation therapy itself. Storage iron, ferritin or hemosiderin, cannot be accessed directly by chelators at a useful rate so that chelation therapy relies on accessing the small fractions of low-molecular-weight body iron that are available for chelation at any moment (see below), often referred to as 'labile iron' pools. Unless chelation therapy begins before clinically significant iron overload develops, it may take several years to bring iron stores into a safe range. DFO chelation therapy has usually been started only after 2–3 years of transfusion or when ferritin exceeds 1,000 g/L, for fear of the unwanted effects of over-chelation by DFO at low levels of body iron (see below). It is not yet clear whether chelation can be commenced sooner with new chelation modalities, but this would be desirable if safety can be demonstrated.

Understanding of what constitutes 'safe' levels of body iron burden is incomplete. The risks of hepatic damage are clearly linked to LIC; LIC values >17 mg/g dry wt [65] are associated with abnormal ALT values, and values >16 mg/g dry wt are associated with progression of fibrosis [35]. The relationship between body iron load and extrahepatic iron distribution to heart and endocrine tissues and body iron load is less clear. Two independent studies in thalassaemia major have demonstrated a link between LIC values above 15 mg/g dry wt and long-term cardiac-event-free survival [33, 34] as well as a possible effect at values >7 mg/g dry wt [34]. However, when single measures are taken, there is a striking lack of correlation between liver and heart T2* measurements [31]. This is in part because once extrahepatic iron has accumulated, it is removed much more slowly from tissues such as the heart by chelation than from the liver [32, 66, 67]. The role of other factors such as the rate of transfusional iron loading, the underlying hematological condition and undefined genetic factors have yet to be elucidated. Furthermore, while it is clear that myocardial iron deposition can be reversed, evidence for removal from endocrine tissues such as pituitary, pancreas and thyroid is not clear. Prevention of extrahepatic iron deposition is therefore a more sensible therapeutic strategy than 'rescue' therapy.

The small magnitude of the rapidly chelatable iron fraction also impacts the dosing strategy for chelation therapy. By increasing the dose of chelators in an attempt to accelerate iron removal from tissues, there is an increasing risk of toxicity from the chelator itself, by chelating iron which is needed for normal tissue metabolism. Plasma NTBI and LPI rebound rapidly after a chelator is cleared from plasma [12, 60] so that in principle, the continuous presence of a chelator is desirable.

5 Origin of Chelatable Iron

5.1 The Intracellular Labile Iron Pool

Current models of iron acquisition, sequestration and storage by mammalian cells are based on a regulated adjustment of membrane iron transport proteins and cytosolic ferritin levels. Iron in transit is believed to exist in a weakly bound low-molecular-weight complex, which is also available for interaction with iron-chelating drugs [68]. This chelatable labile iron pool (LIP) is assumed to be sensed by a cytosolic iron-responsive protein (IRP) that coordinately represses ferritin mRNA translation and increases transferrin receptor mRNA stability [69]. Efficient regulatory mechanisms prevent fluctuations in the size of the labile iron pool under conditions of moderate iron deprivation and iron loading. However, massive iron loading results in uncontrollable expansion of the chelatable pool, which fails to be matched by the sequestrating capacity of cellular ferritin [70]. This expanded LIP is an obvious target of intracellular iron chelation by drugs that are able to cross the barrier of the cytoplasmic membrane.

5.2 Role of Reticuloendothelial and Parenchymal Iron Stores

Although excess iron may be deposited in almost all tissues, most of it is found in association with two cell types: reticuloendothelial (RE) cells (macrophages) in the spleen, hepatic Kupffer cells and bone marrow, or in parenchymal tissues such as the myocardium, liver and endocrine organs. In contrast to RE cells in which iron accumulation is relatively harmless, parenchymal siderosis may result in significant organ damage. The source of iron and the proportion retained in ferritin stores or recycled into the circulation from the two cell types are quite different. RE cells have a limited ability to assimilate transferrin iron, and they derive iron mostly from the catabolism of hemoglobin in non-viable erythrocytes [71]. Most of this catabolic iron is recycled to the plasma within a few hours. In contrast, hepatic parenchymal cells maintain a dynamic equilibrium with plasma transferrin, with iron uptake predominating when transferrin saturation is high, and release when serum iron and transferrin saturation are low. Unlike RE cells, the turnover of parenchymal iron stores is very slow. In general, iron overload associated with increased intestinal absorption such as hereditary hemochromatosis results in predominant parenchymal siderosis, whereas in iron overload caused by multiple blood transfusions, the primary site of siderosis is the RE cells. Considerable redistribution of iron may take place subsequently.

Experimental and clinical observations indicate that the urinary excretion of iron chelated by DFO is derived mainly from RE cells. Studies with DFO in hypertransfused rats have shown that in contrast to hepatocellular radioiron excretion, which is confined entirely to the bile, most of the radioiron excretion derived from RE cells is recovered in the urine. Moreover, when water-soluble synthetic chelators which do not enter cells easily, such as DTPA, are employed in the same experimental model, there is no enhancement at all of hepatocellular iron excretion, but the enhancement of urinary RE radioiron excretion is similar, or higher than that observed previously with DFO [71]. Hence, DFO obtains iron for chelation by one of two alternative mechanisms: (a) in situ interaction with hepatocellular iron and subsequent biliary excretion and (b) chelation of iron derived from RBC catabolism in the RE system directly or following its release into the plasma in the form of non-transferrin-bound iron (NTBI) with subsequent urinary excretion. Iron chelated from myocardial cells, although critically important, represents only a tiny fraction of total excretion. Such iron, once mobilized into the plasma, will be excreted in the urine.

6 Design of Iron Chelators

Iron(III) has six coordination sites that can be accommodated by one large molecule such as deferoxamine (DFO) (hexadentate chelation). Such molecules tend to have high stability once bound to iron(III), but unfortunately it has not been possible to design hexadentate chelators that are small enough to allow efficient oral absorption. Smaller molecules can be absorbed from the gut more effectively and can bind iron(III) in either a 2:1 ratio with each molecule providing three binding sites (tridentate chelation, e.g. deferasirox, DFS) or a 3:1 ratio with each molecule providing two sites (bidentate chelation, e.g. deferiprone, DFP). Chelatable iron occurs both within cells and within the plasma compartment (see above). Access of chelators to intracellular pools is affected by their size, charge, lipid solubility, iron coordination structure and metabolism [72–74]. Thus, in addition to being absorbed more rapidly from the GI tract, small neutrally charged bidentate molecules such as DFP are able to access intracellular iron pools more rapidly than DFO [75, 76]. It is important that the binding of iron to a chelator prevents the further redox cycling of iron. The chelator should also not inhibit essential metalloenzymes such as ribonucleotide reductase within cells [77]. In practice, all chelators exhibit some affinity for other metals such as zinc, copper and aluminum, but clinically available chelators do not appear to be limited in their use by such metal binding. The success of iron chelators is also affected by their pharmacokinetic and pharmacodynamic interactions. Depending on the

Table 28.1 Comparison of the three leading iron-chelating drugs

Compound	Deferoxamine	Deferasirox	Deferiprone
Molecular weight (daltons)	560	373	139
Chelating properties	Hexadentate	Tridentate	Bidentate
Iron-binding affinity (pM)	26.6	22.5	19.9
Delivery	s.c. or i.v.	Oral, once daily	Oral, 3 times daily
Half-life	8–12 h	12–16 h	3–4 h
	5 days/week		
	20–30 min		
Lipid solubility	Low	High	Intermediate
Route of iron excretion	Urinary and fecal	Fecal	Urinary
Recommended dose (mg/kg/day)	30–60	20–30	75–100
Max. plasma levels (μM)	7–10	80	90–450
Min. plasma level (μM)	0	20	0
Chelation efficiency (%)	13	27	7
Adverse effects	Ocular, auditory, growth retardation, local reactions, allergy	Gastrointestinal, increased creatinine, hepatitis	Gastrointestinal, arthralgia, agranulocytosis/neutropenia

rate of absorption, elimination and metabolism, plasma and cellular concentrations of chelators and their iron complexes differ considerably. These considerations will also have a bearing on the balance between cellular iron uptake and iron removal and hence the success of chelation therapy.

In order to identify safe and effective compounds that are orally active, more than one thousand candidate compounds have been screened in animal models. These efforts led to the identification of many interesting compounds, a few of which have been shown to be of clinical value. The present discussion will be limited to the most outstanding of these compounds including deferiprone (DFP, L1), pyridoxal isonicotinoyl hydrazone (PIH), bishydroxyphenyl thiazole (ICL670, deferasirox, Exjade, DFS) and desferrithiocin and its derivatives (DFT). Only three compounds have been shown to be effective in clinical use over a sustained period, however, namely deferoxamine (DFO), deferiprone (DFP) and deferasirox (DFS). A comparison of molecular weights, chelating properties, recommended daily dose, method of delivery and other properties of these three leading chelators is presented in Table 28.1.

7 Deferoxamine (DFO)

Because of its proven efficacy and the extensive experience with its long-term use in many thousands of patients, DFO is still considered the gold standard of iron chelation therapy.

7.1 Chemistry and Pharmacology

DFO is a naturally occurring siderophore chelator where one molecule completely coordinates with the six available sites of iron (III) (hexadentate chelation) (Fig. 28.2). Unfortunately, complete coordination of iron(III) by a single chelate molecule requires a relatively large chelate molecule, thus limiting iron absorption of DFO from the gut. DFO is also highly hydrophilic which retards its entry

Fig. 28.2 Deferoxamine

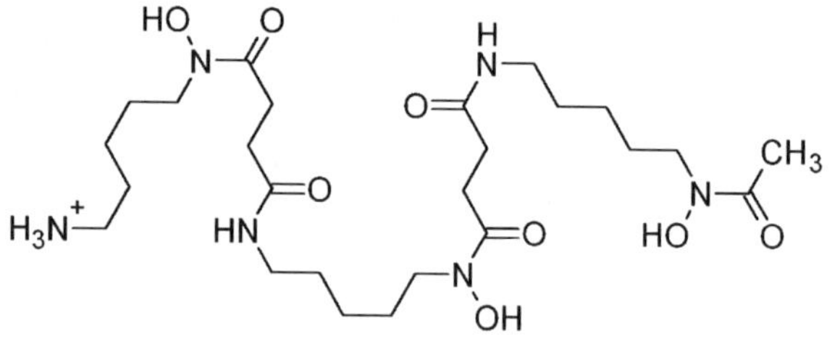

into most cell types with the exception of hepatocytes, for which there appears to be a facilitated uptake mechanism [78]. The free drug is positively charged, as is the iron complex. The latter property partly accounts for the slow egress of the iron complex from cells [77]. The iron complex of DFO is highly stable, giving a high pM value with good iron scavenging properties at low concentrations of iron or chelator. When DFO is infused intravenously at 40–50 mg/kg/day, steady state plasma concentrations are typically no more that 10 μM [60, 79] and due to the short initial half-life of 0.28 h (Table 28.1). Plasma levels fall more slowly following cessation of subcutaneous infusion [78] with an initial T1/2 of 0.56 h. The terminal T1/2 is slower, most likely reflecting the slow egress of the iron complex, ferrioxamine, from cells. The iron-free drug, but not of the iron complex, is metabolized within hepatocytes, so that an increase in metabolites indicates a decrease in the availability of chelatable iron [78, 80]. Removal of NTBI by DFO is usually only partial [78, 81], unless an additional chelator is available to shuttle NTBI subspecies onto DFO [82].

7.2 *Effects on Iron Balance*

Iron balance determination used to require admission to hospital for formal metabolic balance studies. Such studies suggested that daily 12 h infusions at 30 mg/kg could achieve iron balance in thalassaemia major, and that iron excretion is enhanced by oral ascorbic acid at 2–3 mg/kg/day [56]. Current practice typically prescribes 40 mg/kg s.c. DFO five nights a week, unless iron overload is severe or unless myocardial iron has accumulated. However, recent work, using changes in LIC and transfusional iron loading rates to measure iron balance, have shown that the probability of achieving negative iron balance with this regime depends on the transfusional iron loading rate [5, 83] and will be achieved in only about 50% of thalassaemia major patients receiving average transfusional iron loading rates (0.3–0.5 mg/kg/day). By increasing the dose to 50 mg/kg, 5 times a week, >86% of patients achieve negative iron balance, with both average and high (>0.5 mg/kg/day) blood transfusion rates. Thus, commonly prescribed doses of 35–50 mg/kg are insufficient for iron balance in nearly half of patients receiving transfusion at average or high iron loading rates. Under conditions of the study, compliance was likely to have been better than in the general clinical setting, so that an 'intention to treat' dose or frequency of <50 mg/kg 5 times/week may be inadequate in an even higher proportion of patients. Thus, for patients with average or high levels of transfusional iron loading, doses of 50 mg/kg should be considered, with the exception of children where doses >40 mg/kg/day are not recommended, or when ferritin levels are <1,000 μg/L (see below).

7.3 *Effects on Serum Ferritin*

The ability of DFO to control or decrease serum ferritin when used at appropriate doses and frequency has been known since the 1970s. Recent prospective studies have clarified the dose and frequency required to control serum ferritin [83]. In 290 thalassaemia major patients followed up for 1 year, a mean daily dose of 40 mg/kg 5 times/week decreased the mean serum ferritin by approximately 360 μg/L at 1 year, whereas 50 mg/kg decreased serum ferritin by 1,000 μg/L over the same period. These are average effects however, and the findings with LIC (see above) show that the planned dose should be increased if the transfusional iron intake is higher than average. The linking of long-term control of serum ferritin <2,500 μg/L to cardiac complication has only been reported for DFO [16, 34, 48–50], there being inadequate data with other chelators. There is some evidence that long-term control closer to 1,000 μg/L achieves even better results [15].

7.4 *Long-Term Effects on Survival*

The probability of reaching age 25 for thalassaemic patients in the early 1980s was only 25% [84]. The introduction of DFO for iron chelation therapy of transfusional siderosis has changed the life expectancy and life quality of patients with thalassaemia major. Its long-term efficacy has been extensively documented in large multicenter trials in Italy and elsewhere [15]. Only 70% of patients born before 1970 and hence prior to the modern era of iron chelation survived to age 20 compared with 89% of patients born after 1970 and therefore receiving effective chelation from an early age [85]. In a report on thalassaemic patients treated by DFO at a single institution, survival at 40 years was 83%, and in compliant patients born after 1975, survival at 25 years was 100% [50]. The cohort-of-birth-related improvement in survival was reflected in an inverse, mirror-like decrease in cardiac mortality, supporting the assumption that prevention of cardiac mortality is the most important beneficial effect of DFO therapy.

7.5 *Effects on the Heart*

Other than the effects on survival, perhaps the strongest direct evidence supporting the beneficial effect of DFO on hemosiderotic heart disease is the reversal of established myocardiopathy in some far-advanced cases. In former years, the course of established myocardial disease in transfusional hemosiderosis was uniformly fatal. More recent experience indicates that such patients may still be salvaged by intensified chelating treatment. Employing continuous 24-hour i.v. DFO infusion via indwelling catheters, Davis and Porter achieved reversal of cardiac arrhythmias and congestive heart failure [86]. The actuarial survival of their 17 high-risk thalassaemic patients (15 with established cardiac disease) following intensification of iron chelation was 61% at 13 years, and none of the compliant patients died. Reversal of cardiac arrhythmia, previously unresponsive to medical treatment, was achieved in 6 of 6 patients. This occurred in some cases within a few days of starting treatment and therefore cannot be attributed to normalisation of iron stores but to the depletion of a putative limited toxic labile iron pool. Improvements in heart function have also been documented with intermittent therapy. Miskin et al. [87] used intermittent high dose (95 mg/kg/day) of DFO for 8–10 h per day in eight thalassaemic patients with poor compliance, impaired left ventricular function and symptomatic heart disease with an improvement in cardiac function, similar to that obtained by Davis and Porter employing continuous [23] infusion. Improved ejection fraction was achieved in all patients, and all were alive after a follow-up period of 6.5 years (range, 2–12 years). Davis and Porter [86] have suggested that continuous intravenous treatment may be essential for improving cardiac outcome due to the uninterrupted chelation of circulating non-transferrin-bound iron (NTBI). The route of administration may not be critical as good long-term outcome was also achieved with continuous 24-h subcutaneous treatment [50]. Without carefully controlled trials comparing intermittent with continuous therapy at similar total doses in matched populations, the relative contribution of continuous exposure to chelation therapy as compared to general improved compliance cannot be clearly defined. For long-term survival, improved compliance has been maintained even after discontinuation of i.v. therapy [50]. Using continuous infusion, large doses such as those initially used to reverse heart failure and that were associated with severe retinal problems [88, 89] may not be necessary, and the excellent results of Davis and Porter were achieved using doses not exceeding 50–60 mg/kg/day, employing the therapeutic index of DFO to serum ferritin ratio of 0.025 as recommended for conventional subcutaneous DFO treatment [90]. Complications associated with the use of central venous access lines were common, although no toxicity due to DFO itself has been noted. Infection rates (1.2 episodes of local infections and 1.1 episodes of bacteremia per 1,000 days of use) were similar to those described in adult and pediatric cancer patients with central lines. Bacteremia caused by contamination of implantable central venous access devices was also a common problem among the 342 patients described in the North American cross-sectional study [91]. To limit the thrombotic complications of central venous access lines, close monitoring and prophylactic anticoagulant therapy has been suggested. Under such circumstances, the advantages of intensified i.v. DFO in improving survival appear to outweigh the risks of its complications.

Several studies have shown that in addition to improving heart function, DFO can remove myocardial iron effectively [32, 66, 92]. At very high levels of myocardial iron loading with average T2* values of 5 ms, improvement in myocardial T2* was 58% over 1 year [32]. However improvement in heart function preceded these changes in T2*, suggesting a beneficial effect of DFO on toxic labile iron pools independent of the slower improvement in T2*. With continued infusions, improvement continues, but requires up to 5 years to normalise [66]. Other prospective studies have shown improvement of moderately reduced T2* values over 1 year in patients given even low-dose intermittent DFO s.c. [92].

7.6 *Other Long-Term Beneficial Effects*

The other documented improvements with DFO therapy have been reviewed elsewhere and include improvement in liver fibrosis [93], decrease in hypogonadism [94], improved glucose tolerance [95], decreased incidence of diabetes [34], hypothyroidism and hypoparathyroidism in successive birth cohorts of patients [16]. Unlike heart failure, once evidence of advanced endocrine dysfunction has developed, reversal has not been documented.

7.7 *Tolerability and Unwanted Effects*

The unwanted effects of DFO and ways to avoid them have emerged empirically over 4 decades of cumulative experience, rather than from controlled trials that are now required for the licensing of new drugs [91, 96]. Most of the unwanted effects of DFO are dose related. These include effects on growth, skeletal changes, audiometric and retinopathic effects. In an adult, such effects are unlikely, however, if the dose does not exceed 50 mg/kg and if care is taken to reduce the dose as ferritin levels fall (see below). There is no evidence of differences in DFO pharmacokinetics or metabolism between affected and unaffected patients [97] except that predisposed patients have less chelatable iron pools and more of the iron-free drug is available for conversion into metabolite B [80]. Retinal effects that can present with loss of visual acuity, field defects, defects in night or color vision are now very rare, as the doses of 100 mg/kg/day under which these effects were originally described [89] are now hardly ever given. Nevertheless, occasional patients are picked up with retinopathic changes, and if patients on DFO are not routinely monitored, it can be difficult to interpret whether changes are related to DFO. Drug-related ototoxicity is typically symmetrical and of a high-frequency sensorineural nature [76, 98], so that skepticism about the diagnosis should be roused when asymmetric or unilateral effects are found. In patients who develop complications, DFO should be temporarily stopped and reintroduced at lower doses when investigations show improvement.

Some adverse effects are more likely when iron stores are low. This is particularly clear for neurotoxic complications where standard doses have been associated with coma in rheumatoid arthritis patients without iron overload [99] and where audiometric and retinopathic effects are more likely the lower the serum ferritin [98], particularly below 1,000 μg/L (or by not keeping mean daily dose/ferritin ratio <0.025) [90]. Audiometric problems are typically high-frequency sensorineural loss and/or tinnitus. Minor sensorineural deficit may be reversible, but severe hearing loss is usually irreversible [90]. It is advisable to monitor audiometry yearly especially if there has been a marked recent fall in ferritin. Some unwanted effects such as local skin reactions, allergic reactions and *Yersinia enterocolitica* infections are not clearly related to dose or to levels of iron overload, and their management is described elsewhere [91].

Unwanted effects on growth and skeletal development above 40 mg/kg limit the dose that can be administered to children. Growth retardation was seen when treatment was started early (<3 year) and at higher doses [100, 101]. Rickets-like bony lesions and genu valgum in association with metaphyseal changes, particularly in the vertebrae, causing a disproportionately short trunk can also occur, often with vertebral demineralization and flatness of vertebral bodies radiographically [100, 102]. Regular monitoring of growth is recommended, and the dose should not exceed 40 mg/kg until growth has ceased. If we accept the data that 50 mg/kg 5 times a week is a necessary dose to maintain iron balance in about half of thalassaemia major patients (see above), then a similar proportion of children will be under-dosed below 40 mg/kg 5 times/week. Under-dosing is unlikely to cause short-term demonstrable pathology in children but is likely to increase pituitary and myocardial iron loading, which over a period of one to two decades may increase morbidities from iron overload.

7.8 Recommended Dosing Regimes with DFO

7.8.1 Standard Therapy

Guidelines aim to achieve a balance between the unwanted effects of under- or over-chelation as well as advising what is practical for the patient. Because of concerns of the effects of over-chelation, DFO is usually not started until serum ferritin exceeds 1,000 μg/L, which usually occurs after the first 10 or 20 transfusions. Doses are kept below or equal to 40 mg/kg until growth has been completed. DFO is infused via a thin s.c. needle (ideally a Thalaset needle) inserted into the abdomen, arm or lateral thigh region nightly, connected to a portable pump over 8–12 h, 5–7 times per week at a daily dose of 20–60 mg/kg. The infusion site needs to be rotated nightly and a solution infused that is not >10% (1 g in 10 mL) to prevent damage to local tissues. If DFO is infused only 5 nights a week, it is important not to under-dose. In patients with higher transfusional iron intakes

(>0.5 mg/kg/day), doses of 50–60mg/kg/day will be necessary for iron balance if infusions are only given 5 times a week [5].

7.8.2 Rescue Therapy

For patients with heart failure, continuous DFO infusion is recommended. This is usually most conveniently achieved in the acute situation of heart failure by diluting DFO in 500 mL of saline and infusing through a peripheral vein. For longer-term infusions, once the patient has been stabilized, an indwelling line is usually necessary, although 24-h infusion has been successfully achieved by the subcutaneous route in selected cases (see above). Continuous doses above 60 mg/kg are associated with an increased risk of retinal and audiotoxicity and are now not recommended. For patients with evidence of moderately increased myocardial loading (T2* 10–20 ms), improvement in these measures may be achieved by increasing the dose or duration of exposure to subcutaneous DFO above that given for standard therapy. In patients with severe myocardial iron loading (T2* < 10 ms) but without heart failure, intensification of therapy is necessary. This may include increasing the dose and/or duration of DFO exposure with or without the addition of DFP (see below).

8 Development of Orally Effective Chelators

Unfortunately, compliance with the rigorous requirements of daily subcutaneous infusions is still a serious limiting factor in treatment outcome. In the United Kingdom outside expert centers, survival among thalassaemic patients by the age of 35 years was until recently only 50% [103] and mortality was largely attributed to poor compliance. Symptomatic siderotic heart disease was encountered in 23% of North American thalassaemic patients older than 25 years [91], and all patients who are non-compliant with intensified DFO treatment remain at risk of lethal cardiac complications [50]. This has been the rationale behind the intensive efforts to identify alternative, orally effective iron chelators which would be more convenient for use and could improve compliance.

The challenge in developing chelators that are rapidly absorbed from the gut has been to identify compounds that chelate toxic iron pools without accessing physiologically necessary intracellular pools of iron or other metals. Many promising compounds have been discarded because the therapeutic safety margin has been too narrow, either in preclinical studies or during clinical evaluation. Here we discuss four classes of chelators that have been evaluated clinically, with particular emphasis on two compounds, namely deferiprone and deferasirox, with which there is extensive clinical experience.

9 Pyridoxal Isonicotinoyl Hydrazone (PIH)

This compound was introduced by Ponka et al., who recognized its ability to mobilize iron from ^{59}Fe-labeled reticulocytes [104]. PIH is a tridentate chelator (Fig. 28.3) with a molecular weight of 287. At physiologic pH, PIH exists mainly in its neutral form which allows access across cell membranes and absorption from the gut. At pH 7.4 and a ligand concentration of 1 mmol/L, the pM value of PIH is 27.7, which is less than 28.6 for DFO. It would be worthwhile, therefore, to

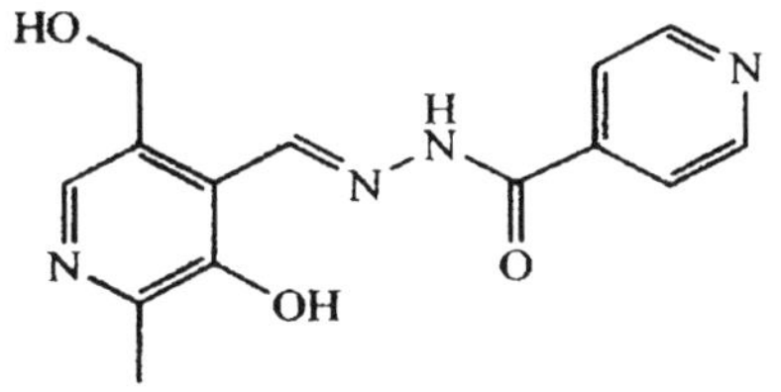

pyridoxal isonicotinoyl hydrazone
(PIH, 111)

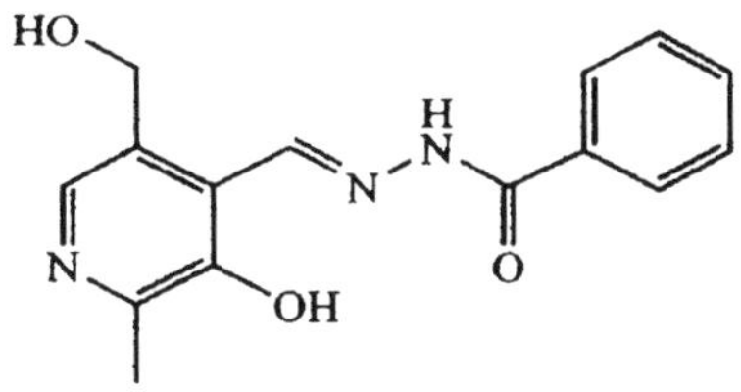

pyridoxal benzoyl hydrazone
(PBH, 101)

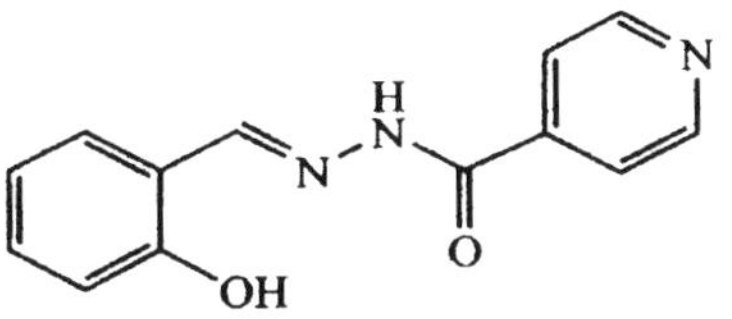

salicylaldehyde isonicotinoyl hydrazone
(SIH, 211)

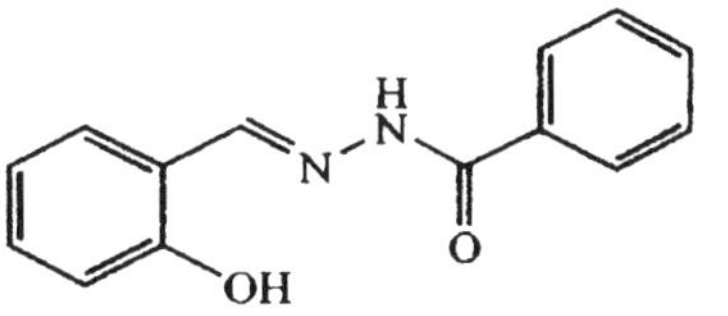

salicylaldehyde benzoyl hydrazone
(SBH, 201)

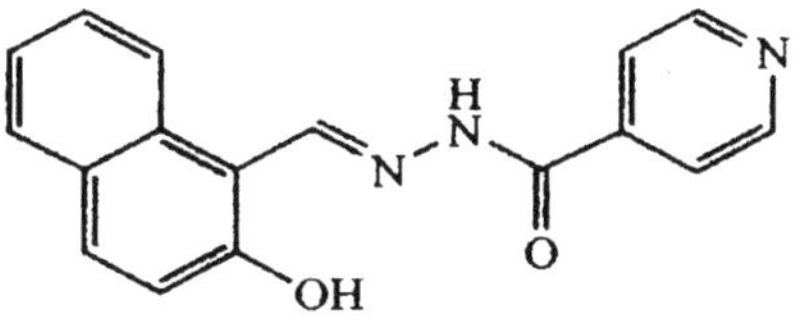

2-hydroxy-1-naphthaldehyde isonicotinoyl hydrazone
(NIH, 311)

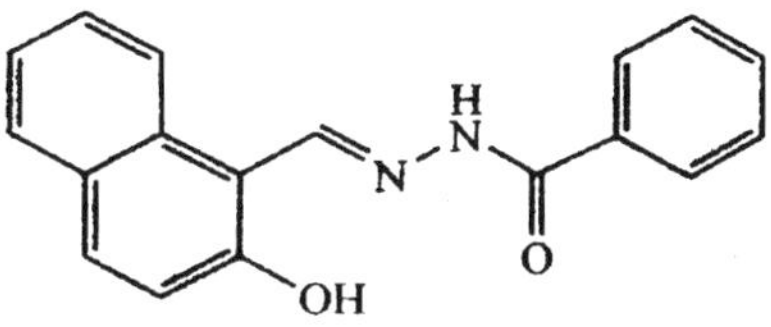

2-hydroxy-1-naphthaldehyde benzoyl hydrazone
(NBH, 301)

Fig. 28.3 Pyridoxal isonicotinoyl hydrazone (*PIH*) and its analogues

examine whether PIH may or may not be able to donate chelated iron to DFO acting as a 'shuttle' when the two chelators are coadministered. The selectivity of PIH for iron is comparable with that of DFO.

Studies in patients with iron overload treated with PIH at a dose of 30 mg/kg/day have shown a modest net iron excretion of 0.12 ± 0.07 mg/kg/d [105], which is much less than the mean value of 0.5 mg/kg/day required to achieve negative iron balance in most cases. Nevertheless, it was estimated that this degree of iron excretion may be sufficient for achieving a negative iron balance in non-transfusion-dependent patients with iron-loading anemias. Although the results of this pilot study in thalassaemic patients were generally regarded as evidence for the limited value of PIH in the treatment of thalassaemia, several arguments have been raised in favor of PIH in a review by Richardson and Ponka [106]. First, the dose of 30 mg/kg used in the above study was much less than the effective doses of 125–500 mg/kg employed in experimental animals. Second, PIH was given to patients after calcium carbonate which could drastically limit its absorption because of the low solubility of PIH in aqueous solution at a neutral pH. Clearly, the therapeutic potential of PIH and its derivatives still awaits extensive and careful evaluation.

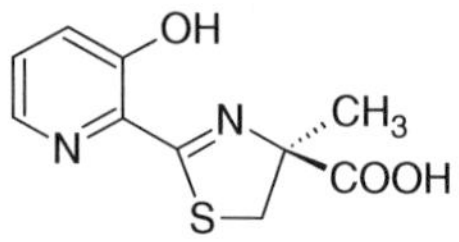

Fig. 28.4 Desferrithiocin (*DFT*)

10 Desferrithiocin (DFT) and Related Compounds

Desferrithiocin (DFT) is a tridentate siderophore (Fig. 28.4) isolated from *1* [107, 108]. It forms a 2:1 complex with Fe(III) and has a formation constant of 4×10^{29} M^{-1}. Desferrithiocin was one of the first iron chelators shown to be orally active in both the bile duct–cannulated rodent model, in which the efficiency was 5.5%, and the iron-overloaded *Cebus apella* primate model, in which the efficiency was 16%, i.e. three times the efficiency of DFO given subcutaneously. However, DFT is severely nephrotoxic. Subsequent studies were designed to assemble DFT analogues which are still orally active, but without the toxicity of the parent molecule. Abstraction of the thiazoline methyl diminished the efficiency substantially in both rodents and primates. Although removal of the pyridine nitrogen attenuated the efficiency in rodents, the efficiency of this compound was increased in primates. Finally, the absence of both the thiazoline methyl and the pyridine nitrogen left a molecule which was considerably less active in the rodent model but was still quite active in the primate. Toxicity studies of these desferrithiocin analogues have shown that it is possible to alter a siderophore in such a way as to ameliorate its toxicity profile while maintaining its iron-clearing properties. A related compound, deferitrin [109, 110], recently underwent evaluation in phase (II/III) trials but was found to have unacceptable renal toxicity. A further desferrithiocin derivative, currently referred to as FBS0701, one of several new derivatives that showed sparing for renal toxicity in preclinical animal studies [111], has recently entered clinical trials. In phase Ib studies in iron-overloaded patients, when given daily for 7 days at doses up to 32 mg/kg, the compound was well tolerated. Pharmacokinetics showed dose proportionality [112]. The maximum plasma concentration (C(max)) was reached within 60–90 min of dosing, and the drug was rapidly distributed at the predicted therapeutic doses. The plasma elimination half-life (*t*(1/2)) was approximately 19 h, and the route of iron excretion is fecal. Phase II studies are currently in progress.

11 Deferiprone (DFP) (L1, Ferriprox, Kelfer)

Deferiprone (Fig. 28.5) was the first orally active chelator to be used in long-term clinical trials, beginning in the 1980s [113]. While these studies were initially small, non-randomized and investigator-led, experience has now been obtained in many thousands of patients and involves several randomized controlled trials, the results of which will be highlighted here. The dose on which long-term safety data have been determined up to 4 years is 75–100 mg/kg p.o. divided into three portions [114].

11.1 Chemistry and Pharmacology

The family of 3-hydroxypyrid-4-one bidentate chelators, designed by Hider and Kontoghiorghes, binds to iron in a 3:1 ratio. The stability constant of 3-hydroxypyrid-4-ones is about six orders of magnitude higher than DFO while the pM of 20 (the –log of the uncoordinated metal (M) (iron)

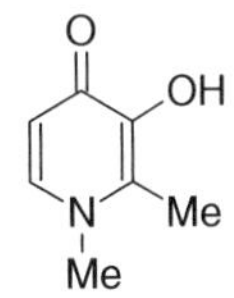

Fig. 28.5 Deferiprone or L1: 1,2-dimethyl-3-hydroxypyrid-4-one

concentration calculated when pH7.4, 10 μM ligand, 1 μM iron(III)) is lower than that of DFO at 27.6 [115]. This indicates that, as with all bidentate ligands, iron coordination is most efficient at higher concentrations relative to hexadentate ligands and that at concentrations of 1 μM iron and 10 μM chelator, DFO will scavenge iron more efficiently than DFP. The most important compound of this family is 1,2-dimethyl-3-hydroxypyrid-4-one (DFP or L1) [116]. The drug has a short plasma half-life of 1.5 h (Table 28.1) [117] and is therefore usually given three times daily. Following a single dose, peak plasma concentration is approximately 100 μM [118]. The drug is rapidly inactivated by glucuronidation in the liver [118].

11.2 Contrasting Cellular Pharmacology with DFO

The pharmacology and clinical efficacy of deferiprone has been the subject of several reviews [119, 120]. Unlike DFO which has a dual route of excretion of its iron-bound forms, deferiprone-induced biliary iron excretion is negligible [117], probably because of the rapid inactivation by glucuronidation of deferiprone within hepatocytes [121], hence the relatively less-impressive effect of DFP on liver iron removal [120]. Outside the liver, however, DFP generally enters cells more rapidly than DFO [122] because it is smaller (m.w. 139) and less hydrophilic than DFO (m.w. 560) (Table 28.1). These properties would favor iron removal from myocytes. These same properties mean that DFO accesses subcellular iron pools more slowly than DFP and related compounds [75, 76, 123].

Another difference of DFO from DFP is the positive charge of DFO and its iron complex, ferrioxamine, which contrasts with the neutral charge of the DFP and its iron complex. Thus, whereas the iron-free form and complex of DFP tends to equilibrate relatively quickly across cell membranes, DFO will slowly accumulate within cells at concentrations above those in the plasma and ferrioxamine will tend to become trapped within cells that lack an excretion mechanism [75, 77, 78]. Studies in iron-loaded rat heart cells have shown that at high chelator/iron molar ratio, the ability of DFP to remove iron from myocardial cells exceeds that of DFO [122]. Peak serum levels of DFP [124] are five to ten times higher than infused DFO [79, 117] (Table 28.1), and such high concentrations, together with a more rapid access to iron in heart cells, may favor the scavenging of chelatable iron by DFP in these cells [125]. Indeed in model systems, clinically relevant concentrations of DFO (10 μM) had a greater effect on preventing uptake of iron into myocytes than removal of iron from intracellular pools, leading to the suggestion that the ability of DFO to decrease heart iron and decrease heart failure may be explained by prevention of iron uptake rather than facilitation of iron release from myocytes [125]. Regardless of whether the clinical effect of DFO on the heart is mainly through prevention of iron uptake or increase in iron release, both of these effects would be enhanced by continuous exposure to chelator. With respect to DFP, the high peak concentrations are punctuated by negligible nocturnal levels. In principle therefore by alternating DFO at night with DFP during the day, both continuous chelation and high levels of a permanent chelator can be achieved [12].

11.3 Effects on Iron Balance

Urinary iron excretion in response to DFP 75 mg/kg is comparable to that with DFO infused subcutaneously over 8–12 h at a dose of 40–50 mg/kg [117]. However, unlike DFO, which elicits significant fecal iron excretion, the increase in fecal iron excretion with DFP is negligible. Thus overall iron balance obtained from metabolic balance studies show that total iron excretion in response to DFP (75 mg/kg) is 62% of that achieved with DFO (50 mg)/kg over 8 h subcutaneously [126].

11.4 Effects on Liver Iron

Combined analysis of randomized studies comparing changes of LIC totaling 143 people has been undertaken [127]. Findings vary considerably between studies, most likely reflecting the heterogeneity of dosing schedules, baseline LIC values and follow-up periods [128–131]. In one study, a mean increase of 5 ng/g dry wt at 33 months ($n=18$) was noted with DFP, compared with an increase of 1 mg/g dry wt with DFO ($n=18$) [128]. By contrast a decrease in LIC was seen with both DFP ($n=21$) and with DFO ($n=15$) at 30 months in an Italian study [129]. In another 1-year study in Italian patients, a mean decrease of 0.93 mg/g dry wt was seen with DFP at the higher dose of 100 mg/kg ($n=27$) compared with a decrease of 1.54 mg/g dry wt with DFO at a dose of 43 mg/kg × 5.7 times a week ($n=30$) [92]. In a fourth study (where baseline LIC values were significantly higher), a greater decrease in LIC was reported with DFP 75 mg/kg (6.6 mg/g dry wt, n=6) than with DFO 30–60 mg/kg 5–7 days/week (2.9 mg/g dry wt, $n=7$) at 6 months [130]. In a recent study, LIC decrease with DFP monotherapy at 1 year (–7%) was less than with combined therapy (–32%) or with DFO monotherapy (–42%) [131]. The transfusion rate was not examined in these studies, which, by analogy with recent findings in DFO and DFS [5], is likely to be an additional factor contributing to variability of LIC response between and within studies.

11.5 Effects on Serum Ferritin

There are numerous non-randomized cohort studies demonstrating a lowering of serum ferritin at doses of 75 mg/kg/day in 3 divided doses (reviewed 119,120). Significant decreases in serum ferritin are seen in patients with baseline values above 2,500 μg/L [132–134] but not with values below 2,500 μg/L [134–136]. The effects of DFP and DFO on serum ferritin have now been examined in several randomized trials (combined total 235 people) [92, 129–131, 137]. The relative effects of the two drugs differ considerably between the studies, which may reflect the different doses of drugs used as well as differences in baseline characteristic of patients both within and between studies. Pooled analysis [127] shows a statistically significant decrease in serum ferritin at 6 months in favor of DFO, with no difference between these drugs at 12 months.

11.6 Effects on Heart Function and Survival

Continued cardiac mortality has been observed in thalassaemic patients treated with DFP. Of 51 patients treated by DFP after failing DFO largely because of poor compliance, four died of cardiac causes and the authors concluded that DFP alone, in the face of pre-existing severe myocardial iron overload and continuing need for blood transfusions, cannot reliably protect patients from death from iron overload [121]. Likewise in the largest study of DFP treatment published so far, of 532 thalassaemic patients nine died of heart failure [138].

Several trials are now available comparing the ability of chelation therapy with either DFO or DFP to prevent heart disease. In a prospective randomized trial, 71 patients treated with DFP and 73 patients treated with DFO for 1 year showed similar and significant improvement in cardiac NMR signal [129]. In another retrospective study, 54 DFP-treated patients were compared with 75 DFO-treated patients for cardiac complications and survival [139]. By the end of the 6-year follow-up period, 3 patients died, all in the DFO group, despite attempted rescue by intensified i.v. therapy. Worsening of pre-existing cardiac disease or new onset of cardiac abnormalities were observed in 4% of the DFP group compared with 20% of the DFO-treated patients. The authors concluded that these findings suggest long-term DFP treatment provides greater protection against the cardiotoxicity of iron than DFO. It should be noted, however, that the 3 patients on DFO who died were 6–8 years older than the mean age of the DFP group. Moreover, five patients in the DFO group had NYHA class II–IV cardiac disease at outset as compared to only one in the DFP group. These difficulties underlined the need for further prospective randomized studies to evaluate the relative merits of the two chelating drugs.

Subsequent studies attempted to compare the effects of DFP on cardiac mortality with those of DFO. The first involved all thalassaemic patients treated at seven Italian hospitals [140], born between 1970 and 1993 and who did not experience cardiac complications prior to 1995. This analysis included 359 patients treated by DFO only, and 157 receiving DFP for a median duration of 4.3 years between 1995 and the end of 2003. There were 52 cardiac events, including ten cardiac deaths, among patients treated with DFO. By contrast, no cardiac event occurred in any of the patients during DFP treatment or within 18 months after stopping DFP. The estimated hazard of a cardiac event on DFP was less than one tenth than in patients on DFO. The dropout rate on DFP was high (46 patients or 31%) including 21 patients with increasing ferritins or liver iron, neutropenia in 8 and agranulocytosis in one patient. Events for each calendar year in patients dropping out of DFP were classed as related to DFO only if treatment had already been switched to DFO by January 1 of that year. This study was subjected to detailed statistical analysis, but the comparator groups were retrospectively allocated an unintentional selection bias, such as differences in duration of chelation or control of iron loading prior to the period of observation cannot be excluded.

Employing their newly developed T2* method for estimating cardiac iron concentrations, Anderson et al. [141] concluded that conventional treatment with DFO did not prevent excess cardiac iron accumulation in more than half the patients with thalassaemia major and that oral DFP was more effective at controlling cardiac iron. This was a retrospective non-randomized study, and although great efforts were made for matching of the two groups using serum ferritin, only 15 patients were treated by DFP whereas the 30 DFO controls had to be selected from a large group of 160 patients receiving DFO. In a subsequent study performed by the same group [92], 61 thalassaemic patients with moderate cardiac siderosis (T2* 8–20 ms) were randomized to continue on DFO 43 mg/kg/day or DFP 92 mg/kg/day. After 1 year of treatment, the improvement in T2* and increase in left ventricular ejection fraction (LVEF) were significantly greater for DFP than for DFO. The authors concluded that DFP monotherapy was significantly more effective than DFO at the doses used in improving asymptomatic myocardial siderosis in beta-thalassaemia major.

11.7 Tolerability and Unwanted Effects

11.7.1 Agranulocytosis and Cytopenias

Agranulocytosis and cytopenias have generally been considered to be the most serious side effect of DFP. In the study designed specifically to establish the frequency of agranulocytosis (neutrophils $0.0–0.5 \times 10^9$/L) involving weekly blood counts with confirmation within 24 h of all neutrophil counts below 1.5×10^9/L and discontinuation of the drug if confirmed, one of 187 patients (0.5%) developed agranulocytosis during 1 year of treatment [122]. Nine patients (4.8%) developed milder neutropenia (absolute neutrophil count $0.5–1.5 \times 10^9$/L). No additional cases of agranulocytosis, but seven new cases of mild neutropenia, occurred during the next 3 years of treatment in this study [114]. In 532 thalassaemic patients treated for a total of 1,154 patient-years, the rates of agranulocytosis and neutropenia were 0.43 and 2.08 per 100 patient-years respectively [142]. Agranulocytosis and milder neutropenia have been reversible on discontinuation of the drug, although some patients required treatment with G-CSF [143]. The mechanism of agranulocytosis is unclear. It has been argued that this is an idiosyncratic toxicity [144], although the incidence has not been compared at different doses clinically and a dose-dependent bone marrow hypoplasia is seen in animal studies [145] as well as dose-dependent inhibition of both DNA synthesis and ribonucleotide reductase [77]. Furthermore agranulocytosis may appear as a late event after more than 1 year of therapy and may be preceded by previous episodes of neutropenia, a pattern not characteristic of idiosyncratic reactions [138]. The involvement of other hemopoietic lineages [146–148] in both animal studies [73] and clinically would also be more consistent with a general effect on hemopoietic progenitors. Milder forms of neutropenia may be related to hypersplenism and intercurrent infections rather than drug toxicity [136]. In view of the risk of agranulocytosis, weekly blood counts are mandatory for all patients on deferiprone therapy. There are very few data on evaluation of DFP in children <6 years old, and a study of 44 patients showed no cases of agranulocytosis, but thrombocytopenia was seen in 45% of patients which was reversible on cessation of treatment [148]. As this was not a randomized study, the significance of this finding is difficult to judge and further studies are needed in this age group.

11.7.2 Hepatotoxicity

The issue of deferiprone-associated liver injury has been particularly contentious following the report of accelerated liver fibrosis in a randomized study comparing deferiprone ($n = 19$) with DFO-treated patients ($n = 20$) over 3.5 years [30, 31]. Progression of liver fibrosis during treatment with DFP has been reported by some additional studies [149, 150], but not others [151]. Variation in the length of treatment [150] and the failure to record baseline values of liver fibrosis [135, 149] have made precise evaluation of the progression and significance of liver fibrosis difficult. In a retrospective study with a median follow-up of 3.5 years, 34 out of 187 patients had both baseline and follow-up biopsies which showed no progression of fibrosis [151]. One prospective randomized study comparing progression of fibrosis with DFO and DFP showed no difference over the relatively short period of 1 year [129]. No long-term prospective data comparing liver fibrosis with DFO have yet been reported nor a study that relates changes in fibrosis to those of liver iron concentration [127], which is known to be a key factor in fibrosis progression in iron overload [35].

11.7.3 Other Toxic Effects

The International Study Group on Oral Chelators found that the complications most frequently associated with treatment with DFP were nausea and other gastrointestinal symptoms, arthralgia, zinc deficiency and fluctuating liver function tests, especially in anti-HCV-positive patients [152]. The prospective, multicenter study of 187 patients, the largest clinical study designed to characterize the safety profile of deferiprone [136], showed a similar range of drug-related effects during the first year of therapy. Nausea and/or vomiting occurred in 24% of patients, abdominal pain in 14% and arthralgia in 13%. Arthralgia and arthropathy seem to vary greatly between locations of studies, with highest incidences 30–40% [133, 153] in the developing world and the lowest in Italy (<5%) [138]. The duration of observation may have a bearing on the incidence of arthropathy as this increased from 6% at 1 year to 13% at 4 year [114]. Small decreases in the mean value of plasma zinc [136] and cases of zinc deficiency [152] not requiring cessation of therapy have been reported. Analysis after 4 years of treatment demonstrated that gastrointestinal symptoms were reported infrequently after the first year of therapy although the dropout rate increased from 15% to 55% between these intervals [114]. Although not reported at conventional doses, overdosing has been associated with neurotoxicities [154].

11.8 Recommended Dosing

The dose at which the safety of DFP has been evaluated over several years is 75 mg/kg in three divided doses. It is likely that patients with poor response at these standard doses have either a higher transfusional requirement or a faster inactivation by glucuronidation, but this has not been formally studied. Licensing in the EU permits doses up to 100 mg/kg daily, but published tolerability data are scarce at this dose, confined to a single one-year prospective study in 32 patients [92]. Because no excess toxicity has been reported in this study, it may be reasonable to increase the dose in otherwise unresponsive patients. However, the study was not large enough or intended to answer whether tolerability issues such as neutropenia and agranulocytosis increase at these higher doses. The effect of dose or levels of iron overload on other tolerability issues has not been studied in prospective trials. There are also few data in young children, and this is reflected in the licensing in the EU which is confined to patients >6 years old.

12 Combined Chelation Therapy

12.1 Pharmacology

In patients where control of iron load or iron distribution is not adequately achieved by monotherapy with one of the above agents, combined use of two chelators may in principle provide an alternative approach. Present clinical experience is largely confined to various combinations of DFP with DFO. There are several ways in which an advantage could result from combined therapy. Firstly, chelators could be alternated so as to provide continuous exposure to chelation, for example, DFO given at night and DFP during the day. In this way labile iron pools can be accessed almost 24 h a day, thereby decreasing toxicity from labile iron as well as maximising interaction with the chelatable iron pool. Given that the unwanted effects of chelators differ somewhat, additive chelation might be achieved without additive toxicity. Chelators could also be given at the same time, allowing the possibility of drug interaction by a so-called shuttle mechanism. Here, iron pools that are inaccessible to one chelator because of its large size or cellular distribution could be accessed by a smaller or more lipid-soluble drug and then donated to the first chelator acting as a 'sink' for the chelatable iron. Such a mechanism was first shown for heavy metal poisoning, and there is experimental evidence for such an effect in animal models of iron overload [155]. If pM values for DFO and DFP are considered, DFP will donate iron to DFO at all clinically relevant concentrations of the two chelators [81]. Furthermore, because DFP gains access to various intracellular iron pools faster than DFO, there is a possibility of increased iron mobilization from these compartments, with potential benefits in iron-overloaded cells. It has recently been shown that chelation of NTBI by DFO is enhanced by low concentrations of DFP and that this is achieved by the shuttling of NTBI iron by DFO to DFO with the formation of FO [82]. The theoretical possibility of increased inhibition of metalloenzymes also exists, however.

12.2 Clinical Regimens Using Combined Therapy

Combined chelation treatment is gaining increasing popularity, in particular in Mediterranean countries [119, 120, 156]. Although at inception its rationale was a shuttle-and-sink hypothesis, there is no compelling evidence that the simultaneous presence of both chelators is necessary to achieve increased chelation. It is quite possible that a simple additive effect resulting from the increased exposure time to chelation may be useful. Although maximal exposure time to chelation could be achieved by alternating DFO every night and DFP every day, in practice many other regimes have been used (Table 28.2). For example, one regime, using DFP for 5 days only and DFO on the other 2 days of the week, showed efficacy similar to conventional DFO for 5–7 days a week, was convenient and not associated with increased toxicity [157]. The choice of combination regime may vary depending on what the reason for adding a second drug is. If the primary aim is to identify a regime that the patient is most likely to comply with in an otherwise low-risk situation, the choice of combination may differ from someone who has extreme levels of iron overload or already has significant cardiac problems.

13 Evidence of Efficacy of Combined Treatment

13.1 Effects of Sequential Use on Serum Ferritin

Several randomized studies have compared effects on serum ferritin of various combinations with that of monotherapy (Table 28.2), and these have been included in a recent systematic review of DFP [127]. This is considerable variability in response between studies which may result from the variety of the regimes and doses used. Differences in study populations with respect to iron loading rates, previous chelation therapy, treatment compliance or population differences in DFP metabolism due to variability in glucuronidation rates are also likely to contribute to these differences. In Lebanese patients, 5 days of DFO monotherapy ($n=14$) produced similar effects to two nights of DFO plus 7 days of DFP at 75 mg/kg ($n=11$) [158]. Thirty patients in India randomized to three different treatments showed the largest decrease with five nights of DFO, the smallest effect with DFP monotherapy and an intermediate effect with combined treatment (DFO two nights a week plus DFP 7 days a week) [137]. In a larger study involving 60 Sardinian patients [157], ferritin changes were similar in patients randomized to combined treatment (2 days desferrioxamine at 33 mg/kg + 7 days DFP at 75 mg/kg) or to DFO at relatively low doses of 33 mg/kg 5 times/week. In a more recent randomized study of 65 patients, serum ferritin was decreased more using combined treatment (DFO 5 days a week plus DFP 7 days a week) than with standard DFO monotherapy (40 mg/kg/x5/week) [159].

13.2 Effects of Sequential Use on Liver Iron

The effects of combined treatment on liver iron were compared with that of DFO monotherapy in a randomized study of 60 patients [157]. The LIC was <7 mg/g dry wt at baseline and was on average maintained in both arms of the study. In a prospective randomized study from Turkey, DFP monotherapy at 75 mg/k daily was compared with a matched group receiving DFP 75 mg/kg daily plus twice weekly DFO [131]. The effect of DFO monotherapy s.c. Five times/week was also examined in an unmatched comparator group (Table 28.2). The decrease in LIC with DFO monotherapy

Table 28.2 Prospective randomized studies comparing monotherapy of DFP or DFO* with combined treatment

Country, Year	*n*	Comparison	DFP (days/week)	DFO (days/week) × dose (mg/kg)	Ferritin change (%)	LIC change	Cardiac changes	Tolerability
Lebanon	14	DFO	0	5×45	−12	Not done	Not done	–
2003 [158]	11	Combo	7	2×45	−32			Arthropathy 27%
India	10	DFO	0	5	−27	Not done	Not done	Injection site
2004 [137]	10	Combo	7	2	+0.9			Arthropathy 10%
	10	DFP	7	0	+28			Raised SPGT
Italy, Greece	30	DFO	0	5×33	−15	−11%	Not done	Injection sites
2006 [161]	30	Combo	7	2×33	−12	−4%		Neutropenia 2
								Alt 3 x baseline > DFO
Italy,	33	DFO	0	5×43	−16	LT2* ratio	cT2* +3 ms	Arthralgia 18%
2007 [159]	32	Combo	7	5×43	−62	1.2	LVEF + 0.6%	Injection site
						LT2* ratio 2.0	cT2* +6 ms	Agranulocytosis 1
							LVEF + 2.6%	Neutropenia 3
								Arthralgia 27%
Turkey	12	DFO$	0	5×45	−35	−42%	LVEF	Injection site
2007 [131]	8	Combo	7	2×45	−32[a]	−32%	−8.9%	Agranulocytosis 1
	12	DFP	7	0	−21	−7%	LVEF + 1.2%	Arthralgia 1 Cerebellar syndrome 1
							LVEF −7%	Neutropenia 1

[a]'Combo' refers to combination treatments. All studies were of 12 months' duration except 139 (6 months), and all doses of DFP were 75 mg/kg/day. DFO doses and frequency of administration varied as shown. Ferritin and LIC are shown as the percentage change from baseline, [−] indicating a decrease. LT2* is the ratio of the final to baseline liver T2*: the larger the ratio, the larger the implied decrease in LIC. cT2* is the cardiac T2*, shown as the average change in ms from baseline. LVEF is the left ventricular ejection fraction, shown as the percentage change from baseline, [+] indicating improvement and [−] deterioration. For the study from India, the tolerability for Combo and DFP monotherapy was reported together. Injection site issues with DFO included pain and occasional abscesses. Arthropathy varied between studies from simple pain to effusions and to joint erosions in some cases

(−42%) or combined treatment (−32%) was significantly greater than with deferiprone monotherapy (−7%) over 1 year. In a randomized study in Italian patients, deferiprone 75 mg/kg/day plus DFO 5 times a week was compared with DFO monotherapy 5 times a week; the improvement in liver T2* (as a surrogate measure of LIC) was greater in the combination arm [159].

13.3 Effects on Heart and Survival

In the above randomized controlled study of 65 patients [159] with baseline LVEF >56%, changes in LVEF improved by approximately 2.6% in the combination arm and 0.6% in the monotherapy arm (Table 28.2). Changes in heart function have also been reported in two observational studies with combined treatment. In 79 patients treated with a variable DFO regime plus deferiprone at 75 mg/kg 7 days a week for a variable time, there was an improvement in LVEF by echocardiography [160]. In an observational study of 42 patients with sequential use of treatment over 3–4 years (deferiprone 75 mg/kg/day plus desferrioxamine 2–6 days a week), the LV shortening fraction improved [161].

In a randomized controlled study of 65 patients with moderate heart iron loading (T2* 8–20 ms), myocardial T2* changes with combined deferiprone 75 mg/kg 7 days a week plus desferrioxamine 5 days were compared with patients who remained on standard desferrioxamine 5 times a week [159]. T2* improved in both groups but was significantly greater 6 ms with combined treatment than with desferrioxamine monotherapy at 3 ms (Table 28.2). In an observational study, the T2 of the heart improved with combined therapy [161].

In thalassaemia major patients from Cyprus, 539 thalassaemic patients born after 1960 and on whom accurate clinical data were available were followed over the period from 1980 to 2004. Overall there were 58 deaths, 53% of which were due to cardiac causes [162]. There was a significant trend of increasing cardiac mortality between 1980 and 2000 and a decline after 2000, which the authors suggested to be due to the introduction of a combined deferiprone–deferoxamine therapy at this time. There were no deaths reported in patients treated with combined therapy between 2000 and 2004 using a regime similar to that employed in Italy [160]. Longer follow-up will be necessary to test the statistical significance of these findings [162].

13.4 Safety of Combined Treatments

Formal safety data on combined treatment are limited. In general, alternating regimes are less likely to be an issue for toxicity compared with regimes where chelation is simultaneous or overlaps. A meta-analysis of the incidence of agranulocytosis with combined regimes compared with deferasirox monotherapy suggested that the risk may be increased several fold although the numbers of evaluable patients are small. The increased incidence appeared to occur mostly in those regimes where the drugs were administered simultaneously. In a recently reported prospective study, one case of agranulocytosis and three of neutropenia were seen at 1 year in the combination arm containing 32 patients [159]. No excess in arthropathy was seen in the combination arm, and no new tolerability entities that were not recognized with monotherapy have been reported. It has been suggested that lower levels of ferritin can be achieved with combined therapy than with monotherapy using DFO of DFP alone. This is based on a retrospective study reporting the attainment of remarkably low ferritin levels without any DFP- or DFO-related toxicities in patients given 'individualized' sequential combinations of DFP and DFO [64].

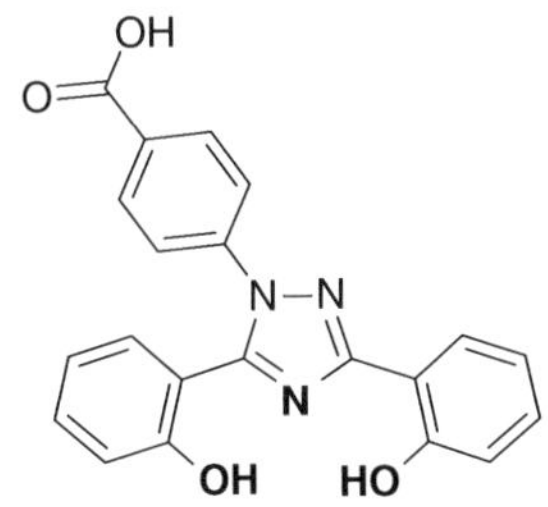

Fig. 28.6 Deferasirox or ICL670, 4-[3,5-bis-(hydroxyphenyl)-[1,2,4] triazol-1-yl]-benzoic acid

14 Deferasirox (Bis-Hydroxyphenyl-Triazole, ICL670, Exjade, DFS)

This compound is a member of a class of tridentate iron-selective synthetic chelators, the bis-hydroxy-phenyl-triazoles developed by Novartis (Fig. 28.6). Deferasirox (DFS) emerged from the screening of over 700 candidate drugs as the most promising compound combining oral effectiveness and low toxicity. The magnitude of efforts invested in the clinical development of DFS is unprecedented in the history of chelator research. Within a few years, over 3,000 patients have been treated in prospective well-controlled trials involving more than 100 medical centers in four continents. Most of these trials were designed to last 1 year, but by now, some have been extended up to 5 years.

14.1 Chemistry and Pharmacology

The pM value of deferasirox for ferric iron is intermediate between DFO and deferiprone, and the ligand is stable both in vivo and in vitro [107] (Table 28.1). Preclinical studies in animal models have shown effective and selective mobilization of tissue iron with greater efficiency than DFO [107]. Studies in cell cultures and in hypertransfused rats with selective radioiron labeling of cellular stores demonstrated the ability of DFS to enter and remove iron from cells including cardiac myocytes [125, 163], and this has been confirmed in studies with gerbils [164]. In iron-overloaded patients, over 90% of plasma drug is unaltered DFS and the concentration of the iron complex is nine times lower. The majority of drug is excreted in the feces, and metabolism is mainly to an acyl glucuronide that retains its ability to bind iron [165]. Iron excretion is almost entirely in the feces, and only 8% of the drug is eliminated in urine [165]. A plasma half-life of 11–19 h supported the use of a once-daily oral dosing employed in subsequent trials [166, 167]. With once-daily repeat dosing at 20 mg/kg, peak plasma levels reach a mean of 80 μM with trough values of 20 μM (Table 28.1) [168].

14.2 Effects on Iron Balance, LIC and Ferritin

In phase I clinical trials, DFS is well tolerated at single oral doses up to 80 mg/kg [166, 167]. Iron excretion was dose-dependent and was almost entirely fecal. Metabolic balance studies showed that excretion averaged 0.13, 0.34 and 0.56 mg/kg/day at DFS doses of 10, 20 and 40 mg/kg/day, respectively, predicting equilibrium or negative iron balance at daily doses of 20 mg and above [167].

Iron balance over 1 year was examined by comparing baseline and end-of-treatment LIC values and accounting for transfusional iron intake. Table 28.3 describes a selection of phase I, II, III and IV clinical trials involving deferasirox. The most extensive and informative of these was a 1-year

Table 28.3 Clinical trials of deferasirox (DFS)

Year / Study / Reference	Phase diagnosis	*N* Total subgroup	Age (years)	Dose (mg/kg/d)	Duration	LIC or iron excretion	Ferritin	Cardiac T2*	Withdrawal
2003	Phase I	24	20–39	10 DFS	12 day	Iron excr. mg/kg/day 0.13	NA	ND	
0104	TM		18–38	20 DFS		0.34			
[167]			19–34	40 DFS		0.56			
2006	Phase II	24	17–33	10 DFS	48 weeks	LIC unchanged	Unchanged	Pilot data effective	–
							Unchanged		2 of 24
0105	TM	24	19–50	20 DFS		Decreased	Unchanged		2 of 24
[166]		23	18–29	40 DFO		Decreased			
2006	Phase II	20	2–12	10 DFS	48 weeks	LIC increased	Increased	ND	2.5%
0106	TM	20	12–17	10 DFS					
[168]									
2006	Phase III	586	2–49	5 DFS	52 weeks	LIC increased	Increased	ND	4.9%
0107	TM	15	2–53	10 DFS	52 weeks	Increased	Increased		
[83]		78		20 DFS		Unchanged	Unchanged		
		84		30 DFS		Decreased	Decreased		
		119		25 DFO		Unchanged	Unchanged		
		14		30 DFO		Unchanged	Unchanged		
		79		40 DFO		Unchanged	Unchanged		
		91		>50DFO		Decreased	Decreased		
		106							
2011	Phase IIIE	555	2–49	20–40 DFS	4–5 years	LIC decreased	Decreased	Pilot data	43%
0107E	TM			22 mean				effective	Stable creatinine
[169]									
2008	Phase II	184	3–81	5–30 DFX range	1 year	LIC decreased at 20–30 mg/kg	Decreased at 30 mg/kg	ND	17% overall
									No disease specific effects
0108	TM	85	4–59						
[6]	MDS	47	20–81						
	DBA	30	3–42						
	RA	22	4–80						

2007 0109 [171]	Phase II SCD	63 132	3–51 3–54	20–60 DFO 10–30 DFS	1 year	Decreased at 35–50 Decreased at 10–30	Decrease NS	ND	DFS 11.4% DFO 11.1%
2011 0109E [172]	Phase IIE SCD	185	3–54	19 DFS mean	4–5 year	ND	Decreased	ND	66% stable creatinine
2010 [170] EPIC	Phase IV	1,744		22 mean [19–39]	1 year	ND	Decreased	See below	19%
2010 [170]	TM	1,115		DFS			Decreased		9.4%
2010 [172]	AA	116		18			Decreased		24%
2010 [173]	MDS	341		19			Decreased		48%
2011 [174]	RA	57		19			Decreased		30%
2009 [173]	Phase IV	114	20.2 mean	20–40 DFS	Baseline	–	–	11.2 ms	7.9%
2010 [176]	TM with	101		33 mean	1 year	Decreased	Decreased	12.9 ms	14.9%
2011 [177]	T2* 5–20ms	71		35 mean	2 year	Decreased	Decreased	14.8 ms	7.0%
				34 mean	3 year	Decreased	Decreased	17.1 ms	
2009 Escalator [180]	Phase IV TM with heavy iron load	252	2–42 range	20–40 DFS 23 mean	1 year	Decreased	Decreased	ND	2%

NA not applicable, *DFO* deferoxamine, *DFS* deferasirox, *LIC* liver iron concentration, *RA* rare anemias, *ND* not done

randomized trial comparing deferoxamine (290 patients) and deferasirox (296 patients) in 586 thalassaemic patients aged 2–53 years [83]. About half the patients were younger than 16 years of age. Discontinuations were rare (5.7% for deferasirox), but the initial selection excluded subjects with a history of non-compliance. A conservative dosing system was applied, adapted to initial liver iron concentrations (LIC). Patients with LIC below 7 mg Fe/g dry weight received DFS dosing of 5–10 mg/kg/day, and those with LIC above seven received 20–30 mg/kg/day. By contrast, patients randomized to DFO were allowed to continue doses closer to those received at baseline, prior to randomization (Table 28.3). The disproportionately low dosing of patients with DFS at 5 and 10 mg/kg/day relative to DFO and the maintenance of high prestudy DFO doses resulted in the failure of DFS to elicit a response equal to the corresponding DFO control groups. By contrast, at dose ranges of 20–30 mg DFS, where a dose relationship of DFS to DFO of 1:2 was maintained, both drugs were equally effective as judged by LIC and ferritin measurements. These results, indicating DFS efficacy at 20–30 mg/kg/day, agree very well with the results of previous studies described in Table 28.3. Further analysis of iron balance based on LIC response over 1 year shows that the dose may be adjusted to the transfusional iron loading rate [4]. For example, the proportion of patients in negative iron balance at 20 mg/kg was 75% at low blood transfusion rates (<0.3 mg/kg/day) but fell to 55% and 47%, respectively, at intermediate (0.3–0.5 mg/kg/day) and high (>0.5 mg/kg/day) blood transfusion rates. This can be increased at 30 mg/kg to 96% in those who have a low transfusional loading, but at intermediate and high transfusional loading rates, the proportion falls to approximately 80% of patients.

The results of extension up to 5 years are now available [169]. In 371 TM patients who completed at least 4 years of treatment (67%), median serum ferritin decreased significantly, as did LIC. The final dosing was 15–25 mg/kg in 32% of patients and 25–35 mg/kg day in the same percentage. Overall 73% patients attained serum ferritin levels ≤2,500 ng/mL and 41% patients achieved serum ferritin levels of ≤1,000 ng/mL, compared with 64% and 12% at baseline respectively. The percentage of patients with LIC values <7 mg/g d wt by biopsy increased from 22% at baseline to 44% at EOS. Creatinine clearance remained stable over this extended period, and the incidence of other common side effects decreased in frequency. There was no adverse effect on pediatric growth or adolescent sexual development in 209 pediatric patients. Four patients died during the extension, one from a road traffic accident and 3 from cardiac complications associated with rising serum ferritin values in two cases. No deaths reported during the extension were attributed to deferasirox toxicity.

A large-scale prospective study (EPIC) has examined the interaction between dose and ferritin response in large-scale studies involving 1,744 transfusion dependent anemias, including 1,115 with TM [170]. The initial dose was 20 mg/kg/day for patients receiving 2–4 packed red blood cell units/month, and 10 or 30 mg/kg/day was recommended for patients receiving less- or more-frequent transfusions, respectively. Dose adjustment was made on the basis of ferritin trends at 3 monthly intervals. A significant though modest overall fall in ferritin was seen at 1 year.

The efficacy and safety has also been examined in a variety of other disease states. The efficiency of chelation (the proportion of administered drug excreted in the iron bound form) is 27–34%, essentially the same across all diagnoses and doses tested [6]. A 1-year randomized study in SCD showed no additional safety issues in this patient group with effective reduction in LIC [171]. In 4–5-year extensions of this study, serum ferritin fell significantly, and creatinine clearance remained within the normal range throughout the study, with no new tolerability issues, at an average dose of 19 mg/kg/day [172]. The efficacy and tolerability of DFS was examined in a variety of other forms of anemia, such as in MDS, DBA and in other rare anemias [6], which showed that differences in transfusional iron intake that were accounted for response of LIC and ferritin to chelation were similar across disease states. In MDS there was a higher study dropout than in other conditions, mainly due to disease progression. More recently, patients with aplastic anemia ($n=116$) [173], MDS ($n=341$) [174] and rare production and hemolytic anemias ($n=57$) [175] have been described in substudies of the EPIC trial. These studies show that responses to chelation in terms of iron balance and serum ferritin are essentially similar across these diagnoses, once the transfusional iron loading rates are taken into account and support a similar approach to dosing. In the aplastic group, concomitant use of cyclosporine had a significant impact on serum creatinine levels, though no cases of progressive renal dysfunction were seen. Mean absolute neutrophil and platelet counts remained stable during treatment, and there were no drug-related cytopenias [173].

14.3 Effects on Heart Iron

A question of vital importance is the effect of DFS on cardiac siderosis and the prevention of cardiac complications. In vitro [125] and animal studies [164] suggested that DFS would be effective at accessing myocyte iron. Initial pilot data from phase II studies suggested that myocardial iron could be removed in TM and other forms of transfusional iron overload [176]. Several prospective studies have examined the effects of DFS on myocardial T2*. The largest prospective study, in 192 patients with TM, has examined effects on myocardial iron at 1 year [177], 2 years [178], with preliminary data now at 3 years [179]. At 1 year, there was an increase in the mT2* geometric mean from 11.2 ms to 12.9 ms (P<.0001) [177] which by 2 years had increased to 14.8 ms [178] and by 3 years to 17.1 ms [179]. Patients with baseline T2* of 10–20 ms normalized the T2* at 2 year (>20 ms). Patients with baseline T2* of 5–10 ms also showed significant increases. The geometric mean T2* reached near moderate-to-mild severity 9.4 ms by 2 years and continued to increase to 10.5 ms at 3 years. Mean actual DFS doses were 33, 35 and 34 mg/kg/day during the first, second and third years, respectively. Tolerability was similar to other DFS studies in TM, and the LVEF remained stable within the reference range throughout the study.

14.4 Effects in Children

This is the first chelator to be formally assessed in children as young as 2 years old. Approximately 50% of patients in the five clinical studies that included 703 patients were children aged <16 years. The drug appears to be tolerated in children similarly to adults. Importantly, no adverse effects on growth or skeletal development have been found [168].

14.5 Tolerability and Unwanted Effects

In general, DFS is well tolerated [83]. Adverse events were generally mild including transient gastrointestinal events in 15%, skin rash in 11% and mild, dose-dependent increases in serum creatinine in 38% of patients which generally remained within the normal range and never exceeded two times the upper limit of normal. Increases in creatinine typically occurred within a few weeks of starting or increasing therapy, were not progressive and reversible or stabilised with dose adjustment when necessary. Increased liver enzymes judged to be related to DFS were observed in two patients only. Audiometric effects and lens opacities did not differ significantly from the control or with DFO. Importantly, no drug-related agranulocytosis has been observed. Evaluation of pediatric patients has shown that growth and development proceeded normally while on DFS, lending support to its use in very young patients. Follow-up data in the five core phase II/III studies have now reached 4–5 years with no evidence of new or progressive toxicities [169]. Understandably, it is too early yet to allow any statements on the impact of DFS on survival. Recommended patient monitoring includes monthly creatinine and liver function and annual auditory and ophthalmic examinations, including slit-lamp examination and fundoscopy.

The tolerability at doses >30 mg/kg has been retrospectively analyzed from studies 107E, 108E, 109E [180] as well as from a further study in patients from the Middle East [181]. In total, 228 patients received doses >30 mg/kg/day with overall median exposure from the first to last administration of >30 mg/kg/day of 36 months. Despite the limited duration of exposure, doses >30 mg/kg/day appeared to effectively reduce SF levels, with a safety profile consistent with previously published data. Of the subjects, 61% experienced AEs, and 16% of these were assessed as possibly drug related. The most common drug-related AEs were gastrointestinal events such as vomiting (3%), abdominal pain and nausea (1.8%) or both. After starting treatment with DFX >30 mg/kg/day, the serum creatinine levels remained close to those seen pre-high-dose level.

14.6 Dosing Regimen

A standard starting dose of 20 mg/kg once daily is recommended for maintenance of iron levels and 30 mg/kg when iron levels need to be decreased. In patients with low transfusion rates (<0.3 mg/kg/day), a daily dose of 20 should be sufficient to maintain iron balance, whereas the respective doses for intermediate (0.3–0.5) and high (>0.5) transfusion loading rates are 25–30 mg respectively [5]. The drug is taken as a suspension in 100–200 mls of water, orange or apple juice stirred with a non-metallic utensil. Recommendations can be fine-tuned on the basis of transfusional iron loading rates and for specific disease categories. Responses in MDS, rare anemias [6] and SCD [171] are consistent with those in TM with respect to dose dependency of LIC and ferritin response. Net iron accumulation from transfusions may be less in MDS and SCD so that lower doses may suffice to maintain iron balance. For patients on doses of 30 mg/kg daily who show an inadequate response, either because of an unusually high transfusion intake or because of as yet unidentified causes, doses up to 40 mg/kg/day have been given, and this is the dose used to treat excess myocardial iron loading. There is some evidence of decreased bioavailability in some patients who lack a clear downward trend in serum ferritin [182]. The timing of the dose, either by giving after food or in divided doses, may improve the response rate. Preliminary evidence suggests that DFS can be combined with DFO without unwanted drug interactions to achieve increased iron mobilization [183], but the precise indications for combined therapy have yet to be defined and are the subject of ongoing studies. The proportion of patients with ferritin values <1,000 μg/L is increasing in patients receiving long-term therapy. Standard recommendations are to stop treatment when ferritin values reach 500 μg/L. However this risks rebound in NTBI and LIP, and in patients who continue to receive blood transfusions, it is preferable to reduce the dose as values fall below 1,000 μg/L so that values can be kept between 500 and 1,000 μg/L without interrupting treatment.

15 Conclusions

The accumulated evidence shows that chelation therapy is a highly effective treatment modality in reducing morbidity and mortality from iron overload. The ability of DFO to prevent damage to the heart and other vital organs and to increase life expectancy in transfusional siderosis is well established. A major limitation of DFO is the inconvenience of parenteral administration resulting in limited compliance. The emergence of orally effective chelators is a very favorable development offering further improvement in quality of life and longevity. The current dilemma is related to the following issues (a) Which chelator is most suitable for first-line therapy? (b) Should patients be switched from DFO only in subjects with unsatisfactory response, or those with significant drug-related complications or failure of compliance? (c) When should chelators be used as monotherapy or in combination? To answer these questions categorically, solid evidence is needed for the impact of each therapeutic option on disease-related morbidity and mortality as well as tolerability [156]. For the practicing clinician, a minimalistic approach would be to adhere to the treatment plan already in use and change treatment only if careful clinical assessment implies unsatisfactory results. At the other end of the spectrum, all patients could be switched to oral chelation. This option offers convenience, improved likelihood of compliance and may be favored by most patients. To take this option, strong evidence would be needed to indicate that upfront treatment with DFP or DFS monotherapy is equal to or exceeds the efficacy of the other options in the medium to long term [156]. For patients inadequately controlled with deferiprone or DFO monotherapy, a combination of DFP and DFO is one option. The advantage of combining DFO with DFP is avoidance of abandoning the old and trusted drug DFO, but limiting its inconvenience by adding an oral drug of reasonable efficacy. On the other hand, the convenience of once-daily monotherapy with DFS is preferred by many patients and the drug is licensed as first-line therapy in young children as well as adults worldwide. The outcome of safety and efficacy data from ongoing 5-year prospective studies as well as the findings from prospective studies on cardiac function with this treatment will be helpful to patients and clinicians in deciding whether this is the best long-term option.

References

1. Andrews NC. A genetic view of iron homeostasis. Semin Hematol. 2002;39:227–34.
2. Ganz T. Hepcidin, a key regulator of iron metabolism and mediator of anemia of inflammation. Blood. 2003;102:783–8.
3. Finch CA, Deubelbeiss K, Cook JD, et al. Ferrokinetics in man. J Clin Invest. 1970;49:17–53.
4. Tanno T, Bhanu NV, Oneal PA, et al. High levels of GDF15 in thalassemia suppress expression of the iron regulatory protein hepcidin. Nat Med. 2007;13:1096–101.
5. Cohen AR, Glimm E, Porter JB. Effect of transfusional iron intake on response to chelation therapy in thalassemia major. Blood. 2008;111:583–7.
6. Porter J, Galanello R, Saglio G, et al. Relative response of patients with myelodysplastic syndromes and other transfusion-dependent anaemias to deferasirox (ICL670): a 1-yr prospective study. Eur J Haematol. 2008;80:168–76.
7. Fung EB, Harmatz P, Milet M, et al. Morbidity and mortality in chronically transfused subjects with thalassemia and sickle cell disease: a report from the multi-center study of iron overload. Am J Hematol. 2007;82:255–65.
8. Hershko C, Graham G, Bates G, Rachmilewitz E. Non-specific serum iron in thalassaemia; an abnormal serum fraction of potential toxicity. Br J Haematol. 1978;40:255–63.
9. Grootveld M, Bell JD, Halliwell B, Aruoma OI, Bomford A, Sadler PJ. Non-transferrin-bound iron in plasma or serum from patients with idiopathic hemochromatosis. Characterization by high performance liquid chromatography and nuclear magnetic resonance spectroscopy. J Biol Chem. 1989;264:4417–22.
10. Evans RW, Rafique R, Zarea A, et al. Nature of non-transferrin-bound iron: studies on iron citrate complexes and thalassemic sera. J Biol Inorg Chem. 2008;13:57–74.
11. Gutteridge J, Rowley D, Griffiths E, Halliwell B. Low molecular weight iron complexes and oxygen radical reactions in idiopathic hemochromatosis. Clin Sci. 1985;68:463–7.
12. Cabantchik ZI, Breuer W, Zanninelli G, Cianciulli P. LPI-labile plasma iron in iron overload. Best Pract Res Clin Haematol. 2005;18:277–87.
13. Oudit GY, Sun H, Trivieri MG, et al. L-type Ca2+ channels provide a major pathway for iron entry into cardiomyocytes in iron-overload cardiomyopathy. Nat Med. 2003;9:1187–94.
14. Zurlo MG, De Stefano P, Borgna-Pignatti C, et al. Survival and causes of death in thalassaemia major. Lancet. 1989;2:27–30.
15. Borgna-Pignatti C, Rugolotto S, De Stefano P, et al. Survival and disease complications in thalassemia major. Ann N Y Acad Sci. 1998;850:227–31.
16. Borgna-Pignatti C, Rugolotto S, De Stefano P, et al. Survival and complications in patients with thalassemia major treated with transfusion and deferoxamine. Haematologica. 2004;89:1187–93.

17. Schafer AI, Cheron RG, Dluhy R, et al. Clinical consequences of acquired transfusional iron overload in adults. N Engl J Med. 1981;304:319–24.
18. Buja LM, Roberts WC. Iron in the heart. Etiology and clinical significance. Am J Med. 1971;51:209–21.
19. Jensen PD, Jensen FT, Christensen T, Eiskjaer H, Baandrup U, Nielsen JL. Evaluation of myocardial iron by magnetic resonance imaging during iron chelation therapy with deferrioxamine: indication of close relation between myocardial iron content and chelatable iron pool. Blood. 2003;101:4632–9.
20. Cazzola M, Malcovati L. Myelodysplastic syndromes – coping with ineffective hematopoiesis. N Engl J Med. 2005;352:536–8.
21. Malcovati L, Della Porta MG, Cazzola M. Predicting survival and leukemic evolution in patients with myelodysplastic syndrome. Haematologica. 2006;91:1588–90.
22. Olivieri NF. Progression of iron overload in sickle cell disease. Semin Hematol. 2001;38:57–62.
23. Darbari DS, Kple-Faget P, Kwagyan J, Rana S, Gordeuk VR, Castro O. Circumstances of death in adult sickle cell disease patients. Am J Hematol. 2006;81:858–63.
24. Vichinsky E, Butensky E, Fung E, et al. Comparison of organ dysfunction in transfused patients with SCD or beta thalassemia. Am J Hematol. 2005;80:70–4.
25. Fung EB, Harmatz PR, Lee PD, et al. Increased prevalence of iron-overload associated endocrinopathy in thalassaemia versus sickle-cell disease. Br J Haematol. 2006;135:574–82.
26. Westwood MA, Shah F, Anderson LJ, et al. Myocardial tissue characterization and the role of chronic anemia in sickle cell cardiomyopathy. J Magn Reson Imaging. 2007;26:564–8.
27. Wood JC, Tyszka JM, Carson S, Nelson MD, Coates TD. Myocardial iron loading in transfusion-dependent thalassemia and sickle cell disease. Blood. 2004;103:1934–6.
28. Porter JB. Concepts and goals in the management of transfusional iron overload. Am J Hematol. 2007;82:1136–9.
29. Cartwright GE, Edwards CQ, Kravitz K, et al. Hereditary hemochromatosis. Phenotypic expression of the disease. N Engl J Med. 1979;301:175–9.
30. Angelucci E, Brittenham GM, McLaren CE, et al. Hepatic iron concentration and total body iron stores in thalassemia major. N Engl J Med. 2000;343:327–31.
31. Anderson LJ, Holden S, Davis B, et al. Cardiovascular T2-star (T2*) magnetic resonance for the early diagnosis of myocardial iron overload. Eur Heart J. 2001;22:2171–9.
32. Anderson LJ, Westwood MA, Holden S, et al. Myocardial iron clearance during reversal of siderotic cardiomyopathy with intravenous desferrioxamine: a prospective study using T2* cardiovascular magnetic resonance. Br J Haematol. 2004;127:348–55.
33. Brittenham GM, Griffith PM, Nienhuis AW, et al. Efficacy of deferoxamine in preventing complications of iron overload in patients with thalassemia major [see comments]. N Engl J Med. 1994;331:567–73.
34. Telfer PT, Prestcott E, Holden S, Walker M, Hoffbrand AV, Wonke B. Hepatic iron concentration combined with long-term monitoring of serum ferritin to predict complications of iron overload in thalassaemia major. Br J Haematol. 2000;110:971–7.
35. Angelucci E, Muretto P, Nicolucci A, et al. Effects of iron overload and hepatitis C virus positivity in determining progression of liver fibrosis in thalassemia following bone marrow transplantation. Blood. 2002;100:17–21.
36. Angelucci E, Giovagnoni A, Valeri G, et al. Limitations of magnetic resonance imaging in measurement of hepatic iron. Blood. 1997;90:4736–42.
37. Brittenham GM, Farrell DE, Harris JW, et al. Magnetic-susceptibility measurement of human iron stores. N Engl J Med. 1982;307:1671–5.
38. Piga A, Fischer R, St Pierre T, et al. Comparison of LIC obtained from biopsy, BLS and R2-MRI in iron overloaded patients with beta-thalassemia, treated with deferasirox (Exjade®, ICL670). Blood 2005;106:Abstract 2689.
39. St Pierre TG, Clark PR, Chua-anusorn W, et al. Noninvasive measurement and imaging of liver iron concentrations using proton magnetic resonance. Blood. 2005;105:855–61.
40. Gandon Y, Olivie D, Guyader D, et al. Non-invasive assessment of hepatic iron stores by MRI. Lancet. 2004;363:357–62.
41. Garbowski M, Carpenter JP, Smith* G, Pennell D, Porter JB. Calibration of improved T2* method for the estimation of liver iron concentration in transfusional iron overload. Blood 2009;114:Abstract 2004.
42. Worwood M, Cragg SJ, Jacobs A, McLaren C, Ricketts C, Economidou J. Binding of serum ferritin to concanavalin a: patients with homozygous beta thalassaemia and transfusional iron overload. Br J Haematol. 1980;46:409–16.
43. Brittenham GM, Cohen AR, McLaren CE, et al. Hepatic iron stores and plasma ferritin concentration in patients with sickle cell anemia and thalassemia major. Am J Hematol. 1993;42:81–5.
44. Porter JB, Huehns ER. Transfusion and exchange transfusion in sickle cell anaemias, with particular reference to iron metabolism. Acta Haematol. 1987;78:198–205.

45. Origa R, Galanello R, Ganz T, et al. Liver iron concentrations and urinary hepcidin in beta-thalassemia. Haematologica. 2007;92:583–8.
46. Fischer R, Longo F, Nielsen P, Engelhardt R, Hider RC, Piga A. Monitoring long-term efficacy of iron chelation therapy by deferiprone and desferrioxamine in patients with beta-thalassaemia major: application of SQUID biomagnetic liver susceptometry. Br J Haematol. 2003;121:938–48.
47. Ang A, Shah F, Davis B, et al. Deferiprone is associated with Lower Serum Ferritin (SF) relative to Liver Iron Concentration (LIC) than Deferoxamine and Deferasirox-implications for clinical practice. Blood 2010;116:Abstract 4246.
48. Olivieri NF, Nathan DG, MacMillan JH, et al. Survival in medically treated patients with homozygous beta-thalassemia. N Engl J Med. 1994;331:574–8.
49. Gabutti V, Piga A. Results of long-term iron-chelating therapy. Acta Haematol. 1996;95:26–36.
50. Davis BA, O'Sullivan C, Jarritt PH, Porter JB. Value of sequential monitoring of left ventricular ejection fraction in the management of thalassemia major. Blood. 2004;104:263–9.
51. Carpenter JP, He T, Kirk P, et al. On t2* magnetic resonance and cardiac iron. Circulation. 2011;123:1519–28.
52. Kirk P, Roughton M, Porter JB, et al. Cardiac T2* magnetic resonance for prediction of cardiac complications in thalassemia major. Circulation. 2009;120:1961–8.
53. Thomas A, Garbowski M, Ang A, et al. A decade follow-up of a Thalassemia Major (TM) cohort monitored by Cardiac Magnetic Resonance Imaging (CMR): Significant reduction in patients with cardiac iron and in total mortality. Blood 2010;116:Abstract 1011.
54. Kirk P, He T, Anderson LJ, et al. International reproducibility of single breathhold T2* MR for cardiac and liver iron assessment among five thalassemia centers. J Magn Reson Imaging. 2010;32:315–9.
55. Sephton-Smith R. Iron excretion in thalassaemia major after administration of chelating agents. Br Med J. 1962;2:1577–80.
56. Pippard M, Johnson D, Callender S, Finch C. Ferrioxamine excretion in iron loaded man. Blood. 1982;60:288–94.
57. Jacobs EM, Hendriks JC, van Tits BL, et al. Results of an international round robin for the quantification of serum non-transferrin-bound iron: need for defining standardization and a clinically relevant isoform. Anal Biochem. 2005;341:241–50.
58. Pootrakul P, Breuer W, Sametband M, Sirankapracha P, Hershko C, Cabantchik ZI. Labile plasma iron (LPI) as an indicator of chelatable plasma redox activity in iron-overloaded beta-thalassemia/HbE patients treated with an oral chelator. Blood. 2004;104:1504–10.
59. Daar S, Taher A, Pathare A, et al. Plasma LPI in thalassemia patients before and after treatment with deferasirox (Exjade®, ICL670). Blood 2005;106:Abstract 2697.
60. Porter JB, Abeysinghe RD, Marshall L, Hider RC, Singh S. Kinetics of removal and reappearance of non-transferrin-bound plasma iron with deferoxamine therapy. Blood. 1996;88:705–13.
61. Shah F, Westwood MA, Evans PJ, Porter JB. Discordance in MRI assessment of iron distribution and plasma NTBI between transfusionally iron loaded adults with sickle cell and thalassaemia syndromes. Blood. 2002;100:468a.
62. Walter PB, Fung EB, Killilea DW, et al. Oxidative stress and inflammation in iron-overloaded patients with beta-thalassaemia or sickle cell disease. Br J Haematol. 2006;135:254–63.
63. Porter J, Cappellini M, El-Beshlawy A, et al. Effect of deferasirox (Exjade®) on labile plasma iron levels in heavily iron-overloaded patients with transfusion-dependent anemias enrolled in the large-scale, prospective 1-year EPIC trial. Blood 2008;112:Abstract 3881.
64. Farmaki K, Tzoumari I, Pappa C, Chouliaras G, Berdoukas V. Normalisation of total body iron load with very intensive combined chelation reverses cardiac and endocrine complications of thalassaemia major. Br J Haematol. 2010;148:466–75.
65. Jensen PD, Jensen FT, Christensen T, Nielsen JL, Ellegaard J. Relationship between hepatocellular injury and transfusional iron overload prior to and during iron chelation with desferrioxamine: a study in adult patients with acquired anemias. Blood. 2003;101:91–6.
66. Porter JB, Davis BA. Monitoring chelation therapy to achieve optimal outcome in the treatment of thalassaemia. Best Pract Res Clin Haematol. 2002;15:329–68.
67. Noetzli LJ, Carson SM, Nord AS, Coates TD, Wood JC. Longitudinal analysis of heart and liver iron in thalassemia major. Blood. 2008;112:2973–8.
68. Rothman RJ, Serroni A, Farber JL. Cellular pool of transient ferric iron, chelatable by deferoxamine and distinct from ferritin, that is involved in oxidative cell injury. Mol Pharmacol. 1992;42:703–10.
69. Klausner R, Rouault T, Harford J. Regulating the fate of mRNA: the control of cellular iron metabolism. Cell. 1993;72:19–28.
70. Breuer W, Epsztejn S, Cabantchik Z. Dynamics of the cytosolic chelatable iron pool of K562 cells. FEBS Lett. 1997;382:304–8.
71. Hershko C, Weatherall D. Iron chelating therapy. CRC Crit Rev Clin Lab Sci. 1988;26:303–45.
72. Porter J, Gyparaki M, Burke L, et al. Iron mobilization from hepatocyte monolayer cultures by Chelators: the importance of membrane permeability and the iron binding constant. Blood. 1988;72:1497–503.

73. Porter JB, Morgan J, Hoyes KP, Burke LC, Huehns ER, Hider RC. Relative oral efficacy and acute toxicity of hydroxypyridin-4-one iron chelators in mice. Blood. 1990;76:2389–96.
74. Porter JB, Singh S, Hoyes KP, Epemolu O, Abeysinghe RD, Hider RC. Lessons from preclinical and clinical studies with 1,2-diethyl-3-hydroxypyridin-4-one, CP94 and related compounds. Adv Exp Med Biol. 1994;356:361–70.
75. Hoyes KP, Porter JB. Subcellular distribution of desferrioxamine and hydroxypyridin-4-one chelators in K562 cells affects chelation of intracellular iron pools. Br J Haematol. 1993;85:393–400.
76. Glickstein H, El RB, Shvartsman M, Cabantchik ZI. Intracellular labile iron pools as direct targets of iron chelators: a fluorescence study of chelator action in living cells. Blood. 2005;106:3242–50.
77. Cooper CE, Lynagh GR, Hoyes KP, Hider RC, Cammack R, Porter JB. The relationship of intracellular iron chelation to the inhibition and regeneration of human ribonucleotide reductase. J Biol Chem. 1996;271:20291–9.
78. Porter JB, Rafique R, Srichairatanakool S, et al. Recent insights into interactions of deferoxamine with cellular and plasma iron pools: implications for clinical use. Ann N Y Acad Sci. 2005;1054:155–68.
79. Lee P, Mohammed N, Abeysinghe RD, Hider RC, Porter JB, Singh S. Intravenous infusion pharmacokinetics of desferrioxamine in thalassaemia patients. Drug Metab Dispos. 1993;21:640–4.
80. Porter JB, Faherty A, Stallibrass L, Brookman L, Hassan I, Howes C. A trial to investigate the relationship between DFO pharmacokinetics and metabolism and DFO-related toxicity. Ann N Y Acad Sci. 1998;850:483–7.
81. Breuer W, Ermers MJ, Pootrakul P, Abramov A, Hershko C, Cabantchik ZI. Desferrioxamine-chelatable iron, a component of serum non-transferrin-bound iron, used for assessing chelation therapy. Blood. 2001;97:792–8.
82. Evans P, Kayyali R, Hider RC, Eccleston J, Porter JB. Mechanisms for the shuttling of plasma non-transferrin-bound iron (NTBI) onto deferoxamine by deferiprone. Transl Res. 2010;156:55–67.
83. Cappellini MD, Cohen A, Piga A, et al. A phase 3 study of deferasirox (ICL670), a once-daily oral iron chelator, in patients with beta-thalassemia. Blood. 2006;107:3455–62.
84. Modell B, Letsky E, Flynn D, Peto R, Weatherall D. Survival and desferrioxamine in thalassaemia major. Br Med J. 1982;284:1081–4.
85. Gabutti V, Borgna-Pignatti C. Clinical manifestations and therapy of transfusional haemosiderosis. Baillieres Clin Haematol. 1994;7:919–40.
86. Davis BA, Porter JB. Long-term outcome of continuous 24-hour deferoxamine infusion via indwelling intravenous catheters in high-risk beta-thalassemia. Blood. 2000;95:1229–36.
87. Miskin H, Yaniv I, Berant M, Hershko C, Tamary H. Reversal of cardiac complications in thalassemia major by long-term intermittent daily intensive iron chelation. Eur J Haematol. 2003;70:398–403.
88. Marcus RE, Davies SC, Bantock HM, Underwood SR, Walton S, Huehns ER. Desferrioxamine to improve cardiac function in iron overloaded patients with thalassaemia major. Lancet. 1984;1:392–3.
89. Davies SC, Marcus RE, Hungerford JL, Miller HM, Arden GB, Huehns ER. Ocular toxicity of high-dose intravenous desferrioxamine. Lancet. 1983;2:181–4.
90. Porter JB, Jaswon MS, Huehns ER, East CA, Hazell JW. Desferrioxamine ototoxicity: evaluation of risk factors in thalassaemic patients and guidelines for safe dosage. Br J Haematol. 1989;73:403–9.
91. Cunningham MJ, Macklin EA, Neufeld EJ, Cohen AR. Complications of beta-thalassemia major in north America. Blood. 2004;104:34–9.
92. Pennell DJ, Berdoukas V, Karagiorga M, et al. Randomized controlled trial of deferiprone or deferoxamine in beta-thalassemia major patients with asymptomatic myocardial siderosis. Blood. 2006;107:3738–44.
93. Barry M, Flynn D, Letsky E, Risdon R. Long term chelation therapy in thalassaemia: effect on liver iron concentration, liver histology and clinical progress. Br Med J. 1974;2:16–20.
94. Bronspiegel-Weintrob N, Olivieri NF, Tyler B, Andrews DF, Freedman MH, Holland FJ. Effect of age at the start of iron chelation therapy on gonadal function in beta-thalassemia major. N Engl J Med. 1990;323:713–9.
95. Fosburg M, Nathan DG. Treatment of Cooley's anaemia. Blood. 1990;76:435–44.
96. Porter JB, Huehns ER. The toxic effects of desferrioxamine. Baillieres Clin Haematol. 1989;2:459–74.
97. Bentur Y, Koren G, Tesoro A, Carley H, Olivieri N, Freedman MH. Comparison of deferoxamine pharmacokinetics between asymptomatic thalassemic children and those exhibiting severe neurotoxicity. Clin Pharmacol Ther. 1990;47:478–82.
98. Olivieri NF, Buncic JR, Chew E, et al. Visual and auditory neurotoxicity in patients receiving subcutaneous deferoxamine infusions. N Engl J Med. 1986;314:869–73.
99. Blake DR, Winyard P, Lunec J, et al. Cerebral and ocular toxicity induced by desferrioxamine. Q J Med. 1985;56:345–55.
100. De Virgillis S, Congia M, Frau F, et al. Desferrioxamine-induced growth retardation in patients with thalassaemia major. J Pediatr. 1988;113:661–9.
101. Piga A, Luzzatto L, Capalbo P, Gambotto S, Tricta F, Gabutti V. High dose desferrioxamine as a cause of growth failure in thalassaemic patients. Eur J Haematol. 1988;40:380–1.
102. Olivieri NF, Koren G, Harris J, et al. Growth failure and bony changes induced by deferoxamine. Am J Pediatr Hematol Oncol. 1992;14:48–56.

103. Modell B, Khan M, Darlison M. Survival in beta-thalassaemia major in the UK: data from the UK thalassaemia register. Lancet. 2000;355:2051–2.
104. Ponka P, Borova J, Neuwirt J, Fuchs O, Necas E. A study of intracellular iron metabolism using pyridoxal isonicotyl hydrazone and other synthetic chelating agents. Biochim Biophys Acta. 1979;586:278–97.
105. Brittenham GM. Pyridoxal isonicotinoyl hydrazone: an effective iron-chelator after oral administration. Semin Hematol. 1990;27:112–6.
106. Richardson DR, Ponka P. Orally effective iron chelators for the treatment of iron overload disease: the case for a further look at pyridoxal isonicotinoyl hydrazone and its analogs. J Lab Clin Med. 1998;132:351–2.
107. Nick H, Acklin P, Lattmann R, et al. Development of tridentate iron chelators: from desferrithiocin to ICL670. Curr Med Chem. 2003;10:1065–76.
108. Bergeron R, Wiegand J, McManis Jea. Structure–activity relationships among desazadesferrithiocin analogues. In hershko C. Iron chelation therapy. Adv Exp Med Biol. 2002;509:167–84.
109. Donovan JM, Plone M, Dagher R, Bree M, Marquis J. Preclinical and clinical development of deferitrin, a novel, orally available iron chelator. Ann N Y Acad Sci. 2005;1054:492–4.
110. Barton JC. Drug evaluation: deferitrin for iron overload disorders. IDrugs. 2007;10:480–90.
111. Anderegg G, Raeber M. Metal complex formation of a new siderophore desferrithiocin and of three related ligands. J Chem Soc, Chem Commun. 1990;17:1194–6.
112. Rienhoff Jr HY, Viprakasit V, Tay L, et al. A phase 1 dose-escalation study: safety, tolerability, and pharmacokinetics of FBS0701, a novel oral iron chelator for the treatment of transfusional iron overload. Haematologica. 2011;96:521–5.
113. Kontoghiorghes GJ, Aldouri MA, Hoffbrand AV, et al. Effective chelation of iron in beta thalassaemia with the oral chelator 1,2-dimethyl-3-hydroxypyrid-4-one. Br Med J (Clin Res Ed). 1987;295:1509–12.
114. Cohen AR, Galanello R, Piga A, De Sanctis V, Tricta F. Safety and effectiveness of long-term therapy with the oral iron chelator deferiprone. Blood. 2003;102:1583–7.
115. Hider RC, Choudhury R, Rai BL, Dehkordi LS, Singh S. Design of orally active iron chelators. Acta Haematol. 1996;95:6–12.
116. Liu ZD, Kayyali R, Hider RC, Porter JB, Theobald AE. Design, synthesis, and evaluation of novel 2-substituted 3-hydroxypyridin-4-ones: structure–activity investigation of metalloenzyme inhibition by iron chelators. J Med Chem. 2002;45:631–9.
117. Olivieri NF, Koren G, Hermann C, et al. Comparison of oral iron chelator L1 and desferrioxamine in iron-loaded patients. Lancet. 1990;336:1275–9.
118. Kontoghiorghes GJ, Goddard JG, Bartlett AN, Sheppard L. Pharmacokinetic studies in humans with the oral iron chelator 1,2-dimethyl-3-hydroxypyrid-4-one. Clin Pharmacol. 1990;48:255–61.
119. Barman Balfour JA, Foster RH. Deferiprone: a review of its clinical potential in iron overload in beta-thalassaemia major and other transfusion-dependent diseases. Drugs. 1999;58:553–78.
120. Hoffbrand AV, Cohen A, Hershko C. Role of deferiprone in chelation therapy for transfusional iron overload. Blood. 2003;102:17–24.
121. Porter JB, Abeysinghe RD, Hoyes KP, et al. Contrasting interspecies efficacy and toxicology of 1,2-diethyl-3- hydroxypyridin-4-one, CP94, relates to differing metabolism of the iron chelating site. Br J Haematol. 1993;85:159–68.
122. Hershko C, Link G, Pinson A, Peter HH, Dobbin P, Hider RC. Iron mobilization from myocardial cells by 3-hydroxypyridin-4-one chelators: studies in rat heart cells in culture. Blood. 1991;77:2049–53.
123. Kayyali R, Porter JB, Liu ZD, et al. Structure-function investigation of the interaction of 1- and 2-substituted 3-hydroxypyridin-4-ones with 5-lipoxygenase and ribonucleotide reductase. J Biol Chem. 2001;15:15.
124. Al-Refaie FN, Sheppard LN, Nortey P, Wonke B, Hoffbrand AV. Pharmacokinetics of the oral iron chelator deferiprone (L1) in patients with iron overload. Br J Haematol. 1995;89:403–8.
125. Glickstein H, El RB, Link G, et al. Action of Chelators in iron-loaded cardiac cells: accessibility to intracellular labile iron and functional consequences. Blood. 2006;108:3195–203.
126. Collins AF, Fassos FF, Stobie S, et al. Iron-balance and dose-response studies of the oral iron chelator 1,2-dimethyl-3-hydroxypyrid-4-one (L1) in iron-loaded patients with sickle cell disease. Blood. 1994;83:2329–33.
127. Roberts D, Brunskill S, Doree C, Williams S, Howard J, Hyde C. Oral deferiprone for iron chelation in people with thalassaemia. Cochrane Database Syst Rev. 2007;18(3):CD004839.
128. Olivieri N, Brittenham G. Final results of the randomised trial of deferiprone and deferoxamine. Blood. 1997;90:264a.
129. Maggio A, D'Amico G, Morabito A, et al. Deferiprone versus deferoxamine in patients with thalassemia major: a randomized clinical trial. Blood Cells Mol Dis. 2002;28:196–208.
130. Ha SY, Chik KW, Ling SC, et al. A randomized controlled study evaluating the safety and efficacy of deferiprone treatment in thalassemia major patients from Hong Kong. Hemoglobin. 2006;30:263–74.
131. Aydinok Y, Ulger Z, Nart D, et al. A randomized controlled 1-year study of daily deferiprone plus twice weekly desferrioxamine compared with daily deferiprone monotherapy in patients with thalassemia major. Haematologica. 2007;92:1599–606.

132. Al-Refaie FN, Wonke B, Hoffbrand AV, Wickens DG, Nortey R, Kontoghiorghes GJ. Efficacy and possible adverse effects of the oral iron chelator 1,2-dimethyl-3-hydroxypyridin-4-one (L1) in thalassemia major. Blood. 1992;80:593–9.
133. Agarwal MB, Gupte SS, Viswanathan C, et al. Long-term assessment of efficacy and safety of L1, an oral iron chelator, in transfusion dependent thalassaemia: Indian trial. Br J Haematol. 1992;82:460–6.
134. Olivieri NF, Brittenham GM, Matsui D, et al. Iron-chelation therapy with oral deferiprone in patients with thalassemia major [see comments]. N Engl J Med. 1995;332:918–22.
135. Hoffbrand AV FA-R, Davis B, et al. Long-term trial of deferiprone in 51 transfusion-dependent iron overloaded patients. Blood. 1998;91:295–300.
136. Cohen AR, Galanello R, Piga A, Dipalma A, Vullo C, Tricta F. Safety profile of the oral iron chelator deferiprone: a multicentre study. Br J Haematol. 2000;108:305–12.
137. Gomber S, Saxena R, Madan N. Comparative efficacy of desferrioxamine, deferiprone and in combination on iron chelation in thalassemic children. Indian Pediatr. 2004;41:21–7.
138. Ceci A, Baiardi P, Felisi M, et al. The safety and effectiveness of deferiprone in a large-scale, 3-year study in Italian patients. Br J Haematol. 2002;118:330–6.
139. Piga A, Gaglioti C, Fogliacco E, Tricta F. Comparative effects of deferiprone and deferoxamine on survival and cardiac disease in patients with thalassemia major: a retrospective analysis. Haematologica. 2003;88:489–96.
140. Borgna-Pignatti C, Cappellini MD, De Stefano P, et al. Cardiac morbidity and mortality in deferoxamine- or deferiprone-treated patients with thalassemia major. Blood. 2006;107:3733–7.
141. Anderson LJ, Wonke B, Prescott E, Holden S, Walker JM, Pennell DJ. Comparison of effects of oral deferiprone and subcutaneous desferrioxamine on myocardial iron concentrations and ventricular function in beta-thalassaemia. Lancet. 2002;360:516–20.
142. Ceci A, Felisi M, De Sanctis V, De Mattia D. Pharmacotherapy of iron overload in thalassaemic patients. Expert Opin Pharmacother. 2003;4:1763–74.
143. Al-Refaie FN, Wonke B, Hoffbrand AV. Deferiprone-associated myelotoxicity. Eur J Haematol. 1994;53:298–301.
144. Cunningham JM, Al-Refaie FN, Hunter AE, Sheppard LN, Hoffbrand AV. Differential toxicity of alpha-keto hydroxypyridine iron chelators and desferrioxamine to human haemopoietic precursors in vitro. Eur J Haematol. 1994;52:176–9.
145. Hoyes KP, Jones HM, Abeysinghe RD, Hider RC, Porter JB. In vivo and in vitro effects of 3-hydroxypyridin-4-one chelators on murine hemopoiesis. Exp Hematol. 1993;21:86–92.
146. Bartlett AN, Hoffbrand AV, Kontoghiorghes GJ. Long-term trial with the oral iron chelator 1,2-dimethyl-3-hydroxypyrid-4-one (L1). II. clinical observations. Br J Haematol. 1990;76:301–4.
147. Cermak J, Brabec V. Treatment of iron overload states with oral administration of the chelator agent, L1 (deferiprone). Vnitr Lek. 1994;40:586–90.
148. Naithani R, Chandra J, Sharma S. Safety of oral iron chelator deferiprone in young thalassaemics. Eur J Haematol. 2005;74:217–20.
149. Tondury P, Zimmermann A, Nielsen P, Hirt A. Liver iron and fibrosis during long-term treatment with deferiprone in Swiss thalassaemic patients. Br J Haematol. 1998;101:413–5.
150. Berdoukas V, Bohane T, Eagle C, et al. The Sydney Children's hospital experience with the oral iron chelator deferiprone (L1). Transfus Sci. 2000;23:239–40.
151. Wanless IR, Sweeney G, Dhillon AP, et al. Lack of progressive hepatic fibrosis during long-term therapy with deferiprone in subjects with transfusion-dependent beta-thalassemia. Blood. 2002;100:1566–9.
152. Al-Refaie FN, Hershko C, Hoffbrand AV, et al. Results of long-term deferiprone (L1) therapy: a report by the international study group on oral iron Chelators. Br J Haematol. 1995;91:224–9.
153. Choudhry VP, Pati HP, Saxena A, Malaviya AN. Deferiprone, efficacy and safety. Indian J Pediatr. 2004;71:213–6.
154. Alert SOS; 2006.
155. Link G, Konijn AM, Breuer W, Cabantchik ZI, Hershko C. Exploring the "iron shuttle" hypothesis in chelation therapy: effects of combined deferoxamine and deferiprone treatment in hypertransfused rats with labeled iron stores and in iron-loaded rat heart cells in culture. J Lab Clin Med. 2001;138:130–8.
156. Hershko C, Link G, Konijn A, Cabantchik Z. Objectives and mechanism of iron chelation therapy. Ann N Y Acad Sci. 2005;1054:124–35.
157. Galanello R, Kattamis A, Piga A, et al. A prospective randomized controlled trial on the safety and efficacy of alternating deferoxamine and deferiprone in the treatment of iron overload in patients with thalassemia. Haematologica. 2006;91:1241–3.
158. Mourad FH, Hoffbrand AV, Sheikh-Taha M, Koussa S, Khoriaty AI, Taher A. Comparison between desferrioxamine and combined therapy with desferrioxamine and deferiprone in iron overloaded thalassaemia patients. Br J Haematol. 2003;121:187–9.
159. Tanner MA, Galanello R, Dessi C, et al. A randomized, placebo-controlled, double-blind trial of the effect of combined therapy with deferoxamine and deferiprone on myocardial iron in thalassemia major using cardiovascular magnetic resonance. Circulation. 2007;115:1876–84.

160. Origa R, Bina P, Agus A, et al. Combined therapy with deferiprone and desferrioxamine in thalassemia major. Haematologica. 2005;90:1309–14.
161. Kattamis A, Ladis V, Berdousi H, et al. Iron chelation treatment with combined therapy with deferiprone and deferioxamine: a 12-month trial. Blood Cells Mol Dis. 2006;36:21–5.
162. Telfer P, Coen P. Christou Sea. Survival of medically treated thalassemia patients in Cyprus. Trends and risk factors over the period 1980–2004. Haematologica. 2006;91:1187–92.
163. Hershko C, Konijn AM, Nick HP, Breuer W, Cabantchik ZI, Link G. ICL670A: a new synthetic oral chelator: evaluation in hypertransfused rats with selective radioiron probes of hepatocellular and reticuloendothelial iron stores and in iron-loaded rat heart cells in culture. Blood. 2001;97:1115–22.
164. Wood JC, Otto-Duessel M, Aguilar M, et al. Cardiac iron determines cardiac T2*, T2, and T1 in the gerbil model of iron cardiomyopathy. Circulation. 2005;112:535–43.
165. Waldmeier F, Bruin GJ, Glaenzel U, et al. Pharmacokinetics, metabolism, and disposition of deferasirox in beta-thalassemic patients with transfusion-dependent iron overload who are at pharmacokinetic steady state. Drug Metab Dispos. 2010;38:808–16.
166. Galanello R, Piga A, Alberti D, Rouan MC, Bigler H, Sechaud R. Safety, tolerability, and pharmacokinetics of ICL670, a new orally active iron-chelating agent in patients with transfusion-dependent iron overload due to beta-thalassemia. J Clin Pharmacol. 2003;43:565–72.
167. Nisbet-Brown E, Olivieri NF, Giardina PJ, et al. Effectiveness and safety of ICL670 in iron-loaded patients with thalassaemia: a randomised, double-blind, placebo-controlled, dose-escalation trial. Lancet. 2003;361: 1597–602.
168. Piga A, Galanello R, Forni GL, et al. Randomized phase II trial of deferasirox (exjade, ICL670), a once-daily, orally-administered iron chelator, in comparison to deferoxamine in thalassemia patients with transfusional iron overload. Haematologica. 2006;91:873–80.
169. Cappellini M, Bejaoui M, Agaoglu L, et al. Iron chelation with deferasirox in adult and pediatric patients with thalassemia major: efficacy and safety during 5 years' follow-up. Blood. 2011;118(4):884–93.
170. Cappellini MD, Porter J, El-Beshlawy A, et al. Tailoring iron chelation by iron intake and serum ferritin: the prospective EPIC study of deferasirox in 1744 patients with transfusion-dependent anemias. Haematologica. 2010;95:557–66.
171. Vichinsky E, Onyekwere O, Porter J, et al. A randomised comparison of deferasirox versus deferoxamine for the treatment of transfusional iron overload in sickle cell disease. Br J Haematol. 2007;136:501–8.
172. Vichinsky E, Bernaudin F, Forni GL, et al. Long-term safety and efficacy of deferasirox (exjade®) for up to 5 years in transfusional iron-overloaded patients with sickle cell disease. Br J Haematol. 2011;154(3):387–97.
173. Lee JW, Yoon SS, Shen ZX, et al. Iron chelation therapy with deferasirox in patients with aplastic anemia: a subgroup analysis of 116 patients from the EPIC trial. Blood. 2010;116(14):2448–54.
174. Gattermann N, Finelli C, Porta MD, et al. Deferasirox in iron-overloaded patients with transfusion-dependent myelodysplastic syndromes: results from the large 1-year EPIC study. Leuk Res. 2010;34:1143–50.
175. Porter J, Lin K, Beris P, et al. Response of iron overload in rare transfusion-dependent anaemias to deferasirox: equivalent effects on serum ferritin and labile plasma iron for haemolytic or production anaemias. Eur J Haematol. 2011;87(4):338–48.
176. Porter JB, Tanner MA, Pennell DJ. Improved myocardial T2* in transfusion dependent anemias receiving ICL670 (Deferasirox). Blood 2005;106:Abstract 3600.
177. Pennell DJ, Porter JB, Cappellini MD, et al. Efficacy of deferasirox in reducing and preventing cardiac iron overload in beta-thalassemia. Blood. 2010;115:2364–71.
178. Pennell DJ, Porter JB, Cappellini MD, et al. Continued improvement in myocardial T2* over two years of deferasirox therapy in beta-thalassemia major patients with cardiac iron overload. Haematologica. 2011;96:48–54.
179. Pennell D, Porter J, Cappellini M, et al. Continued improvement and normalization of myocardial T2* in patients with β thalassemia major treated with deferasirox (Exjade®) for up to 3 years. Blood 2010;116:Abstract #28641.
180. Taher A, Cappellini MD, Vichinsky E, et al. Efficacy and safety of deferasirox doses of >30 mg/kg per d in patients with transfusion-dependent anaemia and iron overload. Br J Haematol. 2009;147:752–9.
181. Taher A, El-Beshlawy A, Elalfy MS, et al. Efficacy and safety of deferasirox, an oral iron chelator, in heavily iron-overloaded patients with beta-thalassaemia: the ESCALATOR study. Eur J Haematol. 2009;82:458–65.
182. Chirnomas D, Smith AL, Braunstein J, et al. Deferasirox pharmacokinetics in patients with adequate versus inadequate response. Blood. 2009;114:4009–13.
183. Lal A, Sweeters N, Ng V, et al. Combined chelation therapy with deferasirox and deferoxamine in transfusion-dependent thalassemia. Blood 2010;116:Abstract 4269.

Section VI
Model Systems for Studying Iron Homeostasis

Chapter 29
Mammalian Models of Iron Homeostasis

Robert S. Britton, Bruce R. Bacon, and Robert E. Fleming

Keywords Anemia • Animal models • Hemochromatosis • Hepcidin • Iron • Mouse • Rat

1 Introduction

Mammalian animal models have proven to be very useful in providing insight into human iron homeostasis and disorders of iron metabolism. Such models provide an integrated picture of the dynamics of iron metabolism in the whole animal, which is not possible in cell culture systems. Both mice and rats provide important models for understanding human iron absorption, distribution, storage, and utilization. Mice have been particularly useful because of the availability of strains with spontaneous or mutagen-induced mutations that affect iron metabolism, and because of the possibility of genetic manipulation (targeted mutagenesis and transgenic gene expression). This chapter will describe existing mammalian models of iron homeostasis, with a particular emphasis on murine models. There are several previous reviews of various aspects of this subject [1–9].

2 Mouse Models of Hereditary Hemochromatosis

Substantial progress has been made in developing mouse models of the major forms of hereditary hemochromatosis (HH). Table 29.1 summarizes the currently available models and their phenotypes.

R.S. Britton, Ph.D. • B.R. Bacon, M.D.
Division of Gastroenterology and Hepatology, Department of Internal Medicine,
Saint Louis University School of Medicine, St. Louis, MO, USA
e-mail: brittonrs100@yahoo.com; baconbr@slu.edu

R.E. Fleming, M.D. (✉)
Department of Pediatrics, Cardinal Glennon Children's Medical Center,

Department of Biochemistry & Molecular Biology, Saint Louis University
School of Medicine, St. Louis, MO, USA
e-mail: flemingr@slu.edu

G.J. Anderson and G. McLaren (eds.), *Iron Physiology and Pathophysiology in Humans*,
Nutrition and Health, DOI 10.1007/978-1-60327-485-2_29,

Table 29.1 Murine models of hereditary hemochromatosis

Classification of human HH (protein)	Mouse genotype	Mouse phenotype	References
HH type 1 (HFE)	*Hfe*$^{-/-}$	Increased body iron, splenic iron sparing, decreased hepcidin	[11–13, 15, 16]
	Hfe$^{C282Y/C282Y}$	Milder phenotype than *Hfe*$^{-/-}$mouse	[12]
	Hfe$^{H63D/H63D}$	Very mild phenotype compared to *Hfe*$^{-/-}$mouse	[14]
HH type 2A (hemojuvelin)	*Hjv*$^{-/-}$	Increased body iron, splenic iron sparing, decreased hepcidin	[25, 26]
HH type 2B (hepcidin)	*Hamp1* $^{-/-}$	Increased body iron, splenic iron sparing, no hepcidin	[33, 38]
HH type 3 (transferrin receptor 2)	*Tfr2*$^{Y245X/Y245X}$	Increased body iron, splenic iron sparing, increased iron absorption, decreased hepcidin	[42, 44, 45]
	Tfr2$^{-/-}$	Similar phenotype to *Tfr2*$^{Y245X/Y245X}$ mouse	[43]
HH type 4 (ferroportin)	Missense mutation (H32R) in *Slc40a1* (flatiron mouse)	Heterozygous mice have iron loading of Kupffer cells, high serum ferritin, and low transferrin saturation	[53]

2.1 *Hfe* Mutant Mice: Model for HH Type 1

The positional cloning of the *HFE* gene which is responsible for HH type 1 triggered intense interest in the function of HFE protein [10]. HFE is an MHC class I-like protein, and a single nucleotide change, resulting in the substitution of tyrosine for cysteine at amino acid 282 of the unprocessed protein (C282Y), is present in nearly all patients with HH type 1. In the original cloning study, a second mutation in *HFE* was also identified which results in the substitution of aspartate for histidine at amino acid 63 (H63D) [10]. Mutant mouse models have been developed to study the in vivo consequences of *Hfe* deletion or mutation.

Five different *Hfe* gene disruptions have been produced in the mouse: an exon 4 knockout [11], an exon 3 disruption/exon 4 knockout [12], an exon 2–3 knockout [13], a C282Y knock-in [12, 14], and an H63D knock-in [14]. In each case, the mutant mice have increased hepatic iron concentrations [11–14]. In *Hfe* knockout mice, decreased hepcidin expression [15, 16], elevated transferrin saturation [11], and increased intestinal iron absorption [13, 17] have also been reported. Like patients with HH type 1, these mice demonstrate relative sparing of iron accumulation in macrophages [17], thought to be due to low hepcidin levels. Interestingly, mice that are homozygous for the C282Y mutation have less-severe iron loading than *Hfe* knockout mice, indicating that the C282Y mutation is not a null allele [12]. The H63D allele, when homozygous or combined with a more consequential mutation like C282Y, leads to very mild hepatic iron accumulation [14]. Iron overload in *Hfe* knockout mice provides proof-of-principle that loss of HFE function underlies HH type 1.

Hepatic expression of bone morphogenetic protein 6 (Bmp6) mRNA is higher in *Hfe* knockout mice, and the level of expression is appropriate for the increased hepatic iron concentrations in these mice [18, 19]. However, levels of hepatic phosphorylated Smad 1/5/8 protein (a mediator of Bmp6 signaling) and Id1 mRNA (a target gene of Bmp6) are inappropriately low for hepatic iron concentration and Bmp6 mRNA levels in *Hfe* knockout mice [18, 19]. These results suggest that Hfe acts to facilitate signal transduction to hepcidin induced by Bmp6.

Hfe knockout mice have been bred to mice carrying mutations in other genes involved in normal iron homeostasis [20]. Studies using these compound mutant animals suggest that divalent metal transporter 1 (Dmt1), hephaestin, β2-microglobulin, and transferrin receptor 1 can all modify the

HH phenotype. A role for naturally occurring strain-dependent gene modifiers has been demonstrated by the variation in iron loading seen when the *Hfe* knockout allele is placed on different background strains [21–24]. Ongoing gene mapping studies are anticipated to identify some of these modifiers in mice, and then it can be determined if the same modifier genes influence the phenotype of C282Y homozygosity in humans.

Hfe knockout mice do not have progressive iron loading throughout their lifespan and do not develop hepatic fibrosis or cirrhosis [2, 11]. Liver iron accumulation in these mice is rapid during the first weeks of life [15, 17]. However, by about 10 weeks of age, the hepatic iron concentration reaches a plateau, accompanied by normalization of hepcidin expression [15] and iron absorption [17].

2.2 Hemojuvelin (Hjv) Knockout Mouse: Model for HH Type 2A

Hjv knockout mice provide a model of HH type 2A. These mice manifest markedly increased iron deposition in the liver, pancreas, and heart, but show sparing of iron accumulation in tissue macrophages [25, 26]. Hepcidin mRNA expression is decreased in these mice [25, 26], and expression of ferroportin protein is increased in both intestinal enterocytes and macrophages [25]. However, *Hjv* knockout mice do not develop diabetes or cardiomyopathy [26]. In these mice, hepcidin expression is not responsive to high iron, but does respond to the inflammatory agent lipopolysaccharide [26], suggesting that hemojuvelin plays a key role in signaling from iron to hepcidin. Hemojuvelin is a co-receptor for BMPs [27], and BMP6 is now recognized as playing a key role in the iron signaling pathway to hepcidin [28, 29].

2.3 Hepcidin Knockout Mouse: Model for HH Type 2B

Hepcidin acts to downregulate ferroportin expression, thereby decreasing intestinal iron absorption and causing iron retention in macrophages [30, 31]. The first evidence that hepcidin is involved in iron homeostasis came from the observation that liver hepcidin mRNA expression is increased in mice with dietary iron loading [32]. This was followed by the fortuitous discovery that coincidental deletion of the hepcidin genes (*Hamp1* and *Hamp2*) in *Usf2* knockout mice led to an HH-like phenotype [33]. This established the critical role of hepcidin as a negative regulator of intestinal iron absorption. It was later discovered that hepcidin mutations are responsible for HH type 2B in several human pedigrees [34]. Transgenic overexpression of hepcidin in mouse hepatocytes leads to a severe form of iron-deficiency anemia [35, 36]. Additionally, liver hepcidin expression is also influenced by factors regulating intestinal iron absorption (iron stores, erythropoietic activity, hemoglobin, oxygen content, and inflammation) [32, 37].

To analyze the consequences of *Hamp1* deletion on iron metabolism without any disturbance due to *Usf2* deficiency, Lesbordes-Brion et al. [38] disrupted the *Hamp1* gene by targeting almost all the coding region. *Hamp1* knockout mice develop early and severe multiorgan iron overload, with sparing of splenic macrophages.

2.4 Transferrin Receptor 2 Mutant Mice: Model for HH Type 3

Hereditary hemochromatosis type 3 is caused by mutations in transferrin receptor 2 (TfR2) [39]. Human TfR2 is 45% identical with the classical transferrin receptor in the extracellular domain, but contains no iron responsive element in its mRNA [40]. The most common mutation found in human

TfR2 is Y250X that introduces a stop codon into the mRNA, resulting in a truncated nonfunctional protein [41]. TfR2 is expressed highly in the liver and is thought to influence iron metabolism by affecting the expression of hepcidin.

Two mouse models have been developed for HH type 3: a mouse that contains the Y245X mutation in *Tfr2* (murine ortholog of the human mutation Y250X) [42], and a *Tfr2* knockout mouse [43]. Both mutant mice demonstrate hepatic iron overload and inappropriately low hepcidin levels [43–45]. In additional studies, *Tfr2*$^{Y245X/Y245X}$ mice were shown to have increased iron absorption, elevated duodenal iron transport gene expression, and increased liver iron uptake [45]. Targeted deletion of *Tfr2* in hepatocytes results in decreased hepcidin expression and hepatic iron overload, indicating that hepatocytes are the site of action of TfR2 on hepcidin [46]. Mice with combined deletion of both *Tfr2* and *Hfe* have a more pronounced decrease in hepcidin expression (relative to hepatic iron levels) than either gene deletion alone [47].

2.5 Ferroportin (Fpn) Mutant Mice: Model for HH Type 4

HH type 4 is autosomal dominant and is caused by missense mutations in the *SLC40A1* gene that encodes ferroportin. It is now considered that there are two categories of *SLC40A1* mutations [48, 49]. The first category includes loss-of-function mutations that reduce the cell surface localization of ferroportin, reducing its ability to export iron. This causes iron deposition primarily in macrophages, and this disorder is sometimes termed ferroportin disease [50]. The second category includes gain-of-function mutations that do not alter cell surface expression but rather abolish hepcidin-induced ferroportin internalization and degradation. In this case, cellular distribution of iron is similar to HH type 1, being primarily parenchymal. In both forms of HH type 4 (unlike other forms of HH), hepcidin expression is elevated rather than decreased [51].

Ferroportin has been targeted for deletion both globally and selectively in mice [52]. Embryonic lethality of *Fpn* knockout animals indicates that ferroportin is essential early in development, especially in the extraembryonic visceral endoderm. Selective knockout of ferroportin in villus enterocytes results in severe iron-deficiency anemia, demonstrating that ferroportin plays a key role in iron absorption [52]. Interestingly, heterozygous mice (*Fpn*$^{+/-}$) do not have iron overload, suggesting that human *SLC40A1* mutations are not simple loss-of-function mutations [52].

The discovery of the flatiron mouse has provided an interesting model for the first category of *SLC40A1* mutations [53]. The flatiron mouse has a missense mutation (H32R) in *Slc40a1* that affects the localization and iron export activity of ferroportin. Similar to patients with ferroportin disease, these mice have iron loading of Kupffer cells, high serum ferritin levels, and low transferrin saturation. Studies in the flatiron mouse support the concept that mutations in ferroportin resulting in protein mislocalization act in a dominant-negative fashion preventing wild-type ferroportin from reaching the cell surface and transporting iron [53]. It is anticipated that new mouse models will also be developed to examine the in vivo effects of putative gain-of-function mutations of ferroportin.

3 Murine Models: Signaling to Hepcidin

Hepcidin is now considered to be the master iron regulatory hormone [54], and several mouse models have been particularly informative regarding the intracellular signaling pathways that regulate hepcidin expression in the liver (Table 29.2).

Table 29.2 Murine models: signaling to hepcidin

Gene	Genotype	Phenotype	References
Bmp6	*Bmp6*$^{-/-}$	Increased body iron, splenic iron sparing, decreased hepcidin	[28, 29]
Tmprss6 (matriptase 2)	*Tmprss6*$^{-/-}$ *Tmprss6*$^{msk/msk}$	Microcytic anemia, low iron stores, low serum iron, increased hepcidin	[55, 56]
Smad4	*Smad4*$^{-/-}$ (hepatocyte-specific)	Increased body iron, splenic iron sparing, decreased hepcidin	[59]

3.1 *Bmp6 Knockout Mice*

Although hemojuvelin was recognized as a co-receptor for BMPs and multiple BMPs regulate hepcidin expression and iron metabolism [27, 31], it was uncertain which endogenous BMP regulates hepcidin in vivo. This situation has been clarified by the demonstration that *Bmp6* knockout mice have an HH-like phenotype with low hepcidin levels and iron overload [28, 29]. This and other evidence have implicated BMP6 as a major regulator of hepcidin expression in vivo.

3.2 *Tmprss6 Mutant Mice*

Characterization of an ethylnitrosourea-induced mutant mouse strain (called *mask*) with microcytic anemia led to the discovery that the protease Tmprss6 plays an important role in signaling to hepcidin [55]. Tmprss6, also known as matriptase-2, is a type II plasma membrane protein whose major site of expression is the liver. Tmprss6 contains an extracellular C-terminal trypsin-like serine protease domain. The mask mutation, an A-to-G transition, eliminates a splice acceptor site, yielding two abnormal splice products that lack the proteolytic domain [55]. Targeted deletion of the *Tmprss6* gene results in a similar high-hepcidin, iron-deficient phenotype [56]. It is proposed that Tmprss6-mediated hepcidin suppression permits adequate absorption of iron from the diet, and that without hepcidin suppression, severe iron deficiency occurs [55, 56]. A key substrate for the proteolytic activity of Tmprss6 is hemojuvelin, and this may explain the dampening effect of Tmprss6 on hepcidin expression [57]. Interestingly, mutations in *TMPRSS6* cause iron-refractory iron-deficiency anemia in humans [58].

3.3 *Smad4 Knockout Mice*

The importance of a Smad4-dependent signaling pathway in regulating hepcidin expression is demonstrated by the phenotype of the hepatocyte-specific *Smad4* knockout mouse: it has low hepcidin expression and iron accumulation in liver, pancreas, and kidney [59]. Of interest, hepcidin expression in this mouse is not responsive to injected interleukin-6 or iron-dextran [59], suggesting possible cross-talk between the inflammatory and iron signaling pathways to hepcidin at the level of Smad4 (or distal to it).

4 Rodent Models of Iron-Deficiency Disorders

Mice and rats with inherited iron deficiency have been very valuable for learning about cellular iron transport. Because iron deficiency leads to anemia, pale mice or rats were easily identified in inbred colonies and the heritability of the trait could be established [60]. With the advances in mouse

Table 29.3 Rodent models of iron-deficiency disorders

Animal	Genetic defect	Phenotype	Mechanism	References
mk mouse	Missense mutation in *Dmt1* gene	Microcytic anemia	Decrease in intestinal and endosomal iron transport	[63]
Belgrade rat	Missense mutation in *Dmt1* gene	Microcytic anemia	Decrease in intestinal and endosomal iron transport	[68]
sla mouse	Deletion in hephaestin gene	Microcytic anemia, low iron stores	Decrease in enterocyte basolateral iron transport	[80]
hbd mouse	Deletion in *Sec15l1* gene	Microcytic hypochromic anemia	Impaired transferrin cycling in reticulocytes	[83]
nm1054 mouse	Deletion of *Steap3* gene	Microcytic hypochromic anemia	Impaired ferrireductase activity in transferrin endosome	[85, 86]
Steap3 knockout mouse		Similar to *nm1054* mouse	Impaired ferric reductase activity in transferrin endosome	[86]

genomics and DNA sequencing, the mutant genes responsible could be readily identified. The genetic defects and phenotypes for some of these informative mutant strains are summarized in Table 29.3.

4.1 Microcytic Anemia (mk) Mouse

Microcytic anemia (*mk*) mice were discovered in a colony at the Jackson Laboratory [61], and are characterized by severe hypochromic, microcytic anemia and poor viability. The *mk* trait was found to be autosomal recessive, and the mice have impaired intestinal iron absorption with decreased apical iron uptake by enterocytes [60]. In addition, iron uptake by reticulocytes is also defective [62]. In 1997, Fleming and coworkers [63] discovered that *mk* mice have a missense mutation in the gene for *Dmt1*. Dmt1 is a proton-coupled metal cation transporter [64], and selective deletion of Dmt1 expression in villus enterocytes demonstrates that it plays a major role in apical iron transport in these cells [65]. The *mk* mutation results in the substitution of an arginine for a glycine (G185R) in transmembrane domain 4 [63], and this impairs Dmt1 localization and activity [66, 67]. Dmt1 is also found in transferrin cycle endosomes where it functions in exporting iron into the cytoplasm, and this explains the reticulocyte defect caused by the *mk* mutation [68, 69].

4.2 Belgrade Rat

Belgrade (*b*) rats were discovered in the former Yugoslavia and have autosomal recessively inherited hypochromic, microcytic anemia and low iron stores [70–73]. Like *mk* mice, these animals have impaired intestinal iron absorption and defective iron uptake by reticulocytes [71, 72, 74, 75]. Interestingly, a glycine-to-arginine missense mutation is present in the *Dmt1* gene of the Belgrade rat, and this G185R amino acid alteration is the same as that seen in the *mk* mouse [68]. Thus, both the *mk* mouse and the Belgrade rat demonstrate the functional consequences of impaired iron transport by Dmt1.

4.3 Sex-Linked Anemia (sla) Mouse

The sex-linked anemia (*sla*) mouse arose in an irradiated mouse colony [76]. The *sla* mouse develops moderate to severe microcytic, hypochromic anemia early in life [77]. Although this mouse strain takes up iron normally from the intestinal lumen into mature epithelial cells, the subsequent egress of iron into the circulation is decreased [78, 79]. Therefore, iron accumulates within enterocytes and is lost during turnover of these cells. Vulpe and colleagues identified the genetic defect in the *sla* mouse as being a large deletion in a gene they called hephaestin (*Heph*), named after the Greek god of metal working [80]. Hephaestin is a multicopper protein that shares 50% homology with ceruloplasmin, but unlike ceruloplasmin, it contains a predicted carboxy-terminal transmembrane domain [80]. Like ceruloplasmin, hephaestin has ferroxidase activity and it may act to facilitate iron egress from intestinal enterocytes [2, 9, 80].

4.4 Hemoglobin-Deficit (hbd) Mouse

The hemoglobin-deficit mouse (*hbd*) arose spontaneously in an inbred colony in Germany [81]. This mouse strain is characterized by a hypochromic, microcytic anemia that is inherited in an autosomal, recessive manner [82]. A deletion in the gene *Sec15l1* is responsible, and *Sec15l1* is specific to hematopoietic cells and has homology to a yeast gene for vesicle docking [82, 83]. Iron trafficking experiments in reticulocytes indicate that transferrin cycling is deficient, and it is proposed that the product of *Sec15l1* is directly involved in vesicular exocytosis [82], docking, fusion, or cargo delivery in erythroid precursors [84].

4.5 nm1054 Mouse and Steap3 Knockout Mouse

The *nm1054* mouse appeared spontaneously in a colony at the Jackson Laboratory [85]. This mouse has the characteristics of moderately severe, congenital, hypochromic, microcytic anemia, with an elevated red cell zinc protoporphyrin, consistent with functional erythroid iron deficiency [85]. However, analysis of serum and tissue iron status indicates that *nm1054* mice are not systemically iron deficient. Fleming and colleagues [86] have identified that deletion of the gene for *Steap3* (6-transmembrane epithelial antigen of the prostate 3) is responsible for this phenotype. *Steap3* knockout mice also share this phenotype. Steap3 is an endosomal ferrireductase required for efficient transferrin-dependent iron uptake in erythroid cells. However, both *nm1054* and *Steap3*$^{-/-}$ erythroid precursors retain some residual ferrireductase as well as iron uptake activity, suggesting that there are other ways of reducing iron in the transferrin-cycle endosome [86]. Steap2 and Steap4 are ferrireductases that are expressed in erythropoietic tissues, which makes them candidates for redundant ferrireductases in the erythroid transferrin-cycle endosome [87]. Interestingly, three Steap proteins (2, 3, and 4) also have cupric reductase activity [87], suggesting the possibility of bifunctional action of these proteins. Use of genetically manipulated mice should clarify the functions of Steap 2 and 4 in vivo.

5 Mice Deficient in Iron-Related Proteins

Table 29.4 summarizes the phenotype of several mouse lines that are deficient in certain iron-related proteins. These mice provide insight into the in vivo functions of these proteins.

Table 29.4 Mice deficient in iron-related proteins

Protein	Mouse and genetic defect	Phenotype	References
Transferrin	Hypotransferrinemic ($Tf^{hpx/hpx}$) mouse, splicing defect	Severe anemia, iron overload	[88–90]
Transferrin receptor 1	*Tfrc* knockout mouse	Embryonic death with anemia and apoptosis of neuroepithelium	[91]
β2-Microglobulin	*B2m* knockout mouse	Increased body iron, splenic iron sparing, decreased hepcidin	[92–94]
Ceruloplasmin	*Cp* knockout mouse	Hepatic and regional CNS iron overload, mild anemia	[97, 101, 102]
Ceruloplasmin/hephaestin	*Cp* and *Heph* double-deficient mouse	Retinal iron accumulation and degeneration	[100, 103]
H-Ferritin	*Fth* knockout mouse	Embryonic lethal in homozygotes, heterozygotes have normal brain iron levels with oxidative stress	[104, 105]
Haptoglobin	*Hp* knockout mouse	Increased duodenal ferroportin and iron transport, increased splenic and renal iron	[106]
Haptoglobin/Hfe	*Hp* and *Hfe* double-knockout mouse	Milder phenotype than $Hfe^{-/-}$ mouse	[107]
Hemopexin	*Hx* knockout mouse	Increased regional CNS iron, increased renal injury after intravascular hemolysis	[109–111]
Irp1	*Irp1* knockout mouse	No overt abnormalities	[114, 115]
Irp2	*Irp2* knockout mouse	Microcytic anemia, increased duodenal and liver iron	[116, 117]
Heme oxygenase 1	*Hmox1* knockout mouse	Anemia, low serum iron, increased hepatic and renal iron	[121]
Flvcr (feline leukemia virus, subgroup C receptor)	*Flvcr* knockout mouse	Macrocytic anemia with proerythroblast maturation arrest	[123]
Duodenal cytochrome B	*Cybrd1* knockout mouse	Little impact on body iron stores	[125]

5.1 *Hypotransferrinemic ($Tf^{hpx/hpx}$) Mouse*

Congenital hypotransferrinemia occurs rarely in humans and a model of this condition is the hypotransferrinemic mouse. The *hpx* mutation in the transferrin gene (*Tf*) occurred spontaneously in an inbred mouse colony [88]. The mice are born alive but die from severe anemia before weaning if they are not treated with exogenous transferrin or red blood cell transfusions [88]. The *hpx* mutation is a point mutation that results in an error in mRNA splicing [89]. Therefore, no normal *Tf* mRNA is made from the *hpx* allele, but a small amount of mRNA containing a 27-base-pair deletion is produced from the use of cryptic splice sites [89]. Consequently, homozygous $Tf^{hpx/hpx}$ mice have less than 1% of normal levels of a shortened transferrin molecule containing a 9-amino-acid deletion near the carboxy terminus [89]. Despite their severe transferrin deficiency, $Tf^{hpx/hpx}$ mice initially given transferrin injections can survive after weaning without any further treatment. They develop massive iron overload in the liver, kidney, heart, and exocrine pancreas, while the spleen is spared [89]. Hepcidin mRNA expression remains low [90], suggesting that the induction of hepcidin by iron is trumped by an inhibitory signal linked to erythropoietic drive. The hepatic iron concentration of *Tf*$^{hpx/hpx}$ mice is approximately 100-fold greater than that of wild-type mice and at least 15-fold higher than *Hfe* knockout mice [89]. However, there is no histologically detectable fibrosis in the liver or pancreas in the *Tf*$^{hpx/hpx}$ mouse [89], suggesting that mice may be resistant to the profibrogenic effects of iron overload.

5.2 *Transferrin Receptor (Tfrc) Knockout Mouse*

Indicative of the key role of the transferrin receptor in early development, Levy et al. [91] demonstrated that *Tfrc* knockout mice undergo embryonic death with anemia and apoptosis of primitive neuroepithelium. It appears that inadequate iron uptake leads to neuronal apoptosis, but that other tissues can obtain sufficient iron for development through mechanisms independent of the transferrin cycle. Haploinsufficiency for *Tfrc* results in microcytic, hypochromic erythrocytes, along with normal hemoglobin and hematocrit values (due to a compensatory increase in the number of red cells) [91]. Although transferrin saturation is normal, *Tfrc* heterozygotes have lower levels of tissue iron [91].

5.3 *β2-Microglobulin (B2m) Knockout Mouse*

β2-Microglobulin (B2M) forms a heterodimer with MHC class I molecules and with many atypical MHC class I–like proteins, including HFE. B2M is involved in the appropriate intracellular trafficking of its partner proteins, and targeted deletion of *B2m* in mice causes immune deficits and iron overload similar to HH type 1 [92, 93]. Like *Hfe* knockout mice, *B2m* knockout mice have decreased hepcidin expression in the liver [94]. The *HFE* C282Y mutation disrupts the binding of HFE to B2M resulting in impaired intracellular transit, accelerated degradation, and failure of the C282Y protein to be presented normally at the cell surface [95]. Therefore, the abrogation of the interaction with B2M provides a basis for the impaired function of the HFE C282Y protein in HH type 1.

5.4 *Ceruloplasmin (Cp) Knockout Mouse*

Hereditary aceruloplasminemia is a rare autosomal recessive disorder characterized by iron overload, anemia, progressive neurodegeneration, diabetes, and retinal degeneration [3, 96, 97]. This condition is caused by mutations in the ceruloplasmin (*CP*) gene, resulting in the absence of ceruloplasmin, a multicopper ferroxidase. *Cp* knockout mice have a progressive increase in iron levels within Kupffer cells and splenic macrophages, as well as in hepatocytes [97]. Ferrokinetic studies in *Cp* knockout mice show no abnormalities in cellular iron uptake but a striking impairment in the egress of iron from macrophages and hepatocytes [97]. These results indicate that ceruloplasmin plays an important role in determining the rate of iron efflux from cells with mobilizable iron stores. It is now appreciated that ceruloplasmin stabilizes ferroportin expression at the cell surface [98] and that glycosylphosphatidylinositol (GPI)-linked ceruloplasmin is the predominant form expressed in brain [99].

Unlike patients with aceruloplasminemia, the original line of *Cp* knockout mice does not manifest significant brain iron overload, retinal degeneration, or neuropathy even at 24 months of age [100]. Another line of *Cp* knockout mice shows increased iron deposition in several brain regions, including the cerebellum and brainstem. Increased lipid peroxidation is also seen in some regions [101]. Of interest, these mice have deficits in motor coordination that are thought to be associated with a loss of brainstem dopaminergic neurons [101]. In the cerebellum of these mice, iron accumulation occurs mainly in astrocytes and is accompanied by a significant loss of these cells [102]. In contrast, Purkinje neurons in *Cp* knockout mice do not accumulate iron but express high levels of Dmt1, suggesting that these cells may be iron deprived: there is also a significant reduction in the number of Purkinje neurons [102]. It has been proposed that neuronal iron starvation with associated astrocyte and microglial iron overload may contribute to the neurodegeneration seen in aceruloplasminemia [99].

In order to examine the effect of combined deficiency of ceruloplasmin and hephaestin on the retina, the *Cp* knockout mouse was crossed with the *sla* mouse. The resulting compound mutant mouse has retinal iron accumulation with secondary increases in ferritin and, ultimately, retinal degeneration [100]. Body iron status has not yet been reported for this mouse strain, but longevity is decreased [100, 103].

5.5 H-Ferritin (Fth) Knockout Mouse

Deletion of the H-ferritin gene (*Fth*) in mice results in early embryonic lethality [104, 105]. Haploinsufficiency for *Fth* does not change brain iron levels, but the levels of H-ferritin are decreased by more than 50% [105]. Interestingly, the brain expression of transferrin, transferrin receptor 1, L-ferritin, Dmt1, and ceruloplasmin are all increased in $Fth^{+/-}$ mice, suggestive of an iron-deficient state. There is also evidence of increased oxidative stress in the brain of these mice [105].

5.6 Haptoglobin (Hp) Knockout Mouse

Haptoglobin is the plasma protein with the highest binding affinity for hemoglobin. It delivers any hemoglobin in the plasma to the reticuloendothelial system, thus reducing loss of hemoglobin through the glomeruli and allowing heme-iron recycling [106]. Analysis of *Hp* knockout mice reveals that they export significantly more iron from the duodenal mucosa to plasma. Increased iron export from the duodenum correlates with increased duodenal expression of ferroportin at both the protein and mRNA levels, whereas hepatic hepcidin expression remains unchanged [106]. Splenic and renal iron concentrations are increased. Marro and coworkers [106] suggest that haptoglobin, by controlling plasma levels of hemoglobin, participates in the regulation of ferroportin expression, thus influencing iron transfer from duodenal mucosa to plasma.

Interestingly, haptoglobin deficiency also influences the phenotype of *Hfe* knockout mice. *Hfe* and *Hg* compound mutant mice accumulate significantly less hepatic iron than *Hfe* knockout mice, suggesting that haptoglobin-mediated heme-iron recovery might contribute to iron loading in *HFE*-associated HH [107].

5.7 Hemopexin (Hx) Knockout Mouse

Hemopexin is an acute-phase plasma glycoprotein produced mainly in the liver and released into plasma where it binds heme with high affinity and delivers it to the liver [108]. The *Hx* knockout mouse was developed to evaluate the in vivo effect of hemopexin deficiency, and an interesting phenotype was observed in the brain [108]. These mice have a twofold increase in the number of iron-loaded oligodendrocytes in the basal ganglia and thalamus, but there is no increase in H-or L-ferritin expression in these regions [109]. However, there is a substantial decrease in the number of ferritin-positive cells in the cerebral cortex of the knockout mouse [109]. These results suggest that hemopexin may play a role in controlling iron distribution within brain. As anticipated from hemopexin's role in heme scavenging, the *Hp* knockout mouse has significantly more renal damage after phenylhydrazine-induced hemolysis [110] and increased endothelial activation and vascular permeability after heme overload [111].

5.8 *Irp1 or 2 Knockout Mice*

The two iron regulatory proteins, IRP1 and IRP2, bind to the mRNAs of ferritin, transferrin receptor, and other target genes to control the expression of these proteins at the posttranscriptional level [3, 4, 7, 112]. In their native conformation, both IRPs have a high binding affinity for stem-loop structures called iron-responsive elements (IREs) present in the mRNAs of their target genes. IRP1 is an iron–sulfur cluster protein that loses its RNA-binding activity in iron-replete conditions, whereas IRP2 is degraded by the proteasome.

Genetic ablation of Irp1 and 2 in mice has been informative about the in vivo functions of these proteins. Complete loss of both Irp1 and 2 prevents viability of murine zygotes beyond the blastocyst stage of embryonic development [113]. *Irp1* knockout mice develop no overt abnormalities [114, 115]. *Irp2* knockout mice develop microcytic anemia [116, 117] and altered body iron distribution with duodenal and hepatic iron loading [118]. In addition, the Ire/Irp system is essential to maintain the structural and functional integrity of the intestine [112]. One line of *Irp2* knockout mice develops adult-onset neurodegeneration [118] while another line does not [119]. Irp2 is sensitive to iron status and can compensate for the loss of Irp1 by increasing its binding activity [114]. Therefore, Irp2 may be the chief physiologic iron sensor in vivo [4].

5.9 *Other Mice Deficient in Iron-Related Proteins*

Heme oxygenase 1 (Hmox1) has been targeted for gene deletion in mice to provide insight into a case of human HMOX1 deficiency that was characterized by growth retardation, hemolytic anemia, liver and kidney iron accumulation, and kidney injury [120] The *Hmox1* knockout mouse has anemia, low serum iron, and increased hepatic and renal iron [121]. These results are consistent with an important role for Hmox1 in the reutilization of heme iron.

As its name connotes, the feline leukemia virus (subgroup C) receptor (FLVCR) was cloned as a viral receptor and was subsequently found to be a heme exporter [3, 122]. *Flvcr* knockout mice develop macrocytic anemia with proerythroblast maturation arrest, which suggests that erythroid precursors must export excess heme to ensure survival [123].

Duodenal cytochrome b (Dcytb, Cybrd1) is an iron-regulated ferric reductase that is highly expressed in duodenal enterocytes [124]. While knockout of *Dcytb* in mice has little effect on their body iron status [125], the potential role in Dcytb in iron absorption is still being evaluated [124].

6 Defects in Mitochondrial Iron Metabolism

The sideroblastic anemias are a group of disorders characterized by a variable population of hypochromic red cells in the blood and by ringed sideroblasts in the bone marrow [3]. The unifying characteristic of all sideroblastic anemias is the ring sideroblast, which is a pathological erythroid

Table 29.5 Murine models of altered mitochondrial iron metabolism

Protein	Mouse genotype	Phenotype	References
Erythroid 5-aminolevulinate synthase (ALAS2)	*Alas2* knockout mouse	Increased iron, but no ring sideroblasts, in primitive erythroid cells. Embryonic lethal by day 11.5	[128]
	Alas2 knockout mouse with transgenic rescue of low activity ALAS2	Ring sideroblasts in primitive erythroid cells	[129]
ATP-binding cassette transporter Abcb7	*Abcb7* knockout mouse	Mid-gestational death	[131]
	$Abcb7^{E433K}$ mouse	Siderocytosis	[132]
Ferrochelatase	$Fech^{m1Pas}$ mouse	Homozygous mouse has microcytic hypochromic anemia and severe porphyria	[135]
	Fech knockout mouse (exon 10 deletion)	Homozygous state is embryonic lethal. Heterozygotes have decreased ferrochelatase activity and mild porphyria	[133]
Frataxin	*Fxn* knockout mouse	Embryonic lethal	[136]
	Knock-in of GAA repeat mutation	No anomalies of motor coordination or iron metabolism	[137]
	Fxn knockout mice with human mutant *FXN* YAC constructs	Progressive neurodegeneration and cardiac pathology	[138]
Mitoferrin 1	*Mfrn1* knockout mouse	Embryonic lethal with profound anemia	[141]

precursor containing iron-loaded mitochondria localized around the nucleus, thereby creating a ring-like appearance [126]. Three forms of hereditary sideroblastic anemia are caused by defects in genes present on the X chromosome (mutations in the *ALAS2*, *ABCB7*, or *GRLX5* gene). For the first two of these forms, mutant mouse models have been created. Mouse models have also been generated for erythropoietic protoporphyria, Friedreich ataxia, and mitoferrin 1 deficiency (Table 29.5).

6.1 Mouse Models of X-Linked Sideroblastic Anemia: Alas2 Mutant Mice

The most frequent form of inherited sideroblastic anemia is X-linked sideroblastic anemia (XLSA), caused by mutations in the erythroid-specific *ALAS2* gene [3]. ALAS2 catalyzes the first step of the heme biosynthetic pathway in erythroid cells. Hemizygous XLSA males have microcytic anemia with iron overload, indicating that XLSA belongs to the group of iron-loading anemias. Various mutations in *ALAS2* cause decreased ALAS2 activity in bone marrow erythroblasts, with resultant impairment of heme biosynthesis and insufficient protoporphyrin IX to use all the available iron (excess iron can be stored as mitochondrial ferritin) [127].

Knockout of the *Alas2* gene in mice results in arrest of erythroid differentiation, and an abnormal hematopoietic cell fraction emerges that accumulates a large amount of iron diffusely in the cytoplasm. Typical ring sideroblasts are not found [128]. Embryonic death occurs by day 11.5. However, when human ALAS2 is expressed in these mice at approximately 50% of normal activity, most of the primitive erythroid cells are transformed into ring sideroblasts while the majority of the circulating definitive erythroid cells become siderocytes [129]. These results suggest that a partially depleted heme supply provokes ring sideroblast formation.

6.2 *Mouse Models of X-Linked Sideroblastic Anemia with Ataxia: Abcb7 Mutant Mice*

XLSA with ataxia is a rare form of inherited sideroblastic anemia of early onset, associated with spinocerebellar ataxia and cerebellar hypoplasia [130]. This form of sideroblastic anemia is due to partial loss-of-function mutations in the ATP-binding cassette transporter ABCB7 which cause mitochondrial accumulation of iron, elevated free erythrocyte protoporphyrin IX levels, and mild hypochromic microcytic anemia: examination of bone marrow shows ringed sideroblasts [3, 130]. ABCB7 is thought to export a mitochondrially derived metabolite required for cytosolic iron–sulfur cluster (ISC) biogenesis. It is an essential protein, as *Abcb7* knockout mice undergo mid-gestational death [131]. To model the severe E433K mutation in humans, an *Abcb7*^{E433K} mutant mouse was created. This strain has siderocytosis but no ring sideroblasts [132]. The absence of ring sideroblasts in these mice led Pondarre et al. [132] to suggest that there is something biologically distinctive with respect to mitochondrial iron handling and/or toxicity between human and murine erythroid precursors.

6.3 *Mouse Model of Erythropoietic Protoporphyria: Fech*^{m1Pas} *Mouse*

Erythropoietic protoporphyria is caused by decreased activity of the mitochondrial enzyme ferrochelatase, the terminal enzyme of the heme biosynthetic pathway, that catalyzes the insertion of iron into protoporphyrin IX to form heme [3]. Clinical symptoms result from an accumulation of protoporphyrin IX behind the partial enzyme block: they include lifelong photosensitivity and, in about 2% of patients, severe liver disease. The inheritance of erythropoietic protoporphyria is usually described as an autosomal dominant disorder with incomplete penetrance: missense, nonsense, and splicing mutations have been identified in the *FECH* gene [3]. Knockout of the murine *Fech* gene results in embryonic lethality, indicating the critical importance of ferrochelatase [133]. Microcytic anemia occurs in 20–60% of patients with erythropoietic protoporphyria [134]. This anemia is not dyserythropoietic, and there is no iron overload but rather iron deficiency. Therefore, ferrochelatase deficiency in erythropoietic protoporphyria appears to result in a steady state in which decreased erythropoiesis is matched by reduced iron absorption and supply [134].

A mouse model of erythropoietic protoporphyria, the homozygous *Fech*^{m1Pas} mouse, develops a similar microcytic anemia, along with accumulation of protoporphyrin IX and liver injury [135]. This mouse has a point mutation in the *Fech* gene resulting in about a 95% decrease in ferrochelatase activity. In this mouse model, there is increased expression of transferrin and redistribution of iron from peripheral tissues to the spleen, while serum iron, ferritin, and hepcidin mRNA levels are normal [135]. Further investigation is needed to understand the cause of microcytic anemia in these mice and in patients with erythropoietic protoporphyria.

6.4 *Mouse Models of Friedreich Ataxia: Fxn Mutant Mice*

Friedreich ataxia, the most common hereditary ataxia, is an autosomal recessive neurodegenerative disease characterized by progressive ataxia associated with cardiomyopathy and increased incidence of diabetes [8]. This condition is caused by reduced levels of frataxin, a highly conserved mitochondrial iron chaperone involved in ISC biogenesis. Most patients are homozygous for a large GAA triplet expansion within the first intron of the frataxin (*FXN*) gene. The pathophysiologic consequences of frataxin deficiency are a disruption of ISC biosynthesis, mitochondrial iron overload coupled with cellular iron dysregulation, and increased sensitivity to oxidative stress [8].

Knockout of *Fxn* in the mouse leads to early embryonic lethality, demonstrating an important role for frataxin during mouse development [136]. Heterozygous *Fxn*$^{+/-}$mice express about 50% of wild-type frataxin levels but do not have a phenotype [8]. Using a conditional gene-targeting approach, Puccio et al. [136] generated a striated muscle *Fxn*–deficient mouse and a neuron/cardiac muscle *Fxn*–deficient mouse, which together reproduce some features of the human disease: cardiac hypertrophy without skeletal muscle involvement, large sensory neuron dysfunction, and low activities of mitochondrial and extramitochondrial ISC proteins. Another mouse model contains a knock-in of the GAA repeat *Fxn* mutation [137]. These GAA repeat knock-in mice were crossed with *Fxn* knockout mice to obtain double heterozygous mice expressing 25–36% of wild-type frataxin levels. However, these mice do not develop anomalies of motor coordination or iron metabolism [137], suggesting that their frataxin levels are sufficient to preserve ISC biogenesis. Using an innovative approach, Al-Mahdawi et al. [138] generated "humanized" GAA repeat expansion mice by combining the constitutive *Fxn* knockout with the transgenic expression of a yeast artificial chromosome (YAC) carrying the human *FXN* gene with GAA triplet expansion. These mice have coordination defects and progressive neuronal and cardiac pathology, and should serve as a useful model to test potential therapeutic agents.

6.5 Mitoferrin 1 (Mfrn1) Knockout Mouse

Mitoferrin 1 is involved in the transport of iron into the mitochondrion [139, 140]. It is located in the inner mitochondrial membrane and is a member of the mitochondrial solute carrier family (SLC25A37). Knockout of *Mfrn1* in mice results in embryonic lethality with profound anemia, demonstrating the essential role of mitoferrin 1 [141]. Mitoferrin 1 is expressed mainly in erythroid cells, but its homolog mitoferrin 2 is expressed in non-erythroid tissues, and may play a similar transport role there [139, 140].

7 Mice with Floxed Iron-Related Genes

It is of great interest to be able to selectively delete iron-related genes in various cell types to assess their function and impact. This can be accomplished using the Cre–loxP system, and this approach has already been applied to several iron-related genes (Table 29.6). The Cre–loxP system utilizes the ability of Cre recombinase to catalyze recombination between two loxP sites in DNA [142, 143]. To accomplish cell-selective gene deletion, transgenic mice containing an iron-related gene flanked by loxP sites are crossed with transgenic mice containing a *Cre* gene construct with a cell-selective promoter. The resulting mice contain both the *Cre* gene construct and the loxP-flanked iron-related gene (floxed gene). In cells where Cre recombinase is expressed, the floxed iron-related gene will be deleted. There are now a substantial number of available mouse strains that already contain the *Cre* gene driven by either ubiquitous or cell-selective promoters. When using the Cre–loxP system, it is important to evaluate the specificity and efficiency of gene deletion [142].

Using the Cre–loxP approach, studies have found that hepatocyte-selective deletion of *Hfe* [144] or *Tfr2* [46] results in an HH phenotype, suggesting that Hfe and Tfr2 act in hepatocytes to regulate hepcidin expression. Deletion of either *Dmt1* or *Fpn* in villus enterocytes results in iron-deficiency anemia, highlighting the importance of these transporters in dietary iron absorption [52, 65]. The developing hippocampus may be particularly susceptible to iron deficiency, and selective knockout

Table 29.6 Mice with floxed iron-related genes

Gene	Observations	References
Hfe	Selective knockout in hepatocytes (but not in villus enterocytes) produces HH phenotype	[144, 160]
Tfr2	Selective knockout in hepatocytes produces HH phenotype	[46]
Dmt1 (Slc11a2)	Selective knockout in intestine produces iron-deficiency anemia	[65]
	Selective knockout in hippocampus disrupts hippocampal neuronal development and spatial memory behavior	[145]
Fpn (Slc40a1)	Selective knockout in intestine produces iron-deficiency anemia	[52]
Irp2	Selective knockout in liver or intestine causes tissue-specific iron loading	[115, 146]
Irp1 and 2	Selective knockout of both *Irp1* and *Irp2* in intestine causes malabsorption and death	[112]
Abcb7	Selective knockout in hepatocytes impairs cytosolic iron–sulfur cluster assembly	[131]
Fxn	Selective knockout in neurons/cardiac muscle, liver, or striated muscle is useful to model different aspects of Friedreich ataxia	[136, 161]

of *Dmt1* in hippocampal neurons provides the first conditionally targeted model of iron uptake in the brain [145]. Deletion of *Dmt1* in these mice disrupts hippocampal neuronal development and spatial memory behavior. Cell-selective deletion of *Irp2* (with or without *Irp1*) has been used to investigate its action in the intestine and liver [112, 146]. Some mouse models of Friedreich ataxia have used cell-selective deletion of the frataxin gene [136]. In the future, it is likely that more mice with floxed iron-related genes will be generated, thus allowing investigation of the in vivo consequences of cell-selective deletion of these genes.

8 Animal Models of Dietary Iron Deficiency

Iron deficiency is the most prevalent micronutrient deficiency in the world, and infants and young children are particularly vulnerable [147, 148]. The effects of iron deficiency on iron metabolism, brain function, and behavior have been widely studied in animal models, often using rodents [149–151]. Iron deficiency is usually induced by dietary iron restriction, and such models provide convincing evidence that, despite iron repletion, iron deficiency during the brain growth spurt alters neurotransmission, myelination, and gene and protein profiles [150, 151]. Impaired developmental outcome has also been shown in human and monkey infants with fetal/neonatal iron deficiency [149]. Therefore, cross-species studies indicate that there is a vulnerable period in early development that may result in long-lasting neurobehavioral damage [150].

9 Animal Models of Iron Overload Produced by Exogenous Iron

In order to study the effects of iron overload, animal models have been developed using dietary iron supplementation (e.g., carbonyl iron, ferrocene) or parental iron administration (e.g., iron-dextran, iron-sorbitol). Many species have been used, but studies in rodents are most common. Dietary carbonyl iron supplementation produces substantial hepatic iron overload in a periportal distribution with iron deposition predominantly in hepatocytes [152], which mimics the pattern of iron loading in HH type 1. Parenteral administration of iron chelates produces hepatic iron overload with predominant accumulation in Kupffer cells [153]. There is an extensive body of literature describing the hepatotoxicity of iron overload in animal models [5, 6, 154–156]. To summarize, iron overload in experimental animals can result in oxidative damage to lipids in vivo, once the concentration of iron exceeds a threshold level. In the liver, this lipid peroxidation is associated with impairment of membrane-dependent functions of mitochondria (oxidative metabolism) and lysosomes (membrane integrity, pH). Iron overload diminishes hepatic mitochondrial respiration primarily through a decrease in cytochrome C oxidase activity. In iron overload, hepatocellular calcium homeostasis may also be impaired through damage to mitochondrial and microsomal calcium sequestration. DNA is also a target of iron-induced damage, and this may have consequences regarding malignant transformation. Levels of some antioxidants in the liver are decreased in rodents with iron overload, which is also suggestive of ongoing oxidative stress. Therefore, reduced cellular ATP levels, lysosomal fragility, impaired cellular calcium homeostasis, and damage to DNA may all contribute to hepatocellular injury in iron overload. One limitation of rodent models of iron overload is the difficulty in producing histologic hepatic fibrosis and cirrhosis, despite achieving high hepatic iron levels [5, 89, 155]. However, there is evidence of increased hepatic collagen gene expression and early activation of hepatic stellate cells, the key cell type involved in hepatic fibrogenesis [5].

In humans, elevated cardiac iron leads to diastolic dysfunction, arrhythmias, and dilated cardiomyopathy. These are major risk factors in patients with secondary iron overload [157, 158]. The effects of iron overload on the heart have been examined in several animal models [157]. One such model involves chronic treatment of mice with iron-dextran, which results in myocardial iron deposition, alterations in myocardial ultrastructure, and impaired cardiac function [159]. L-type calcium channels may be involved in ferrous iron uptake into cardiomyocytes, and pharmacological blockade of these channels decreases iron accumulation and associated cardiac dysfunction [159]. In addition, enzymes in the plasma membrane such as $Na^{+}+K^{+}$-ATPase may be key targets of damage by non-transferrin-bound iron in cardiac myocytes [157].

10 Concluding Remarks

Mammalian models continue to make valuable contributions to our understanding of iron metabolism. Murine models are now available for the major forms of HH, and findings in these mice support the concept that the pathogenesis of HH types 1, 2, and 3 involves inappropriately low expression of hepcidin. Altered hepcidin expression in mice deficient in Bmp6, Tmprss6, or Smad4 has focused attention on the role that these molecules play in iron signaling to hepcidin. Investigation of mice with inherited forms of anemia has led to the discovery of novel proteins involved in iron homeostasis (e.g., hephaestin, Steap3). A growing number of murine models are being developed to investigate mitochondrial iron metabolism. Although not emphasized in this chapter, murine transgenic technology allows the overexpression of iron-related proteins either globally or in a cell-selective manner. The neurobehavioral consequences of dietary iron deficiency have been widely studied in animal models and indicate that there is a vulnerable period in early development that may result in long-lasting changes. Exogenous iron administration has been used to study the pathophysiologic effects of iron overload, particularly in the liver and heart. In the future, it is anticipated that the production of mice with floxed iron-related genes will accelerate, thus allowing the study of the in vivo consequences of cell-selective deletion of these genes. Transgenic expression of selectively mutated and tagged iron-related proteins in mice is also expected to be a powerful tool to further unravel the mechanisms of iron homeostasis.

Acknowledgments The research work of the authors was supported by United States Public Health Service NIH grants DK41816 (B.R.B.) and HL66225 (R.E.F.).

References

1. Andrews NC. Iron homeostasis: insights from genetics and animal models. Nat Rev Genet. 2000;1:208–17.
2. Andrews NC. Animal models of hereditary iron transport disorders. Adv Exp Med Biol. 2002;509:1–17.
3. Iolascon A, De Falco L, Beaumont C. Molecular basis of inherited microcytic anemia due to defects in iron acquisition or heme synthesis. Haematologica. 2009;94:395–408.
4. Rouault TA. The role of iron regulatory proteins in mammalian iron homeostasis and disease. Nat Chem Biol. 2006;2:406–14.
5. Ramm GA, Ruddell RG. Hepatotoxicity of iron overload: mechanisms of iron-induced hepatic fibrogenesis. Semin Liver Dis. 2005;25:433–49.
6. Britton RS, Leicester KL, Bacon BR. Iron toxicity and chelation therapy. Int J Hematol. 2002;76:219–28.
7. Muckenthaler MU, Galy B, Hentze MW. Systemic iron homeostasis and the iron-responsive element/iron-regulatory protein (IRE/IRP) regulatory network. Annu Rev Nutr. 2008;28:197–213.
8. Puccio H. Multicellular models of Friedreich ataxia. J Neurol. 2009;256(Suppl. 1):18–24.
9. Anderson GJ, Vulpe CD. Mammalian iron transport. Cell Mol Life Sci. 2009;66:3241–61.
10. Feder JN, Gnirke A, Thomas W, et al. A novel MHC class I-like gene is mutated in patients with hereditary haemochromatosis. Nat Genet. 1996;13:399–408.
11. Zhou XY, Tomatsu S, Fleming RE, et al. HFE gene knockout produces mouse model of hereditary hemochromatosis. Proc Natl Acad Sci USA. 1998;95:2492–7.
12. Levy JE, Montross LK, Cohen DE, Fleming MD, Andrews NC. The C282Y mutation causing hereditary hemochromatosis does not produce a null allele. Blood. 1999;94:9–11.
13. Bahram S, Gilfillan S, Kuhn LC, et al. Experimental hemochromatosis due to MHC class I HFE deficiency: immune status and iron metabolism. Proc Natl Acad Sci USA. 1999;96:13312–7.
14. Tomatsu S, Orii KO, Fleming RE, et al. Contribution of the H63D mutation in HFE to murine hereditary hemochromatosis. Proc Natl Acad Sci USA. 2003;100:15788–93.
15. Ahmad KA, Ahmann JR, Migas MC, et al. Decreased liver hepcidin expression in the Hfe knockout mouse. Blood Cells Mol Dis. 2002;29:361–6.
16. Bridle KR, Frazer DM, Wilkins SJ, et al. Disrupted hepcidin regulation in HFE-associated haemochromatosis and the liver as a regulator of body iron homoeostasis. Lancet. 2003;361:669–73.
17. Ajioka RS, Levy JE, Andrews NC, Kushner JP. Regulation of iron absorption in Hfe mutant mice. Blood. 2002;100:1465–9.
18. Corradini E, Garuti C, Montosi G, et al. Bone morphogenetic protein signaling is impaired in an HFE knockout mouse model of hemochromatosis. Gastroenterology. 2009;137:1489–97.
19. Kautz L, Meynard D, Besson-Fournier C, et al. BMP/Smad signaling is not enhanced in Hfe-deficient mice despite increased Bmp6 expression. Blood. 2009;114:2515–20.
20. Levy JE, Montross LK, Andrews NC. Genes that modify the hemochromatosis phenotype in mice. J Clin Invest. 2000;105:1209–16.
21. Fleming RE, Holden CC, Tomatsu S, et al. Mouse strain differences determine severity of iron accumulation in Hfe knockout model of hereditary hemochromatosis. Proc Natl Acad Sci USA. 2001;98:2707–11.
22. Dupic F, Fruchon S, Bensaid M, et al. Inactivation of the hemochromatosis gene differentially regulates duodenal expression of iron-related mRNAs between mouse strains. Gastroenterology. 2002;122:745–51.
23. Courselaud B, Troadec MB, Fruchon S, et al. Strain and gender modulate hepatic hepcidin 1 and 2 mRNA expression in mice. Blood Cells Mol Dis. 2004;32:283–9.
24. Bensaid M, Fruchon S, Mazeres C, Bahram S, Roth MP, Coppin H. Multigenic control of hepatic iron loading in a murine model of hemochromatosis. Gastroenterology. 2004;126:1400–8.
25. Huang FW, Pinkus JL, Pinkus GS, Fleming MD, Andrews NC. A mouse model of juvenile hemochromatosis. J Clin Invest. 2005;115:2187–91.
26. Niederkofler V, Salie R, Arber S. Hemojuvelin is essential for dietary iron sensing, and its mutation leads to severe iron overload. J Clin Invest. 2005;115:2180–6.
27. Babitt JL, Huang FW, Wrighting DM, et al. Bone morphogenetic protein signaling by hemojuvelin regulates hepcidin expression. Nat Genet. 2006;38:531–9.
28. Meynard D, Kautz L, Darnaud V, Canonne-Hergaux F, Coppin H, Roth MP. Lack of the bone morphogenetic protein BMP6 induces massive iron overload. Nat Genet. 2009;41:478–81.
29. Andriopoulos Jr B, Corradini E, Xia Y, et al. BMP6 is a key endogenous regulator of hepcidin expression and iron metabolism. Nat Genet. 2009;41:482–7.
30. Nemeth E, Tuttle MS, Powelson J, et al. Hepcidin regulates cellular iron efflux by binding to ferroportin and inducing its internalization. Science. 2004;306:2090–3.
31. Nemeth E, Ganz T. The role of hepcidin in iron metabolism. Acta Haematol. 2009;122:78–86.

32. Pigeon C, Ilyin G, Courselaud B, et al. A new mouse liver-specific gene, encoding a protein homologous to human antimicrobial peptide hepcidin, is overexpressed during iron overload. J Biol Chem. 2001;276:7811–9.
33. Nicolas G, Bennoun M, Devaux I, et al. Lack of hepcidin gene expression and severe tissue iron overload in upstream stimulatory factor 2 (USF2) knockout mice. Proc Natl Acad Sci USA. 2001;98:8780–5.
34. Roetto A, Papanikolaou G, Politou M, et al. Mutant antimicrobial peptide hepcidin is associated with severe juvenile hemochromatosis. Nat Genet. 2003;33:21–2.
35. Nicolas G, Bennoun M, Porteu A, et al. Severe iron deficiency anemia in transgenic mice expressing liver hepcidin. Proc Natl Acad Sci USA. 2002;99:4596–601.
36. Roy CN, Mak HH, Akpan I, Losyev G, Zurakowski D, Andrews NC. Hepcidin antimicrobial peptide transgenic mice exhibit features of the anemia of inflammation. Blood. 2007;109:4038–44.
37. Nicolas G, Chauvet C, Viatte L, et al. The gene encoding the iron regulatory peptide hepcidin is regulated by anemia, hypoxia, and inflammation. J Clin Invest. 2002;110:1037–44.
38. Lesbordes-Brion JC, Viatte L, Bennoun M, et al. Targeted disruption of the hepcidin 1 gene results in severe hemochromatosis. Blood. 2006;108:1402–5.
39. Pietrangelo A. Non-HFE hemochromatosis. Semin Liver Dis. 2005;25:450–60.
40. Kawabata H, Yang R, Hirama T, et al. Molecular cloning of transferrin receptor 2. A new member of the transferrin receptor-like family. J Biol Chem. 1999;274:20826–32.
41. Camaschella C, Roetto A, Cali A, et al. The gene TFR2 is mutated in a new type of haemochromatosis mapping to 7q22. Nat Genet. 2000;25:14–5.
42. Fleming RE, Ahmann JR, Migas MC, et al. Targeted mutagenesis of the murine transferrin receptor-2 gene produces hemochromatosis. Proc Natl Acad Sci USA. 2002;99:10653–8.
43. Wallace DF, Summerville L, Lusby PE, Subramaniam VN. First phenotypic description of transferrin receptor 2 knockout mouse, and the role of hepcidin. Gut. 2005;54:980–6.
44. Kawabata H, Fleming RE, Gui D, et al. Expression of hepcidin is down-regulated in TfR2 mutant mice manifesting a phenotype of hereditary hemochromatosis. Blood. 2005;105:376–81.
45. Drake SF, Morgan EH, Herbison CE, et al. Iron absorption and hepatic iron uptake are increased in a transferrin receptor 2 (Y245X) mutant mouse model of hemochromatosis type 3. Am J Physiol Gastrointest Liver Physiol. 2007;292:G323–8.
46. Wallace DF, Summerville L, Subramaniam VN. Targeted disruption of the hepatic transferrin receptor 2 gene in mice leads to iron overload. Gastroenterology. 2007;132:301–10.
47. Wallace DF, Summerville L, Crampton EM, Frazer DM, Anderson GJ, Subramaniam VN. Combined deletion of Hfe and transferrin receptor 2 in mice leads to marked dysregulation of hepcidin and iron overload. Hepatology. 2009;50:1992–2000.
48. Olynyk JK, Trinder D, Ramm GA, Britton RS, Bacon BR. Hereditary hemochromatosis in the post-HFE era. Hepatology. 2008;48:991–1001.
49. Fernandes A, Preza GC, Phung Y, et al. The molecular basis of hepcidin-resistant hereditary hemochromatosis. Blood. 2009;114:437–43.
50. Pietrangelo A. The ferroportin disease. Blood Cells Mol Dis. 2004;32:131–8.
51. Pietrangelo A. Hemochromatosis: an endocrine liver disease. Hepatology. 2007;46:1291–301.
52. Donovan A, Lima CA, Pinkus JL, et al. The iron exporter ferroportin/Slc40a1 is essential for iron homeostasis. Cell Metab. 2005;1:191–200.
53. Zohn IE, De Domenico I, Pollock A, et al. The flatiron mutation in mouse ferroportin acts as a dominant negative to cause ferroportin disease. Blood. 2007;109:4174–80.
54. Ganz T. Hepcidin, a key regulator of iron metabolism and mediator of anemia of inflammation. Blood. 2003;102:783–8.
55. Du X, She E, Gelbart T, et al. The serine protease TMPRSS6 is required to sense iron deficiency. Science. 2008;320:1088–92.
56. Folgueras AR, de Lara FM, Pendas AM, et al. Membrane-bound serine protease matriptase-2 (Tmprss6) is an essential regulator of iron homeostasis. Blood. 2008;112:2539–45.
57. Silvestri L, Pagani A, Nai A, De Domenico I, Kaplan J, Camaschella C. The serine protease matriptase-2 (TMPRSS6) inhibits hepcidin activation by cleaving membrane hemojuvelin. Cell Metab. 2008;8:502–11.
58. Finberg KE, Heeney MM, Campagna DR, et al. Mutations in TMPRSS6 cause iron-refractory iron deficiency anemia (IRIDA). Nat Genet. 2008;40:569–71.
59. Wang RH, Li C, Xu X, et al. A role of SMAD4 in iron metabolism through the positive regulation of hepcidin expression. Cell Metab. 2005;2:399–409.
60. Bannerman RM, Edwards JA, Kreimer-Birnbaum M, McFarland E, Russell ES. Hereditary microcytic anaemia in the mouse; studies in iron distribution and metabolism. Br J Haematol. 1972;23:235–45.
61. Nash DJ, Kent E, Dickie MM, Russell ES. The inheritance of "mick", a new anemia in the house mouse. Am Zool. 1964;4:404–5.
62. Edwards JA, Hoke JE. Red cell iron uptake in hereditary microcytic anemia. Blood. 1975;46:381–8.

63. Fleming MD, Trenor 3rd CC, Su MA, et al. Microcytic anaemia mice have a mutation in Nramp2, a candidate iron transporter gene. Nat Genet. 1997;16:383–6.
64. Gunshin H, Mackenzie B, Berger UV, et al. Cloning and characterization of a mammalian proton-coupled metal-ion transporter. Nature. 1997;388:482–8.
65. Gunshin H, Fujiwara Y, Custodio AO, Direnzo C, Robine S, Andrews NC. Slc11a2 is required for intestinal iron absorption and erythropoiesis but dispensable in placenta and liver. J Clin Invest. 2005;115:1258–66.
66. Su MA, Trenor CC, Fleming JC, Fleming MD, Andrews NC. The G185R mutation disrupts function of the iron transporter Nramp2. Blood. 1998;92:2157–63.
67. Canonne-Hergaux F, Fleming MD, Levy JE, et al. The Nramp2/DMT1 iron transporter is induced in the duodenum of microcytic anemia mk mice but is not properly targeted to the intestinal brush border. Blood. 2000;96:3964–70.
68. Fleming MD, Romano MA, Su MA, Garrick LM, Garrick MD, Andrews NC. Nramp2 is mutated in the anemic Belgrade (b) rat: evidence of a role for Nramp2 in endosomal iron transport. Proc Natl Acad Sci USA. 1998;95:1148–53.
69. Gruenheid S, Canonne-Hergaux F, Gauthier S, Hackam DJ, Grinstein S, Gros P. The iron transport protein NRAMP2 is an integral membrane glycoprotein that colocalizes with transferrin in recycling endosomes. J Exp Med. 1999;189:831–41.
70. Sladic-Simic D, Martinovitch PN, Zivkovic N, et al. A thalassemia-like disorder in Belgrade laboratory rats. Ann N Y Acad Sci. 1969;165:93–9.
71. Edwards JA, Sullivan AL, Hoke JE. Defective delivery of iron to the developing red cell of the Belgrade laboratory rat. Blood. 1980;55:645–8.
72. Bowen BJ, Morgan EH. Anemia of the Belgrade rat: evidence for defective membrane transport of iron. Blood. 1987;70:38–44.
73. Farcich EA, Morgan EH. Diminished iron acquisition by cells and tissues of Belgrade laboratory rats. Am J Physiol. 1992;262:R220–4.
74. Garrick MD, Gniecko K, Liu Y, Cohan DS, Garrick LM. Transferrin and the transferrin cycle in Belgrade rat reticulocytes. J Biol Chem. 1993;268:14867–74.
75. Oates PS, Morgan EH. Defective iron uptake by the duodenum of Belgrade rats fed diets of different iron contents. Am J Physiol. 1996;270:G826–32.
76. Falconer DS, Isaacson JH. The genetics of sex-linked anaemia in the mouse. Genet Res. 1962;3:248–50.
77. Grewal MD. A sex-linked anaemia in the mouse. Genet Res. 1962;3:238–47.
78. Edwards JA, Bannerman RM. Hereditary defect of intestinal iron transport in mice with sex-linked anemia. J Clin Invest. 1970;49:1869–71.
79. Manis J. Intestinal iron-transport defect in the mouse with sex-linked anemia. Am J Physiol. 1971;220:135–9.
80. Vulpe CD, Kuo YM, Murphy TL, et al. Hephaestin, a ceruloplasmin homologue implicated in intestinal iron transport, is defective in the sla mouse. Nat Genet. 1999;21:195–9.
81. Scheufler H. An additional house mouse mutant with anemia (hemoglobin deficiency). Z Versuchstierkd. 1969;11:348–53.
82. Lim JE, Jin O, Bennett C, et al. A mutation in Sec15l1 causes anemia in hemoglobin deficit (hbd) mice. Nat Genet. 2005;37:1270–3.
83. White RA, Boydston LA, Brookshier TR, et al. Iron metabolism mutant hbd mice have a deletion in Sec15l1, which has homology to a yeast gene for vesicle docking. Genomics. 2005;86:668–73.
84. Zhang AS, Sheftel AD, Ponka P. The anemia of "haemoglobin-deficit" (hbd/hbd) mice is caused by a defect in transferrin cycling. Exp Hematol. 2006;34:593–8.
85. Ohgami RS, Campagna DR, Antiochos B, et al. nm1054: a spontaneous, recessive, hypochromic, microcytic anemia mutation in the mouse. Blood. 2005;106:3625–31.
86. Ohgami RS, Campagna DR, Greer EL, et al. Identification of a ferric reductase required for efficient transferrin-dependent iron uptake in erythroid cells. Nat Genet. 2005;37:1264–9.
87. Ohgami RS, Campagna DR, McDonald A, Fleming MD. The Steap proteins are metalloreductases. Blood. 2006;108:1388–94.
88. Bernstein SE. Hereditary hypotransferrinemia with hemosiderosis, a murine disorder resembling human atransferrinemia. J Lab Clin Med. 1987;110:690–705.
89. Trenor 3rd CC, Campagna DR, Sellers VM, Andrews NC, Fleming MD. The molecular defect in hypotransferrinemic mice. Blood. 2000;96:1113–8.
90. Roy CN, Weinstein DA, Andrews NC. 2002 E. Mead Johnson Award for Research in Pediatrics Lecture: the molecular biology of the anemia of chronic disease: a hypothesis. Pediatr Res. 2003;53:507–12.
91. Levy JE, Jin O, Fujiwara Y, Kuo F, Andrews NC. Transferrin receptor is necessary for development of erythrocytes and the nervous system. Nat Genet. 1999;21:396–9.
92. de Sousa M, Reimao R, Lacerda R, Hugo P, Kaufmann SH, Porto G. Iron overload in beta 2-microglobulin-deficient mice. Immunol Lett. 1994;39:105–11.

93. Rothenberg BE, Voland JR. beta2 knockout mice develop parenchymal iron overload: a putative role for class I genes of the major histocompatibility complex in iron metabolism. Proc Natl Acad Sci USA. 1996;93:1529–34.
94. Muckenthaler MU, Rodrigues P, Macedo MG, et al. Molecular analysis of iron overload in beta2-microglobulin-deficient mice. Blood Cells Mol Dis. 2004;33:125–31.
95. Waheed A, Parkkila S, Zhou XY, et al. Hereditary hemochromatosis: effects of C282Y and H63D mutations on association with beta2-microglobulin, intracellular processing, and cell surface expression of the HFE protein in COS-7 cells. Proc Natl Acad Sci USA. 1997;94:12384–9.
96. Harris ZL, Takahashi Y, Miyajima H, Serizawa M, MacGillivray RT, Gitlin JD. Aceruloplasminemia: molecular characterization of this disorder of iron metabolism. Proc Natl Acad Sci USA. 1995;92:2539–43.
97. Harris ZL, Durley AP, Man TK, Gitlin JD. Targeted gene disruption reveals an essential role for ceruloplasmin in cellular iron efflux. Proc Natl Acad Sci USA. 1999;96:10812–7.
98. De Domenico I, Ward DM, di Patti MC, et al. Ferroxidase activity is required for the stability of cell surface ferroportin in cells expressing GPI-ceruloplasmin. EMBO J. 2007;26:2823–31.
99. Texel SJ, Xu X, Harris ZL. Ceruloplasmin in neurodegenerative diseases. Biochem Soc Trans. 2008;36:1277–81.
100. Hahn P, Qian Y, Dentchev T, et al. Disruption of ceruloplasmin and hephaestin in mice causes retinal iron overload and retinal degeneration with features of age-related macular degeneration. Proc Natl Acad Sci USA. 2004;101:13850–5.
101. Patel BN, Dunn RJ, Jeong SY, Zhu Q, Julien JP, David S. Ceruloplasmin regulates iron levels in the CNS and prevents free radical injury. J Neurosci. 2002;22:6578–86.
102. Jeong SY, David S. Age-related changes in iron homeostasis and cell death in the cerebellum of ceruloplasmin-deficient mice. J Neurosci. 2006;26:9810–9.
103. Hadziahmetovic M, Dentchev T, Song Y, et al. Ceruloplasmin/hephaestin knockout mice model morphologic and molecular features of AMD. Invest Ophthalmol Vis Sci. 2008;49:2728–36.
104. Ferreira C, Bucchini D, Martin ME, et al. Early embryonic lethality of H ferritin gene deletion in mice. J Biol Chem. 2000;275:3021–4.
105. Thompson K, Menzies S, Muckenthaler M, et al. Mouse brains deficient in H-ferritin have normal iron concentration but a protein profile of iron deficiency and increased evidence of oxidative stress. J Neurosci Res. 2003;71:46–63.
106. Marro S, Barisani D, Chiabrando D, et al. Lack of haptoglobin affects iron transport across duodenum by modulating ferroportin expression. Gastroenterology. 2007;133:1261–71.
107. Tolosano E, Fagoonee S, Garuti C, et al. Haptoglobin modifies the hemochromatosis phenotype in mice. Blood. 2005;105:3353–5.
108. Tolosano E, Altruda F. Hemopexin: structure, function, and regulation. DNA Cell Biol. 2002;21:297–306.
109. Morello N, Tonoli E, Logrand F, et al. Haemopexin affects iron distribution and ferritin expression in mouse brain. J Cell Mol Med. 2009;13:4192–204.
110. Tolosano E, Hirsch E, Patrucco E, et al. Defective recovery and severe renal damage after acute hemolysis in hemopexin-deficient mice. Blood. 1999;94:3906–14.
111. Vinchi F, Gastaldi S, Silengo L, Altruda F, Tolosano E. Hemopexin prevents endothelial damage and liver congestion in a mouse model of heme overload. Am J Pathol. 2008;173:289–99.
112. Galy B, Ferring-Appel D, Kaden S, Grone HJ, Hentze MW. Iron regulatory proteins are essential for intestinal function and control key iron absorption molecules in the duodenum. Cell Metab. 2008;7:79–85.
113. Smith SR, Ghosh MC, Ollivierre-Wilson H, Hang Tong W, Rouault TA. Complete loss of iron regulatory proteins 1 and 2 prevents viability of murine zygotes beyond the blastocyst stage of embryonic development. Blood Cells Mol Dis. 2006;36:283–7.
114. Meyron-Holtz EG, Ghosh MC, Iwai K, et al. Genetic ablations of iron regulatory proteins 1 and 2 reveal why iron regulatory protein 2 dominates iron homeostasis. EMBO J. 2004;23:386–95.
115. Galy B, Ferring D, Hentze MW. Generation of conditional alleles of the murine Iron Regulatory Protein (IRP)-1 and -2 genes. Genesis. 2005;43:181–8.
116. Cooperman SS, Meyron-Holtz EG, Olivierre-Wilson H, Ghosh MC, McConnell JP, Rouault TA. Microcytic anemia, erythropoietic protoporphyria, and neurodegeneration in mice with targeted deletion of iron-regulatory protein 2. Blood. 2005;106:1084–91.
117. Galy B, Ferring D, Minana B, et al. Altered body iron distribution and microcytosis in mice deficient in iron regulatory protein 2 (IRP2). Blood. 2005;106:2580–9.
118. LaVaute T, Smith S, Cooperman S, et al. Targeted deletion of the gene encoding iron regulatory protein-2 causes misregulation of iron metabolism and neurodegenerative disease in mice. Nat Genet. 2001;27:209–14.
119. Galy B, Holter SM, Klopstock T, et al. Iron homeostasis in the brain: complete iron regulatory protein 2 deficiency without symptomatic neurodegeneration in the mouse. Nat Genet. 2006;38:967–9.
120. Yachie A, Niida Y, Wada T, et al. Oxidative stress causes enhanced endothelial cell injury in human heme oxygenase-1 deficiency. J Clin Invest. 1999;103:129–35.

121. Poss KD, Tonegawa S. Heme oxygenase 1 is required for mammalian iron reutilization. Proc Natl Acad Sci USA. 1997;94:10919–24.
122. Quigley JG, Yang Z, Worthington MT, et al. Identification of a human heme exporter that is essential for erythropoiesis. Cell. 2004;118:757–66.
123. Keel SB, Doty RT, Yang Z, et al. A heme export protein is required for red blood cell differentiation and iron homeostasis. Science. 2008;319:825–8.
124. McKie AT. The role of Dcytb in iron metabolism: an update. Biochem Soc Trans. 2008;36:1239–41.
125. Gunshin H, Starr CN, Direnzo C, et al. Cybrd1 (duodenal cytochrome b) is not necessary for dietary iron absorption in mice. Blood. 2005;106:2879–83.
126. Sheftel AD, Richardson DR, Prchal J, Ponka P. Mitochondrial iron metabolism and sideroblastic anemia. Acta Haematol. 2009;122:120–33.
127. Camaschella C. Recent advances in the understanding of inherited sideroblastic anaemia. Br J Haematol. 2008;143:27–38.
128. Yamamoto M, Nakajima O. Animal models for X-linked sideroblastic anemia. Int J Hematol. 2000;72:157–64.
129. Nakajima O, Okano S, Harada H, et al. Transgenic rescue of erythroid 5-aminolevulinate synthase-deficient mice results in the formation of ring sideroblasts and siderocytes. Genes Cells. 2006;11:685–700.
130. Allikmets R, Raskind WH, Hutchinson A, Schueck ND, Dean M, Koeller DM. Mutation of a putative mitochondrial iron transporter gene (ABC7) in X-linked sideroblastic anemia and ataxia (XLSA/A). Hum Mol Genet. 1999;8:743–9.
131. Pondarre C, Antiochos BB, Campagna DR, et al. The mitochondrial ATP-binding cassette transporter Abcb7 is essential in mice and participates in cytosolic iron-sulfur cluster biogenesis. Hum Mol Genet. 2006;15:953–64.
132. Pondarre C, Campagna DR, Antiochos B, Sikorski L, Mulhern H, Fleming MD. Abcb7, the gene responsible for X-linked sideroblastic anemia with ataxia, is essential for hematopoiesis. Blood. 2007;109:3567–9.
133. Magness ST, Maeda N, Brenner DA. An exon 10 deletion in the mouse ferrochelatase gene has a dominant-negative effect and causes mild protoporphyria. Blood. 2002;100:1470–7.
134. Holme SA, Worwood M, Anstey AV, Elder GH, Badminton MN. Erythropoiesis and iron metabolism in dominant erythropoietic protoporphyria. Blood. 2007;110:4108–10.
135. Lyoumi S, Abitbol M, Andrieu V, et al. Increased plasma transferrin, altered body iron distribution, and microcytic hypochromic anemia in ferrochelatase-deficient mice. Blood. 2007;109:811–8.
136. Puccio H, Simon D, Cossee M, et al. Mouse models for Friedreich ataxia exhibit cardiomyopathy, sensory nerve defect and Fe-S enzyme deficiency followed by intramitochondrial iron deposits. Nat Genet. 2001;27:181–6.
137. Miranda CJ, Santos MM, Ohshima K, et al. Frataxin knockin mouse. FEBS Lett. 2002;512:291–7.
138. Al-Mahdawi S, Pinto RM, Varshney D, et al. GAA repeat expansion mutation mouse models of Friedreich ataxia exhibit oxidative stress leading to progressive neuronal and cardiac pathology. Genomics. 2006;88:580–90.
139. Shaw GC, Cope JJ, Li L, et al. Mitoferrin is essential for erythroid iron assimilation. Nature. 2006;440:96–100.
140. Paradkar PN, Zumbrennen KB, Paw BH, Ward DM, Kaplan J. Regulation of mitochondrial iron import through differential turnover of mitoferrin 1 and mitoferrin 2. Mol Cell Biol. 2009;29:1007–16.
141. Chen W, Paradkar PN, Li L, et al. Abcb10 physically interacts with mitoferrin-1 (Slc25a37) to enhance its stability and function in the erythroid mitochondria. Proc Natl Acad Sci USA. 2009;106:16263–8.
142. Le Y, Sauer B. Conditional gene knockout using cre recombinase. Methods Mol Biol. 2000;136:477–85.
143. Nagy A. Cre recombinase: the universal reagent for genome tailoring. Genesis. 2000;26:99–109.
144. Vujic Spasic M, Kiss J, Herrmann T, et al. Hfe acts in hepatocytes to prevent hemochromatosis. Cell Metab. 2008;7:173–8.
145. Carlson ES, Tkac I, Magid R, et al. Iron is essential for neuron development and memory function in mouse hippocampus. J Nutr. 2009;139:672–9.
146. Ferring-Appel D, Hentze MW, Galy B. Cell-autonomous and systemic context-dependent functions of iron regulatory protein 2 in mammalian iron metabolism. Blood. 2009;113:679–87.
147. Lutter CK. Iron deficiency in young children in low-income countries and new approaches for its prevention. J Nutr. 2008;138:2523–8.
148. Borgna-Pignatti C, Marsella M. Iron deficiency in infancy and childhood. Pediatr Ann. 2008;37:329–37.
149. Lozoff B, Georgieff MK. Iron deficiency and brain development. Semin Pediatr Neurol. 2006;13:158–65.
150. Beard J. Recent evidence from human and animal studies regarding iron status and infant development. J Nutr. 2007;137:524S–30S.
151. Lozoff B. Iron deficiency and child development. Food Nutr Bull. 2007;28:S560–71.
152. Bacon BR, Tavill AS, Brittenham GM, Park CH, Recknagel RO. Hepatic lipid peroxidation in vivo in rats with chronic iron overload. J Clin Invest. 1983;71:429–39.

153. Fletcher LM, Roberts FD, Irving MG, Powell LW, Halliday JW. Effects of iron loading on free radical scavenging enzymes and lipid peroxidation in rat liver. Gastroenterology. 1989;97:1011–8.
154. Britton RS, Bacon BR. Role of free radicals in liver diseases and hepatic fibrosis. Hepatogastroenterology. 1994;41:343–8.
155. Britton RS. Metal-induced hepatotoxicity. Semin Liver Dis. 1996;16:3–12.
156. Pietrangelo A. Mechanism of iron toxicity. Adv Exp Med Biol. 2002;509:19–43.
157. Hershko C, Link G, Cabantchik I. Pathophysiology of iron overload. Ann N Y Acad Sci. 1998;850:191–201.
158. Oudit GY, Trivieri MG, Khaper N, Liu PP, Backx PH. Role of L-type Ca2+ channels in iron transport and iron-overload cardiomyopathy. J Mol Med. 2006;84:349–64.
159. Oudit GY, Sun H, Trivieri MG, et al. L-type Ca2+ channels provide a major pathway for iron entry into cardiomyocytes in iron-overload cardiomyopathy. Nat Med. 2003;9:1187–94.
160. Vujic Spasic M, Kiss J, Herrmann T, et al. Physiologic systemic iron metabolism in mice deficient for duodenal Hfe. Blood. 2007;109:4511–7.
161. Thierbach R, Schulz TJ, Isken F, et al. Targeted disruption of hepatic frataxin expression causes impaired mitochondrial function, decreased life span and tumor growth in mice. Hum Mol Genet. 2005;14:3857–64.

Chapter 30
Yeast Iron Metabolism

Caroline C. Philpott

Keywords Copper • Hem • Iron • Iron–sulfur cluster • Siderophore • Transport • Yeast

1 Introduction

The budding yeast *Saccharomyces cerevisiae* has served as a model eukaryote for the study of basic cellular processes common to all eukaryotic cells, including the uptake and utilization of transition metals, such as iron. Proteins found in higher or multicellular eukaryotes usually are functionally similar to the orthologous proteins in yeast and can frequently be substituted for the yeast protein without deleterious effects on the yeast cell. This functional similarity coupled with the genetic tractability of yeast have allowed researchers studying human proteins of iron metabolism to quickly focus their efforts based on the known functions of the yeast ortholog.

There are, of course, limitations to the use of yeast as a model organism for the study of human iron metabolism. The most obvious difference is that, as a single-celled organism, yeast has not developed systems for the communication of iron balance or the delivery of iron compounds between cells. Other differences are more subtle. Fungi acquire iron directly from the environment and have evolved strategies for the solubilization of iron that is largely present as insoluble colloidal aggregates of ferric oxyhydroxides. Humans acquire dietary iron from plant and animal sources and thus may bypass the solubilization steps required to make iron bioavailable. In the extracellular milieu of yeast, soluble iron is found in a variety of chemical forms, and the uptake systems of yeast reflect this variety. Yeast does not express ferritins and stores excess cellular iron within the vacuole, a membrane-bound organelle similar to the mammalian lysosome. Yeast largely relies on transcriptional systems to regulate the uptake and utilization of iron. In contrast, mammalian cells largely rely on translational or posttranslational regulatory systems for cellular iron homeostasis.

This chapter will summarize the molecular biology of iron uptake and utilization in *S. cerevisiae*. Where possible, similarities between yeast and humans will be discussed.

C.C. Philpott, M.D. (✉)
Genetics and Metabolism Section, Liver Diseases Branch, NIDDK, NIH, National Institute of Diabetes and Digestive and Kidney Diseases, National Institutes of Health, Bethesda, MD, USA
e-mail: carolinep@intra.niddk.nih.gov

G.J. Anderson and G. McLaren (eds.), *Iron Physiology and Pathophysiology in Humans*, Nutrition and Health, DOI 10.1007/978-1-60327-485-2_30,

2 Iron Uptake at the Cell Surface

Most of the proteins involved in the uptake of iron in yeast are homeostatically regulated; that is, they are expressed at high levels when cellular iron levels are low and they are expressed at low levels when cellular iron levels are high. Examination of the set of proteins that are homeostatically regulated by iron reveals the major strategies that yeast cells employ to maintain iron balance. When cellular iron levels fall, yeast responds by (1) activating systems of iron uptake, (2) mobilizing intracellular stores of iron, and (3) adjusting cellular metabolism to optimize the use of iron. The genes that are activated by intracellular iron depletion are presented in Table 30.1 and Fig. 30.1 [1–4].

S. cerevisiae takes up iron in the form of ferric and ferrous salts, low-affinity ferric chelates (such as ferric citrate), and high-affinity ferric chelates (such as ferric siderophores). Siderophores are a heterogeneous group of low-molecular-weight organic compounds that bind ferric iron with extremely high affinity and specificity. These molecules are synthesized and secreted in their iron-free form by many species of bacteria and fungi, and graminaceous plants. After secretion, siderophores can bind and solubilize ferric iron, thereby making it available to cellular uptake systems [5].

Table 30.1 Aft1p/Aft2p target genes and their subcellular location and function

ORF name	Gene name	Location	Function
Uptake of iron at the cell surface			
YDR534C	FIT1	Cell wall	Siderophore binding/uptake
YOR382W	FIT2	Cell wall	Siderophore binding/uptake
YOR383C	FIT3	Cell wall	Siderophore binding/uptake
YLR214W	FRE1	Plasma membrane	Metalloreductase
YKL220C	FRE2	Plasma membrane	Metalloreductase
YOR381W	FRE3	Plasma membrane	Siderophore reductase
YNR060W	FRE4	?	? reductase
YOR384W	FRE5	?	? reductase
YMR058W	FET3	Plasma membrane	Multicopper oxidase, Fe(II) uptake
YER145C	FTR1	Plasma membrane	Permease, Fe(II) uptake
YNL259C	ATX1	Cytosol	Cu chaperone, deliver Cu to Ccc2p
YDR270W	CCC2	Post-Golgi vesicle	Cu transport into vesicles
YHL040C	ARN1	Endosome, plasma membrane	Ferrichrome transport
YHL047C	ARN2/TAF1	?	TAFC transport
YEL065W	ARN3/SIT1	Endosome, plasma membrane	Hydroxamate siderophore transport
YOL158C	ARN4/ENB1	Plasma membrane	Enterobactin transport
Efflux of iron from vacuole to cytosol			
YLL051C	FRE6	Vacuole	Metalloreductase
YLR034C	SMF3[a]	Vacuole	Fe(II) transport
YFL041W	FET5	Vacuole	Multicopper oxidase, Fe(II) transport
YBR207W	FTH1	Vacuole	Permease, Fe(II) transport
Other transporters			
YGR065C	VHT1	Plasma membrane	Biotin transporter
YOR316C	COT1	Vacuole	Zn, Co storage/detoxification
YKR052C	MRS4[a]	Mitochondria	Mitochondrial iron import
Metabolic adaptation to low iron			
YLR205C	HMX1	Endoplasmic reticulum	Heme oxygenase
YLR136C	CTH2/TIS11	Cytosol	mRNA degradation

[a] Predominately regulated by Aft2p. All others predominately regulated by Aft1p. Reproduced with permission from [77]

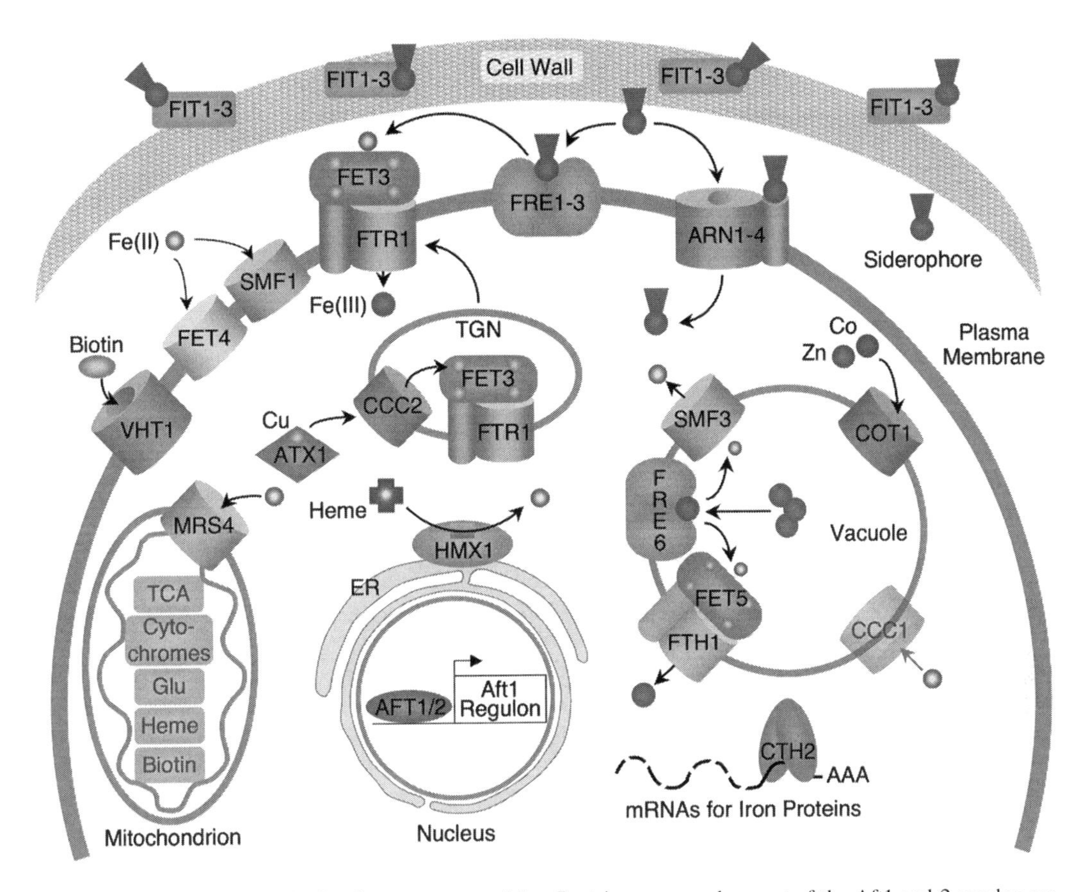

Fig. 30.1 Iron homeostasis in *Saccharomyces cerevisiae*. Proteins expressed as part of the Aft1 and 2 regulon are labeled in *black text*. The low affinity iron transporters Smf1 and Fet4 are also shown. Genes that are downregulated during iron deficiency are indicated in *gray text*. Modified and reproduced with permission from [77]

S. cerevisiae is somewhat unusual in that it does not synthesize siderophores, but, similar to most fungi, it can take up iron bound to a variety of these iron chelates [6]. More than half of the genes that are activated during intracellular iron depletion are involved directly or indirectly with the uptake of siderophore-bound iron. Clearly, these systems allow *S. cerevisiae* to compete with other organisms for available environmental iron.

2.1 Siderophores and the Cell Wall

Before iron compounds can reach the plasma membrane of yeast, they must first pass through the cell wall. The cell wall of yeast is a rigid structure consisting of layers of interlinked ß-1,3 glucan, ß-1,6 glucan, chitin and mannoproteins [7]. The cell wall is a highly dynamic, porous structure, but the passage of higher molecular weight molecules is restricted. As cellular iron levels fall, yeast expresses a family of three GPI-linked cell wall mannoproteins called Fit1, 2, and 3 [8]. The *FIT* genes are the most strongly induced of all the genes expressed during cellular iron depletion, but their exact function is unclear. Expression of the *FIT* proteins enhances the retention of ferrichrome, a hydroxamate siderophore, in the cell wall and enhances the uptake of ferrichrome and ferrioxamine B at the cell surface. The *FIT* proteins may function by increasing the permeability of the cell wall to siderophores or by enhancing their retention in the periplasmic space.

2.2 The Reductive System of Iron Uptake

Iron compounds that reach the cell surface can become substrates for two genetically separate systems of iron uptake, the reductive and the nonreductive systems. In the reductive system, the ferric substrate is reduced at the cell surface prior to uptake of the free ferrous iron ion. This reduction step is carried out by a family of broad-specificity metalloreductases, the *FRE* family. *FRE1* and *FRE2* encode the majority of the cell surface reductase activity and are strongly induced by cellular iron depletion, or, in the case of *FRE1*, copper depletion [9–15]. The *FRE* reductases are polytopic integral membrane proteins with binding sites for heme, FAD, and NADPH, and Fre1 has been shown to bind heme as a b-type flavocytochrome [16]. Fre1 and Fre2 can catalyze the reduction of oxidized forms of iron and copper, as well as a variety of one-electron acceptors. Although they were initially characterized as ferric citrate reductases, Fre1 and Fre2 can also reduce the ferric iron in siderophore chelates, such as ferric enterobactin, ferrichrome, and ferrioxamine B [17]. Because the siderophores only bind ferric iron with high affinity and bind ferrous iron with much lower affinity, this reduction of the bound ferric iron to the ferrous form leads to the dissociation of the ferrous iron from the siderophore, making the ferrous iron available to ferrous-specific transporters. Additional paralogs of the *FRE* family are expressed during cellular iron depletion [18], and two of these, Fre3 and Fre4, exhibit the capacity to reduce ferric hydroxamate siderophores. The *FRE* family of reductases exhibits sequence conservation with the STEAP family of proteins found in mammals. Recent studies have shown that Steap3 is also a ferric reductase that is required for transferrin-dependent iron uptake in erythroid cells [19]. Steap2, 3, and 4 are both ferric and cupric reductases and are predicted to require flavin, heme, and NADPH cofactors [20].

Uptake of reduced iron at the cell surface occurs through both high-affinity and low-affinity transporters. The high-affinity ferrous iron transport complex is strongly induced during iron depletion and is composed of a copper-dependent oxidase encoded by *FET3* [21] and a permease encoded by *FTR1* [22]. Ferrous iron is the only known substrate for this complex, and the iron must be oxidized prior to uptake in a reaction that requires copper metallation of Fet3 and the consumption of oxygen [23–26]. The ferric iron is then delivered to the cytosol by the Ftr1 permease. The advantage gained by this curious coupling of oxidation and transport is not clear, but this mechanism may contribute to the high affinity of the complex or to its specificity for ferrous ions. Copper insertion into Fet3 occurs intracellularly in the lumen of the late secretory pathway [27], and two proteins required for this process are the copper ATPase Ccc2 [28] and the cytosolic copper chaperone Atx1 [29]. Atx1 binds cytosolic copper and delivers it to a methionine-rich domain of Ccc2, which then pumps the copper into the post-Golgi vesicle. Both *ATX1* and *CCC2* are transcriptionally regulated by iron rather than by copper, supporting their primary role in iron rather than copper homeostasis.

Cells containing adequate levels of intracellular iron transcriptionally downregulate the high-affinity ferrous iron uptake complex, and uptake of iron under these conditions occurs through low-affinity transporters with broader transition metal specificity. Yeast expresses three members of the Nramp family of divalent metal transporters, called Smf1, 2, and 3 [30]. Smf1 is primarily a plasma membrane transporter of manganese, but it can also transport iron and cobalt, and yeast overexpressing Smf1 accumulates higher levels of intracellular iron [31]. A second low-affinity transporter of broad metal ion specificity is encoded by *FET4*. Fet4 exhibits transport activity for ferrous iron, zinc, copper, and cadmium [32–34]. This transporter is strongly induced under conditions of reduced oxygen tension and may constitute the major source of iron transport activity during hypoxic or anaerobic growth, when the oxygen-dependent Fet3/Ftr1 complex is inactive [26, 35].

Although the reductive iron uptake system of yeast is not precisely duplicated in human cells, several orthologous proteins are involved in human iron transport. Members of the yeast SMF family of divalent metal transporters are homologous to the major ferrous iron transporter of humans, DMT1 [36]. Transporters of this family are present in most eukaryotes and primarily function in the

Table 30.2 Siderophore substrates of ARN/SIT family of transporters

Transporter	Siderophore substrate	K_t (μM)
Arn1p	Ferrichromes[a]	0.9
Arn2p/Taf1p	Triacetylfusarinine C	1.6
Arn3p/Sit1p	Ferrioxamine B	0.5
	Ferrichromes[a]	2.3
Arn4p/Enb1p	Enterobactin	1.9

[a]Ferrichromes include ferrichrome, ferrichrome A, ferricrocin, ferrichrycin, ferrirhodin, and ferrirubin. Some strain-specific variation in the specificity of Arn1 and Arn3 for different ferrichromes has been reported. Reproduced with permission from [77]

uptake of either manganese or iron (and sometimes both). Although humans are not known to express a transport complex similar to Fet3/Ftr1, multicopper oxidases homologous to Fet3 have a clear role in iron homeostasis. Ceruloplasmin is a multicopper oxidase found in human serum and on the surface of glial cells and appears to be required for cellular iron efflux, rather than uptake, as is the case with Fet3 [37]. Hephaestin, another membrane-bound multicopper oxidase, is involved in the efflux of iron from the basolateral surface of the enterocyte [38]. For both ceruloplasmin and hephaestin, recent evidence suggests that their role in cellular iron efflux occurs through an interaction with ferroportin, the mammalian ferrous iron efflux pump [39]. The ferroxidase activity is required to transfer the ferrous iron from ferroportin to the circulating ferric iron carrier transferrin. Human orthologs of Atx1 and Ccc2 share activities similar to the yeast proteins, that is, binding and transporting copper [40, 41]. However, the primary role of the human copper-transporting ATPases is not in iron homeostasis, but in copper efflux. Mutations in ATP7A and ATP7B lead to Menkes and Wilson diseases, respectively. In the case of Menkes disease, defects in ATP7A result in poor absorption of dietary copper and deficiencies of copper-dependent enzymes, while in the case of Wilson disease, mutations in ATP7B result in cellular copper overload, especially in the liver.

2.3 *Nonreductive Uptake of Iron*

The nonreductive iron uptake system of yeast is specific for siderophore–iron chelates. Under conditions of iron depletion, *S. cerevisiae* expresses a family of four homologous transporters of the ARN/SIT subfamily of the major facilitator superfamily [42]. These transporters are unique to fungi, are predicted to have 14 membrane-spanning domains, and are likely energized by proton symport. Each of these transporters exhibits specificity for a group of fungal and/or bacterial siderophores (Table 30.2). Siderophores can be broadly grouped into two classes based on the moieties that coordinate the iron. Fungi generally produce hydroxamate-type siderophores, such as ferrichromes, while gram-negative bacteria produce catecholate-type siderophores, such as enterobactin. Arn1, 2, and 3 transport a variety of trihydroxamate siderophores, while Arn4 transports only catecholate siderophore [43–49]. The siderophore substrates for an individual transporter can be structurally heterogeneous. For example, Arn3/Sit1 transports several types of ferrichromes, which are cyclic, peptide-linked trihydroxamates, as well as ferrioxamine B, which is a linear, peptide-linked trihydroxamate that is about half the size of ferrichrome. Siderophores that lack bound iron do not compete with ferric siderophores for uptake and thus are not substrates for the transporters [50]. This substrate diversity and specificity for the iron-bound form suggest that the ARN transporter primarily recognizes the hexadentate iron coordination site of the siderophore and that the remaining side chains have lesser influence on substrate recognition.

Two members of the ARN/SIT transporter family exhibit posttranslational regulation through their localization in the late secretory pathway. While Arn4 traffics directly to the plasma membrane after synthesis, the ferrichrome transporters, Arn1 and Arn3, are sorted directly from the trans-Golgi network (TGN) to the vacuole for degradation when their respective siderophore substrates are not present in the extracellular medium [51, 52]. Arn1 is recognized at the TGN by Gga2, a clathrin adaptor protein that directs cargo to the endosomal pathway [53]. In the late endosome, Arn1 is ubiquitinated by Rsp5, which allows Arn1 to be captured by the multivesicular body for delivery to the vacuolar lumen. Thus, in the absence of ferrichrome, Arn1 is never expressed on the cell surface and is degraded with a half-life of approximately 10 min. In the presence of siderophore substrates, however, Arn1 and Arn3 are captured at the TGN and diverted to the plasma membrane. In the case of Arn1, this is triggered by the binding of ferrichrome to a high-affinity receptor site on the extracytosolic face of the transporter, and ferrichrome is thought to gain access to intracellular Arn1 through fluid-phase endocytosis [54]. Uptake of siderophore substrates at the plasma membrane is accompanied by the endocytic cycling of Arn1 and Arn3, which also requires ubiquitination by Rsp5. The purpose of this intracellular trafficking is not clear, but this may have evolved to protect the cell from potentially toxic small molecules that could also be transported nonspecifically by Arn1 and Arn3. Degradation of the transporters in the absence of their siderophore substrates could ensure that yeast cells do not inadvertently take up toxic compounds masquerading as siderophores.

Siderophore transporters of the ARN/SIT family are not present in the genomes of higher eukaryotes, but the regulated intracellular trafficking of these transporters is similar in some ways to the regulation of ferroportin, the basolateral iron efflux pump of mammals. Ferroportin activity is regulated by hepcidin, a peptide hormone that controls iron homeostasis in mammals. Hepcidin binds to a receptor domain on the extracellular face of ferroportin, which triggers the endocytosis and eventual degradation of the transporter [55].

Humans are not known to utilize siderophores as nutritional sources of iron, although these are certainly secreted by the intestinal flora of humans. Humans do, however, express siderophore-binding proteins, called lipocalins or siderocalins, that appear to function primarily in innate immunity by withholding iron–siderophore complexes from microbial pathogens [56–58]. Additional evidence suggests that the siderophore-binding proteins have a role in human physiology beyond their role in innate immunity, and this role may involve binding an endogenously produced siderophore-like ligand. Two reports indicate that catechol-like molecules serve as iron ligands both within cells and in the systemic circulation, enabling the iron:catechol complex to be bound by siderocalin [59, 60].

2.4 Heme Iron Uptake

S. cerevisiae differs from pathogenic yeast, such as *Candida albicans*, in that it does not use heme as a nutritional source of iron. Under conditions of cellular iron depletion, *S. cerevisiae* does not take up significant quantities of heme iron [61, 62]. This yeast does have the capacity to take up heme iron, however, and heme transport is activated under conditions of heme deficiency [63]. Heme deficiency occurs naturally during periods of hypoxic growth, as heme synthesis is highly dependent on molecular oxygen. Laboratory strains of yeast with defects in heme biosynthesis have been engineered, and these strains also exhibit inducible heme uptake. No high-affinity transporters for heme have been identified in any fungal species, and indirect evidence suggests that heme uptake may be a genetically complex trait in this species. Pug1, a transporter with limited capacity for the efflux of heme and the uptake of protoporphyrin IX, has been identified in yeast, but this protein bears no homology with the heme efflux pump of mammals, FLVCR [64].

3 Iron Storage

Yeast stores excess iron in the vacuole, and although the molecular form of the iron is unknown, the vacuole also contains amino acids and polyphosphate that could potentially interact with iron to maintain its solubility. When yeasts are grown in media containing high concentrations of iron, vacuoles accumulate iron through the activity of Ccc1, a transporter specific for iron and manganese located on the vacuolar membrane [65, 66]. Yeast lacking *CCC1* exhibits sensitivity to high concentrations of iron, indicating that sequestration of iron in the vacuole is important for detoxification of the metal. *CCC1* is transcriptionally activated under iron-replete conditions by the transcription factor Yap5 [67]. Yap5 is a member of a family of yeast transcription factors with similarity to mammalian AP-1. Other members of this family respond to oxidative stress and cadmium, while Yap5 appears to be the only family member that responds to excess iron.

3.1 Mobilization of Iron Stores

Yeast can grow for several generations in iron-free medium, indicating that iron stored within the cell can be mobilized for use in iron-dependent processes. Growth in iron-poor medium activates the expression of several genes involved in vacuolar iron mobilization, and these genes essentially duplicate the reductive transport system found on the plasma membrane. Fre6, a member of the *FRE* family of metalloreductases, is activated during iron depletion and is expressed exclusively on the vacuolar membrane [68, 69]. Fre6 activity is required for the reduction of vacuolar iron prior to its export from the organelle to the cytosol. Fet5 and Fth1 are paralogs of the high-affinity plasma membrane ferrous iron transport complex, Fet3 and Ftr1, and are also expressed as a complex on the vacuolar membrane [70]. Smf3 is a paralog of Smf1 and 2 and is also found exclusively on the vacuolar membrane [69]. Together, Fet5/Fth1 and Smf3 can transport ferrous iron produced by the reductase activity of Fre6, mobilizing the iron from the vacuole to the cytosol. The requirement of Fre6 in this process suggests that the majority of the iron stored in the vacuole is in the ferric form.

The vacuole is a site of storage for metal ions other than iron, such as zinc, copper, manganese, and cobalt. Yeast cells grown in iron-poor medium exhibit greater sensitivity to the toxic effects of these other metals than yeast grown in iron-rich medium. Cells grown in iron-poor medium also induce the expression of Cot1, a vacuolar transporter primarily involved in the vacuolar accumulation of zinc and cobalt [71, 72]. Expression of Cot1 during iron deficiency is thought to protect cells by sequestering these metals in the lumen of the vacuole [73].

Although the vacuole appears to be the primary site of iron storage in yeast, substantial quantities of iron are present in the mitochondria. Mitochondria are the sites of heme biosynthesis and iron–sulfur cluster assembly as well as the location of the respiratory enzymes, which are rich in heme and iron–sulfur clusters. Although no evidence exists for the mobilization of iron from mitochondria during growth in iron-poor medium, heme and iron–sulfur proteins represent a large pool of cellular iron that could potentially be mobilized for other purposes during iron deficiency. Yeast cells growing on iron-poor medium induce the expression of Hmx1, the yeast heme oxygenase, and can degrade heme to liberate the iron for other metabolic purposes [74]. Heme is also an important regulatory molecule in yeast and, in conjunction with the Hap1 and Hap2/3/4/5 transcription factors, can activate the expression of a number of genes involved in aerobic growth, including the iron-rich respiratory cytochromes. Thus, expression of Hmx1 during iron deficiency also serves to degrade heme and downregulate the expression of iron-containing proteins.

3.2 *Mitochondrial Iron for the Synthesis of Heme and Iron–Sulfur Clusters*

Much of the iron taken up by the yeast cell is dedicated to the synthesis of heme and the assembly of iron–sulfur clusters (ISCs), both of which occur within mitochondria. While a detailed description of the machinery dedicated to the synthesis of these cofactors is beyond the scope of this chapter, the influence of these systems on cellular iron homeostasis will be described (see also Chap. 2). Iron can enter mitochondria through multiple mechanisms, not all of which have been identified. Mrs3 and Mrs4 encode mitochondrial carrier proteins that can transport iron into the mitochondrial matrix [75]. Mrs4 is transcriptionally activated by iron depletion, suggesting that cells attempt to maintain the import of iron into mitochondria in the face of falling intracellular iron levels. A murine ortholog of Mrs3 and 4, termed mitoferrin, is required for the insertion of iron into heme, and mutation of the zebrafish ortholog results in a profound defect in heme and ISC synthesis [76].

4 Iron and Cellular Metabolism

The nutritional requirement of yeast for iron changes according the metabolic state of the cell, and changes in iron availability can result in changes in cellular metabolism. Glucose is the preferred carbon source for *S. cerevisiae*, and this species can metabolize the products of glycolysis through either fermentation or respiration. Happily, yeast preferentially ferment glucose to ethanol, but when glucose is limiting, nonfermentable carbon sources, such as ethanol, acetate, or lactate, can be converted to carbon dioxide and water through the TCA cycle and oxidative phosphorylation. When yeasts are grown in iron-poor media, they rely exclusively on the fermentation of glucose, as cells cannot grow on iron-poor media containing only nonfermentable carbon sources [77]. Similarly, yeast lacking high-affinity iron uptake also cannot grow on nonfermentable carbon sources [78]. Presumably, this respiratory defect is due to a lack of activity of iron-dependent respiratory enzymes, but this has not been rigorously tested. Conversely, yeasts grown on nonfermentable carbon sources accumulate larger amounts of intracellular iron than do yeasts grown on glucose, and transcription of the high-affinity ferrous transport complex is increased upon a shift to respiration [79]. This increased expression requires the Snf1/Snf4 kinase complex. Iron limitation has been shown to increase the phosphorylation of Snf1 [80], which activates the expression of genes involved in glucose uptake and metabolism.

4.1 *Metabolic Alterations Controlled by Cth2/Tis11*

Several lines of evidence suggest that under conditions of iron deficiency, yeasts alter their utilization of iron by downregulating nonessential iron-requiring metabolic pathways and shifting to iron-independent metabolic pathways. Analysis of the transcriptome of yeast indicates that mRNAs encoding heme and iron–sulfur proteins are downregulated in iron-deficient cells [2, 4]. The transcripts encode proteins of the TCA cycle, respiratory cytochromes, heme and biotin biosynthetic pathways, and ISC proteins involved in the synthesis of amino acids. Many of these changes are mediated in part by the activities of RNA-binding proteins expressed during iron deficiency. Cth2 and Cth1 are members of the tristetraprolin family of RNA-binding proteins, and they recognize AU-rich elements in the 3′UTR of specific mRNA transcripts [2, 80]. Mammalian versions of these proteins are involved in the regulation of the immune response. Expression of Cth2 is greatly increased during iron deficiency, and Cth1 expression also increases slightly in milder iron deficiency.

Binding of Cth2 to mRNA transcripts leads to destabilization and degradation of the mRNA. This has been specifically shown for *SHD4* and *ACO1* mRNAs, which encode the heme-binding subunit of succinate dehydrogenase and aconitase, respectively. Thus, during iron deficiency, yeast cells synthesize a protein that downregulates the expression of many genes involved in iron utilization.

4.2 *Alteration of Biotin Acquisition*

Under conditions of iron deficiency, yeast shifts from biosynthesis of biotin to uptake of exogenous biotin from the medium [4]. *S. cerevisiae* can synthesize biotin from 7-keto, 8-amino-, and 7, 8-diamino-pelargonic acid precursors, and the ultimate step of this pathway is catalyzed by Bio2, an iron–sulfur protein [81, 82]. The biosynthetic enzymes Bio2, Bio3, and Bio4 are expressed when cells are grown in iron-rich medium, but transcription is shut off in iron deficiency. Iron deficiency also activates the transcription of *VHT1*, which encodes the plasma membrane high-affinity transporter for biotin. Thus, yeast reciprocally regulates the uptake and biosynthesis of biotin, relying exclusively on uptake when iron is low and shifting to biosynthesis when iron is high.

5 Regulators of the Iron Deficiency Response: Aft1 and 2

Yeast iron homeostasis is primarily controlled by the transcription factor Aft1 and, to a lesser extent, Aft2 (Fig. 30.2) [78, 83–85]. These transcription factors activate the set of genes that constitute the major response to iron deficiency in yeast [1, 3, 4]. No mammalian orthologs of these proteins have been identified, and they do not appear to be conserved among other fungal species. Aft1 and Aft2 recognize and bind to consensus sequences (PyPuCACCC) present in one or more copies in the upstream region of their respective target genes. Aft2 is 39% identical to Aft1 and recognizes a partially overlapping set of genes with similar consensus sequences, but the effects of Aft2 are largely unapparent unless Aft1 is deleted. An exception to this is the transcriptional activation of *SMF3* and *MRS4*, which are targets for Aft2, but not Aft1.

Aft1 is constitutively expressed in growing yeast cells, and under conditions of iron depletion, Aft1 accumulates in the nucleus, where it binds DNA and activates the transcription of the set of genes described in Table 30.1 [86]. Under conditions of iron sufficiency, Aft1 is predominately located in the cytosol, where it is inactive. Aft1 may be continuously cycling in and out of the nucleus, and some evidence suggests that iron exerts its effects at the level of nuclear export. Aft1 requires the karyopherin Pse1 for import into the nucleus and the nuclear exportin Msn5 for export to the cytosol [87, 88]. Some investigators report that Aft1 undergoes an intermolecular interaction in the presence of iron that leads to the formation of Aft1 dimers, which are exported from the nucleus.

Aft1 appears to sense the levels of intracellular iron, but whether it directly binds iron is not known. Several components of the mitochondrial iron–sulfur cluster assembly system are required for the inactivation of Aft1 in the presence of iron, leading to the hypothesis that Aft1 senses cellular iron levels in the form of a product of the ISC assembly system. Deletion of the monothiol glutaredoxin Grx5; depletion of the yeast frataxin homologue, Yfh1; or depletion of glutathione all lead to loss of both ISC assembly and iron-dependent Aft1 inactivation [89–91]. Aft1 inactivation also requires Atm1, a mitochondrial inner membrane transporter that is thought to export a product of the ISC assembly system. The components of the cytosolic ISC machinery appear not to be required for the inactivation of Aft1, as their depletion does not result in the constitutive expression of the Aft1-regulated genes. These observations suggest that Aft1 responds to changes in the levels of a product

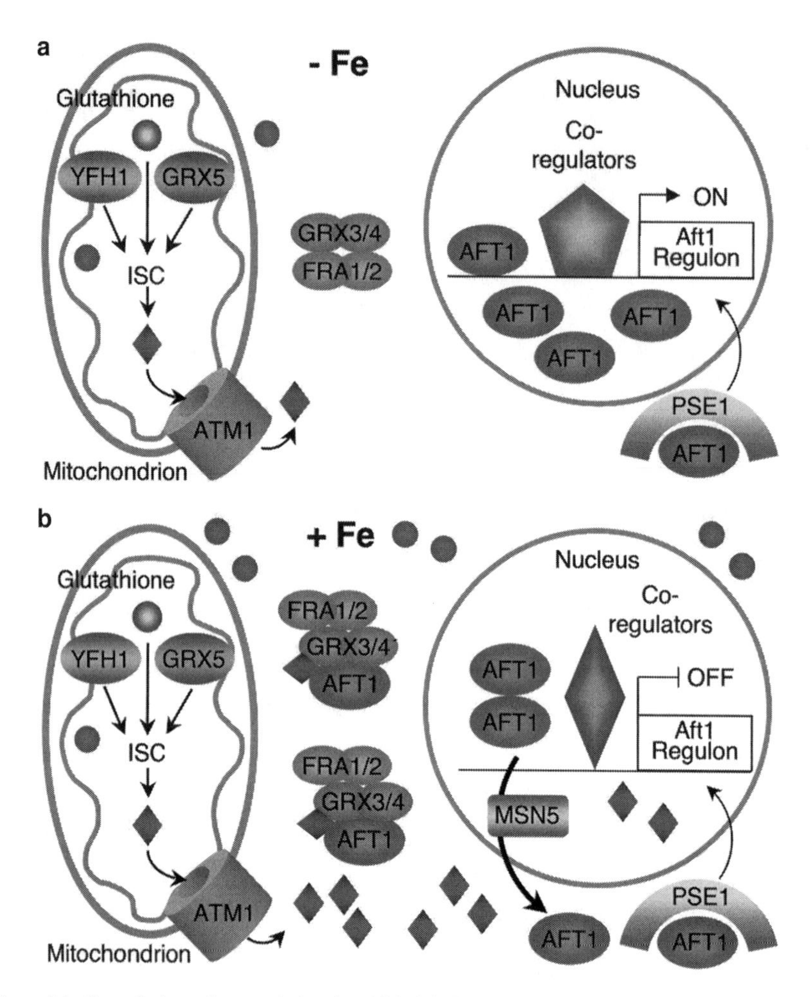

Fig. 30.2 A model of regulation of transcription by Aft1. (**a**). In cells lacking iron, production of ISCs is low. Aft1 continuously cycles between the nucleus and cytosol, and in the absence of ISCs, Aft1 accumulates in the nucleus and activates transcription. (**b**). In cells replete with iron, production of ISCs is high. ISCs bind to the Grx3/4 and Fra1/2 complex, which interacts with Aft1 to promote its retention in the cytosol. Aft1 may form a dimer in iron-replete cells. Modified and reproduced with permission from [77]

of the mitochondrial ISC assembly machinery and that the levels of this ISC product are proportional to the levels of metabolically available cellular iron.

Iron-dependent inactivation of Aft1 requires the activities of several additional proteins that directly interact with the transcription factor. Grx3 and Grx4 are monothiol glutaredoxins required for the inactivation and cytosolic accumulation of Aft1 [92, 93]. Both glutaredoxins can bind to Aft1, and a conserved cysteine residue in the glutaredoxin active site is required for both binding and inactivation. Fra1 and Fra2 are two additional proteins that are individually required for the inactivation of Aft1 [94]. Fra1 and Fra2 interact in the cytosol as a complex, and the complex can directly bind to Grx3 and Grx4. In vitro, Grx3 and Grx4 can form heterodimers with Fra2 that bind a [2Fe–2S] cluster, and the presence of the ISC may be communicated to Aft1 as it cycles through the cytosol [95]. A clearer picture of the molecular events controlling the response of Aft1 to iron must await further research.

Several coregulators of Aft1 have been identified. Heme is required for the activation of a subset of the Aft1 regulon, as some of these genes, such as Fet3, are repressed in the absence of heme [96].

This repression is mediated by the coregulators Tup1 and Hda1 [97]. Other genes in the Aft1 regulon are not repressed in the absence of heme, such as Arn1, and Cti6 is required to escape this repression [97, 98]. This regulation by heme may allow the cells to coordinate iron uptake with oxygen availability. Activation of some Aft1 target genes requires the Tup1, Ssn6, and Nhp6 coregulators, and the mediator complex has also been reported to specifically repress the Aft1 regulon [46, 99, 100].

6 Yeast as a System for Xenoprotein Expression

Much of the utility of yeast as a model system for human iron metabolism has been based on the shared functions of the endogenous yeast proteins and their human orthologs. However, yeast can also serve as a model organism for expression and functional characterization of xenoproteins, thus allowing the investigator to exploit the genetic tractability of *S. cerevisiae*. This genetic tractability was used to identify poly r(C)-binding protein (PCBP1) as a human protein that functions as an iron chaperone for the delivery of iron to ferritin [101]. Human ferritins were expressed in a yeast strain that contained an iron-sensing reporter gene, and PCBP1 was selected from a human cDNA library on the basis of its capacity to deliver iron to ferritin and thereby activate the iron-sensing reporter. The utility of the yeast system can be expanded to include the study of human proteins that confer functions that do not naturally occur in yeast but can be measured and studied. Thus, yeast may prove useful in identifying additional human genes involved in iron homeostasis.

Acknowledgments This work was supported by the Intramural Research Program of the National Institutes of Diabetes and Digestive and Kidney Diseases of the National Institutes of Health, USA.

References

1. Courel M, Lallet S, Camadro JM, Blaiseau PL. Direct activation of genes involved in intracellular iron use by the yeast iron-responsive transcription factor Aft2 without its paralog Aft1. Mol Cell Biol. 2005;25:6760–71.
2. Puig S, Askeland E, Thiele DJ. Coordinated remodeling of cellular metabolism during iron deficiency through targeted mRNA degradation. Cell. 2005;120:99–110.
3. Rutherford JC, Jaron S, Winge DR. Aft1p and Aft2p mediate iron-responsive gene expression in yeast through related promoter elements. J Biol Chem. 2003;278:27636–43.
4. Shakoury-Elizeh M, Tiedeman J, Rashford J, et al. Transcriptional remodeling in response to iron deprivation in *Saccharomyces cerevisiae*. Mol Biol Cell. 2004;15:1233–43.
5. Neilands JB. Siderophores: structure and function of microbial iron transport compounds. J Biol Chem. 1995;270:26723–6.
6. Philpott CC, Protchenko O, Kim YW, Boretsky Y, Shakoury-Elizeh M. The response to iron deprivation in *Saccharomyces cerevisiae*: expression of siderophore-based systems of iron uptake. Biochem Soc Trans. 2002;30:698–702.
7. Orlean P. Biogenesis of yeast wall and surface components. In: Pringle JR, Broach JR, Jones EW, editors. The molecular and cellular biology of the yeast saccharomyces: cell cycle and cell biology. Cold Spring Harbor: Cold Spring Harbor Laboratory Press; 1997. p. 229–362.
8. Protchenko O, Ferea T, Rashford J, et al. Three cell wall mannoproteins facilitate the uptake of iron in *Saccharomyces cerevisiae*. J Biol Chem. 2001;276:49244–50.
9. Dancis A, Klausner RD, Hinnebusch AG, Barriocanal JG. Genetic evidence that ferric reductase is required for iron uptake in Saccharomyces cerevisiae. Mol Cell Biol. 1990;10:2294–301.
10. Dancis A, Roman DG, Anderson GJ, Hinnebusch AG, Klausner RD. Ferric reductase of *Saccharomyces cerevisiae*: molecular characterization, role in iron uptake, and transcriptional control by iron. Proc Natl Acad Sci USA. 1992;89:3869–73.
11. Georgatsou E, Alexandraki D. Two distinctly regulated genes are required for ferric reduction, the first step of iron uptake in *Saccharomyces cerevisiae*. Mol Cell Biol. 1994;14:3065–73.

12. Georgatsou E, Mavrogiannis LA, Fragiadakis GS, Alexandraki D. The yeast Fre1p/Fre2p cupric reductases facilitate copper uptake and are regulated by the copper-modulated Mac1p activator. J Biol Chem. 1997;272:13786–92.
13. Hassett R, Kosman DJ. Evidence for Cu(II) reduction as a component of copper uptake by *Saccharomyces cerevisiae*. J Biol Chem. 1995;270:128–34.
14. Jungmann J, Reins HA, Lee J, et al. MAC1, a nuclear regulatory protein related to Cu-dependent transcription factors is involved in Cu/Fe utilization and stress resistance in yeast. EMBO J. 1993;12:5051–6.
15. Lesuisse E, Labbe P. Reductive iron assimilation in *Saccharomyces cerevisiae*. In: Winkelmann G, Winge DR, editors. Metal ions in fungi. New York: Marcel Dekker; 1994. p. 149–78.
16. Finegold AA, Shatwell KP, Segal AW, Klausner RD, Dancis A. Intramembrane bis-heme motif for transmembrane electron transport conserved in a yeast iron reductase and the human NADPH oxidase. J Biol Chem. 1996;271:31021–4.
17. Yun CW, Bauler M, Moore RE, Klebba PE, Philpott CC. The role of the FRE family of plasma membrane reductases in the uptake of siderophore-iron in *Saccharomyces cerevisiae*. J Biol Chem. 2001;276:10218–23.
18. Martins LJ, Jensen LT, Simon JR, Keller GL, Winge DR, Simons JR. Metalloregulation of FRE1 and FRE2 homologs in *Saccharomyces cerevisiae*. J Biol Chem. 1998;273:23716–21.
19. Ohgami RS, Campagna DR, Greer EL, et al. Identification of a ferrireductase required for efficient transferrin-dependent iron uptake in erythroid cells. Nat Genet. 2005;37:1264–9.
20. Ohgami RS, Campagna DR, McDonald A, Fleming MD. The Steap proteins are metalloreductases. Blood. 2006;108:1388–94.
21. Askwith C, Eide D, Van Ho A, et al. The FET3 gene of *S. cerevisiae* encodes a multicopper oxidase required for ferrous iron uptake. Cell. 1994;76:403–10.
22. Stearman R, Yuan DS, Yamaguchi-Iwai Y, Klausner RD, Dancis A. A permease-oxidase complex involved in high-affinity iron uptake in yeast. Science. 1996;271:1552–7.
23. de Silva D, Davis-Kaplan S, Fergestad J, Kaplan J. Purification and characterization of Fet3 protein, a yeast homologue of ceruloplasmin. J Biol Chem. 1997;272:14208–13.
24. De Silva DM, Askwith CC, Eide D, Kaplan J. The FET3 gene product required for high affinity iron transport in yeast is a cell surface ferroxidase. J Biol Chem. 1995;270:1098–101.
25. Hassett RF, Romeo AM, Kosman DJ. Regulation of high affinity iron uptake in the yeast *Saccharomyces cerevisiae*. Role of dioxygen and Fe. J Biol Chem. 1998;273:7628–36.
26. Hassett RF, Yuan DS, Kosman DJ. Spectral and kinetic properties of the Fet3 protein from *Saccharomyces cerevisiae*, a multinuclear copper ferroxidase enzyme. J Biol Chem. 1998;273:23274–82.
27. Yuan DS, Dancis A, Klausner RD. Restriction of copper export in *Saccharomyces cerevisiae* to a late Golgi or post-Golgi compartment in the secretory pathway. J Biol Chem. 1997;272:25787–93.
28. Yuan DS, Stearman R, Dancis A, Dunn T, Beeler T, Klausner RD. The Menkes/Wilson disease gene homologue in yeast provides copper to a ceruloplasmin-like oxidase required for iron uptake. Proc Natl Acad Sci USA. 1995;92:2632–6.
29. Lin SJ, Pufahl RA, Dancis A, O'Halloran TV, Culotta VC. A role for the *Saccharomyces cerevisiae* ATX1 gene in copper trafficking and iron transport. J Biol Chem. 1997;272:9215–20.
30. Culotta VC, Yang M, Hall MD. Manganese transport and trafficking: lessons learned from *Saccharomyces cerevisiae*. Eukaryot Cell. 2005;4:1159–65.
31. Cohen A, Nelson H, Nelson N. The family of SMF metal ion transporters in yeast cells. J Biol Chem. 2000;275:33388–94.
32. Dix D, Bridgham J, Broderius M, Eide D. Characterization of the FET4 protein of yeast. Evidence for a direct role in the transport of iron. J Biol Chem. 1997;272:11770–7.
33. Dix DR, Bridgham JT, Broderius MA, Byersdorfer CA, Eide DJ. The FET4 gene encodes the low affinity Fe(II) transport protein of *Saccharomyces cerevisiae*. J Biol Chem. 1994;269:26092–9.
34. Hassett R, Dix DR, Eide DJ, Kosman DJ. The Fe(II) permease Fet4p functions as a low affinity copper transporter and supports normal copper trafficking in *Saccharomyces cerevisiae*. Biochem J. 2000;351:477–84.
35. Jensen LT, Culotta VC. Regulation of *Saccharomyces cerevisiae* FET4 by oxygen and iron. J Mol Biol. 2002;318:251–60.
36. Nevo Y, Nelson N. The NRAMP family of metal-ion transporters. Biochim Biophys Acta. 2006;1763:609–20.
37. Cherukuri S, Potla R, Sarkar J, Nurko S, Harris ZL, Fox PL. Unexpected role of ceruloplasmin in intestinal iron absorption. Cell Metab. 2005;2:309–19.
38. Vulpe CD, Kuo YM, Murphy TL, et al. Hephaestin, a ceruloplasmin homologue implicated in intestinal iron transport, is defective in the sla mouse. Nat Genet. 1999;21:195–9.
39. De Domenico I, Ward DM, di Patti MC, et al. Ferroxidase activity is required for the stability of cell surface ferroportin in cells expressing GPI-ceruloplasmin. EMBO J. 2007;26:2823–31.
40. Huffman DL, O'Halloran TV. Function, structure, and mechanism of intracellular copper trafficking proteins. Annu Rev Biochem. 2001;70:677–701.

41. Lutsenko S, Barnes NL, Bartee MY, Dmitriev OY. Function and regulation of human copper-transporting ATPases. Physiol Rev. 2007;87:1011–46.
42. Philpott CC. Iron uptake in fungi: a system for every source. Biochim Biophys Acta. 2006;1763:636–45.
43. Heymann P, Ernst JF, Winkelmann G. Identification of a fungal triacetylfusarinine C siderophore transport gene (TAF1) in *Saccharomyces cerevisiae* as a member of the major facilitator superfamily. Biometals. 1999;12:301–6.
44. Heymann P, Ernst JF, Winkelmann G. A gene of the major facilitator superfamily encodes a transporter for enterobactin (Enb1p) in *Saccharomyces cerevisiae*. Biometals. 2000;13:65–72.
45. Heymann P, Ernst JF, Winkelmann G. Identification and substrate specificity of a ferrichrome-type siderophore transporter (Arn1p) in *Saccharomyces cerevisiae*. FEMS Microbiol Lett. 2000;186:221–7.
46. Lesuisse E, Blaiseau PL, Dancis A, Camadro JM. Siderophore uptake and use by the yeast *Saccharomyces cerevisiae*. Microbiology. 2001;147:289–98.
47. Lesuisse E, Simon-Casteras M, Labbe P. Siderophore-mediated iron uptake in *Saccharomyces cerevisiae*: the SIT1 gene encodes a ferrioxamine B permease that belongs to the major facilitator superfamily. Microbiology. 1998;144:3455–62.
48. Yun CW, Ferea T, Rashford J, et al. Desferrioxamine-mediated iron uptake in *Saccharomyces cerevisiae*. Evidence for two pathways of iron uptake. J Biol Chem. 2000;275:10709–15.
49. Yun CW, Tiedeman JS, Moore RE, Philpott CC. Siderophore-iron uptake in saccharomyces cerevisiae. Identification of ferrichrome and fusarinine transporters. J Biol Chem. 2000;275:16354–9.
50. Moore RE, Kim Y, Philpott CC. The mechanism of ferrichrome transport through Arn1p and its metabolism in *Saccharomyces cerevisiae*. Proc Natl Acad Sci USA. 2003;100:5664–9.
51. Erpapazoglou Z, Froissard M, Nondier I, Lesuisse E, Haguenauer-Tsapis R, Belgareh-Touze N. Substrate- and Ubiquitin-dependent trafficking of the yeast siderophore transporter Sit1. Traffic. 2008;9:1372–91.
52. Kim Y, Yun CW, Philpott CC. Ferrichrome induces endosome to plasma membrane cycling of the ferrichrome transporter, Arn1p, in *Saccharomyces cerevisiae*. EMBO J. 2002;21:3632–42.
53. Kim Y, Deng Y, Philpott CC. GGA2- and ubiquitin-dependent trafficking of Arn1, the ferrichrome transporter of *Saccharomyces cerevisiae*. Mol Biol Cell. 2007;18:1790–802.
54. Kim Y, Lampert SM, Philpott CC. A receptor domain controls the intracellular sorting of the ferrichrome transporter, ARN1. EMBO J. 2005;24:952–62.
55. De Domenico I, McVey Ward D, Kaplan J. Regulation of iron acquisition and storage: consequences for iron-linked disorders. Nat Rev Mol Cell Biol. 2008;9:72–81.
56. Flo TH, Smith KD, Sato S, et al. Lipocalin 2 mediates an innate immune response to bacterial infection by sequestrating iron. Nature. 2004;432:917–21.
57. Goetz DH, Holmes MA, Borregaard N, Bluhm ME, Raymond KN, Strong RK. The Neutrophil Lipocalin NGAL is a bacteriostatic agent that interferes with siderophore-mediated iron acquisition. Mol Cell. 2002;10:1033–43.
58. Yang J, Goetz D, Li JY, et al. An iron delivery pathway mediated by a lipocalin. Mol Cell. 2002;10:1045–56.
59. Devireddy LR, Hart DO, Goetz DH, Green MR. A mammalian siderophore synthesized by an enzyme with a bacterial homolog involved in enterobactin production. Cell. 2010;141:1006–17.
60. Bao G, Clifton M, Hoette T. Siderocalin (Ngal) traffics Iron with catechols, products of intestinal bacteria. Nat Chem Biol. 2010;6:602–9.
61. Protchenko O, Rodriguez-Suarez R, Androphy R, Bussey H, Philpott CC. A screen for genes of heme uptake identifies the FLC family required for import of FAD into the endoplasmic reticulum. J Biol Chem. 2006;281:21445–57.
62. Weissman Z, Kornitzer D. A family of Candida cell surface haem-binding proteins involved in haemin and haemoglobin-iron utilization. Mol Microbiol. 2004;53:1209–20.
63. Protchenko O, Shakoury-Elizeh M, Keane P, Storey J, Androphy R, Philpott CC. Role of PUG1 in inducible porphyrin and heme transport in *Saccharomyces cerevisiae*. Eukaryot Cell. 2008;7:859–71.
64. Quigley JG, Yang Z, Worthington MT, et al. Identification of a human heme exporter that is essential for erythropoiesis. Cell. 2004;118:757–66.
65. Chen OS, Kaplan J. CCC1 suppresses mitochondrial damage in the yeast model of Friedreich's ataxia by limiting mitochondrial iron accumulation. J Biol Chem. 2000;275:7626–32.
66. Lapinskas PJ, Lin SJ, Culotta VC. The role of the *Saccharomyces cerevisiae* CCC1 gene in the homeostasis of manganese ions. Mol Microbiol. 1996;21:519–28.
67. Li L, Bagley D, Ward DM, Kaplan J. Yap5 is an iron-responsive transcriptional activator that regulates vacuolar iron storage in yeast. Mol Cell Biol. 2008;28:1326–37.
68. Rees EM, Thiele DJ. Identification of a vacuole-associated metalloreductase and its role in Ctr2-mediated intracellular copper mobilization. J Biol Chem. 2007;282:21629–38.
69. Singh A, Kaur N, Kosman DJ. The metalloreductase Fre6p in Fe-efflux from the yeast vacuole. J Biol Chem. 2007;282:28619–26.

70. Urbanowski JL, Piper RC. The iron transporter Fth1p forms a complex with the Fet5 iron oxidase and resides on the vacuolar membrane. J Biol Chem. 1999;274:38061–70.
71. Conklin DS, McMaster JA, Culbertson MR, Kung C. COT1, a gene involved in cobalt accumulation in *Saccharomyces cerevisiae*. Mol Cell Biol. 1992;12:3678–88.
72. MacDiarmid CW, Gaither LA, Eide D. Zinc transporters that regulate vacuolar zinc storage in *Saccharomyces cerevisiae*. EMBO J. 2000;19:2845–55.
73. Li L, Kaplan J. Defects in the yeast high affinity iron transport system result in increased metal sensitivity because of the increased expression of transporters with a broad transition metal specificity. J Biol Chem. 1998;273:22181–7.
74. Protchenko O, Philpott CC. Regulation of intracellular heme levels by HMX1, a homologue of heme oxygenase, in *Saccharomyces cerevisiae*. J Biol Chem. 2003;278:36582–7.
75. Foury F, Roganti T. Deletion of the mitochondrial carrier genes MRS3 and MRS4 suppresses mitochondrial iron accumulation in a yeast frataxin-deficient strain. J Biol Chem. 2002;277:24475–83.
76. Shaw GC, Cope JJ, Li L, et al. Mitoferrin is essential for erythroid iron assimilation. Nature. 2006;440:96–100.
77. Philpott CC, Protchenko O. Response to iron deprivation in *Saccharomyces cerevisiae*. Eukaryot Cell. 2008;7:20–7.
78. Blaiseau PL, Lesuisse E, Camadro JM. Aft2p, a novel iron-regulated transcription activator that modulates, with Aft1p, intracellular iron use and resistance to oxidative stress in yeast. J Biol Chem. 2001;276:34221–6.
79. Haurie V, Boucherie H, Sagliocco F. The Snf1 protein kinase controls the induction of genes of the iron uptake pathway at the diauxic shift in *Saccharomyces cerevisiae*. J Biol Chem. 2003;278:45391–6.
80. Puig S, Vergara SV, Thiele DJ. Cooperation of two mRNA-binding proteins drives metabolic adaptation to iron deficiency. Cell Metab. 2008;7:555–64.
81. Marquet A, Bui BT, Florentin D. Biosynthesis of biotin and lipoic acid. Vitam Horm. 2001;61:51–101.
82. Stolz J, Hoja U, Meier S, Sauer N, Schweizer E. Identification of the plasma membrane H+-biotin symporter of *Saccharomyces cerevisiae* by rescue of a fatty acid-auxotrophic mutant. J Biol Chem. 1999;274:18741–6.
83. Rutherford JC, Jaron S, Ray E, Brown PO, Winge DR. A second iron-regulatory system in yeast independent of Aft1p. Proc Natl Acad Sci USA. 2001;98:14322–7.
84. Yamaguchi-Iwai Y, Dancis A, Klausner RD. AFT1: a mediator of iron regulated transcriptional control in *Saccharomyces cerevisiae*. EMBO J. 1995;14:1231–9.
85. Yamaguchi-Iwai Y, Stearman R, Dancis A, Klausner RD. Iron-regulated DNA binding by the AFT1 protein controls the iron regulon in yeast. EMBO J. 1996;15:3377–84.
86. Yamaguchi-Iwai Y, Ueta R, Fukunaka A, Sasaki R. Subcellular localization of Aft1 transcription factor responds to iron status in *Saccharomyces cerevisiae*. J Biol Chem. 2002;277:18914–8.
87. Ueta R, Fujiwara N, Iwai K, Yamaguchi-Iwai Y. Mechanism underlying the iron-dependent nuclear export of the iron-responsive transcription factor Aft1p in *Saccharomyces cerevisiae*. Mol Biol Cell. 2007;18:2980–90.
88. Ueta R, Fukunaka A, Yamaguchi-Iwai Y. Pse1p mediates the nuclear import of the iron-responsive transcription factor Aft1p in *Saccharomyces cerevisiae*. J Biol Chem. 2003;278:50120–7.
89. Belli G, Molina MM, Garcia-Martinez J, Perez-Ortin JE, Herrero E. *Saccharomyces cerevisiae* glutaredoxin 5-deficient cells subjected to continuous oxidizing conditions are affected in the expression of specific sets of genes. J Biol Chem. 2004;279:12386–95.
90. Chen OS, Crisp RJ, Valachovic M, Bard M, Winge DR, Kaplan J. Transcription of the yeast iron regulon does not respond directly to iron but rather to iron–sulfur cluster biosynthesis. J Biol Chem. 2004;279:29513–8.
91. Rutherford JC, Ojeda L, Balk J, Muhlenhoff U, Lill R, Winge DR. Activation of the iron regulon by the yeast Aft1/Aft2 transcription factors depends on mitochondrial but not cytosolic iron-sulfur protein biogenesis. J Biol Chem. 2005;280:10135–40.
92. Ojeda L, Keller G, Muhlenhoff U, Rutherford JC, Lill R, Winge DR. Role of glutaredoxin-3 and glutaredoxin-4 in the iron regulation of the Aft1 transcriptional activator in *Saccharomyces cerevisiae*. J Biol Chem. 2006;281:17661–9.
93. Pujol-Carrion N, Belli G, Herrero E, Nogues A, de la Torre-Ruiz MA. Glutaredoxins Grx3 and Grx4 regulate nuclear localisation of Aft1 and the oxidative stress response in *Saccharomyces cerevisiae*. J Cell Sci. 2006;119:4554–64.
94. Kumanovics A, Chen OS, Li L, et al. Identification of FRA1 and FRA2 as genes involved in regulating the yeast iron regulon in response to decreased mitochondrial iron–sulfur cluster synthesis. J Biol Chem. 2008;283:10276–86.
95. Li H, Mapolelo DT, Dingra NN, et al. The yeast iron regulatory proteins Grx3/4 and Fra2 form heterodimeric complexes containing a [2Fe–2S] cluster with cysteinyl and histidyl ligation. Biochemistry. 2009;48:9569–81.
96. Crisp RJ, Pollington A, Galea C, Jaron S, Yamaguchi-Iwai Y, Kaplan J. Inhibition of heme biosynthesis prevents transcription of iron uptake genes in yeast. J Biol Chem. 2003;278:45499–506.
97. Crisp RJ, Adkins EM, Kimmel E, Kaplan J. Recruitment of Tup1p and Cti6p regulates heme-deficient expression of Aft1p target genes. EMBO J. 2006;25:512–21.

98. Puig S, Lau M, Thiele DJ. Cti6 is an Rpd3-Sin3 histone deacetylase-associated protein required for growth under iron-limiting conditions in *Saccharomyces cerevisiae*. J Biol Chem. 2004;279:30298–306.
99. Fragiadakis GS, Tzamarias D, Alexandraki D. Nhp6 facilitates Aft1 binding and Ssn6 recruitment, both essential for FRE2 transcriptional activation. EMBO J. 2004;23:333–42.
100. van de Peppel J, Kettelarij N, van Bakel H, Kockelkorn TT, van Leenen D, Holstege FC. Mediator expression profiling epistasis reveals a signal transduction pathway with antagonistic submodules and highly specific downstream targets. Mol Cell. 2005;19:511–22.
101. Shi H, Bencze KZ, Stemmler TL, Philpott CC. A cytosolic iron chaperone that delivers iron to ferritin. Science. 2008;320:1207–10.

Chapter 31
Zebrafish Models of Heme Synthesis and Iron Metabolism

Paula Goodman Fraenkel

Keywords Anemia • Ferroportin1 • Glutaredoxin5 • Heme • Hepcidin • Mitoferrin • Porphyria • Transferrin • Zebrafish

1 Zebrafish as a Model for Human Erythropoiesis

Zebrafish are small freshwater fish in the teleost infraclass of ray-finned fishes, which have been developed as a laboratory model for the study of genetics and developmental biology. Zebrafish hematopoiesis, like human hematopoiesis, occurs in two phases, a short-lived primitive or embryonic phase, which primarily generates erythrocytes and macrophages, followed by a definitive or adult phase, which continues to produce all the blood lineages throughout the life of the organism (reviewed in [1]). Similar to mammalian embryos, the primary sites of hematopoiesis shift in the zebrafish embryo. During development, the location of mammalian hematopoiesis shifts location from ventral blood islands in the yolk sac, to the liver, and then to the bone marrow. In the zebrafish, hematopoiesis transitions from the embryonic rostral blood islands and intermediate cell mass (ICM) to the aorto-gonado-mesonephric region and posterior blood island [1]. In the adult zebrafish, hematopoiesis occurs in the kidney and thymus [1, 2].

Similar to human hematopoietic stem cells, zebrafish hematopoietic stem cells follow a conserved genetic program and differentiate into three major lineages: erythroid, myeloid, and lymphoid. Zebrafish primitive hematopoietic progenitors (Fig. 31.1) express transcription factors such as *scl*, *fli1*, *gata-2*, *hhex*, *lmo2*, and *tif1γ* [3–6]. A group of *scl*+progenitor cells express *gata-1* and are destined to become erythrocytes [5–7]. As the erythrocytes develop, they begin to express the genes required for hemoglobin synthesis and iron uptake [1]. Resembling human hemoglobin, zebrafish hemoglobin contains four globin chains ($\alpha_2\beta_2$) and a switch occurs from expression of embryonic globin genes to adult globin genes [8, 9]. Unlike human definitive erythrocytes, which lack nuclei, zebrafish erythrocytes retain their nuclei in both the primitive and definitive stages of hematopoiesis.

Zebrafish embryos are transparent, facilitating observation of erythrocyte development and identification of embryos with deficiencies in iron metabolism and hemoglobin production. Embryonic erythrocytes begin to circulate at 36 h post-fertilization (hpf). Three criteria may be used to determine that zebrafish embryos are anemic (1) a decrease in the estimated number of circulating erythrocytes, (2) increased pallor of erythrocytes, and (3) decreased hemoglobin staining with *o*-dianisidine.

P.G. Fraenkel, M.D. (✉)
Division of Hematology/Oncology, Department of Medicine, Beth Israel Deaconess Medical Center and Harvard Medical School, Boston, MA, USA
e-mail: pfraenke@bidmc.harvard.edu

G.J. Anderson and G. McLaren (eds.), *Iron Physiology and Pathophysiology in Humans*, Nutrition and Health, DOI 10.1007/978-1-60327-485-2_31,

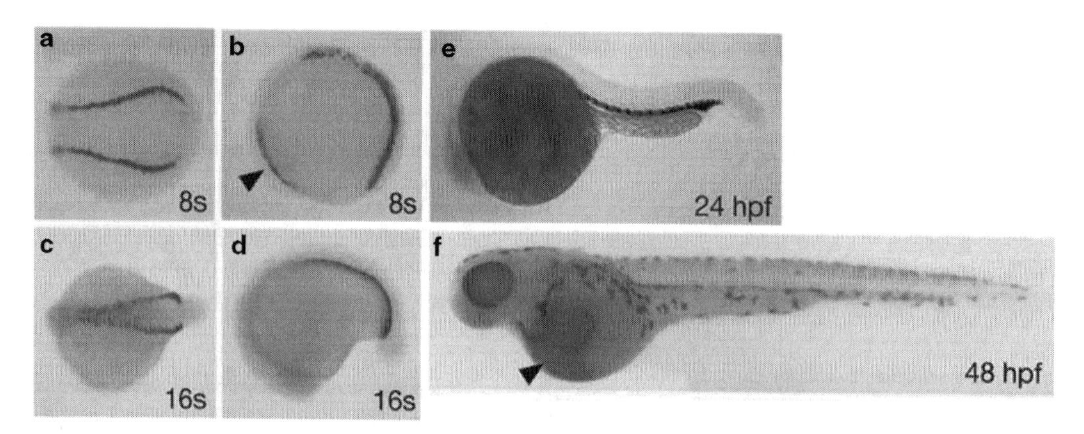

Fig. 31.1 Formation of early blood precursors in the zebrafish embryo. (**a** and **b**) Whole-mount in situ hybridization with *scl* at the 8 somite stage, marking the bilateral stripes of mesoderm, which will migrate to form the ICM. Anterior hematopoietic precursors are evident in the rostral blood island (RBI) (*arrow*). (**c** and **d**) Whole-mount in situ hybridization with *gata-1* at the 16 somite stage. (**e**) Whole-mount in situ hybridization with *gata-1* at 24 hpf, marking erythroid precursors in the ICM, preceding the onset of circulation. (**f**) *o*-dianisine staining of hemoglobin at 48 hpf in circulating erythrocytes, noted prominently in the ducts of Cuvier over the yolk sac (*arrow*). Reprinted, with permission, from [1] ©2005 by Annual Reviews (www.annualreviews.org)

2 Genetic Screens

Large-scale chemical mutagenesis screens, performed in Tübingen, Germany, and Boston, Massachusetts [10, 11], were used to identify a variety of zebrafish mutants with defects in embryonic erythropoiesis [12, 13]. Male founder fish (P generation) were treated with ethylnitrosourea (ENU) to introduce germline mutations in their gametes (Fig. 31.2). The F_1-progeny of these males were bred to generate a second generation (F_2). Fish in the F_2-generation were bred to their siblings in order to uncover recessive mutations causing anemia in the F_3-progeny (reviewed in [14]). In this manner, more than 20 complementation groups were identified, with the majority named for varieties of wine.

3 Microinjection Techniques

An advantage of the zebrafish system is the ease with which gene expression may be modified in the embryo via microinjection at the unicellular stage. Injection of cRNA or cDNA may be used to overexpress a gene of interest and assess the effect on a particular mutant. This technique has been particularly helpful in confirming the function of mutated genes. In addition, DNA constructs containing promoters, linked to sequences encoding fluorescent proteins, have been injected into zebrafish embryos to generate transgenic lines of zebrafish with fluorescent labeling of particular cells. This technique has been used to study erythroid development [15] and hematopoietic stem cell transplantation [16, 17].

Morpholino knockdown technology [18] has been used extensively to validate observations in zebrafish mutants and has provided critical data where mutants are not available. Morpholinos are chemically synthesized antisense oligonucleotides, modified to resist cellular degradation, which either inhibit translation or splicing of a specific mRNA. After injection into the unicellular embryo, the morpholino is distributed to the daughter cells and may continue to be effective for up to 3 days post-fertilization (dpf). Epistatic relationships between genes may be assessed by co-injecting a particular morpholino with cRNA or cDNA encoding another gene.

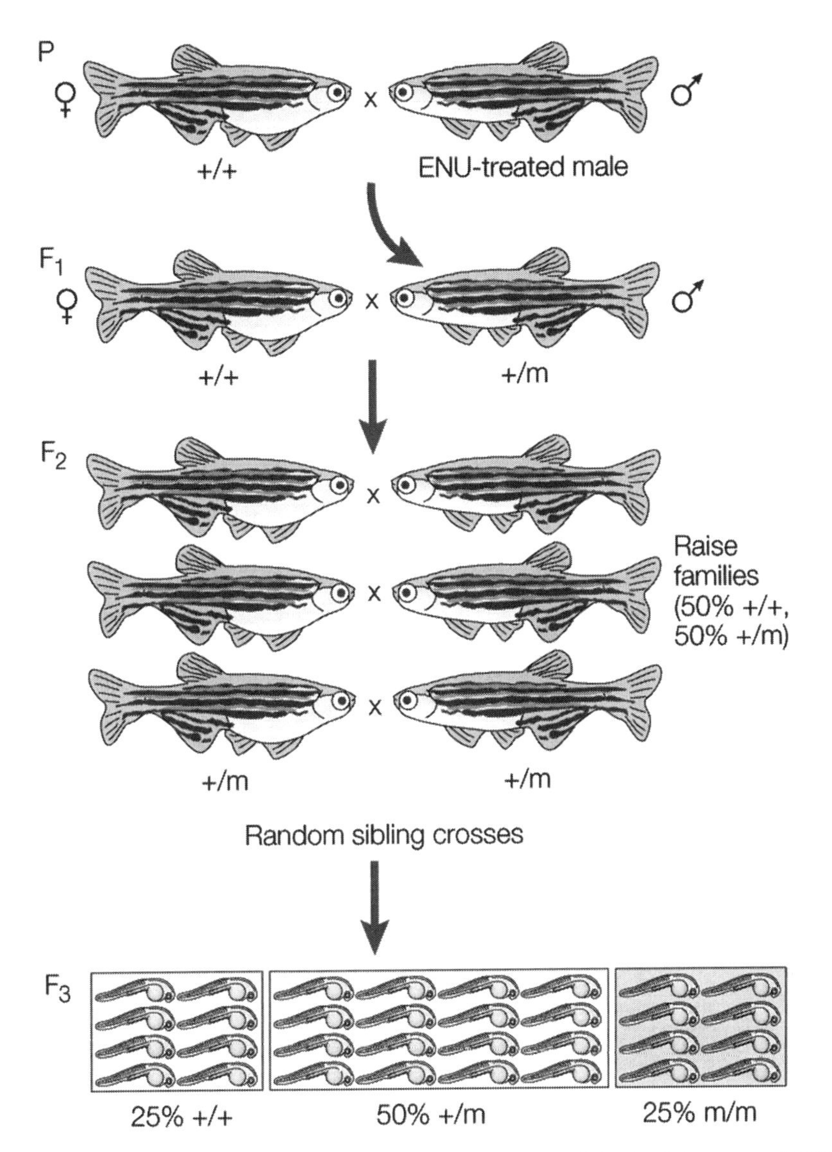

Fig. 31.2 Schematic of large-scale screen for recessive mutations in zebrafish. Ethylnitrosourea (ENU) is used to generate mutations in the premeiotic germ cells of male founders, which are crossed to wild-type females to produce the F_1 progeny. F_1 fish are bred to create F_2 families. F_2 siblings are incrossed. The resulting F_3 progeny are 25% wild-type (+/+), 50% heterozygous (+/m), and 25% homozygous (m/m) for a recessive mutation. Reprinted, with permission of Macmillan Publishers, Ltd., from [14]

4 Zebrafish Models with Deficiencies in Heme Synthesis

Hemoproteins are essential for cellular functions including oxygen binding, oxygen metabolism, and electron transfer (reviewed in [19]). Hemoglobin, the most abundant hemoprotein in human adults, is produced in developing erythrocytes. Production of hemoglobin requires synthesis of the heme prosthetic group, insertion of iron into its center, and synthesis of the globin protein. Synthesis of heme occurs in mammalian cells via the actions of eight enzymes (reviewed in [19]). Analysis of zebrafish anemia mutants indicates that the same process is conserved in the zebrafish.

4.1 Alas2

Positional cloning of *sauternes* (*sau*), the first zebrafish anemia mutant to be characterized genetically [20], revealed that each of the two *sau* alleles exhibits a mutation in *alas2*, the ortholog of the human gene encoding the erythroid-specific isoform of the enzyme δ-aminolevulinate synthase 2 (ALAS2 or ALAS-E). This enzyme catalyzes the condensation of glycine and succinyl CoA to yield δ-aminolevulinic acid, the first step in heme biosynthesis. Similar to mammalian models, *alas2* was specifically expressed in zebrafish erythrocytes while *alas1*, the ortholog of δ-aminolevulinate synthase 1 (ALAS1 or ALAS-N), was expressed ubiquitously [20]. The protein sequence encoded by zebrafish *alas2* was highly conserved in comparison to mouse, rat, human, and toadfish ALAS2. As expected, the erythrocytes in *sau* mutants exhibited lower levels of heme and experimental overexpression of *alas2* rescued hemoglobin production in the *sau* mutants, confirming that the anemia was due to ALAS2 deficiency [20].

The *sau* phenotype demonstrates both similarities and differences to mammalian models of ALAS2 deficiency. *Sau* mutant erythrocytes exhibited maturation arrest, characterized by persistent expression of *gata-1* and β_{e2}, an embryonic β-globin gene [20]. Similarly, defects in erythrocyte maturation and globin expression have been observed in erythrocyte differentiation experiments utilizing ALAS2-deficient mouse embryonic stem cells [21, 22]. Mutations in ALAS2 in humans [23–25] result in the disease congenital sideroblastic anemia (CSA). Although *sau* zebrafish, like CSA patients, exhibit hypochromic microcytic anemia, they do not display the characteristic ring sideroblasts caused by iron deposition in the mitochondria of erythrocytes in affected patients. The reason for this difference is not known, although it has been proposed that it may be due to differences in iron metabolism in zebrafish embryos [20].

4.2 Porphyria Models

Zebrafish mutants have been identified with defects in the enzymes that follow ALAS2 in the heme biosynthetic pathway. These mutants exhibit autofluorescence in erythrocytes, hepatocytes, or yolk sac and are models for human porphyrias, diseases in which fluorescent porphyrin intermediates accumulate due to deficiencies in heme synthetic enzymes. In *yqem*, which exhibits a mutation in uroporphyrinogen III decarboxylase (*UROD*) [26], homozygous mutant zebrafish embryos exhibit fluorescent erythrocytes, which hemolyze when exposed to light [12]. Photosensitivity is a characteristic of the human disease hepatoerythropoietic porphyria (HEP), which is caused by deficiency of *UROD*. *Montalcino* exhibits hypochromic anemia and yolk sac fluorescence due to a mutation in protoporphyrinogen III oxidase (*PPO*) [27] and is a model for the human disease variegate porphyria (VP), which is caused by mutations in *PPO*. Overexpression of the human ortholog for *PPO* resulted in partial rescue of the embryonic anemia in *montalcino* mutants, consistent with a conserved function for the enzyme [27]. A mutation in *ferrochelatase*, the final enzyme in the heme biosynthetic pathway, which inserts iron into protoporphyrin IX, results in the zebrafish mutant *dracula* [28]. This mutant exhibits autofluorescent erythrocytes and hepatocytes [28], reminiscent of the human disease erythropoietic porphyria (EP), in which patients exhibit mutations in *ferrochelatase*, erythrocytes are autofluorescent, and toxic porphyrins accumulate in the liver.

4.3 Glutaredoxin5

Positional cloning of the gene affected in the zebrafish mutant *shiraz* (*sir*) resulted in the identification of a new gene regulating heme synthesis (Fig. 31.3). *Sir* homozygotes exhibit severe hypochromic anemia and impaired hemoglobin production, yet morpholino knockdown of *UROD* or *ferrochelatase*

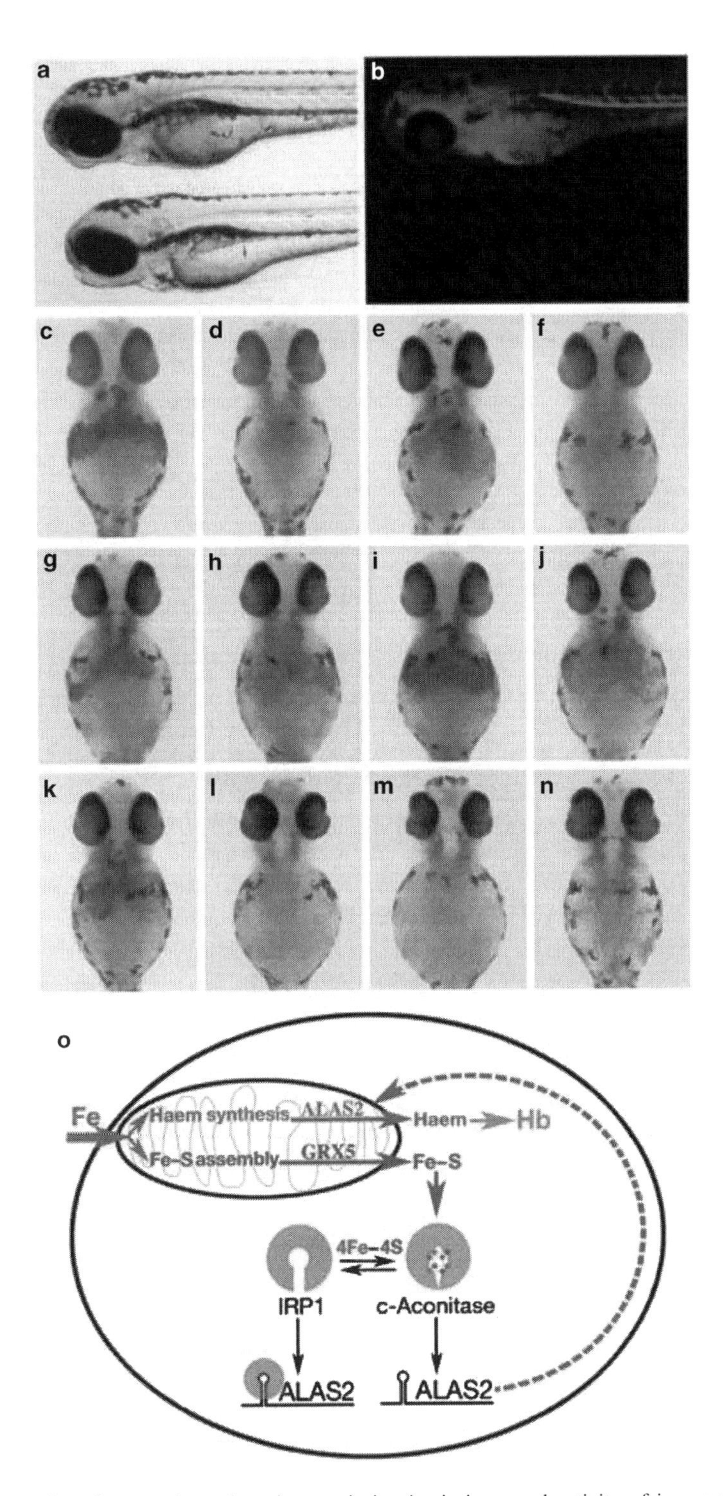

Fig. 31.3 Deletion of *grx5* causes hypochromic anemia in *sir* via increased activity of iron regulatory protein 1 (IRP1). (**a**, **b**) Photomicrographs in bright field (**a**) or dark field with epifluorescent light source (**b**) of wild-type embryos injected with *ferrochelatase* morpholino, which causes erythrocyte autofluorescence (*top*), while *sir* (*bottom*) embryos are unaffected. (**c–n**) *o*-dianisidine staining in embryos at 48 hpf (**c**) wild type; (**d**) *sir* mutant. (**e–j**) *sir* mutants injected with *alas2* cDNA constructs: (**e**) *alas2* cDNA lacking the 5'UTR; (**f**) *alas2* cDNA with the entire 5'UTR; (**g**) *alas2* cDNA with 5' IRE six-base loop (CAGUGC) deleted; (**h**) *alas2* cDNA loop 5'-GCTCGG-3'; (**i**) *alas2* cDNA loop 5'-CCGAGC-3'; (**j**) *alas2* cDNA loop 5'-CAGΔGC-3'. (**k–n**) *sir* mutants injected with *IRP1* morpholino (**k**) or *IRP1* four-base morpholino mismatch (**l**), injected with both *IRP1* morpholino and *IRP1* cDNA (**m**), and injected with *IRP2* morpholino (**n**). Mutated nucleotides are underlined. (**o**) Model for the role of Fe-S cluster production in erythroid heme synthesis. Reprinted, with permission of Macmillan Publishers, Ltd., from [29]

failed to produce autofluorescence. This indicated an absence of porphyrin intermediates and suggested that the first step in heme synthesis, catalyzed by ALAS2, was impaired [29]. While most of the mutants identified in the Tübingen and Boston screens were due to point mutations, positional cloning of *sir* revealed a deletion of approximately 150 kb on linkage group 20 [29]. Glutaredoxin5 (*grx5*), previously characterized in yeast as a gene required for Fe-S cluster biosynthesis in mitochondria [30, 31], was identified as a candidate gene in the deleted region. *Grx5* expression was absent in *sir*, while overexpression of either yeast, mouse, zebrafish, or human *grx5* rescued the anemia phenotype [29]. Furthermore, zebrafish *grx5* rescued aconitase activity and lysine auxotrophy in a *grx5*-deletion strain of yeast [29]. Taken together, these data indicate that deletion of *grx5* caused the *sir* anemia phenotype and that zebrafish *grx5* has a conserved function in Fe-S cluster biosynthesis.

The genetic interaction between *grx5* and *IRP1* in the zebrafish embryo was demonstrated by a series of microinjection experiments [29]. Iron regulatory proteins (IRPs) bind stem-loop motifs, termed iron-responsive elements (IREs), in the 5′ or 3′ untranslated regions (UTRs) of RNAs. IRPs binding IREs in the 5' UTR repress translation, while those binding in the 3′ UTR stabilize the message. When iron regulatory protein 1 (IRP1) binds a 4Fe–S cluster, it loses IRE-binding activity and transforms to a cytosolic aconitase (reviewed in [32]). Overexpression of *alas2* lacking the 5′-IRE rescued *sir*, while overexpression of *alas2* with an intact 5′-IRE failed to rescue the phenotype. In addition, morpholino knockdown of *IRP1* rescued the anemia phenotype in *sir*, while morpholino knockdown of *IRP2* did not. Thus, it appears that *sir* is required to generate the Fe-S cluster that inactivates IRP1 [29]. A mutation in *grx5* has subsequently been identified in a patient with sideroblastic anemia and biochemical evidence for increased IRP1 activity, similar to that seen in *sir* [33].

5 Zebrafish Models with Deficiencies in Iron Metabolism

5.1 *DMT1*

Chardonnay was the first zebrafish anemia mutant identified with a defect in an erythroid iron transporter. The *chardonnay* mutation was mapped to the *DMT1* locus, and a point mutation (K264X) was identified in the mutants [34]. DMT1 has been proposed to have two vital roles in cellular iron transport (1) at the apical surface of the enterocyte mediating iron entry into the cell [35, 36] and (2) facilitating exit of iron from the endosome following endocytosis of the holotransferrin/transferrin receptor complex [37, 38]. In zebrafish embryos, *DMT1* is expressed in blood precursors as early as the 4 somite stage, in circulating erythrocytes at 48 hpf, and subsequently in the intestine at 5 days post-fertilization. Functional analysis of zebrafish *DMT1* transfected into 293 T cells revealed that the wild-type gene encodes a functional iron transporter, while the mutant variant does not [34]. Despite the impaired function of K264X DMT1, *chardonnay* mutants are viable. These resemble the *mk* mouse [39] and Belgrade rat [37], mutants with impaired DMT1 function, which exhibit hypochromic anemia but are still viable. This suggests that DMT1-independent pathways exist for iron transport in vivo.

5.2 *Ferroportin1*

The existence of a vertebrate iron exporter had been postulated, but was not identified until the positional cloning of *ferroportin1* (*fpn1*), the gene affected in the zebrafish hypochromic anemia mutant, *weissherbst* (*weh*). *Weh* mutants exhibit severe hypochromic anemia and are not viable beyond 14 dpf. Erythrocyte iron levels, measured by atomic absorption spectroscopy, were decreased in *weh* mutants, while intravenous injection of iron dextran rescued the anemia, suggesting that the mutants had a defect in iron transport [40]. The mutation was mapped to a previously unidentified gene with ten predicted transmembrane domains. Two alleles of *weh* were identified, *weh*^{Tp85c} and *weh*^{Th238}, with a missense mutation (L167F) and a nonsense mutation (C361X), respectively [40]. The cause of the anemia phenotype was deemed to be due to impaired transport of iron from maternal iron stores to the embryo for the following reasons [40] (1) *fpn1* is specifically expressed in the yolk syncytial layer (YSL), which separates the yolk from the developing embryo; (2) injection of *fpn1-GFP* cRNA into the yolk of zebrafish embryos at the 256-cell stage resulted in localization of the protein to the YSL and rescue of the anemia phenotype; and (3) zebrafish *fpn1* was shown to function as an iron exporter when expressed in *Xenopus* oocytes [40]. Mammalian orthologs of zebrafish fpn1 (also known as IREG1 or MTP1) were identified and localized to the basolateral surface of enterocytes, as well as placenta and liver cells [40]. Mammalian FPN1 was upregulated in enterocytes in response to iron deficiency and shown to export iron [41, 42].

The *weh*^{Tp85c} allele is of particular interest because it encodes a missense mutation (L167F) at a conserved residue between the third and fourth predicted transmembrane domains of fpn1, in the same region as a cluster of missense mutations identified in patients with an iron overload syndrome, termed type 4 hemochromatosis [43–49]. Type 4 hemochromatosis is characterized by an autosomal dominant pattern of inheritance, accumulation of iron in the reticuloendothelial system, absence of hepatic fibrosis, and a tendency for affected patients to develop anemia following venesection [50, 51]. To determine if the zebrafish model of fpn1 deficiency could provide insight into the FPN1-related iron overload syndrome, *weh*$^{Tp85c-/-}$, as well as *weh*$^{Tp85c+/-}$ and *weh*$^{Tp85c+/+}$ siblings, were treated with a series of intramuscular iron dextran injections at 3 days, 5 weeks, 8 weeks, and 16 weeks post-fertilization, enabling the mutant animals to reach adult size [52]. Two months after iron injections were discontinued, *weh*$^{Tp85c-/-}$ erythrocytes exhibited normal size (mean corpuscular volume) and hemoglobin content; however, 8 months after the discontinuation of the iron injections, *weh*$^{Tp85c-/-}$ exhibited profound microcytic, hypochromic anemia and impairment in erythroid maturation [52]. Histologic evaluation with Perls' staining revealed iron accumulation in the tips of the intestinal villi [52], specifically in *weh*$^{Tp85c-/-}$, consistent with a block in iron export from the enterocytes into the circulation (Fig. 31.4). This pattern of iron accumulation resembles the *sla* mouse [53, 54], which has a defect in intestinal iron export due to a mutation in *hephaestin*, the basolateral ferroxidase [55]. Furthermore, even 8 months after iron injections were discontinued, the *weh*$^{Tp85c-/-}$ zebrafish exhibited increased iron staining in kidney marrow macrophages and hepatic Kupffer cells, consistent with impaired iron export from the reticuloendothelial system. Thus, the iron injections were effective initially in treating the anemia, but the impairment in iron export resulted in an inability to mobilize stored iron. Despite accumulation of iron in the reticuloendothelial system, *weh*$^{Tp85c-/-}$ adult zebrafish exhibited severely impaired hepatic expression of the iron regulatory hormone *hepcidin* [52].

Reduction of *hepcidin* expression in *weh*$^{Tp85c-/-}$ zebrafish represents a homeostatic response to fpn1 deficiency. Recently, it has been shown that fpn1 is the receptor for hepcidin: hepcidin modulates iron absorption and iron delivery to erythrocytes by binding fpn1, resulting in its internalization and degradation [56]. The zebrafish hepcidin peptide is 52% identical to human hepcidin and has been shown to mediate degradation of ferroportin and cellular iron retention in vitro [57]. In mammalian models, *hepcidin* is transcriptionally upregulated in response to inflammation [58, 59] or iron overload [60], and downregulated in response to anemia, iron deficiency, or hypoxia [58]. In the zebrafish, *hepcidin* has been shown to be induced by bacterial infection [59] and iron loading [52].

The zebrafish has proved a useful tool for evaluating mutations in fpn1. Mutant forms of fpn1 have been overexpressed in zebrafish embryos to assess the effects of the mutations on iron transport, using embryonic hemoglobin production as a read-out. Overexpression of H32R or N174I in zebrafish embryos resulted in severe hypochromic anemia, while overexpression of N144H did not [61]. This correlates with differences in mammalian phenotypic and biochemical data. H32R

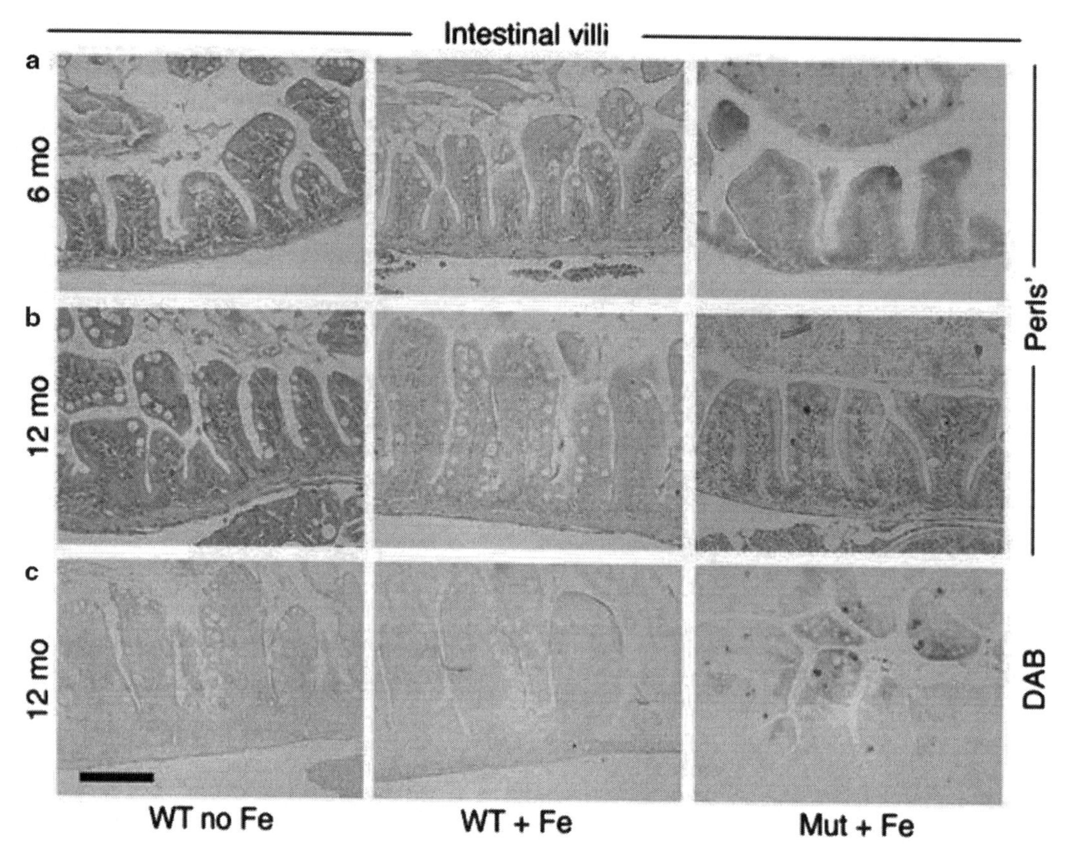

Fig. 31.4 Fpn1 is required for intestinal iron export in zebrafish. Histology of intestinal villi in uninjected wild type (WT) (*left*), WT injected with iron (*center*), and *weh*$^{Tp85c-/-}$ zebrafish injected with iron (*right*). Perls' stain, performed at 6 months of age (**a**) and 12 months of age (**b**) revealed nonheme-iron accumulation in the intestinal villi of *weh*$^{Tp85c-/-}$ zebrafish, but not in controls. (**c**) DAB-enhanced Perls' staining for nonheme iron at 12 months, for the same specimens as shown in (**b**). *Scale bar* represents 100 μm (Reprinted, with permission, from [52])

(the mutation observed in the *flatiron* mouse) [62] and the human mutation N174I [63] result in loss of iron export function in vitro and are associated with iron accumulation, predominantly in macrophages [62, 63], while N144H is associated with hepatocyte-dominant iron accumulation [64], normal iron export function [65], and resistance to hepcidin-mediated impairment in iron export [66].

5.3 Transferrin Receptors and Transferrin

Most vertebrate cells absorb iron primarily via the interaction of transferrin with transferrin receptor 1 (TfR1) [67]. Transferrin-mediated iron uptake is particularly important for erythroid development, as demonstrated by the TfR1 knockout mouse, which is embryonically lethal due to severe anemia, growth retardation, and neuronal apoptosis [68]. The zebrafish hypochromic anemia mutant, *chianti* (*cia*), mapped to a zebrafish ortholog of *TfR1* on linkage group 2, which was named *TfR1a*. Four alleles of *cia* were identified, each with a different mutation in *TfR1a*. The most severe alleles, *cia*^{hp327} and *cia*^{hs019}, were embryonically lethal and exhibited mutations in the proposed transferrin-binding domain [69]. In contrast to *fpn1*-deficient *weh*^{l}, intravenous iron injection into *cia* mutant embryos failed to reverse the anemia, demonstrating that *TfR1a* is required for erythroid iron uptake from the circulation [69]. Further supporting the requirement of *TfR1a* for erythroid iron uptake, *TfR1a* was expressed specifically in hematopoietic cells, knockdown of *TfR1a* reproduced the anemia phenotype, and overexpression of *TfR1a* or mouse *TfR1* decreased the severity of the anemia [69].

A peculiarity of the teleost genome is the existence of duplicated genes, which are hypothesized to have arisen during a genome duplication event following the divergence of teleosts and tetrapods [70, 71]. *TfR1b*, a homolog of *TfR1a*, appears to be the result of such a duplication. *TfR1b* maps to zebrafish linkage group 24; however, the regions surrounding both *TfR1a* and *TfR1b* exhibit synteny with human chromosome 3, the location of human *TfR1* [69]. In contrast to the erythroid-specific expression of *TfR1a*, *TfR1b* was expressed ubiquitously in the developing embryo [69]. Morpholino knockdown of *TfR1b* resulted in growth retardation and brain necrosis, which was ameliorated by overexpression of *TfR1b* [69]. Interestingly, although overexpression of *TfR1b* improved the anemia phenotype in *TfR1a* morphants, knockdown of *TfR1b* failed to produce anemia [69]. Thus, in the zebrafish, the hematologic and neurologic effects of *TfR1* deficiency observed in the *TfR1* knockout mouse [68] are separable due to the differential expression pattern of the zebrafish orthologs, *TfR1a* and *TfR1b*.

The requirement of *TfR1a* for hemoglobin synthesis in the zebrafish presupposes that transferrin transports iron in the zebrafish. Recently, a zebrafish strain, *gavi*, was identified with mutations in zebrafish *transferrin* (*transferrin-a*), exhibiting reduced *transferrin-a* expression and hypochromic anemia [72], which may be considered a model for the rare human condition atransferrinemia [73]. In zebrafish embryos, *transferrin-a* is expressed in the yolk and developing liver [72]. *Gavi* mutant embryos exhibited decreased iron stores in the somites and terminal gut, consistent with impaired iron transport from the yolk to the embryo [72]. Furthermore, *gavi* mutant embryos displayed decreased levels of *hepcidin* expression, which failed to recover following iron injection [72].

Although a zebrafish mutant in *TfR2* has not been identified, it has now been shown that *TfR2* is expressed specifically [72] in the liver of the developing embryo and that morpholino knockdown of *TfR2* decreases hepcidin expression, while embryonic deficiency of *fpn1* [52], *TfR1a*, *TfR1b*, or *DMT1* [72] did not produce significant effects. Analysis of *hepcidin* expression in zebrafish models, consistent with observations in mouse models of transferrin [74] and TfR2 deficiency [75], provides strong support for the hypothesis that transferrin-bound iron regulates transcriptional expression of *hepcidin* via interactions with *TfR2*.

5.4 Mitoferrin

The first erythroid mitochondrial iron transporter was discovered by cloning the mutated gene in the zebrafish anemia mutant *frascati* (*frs*) [76]. *Mitoferrin* (*mfrn*), a member of the SLC25 family of mitochondrial solute transporters, is mutated in several alleles of *frascati* (Fig. 31.5). *Mfrn* is highly expressed in erythropoietic tissues in zebrafish and mouse embryos, upregulated during maturation of Friend mouse erythroleukemia (MEL) cells, and rescues the *frascati* phenotype when overexpressed in mutant embryos [76]. *Mfrn*-null mouse erythroblasts incubated with ^{55}Fe-saturated transferrin failed to incorporate ^{55}Fe into heme [76]; thus, it has been proposed that *mfrn* transports iron into the mitochondrion for insertion into protoporphyrin IX by ferrochelatase.

Mfrn's function as a mitochondrial iron transporter was further supported by its ability to rescue mitochondrial iron transport in the *Δmrs3/4* yeast strain, which lacks both yeast orthologs of *mfrn* [76]. A second mitoferrin gene, *mitoferrin2* (*mfrn2*), maps to a different locus in the zebrafish and is ubiquitously expressed, both in zebrafish and mouse embryos. While *mfrn2* complements the *Δmrs3/4* yeast strain, it is unable to rescue *frs*, and thus has been proposed as a mitochondrial iron transporter for nonerythroid cells [76].

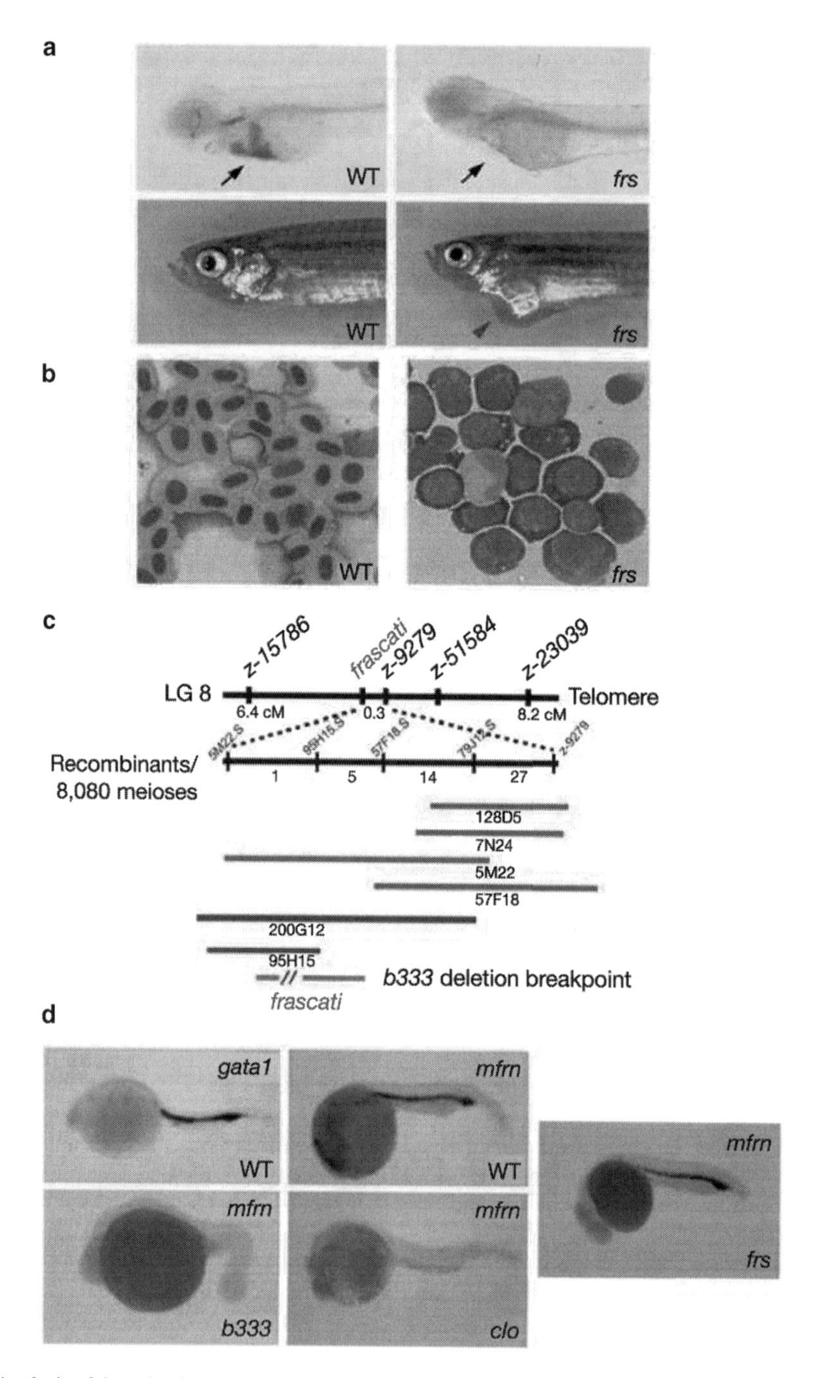

Fig. 31.5 Analysis of the zebrafish *frs* mutation, the *frs* locus, and expression of *mfrn*. (**a**) Wild-type and *frs* embryos were stained to detect hemoglobinized cells (top). Juvenile *frs* zebrafish (bottom right) show cardiomegaly (*arrowhead*) from chronic anemia. (**b**) *frs* blood erythrocytes show maturation arrest (*right*), compared with erythrocytes from wild-type fish (*left*). (**c**) Map of the *frs* locus on linkage group 8. The critical bacterial artificial chromosome (BAC) clones encompassing the *frs* locus and the location of the deletion breakpoint for the deficiency allele spt^{b333} are shown below. (**d**) Whole-mount embryo in situ hybridization at 24 hpf demonstrates expression of *gata-1* and *mfrn* in the intermediate cell mass, the site of embryonic hematopoiesis in the zebrafish. In contrast, *mfrn* expression is absent in spadetail (spt^{b333}) and *cloche* embryos, mutants with defective hematopoiesis. *Mfrn* RNA expression is normal in *frs* alleles because the missense mutations would not be expected to affect RNA stability. Reprinted, with permission of Macmillan Publishers, Ltd., from [76]

5.5 *Huntingtin*

The zebrafish has been used to identify a role for *hd*, the gene affected in Huntington's disease, in iron metabolism [77]. Huntington's disease is an autosomal dominant neurodegenerative condition caused by the expansion of a trinucleotide CAG repeat in *hd*, resulting in an expanded polyglutamine (poly-Q) tract in the Huntingtin protein [78]. Huntingtin has been implicated in a variety of cellular processes, including dendrite development, endocytosis, vesicle trafficking, and apoptosis (reviewed in [78, 79]). The striatum, a particularly vulnerable part of the brain in Huntington's disease [80, 81], has been noted, in affected patients, to exhibit iron accumulation [82, 83], biochemical evidence of oxidative stress [84], and decreased activity of iron-requiring enzymes, such as aconitase [85] and mitochondrial complexes II–IV [86, 87].

In the zebrafish embryo, *hd* is expressed ubiquitously, but more prominently, at 36 hpf in the ICM [77], the site of primitive hematopoiesis. Morpholino knockdown of *hd* resulted in a transient decrease in hemoglobin production, as well as morphologic defects, including a thin yolk extension and brain necrosis [77]. Diaminobenzidine (DAB)-enhanced Perls' staining revealed normal amounts of nonheme iron in *hd*-deficient erythrocytes, suggesting that erythroid iron uptake was preserved [77]. Injection of iron dextran into the cytoplasm of unicellular embryos has been shown to rescue *cia* by providing iron to the embryo [69], without requiring transferrin receptor-mediated endocytosis. This technique was applied to *hd*-deficient embryos, resulting in improvement in anemia and the yolk extension abnormality [77]. A model was proposed for *hd* to act downstream of *TfR1a*, participating in the release of iron from endosomes [77]. The role of *Hd* in cellular iron utilization may help to explain the iron accumulation and metabolic abnormalities observed in the striatal neurons of patients with Huntington's disease.

6 Future Directions

6.1 *HFE and Hemojuvelin (HFE2)*

The most common form of hemochromatosis occurs in middle age and is associated with mutations in *HFE*, an atypical MHC class I protein (reviewed in [50]), while a rarer form of severe, early onset hemochromatosis is caused by mutations in *hemojuvelin* (*HFE2*), a repulsive guidance molecule (RGM) family member [88]. Genomic analysis has failed to identify a close ortholog for human *HFE* in the zebrafish [89] or in other fish species, although nine orthologs of MHC class I with distant homology to HFE have been identified (P. Fraenkel and Y. Gibert, April 14, 2008, unpublished data). A zebrafish ortholog for *hemojuvelin* has been identified by sequence homology [88]; which does not regulate *hepcidin* expression in zebrafish embryos [90].

6.2 *Screens for Small Molecules Affecting Iron Metabolism*

The potential use of zebrafish to identify pharmacologic agents has begun to be exploited by performing chemical screens. In a chemical screen, zebrafish embryos are cultured in wells of microtiter plates, each containing a different small molecule or a combination of small molecules. After a specified period of incubation, embryos are evaluated for changes in development, gene expression, or protein modifications. Using this technology, chemical screens have identified small molecules affecting the cell cycle [91], hematopoietic stem cell proliferation [92], vascular development [93], and fin regeneration [94]. A screen for chemicals affecting iron metabolism has not yet been performed, although a screen for chemicals affecting copper metabolism identified small molecules with copper-chelating effects [95], proving the principle that chemical screens may be used to study metal metabolism in zebrafish.

Although screens for genes affecting hemoglobin production in the zebrafish have revealed much about iron metabolism, screens for other phenotypes may be useful to identify molecules that affect iron homeostasis. For example, a screen for molecules that disturb dorsoventral axis formation uncovered dorsomorphin [96] as a specific inhibitor of BMP signaling and *hepcidin* expression. Exposing zebrafish embryos to dorsomorphin prior to 8 hpf recapitulated the dorsalized phenotype seen in zebrafish models of impaired BMP signaling. Injection of dorsomorphin into adult zebrafish lowered hepatic *hepcidin* expression, while injection of dorsomorphin into mice resulted in decreased hepatic *hepcidin* expression and increased serum iron levels [96].

7 Conclusion

The past decade has provided a wealth of zebrafish models affecting heme synthesis and iron metabolism, and these are relevant to the pathophysiology of a variety of human diseases, including sideroblastic anemia, porphyria, atransferrinemia, type 4 hemochromatosis, and Huntington's disease. The use of transposon-based mutagenesis [97], which eliminates the need for positional cloning, is accelerating the identification of mutated genes. While, in the past, it has not been possible to perform gene-targeted knockdowns with germline transmission in the zebrafish, new technology using zinc finger nucleases has made this feasible [98]. The next stage of scientific discovery will utilize zebrafish models to develop better approaches to treating anemia, porphyria, and disorders of iron metabolism.

References

1. de Jong JL, Zon LI. Use of the zebrafish system to study primitive and definitive hematopoiesis. Annu Rev Genet. 2005;39:481–501.
2. Bertrand JY, Kim AD, Violette EP, Stachura DL, Cisson JL, Traver D. Definitive hematopoiesis initiates through a committed erythromyeloid progenitor in the zebrafish embryo. Development. 2007;134:4147–56 (Cambridge).
3. Liao W, Ho CY, Yan YL, Postlethwait J, Stainier DY. Hhex and scl function in parallel to regulate early endothelial and blood differentiation in zebrafish. Development. 2000;127:4303–13 (Cambridge).
4. Ransom DG, Bahary N, Niss K, et al. The zebrafish moonshine gene encodes transcriptional intermediary factor 1gamma, an essential regulator of hematopoiesis. PLoS Biol. 2004;2:E237.
5. Thompson MA, Ransom DG, Pratt SJ, et al. The cloche and spadetail genes differentially affect hematopoiesis and vasculogenesis. Dev Biol. 1998;197:248–69.
6. Dooley KA, Davidson AJ, Zon LI. Zebrafish scl functions independently in hematopoietic and endothelial development. Dev Biol. 2005;277:522–36.
7. Detrich 3rd HW, Kieran MW, Chan FY, et al. Intraembryonic hematopoietic cell migration during vertebrate development. Proc Natl Acad Sci USA. 1995;92:10713–7.
8. Chan FY, Robinson J, Brownlie A, et al. Characterization of adult alpha- and beta-globin genes in the zebrafish. Blood. 1997;89:688–700.
9. Brownlie A, Hersey C, Oates AC, et al. Characterization of embryonic globin genes of the zebrafish. Dev Biol. 2003;255:48–61.
10. Driever W, Solnica-Krezel L, Schier AF, et al. A genetic screen for mutations affecting embryogenesis in zebrafish. Development. 1996;123:37–46 (Cambridge).
11. Haffter P, Granato M, Brand M, et al. The identification of genes with unique and essential functions in the development of the zebrafish, Danio rerio. Development. 1996;123:1–36 (Cambridge).

12. Ransom DG, Haffter P, Odenthal J, et al. Characterization of zebrafish mutants with defects in embryonic hematopoiesis. Development. 1996;123:311–9 (Cambridge).
13. Weinstein BM, Schier AF, Abdelilah S, et al. Hematopoietic mutations in the zebrafish. Development. 1996; 123:303–9 (Cambridge).
14. Patton EE, Zon LI. The art and design of genetic screens: zebrafish. Nat Rev Genet. 2001;2:956–66.
15. Long Q, Meng A, Wang H, Jessen JR, Farrell MJ, Lin S. GATA-1 expression pattern can be recapitulated in living transgenic zebrafish using GFP reporter gene. Development. 1997;124:4105–11 (Cambridge).
16. Langenau DM, Ferrando AA, Traver D, et al. In vivo tracking of T cell development, ablation, and engraftment in transgenic zebrafish. Proc Natl Acad Sci USA. 2004;101:7369–74.
17. Traver D, Paw BH, Poss KD, Penberthy WT, Lin S, Zon LI. Transplantation and in vivo imaging of multilineage engraftment in zebrafish bloodless mutants. Nat Immunol. 2003;4:1238–46.
18. Nasevicius A, Ekker SC. Effective targeted gene 'knockdown' in zebrafish. Nat Genet. 2000;26:216–20.
19. Ponka P. Tissue-specific regulation of iron metabolism and heme synthesis: distinct control mechanisms in erythroid cells. Blood. 1997;89:1–25.
20. Brownlie A, Donovan A, Pratt SJ, et al. Positional cloning of the zebrafish sauternes gene: a model for congenital sideroblastic anaemia. Nat Genet. 1998;20:244–50.
21. Yin X, Dailey HA. Erythroid 5-aminolevulinate synthase is required for erythroid differentiation in mouse embryonic stem cells. Blood Cells Mol Dis. 1998;24:41–53.
22. Harigae H, Suwabe N, Weinstock PH, et al. Deficient heme and globin synthesis in embryonic stem cells lacking the erythroid-specific delta-aminolevulinate synthase gene. Blood. 1998;91:798–805.
23. Cotter PD, Baumann M, Bishop DF. Enzymatic defect in "X-linked" sideroblastic anemia: molecular evidence for erythroid delta-aminolevulinate synthase deficiency. Proc Natl Acad Sci USA. 1992;89:4028–32.
24. Cox TC, Bottomley SS, Wiley JS, Bawden MJ, Matthews CS, May BK. X-linked pyridoxine-responsive sideroblastic anemia due to a Thr388-to-Ser substitution in erythroid 5-aminolevulinate synthase. N Engl J Med. 1994;330:675–9.
25. Cotter PD, Rucknagel DL, Bishop DF. X-linked sideroblastic anemia: identification of the mutation in the erythroid-specific delta-aminolevulinate synthase gene (ALAS2) in the original family described by Cooley. Blood. 1994;84:3915–24.
26. Wang H, Long Q, Marty SD, Sassa S, Lin S. A zebrafish model for hepatoerythropoietic porphyria. Nat Genet. 1998;20:239–43.
27. Dooley KA, Fraenkel PG, Langer NB, et al. montalcino, a zebrafish model for variegate porphyria. Exp Hematol. 2008;36:1132–42.
28. Childs S, Weinstein BM, Mohideen MA, Donohue S, Bonkovsky H, Fishman MC. Zebrafish dracula encodes ferrochelatase and its mutation provides a model for erythropoietic protoporphyria. Curr Biol. 2000;10:1001–4.
29. Wingert RA, Galloway JL, Barut B, et al. Deficiency of glutaredoxin 5 reveals Fe-S clusters are required for vertebrate haem synthesis. Nature. 2005;436:1035–9.
30. Belli G, Polaina J, Tamarit J, et al. Structure–function analysis of yeast Grx5 monothiol glutaredoxin defines essential amino acids for the function of the protein. J Biol Chem. 2002;277:37590–6.
31. Rodriguez-Manzaneque MT, Tamarit J, Belli G, Ros J, Herrero E. Grx5 is a mitochondrial glutaredoxin required for the activity of iron/sulfur enzymes. Mol Biol Cell. 2002;13:1109–21.
32. Hentze MW, Muckenthaler MU, Andrews NC. Balancing acts: molecular control of mammalian iron metabolism. Cell. 2004;117:285–97.
33. Camaschella C, Campanella A, De Falco L, et al. The human counterpart of zebrafish shiraz shows sideroblastic-like microcytic anemia and iron overload. Blood. 2007;110:1353–8.
34. Donovan A, Brownlie A, Dorschner MO, et al. The zebrafish mutant gene chardonnay (cdy) encodes divalent metal transporter 1 (DMT1). Blood. 2002;100:4655–9.
35. Gunshin H, Mackenzie B, Berger UV, et al. Cloning and characterization of a mammalian proton-coupled metal-ion transporter. Nature. 1997;388:482–8.
36. Fleming MD, Trenor 3rd CC, Su MA, et al. Microcytic anaemia mice have a mutation in Nramp2, a candidate iron transporter gene. Nat Genet. 1997;16:383–6.
37. Fleming MD, Romano MA, Su MA, Garrick LM, Garrick MD, Andrews NC. Nramp2 is mutated in the anemic Belgrade (b) rat: evidence of a role for Nramp2 in endosomal iron transport. Proc Natl Acad Sci USA. 1998;95:1148–53.
38. Garrick MD, Gniecko K, Liu Y, Cohan DS, Garrick LM. Transferrin and the transferrin cycle in Belgrade rat reticulocytes. J Biol Chem. 1993;268:14867–74.
39. Su MA, Trenor CC, Fleming JC, Fleming MD, Andrews NC. The G185R mutation disrupts function of the iron transporter Nramp2. Blood. 1998;92:2157–63.
40. Donovan A, Brownlie A, Zhou Y, et al. Positional cloning of zebrafish ferroportin1 identifies a conserved vertebrate iron exporter. Nature. 2000;403:776–81.
41. McKie AT, Marciani P, Rolfs A, et al. A novel duodenal iron-regulated transporter, IREG1, implicated in the basolateral transfer of iron to the circulation. Mol Cell. 2000;5:299–309.

42. Abboud S, Haile DJ. A novel mammalian iron-regulated protein involved in intracellular iron metabolism. J Biol Chem. 2000;275:19906–12.
43. Wallace DF, Pedersen P, Dixon JL, et al. Novel mutation in ferroportin1 is associated with autosomal dominant hemochromatosis. Blood. 2002;100:692–4.
44. Roetto A, Merryweather-Clarke AT, Daraio F, et al. A valine deletion of ferroportin 1: a common mutation in hemochromastosis type 4. Blood. 2002;100:733–4.
45. Devalia V, Carter K, Walker AP, et al. Autosomal dominant reticuloendothelial iron overload associated with a 3-base pair deletion in the ferroportin 1 gene (SLC11A3). Blood. 2002;100:695–7.
46. Njajou OT, Vaessen N, Joosse M, et al. A mutation in SLC11A3 is associated with autosomal dominant hemochromatosis. Nat Genet. 2001;28:213–4.
47. Hetet G, Devaux I, Soufir N, Grandchamp B, Beaumont C. Molecular analyses of patients with hyperferritinemia and normal serum iron values reveal both L ferritin IRE and 3 new ferroportin (slc11A3) mutations. Blood. 2003;102:1904–10.
48. Arden KE, Wallace DF, Dixon JL, et al. A novel mutation in ferroportin1 is associated with haemochromatosis in a Solomon Islands patient. Gut. 2003;52:1215–7.
49. Wallace DF, Clark RM, Harley HA, Subramaniam VN. Autosomal dominant iron overload due to a novel mutation of ferroportin1 associated with parenchymal iron loading and cirrhosis. J Hepatol. 2004;40:710–3.
50. Pietrangelo A. Hereditary hemochromatosis – a new look at an old disease. N Engl J Med. 2004;350:2383–97.
51. Montosi G, Donovan A, Totaro A, et al. Autosomal-dominant hemochromatosis is associated with a mutation in the ferroportin (SLC11A3) gene. J Clin Invest. 2001;108:619–23.
52. Fraenkel PG, Traver D, Donovan A, Zahrieh D, Zon LI. Ferroportin1 is required for normal iron cycling in zebrafish. J Clin Invest. 2005;115:1532–41.
53. Edwards JA, Bannerman RM. Hereditary defect of intestinal iron transport in mice with sex-linked anemia. J Clin Invest. 1970;49:1869–71.
54. Manis J. Intestinal iron-transport defect in the mouse with sex-linked anemia. Am J Physiol. 1971;220:135–9.
55. Vulpe CD, Kuo YM, Murphy TL, et al. Hephaestin, a ceruloplasmin homologue implicated in intestinal iron transport, is defective in the sla mouse. Nat Genet. 1999;21:195–9.
56. Nemeth E, Tuttle MS, Powelson J, et al. Hepcidin regulates cellular iron efflux by binding to ferroportin and inducing its internalization. Science. 2004;306:2090–3.
57. Nemeth E, Preza GC, Jung CL, Kaplan J, Waring AJ, Ganz T. The N-terminus of hepcidin is essential for its interaction with ferroportin: structure–function study. Blood. 2006;107:328–33.
58. Nicolas G, Chauvet C, Viatte L, et al. The gene encoding the iron regulatory peptide hepcidin is regulated by anemia, hypoxia, and inflammation. J Clin Invest. 2002;110:1037–44.
59. Shike H, Shimizu C, Lauth X, Burns JC. Organization and expression analysis of the zebrafish hepcidin gene, an antimicrobial peptide gene conserved among vertebrates. Dev Comp Immunol. 2004;28:747–54.
60. Pigeon C, Ilyin G, Courselaud B, et al. A new mouse liver-specific gene, encoding a protein homologous to human antimicrobial peptide hepcidin, is overexpressed during iron overload. J Biol Chem. 2001;276:7811–9.
61. De Domenico I, Vaughn MB, Yoon D, Kushner JP, Ward DM, Kaplan J. Zebrafish as a model for defining the functional impact of mammalian ferroportin mutations. Blood. 2007;110:3780–3.
62. Zohn IE, De Domenico I, Pollock A, et al. The flatiron mutation in mouse ferroportin acts as a dominant negative to cause ferroportin disease. Blood. 2007;109:4174–80.
63. De Domenico I, McVey Ward D, Nemeth E, et al. Molecular and clinical correlates in iron overload associated with mutations in ferroportin. Haematologica. 2006;91:1092–5.
64. Njajou OT, de Jong G, Berghuis B, et al. Dominant hemochromatosis due to N144H mutation of SLC11A3: clinical and biological characteristics. Blood Cells Mol Dis. 2002;29:439–43.
65. Schimanski LM, Drakesmith H, Merryweather-Clarke AT, et al. In vitro functional analysis of human ferroportin (FPN) and hemochromatosis-associated FPN mutations. Blood. 2005;105:4096–102.
66. Drakesmith H, Schimanski LM, Ormerod E, et al. Resistance to hepcidin is conferred by hemochromatosis-associated mutations of ferroportin. Blood. 2005;106:1092–7.
67. Aisen P. Transferrin receptor 1. Int J Biochem Cell Biol. 2004;36:2137–43.
68. Levy JE, Jin O, Fujiwara Y, Kuo F, Andrews NC. Transferrin receptor is necessary for development of erythrocytes and the nervous system. Nat Genet. 1999;21:396–9.
69. Wingert RA, Brownlie A, Galloway JL, et al. The chianti zebrafish mutant provides a model for erythroid-specific disruption of transferrin receptor 1. Development. 2004;131:6225–35 (Cambridge).
70. Postlethwait JH, Yan YL, Gates MA, et al. Vertebrate genome evolution and the zebrafish gene map. Nat Genet. 1998;18:345–9.
71. Postlethwait JH, Woods IG, Ngo-Hazelett P, et al. Zebrafish comparative genomics and the origins of vertebrate chromosomes. Genome Res. 2000;10:1890–902.
72. Fraenkel PG, Gibert Y, Holzheimer JL, et al. Transferrin-a modulates hepcidin expression in zebrafish embryos. Blood. 2009;113:2843–50.

73. Goya N, Miyazaki S, Kodate S, Ushio B. A family of congenital atransferrinemia. Blood. 1972;40:239–45.
74. Roy CN, Weinstein DA, Andrews NC. 2002 E. Mead Johnson Award for Research in Pediatrics Lecture: the molecular biology of the anemia of chronic disease: a hypothesis. Pediatr Res. 2003;53:507–12.
75. Kawabata H, Fleming RE, Gui D, et al. Expression of hepcidin is down-regulated in TfR2 mutant mice manifesting a phenotype of hereditary hemochromatosis. Blood. 2005;105:376–81.
76. Shaw GC, Cope JJ, Li L, et al. Mitoferrin is essential for erythroid iron assimilation. Nature. 2006;440:96–100.
77. Lumsden AL, Henshall TL, Dayan S, Lardelli MT, Richards RI. Huntingtin-deficient zebrafish exhibit defects in iron utilization and development. Hum Mol Genet. 2007;16:1905–20.
78. Harjes P, Wanker EE. The hunt for huntingtin function: interaction partners tell many different stories. Trends Biochem Sci. 2003;28:425–33.
79. Cattaneo E, Zuccato C, Tartari M. Normal huntingtin function: an alternative approach to Huntington's disease. Nat Rev Neurosci. 2005;6:919–30.
80. Graveland GA, Williams RS, DiFiglia M. Evidence for degenerative and regenerative changes in neostriatal spiny neurons in Huntington's disease. Science. 1985;227:770–3.
81. Vonsattel JP, Myers RH, Stevens TJ, Ferrante RJ, Bird ED, Richardson Jr EP. Neuropathological classification of Huntington's disease. J Neuropathol Exp Neurol. 1985;44:559–77.
82. Chen JC, Hardy PA, Kucharczyk W, et al. MR of human postmortem brain tissue: correlative study between T2 and assays of iron and ferritin in Parkinson and Huntington disease. Am J Neuroradiol. 1993;14:275–81.
83. Bartzokis G, Cummings J, Perlman S, Hance DB, Mintz J. Increased basal ganglia iron levels in Huntington disease. Arch Neurol. 1999;56:569–74.
84. Browne SE, Ferrante RJ, Beal MF. Oxidative stress in Huntington's disease. Brain Pathol. 1999;9:147–63.
85. Tabrizi SJ, Cleeter MW, Xuereb J, Taanman JW, Cooper JM, Schapira AH. Biochemical abnormalities and excitotoxicity in Huntington's disease brain. Ann Neurol. 1999;45:25–32.
86. Gu M, Gash MT, Mann VM, Javoy-Agid F, Cooper JM, Schapira AH. Mitochondrial defect in Huntington's disease caudate nucleus. Ann Neurol. 1996;39:385–9.
87. Browne SE, Bowling AC, MacGarvey U, et al. Oxidative damage and metabolic dysfunction in Huntington's disease: selective vulnerability of the basal ganglia. Ann Neurol. 1997;41:646–53.
88. Papanikolaou G, Samuels ME, Ludwig EH, et al. Mutations in HFE2 cause iron overload in chromosome 1q-linked juvenile hemochromatosis. Nat Genet. 2004;36:77–82.
89. Sambrook JG, Figueroa F, Beck S. A genome-wide survey of Major Histocompatibility Complex (MHC) genes and their paralogues in zebrafish. BMC Genomics. 2005;6:152.
90. Gibert Y, Lattanzi VJ, Zhen AW, et al. BMP signaling modulates hepcidin expression in zebrafish embryos independent of hemojuvelin. 2011;PLoS ONE 6(1):e14553. doi:10.1371/journal.pone.0014553.
91. Stern HM, Murphey RD, Shepard JL, et al. Small molecules that delay S phase suppress a zebrafish bmyb mutant. Nat Chem Biol. 2005;1:366–70.
92. North TE, Goessling W, Walkley CR, et al. Prostaglandin E2 regulates vertebrate haematopoietic stem cell homeostasis. Nature. 2007;447:1007–11.
93. Peterson RT, Shaw SY, Peterson TA, et al. Chemical suppression of a genetic mutation in a zebrafish model of aortic coarctation. Nat Biotechnol. 2004;22:595–9.
94. Mathew LK, Sengupta S, Kawakami A, et al. Unraveling tissue regeneration pathways using chemical genetics. J Biol Chem. 2007;282:35202–10.
95. Mendelsohn BA, Yin C, Johnson SL, Wilm TP, Solnica-Krezel L, Gitlin JD. Atp7a determines a hierarchy of copper metabolism essential for notochord development. Cell Metab. 2006;4:155–62.
96. Yu PB, Hong CC, Sachidanandan C, et al. Dorsomorphin inhibits BMP signals required for embryogenesis and iron metabolism. Nat Chem Biol. 2008;4:33–41.
97. Sivasubbu S, Balciunas D, Davidson AE, et al. Gene-breaking transposon mutagenesis reveals an essential role for histone H2afza in zebrafish larval development. Mech Dev. 2006;123:513–29.
98. Meng X, Noyes MB, Zhu LJ, Lawson ND, Wolfe SA. Targeted gene inactivation in zebrafish using engineered zinc-finger nucleases. Nat Biotechnol. 2008;26:695–701.

Index

G.J. Anderson and G. McLaren (eds.), *Iron Physiology and Pathophysiology in Humans*, Nutrition and Health, DOI 10.1007/978-1-60327-485-2, © Springer Science+Business Media, LLC 2012

B

C

N

About the Editors

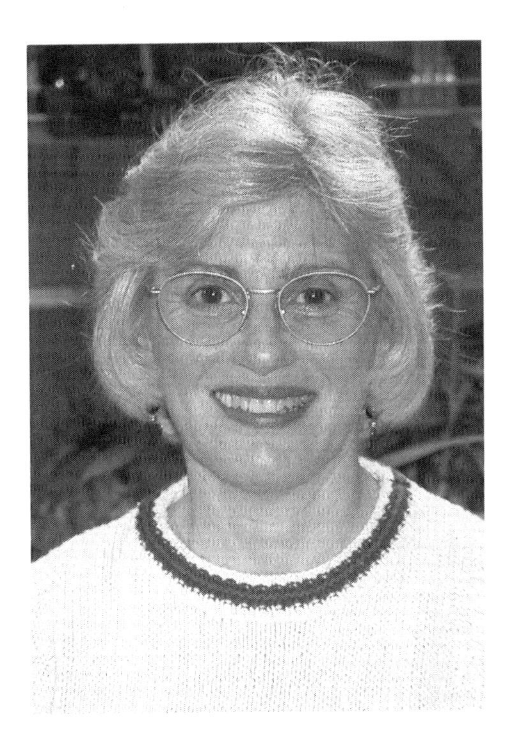

Dr Adrianne Bendich has recently retired as Director of Medical Affairs at GlaxoSmithKline (GSK) Consumer Healthcare where she was responsible for leading the innovation and medical programs in support of many well-known brands including TUMS and Os-Cal. Dr. Bendich had primary responsibility for GSK's support for the Women's Health Initiative (WHI) intervention study. Prior to joining GSK, Dr. Bendich was at Roche Vitamins Inc. and was involved with the groundbreaking clinical studies showing that folic acid–containing multivitamins significantly reduced major classes of birth defects. Dr. Bendich has coauthored over 100 major clinical research studies in the area of preventive nutrition. Dr Bendich is recognized as a leading authority on antioxidants, nutrition and immunity and pregnancy outcomes, vitamin safety and the cost-effectiveness of vitamin/mineral supplementation.

Dr Bendich, who is now President of Consultants in Consumer Healthcare LLC, is the editor of ten books including *Preventive Nutrition: The Comprehensive Guide For Health Professionals*, Fourth Edition coedited with Dr. Richard Deckelbaum, and is series editor of *Nutrition and Health* for Springer/Humana Press (www.springer.com/series/7659). The series contains 40 published volumes – major new editions in 2010–2011 include *Vitamin D*, Second Edition edited by Dr. Michael Holick; *Dietary Components and Immune Function* edited by Dr. Ronald Ross Watson, Dr. Sherma Zibadi, and Dr. Victor R. Preedy; *Bioactive Compounds and Cancer* edited by Dr. John A. Milner and Dr. Donato F. Romagnolo; *Modern Dietary Fat Intakes in Disease Promotion* edited by Dr. Fabien DeMeester, Dr. Sherma Zibadi, and Dr. Ronald Ross Watson; *Iron Deficiency and Overload* edited by Dr. Shlomo Yehuda and Dr. David Mostofsky; *Nutrition Guide for Physicians* edited by Dr. Edward Wilson, Dr. George A. Bray, Dr. Norman Temple, and Dr. Mary Struble; *Nutrition and Metabolism* edited by Dr. Christos Mantzoros; and *Fluid and Electrolytes in Pediatrics* edited by Leonard Feld and Dr. Frederick Kaskel. Recent volumes include: *Handbook of Drug-Nutrient Interactions* edited by Dr. Joseph Boullata and Dr. Vincent Armenti; *Probiotics in Pediatric Medicine* edited by Dr. Sonia Michail and Dr. Philip Sherman; *Handbook of Nutrition and Pregnancy* edited by Dr. Carol Lammi-Keefe, Dr. Sarah Couch, and Dr. Elliot Philipson; *Nutrition and Rheumatic Disease* edited by Dr. Laura Coleman; *Nutrition and Kidney Disease* edited by Dr. Laura Byham-Grey, Dr. Jerrilynn Burrowes, and Dr. Glenn Chertow; *Nutrition and Health in Developing Countries* edited by Dr. Richard Semba and Dr. Martin Bloem; *Calcium in Human Health* edited by Dr. Robert Heaney and Dr. Connie Weaver; and *Nutrition and Bone Health* edited by Dr. Michael Holick and Dr. Bess Dawson-Hughes.

Dr Bendich served as Associate Editor for *Nutrition* the International Journal; served on the Editorial Board of the *Journal of Women's Health and Gender-Based Medicine*; and was a member of the Board of Directors of the American College of Nutrition.

Dr Bendich was the recipient of the Roche Research Award, is a *Tribute to Women and Industry* Awardee, and was a recipient of the Burroughs Wellcome Visiting Professorship in Basic Medical Sciences, 2000–2001. In 2008, Dr. Bendich was given the Council for Responsible Nutrition (CRN) Apple Award in recognition of her many contributions to the scientific understanding of dietary supplements. Dr Bendich holds academic appointments as Adjunct Professor in the Department of Preventive Medicine and Community Health at UMDNJ and has an adjunct appointment at the Institute of Nutrition, Columbia University P&S, and is an Adjunct Research Professor, Rutgers University, Newark Campus. She is listed in Who's Who in American Women.

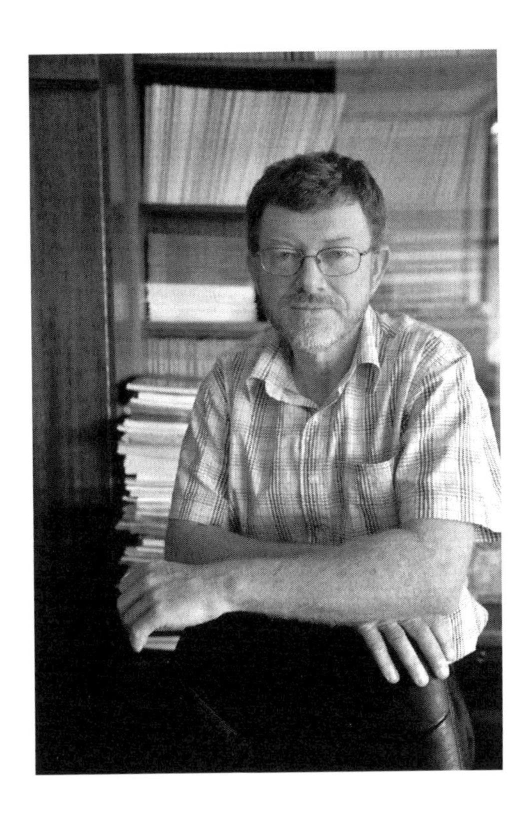

Professor Greg Anderson is Head of the Iron Metabolism Laboratory at the Queensland Institute of Medical Research in Brisbane, Australia, and has worked in the area of iron homeostasis for over 25 years. He also has adjunct appointments in the School of Chemical and Molecular Biosciences and the School of Medicine at the University of Queensland, and at Griffith University. After gaining a BSc with Honors at the University of Newcastle in Australia and an MSc in biochemistry at McMaster University in Canada, he commenced his iron career by completing a PhD under the tutelage of June Halliday and Lawrie Powell at the University of Queensland on the role of transferrin receptors in the small intestine. This was followed by postdoctoral studies on yeast iron uptake in Rick Klausner's group at the US National Institutes of Health. Thereafter, he returned to Australia and has been directing his own research laboratory since 1995.

Dr Anderson has had long-term interests in basic mechanisms of mammalian iron transport, the regulation of iron homeostasis, and disorders of iron metabolism. He is particularly well known for his work on intestinal iron absorption and hemochromatosis and has published widely in these areas. His group was one of the first to apply a genetic approach to understanding the mechanisms of intestinal iron transport, and this led to the cloning of the gene encoding hephaestin, an iron oxidase that is required for efficient dietary iron absorption. He has also made significant contributions to the understanding of the biology of the iron regulatory hormone hepcidin and showed that hepcidin was a target of HFE, the gene mutated in the most common form of hereditary iron loading. In addition to providing basic information on the mechanisms underlying iron loading in HFE-related hemochromatosis, Dr Anderson's group has also contributed to studies on clinical aspects of the disorder, population prevalence, and disease penetrance. His group also has a long-term interest in iron metabolism during pregnancy and in early infancy.

Dr Anderson was an inaugural member of the Board of Directors of the International BioIron Society (2003–2007) and returned to the Board in 2011 as President-Elect of the Society. He has been involved in the organization of several international BioIron meetings and has received the

Society's Marcel Simon Prize for his contributions to the field. He is also currently a member of the Board of the International Biometals Society and heads the Australian Biometals Group. Outside the iron area, he is a member of the Council of the Australian Society for Biochemistry and Molecular Biology and has served on the Research Committee of the Gastroenterological Society of Australia for a number of years.

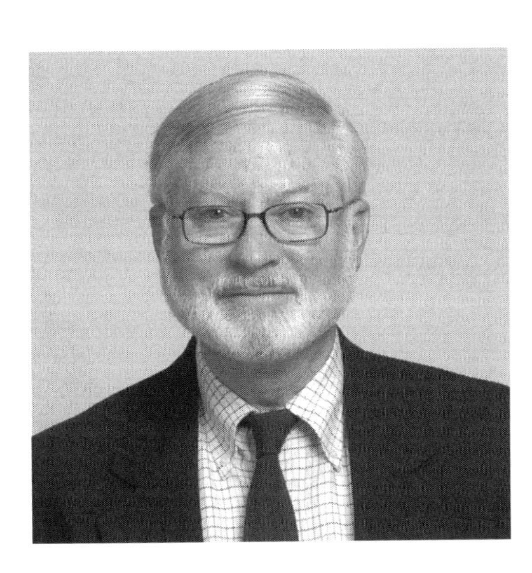

Gordon D. McLaren is a practicing hematologist and oncologist at the Department of Veterans Affairs Long Beach Healthcare System, Long Beach, California and a professor in the Division of Hematology/Oncology and the Chao Family Comprehensive Cancer Center at the University of California, Irvine. He previously held faculty appointments at Case Western Reserve University, Cleveland, Ohio and at the University of North Dakota School of Medicine and Health Sciences, where he served as Chief of the Division of Hematology and Oncology at the University and at the VA Medical Center in Fargo. He received a BA in chemistry from the University of Missouri and an MD from Stanford University School of Medicine. He began his training in internal medicine at the Mary Imogene Bassett Hospital (affiliated with Columbia University) in Cooperstown, NY, followed by 2 years at the Centers for Disease Control and Prevention in Atlanta. While at the CDC, he adapted and validated an erythrocyte protoporphyrin assay for use in the detection of iron deficiency as part of the National Health and Nutrition Examination Survey (NHANES) and received the Commendation Medal of the U.S. Public Health Service. He completed his internal medicine residency and hematology/oncology fellowship at the University Hospitals of Cleveland and Case Western Reserve University.

After completing his medical training, Dr. McLaren spent a year as a British-American Research Fellow at the Welsh National School of Medicine, Cardiff, where he studied iron metabolism under the guidance of the late Allan Jacobs. After returning to Case Western Reserve University, he developed a clinical and laboratory research program with colleagues in the area of iron overload disorders, including studies of the regulation of intestinal iron absorption using a novel mathematical model of iron kinetics. He continued these studies at the University of North Dakota, and this work provided the first demonstration that the defective regulation of iron absorption in hemochromatosis is mediated at the level of mucosal iron transfer. He was later Visiting Scientist in the laboratories of Lawrie Powell and June Halliday at the Queensland Institute of Medical Research, where he collaborated with Greg Anderson on mapping the *sla* gene in mice. After moving to the University of California, Irvine, he became Co-Principal Investigator and Medical Director of the University's Field Center for the National Institutes of Health-sponsored Hemochromatosis and Iron Overload Screening (HEIRS) Study. He has continued to pursue his interests in gene discovery, and current efforts are focused on identification of single nucleotide polymorphisms associated with iron status.

Dr McLaren is a member of several professional societies, including the International BioIron Society. He is a Fellow of the American College of Physicians and previously served as the medical school representative for the University of North Dakota to the American Federation for Medical Research. He is a member of the American Society of Hematology's Scientific Committee on Iron and Heme, serving as Vice-Chair in 2011 and Chair in 2012. He is also a member of the Medical and Scientific Advisory Board of the Iron Disorders Institute.